Anatomic Basis of Echocardiographic Diagnosis

Kwan-Leung Chan
John P. Veinot

Anatomic Basis of Echocardiographic Diagnosis

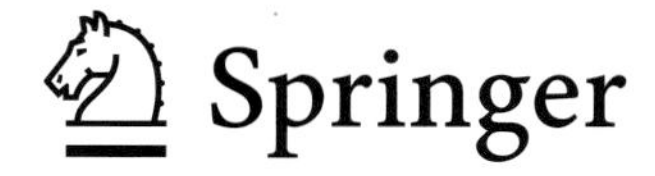

Authors
Dr. Kwan-Leung Chan
University of Ottawa
Heart Institute
Division of Cardiology
Ruskin Street
40 K1Y 4W7 Ottawa Ontario
Canada
kchan@ottawaheart.ca

Dr. John P. Veinot
Ottawa Hospital
Department of Laboratory Medicine
Carling Ave.
1053 K1Y 4E9 Ottawa Ontario
Civic Campus
Canada
jpveinot@ottawahospital.on.ca

ISBN 978-1-84996-386-2 e-ISBN 978-1-84996-387-9
DOI 10.1007/978-1-84996-387-9
Springer London Dordrecht Heidelberg New York

A catalogue record for this book is available from the British Library

Library of Congress Control Number: 2010938219

Cover design: eStudio Calamar, Figueres/Berlin

Printed on acid-free paper

Springer is part of Springer Science+Business Media (www.springer.com)

Foreword

It is my pleasure and honor to write a Foreword for this most informative book on a technology that has become essential to the diagnosis, prognosis, and treatment of many disorders, in particular, cardiovascular diseases. Echocardiography, the subject of this book, has for decades been pivotal in the diagnostic and prognostic assessment of cardiovascular diseases. In addition to its safety (lack of radiation) and portability, it has the capability to illustrate at the bedside and in real-time cardiac anatomy while simultaneously demonstrating all aspects of cardiac function. It is relatively user-friendly; however, the expertise of an experienced echocardiographer is often required. This too has recently been facilitated with the development of high-resolution picture archiving and communication system (PACS) whereby echocardiographic images can be transferred almost immediately to the central laboratory not just from the operating room, but also from areas hundreds and even thousands of miles away. Such developments have enabled the cardiologist, the anesthesiologist, and the surgeon to utilize it not just for diagnosis and prognosis, but also for on-site real-time assessment of procedures in the operating room.

This book is carefully written by, not just a world renowned expert in echocardiography but, someone with extensive experience in all aspects of cardiovascular diseases over more than 3 decades. Dr. Kwan Chan has been Head of the Echocardiography Laboratory and supervised this technology in many different settings from the operating room at University of Ottawa Heart Institute to Canada's northland – Baffin Island. His knowledge of cardiovascular diseases is vast and he has also had the privilege of correlating echocardiographic imaging with other sophisticated imaging techniques in his own Institution including Nuclear and Positron technologies. This book is written by just two authors, very unusual in today's era, who have worked together in the same Institution. His coauthor (Dr. J.P. Veinot) is a renowned cardiac pathologist. Dr. Chan, as Director of the Echocardiography Laboratory, has directed national and international studies, the most recent being Aortic Stenosis Progression Observation: Measuring Effects of Rosuvastatin (ASTRONOMER) trial. The book is an enriched resource of high-resolution images of normal and abnormal pathology as detected and quantified by echocardiography. The text is extremely up to date while at the same time written in the style of a masterful teacher. Since the book is written by only two authors, it comprehensively and seamlessly moves from one topic to the next in continuity without redundancy. The prose and the abundant illustrations have been selected to be appreciated by the novice as well as the most advanced echocardiographer.

My congratulations to Dr. Kwan Chan and Dr. John Veinot for a job well done.

Dr Robert Roberts
President and CEO
University of Ottawa Heart Institute
40 Ruskin Street,Ottawa
Ontario, Canada

Preface

Echocardiography is a widely used imaging modality for the assessment of patients with heart disease. It is versatile and can be performed at the bedside to promptly provide reliable anatomic and functional information useful for the management of the patient. It involves no ionizing radiation and is therefore ideally suited for serial studies in the follow-up of patients with chronic heart diseases.

There have been many technological advances in echocardiography, resulting in an improvement in image quality and new insights into cardiac mechanics. New indices such as tissue velocities, torsion, strain, and strain rate open new avenues to assess global and regional myocardial performance. Real-time three-dimensional echocardiography has recently become a reality and provides unique anatomic perspectives unobtainable heretofore. Further technological improvement will likely ensure that three-dimensional echocardiography becomes an integral part of the echocardiographic examination. In order to fully appreciate and utilize these advances, it is crucial to have an in-depth understanding of the cardiac anatomy, which is the basis of echocardiography. For instance, mitral valve repair is now the surgical method of choice for the treatment of patients with degenerative mitral valve disease and severe mitral regurgitation. Repair is also increasingly used for other etiologies of mitral regurgitation. An excellent understanding of the mitral valvular and subvalvular anatomy is a prerequisite to the selection of appropriate patients and the detection of complications associated with the surgical repair.

The aim of this book is to provide a systematic approach in the clinical application of echocardiography, which is based on a comprehensive understanding of cardiac anatomy and pathology. We have included many three-dimensional echocardiographic images to highlight normal and abnormal findings, as well as numerous pathologic images to provide anatomic correlates of the echocardiographic findings. All the images are carefully selected to illustrate the key findings of the conditions under discussion. There are a total of 680 figures, many of which are composites of two to six images covering a wide spectrum of cardiac diseases, and therefore the book can serve very well as an atlas and should be useful to sonographers, cardiology trainees, internists, and cardiologists.

The book is divided into three sections. The first section discusses the cardiac anatomy and normal variants, which need to be appreciated and differentiated from abnormal findings. The ability to obtain optimal images requires an understanding of the orientation of the heart in the thorax and its effect on the acoustic windows. The impact of aging on cardiac structure and function is also included in this section. The second section covers diseases that affect various cardiac structures such as the valves, the myocardium, and the pericardium. The last section of the book examines specific

General Anatomy of the Heart in the Chest

1

The heart is located in the chest between the lungs and in front of the esophagus (Fig. 1.1). It has four chambers – two atria and two ventricles (Fig. 1.2). The right atrium receives blood from the head and neck via the superior vena cava, while the blood from the body and lower limbs enters the right atrium via the inferior vena cava. The blood passes through the tricuspid valve into the right ventricle which pumps it to the pulmonary trunk to the lungs. After oxygenation, the oxygenated blood from the lungs returns to the left atrium via the pulmonary veins. From the left atrium the blood enters the left ventricle and is pumped out the aorta to be distributed to the entire body via the aorta and its arterial branches.

The heart is normally in a sac of fibrous pericardium (Fig. 1.3). This sac contains the entire heart and extends into the proximal few centimeters of the great vessels. In the base of the heart between the four pulmonary veins there is a space termed the oblique sinus.

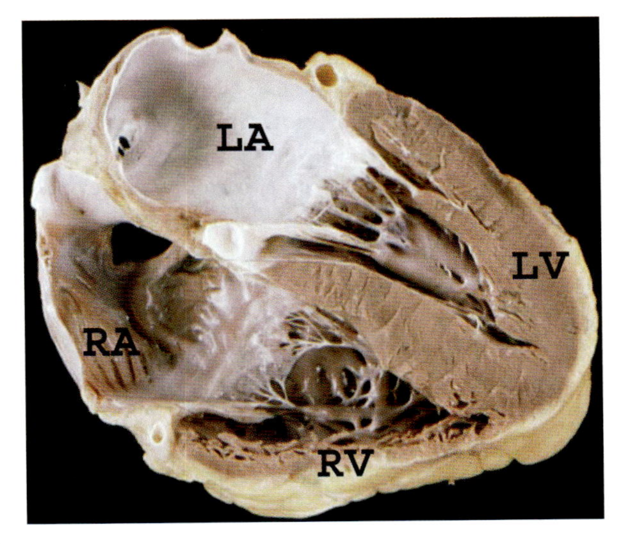

Fig. 1.2 The heart has been cut in a four-chamber view illustrating the right atrium (*RA*), left atrium (*LA*), right ventricle (*RV*) and left ventricle (*LV*)

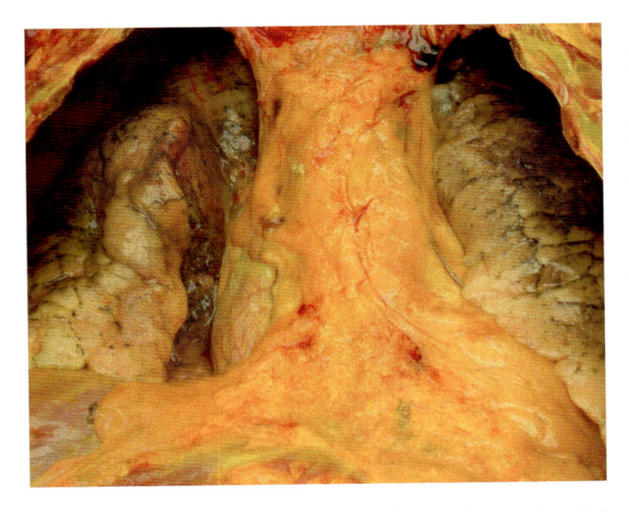

Fig. 1.1 The chest is open and the heart is seen in its pericardial sac between the two lungs

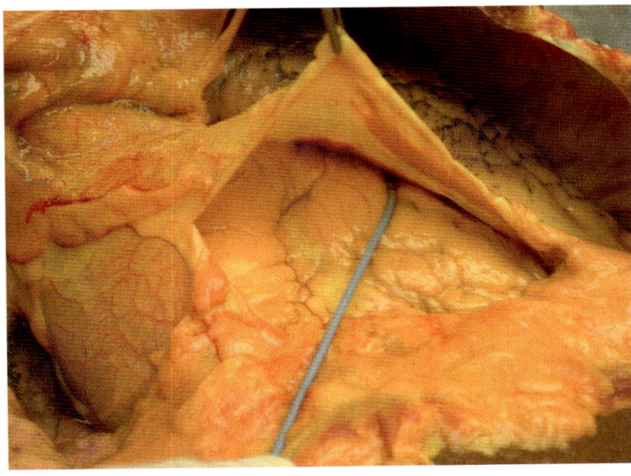

Fig. 1.3 The heart is covered by visceral pericardium on the epicardial surface and parietal pericardium which is lifted up in the picture. The fibrous parietal pericardium forms the pericardial sac

K.-L. Chan and J.P. Veinot, *Anatomic Basis of Echocardiographic Diagnosis*,
DOI: 10.1007/978-1-84996-387-9_1,

Another pericardial sinus exists, the transverse sinus, just behind the great arteries.

The heart apex is normally present in the left chest. This usual position is termed levocardia. If the heart is vertical midline in the chest, this is termed mesocardia and may be seen in tall thin individuals. If the apex points to the right side of the chest, this is termed dextrocardia. The term dextrocardia has nothing to do with the side of the chambers and does not mean the same as situs inversus where the chambers and sometimes viscera are "flipped" as compared to normal.

The sidedness or situs of the heart refers only to where the right atrium is in relation to what is the normal right-sided right atrial location. If the morphological right atrium is right sided, as is usual, this is termed situs solitus. If the morphological right atrium is left sided, this is termed situs inversus. If there are bilateral morphological right atria or two morphological left atria then it is impossible to determine which one is correct. This is termed situs ambiguous, and subclassified as right atrial isomerism or left atrial isomerism. Knowing what anatomically constitutes a morphological right atrium, right ventricle, left atrium, or left ventricle becomes important.

The heart does not usually lie in a vertical plane in the body but is somewhat rotated to the left and rests on the diaphragm. The mid to apical portion of the left ventricle resting on the diaphragm is termed the inferior wall and gives it a flat contour, as compared to the anterior wall of the heart.

The most anterior chamber of the heart is the right ventricle which lies under the anterior chest wall and sternum. This explains the propensity for right ventricle and tricuspid valve to sustain injury following blunt force trauma to the anterior chest. The right atrium is a posterior right chamber. The left ventricle is a left lateral chamber. The left atrium is a posterior left-sided chamber. Its posterior location makes it accessible for imaging via the esophagus which is another posterior mediastinal structure.

Atrial Anatomy

The right atrium is derived from the primitive sinus venosus and primitive atrium of the embryological heart. The sinus venosus gives rise to the smooth part of the atrium between the vena caval orifices. The right sinus horn contributes to the formation of the right atrium wall. The left sinus horn becomes part of the coronary sinus which normally enters into the right atrium. The primitive atrium becomes the rough muscular part of the right atrium and contributes to the left atrial appendage. The division between the two parts of the atrium is a band of muscle on the lateral atrial wall termed the crista terminalis or the terminal band (Fig. 1.4). This band extends inside the heart from the region of the sinoatrial node near the superior vena cava down the right lateral wall. On the outside epicardium of the right atrium, the terminal band has a corresponding epicardial depression on the lateral right atrial wall known as the sulcus terminalis. From this muscular band the pectinate muscles, which resemble a comb, radiate out in the same direction. At the entrance of the right atrial appendage, there is a particularly large pectinate muscle termed the taenia sagittalis. It is important to know the existence of this structure so as not to confuse it with a thrombus by imaging.

The free wall of the left atrium is smooth and has no cristae terminalis or free wall pectinate muscles (Fig. 1.5). The only pectinate muscles on the left side are small and are located in the left atrial appendage. These appendageal pectinate muscles are usually 1–2 mm in thickness and may be confused with a space occupying atrial thrombus if their existence is not recognized. The left atrium derives from the primitive atrium in part, but mostly derives its structure from a vein. The primitive pulmonary vein develops with the lung buds and, if the heart is in the correct position, grows downward to join with the heart and form the left atrium with its adjacent

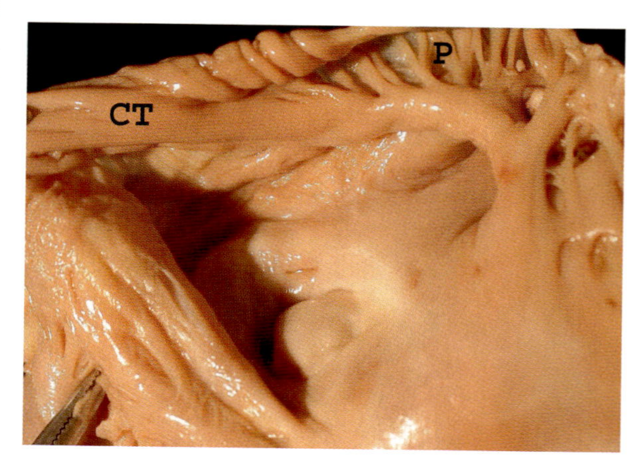

Fig. 1.4 The right atrial free wall with the crista terminalis (*CT*) and the multiple pectinate muscles (*P*)

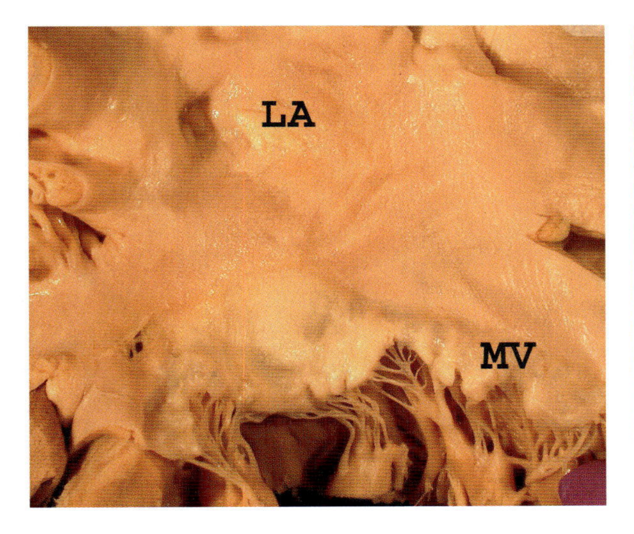

Fig. 1.5 The left heart is opened demonstrating the left atrium (*LA*) and the adjacent mitral valve (*MV*)

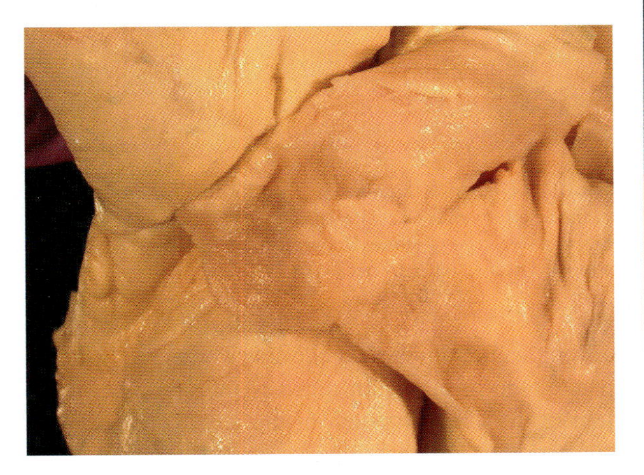

Fig. 1.6 Triangular right atrial appendage

pulmonary veins that enter the atrium. If the heart is embryologically not in the correct position, the pulmonary veins may join with other structures, thus giving rise to the condition known as partial or total anomalous pulmonary venous drainage.

The right and left atrial appendages differ in gross external structure. The right appendage has a broad based origin and tapers in a triangular shape (Fig. 1.6). In contrast, the left atrial appendage has a narrower origin and is multilobulated resembling a cock's comb (Fig. 1.7). These left appendage lobulations are variable in number, mostly one to two, but there may be up to five lobes normally [1].

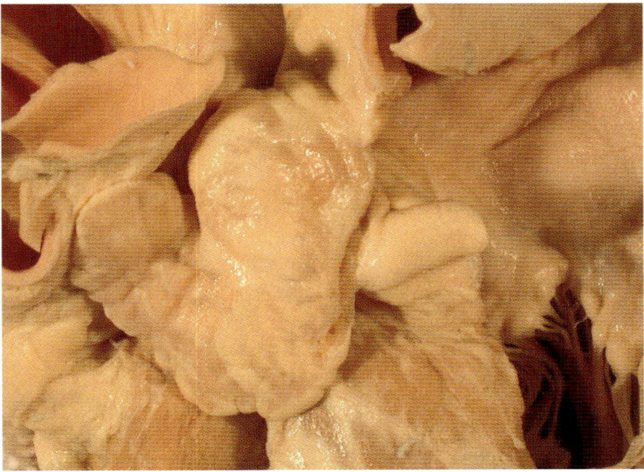

Fig. 1.7 Irregular left atrial appendage

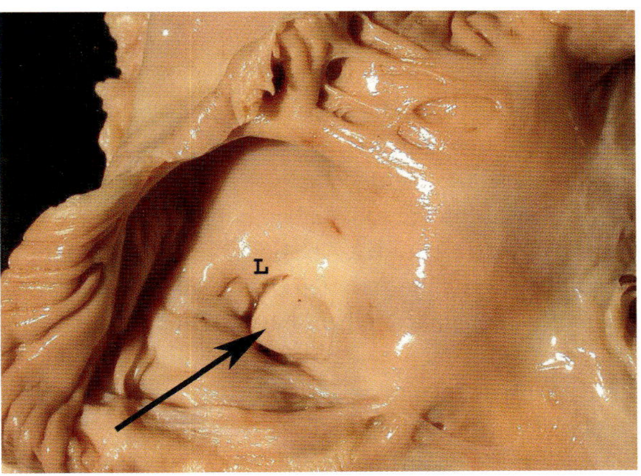

Fig. 1.8 The right atrium is opened demonstrating the fossa ovale (*arrow*). The raised edge is the limbus of the fossa (*L*)

The right and left sides of the inter-atrial septum also differ substantially. The right side has an oval raised region with a central depression termed the fossa ovale (Fig. 1.8). This is the residua of the septum primum. In this fossa there is often a residual hole termed the foramen ovale (Fig. 1.9). This is a patent structure during fetal life that is usually closed after birth. Surprisingly, it can remain open for many decades; up to 40% of those under the age of 30 years have a patent foramen ovale, while the percentage drops to 10–15 % after the age of 50 years [2]. In the fetal life this communication is important for blood distribution of the oxygenated blood from the placenta until the lungs become functional. Despite being patent, the foramen ovale is normally closed as the left sided atrial pressure is greater

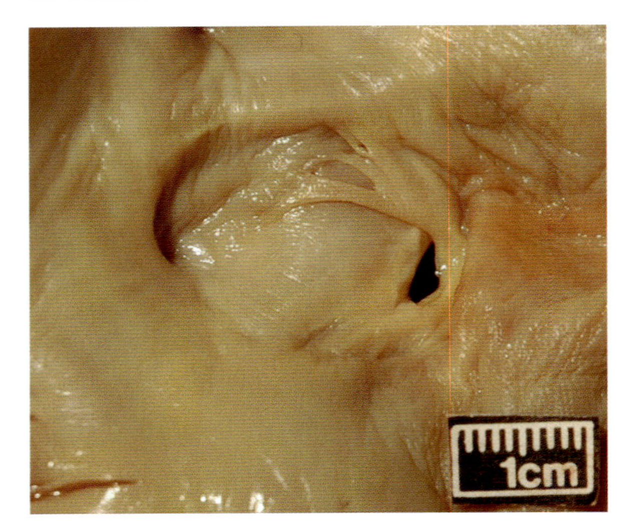

Fig. 1.9 A patent foramen ovale

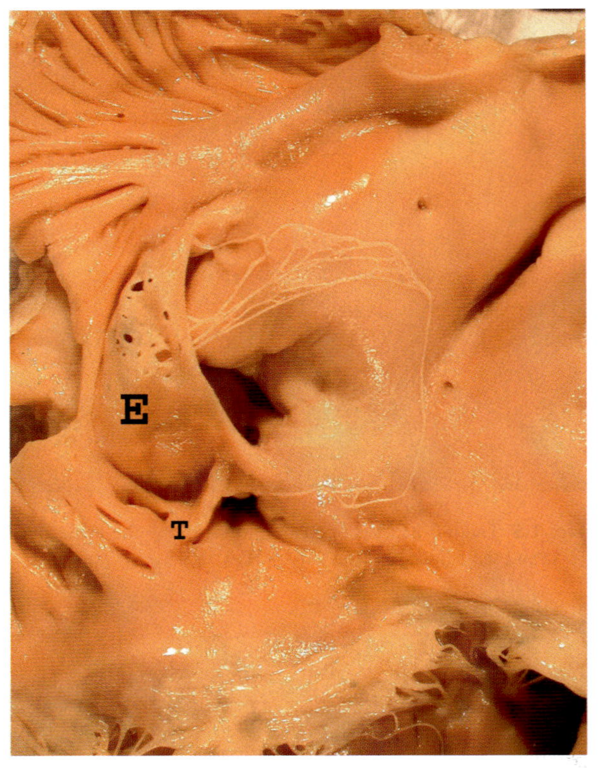

Fig. 1.10 The eustachian valve (*E*) is located near the opening of the inferior vena cava. The Thebesian valve (*T*) is at the opening of the coronary sinus. Between the two there is a net-like structure termed a Chairi net

than the right atrial pressure. If this pressure situation reverses, in such conditions as congenital heart disease, pulmonary hypertension, or with pulmonary thromboembolism, the foramen may open and shunting of blood may occur. Paradoxical emboli traveling from the right to left atria would also be possible. If the left atrium greatly enlarges, the foramen ovale can become a permanently open hole and become an acquired secundum atrial septal defect – a clinical condition known as Lutembacher's syndrome when associated with intral stenosis. Surrounding the fossa ovalis there is a ridge termed the limbus of the fossa (Fig. 1.8). The anterior and posterior limbs of the limbus are important anterior and posterior interatrial conduction pathways, as is the cristae terminalis. The left atrial side of the interatrial septum is usually flat, without a limbus or a fossa. A few muscular endocardial ridges or chords may exist where the foramen ovale communicates, or previously communicated, but generally the contour is relatively flat in comparison to the right side of the septum.

Thus a morphological right atrium has a rough free wall with pectinate muscles, a triangular appendage and a depressed region of the fossa ovalis on the interatrial septum. In contrast, the left atrium has a smooth, free wall, a complex, multilobulated appendage, and the inter-atrial septal contour is simple and flat.

The sinoatrial node is located at the junction of the superior vena cava and the summit of the right atrial appendage. It is an epicardial structure, not visible to the naked eye, except for its occasionally visible accompanying sinoatrial node artery branch. The lower part of the right atrium receives the coronary sinus, part of the venous system of the heart. The coronary sinus orifice is guarded by a small Thebesian valve (Fig. 1.10). There is often a web like structure extending from the orifice of the inferior vena cava to the Thebesian valve. This web is known as a Chairi web. The orifice of the inferior vena cava has a variably sized Eustachian valve.

The atrioventricular node is located in Koch's triangle (Fig. 1.11). This triangle is bordered by the opening of the coronary sinus on one side, and the tricuspid valve annulus from this coronary sinus orifice region to the area of the membranous septum (above the septal posterior commissure of the tricuspid valve). The roof of the triangle, completed by an oblique line between the top of the sinus and the membranous septum region, corresponds to the deep tendon of Todaro, a structure not visible as it lies beneath

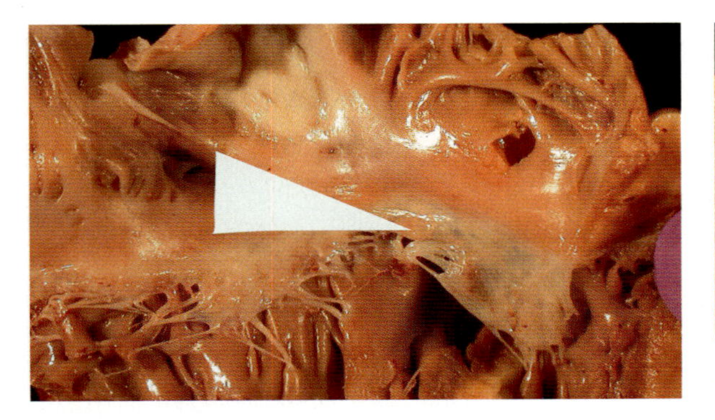

Fig. 1.11 The right atrium and the tricuspid valve are open. The atrioventricular node is located in Koch's triangle depicted in the illustration

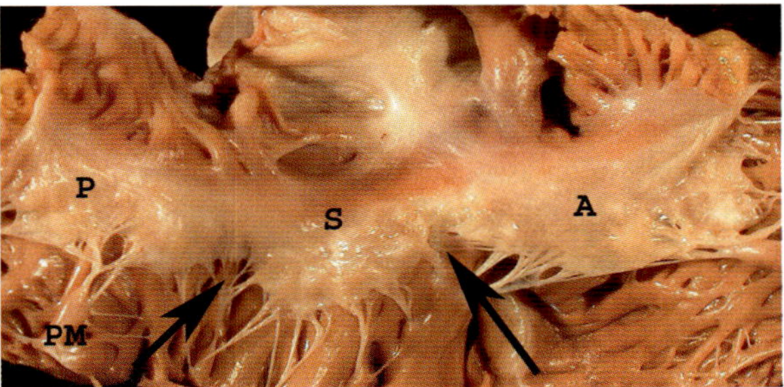

Fig. 1.12 The tricuspid valve has three leaflets – anterior (*A*), posterior (*P*), and septal (*S*). These are separated by commissures (*arrows*). Chordae tendonae connect the valve leaflets to the septum and the papillary muscles (*PM*)

the endocardium. Some extension of the atrioventricular node extends into the coronary sinus for variable lengths. The node lies on top of the ventricular septum and becomes the atrioventricular bundle – the bundle of His, at the membranous septum. The His bundle subsequently divides into the right bundle which travels to the right ventricle in the moderator band, as will be described, and the left bundle disperses into numerous subendocardial Purkinji fibers in the left ventricle subendocardium.

The conduction pathways from the sinoatrial node to the atrioventricular node and the left atrium include the following potential pathways: the crista terminalis, the anterior and posterior pathways on either side of the atrial septum fossa ovalis and an epicardial Bachmann's bundle. This bundle extends from the left side of the superior vena cava across the atrium over to the left atrial appendage, thus allowing coordination of both atria with conduction.

Tricuspid Valve Anatomy

The tricuspid valve is an atrioventricular valve, as is the mitral valve. However, the similarity ends there as these valves have completely different structures. The atrioventricular valves delaminate from their ventricles, thus the atrioventricular valves are invariably associated with their respective underlying ventricles. The tricuspid valve is associated with the right ventricle and the mitral valve with the left ventricle. The ventricle is also defined by its association with its atrioventricular valve. The same relationship does not exist with the ventricle and its atrium or with its great vessel.

The tricuspid valve has three leaflets, the anterior, the septal, and the posterior (Fig. 1.12). The anterior leaflet is the largest of the three. As with all cardiac valves, there is a free edge and a line of closure, located on the atrial side of the tricuspid valve. There are three commissures separating the leaflets. Each leaflet has chordae tendonae attaching to ventricular papillary muscles. One of the defining characteristics of a tricuspid valve is that the septal leaflet chordae attach directly to the underlying adjacent ventricular septum. No such relationship exists on the left side of the heart, otherwise the left ventricle outflow tract would be obstructed.

The anterior papillary muscle is large and has multiple heads, as is also common with the posterior muscle. The septal papillary muscle is also termed the muscle of Lanusic. The annulus of the tricuspid valve is discontinuous and not as well formed as the mitral annulus. The tricuspid valve delaminates from its underlying ventricle as part of normal development. If it fails to do so a condition known as Ebstein's anomaly may exist. The anomaly is characterized by the failure of the posterior leaflet to detach from the ventricle beyond 1 cm from the atrioventricular ring. Thus 1 cm of attachment of the leaflet is considered within normal limits. The tricuspid valve also is different than the mitral valve as it is separate from the corresponding semilunar valve, the pulmonary valve. The separation is due to the presence of the infundibular septum of the morphological right ventricle.

Right Ventricle Anatomy

The right ventricle is a morphological right ventricle firstly due to its association with a tricuspid atrioventricular valve with septal chordal attachments and discontinuity with the pulmonary valve. The normal right ventricle is a crescent shaped chamber located anterior and to the right in the chest (Fig. 1.13). It is behind the sternum and it is the most anterior chamber. The ventricle is usually 0.3–0.4 cm thick, but it may hypertrophy in pulmonary hypertension or pressure overload situations. Therefore, the wall thickness of the ventricle is not a good criterion to identify it. It characteristically has large prominent trabecular muscle termed trabeculae carnae. Trabecular muscles also exist in the left ventricle, but they are small compared to those of the right ventricle. The tricuspid and the pulmonary valves are separated by the infundibular septum. This is an arch-like structure composed of the parietal band, the infundibulum, and the septomarginal band, which terminates in the moderator band. This band contains the aforementioned right bundle branch.

Pulmonary Valve Anatomy

The pulmonary valve and the aortic valve are both semilunar valves, a name derived from their half moon cusp shape (Fig. 1.14). They both have a corona shaped annulus like a crown. The pulmonary valve is separate from its atrioventricular valve, the tricuspid valve. There are normally three cusps. These are separated from each other at three commissures. The cusps are the anterior, left, and right cusps. The cusps have a free edge and a line of closure, which is along the ventricular surface. This arrangement, as exists in all the valves, allows for some redundancy and prevents regurgitation with normal physiological events. The cusps are thinner then the aortic valve cusps, mainly reflecting the lower right-sided pressures.

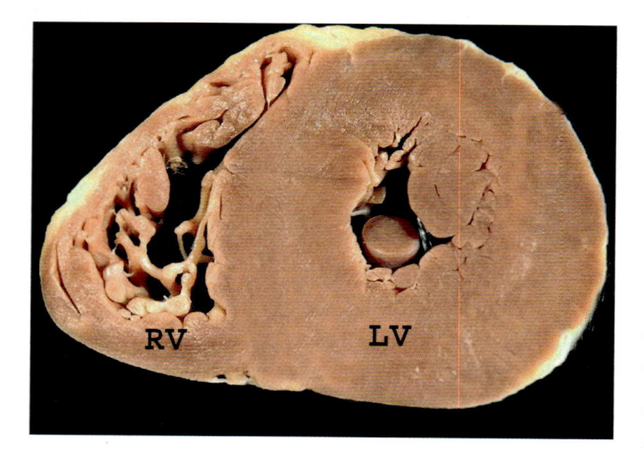

Fig. 1.13 Short axis cut of the heart showing the typical right ventricle (*RV*) crescent shape and the round left ventricle (*LV*) shape

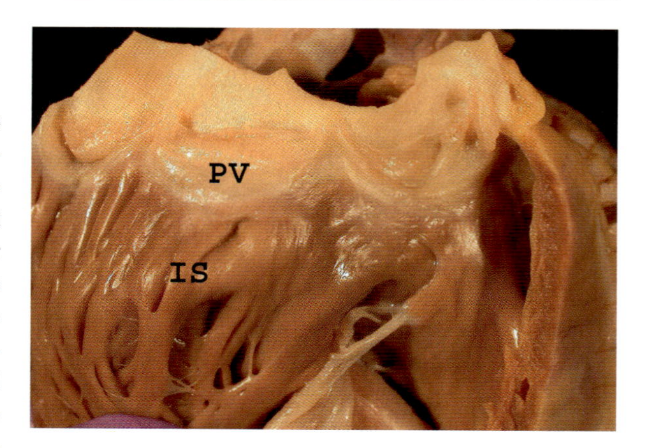

Fig. 1.14 Opened right ventricle outflow tract demonstrating the pulmonary valve (*PV*) cusps. The infundibular septum (*IS*) lies before the valve

Mitral Valve Anatomy

The mitral valve is an atrioventricular valve. Like the tricuspid valve it has leaflets and chordae which attach to papillary muscles. It is invariably associated with a left ventricle, similar to the association of the tricuspid valve with the right ventricle. There are two leaflets – the anterior and the posterior (Fig. 1.15). Although the posterior occupies more of the circumference of the annulus, the actual surface areas occupied by each of the leaflets is about equal, as the anterior leaflet is longer in length. On either side of the leaflets there are commissures, the posteromedial and the anterolateral. The mitral valve has no septal chordal attachments. The anterior leaflet is in fibrous continuity with the aortic valve (Fig. 1.16). This defines the mitral valve and the left ventricle and is a distinctive feature of this ventricle. The leaflets have free edges and closing margins, approximately a few mm from the edge. These

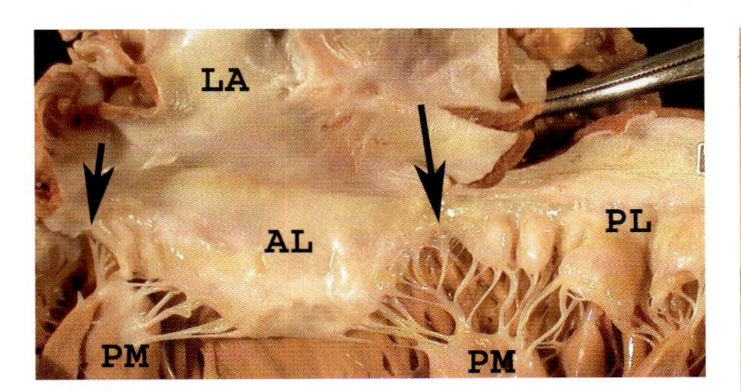

Fig. 1.15 Mitral valve with anterior leaflet (*AL*) and the posterior leaflet (*PL*), which has been cut through with heart opening. Two commissures are present on either side of the leaflets (*arrows*). Left atrium is above (*LA*) the valve and the left ventricle papillary muscles are below (*PM*), connected by the chordae tendonae

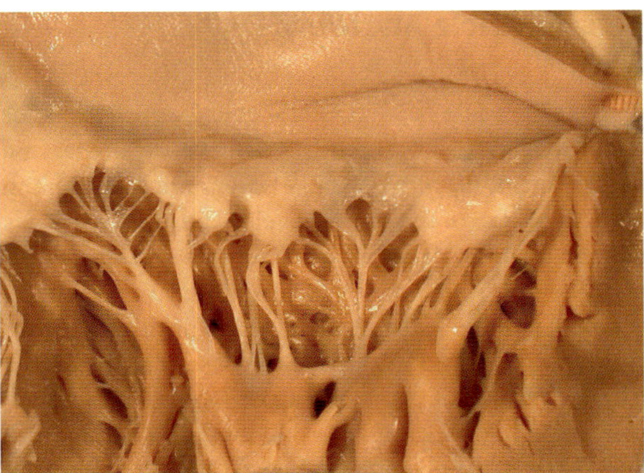

Fig. 1.17 Posterior mitral valve with numerous complex chordae

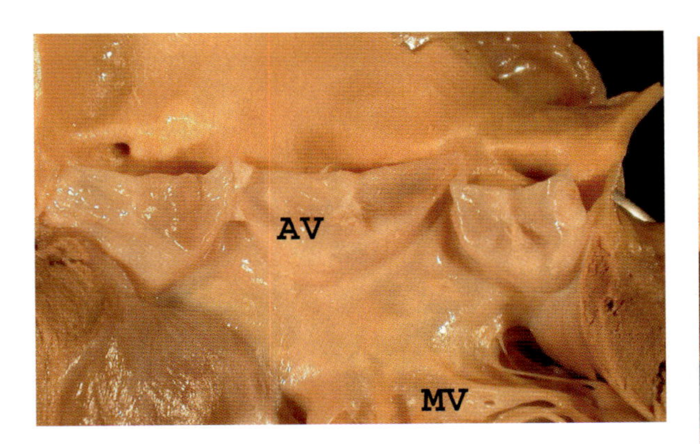

Fig. 1.16 The left ventricle outflow tract opened to show the continuity between the aortic valve (*AV*) and the anterior mitral leaflet (*MV*)

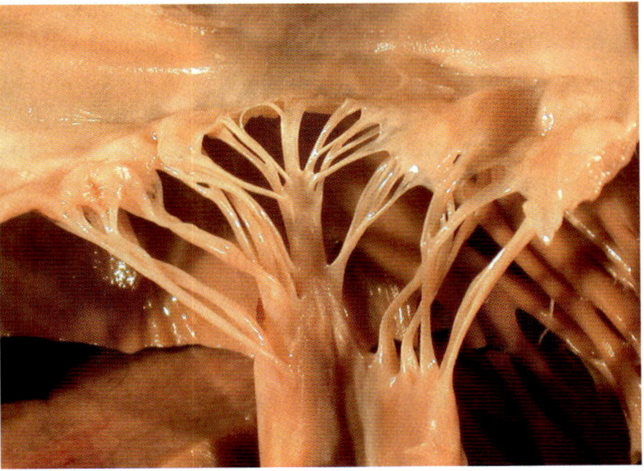

Fig. 1.18 Commissural chordae noted

lines are more distinctive than the closing margins on the right sided valves due to the higher pressures on the left side of the heart. The mitral valve annulus is better defined and a fibrous annular band can be seen. The posterior leaflet has three scallops that are formed to variable degrees. These small leaflet indentations allow some redundancy to the valve, which is important for competency. The chordae are complex and different anatomical or surgical classifications exist (Fig. 1.17). Some investigators divide the chordae into first order (attached to free edge of leaflet), second order (attached mid leaflet), and third order (attached to papillary muscle). Others have assigned specific names to the chords. These include strut chords, commissural chords (Fig. 1.18), basal chords, and rough zone chords. Only the posterior leaflet has basal chords which run between the leaflet and the adjacent left ventricle wall. Only the anterior leaflet has strut chords – these are two large chords on either side of the anterior leaflet. The chords are responsible for different functions. Some are important for the basic integrity and structure of the valve, some ensure good leaflet coaptation, while others prevent leaflet prolapse. Rupture of a chord may thus have very different consequences depending upon the type involved.

The chords attach to two left ventricle papillary muscles, the anterolateral and the posteromedial papillary muscles (Fig. 1.15). These are much larger than the right sided analogous structures. The anterior muscle usually has one head while the posteromedial papillary muscle is usually bifid. The papillary muscles contract and ensure good opposition of the mitral valve leaflets.

Left Ventricle Anatomy

The left ventricle is a left lateral chamber. It is cone or bullet shaped (Fig. 1.13). It is the thickest chamber in a normal heart, usually about 1–1.5 cm thick depending upon the phase of the cardiac cycle. The left ventricle is defined by its association with a mitral valve, the continuity between its atrioventricular mitral valve and its semilunar aortic valve and its thin inner trabeculae. Conventionally, the left ventricle is described to have an anterior wall, a lateral wall between the papillary muscles, and an inferior wall. As previously mentioned, the inferior wall (mid to apical level) rests on the diaphragm, whereas the posterior or basal wall is located toward the left atrium junction. The ventricle relaxes during diastole and fills with blood from the left atrium. During contraction or systole the ventricle motion is complex. The ventricle shortens, squeezes, and wrings itself out with a twisting motion with the apex rotating counter clockwise and the base rotating clockwise. The ventricular shortening can be understood as the longitudinal superficial muscle fibers extend to the apex and then do a sharp turn and form the inner papillary muscles. Contraction of these sinospiral and bulbospiral superficial layers pulls up the ventricle during systolic contraction. The middle layer of circular scroll muscles is responsible for the squeezing and wringing actions. The fibers of the right and left ventricles interdigitate at either end of the interventricular septum. The left ventricular outflow tract has no obstruction as there are no septal chordal attachments (Fig. 1.16). At the apex, due to the abrupt changes in fiber direction, the thickness of the muscle is usually less than a few millimeters. Surgeons take advantage of this fact to use the apex for an easy site to vent the ventricle and remove air after the heart has been opened.

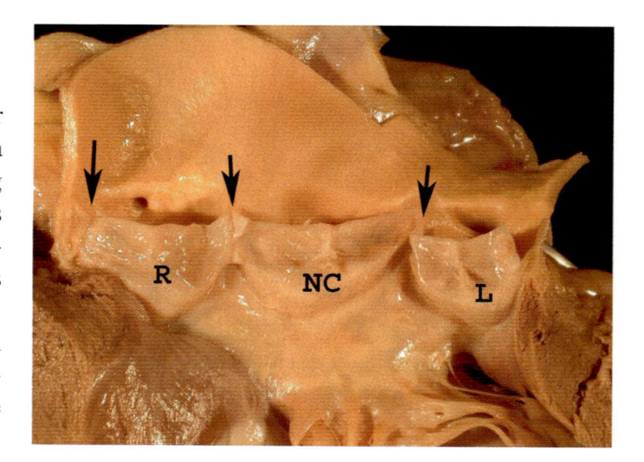

Fig. 1.19 Opened aortic valve with right (*R*), non-coronary (*NC*) and left (*l*) cusps. Commissures separate the cusps (*arrows*)

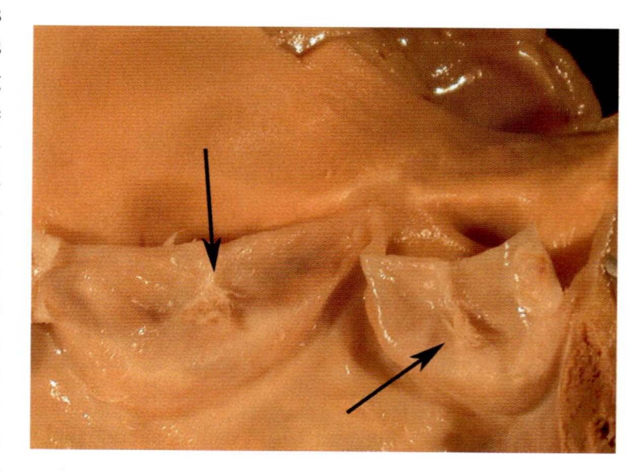

Fig. 1.20 Aortic valve cusp with raised line of closure or coaptation, and a mid cusp nodule of Ariantus with Lambl's excrescences which are whisker like (*arrows*)

Aortic Valve Anatomy

The aortic valve is a semilunar valve. It has three cusps – the right, left, and posterior or non-coronary cusp (Fig. 1.19). The non-coronary cusp is usually slightly larger than the other two cusps. Between each cusp and its adjacent cusp there is a commissure which separates them. The cusps have free edges and lines of closure which are well developed due to the higher pressure on the left side of the heart. The area between the line of closure and the free edge of the cusp has been termed the lunula. Near the commissures there are often horizontal cusp defects termed fenestrations. These are normal structures that become more prominent with age. These are not normally in the line of closure so they do not cause insufficiency unless the valve annulus enlarges and they move into the line of closure. In the middle of each cusp there is a well developed nodule or protrusion on the ventricular side along the line of closure termed the nodule of Ariantus (Fig. 1.20). All along the closure line, and especially at the nodule, small whisker like fronds termed Lambl's excrescences may develop. Beneath the right and non-coronary cusps, the interventricular septum is at its thinnest point – the membranous septum. In this septum, the atrioventricular His bundle penetrates and the left bundle branch Purkinji fibers then extend along the left ventricle endocardial surface.

The annulus of the aortic valve is not a simple ring but is shaped like a crown or a corona, similar to the annulus of the pulmonary valve. Each cusp is attached along this fibrous crown leaving intercommissural spaces between the cusps. At the back of each cusp, there is an out pouched region termed the aortic sinus. This fills with blood during diastole when the valve is closed. The proximal aortic structure thus has large proximal sinuses and then tapers on its way out to the ascending aorta, similar to a vase or a flask. Just above the aortic valve and sinus, there is a tapered area with an intimal ridge termed the sinotubular junction. The right and non-coronary cusps of the aortic valve are in fibrous continuity with the anterior mitral leaflet. The fibrous area between the aortic and mitral valves has been termed the fibrous subaortic curtain by some investigators. The continuity of the valves is important in disease processes such as infective endocarditis where an infection can easily spread between the two adjacent valve structures.

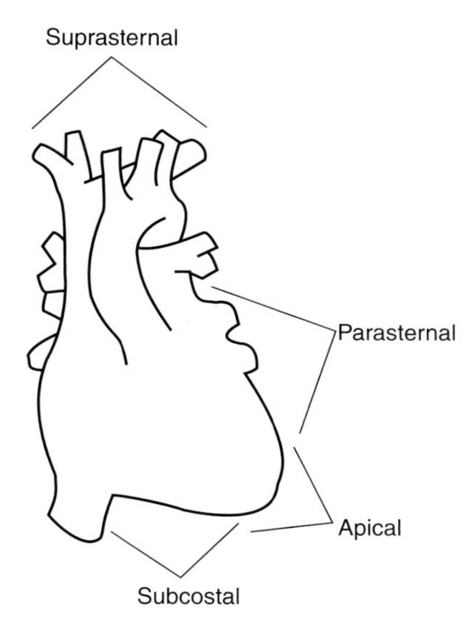

Fig. 1.21 This diagram illustrates the standard windows in the echocardiographic assessment of the heart

Echocardiography Considerations

In most echocardiographic laboratories a detailed stepwise protocol is generally followed to obtain a comprehensive echocardiographic assessment of cardiac structure and function. This involves imaging the heart from four acoustic windows namely parasternal, apical, subcostal, and suprasternal windows (Fig. 1.21). Since the early development of echocardiography, it is recognized that the passage of ultrasound is impeded by bone and air, such that adequate images would not be obtained if there is intervening bone or air containing lung tissue between the transducer and heart. The four standard acoustic windows are areas on the chest wall that provide good passage of ultrasound and thus diagnostic echo images in most subjects.

The parasternal window generally refers to the fourth and fifth intercostal space just to the left of the sternum (Fig. 1.22). It has the least distance between the body surface and the cardiac valves. Multiple imaging planes can be obtained to provide long and short-axis views of cardiac structures, particularly the aortic and mitral valves. It is also the preferred window to assess the left ventricle, as multiple short axis views of the left ventricle from its base to apex can frequently be obtained. To obtain a short-axis image of the left ventricular apex, the transducer may need to be moved down an intercostal space and further lateral with the patient lying in a more shallow left decubitus position and sometime even supine (Fig. 1.23). What is not frequently done, but is again feasible in most subjects, are multiple short axis cuts of the right ventricle from this window (Fig. 1.24). The transducer is positioned near the sternum and angled rightward, so as to image the entire right ventricle. A sweep from the base of the heart to the ventricular apex with multiple short-axis images of the right ventricle provides a comprehensive assessment of right ventricular size and function.

The apical window is located at or near the cardiac apical impulse (Fig. 1.25). The left and right ventricles are well imaged from this window. Volumetric and topographic assessment of the left ventricle is best obtained using this window. The subcostal and suprasternal windows may not be routinely used in some echocardiographic laboratories as they yield less information and adequate images are more difficult to obtain, as compared to the parasternal and apical windows.

The subcostal window is versatile, and almost all the standard views can be obtained in many patients

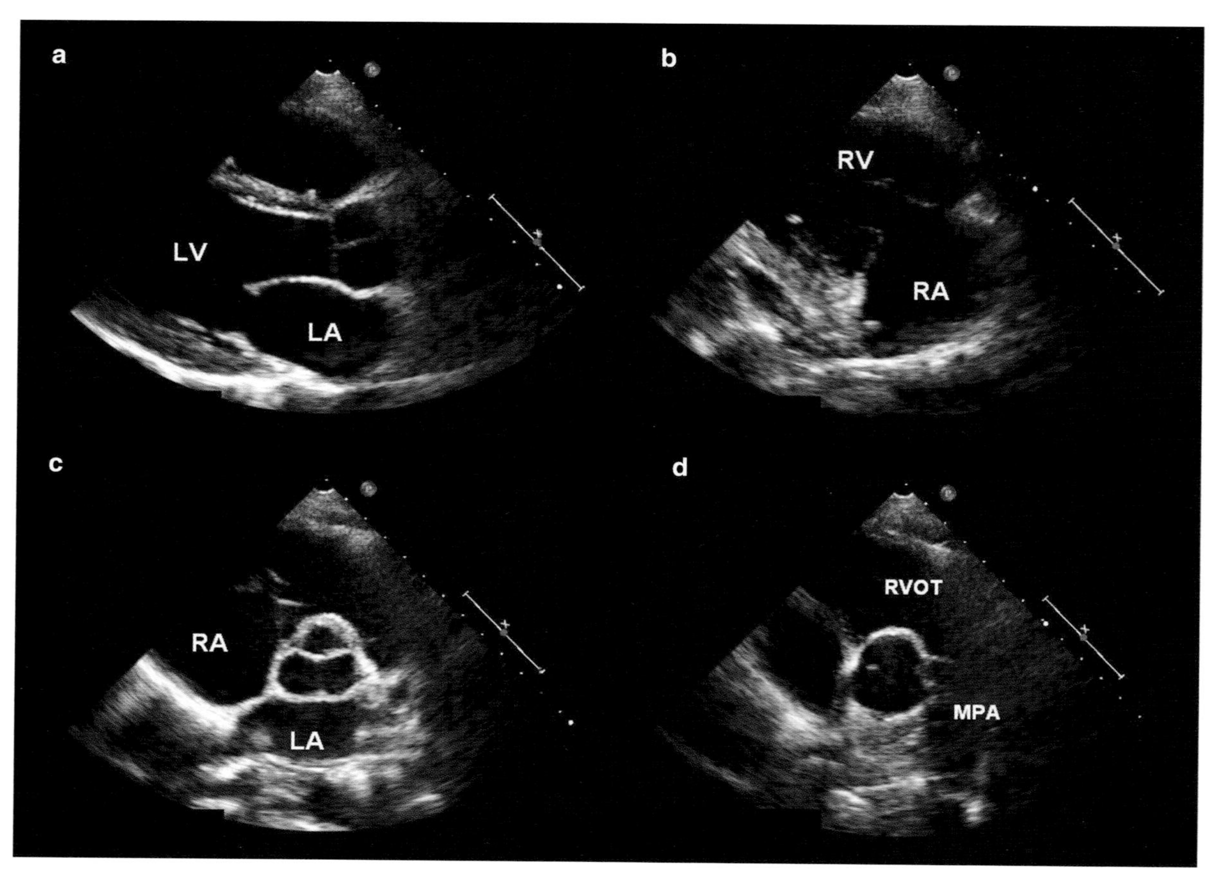

Fig. 1.22 (**a**) This is the parasternal long-axis view which is used to obtain 2D measurements of the left ventricle. The excursion of the aortic and mitral valves is well seen in this view. (**b**) This is the right ventricular inflow view showing the right atrium, tricuspid valve and right ventricle. (**c**) The aortic valve is the focus in the aortic short-axis view. (**d**) The right ventricular outflow tract, pulmonic valve and main pulmonary artery can be imaged by scanning more superiorly from the aortic short axis view. *LA* left atrium, *LV* left ventricle, *MPA* main pulmonary artery, *RA* right atrium, and *RV* right ventricle

particularly those with obstructive lung diseases (Figs. 1.26–1.28). Four-chamber view can be obtained, although the true left ventricular apex may be difficult to visualize. With the patient in held inspiration, it is feasible to obtain multiple short-axis images of the left ventricle from the level of the mitral valve to the apex (Fig. 1.27). This is also a preferred window to assess the right ventricular outflow tract which is usually in good alignment with the Doppler beam to provide accurate assessment of pulmonary valvular or infundibular stenosis (Fig. 1.28). The aortic arch and right pulmonary artery are generally well seen in the suprasternal window (Fig. 1.29). It can be the optimal window for Doppler interrogation of the aortic stenotic jet velocity in patients with aortic stenosis. Our view is that these two windows should be routinely explored so that skills needed to obtain images from these windows are retained, since images from these two windows can be essential in specific circumstances. For instance, detection of atrial septal defect is very much dependent on visualization of the atrial septum using the subcostal window, and the hint of patent ductus arteriosus in adult patients may be present only in the suprasternal views.

It is our practice to routinely perform and obtain the pulsed wave Doppler recordings of the right and left ventricular outflow tracts to assess the stroke volumes of the two ventricles (Fig. 1.30). In the absence of intracardiac shunt and valvular regurgitation (aortic or pulmonary), the stroke volumes of the two ventricles should be identical. The systolic flow in the left ventricular outflow tract has a higher peak velocity and time integral, compared to the right ventricular outflow

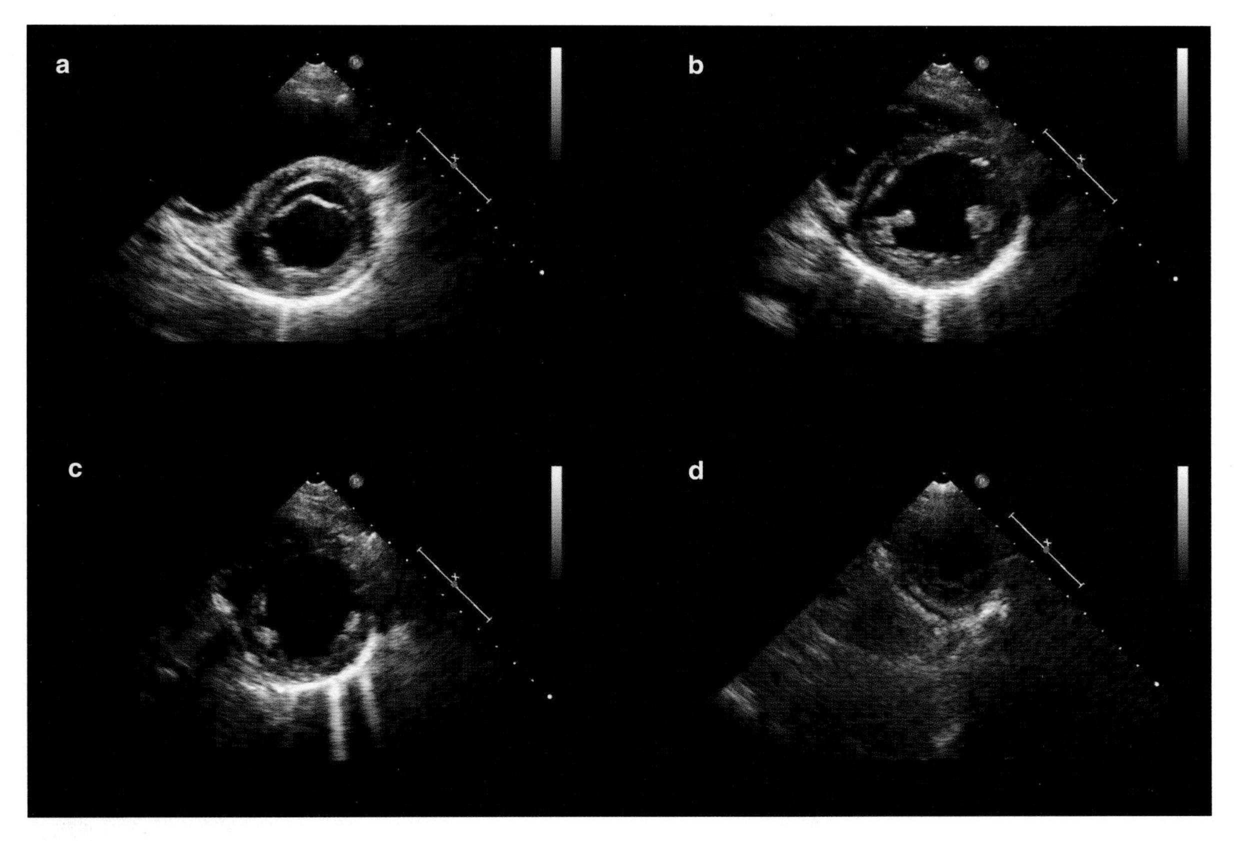

Fig. 1.23 The parasternal short axis views of the left ventricle are shown at the level of the mitral leaflets in (**a**), the papillary muscles in (**b**), below the papillary muscle in (**c**) and the apex in (**d**)

tract which has a large annular area. When the flow velocity in the right ventricular outflow tract has a high velocity or time integral, left to right shunt should be suspected. Knowledge of the stroke volume can be useful in patient management. A small stroke volume in the setting of normal systolic function suggests hypovolemia and should be considered in the assessment of aortic stenosis severity in patients with low transvalvular gradients [3] (Fig. 1.31).

Although a diagnostic study can be generated by the acquisition of predefined imaging planes from the four standard windows, strict adherence to such an approach may undermine the principle underlying the development of these conventional windows. In the early days of two-dimensional echocardiography, imaging from multiple surface locations provided information of the orientation of the heart within the chest cavity. This knowledge provided the essential framework for the proper interpretation of the images and led to the recognition that certain body surface locations were more useful in consistently yielding adequate images and diagnostic information. These surface locations became the standard echocardiographic windows. However these standard windows are by no means the only useful windows. Other non-standard windows may be critically important in specific clinical situations. They may be particularly useful when extracardiac conditions such as pectus excavatum and anterior mediastinal tumors are present to cause the heart to shift from its normal position and orientation. In subjects with severe pectus excavatum, the heart may shift leftward. In fact, an extreme leftward and posterior shift of the cardiac apex is probably the best indication of the presence of the complete absence of the pericardium.

It is essential to have a good working knowledge of the cardiac chambers within the thoracic cavity after one has reviewed the acquired images. Based on this knowledge, the echocardiographer may wish to acquire additional images using the different imaging planes from the standard windows, together with any available

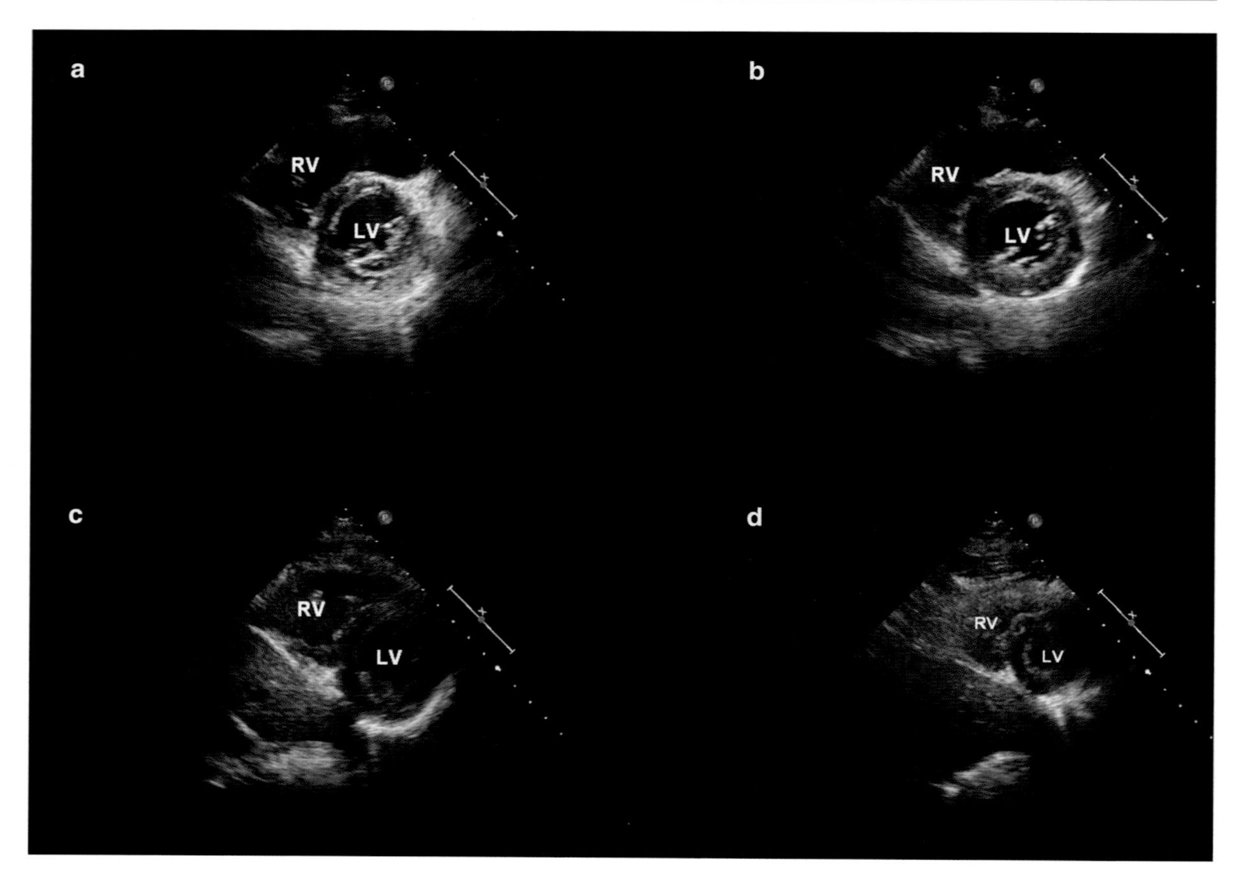

Fig. 1.24 Multiple short axis views (**a–d**) of the right ventricle can be obtained from the parasternal window by tilting the image plane more rightward from the usual orientation. *LV* left ventricle, *RV* right ventricle

images from additional non-standard windows. The locations of non-standard imaging windows are determined by the position of the heart within the thoracic cavity and less influenced by surface anatomy. In fact any surface location can be, and should be, considered a potential image window depending upon the specific clinical question and the position of the cardiac structures within the thorax. An effective echocardiographer is one who not only can integrate the images from multiple windows, but also has the technical ability to perform and acquire images from conventional and unusual windows.

There are specific clinical situations where the use of non-conventional imaging windows should be an integral part of the echocardiographic examinations as there is a high likelihood of additional information provided by these additional windows. The following additional windows are highlighted because of their usefulness in specific situations. Prior knowledge of the results of other imaging investigations such as chest x-ray, computed tomogram scan or angiogram are useful to consider when additional imaging windows should be sought and where the additional windows will be obtained.

The right parasternal window should be used in subjects with dilatation of the ascending aorta, which takes a more rightward and anterior course such that the mid and distal ascending aorta can frequently be imaged from this window (Fig. 1.32). Imaging from the back is feasible in the presence of pleural effusion [4, 5] (Figs. 1.33, 1.34). When a left pleural effusion is present, the left paraspinal window should be used as it can provide multiple imaging planes to assess cardiac chambers and valves. Another situation where the left spinal window is useful is in the setting of tortuous and dilated descending thoracic aorta which abuts against the posterior chest wall [6]. Aortic aneurysms and aortic dissection can be diagnosed using this

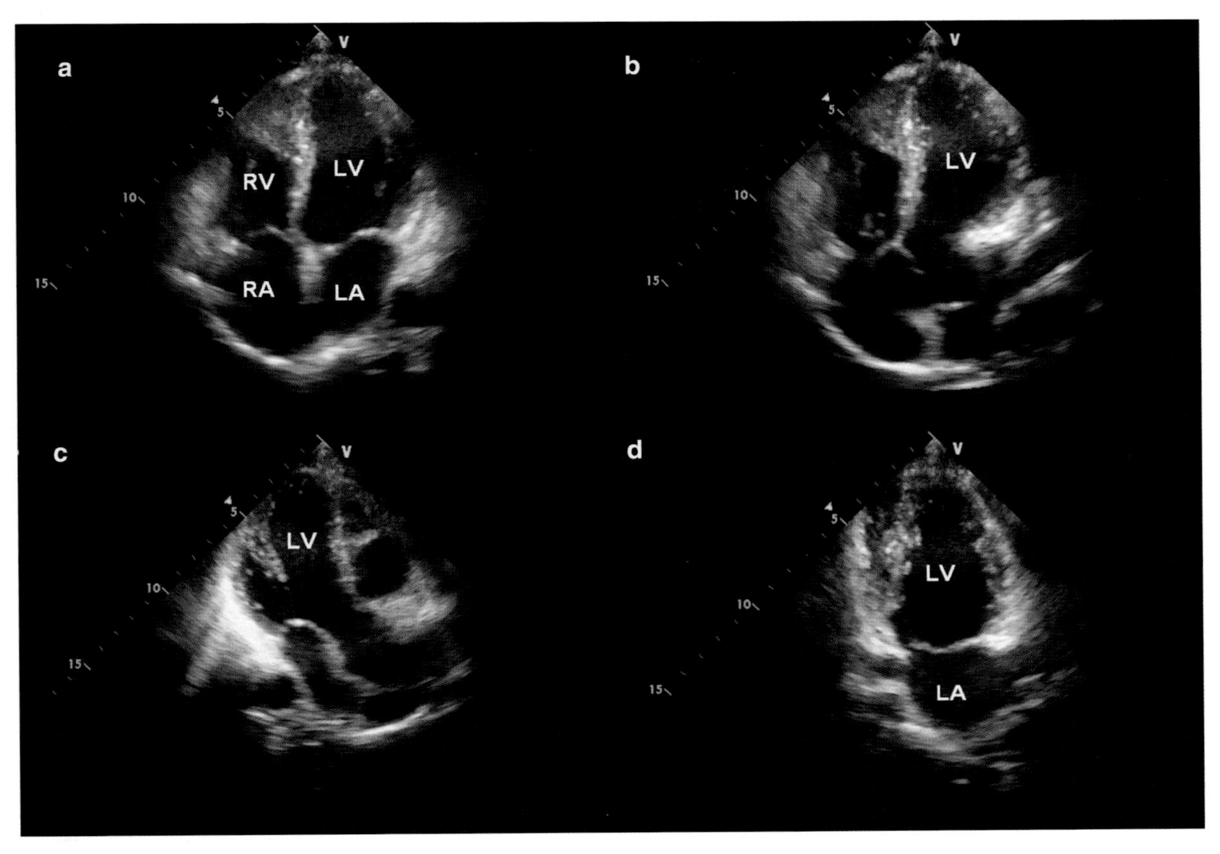

Fig. 1.25 Multiple views can be obtained from the apical window with the four chamber view shown in (**a**), five chamber view in (**b**), long axis view in (**c**), and two chamber view in (**d**). *LA* left atrium, *LV* left ventricle, *RA* right atrium, *RV* right ventricle

window. In patients with chronic obstructive lung disease, the subcostal window should be exploited because in these patients almost all the imaging planes from the parasternal and apical windows can be obtained (Figs. 1.26–1.28). In this clinical setting, it is important to utilize the entire subcostal region because frequently the transducer needs to be positioned considerably leftward to provide a comprehensive assessment of the left ventricular cavity and apex.

In some patients no optimal acoustic windows can be obtained from the body surface. These may include obese patients, patients with severe emphysema, patients with chest wall deformities, and patients who have had recent cardiac surgery. Transesophageal echocardiography provides high quality images due to the use of a high frequency transducer and little soft tissue separating the ultrasound transducer in the esophagus from the cardiac chambers (Fig. 1.35). In clinical situations such as endocarditis, the diagnostic yield in terms of detection of vegetations and abscess is higher with transesophageal echocardiography, which is frequently indicated despite adequate transthoracic images. The posterior vantage point of this imaging approach allows a novel and detailed view of posteriorly located structures such as the atria, atrial septum, and mitral valve. The superior vena cava and pulmonary veins, which cannot be imaged from the chest surface, can be routinely assessed using the esophageal window. This window is ideal in the intra-operative setting in which transthoracic windows are unavailable. The indications for transesophageal echocardiography are summarized in Table 1.1.

High quality echocardiographic images can be obtained by placing the transducer directly onto the beating heart during an open heart procedure (Fig 1.36). This approach, epicardial echocardiography, can provide information not obtainable by other means but essential to the management of patients with unusual

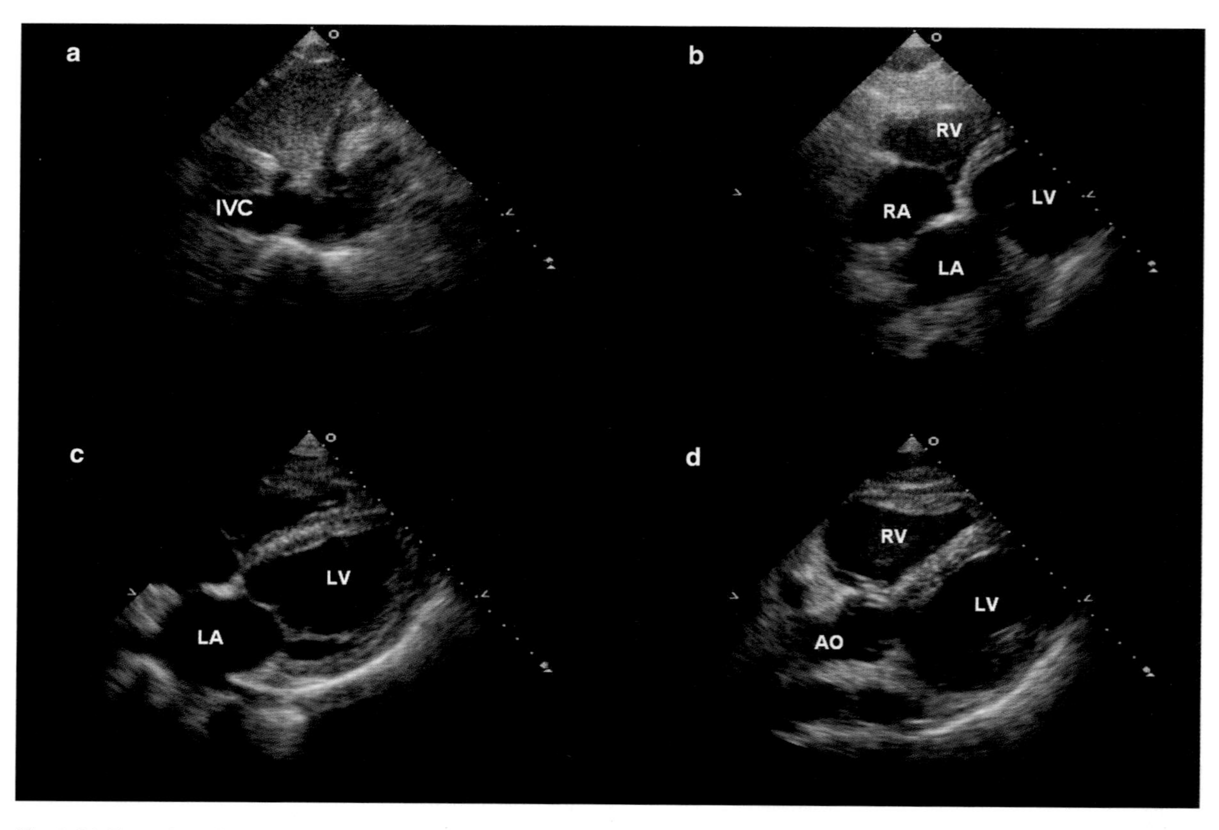

Fig. 1.26 From the subcostal window, the inferior vena cava can be imaged as show in (**a**). Modified four chamber views are shown in (**b**) and (**c**). In (**c**) the atrial septum is well seen. In (**d**) the left ventricular outflow tract and aortic valve are imaged by tilting the imaging plane anteriorly. *Ao* aorta, *IVC* inferior vena cava, *LA* left atrium, *LV* left ventricle, *RA* right atrium, *RV* right ventricle

cardiac anatomy and patients following complex surgical repair, such as patients with complex congenital heart disease following a complicated intracardiac procedure. Epicardial echocardiography underscores the versatility of echocardiography in exploiting any available acoustic windows.

External Versus Internal Landmarks

The standard imaging windows are practical landmarks for the echocardiographic examination. Images acquired from these windows should provide a good conceptual framework of the position of the heart in relation to the thoracic cavity. Together with results from other imaging modalities, images from these standard windows are the basis for additional images from other windows. There is an almost limitless number of imaging planes that can be obtained from the standard and non-standard windows. A set of standard imaging planes has been proposed and generally adopted in the practice of echocardiography. This relatively small number of imaging planes was chosen as they have been found to be useful to illustrate specific cardiac anatomy such as cardiac valves. As indicated above, these imaging planes can be obtained in most patients and provide most of the echocardiographic data relating to cardiac structure and function.

With the body surface landmarks as the starting point, additional landmarks are needed for the proper framing of the individual imaging planes. The use of internal landmarks can ensure that the cardiac structure is properly displayed. In the parasternal long-axis view, the imaging plane should be adjusted to maximize the internal diameter of the left ventricle to ensure that it transects the long-axis of the left ventricle. Although the true long-axis of the ascending aorta and the long-axis of the left ventricle can be imaged at the same time in one imaging plane, this is not necessarily the case in all

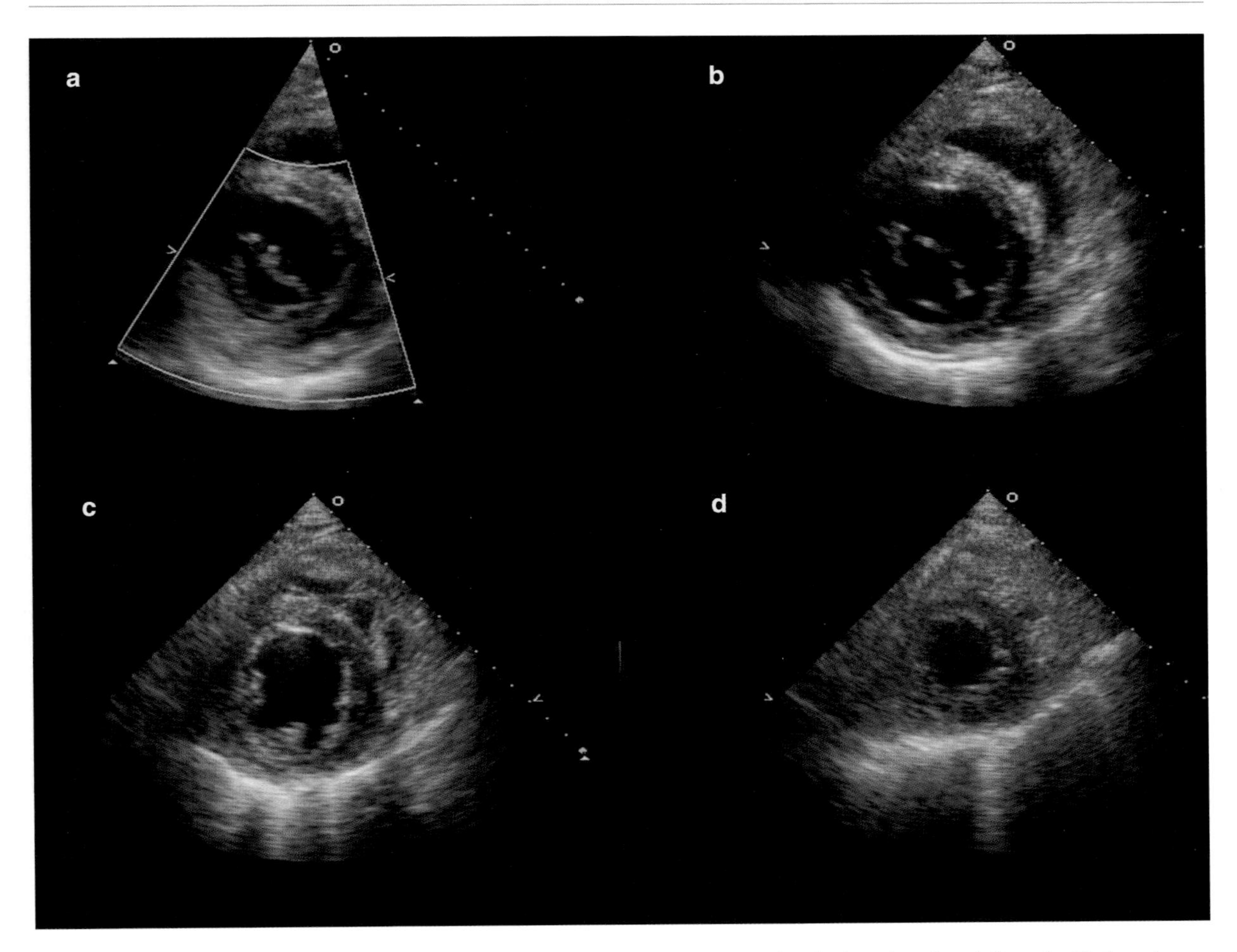

Fig. 1.27 The left ventricle can be imaged from the base to the apex (**a–d**) by moving the imaging plane leftward with the echocardiographic transducer at the subcostal region

subjects. Fine adjustment of the imaging plane to ensure that the ascending aorta is optimally imaged is evidenced by achieving parallel alignment of the anterior and posterior aortic walls in the same view. Attention to this anatomic detail is essential when comparing the measurement of the ascending aorta during serial follow-up of patients with ascending aortic aneurysm. To achieve these internal landmarks may require modifying the transducer location from one intercostal space to another. In the parasternal short-axis view, the papillary muscles serve a useful landmark for localizing the mid left ventricular segments. In addition, a normal left ventricle should assume a symmetric circular geometry in this view. There are no good internal landmarks to guide the optimal image of the left ventricle from the apical window, such that foreshortening the left ventricular apex should be a constant concern. The position of the transducer should be carefully adjusted to maximize the length of the left ventricle (Fig. 1.37). The recent development of three-dimensional imaging should address this technical concern. Subcostal images are particularly useful to image the atrial septum, but the left ventricular apex is frequently not imaged from this window (Fig. 1.26). Another structure that is well seen from the subcostal window is the right ventricular outflow tract and the pulmonic valve (Fig. 1.27). From the suprasternal window, the aortic arch and proximal descending aorta are well seen particularly in young individuals. Excessive pressure on the transducer should be avoided so as to not compress the inominate vein making its recognition difficult (Fig. 1.38). In subjects with unfolded aortic arch, imaging from the right and left supraclavicular fossae may provide better images of the aortic arch.

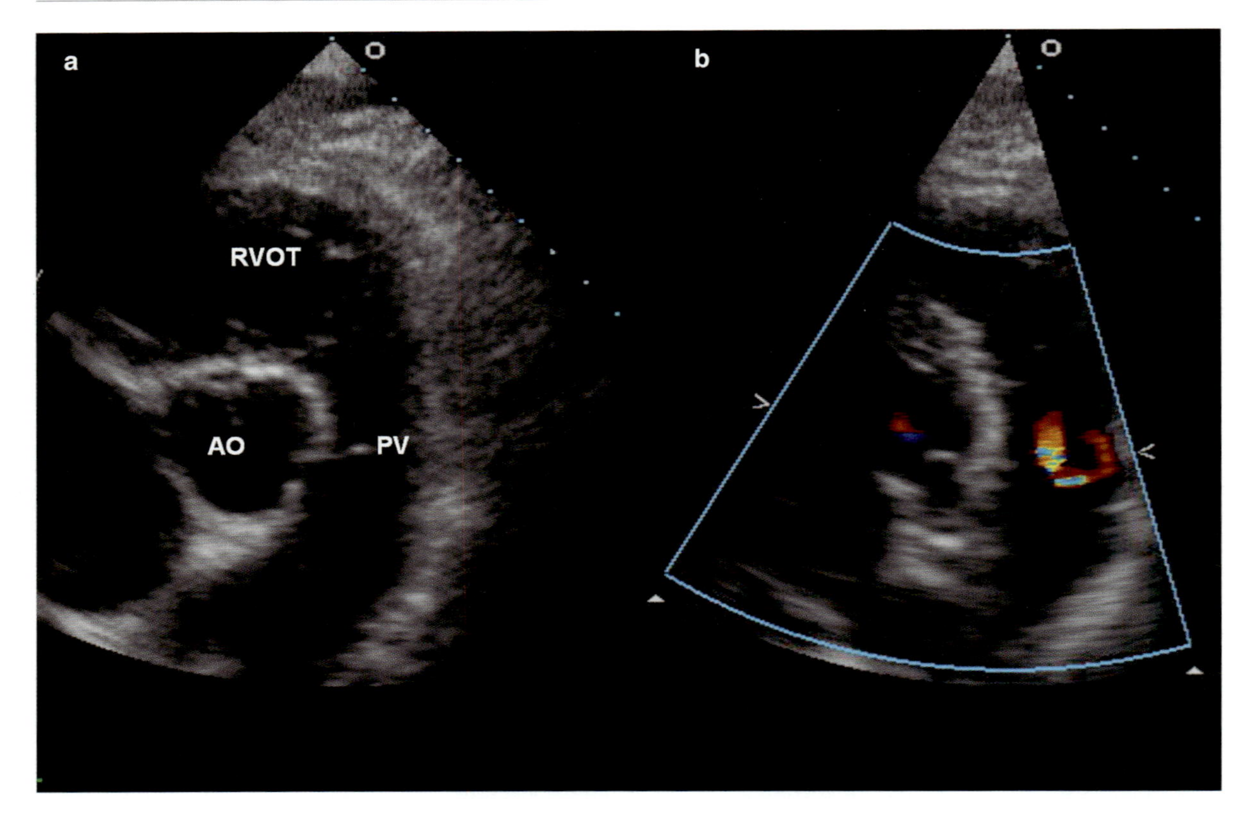

Fig. 1.28 (**a**) The subcostal window also provides assessment of the right ventricular outflow tract and the pulmonic valve, because there is good alignment of these structures with the ultrasound beam. The color flow image in (**b**) shows mild physiological pulmonic regurgitation. *Ao* aorta, *PV* pulmonic valve, *RVOT* right ventricular outflow tract

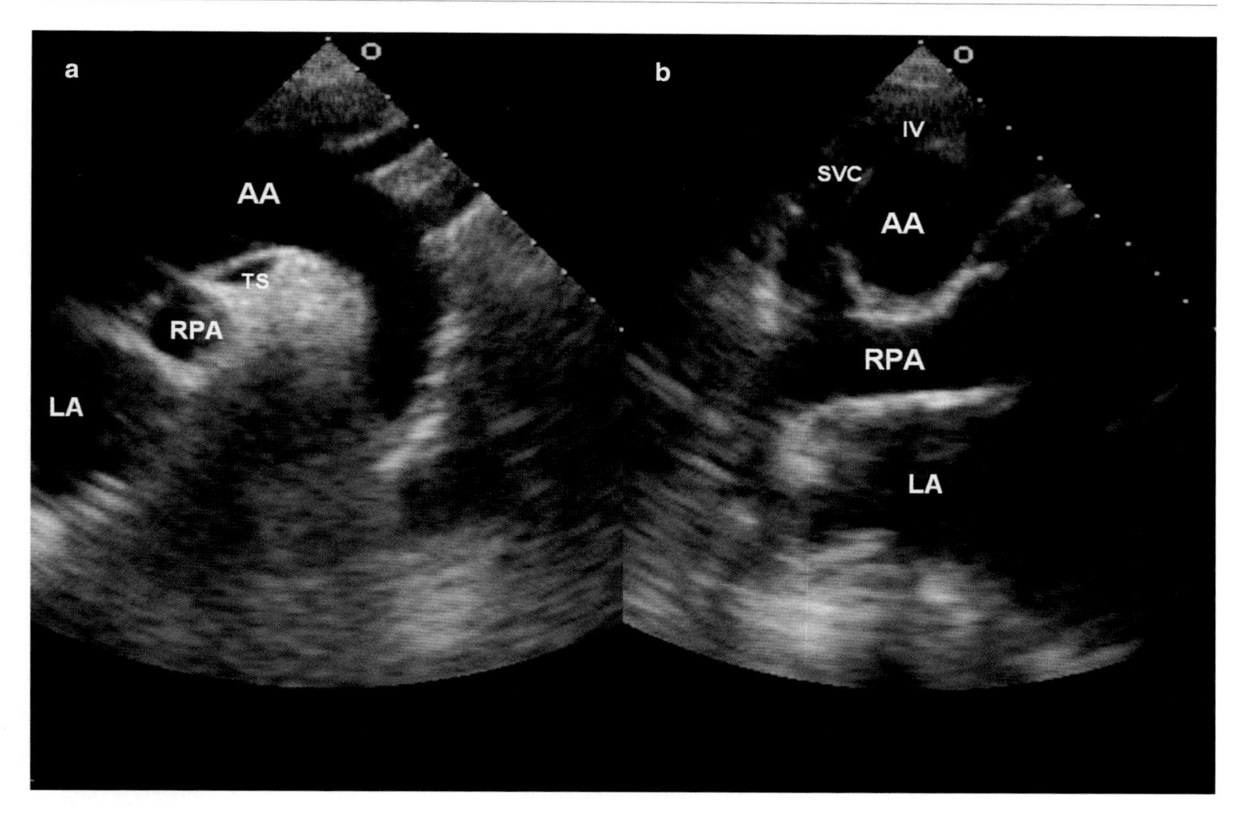

Fig. 1.29 Both the long axis (**a**) and short axis (**b**) views of the aortic arch can be obtained from the suprasternal window. *AA* aortic arch, *IV* innominate vein, *LA* left atrium, *RPA* right pulmonary artery, *SVC* superior vena cava, *TS* transverse sinus

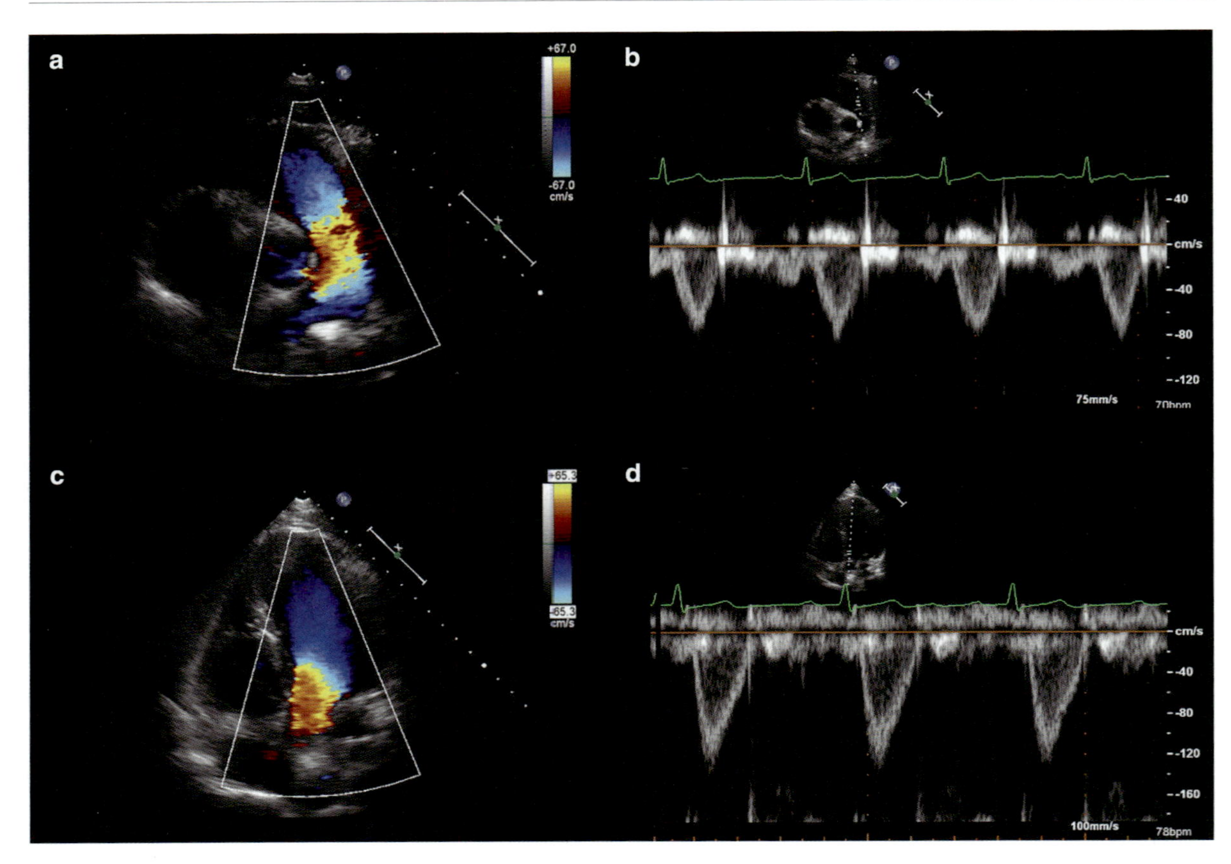

Fig. 1.30 The systolic flow in the right ventricular outflow tract by color flow imaging is shown in (**a**), and the pulsed wave spectral signals in (**b**). The same assessments of the left ventricular outflow tract are shown in (**c**) and (**d**). In normal individuals, the pulsed wave spectral signals in the left ventricular outflow tract have high peak velocity and time integrals than those of the right ventricular outflow tract which has a large annular area

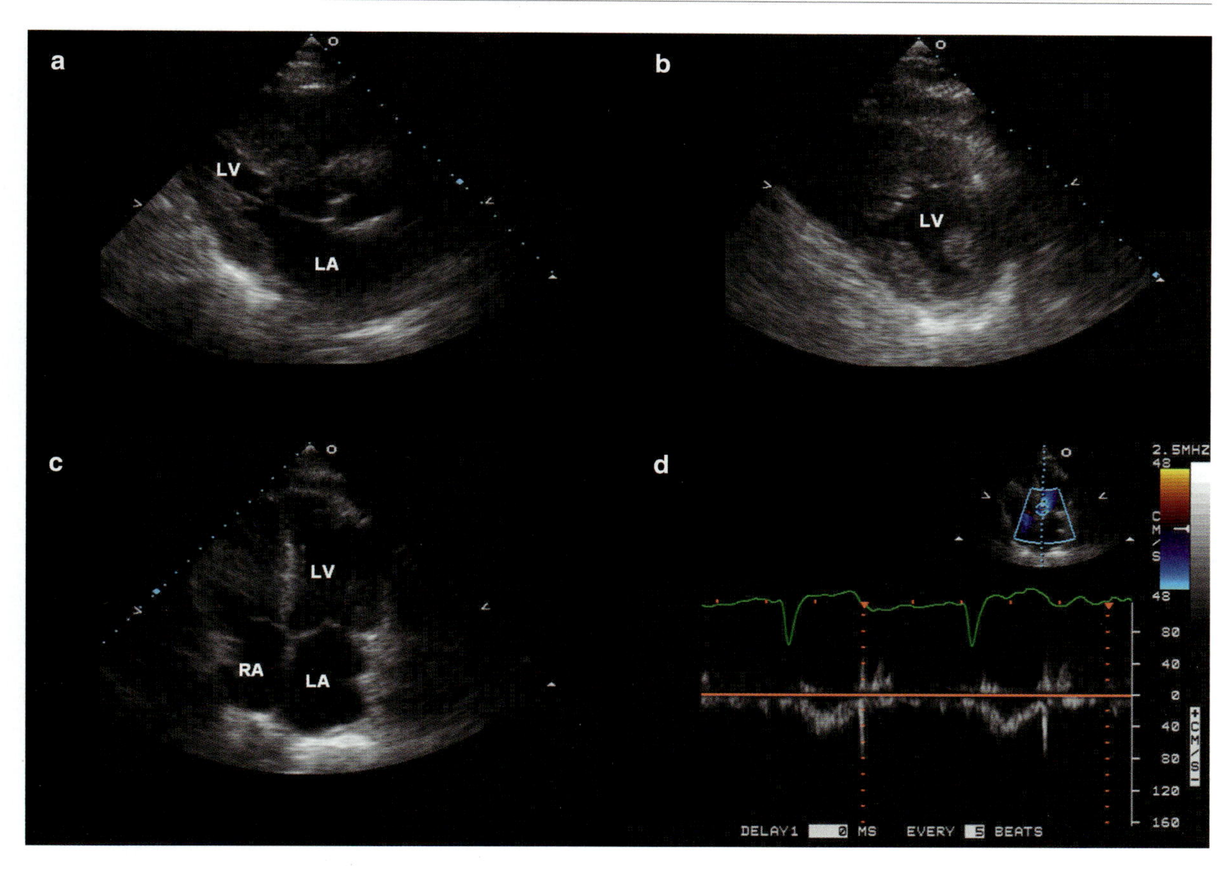

Fig. 1.31 This 94-year-old man has an increased left ventricular wall thickness and a small cavity. This is illustrated in the parasternal long-axis (**a**), short axis (**b**), and apical four chamber (**c**) views. The flow in the left ventricular outflow tract (**d**) has a low velocity and time integral, indicating a small stroke volume despite a normal ejection fraction. *LA* left atrium, *LV* left ventricle, *RA* right atrium

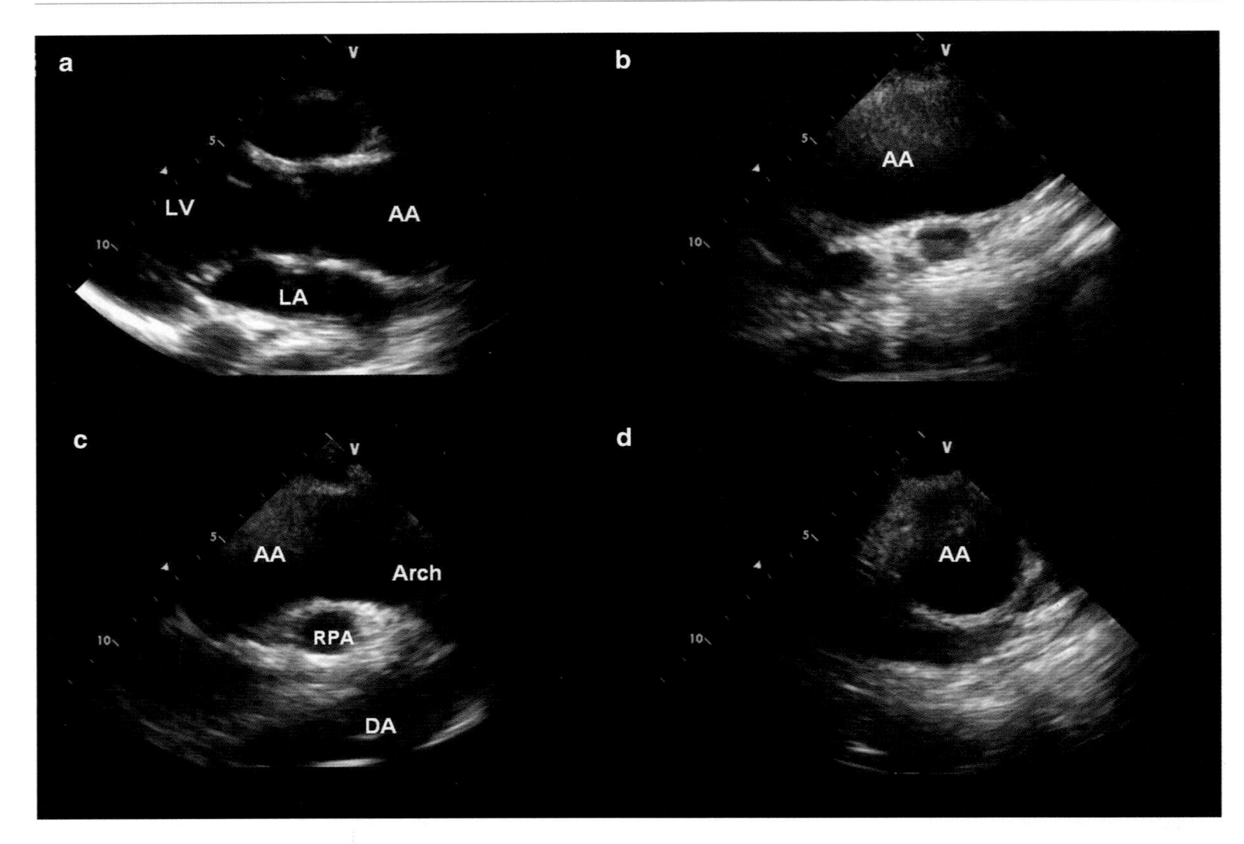

Fig. 1.32 The right sternal border can be very useful in imaging the ascending aorta in the patients with a dilated aorta. The standard left parasternal long axis view is shown in (**a**). (**b**) Is obtained from the right sternal border at the fourth intercostal space near the sternum, showing the dilated ascending aorta. By moving the transducer to the right third intercostal space, the distal ascending aorta, aortic arch and descending aorta can be imaged. (**c**) The short-axis view of ascending aorta from the right sternal border is shown in (**d**). *AA* ascending aorta, *Arch* aortic arch, *DA* descending aorta, *LA* left atrium, *LV* left ventricle, *RPA* right pulmonary artery

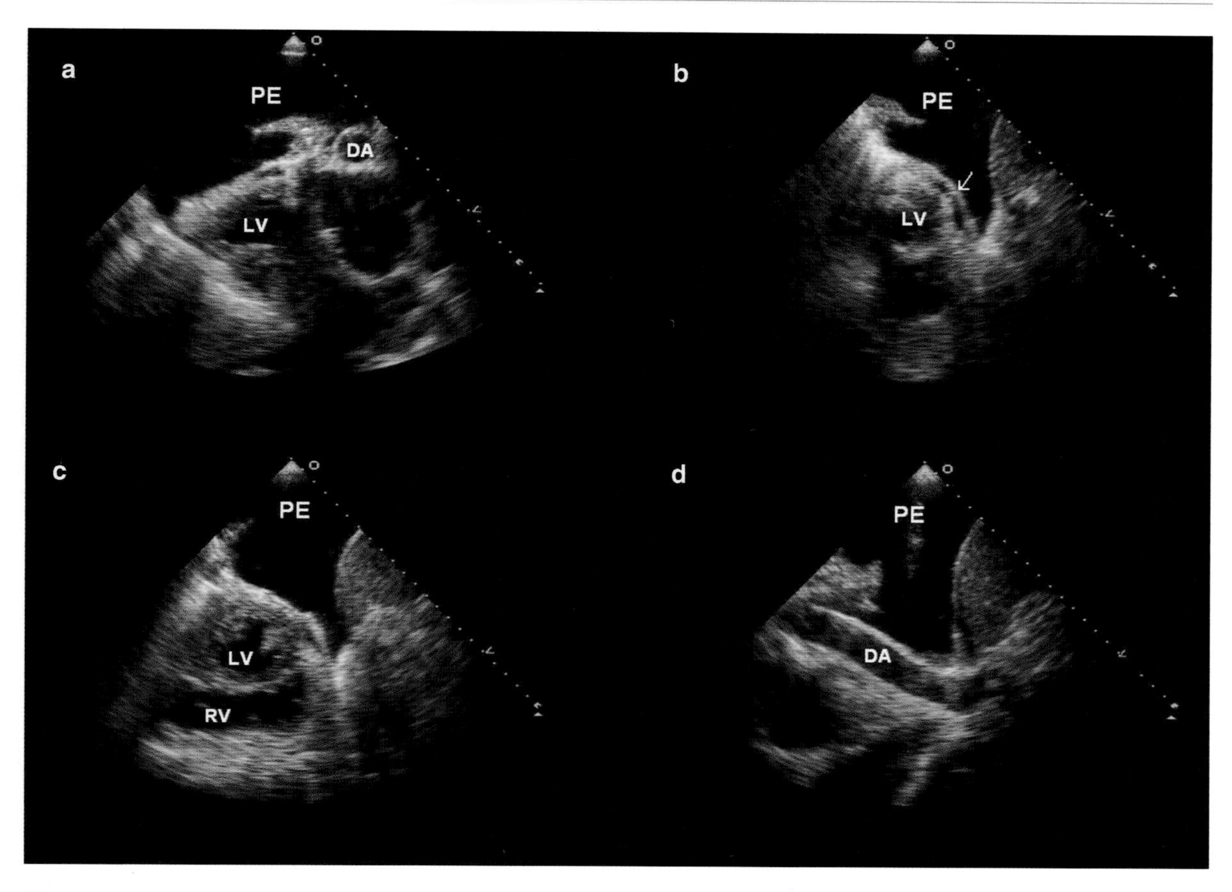

Fig. 1.33 The presence of a large left pleural effusion allows the use of the left paraspinal window to image the heart. In (**a**) the left ventricle is imaged in long axis and in (**b**) in short-axis. The pericardium (*arrow*) is well seen due to the presence of a small pericardial effusion. The left ventricle and the two papillary muscle are imaged in (**c**). The descending thoracic aorta is imaged in (**d**). *DA* descending aorta, *LV* left ventricle, *PE* pleural effusion, *RV* right ventricle

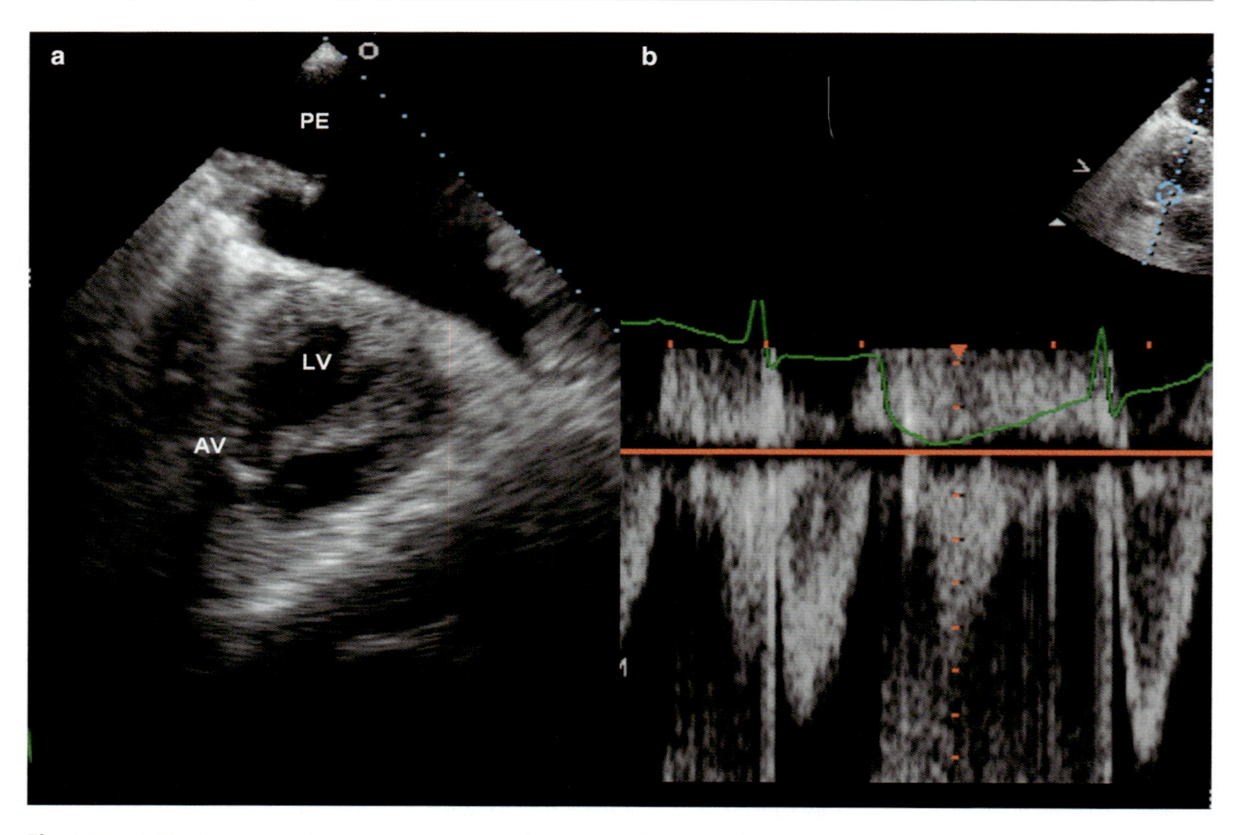

Fig. 1.34 (**a**) The left ventricular outflow tract and aortic valve are imaged in the view from the left paraspinal window. The aortic flow can be assessed by pulsed wave Doppler as shown in (**b**). *AV* aortic valve, *LV* left ventricle, *PE* pleural effusion

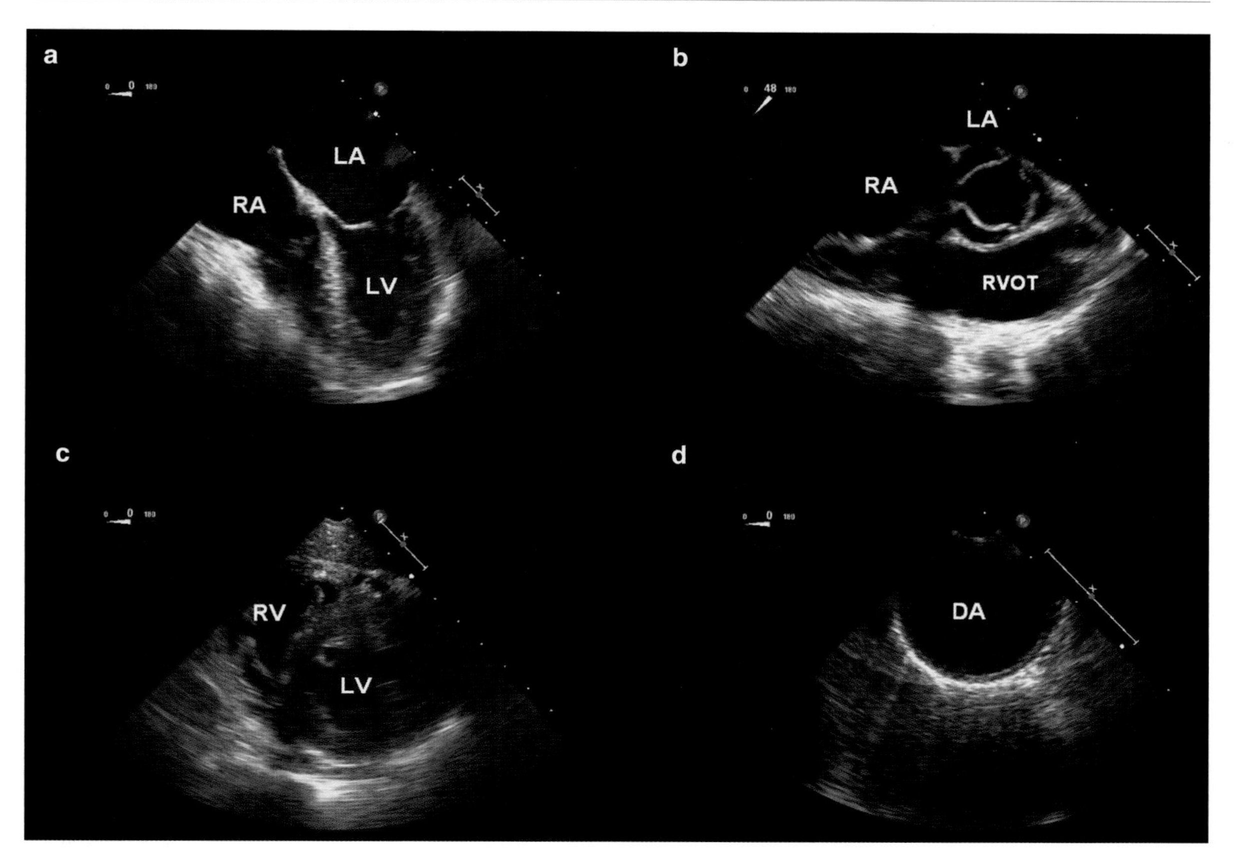

Fig. 1.35 Transesophageal echocardiography provides many views which can be divided into groups of views represented by the four chamber view shown in (**a**), the basal aortic valve view in (**b**), the transgastric view in (**c**) and the aortic views in (**d**)

Table 1.1 Indications of transesophageal echocardiography

Suboptimal or unavailable transthoracic images: • Obesity, emphysema, ventilator, chest wall deformities, post sternotomy • Intraoperative assessment
Additional anatomic details despite adequate transthoracic images: • Mechanism of valvular regurgitation • Detection of small vegetations • Detection of perivalvular abscess • Aortic plaques
Structures not imaged by transthoracic echocardiography • Superior vena cava • Left atrial appendage • Pulmonary veins • Descending thoracic aorta

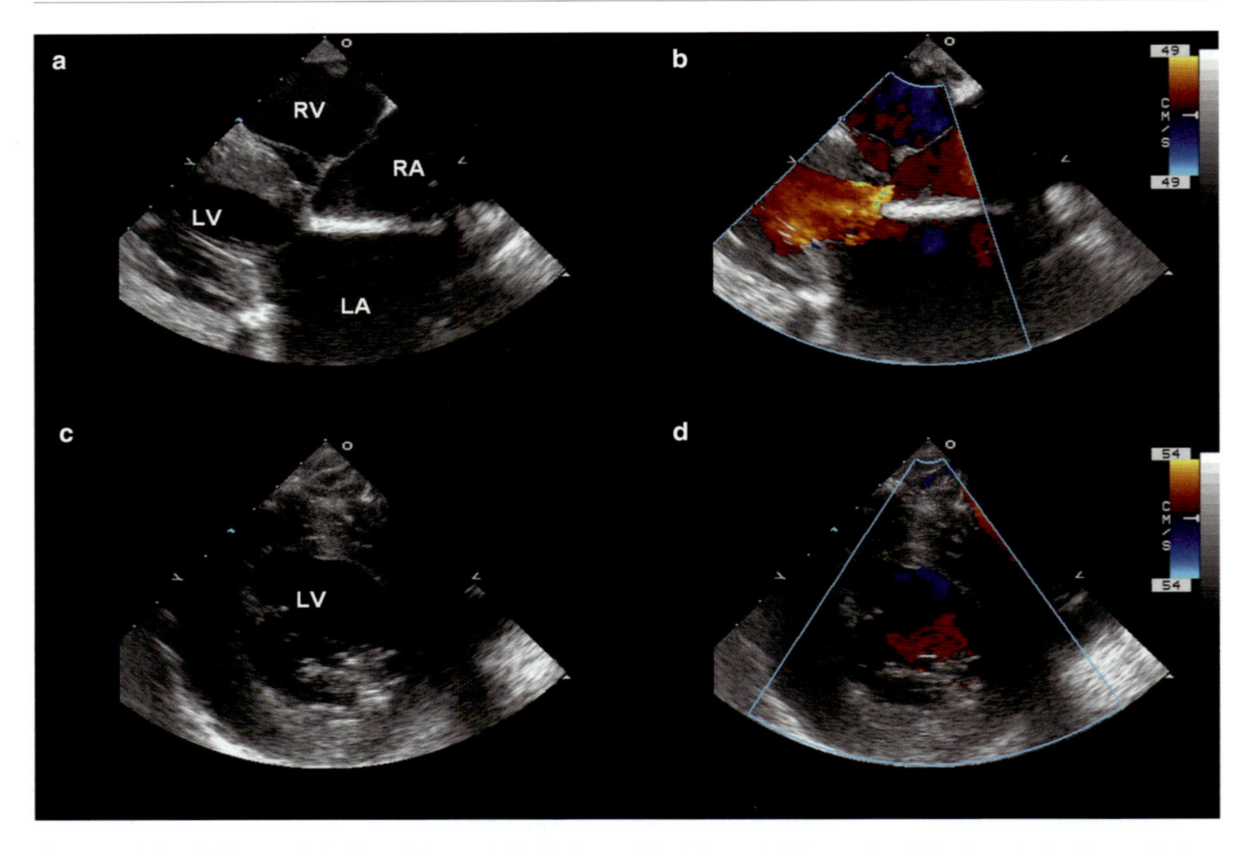

Fig. 1.36 Epicardial long-axis (**a**, **b**) and short-axis (**c**, **d**) views of the left ventricle in a patient following mitral valve repair show thickening of the posterior mitral leaflet consistent with repair and no mitral regurgitation. *LA* left atrium, *LV* left ventricle, *RA* right atrium, *RV* right ventricle

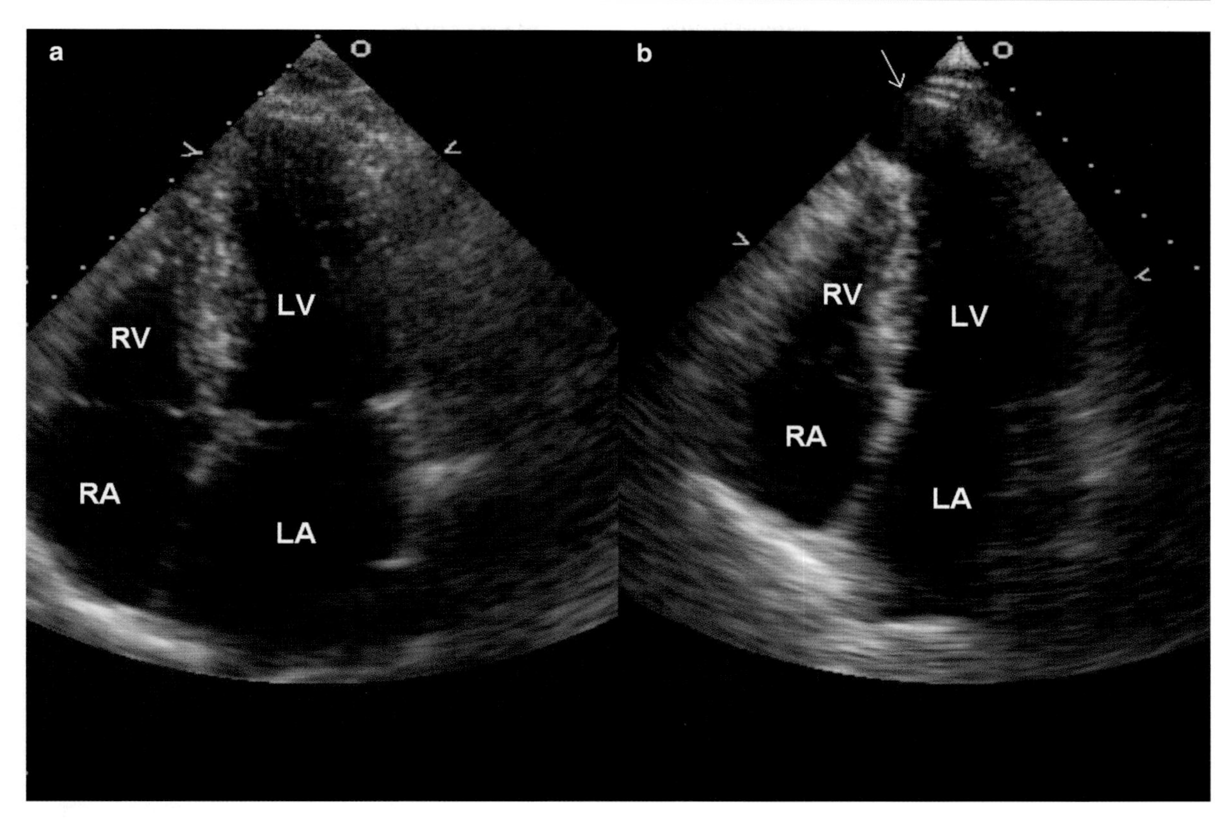

Fig. 1.37 The true apex of the left ventricle may not be imaged if the apical views are foreshortened. This patient has a small left ventricular apical aneurysm which is missed in the foreshortened four chamber view in (**a**) and nicely demonstrated in (**b**) when the transducer is positioned more laterally. *LA* left atrium, *LV* left ventricle, *RA* right atrium, *RV* right ventricle

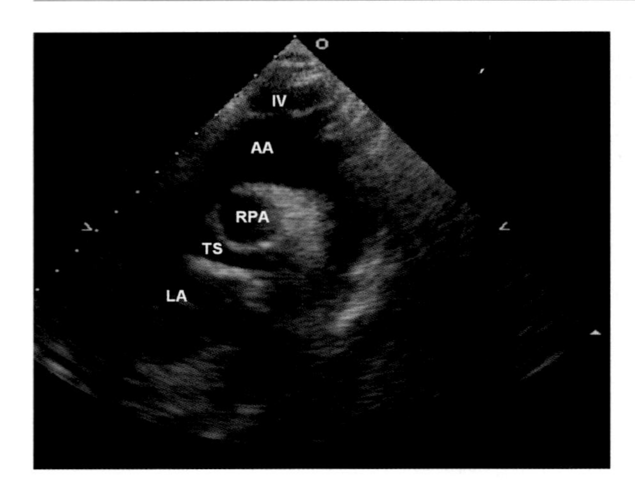

Fig. 1.38 The suprasternal long axis view of the aortic arch shows the innominate vein superior to the arch. Excessive transducer pressure at the suprasternal window may obliterate the innominate vein. *AA* aortic arch, *IV* innominate vein; *LA* left atrium, *RPA* right pulmonary artery, *TS* transverse sinus

Summary

A good understanding of the position of the heart in relation to the thoracic cavity can be obtained from images acquired from imaging windows on the body surface and the results from other imaging modalities. This information is helpful in the assessment of intrinsic cardiac abnormalities and extrinsic cardiac conditions. It also provides the necessary framework for the use of additional non-standard windows which can provide valuable information in specific clinical situations. The non-invasive nature and versatility of echocardiography can provide almost limitless number of imaging planes from many locations on the body surface. The proper display of cardiac structures requires careful attention to internal landmarks. The development of 3D echocardiography will likely further enhance the diagnostic capability of echocardiography.

References

1. Veinot JP, Harrity PJ, Gentile F, et al. Anatomy of the normal left atrial appendage: a quantitative study of age-related changes in 500 autopsy hearts: implications for echocardiographic examination. *Circulation*. 1997 Nov 4;96(9): 3112-3115.
2. Hagen PT, Scholz DG, Edwards WD. Incidence and size of patent foramen ovale during the first 10 decades of life: an autopsy study of 965 normal hearts. *Mayo Clin Proc*. 1984 Jan;59(1):17-20.
3. Hachicha Z, Dumesnil JG, Bogaty P, Pibarot P. Paradoxical low-flow, low-gradient severe aortic stenosis despite preserved ejection fraction is associated with higher afterload and reduced survival. *Circulation*. 2007;115:2856-2864.
4. Waggoner AD, Baumann CM, Stark PA. Views from the back by subscapular retrocardiac imaging: technique and clinical application. *J Am Soc Echocardiogr*. 1995; 8:257-262.
5. Naqvi TZ, Huynh HK. A new window of opportunity in echocardiography. *J Am Soc Echocardiogr*. 2006;19: 569-577.
6. Klein A, Chan K, Walley W. A new paraspinal window in the echocardiographic diagnosis of descending aortic dissection. *Am Heart J*. 1987;114:902-904.

2 Age-Related Cardiac Changes

Like all visceral organs, the heart ages. The fibrous skeleton of the heart becomes sclerotic and calcifies, the valve closing margins thicken, the aorta dilates and tilts rightward on the interventricular septum making the latter seem prominent, the ventricles decrease in size, the left atrium enlarges, valves calcify and/or become myxomatous and amyloid may deposit in the heart.

Fenestrations

Fenestrations of semilunar valve cusps are very commonly noted at pathology examination and at surgery and may be detected by imaging studies. Fenestrations are an acquired degenerative change whose frequency increases with age. Fenestrations are typically found in the region of the lunula, which is the portion of the valve cusp between the line of closure and the free edge of the cusp (Figs. 2.1, 2.2). They may extend from the region of the commissures all the way to the nodule of Arantius in the middle of the cusp. Fenestrations are not usually associated with aortic regurgitation as they are located distal to the line of closure. Acute aortic insufficiency due to rupture of fenestrated aortic valve cusp has been reported [1]. This occurs when the fenestration is large and extends beyond the line of closure into the body of the cusp, or the fenestration is located at the commissure and its rupture leads to cusp prolapse. If dilation of the aortic root moves the line of valve closure towards the cusp free edge, the fenestration may be incorporated into the functional portion of the valve, and regurgitation through the fenestration may develop [2].

Un-ruptured aortic fenestrations are not detectable echocardiographically, because they are located in the lunula region beyond the line of closure. Ruptured fenestrations can be identified as long linear strands arising from the aortic cusps. They are best seen in the left ventricular outflow tract during aortic valve closure (Fig. 2.2). They are differentiated from vegetations by their long linear appearance and the absence of aortic regurgitation as previously discussed.

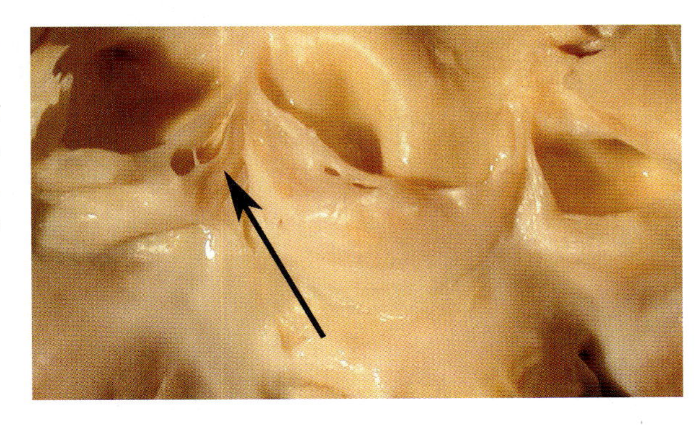

Fig. 2.1 Opened aortic valve with fenestrations (*arrow*) visible. Note they are above the line of valve closure near the commissures laterally

Lambl's Excresences

Lambl's excrescences and fibrous tags are thought to represent a common valvular degenerative or age-related lesion, often thought to reflect wear and tear. Some consider these to represent repetitive trauma-related endothelial proliferations or organized thrombi. They may occasionally be found in much younger patients, including children. Thrombi have a tendency to form on these areas of endocardial roughening (non-bacterial thrombotic endocarditis). On gross examination Lambl's excrescences commonly occur at lines of valve closure and are most common on the left sided

K.-L. Chan and J.P. Veinot, *Anatomic Basis of Echocardiographic Diagnosis*,
DOI: 10.1007/978-1-84996-387-9_2,

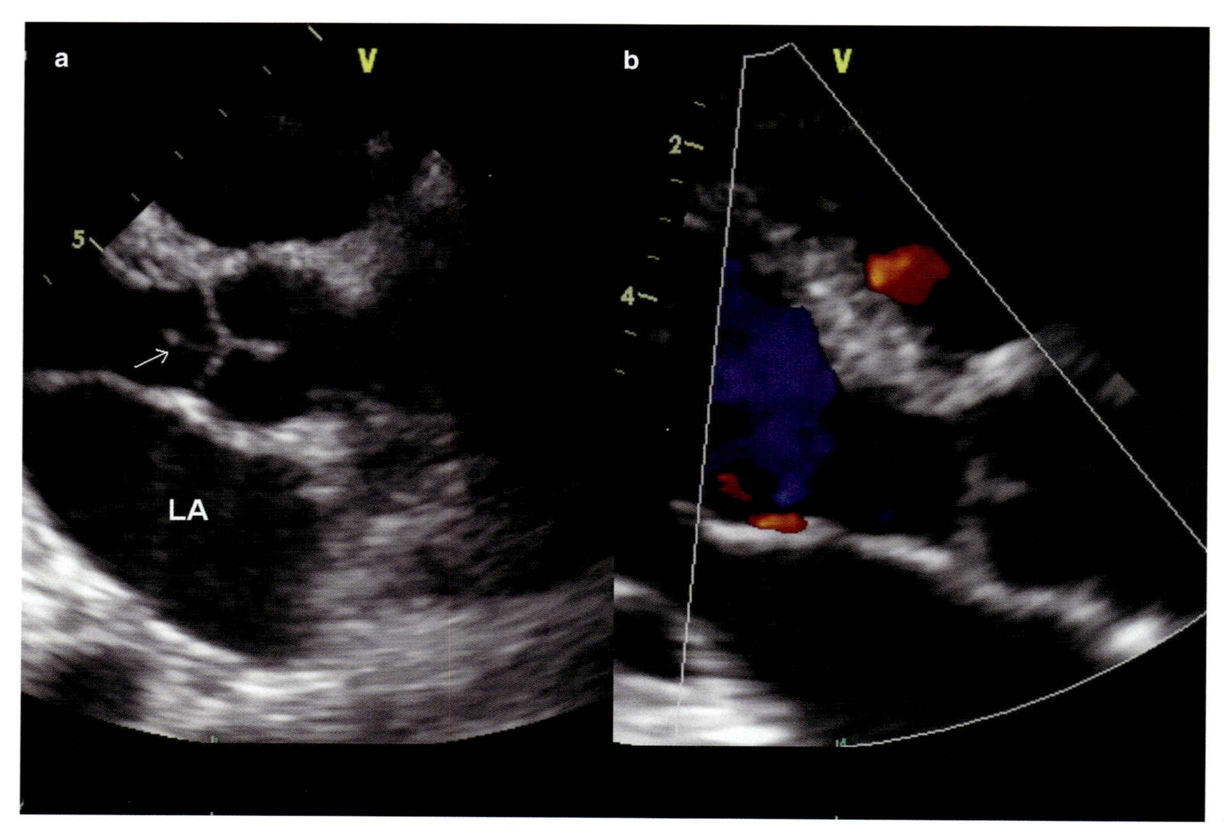

Fig. 2.2 The parasternal long-axis view (**a**) of a 43-year-old woman shows that there is long linear density (*arrows*) attaching to the tip of the aortic valve and prolapsing into the left ventricular outflow tract in diastole. Color flow imaging shows no aortic regurgitation (**b**). This linear mobile density likely represents a ruptured aortic fenestration. *LA* left atrium

valves, including the aortic valve near the nodulus of Arantius. The excrescences appear as tiny tags of fibrous material and are best visualized immersed under water (Fig. 2.3). These morphologic features have been observed on echocardiography (Fig. 2.4). These excrescences are grossly similar to papillary fibroelastoma neoplasms, but differ in size and location. On microscopic examination they are similar to papillary fibroelastomas with endothelial covered fibroelastic cores, sometimes associated with adherent thrombi. They can cause turbulence, and are a site of relative stasis where thrombosis may occur and thus may provide a site for the development of infective endocarditis. Coronary ostial obstruction and embolization of fragments or excrescences have been reported. It is probable that the emboli originate from thrombus on the Lambl's, rather than the fibroelastic material itself.

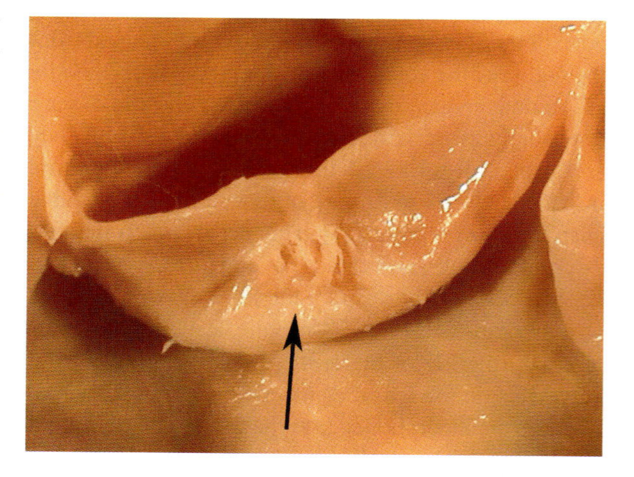

Fig. 2.3 Close up view of an aortic valve cusp. In the center of the cusp, midline, along the line of closure, there are multiple small whisker like Lambl's excrescences (*arrow*)

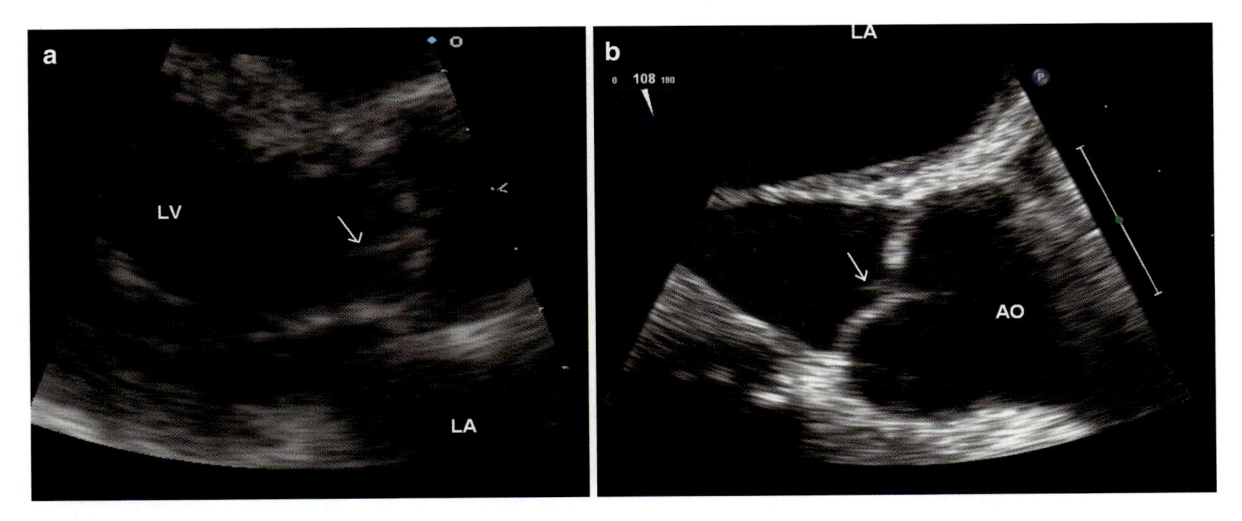

Fig. 2.4 (a) Small whisker-like mobile densities (*arrow*) consistent with Lambl's excrescences are seen on the aortic valve in this 87-year-old woman. (b) These are more clearly demonstrated (*arrow*) by transesophageal echocardiography. *Ao* aorta, *LA* left atrium, *LV* left ventricle

Mitral Annular Calcification

Mitral annular calcification (MAC) is a common finding in the hearts of elderly patients, especially females. Although MAC has been considered to be an age-related finding, it probably is a pathological process due to degenerative changes in the mitral annulus. Its incidence is low in those under the age of 50 years; however, the incidence of MAC increases to become common in the elderly. It is a progressive process, albeit at a slow pace in most patients. In association with mitral valve disease, especially mitral valve prolapse (myxomatous/floppy mitral valve), the condition may occur in younger patients. MAC occurs at an earlier age, is more exaggerated and has a more rapid progression in those with calcium metabolic abnormalities such as hyperparathyroidism and chronic renal failure, especially in those who are dialysis dependent.

Mitral annular calcification is usually localized to the mitral ring, invariably the most common site being the base of the posterior mitral leaflet (Fig. 2.5). Rarely the calcium extends onto the mitral leaflet (Fig. 2.6). This process generally starts at the base of the leaflets and the tips of leaflets remain mobile (Fig. 2.7). MAC may be distinguished from post-rheumatic changes by the lack of leaflet commissural fusion and the fact that the leaflet is not diffusely diseased. MAC may also fix or tether the posterior leaflet

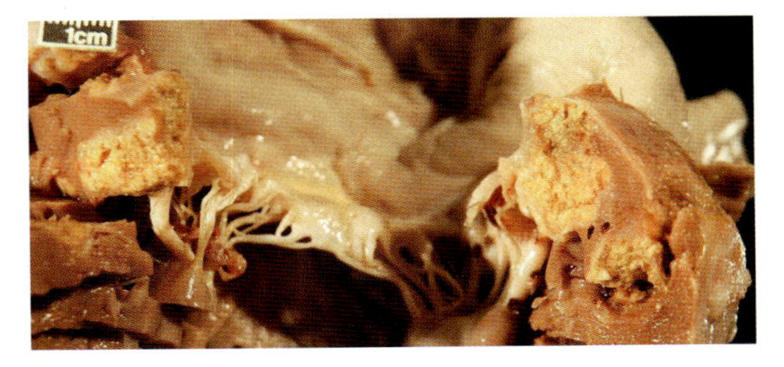

Fig. 2.5 The mitral valve has been opened laterally demonstrating severe calcification of the posterior annulus between the left atrium and the left ventricle

to the underlying calcified mass, restricting the leaflet motion and contributing to valve insufficiency. Loss of the normal left ventricle squeezing motion during systole due to rigidity, also contributes to mitral insufficiency. When liquefactive degeneration of the calcific mass occurs, extension to the posterior left atrial wall has been described (Figs. 2.8, 2.9). In these cases, the mass may mimic a valvular mass (Fig. 2.10). MAC with liquefaction necrosis may grossly mimic a gumma, an abscess or more commonly a necrotizing granuloma (Fig. 2.9). MAC may also ulcerate with thrombus deposition with the potential for embolization (Fig. 2.11). MAC was associated with a doubled risk of stroke, independent of traditional risk factors for stroke, in longitudinally followed population-based cohort (Framingham Heart Study). MAC may

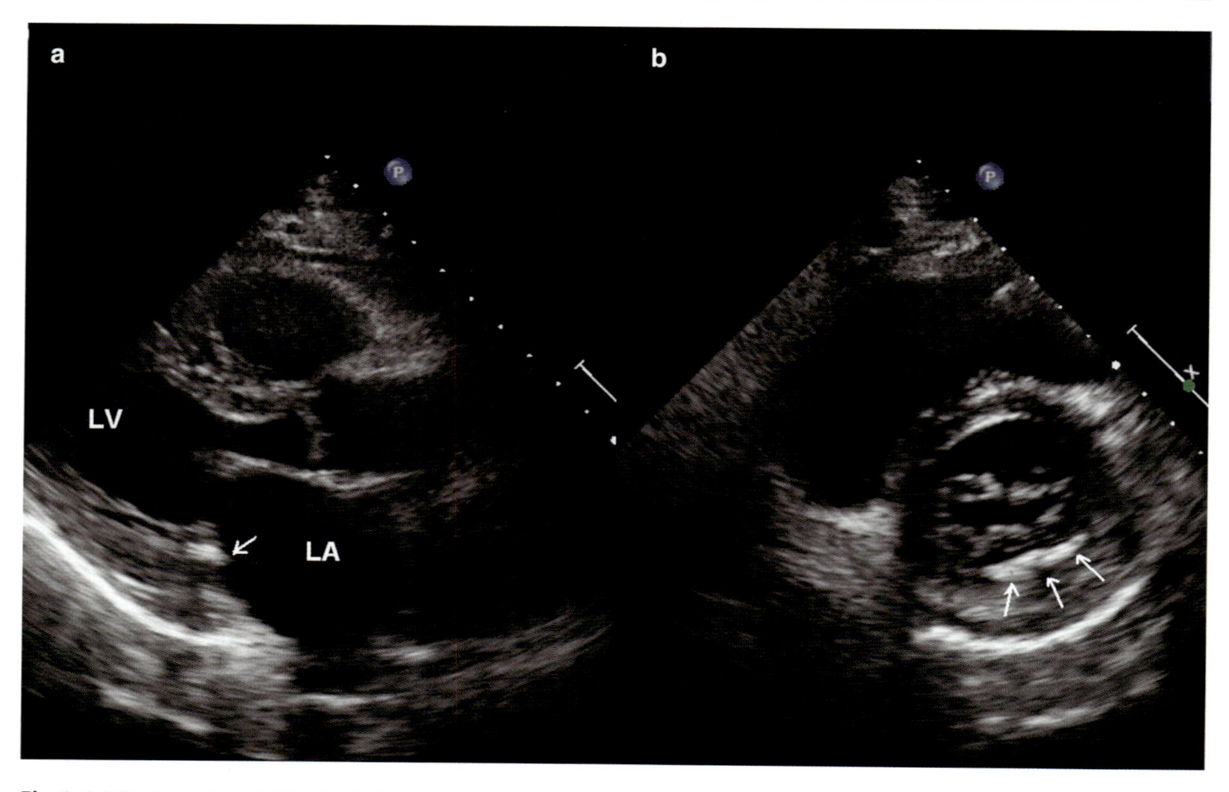

Fig. 2.6 Mitral annular calcification is demonstrated in the parasternal long- (**a**) and short-axis (**b**) views as localized, bright density at the base of the posterior mitral leaflet (*arrow*). The circumferential extent is clearly shown on the short-axis view (*arrows*). *LA* left atrium, *LV* left ventricle

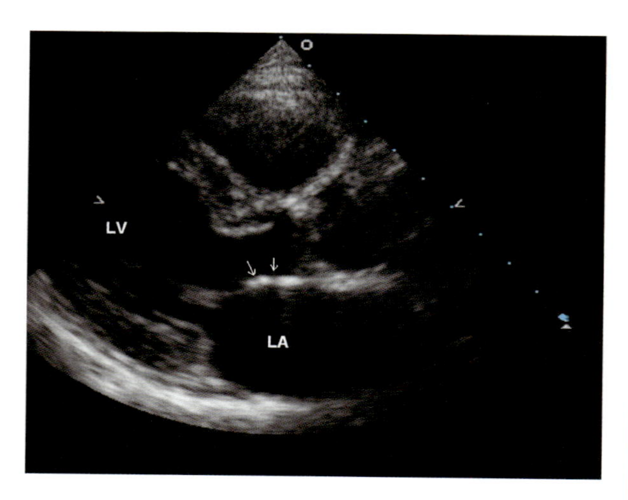

Fig. 2.7 In this 86-year-old woman, the sclerotic changes involve the aortic root and extend to involve the basal two thirds of the anterior mitral leaflet. Mitral stenosis should be suspected when both mitral annular calcification and sclerotic involvement of the mitral leaflets are present. *LA* left atrium, *LV* left ventricle

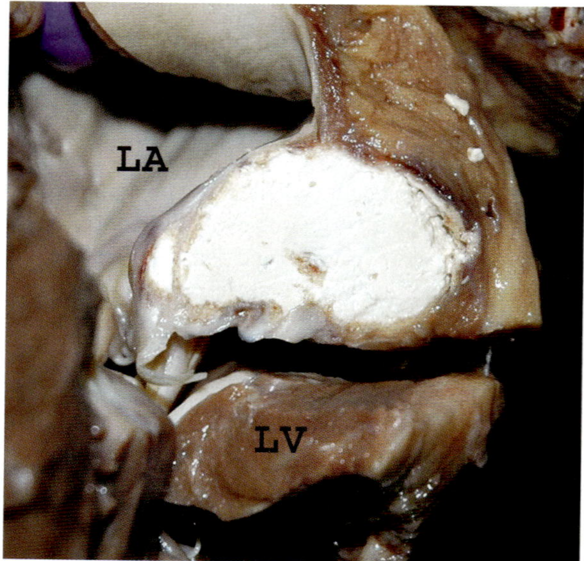

Fig. 2.8 Liquefaction of a large mitral annular calcific deposit. It extends under the left atrium (*LA*) wall and fixes the posterior mitral leaflet to it. *LV* left ventricle

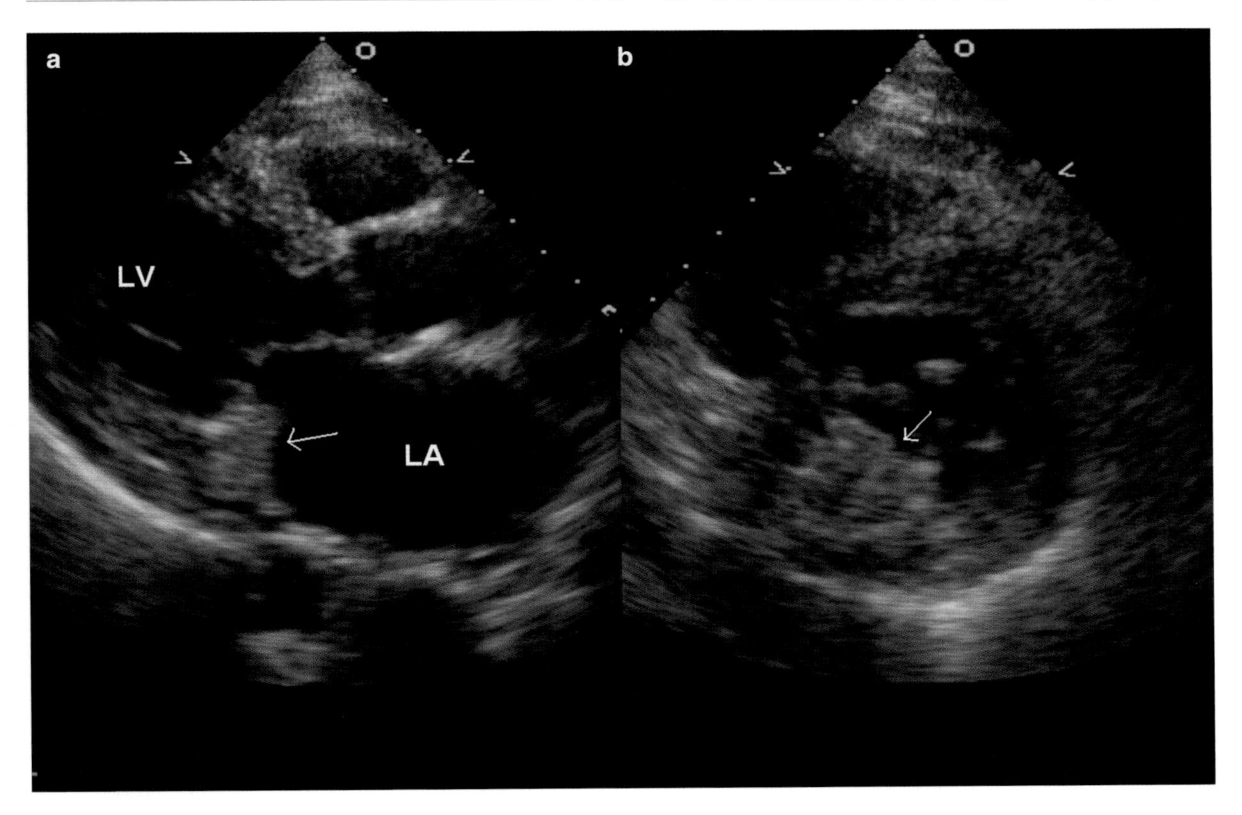

Fig. 2.9 This 88-year-old woman has a large calcific mass at the posterior mitral annulus which may be confused with an abscess or necrotizing granuloma. The mitral annular calcification is less echo dense in keeping with liquefaction, and is shown (*arrows*) in the parasternal long-axis (**a**) and short-axis (**b**) views. *LA* left atrium, *LV* left ventricle

also become ulcerated and infected, giving rise to emboli. If infected, there is usually leaflet perforation and myocardial abscess formation. Thus when MAC is noted in an echocardiographic examination to assess for a source of emboli, it should be remembered that MAC is not only a risk factor for thromboembolism but may have a direct causative role.

Calcific Aortic Valve Changes

Age-related "degenerative change" of aortic valves is the most common cause of adult aortic valve stenosis encountered in North America. Traditionally valve "degenerative" calcification was thought to be passive in nature representing dystrophic calcification of degenerated material from wear and tear of the valve tissue. Increasingly, this theory has been shown to be incomplete. Early there is endothelial dysfunction from wear and tear, and hemodynamic shear stresses, followed by lipid accumulation, inflammation, alteration of cytokines, growth factors and valve matrix metalloproteinases [3]. The process of valve calcification has much in common with atherosclerosis and bone formation [4–6]. Progression of aortic valvular disease in patients from the general population has been associated with many of the traditional risk factors for atherosclerotic disease including systemic arterial hypertension, hyperlipidemia, and diabetes mellitus [7–10]. Stenotic aortic valves have a larger amount of lipid compared to non-stenotic valves [11]. The lipid may oxidize and attract inflammatory cells. Early cusp yellow discoloration and fibrosis eventually evolves into an arch of calcium extending from the base of each cusp like an inverted "u" (Fig. 2.12). With repetitive valve deformation, endothelial damage, inflammation and lipid oxidation, nodules of calcium form and the cusp becomes sclerotic.

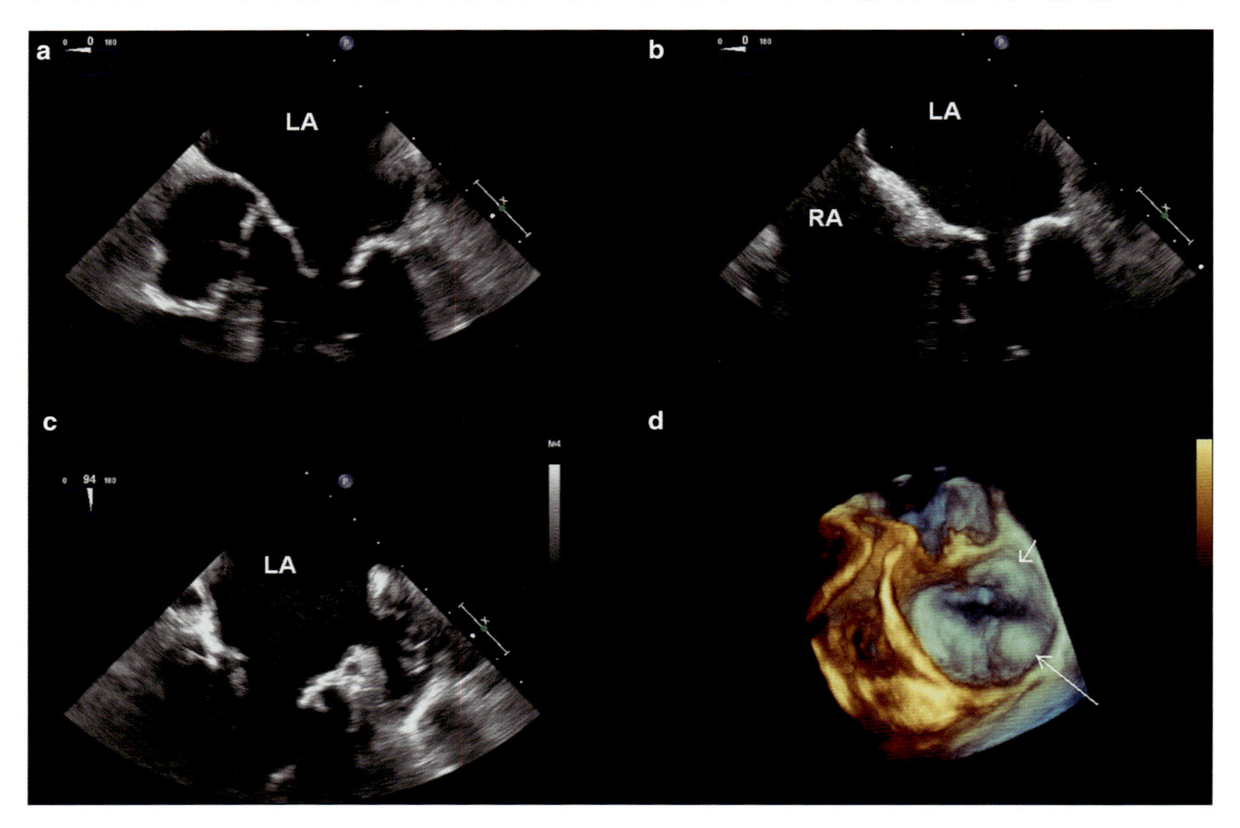

Fig. 2.10 The extent of mitral annular calcification and involvement of the mitral leaflet are shown in these transesophageal echo views (**a–c**). The calcification extends and limits the excursion of both leaflets. The 3D view of the mitral orifice from the left atrial perspective (**d**) shows that the calcification involves the basal half of the entire anterior mitral leaflet (*short arrow*), and a large calcific mass in the medial aspect of the annulus (*long arrow*) *LA* left atrium, *RA* right atrium

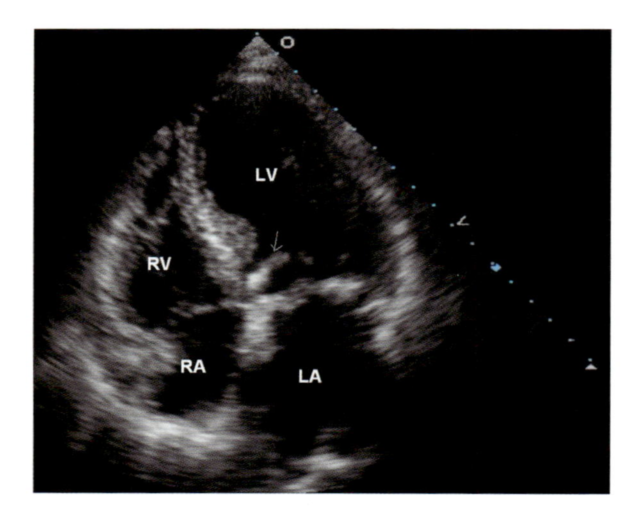

Fig. 2.11 There is a mobile mass (*arrow*) attaching to the ventricular surface of the mitral annulus calcification in this 73-year-old man with coronary artery disease. The mass is likely a thrombus because it resolves following anticoagulation treatment. *LA* left atrium, *LV* left ventricle, *RA* right atrium, *RV* right ventricle

Nodular thickening of one or more of the aortic cusps is an early sign of age-related degeneration [12]. The thickening is usually located at the nodule of Arantius or the base of the commissures (Fig. 2.13). In a follow-up of 3–5 years, about 10% of individuals with aortic sclerosis will progress to develop aortic stenosis. Aortic stenosis is also a progressive process, and individuals with more extensive valvular calcification have a more rapid rate of progression. Recent trials have showed that cholesterol lowering with statin does not have an effect on the progression of aortic stenosis.

When aortic valve cusp calcification is present, it is not unusual to note calcification of the sinotubular junction above the aortic valve (Figs. 2.14, 2.15). Pathologically, the sinotubular calcium deposits are similar to those observed in MAC. This calcification is usually benign and clinically silent. However, if the deposit becomes large it may extend to and obstruct the coronary arterial ostia.

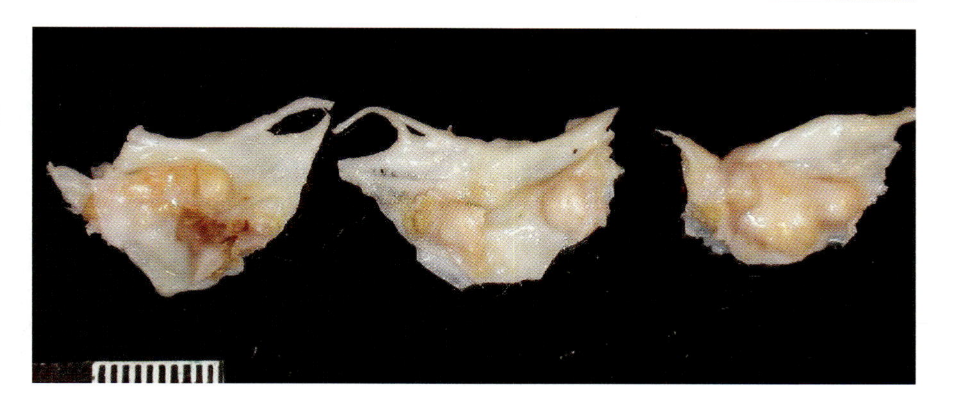

Fig. 2.12 Excised aortic valve with degenerative calcification. The calcium is localized and the free edge of the cusp is relatively spared. Small fenestrations at the lateral area of each cusp are also evident

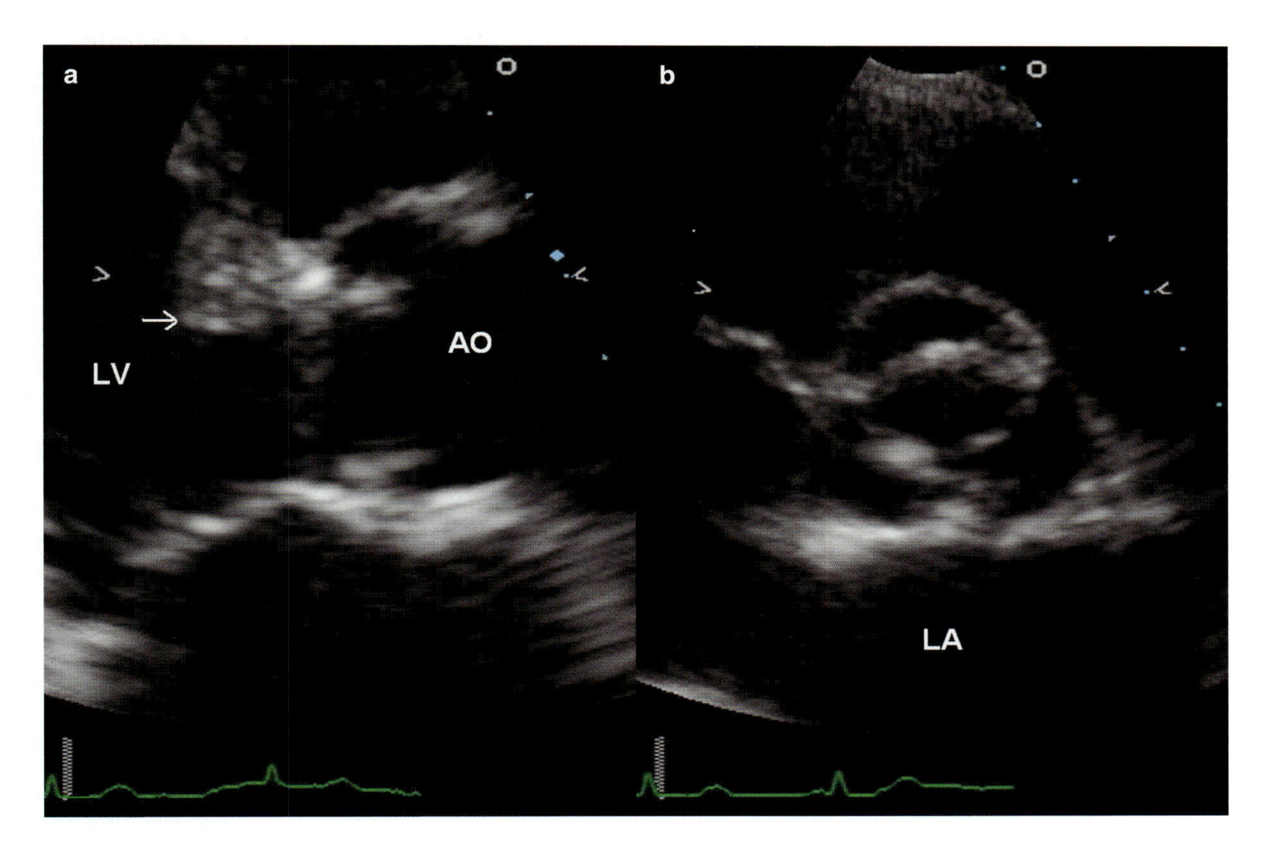

Fig. 2.13 The age-related sclerotic changes are shown in the parasternal long-axis (**a**) and short-axis (**b**) views. The aortic valve is tricuspid with diffuse thickening of the right cusp and thickening of the nodule of Arantius of the non-coronary cusp. The left cusp is relatively unaffected. There is mild restriction in excursion of the aortic cusps. The aortic root is also involved, as it has increased thickness. *Ao* aorta, *LA* left atrium, *LV* left ventricle

Age-Related Amyloidosis

Amyloid deposition is common in the elderly heart. Amyloidosis is a disease process, with a common staining characteristic – eosinophilic amorphous on routine stains, and birefringence with polarized light using a Congo red stain. The heart may be involved by primary amyloid, secondary amyloid, and senile or age-related systemic and familial transthyretin types. The prevalence of cardiac involvement and the resultant clinical consequences vary considerably between the groups. Amyloid may be clinically silent, or may

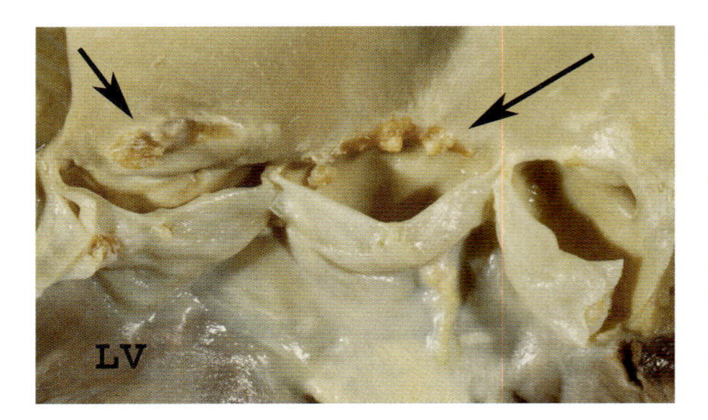

Fig. 2.14 Calcification of the sinotubular junction (*arrows*) above the aortic valve and the aortic sinuses. *LV* left ventricle

be associated with arrhythmias, diastolic dysfunction and restrictive myocardial findings, asymmetrical septal hypertrophy, systolic dysfunction, conduction disturbances, and coronary insufficiency [13].

Senile or age-related transthyretin amyloid is often without clinical complication. Histologically it cannot be distinguished on routine stains from the other amyloid types, so immunostaining is informative. Age-related amyloid may be found in any chamber, the coronary arteries, the valves and the pericardium. Commonly it deposits in a pericellular location around the myocytes, and if significant, it may contribute to diastolic dysfunction. Endocardial and valve amyloid deposits may cause stiffening. Epicardial vascular amyloid is often silent, but the small vessel disease may cause microinfarcts. The fibrosis associated with these infarcts aggravates the diastolic dysfunction.

Age-Related Cardiac Chamber Changes

With age, studies have found that the heart weight remains relatively constant in men but the heart weight increases in women, up to about the tenth decade and then the heart weight decreases in both men and women [14]. The heart stiffens and the volume of the left ventricle decreases with a decrease in base to apex dimension [15–20]. The interventricular septum may slightly

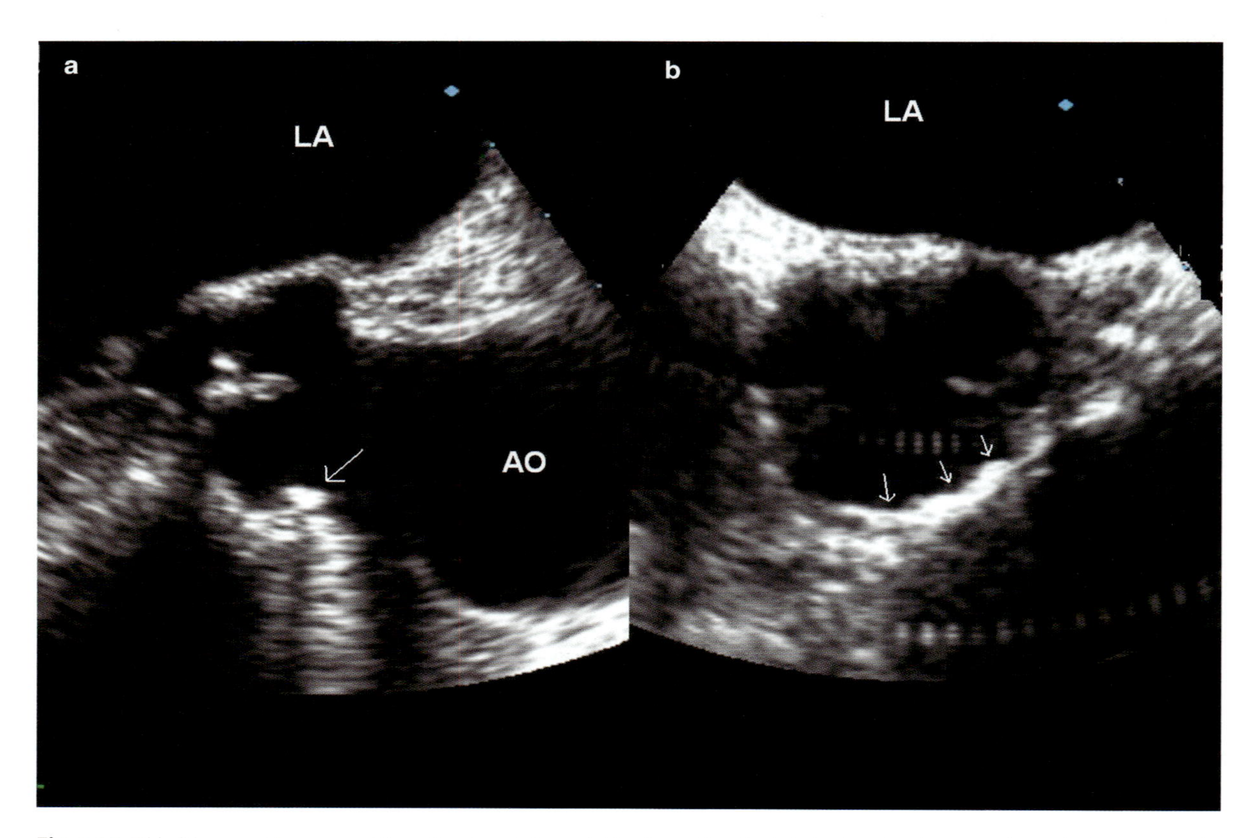

Fig. 2.15 This 84-year-old woman with aortic stenosis has calcification at the sinotubular junction (*arrows*) shown in the transesophageal aortic long-axis (**a**) and short-axis (**b**) views. *Ao* aorta, *LA* left atrium

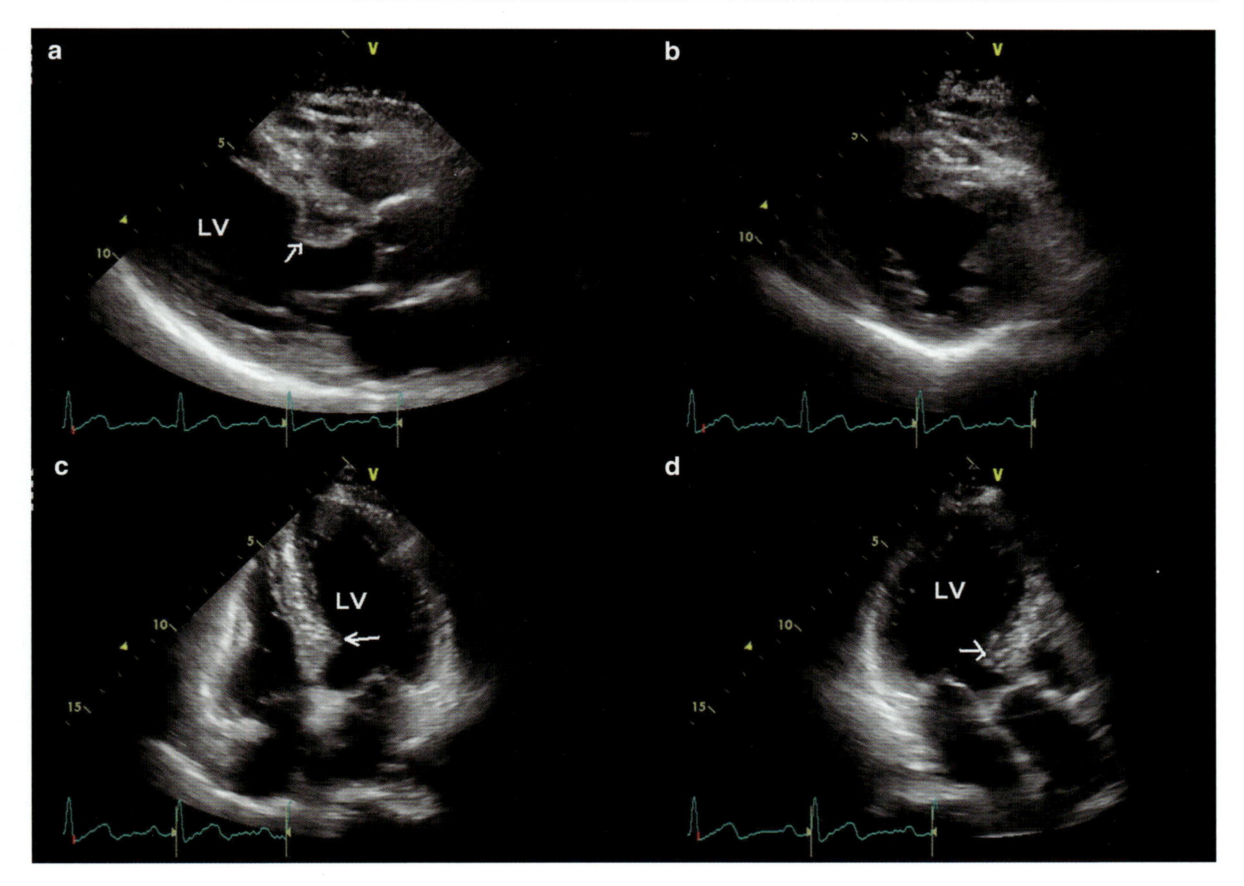

Fig. 2.16 These are the parasternal long-axis (**a**), short-axis (**b**), apical four chamber (**c**) and apical long-axis (**d**) views of a 71-year-old woman. The ventricular septum is angulated with a sigmoid shape (*arrow*) and the left ventricular wall thickness is mildly increased. *LV* left ventricle

increase in thickness (Fig. 2.16). This needs to be considered in the assessment of patients suspected to have hypertrophic cardiomyopathy [14, 21] The left atrium increases in volume and dilates with age [21, 22]

With age, the aorta dilates and tilts to the right on the interventricular septum, thus the ventricular septum under the aortic valve becomes protuberant or prominent in the left ventricle outflow tract (Figs. 2.16, 2.17). This has been termed the "sigmoid" septum due to the shape of the left ventricle outflow tract. It is generally not clinically significant but it can contribute to systolic anterior motion of the mitral valve leaflet and may contribute to left ventricle outflow obstruction in hearts with significant left ventricular hypertrophy (Fig. 2.18). It is sometimes removed as a surgical myomectomy specimen during aortic valve replacement (as the individuals have aortic stenosis related left ventricular hypertrophy exacerbating the prominence of the septum).

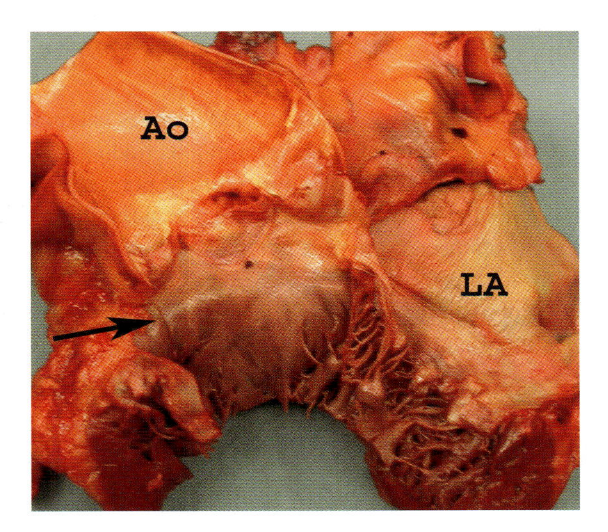

Fig. 2.17 The heart has been opened to show the left ventricle outflow tract. The upper part of the ventricle septum is prominent (*arrow*), as the aorta (*Ao*) has shifted slightly rightward with age. *LA* left atrium

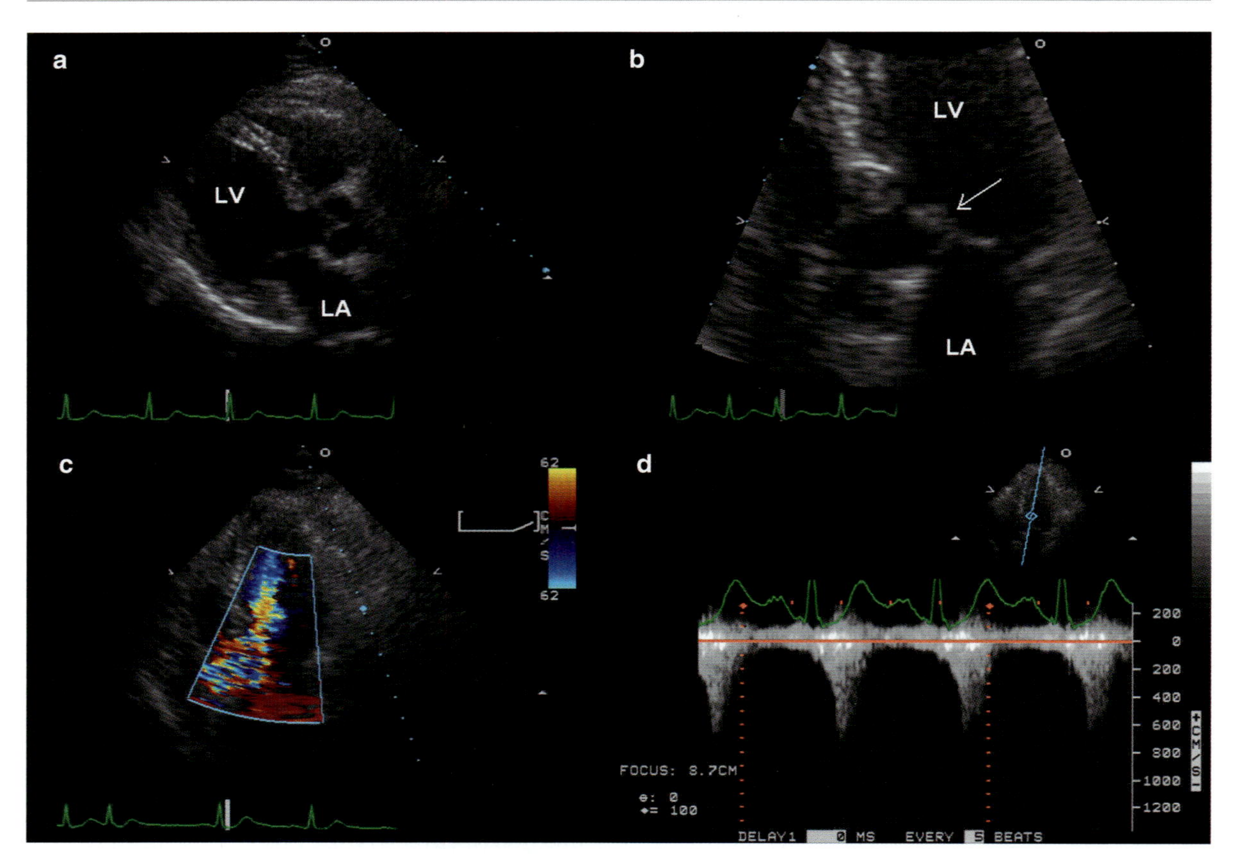

Fig. 2.18 This 69-year-old woman undergoes dobutamine stress echocardiography because of exertional dyspnea and tiredness. The parasternal long-axis view is shown in (**a**), apical long-axis view in (**b**), color flow imaging of the apical long-axis view in (**c**) and continuous wave Doppler assessment of the left ventricular outflow tract in (**d**). During dobutamine infusion, systolic anterior motion of the mitral valve (*arrow*) develops associated with a high subaortic gradient. *LA* left atrium, *LV* left ventricle

Summary

An understanding of the age-related changes is crucial to the interpretation of echocardiographic findings. The presence of a sigmoid septum is likely normal in an elderly individual but should raise the possibility of hypertrophic cardiomyopathy in a young person. Sclerotic changes and calcification of cardiac structures are common in the elderly, and should not be confused with abnormalities such as tumors.

References

1. Blaszyk H, Witkiewicz AJ, Edwards WD. Acute aortic regurgitation due to spontaneous rupture of a fenestrated cusp: report in a 65-year-old man and review of seven additional cases. *Cardiovasc Pathol*. 1999 July;8(4):213-216.
2. Lee AP, Walley VM, Ascah KJ, Veinot JP, Davies RA, Keon WJ. A fenestrated aortic valve contributing to iatrogenic aortic insufficiency post mitral valve replacement. *Cardiovasc Pathol*. 1996;5(2):81-83.
3. Mohler ER III. Mechanisms of aortic valve calcification. *Am J Cardiol*. 2004 Dec 1;94(11):1396-1402.
4. Rajamannan NM, Subramaniam M, Rickard D, et al. Human aortic valve calcification is associated with an osteoblast phenotype. *Circulation*. 2003;107(17):2181-2184.
5. Wallby L, Janerot-Sjoberg B, Steffensen T, Broqvist M. T lymphocyte infiltration in non-rheumatic aortic stenosis: a comparative descriptive study between tricuspid and bicuspid aortic valves. *Heart*. 2002;88(4):348-351.
6. Mohler ER III, Gannon F, Reynolds C, Zimmerman R, Keane MG, Kaplan FS. Bone formation and inflammation in cardiac valves. *Circulation*. 2001;103(11):1522-1528.
7. Wierzbicki A, Shetty C. Aortic stenosis: an atherosclerotic disease? *J Heart Valve Dis*. 1999 July;8(4):416-423.
8. Palta S, Pai AM, Gill KS, Pai RG. New insights into the progression of aortic stenosis: implications for secondary prevention. *Circulation*. 2000;101(21):2497-2502.
9. Aronow WS, Ahn C, Kronzon I, Goldman ME. Association of coronary risk factors and use of statins with progression

of mild valvular aortic stenosis in older persons. *Am J Cardiol*. 2001 Sept 15;88(6):693-695.
10. Iivanainen AM, Lindroos M, Tilvis R, Heikkila J, Kupari M. Calcific degeneration of the aortic valve in old age: is the development of flow obstruction predictable? *J Intern Med*. 1996 Mar;239(3):269-273.
11. Nissen SE, Tuzcu EM, Schoenhagen P, et al. Statin therapy, LDL cholesterol, C-reactive protein, and coronary artery disease. *N Engl J Med*. 2005 Jan 6;352(1):29-38.
12. Sahasakul Y, Edwards WD, Naessens JM, Tajik AJ. Age-related changes in aortic and mitral valve thickness: implications for two-dimensional echocardiography based on an autopsy study of 200 normal human hearts. *Am J Cardiol*. 1988 Sept 1;62(7):424-430.
13. Stamato N, Cahill J, Goodwin M, Winters G. Cardiac amyloidosis causing ventricular tachycardia: diagnosis made by endomyocardial biopsy. *Chest*. 1989;96:1431-1433.
14. Kitzman DW, Scholz DG, Hagen PT, Ilstrup DM, Edwards WD. Age-related changes in normal human hearts during the first 10 decades of life. Part II (Maturity): a quantitative anatomic study of 765 specimens from subjects 20 to 99 years old. *Mayo Clin Proc*. 1988 Feb;63(2):137-146.
15. Okura H, Takada Y, Yamabe A, et al. Age- and gender-specific changes in the left ventricular relaxation: a Doppler echocardiographic study in healthy individuals. *Circ Cardiovasc Imaging*. 2009 Jan;2(1):41-46.
16. Lieb W, Xanthakis V, Sullivan LM, et al. Longitudinal tracking of left ventricular mass over the adult life course: clinical correlates of short- and long-term change in the framingham offspring study. *Circulation*. 2009 June 23;119(24):3085-3092.
17. Salmasi AM, Alimo A, Jepson E, Dancy M. Age-associated changes in left ventricular diastolic function are related to increasing left ventricular mass. *Am J Hypertens*. 2003 June;16(6):473-477.
18. Lindroos M, Kupari M, Heikkila J, Tilvis R. Echocardiographic evidence of left ventricular hypertrophy in a general aged population. *Am J Cardiol*. 1994 Aug 15; 74(4):385-390.
19. Shub C, Klein AL, Zachariah PK, Bailey KR, Tajik AJ. Determination of left ventricular mass by echocardiography in a normal population: effect of age and sex in addition to body size. *Mayo Clin Proc*. 1994 Mar;69(3):205-211.
20. Grandi AM, Venco A, Barzizza F, Scalise F, Pantaleo P, Finardi G. Influence of age and sex on left ventricular anatomy and function in normals. *Cardiology*. 1992;81(1):8-13.
21. Kitzman DW, Edwards WD. Age-related changes in the anatomy of the normal human heart. *J Gerontol*. 1990 Mar; 45(2):M33-M39.
22. Waller BF, Bloch T, Barker BG, et al. The old-age heart: aging changes of the normal elderly heart and cardiovascular disease in 12 necropsy patients aged 90 to 101 years. *Cardiol Clin*. 1984;2:753-779.

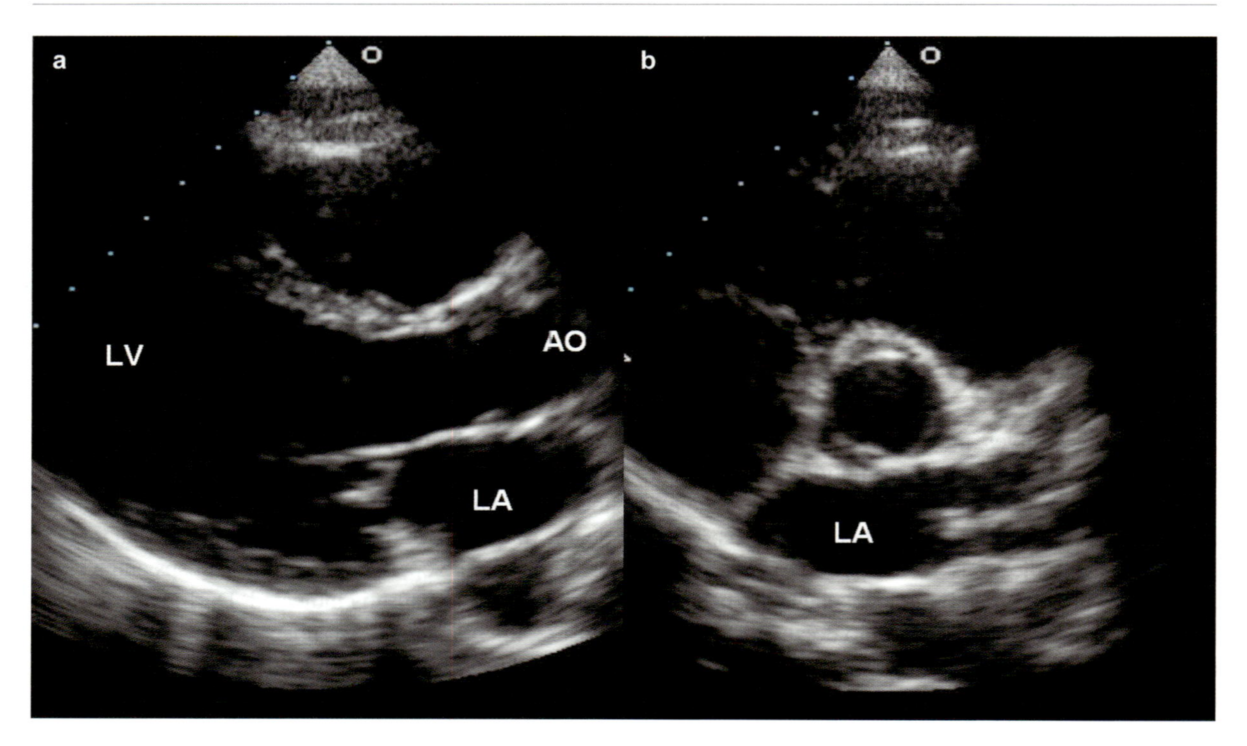

Fig. 3.1 A normal tricuspid aortic valve in a young individual is shown in the long-axis (**a**) and short axis (**b**) views in systole. The aortic cusps open fully parallel to and almost abutting the aortic walls, with a circular orifice in the short-axis view. *Ao* aorta, *LA* left atrium, *RA* right atrium, *RVOT* right ventricular outflow tract

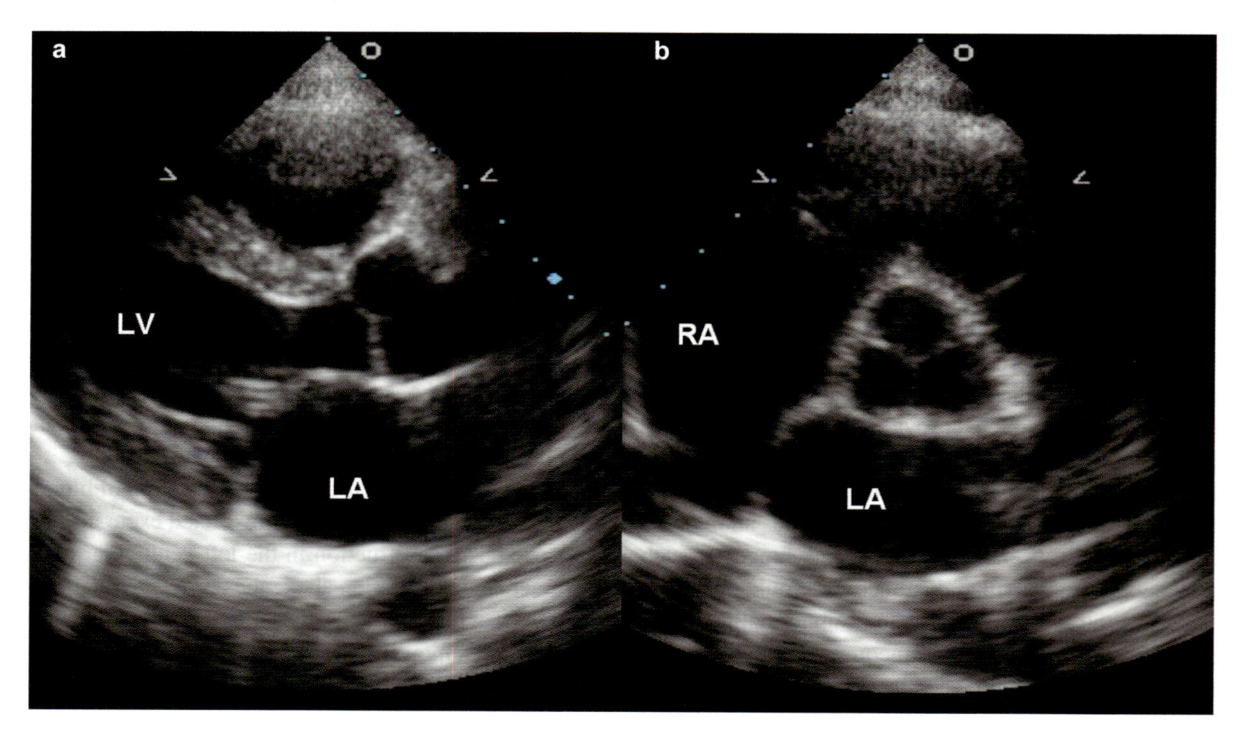

Fig. 3.2 These are the parasternal long-axis (**a**) and short-axis (**b**) views in diastole of the same subject shown in Fig. 3.1. The three symmetrical aortic cusps are clearly seen. *LA* left atrium, *LV* left ventricle

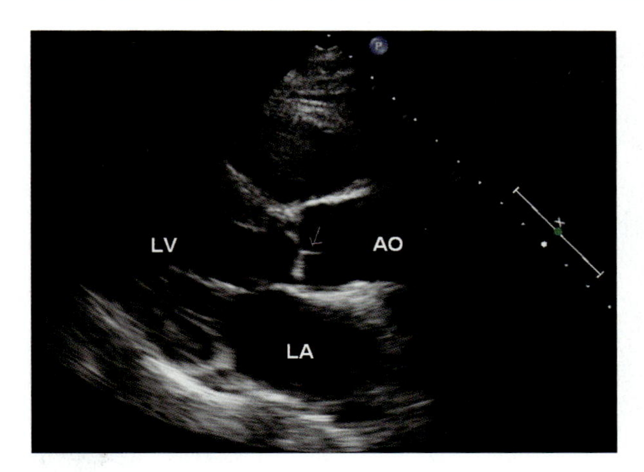

Fig. 3.3 Proper aortic cusp coaptation (*arrow*) in diastole is shown in the parasternal long-axis view. The aortic cusps oppose over a length of 1–2 mm

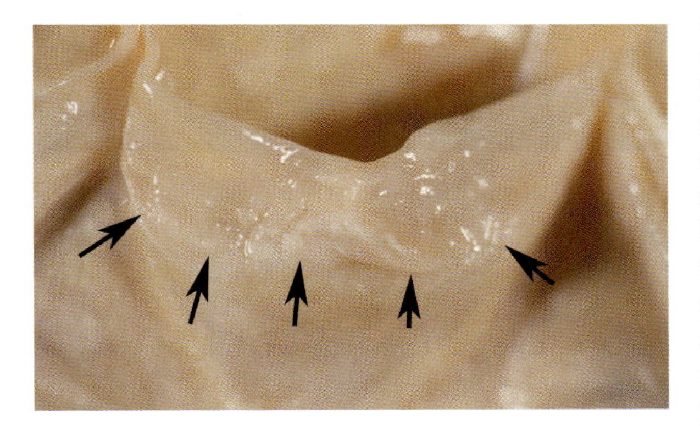

Fig. 3.4 Aortic valve cusp with line of closure indicated (*arrows*)

of aortic valve stenosis is increasing with the aging of the population.

Stenosis of the aortic valve is usually due to pathology of the valve cusps, most commonly cusp fibrosis, calcification and commissural fusion. The most common causes of aortic valve stenosis include: age-related calcific degenerative (senile) changes, post-inflammatory changes – usually rheumatic, and congenitally bicuspid valve [2]. Another cause of valvular aortic stenosis is congenitally unicuspid valve. In general, age-related calcific degenerative disease is increasing in incidence, congenital valve disease remains stable at about 1–2% of the population and post-inflammatory and rheumatic valve disease is on the decline in North America. Rheumatic disease remains a major cause of valve disease in the developing world.

Age-Related Calcific Valve Stenosis

Due to the increasing age of the population, age-related degenerative aortic valve changes might have important implications for future health care costs. Age-related degenerative change of aortic valves is the most common cause of adult aortic valve stenosis encountered in North America [2]. In age-related degeneration there are three cusps that only undergo degeneration after many decades of normal function. The cusps are separate and the commissures are not fused. The process probably begins with lipid accumulation, but eventually calcium and sometimes bone are deposited in an arch-like configuration in each cusp. The lipid may oxidize and attract inflammatory cells. The top of each arch is directed at the free edge of the cusp with the calcium ridge extending to the base of each cusp (Figs. 3.6, 3.7). Traditionally valve calcification was thought to be passive in nature representing dystrophic calcification of degenerated material. Wear and tear of the valve tissue was postulated. Increasingly, this theory has been shown to be incomplete. An early event appears to be endothelial dysfunction from wear and tear and hemodynamic shear stresses. After this, numerous active mechanisms ensue including lipid accumulation, inflammation, alteration of cytokines, growth factors, and valve matrix metalloproteinases [3]. The process of valve calcification has much in common with atherosclerosis and bone formation [4–6]. Progression of aortic valvular disease in patients from the general population has been associated with many of the traditional risk factors for atherosclerotic disease, including systemic arterial hypertension, hyperlipidemia, and diabetes mellitus [7–9].

The calcified aortic valves commonly have variable degrees of inflammation including macrophages, plasma cells, and lymphocytes [6, 10]. These cells are capable of synthesizing osteopontin, which may act to hold surrounding cells to the calcified deposits [11]. Bone with osteoblast-like cells may be observed. Aortic valve stenosis from degenerative or age-related changes is commonly seen in individuals over the age of 50 years. A sclerotic valve may eventually become a stenotic calcified valve given time and the right environment. Earlier calcification is seen if the valve has been damaged, such as previous surgical manipulation or radiation. The internal milieu may also accelerate calcification. Patients with hyperparathyroidism and chronic renal failure, especially those who are dialysis dependent, have accelerated valve disease [12]. Finally some storage diseases,

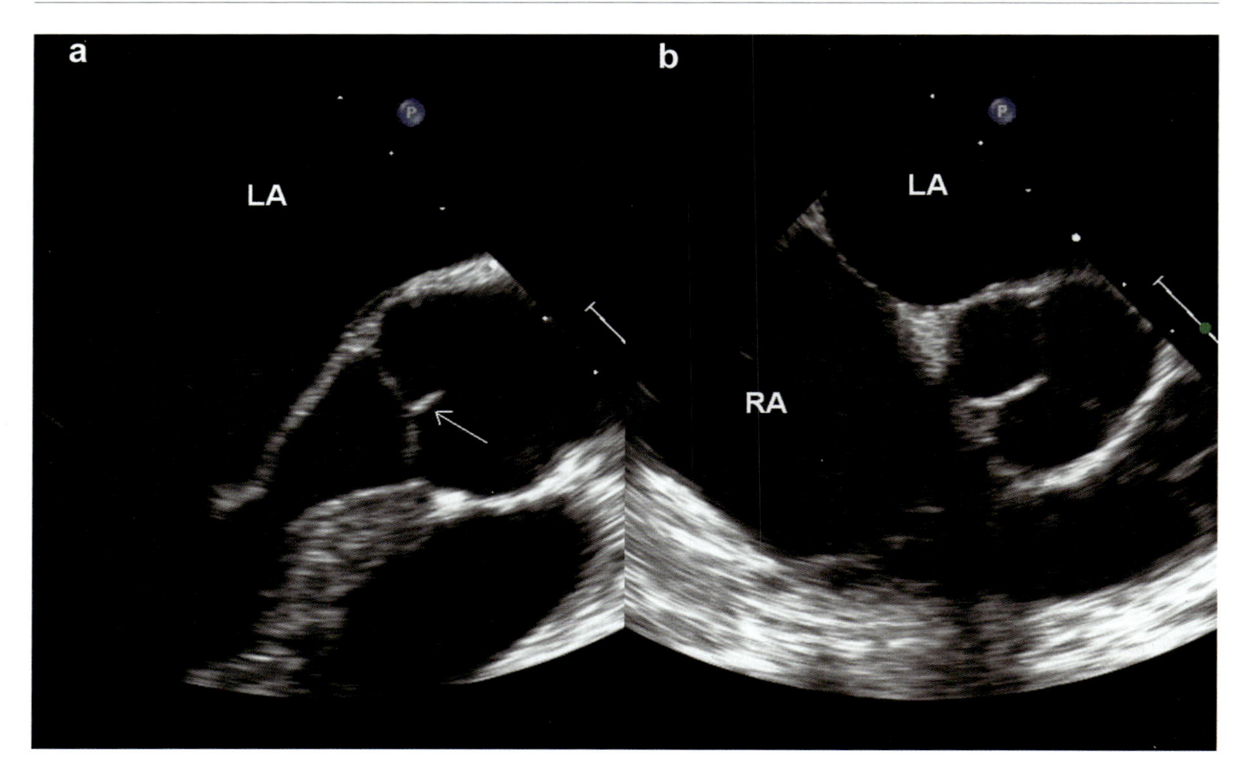

Fig. 3.5 The aortic cusp coaptation (**a**) and valve morphology (**b**) are shown in the transesophageal echocardiograms, showing a normal tricuspid aortic valve

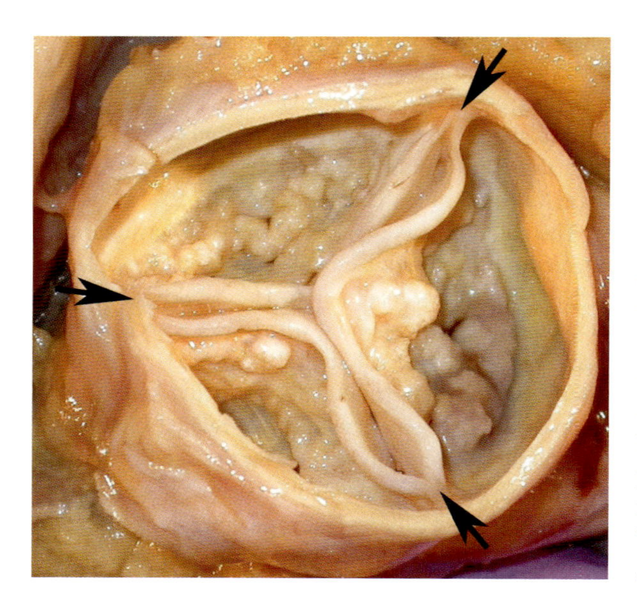

Fig. 3.6 Closed aortic valve with calcific degenerative changes – age-related degeneration. The three cusps are of almost equal size and the commissures are not fused (*arrows*)

such as certain types of Gaucher's disease, lead to aortic valve disease in young individuals [13].

Congenitally Bicuspid Aortic Valve

Congenitally bicuspid valve is present in 1–2% of the population. Some of these valves calcify and are stenotic, while others become regurgitant, as will be discussed. The bicuspid valve forms as two of the cusps fail to split during development. The resulting cusp is termed the conjoined cusp. The two congenitally bicuspid valve cusps are usually about equal in the circumference they occupy in the aorta, but are rarely identical. They often occupy some combination of 40–60% of the circumference each. The conjoined cusp has a flat free edge and a ridge at the base of the cusp near the aorta. This ridge is perpendicular to the aorta and is termed the raphe and represents the area of failed cusp division.

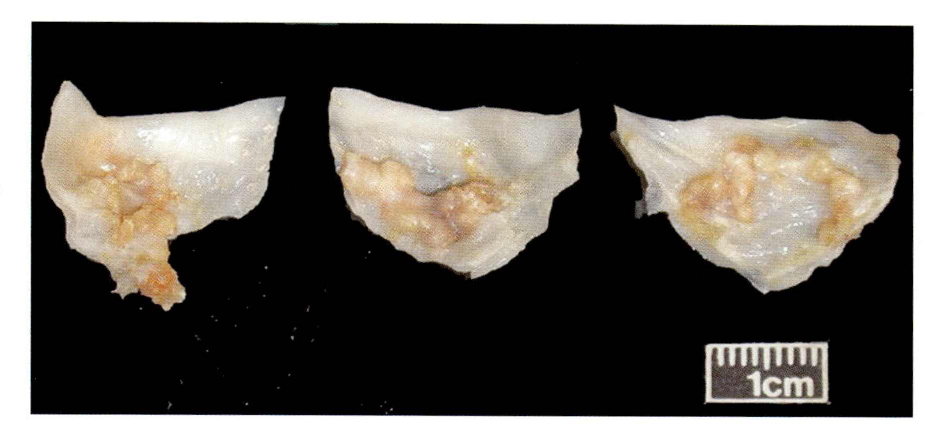

Fig. 3.7 Excised aortic valve with age-related degenerative changes. The valve is not fused at the commissures and therefore can be removed in three pieces. The free edges are flat and the calcification is arch like causing cusp rigidity

The raphe usually only reaches about half way up the cusp and is of variable size and shape (Figs. 3.8, 3.9). Some raphes are fibrotic and calcified. Bicuspid aortic valve is the most common predisposing condition for the development of aortic stenosis. It is more prevalent than tricuspid aortic valve in patients with aortic stenosis who are in or below the sixth decade of life. It should be remembered that the congenitally bicuspid valve may be associated with an aortopathy in many cases, as the ascending aorta and the aortic valve have the same cells of origin and develop from the same embryological truncus arteriosus. In a patient with a congenitally bicuspid valve, the aorta must be observed for dilatation, as there is a risk of aneurysm or dissection [14].

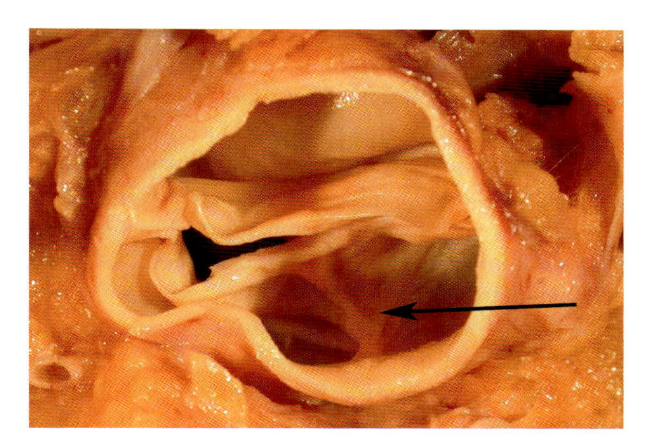

Fig. 3.9 Congenitally bicuspid aortic valve in situ from above. The raphe is noted (*arrow*)

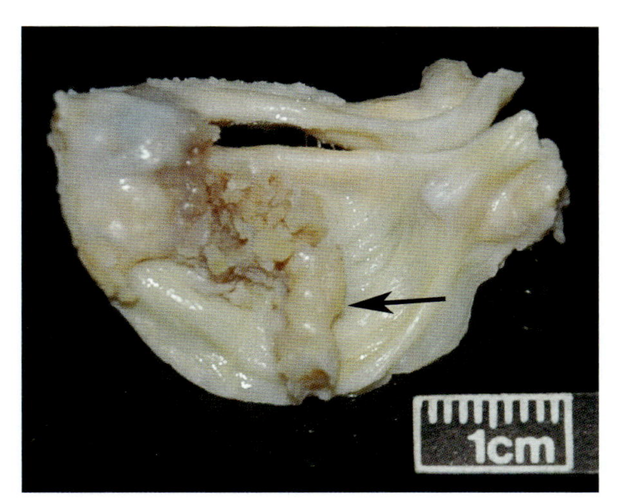

Fig. 3.8 Congenitally bicuspid valve surgically excised. On the conjoined cusp there is a flat free edge and a ridge at the cusp base termed the raphe (*arrow*). This is the area where the cusp failed to divide

Congenitally unicuspid valves are usually stenotic and are invariably symptomatic before the third decade of age. There is failure of the cusps to split, and one finds a valve with a tear drop-like orifice unicuspid unicommissural valve, or with no commissures as a dome- or hole-shaped unicuspid acommissural valve.

Post-inflammatory Rheumatic Aortic Stenosis

Rheumatic valve disease, a chronic result of rheumatic fever, is the disease most associated with "post-inflammatory" valve disease. Rheumatic disease still remains an important cause of valve disease in the global perspective. The acutely involved rheumatic valve is not seen by the pathologist, but the chronically scarred, inflamed, and neovascularized valves are. Chronically, rheumatic fever leads to valve neovascularization, chronic inflammation, commissural fusion, valve thickening, and calcification. Scarring, important in the progression of valvular disease, is accompanied by neovascularization. Once the valve is inflamed and there is neovascularization, lymphocytes can infiltrate the valve, both through the valve surface as well as through the neovascularization channels. Even in old calcified rheumatic valves, lymphocytes and neovascularization are still present, indicating progression or persistence of disease in the valve [15].

Chronic rheumatic aortic valves have three cusps with fibrosis, with or without calcification. The commissures are often fused. Valves may be thickened and show scar cusp retraction resulting in a combination of aortic stenosis and regurgitation. If the cusps fuse into an acquired bicuspid valve, the distinction from a congenitally bicuspid valve is sometimes difficult. In a post-inflammatory fused cusp, one cusp should be twice the circumference and size of the other cusp, as it represents fusion of two previously normally sized cusps. The free edge of the fused cusp usually is "v" shaped rather than flat. No raphe is seen (Fig. 3.10a, b). If there is a ridge in the area of commissural fusion, this ridge often extends all the way to the cusp free edge.

Sub-aortic Valve Stenosis

Subaortic stenosis is usually due to fibromuscular ridges or membranes. Three pathological types are recognized. Membranous subaortic stenosis is due to a discrete fibrous membrane beneath the valve. Fibromuscular obstruction may be a discrete ridge of muscle or the process may be a diffuse muscular hypertrophy as a tunnel stenosis. In all cases, the aortic valve above the area of stenosis is often damaged by the valve turbulence and often the valve, the ridge, and the outflow tract have to be dealt with at surgery. The subaortic stenosis may slowly reoccur after surgery.

Subvalvular aortic stenosis can be categorized into two main groups by echocardiography: fixed and dynamic stenosis. This is best assessed using the parasternal long axis view. There are three types of fixed subaortic stenosis. The subaortic membrane is the most common variety (Figs. 3.11, 3.12). It is typically located about 1 cm from the aortic annulus within the left ventricular outflow tract. The severe form shows extension onto the ventricular surface of the anterior mitral leaflet within 1 cm of the posterior aortic annulus. The membrane is visualized as a thin linear echo density within the left ventricular outflow tract. In the mild form, it appears as a crescentric curtain at the superior aspect of the left ventricular outflow tract in the short axis view. The severe variety will have an appearance of a circumferential curtain within the left

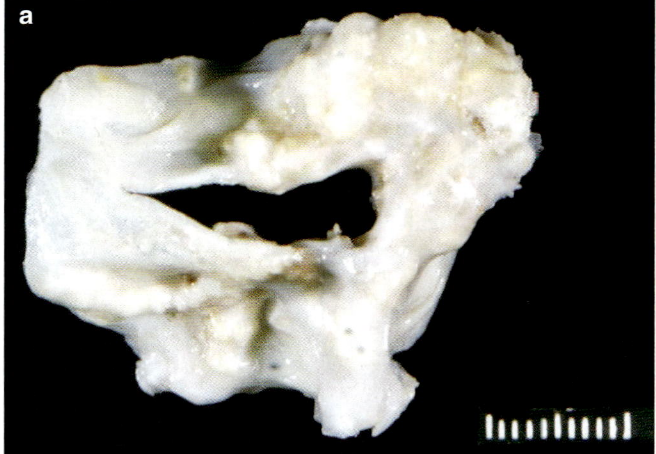

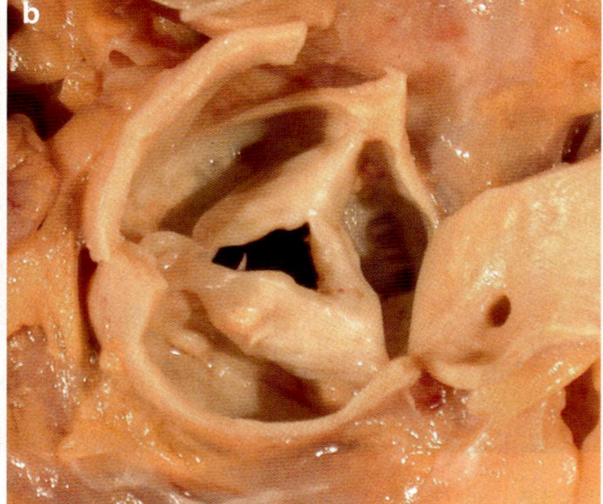

Fig. 3.10 (**a**) Chronic rheumatic aortic valve disease surgical specimen. The three commissures are fused and there is fibrosis. The valve orifice is stenotic (and would also remain open) and the cusps are rigid. (**b**) An in situ aortic valve demonstrating the commissural fusion of the three valve cusps in the aorta

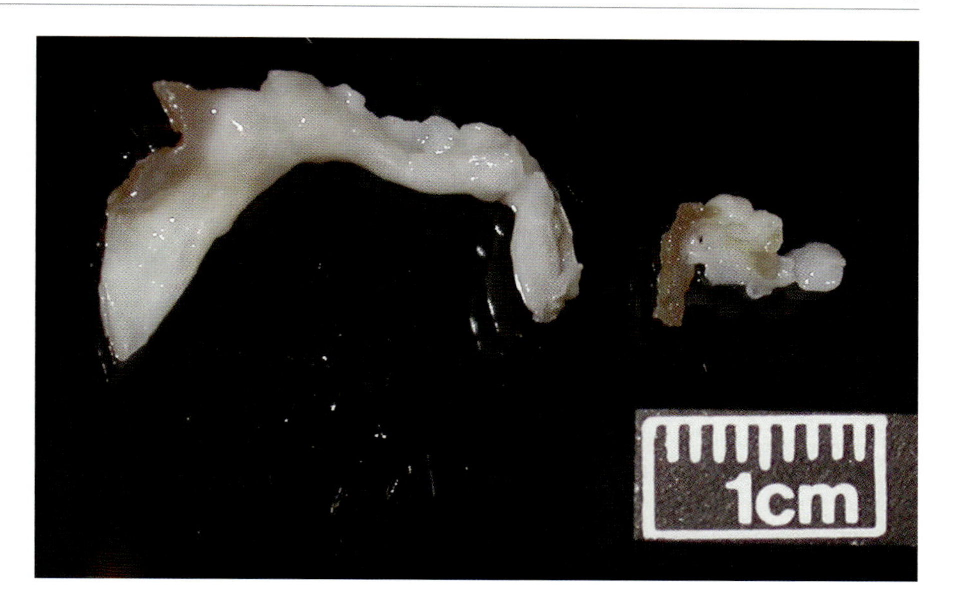

Fig. 3.11 Excised subaortic fibrous membrane from a patient with subaortic stenosis

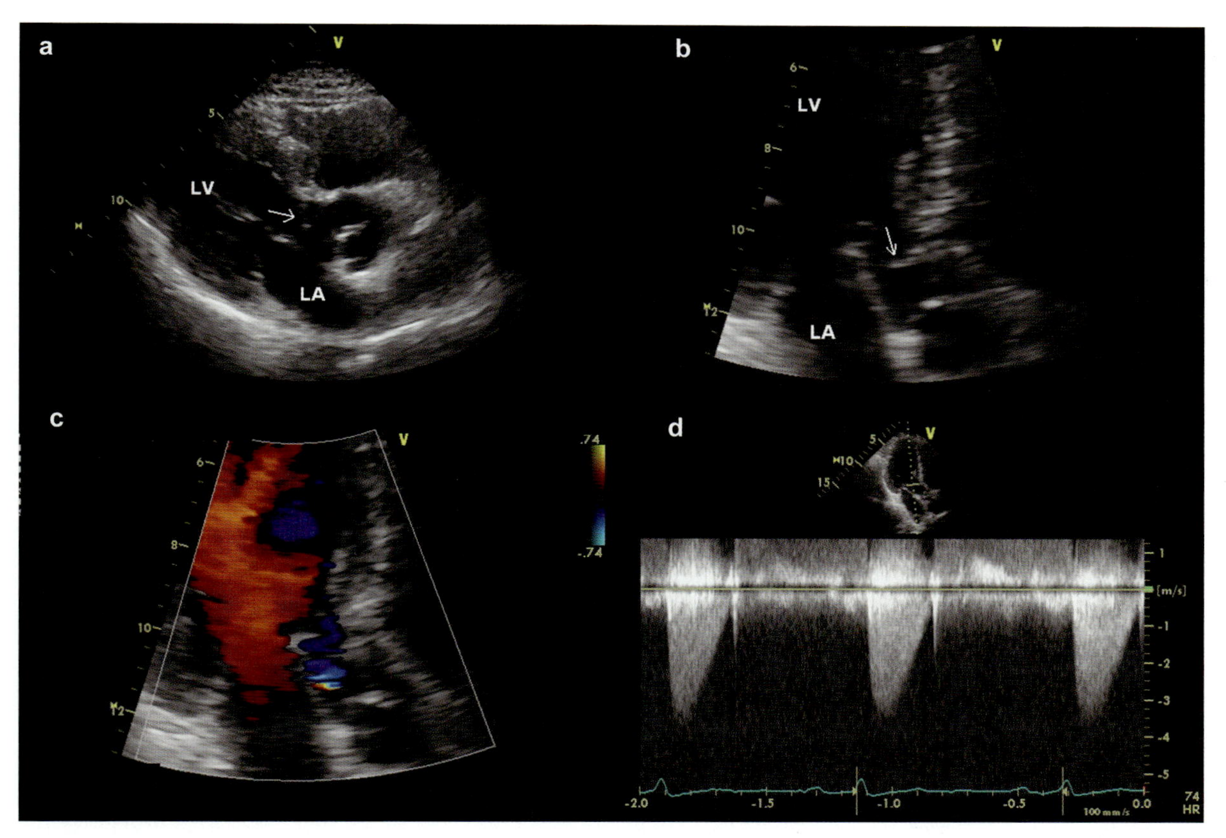

Fig. 3.12 The subaortic membrane is usually imaged in the parasternal long-axis view (**a**) and located about one centimeter from the aortic annulus frequently extending onto the anterior mitral leaflet. The apical long-axis is view (**b**) is also a good view to show the subaortic membrane which is orthogonal to the ultrasound beam in this view. The color flow image of the apical long-axis view (**c**) shows flow acceleration at the site of the membrane, and the continuous wave Doppler (**d**) shows a peak gradient of 50 mmHg. *LA* left atrium, *LV* left ventricle

ventricular outflow tract. Mild aortic regurgitation is usually present. The subaortic membrane may be better seen from the apical window because the membrane is orthogonal to the ultrasound beam in this window. When a subaortic membrane is present, additional left heart obstructive lesions such as supra-mitral valvular ring, bicuspid aortic valve, and coarctation should be sought. In the adult population, there is little or no progression of the subaortic membrane with time [16, 17]. Aortic regurgitation usually does not progress rapidly and resection of subaortic membrane to preserve aortic valvular function may not be indicated.

Fibromuscular subaortic stenosis also involves the left ventricular outflow tract adjacent to the aortic annulus. It has a thick profile with a larger base. It has a higher recurrence rate following surgical resection. Diffuse narrowing of the left ventricular outflow tract giving rise to the subaortic tunnel is the least common type of fixed subaortic stenosis. Amelioration of the tunnel obstruction is difficult and requires complex patch enlargement of the left ventricular outflow tract.

Dynamic Subaortic Obstruction

This type of obstruction is due the development of dynamic obstruction related to hypertrophy and protrusion of the basal anterior septum. It is most commonly seen in patients with hypertrophic cardiomyopathy in whom systolic anterior motion of the mitral leaflet is a common associated finding (Fig. 3.13). However, dynamic left ventricular outflow tract obstruction is not restricted to patients with hypertrophic cardiomyopathy. It is

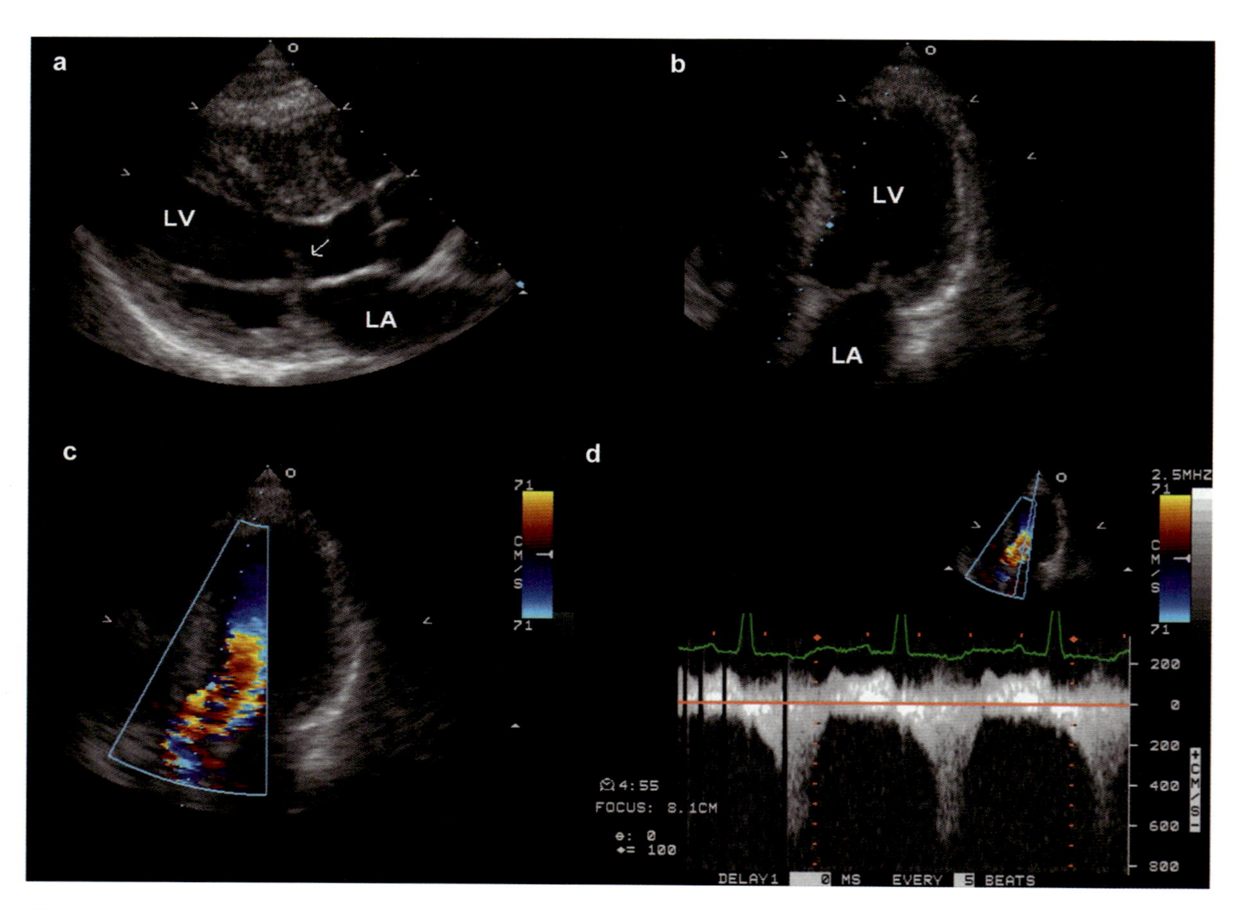

Fig. 3.13 In this patient with obstructive hypertrophic cardiomyopathy, there is severe hypertrophy involving the anterior septum clearly shown in the parasternal long-axis (**a**) and apical four-chamber (**b**) views. In the long-axis view (**a**), systolic anterior motion of the mitral valve is present (*arrow*). The color flow image of the apical long-axis view (**c**) shows flow acceleration in the left ventricular outflow tract indicative of subaortic obstruction which is assessed by continuous wave Doppler (**d**) showing a late peak signal with a peak velocity of exceeding 6 m/s. *LA* left atrium, *LV* left ventricle

also seen in patients with anterior wall myocardial infarction with sparing of the basal septum [18]. This is an important phenomenon to recognize as proper management with fluid replacement and beta-blockade can frequently ameliorate the subaortic obstruction. On the other hand, inotropic support and diuretics may exacerbate the subaortic obstruction leading to more profound hypotension.

Dynamic subaortic stenosis can also be detected in the elderly, particularly in those with concentric hypertrophy due to longstanding hypertension (Fig. 3.14). With age the aorta shifts right-ward making the top of the interventricular septum prominent [19]. Hypovolemia due to dehydration or blood loss may accentuate the subaortic stenosis and bring this to clinical attention. This finding may be the basis of the development of a heart murmur in these patients, and may be the reason for limited physical endurance in some of these patients. Exercise stress echocardiography with the bicycle protocol allows the assessment of the severity of dynamic subaortic stenosis at different stages of exercise providing useful insights to the management of these patients.

Supravalvular Aortic Stenosis

Supravalvular aortic stenosis may be associated with syndromes such as Williams's syndrome. This syndrome has serum calcium metabolic abnormalities, a characteristic facies, and dysplasia and thickening of the aorta [20]. The arterial thickening process may even extend into the proximal coronary arteries

By echocardiography this can be recognized as focal narrowing of the ascending aorta at the

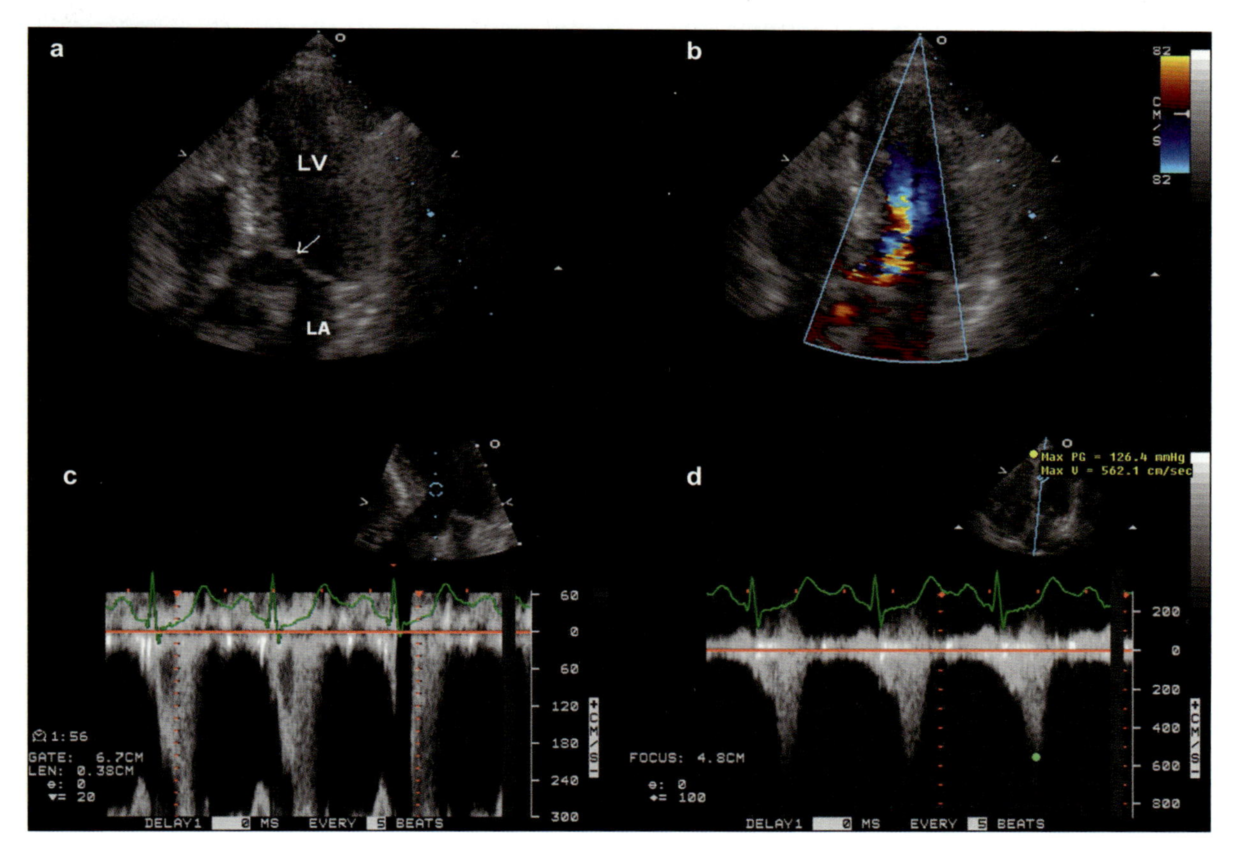

Fig. 3.14 This is a 76-year-old woman admitted for gastrointestinal bleeding. She was noted to have a heart murmur. The apical long-axis view (**a**) shows small left ventricular cavity and the presence of systolic anterior motion of the mitral valve (arrow). Color flow imaging (**b**) of the same view shows flow acceleration in the left ventricular outflow tract, confirmed by pulsed wave Doppler (**c**) and continuous wave Doppler (**d**) shows a high subaortic gradient. She responded favorably to volume replacement. *LA* left atrium, *LV* left ventricle

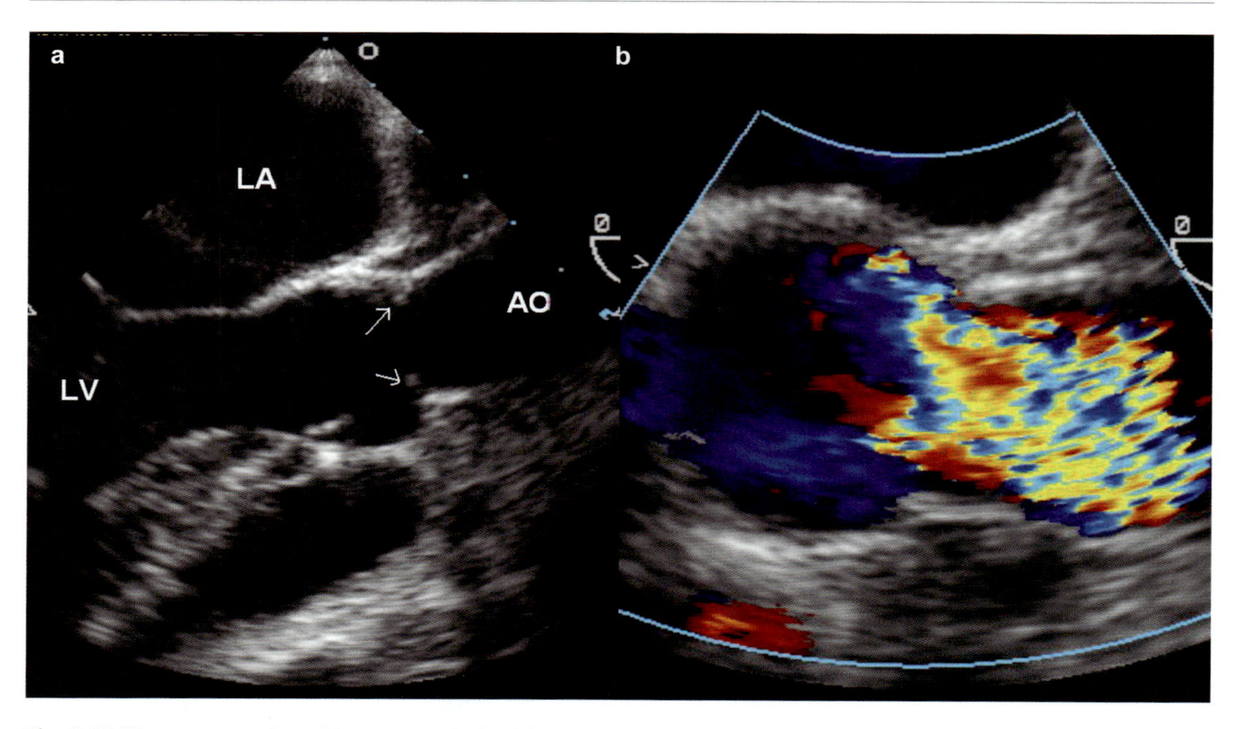

Fig. 3.15 These transesophageal images are obtained from an 18-year-old woman with discrete supravalvular aortic stenosis (**a**), and the presence of stenosis is confirmed by the color flow image in (**b**). *Ao* aorta, *LA* left atrium, *LV* left ventricle

sinotubular junction in the parasternal long axis view (Fig. 3.15). Although this is usually a condition associated with congenital heart disease, this can be an acquired condition in patients with familial hypercholesterolemia. With the congenital variety, other cardiac congenital anomalies are common.

Echocardiographic Assessment of Aortic Valve Morphology

In the Western world, rheumatic aortic stenosis has become rare. The most common underlying predisposing condition for aortic stenosis is congenital bicuspid aortic valve [21, 22]. In most surgical series of explanted stenotic aortic valves, bicuspid aortic valves accounts for about half of the cases. Under the age of 65, bicuspid aortic valve is much more likely to be the underlying valve morphology in patients with severe AS, whereas tricuspid aortic valve is more common in AS patients more than 70 years of age. The determination of aortic morphology in patients with aortic stenosis is clinically important, as familial clustering has been reported in patients with bicuspid aortic valve who frequently have associated findings which need to be looked for. In the short axis view, the bicuspid aortic valve has a fish-mouth appearance during systole (Figs. 3.16–3.19). A raphe is present in many of these patients and can be confused for a commissure. This is particularly problematic in patients with a cleft of the conjoined cusp near the raphe. Moving the imaging plane slightly more cephalic is important to differentiate a raphe from a commissure, which demonstrates opening right up to the aortic wall, as opposed to a raphe. Determination of the orientation of the commissure may be useful, as associated findings such as aortic dilatation appear to have a predilection to a particular commissural orientation. Whether 3D imaging can enhance ability in correctly identifying the commissural orientation remains to be evaluated (Fig. 3.20).

In young people with aortic stenosis, unicommissural unicuspid aortic valve is uncommon but not rare [22]. It may account for 5% of the cases with aortic stenosis under the age of 50. It is frequently confused with bicuspid aortic valve. This condition should be suspected, when the commissure of a suspected bicuspid

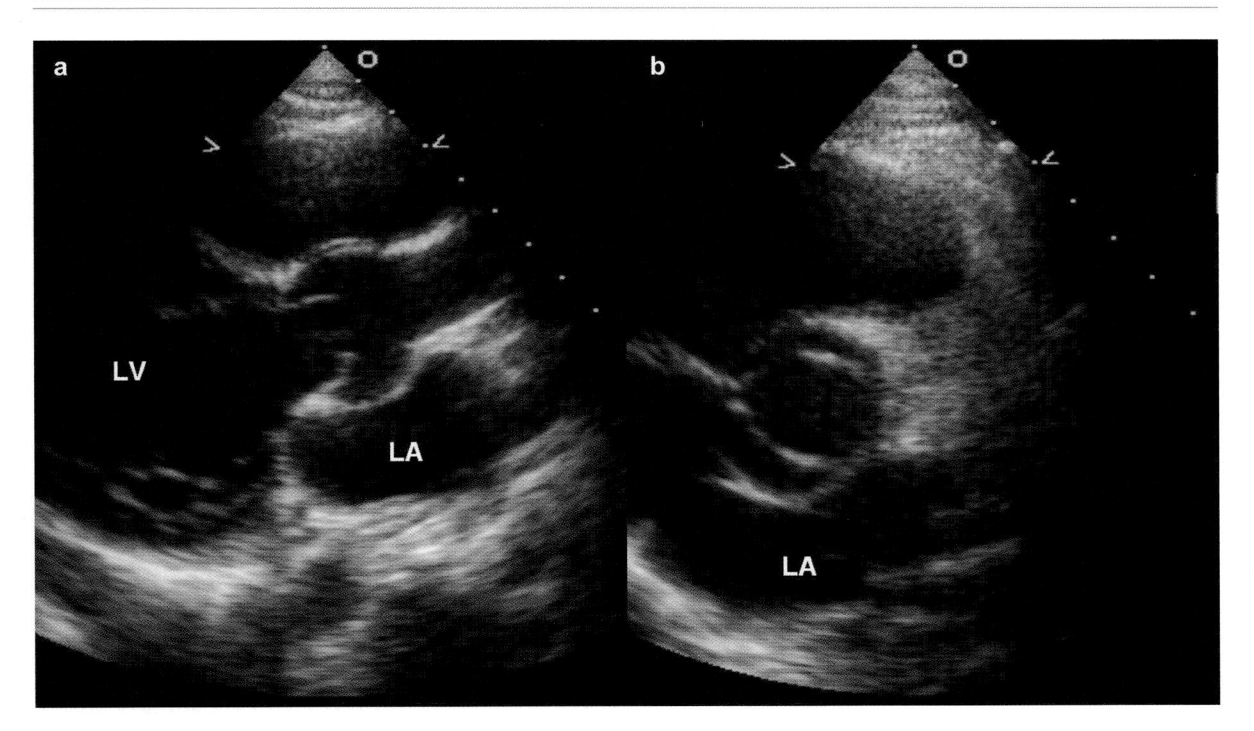

Fig. 3.16 The parasternal long-axis (**a**) and short-axis (**b**) views in systole show that the aortic valve demonstrates systolic doming consistent with restricted cusp excursion and the aortic valve is bicuspid with the commissure from about 9 o'clock to 5 o'clock. This can also be described as fusion of the right and left cusp, and is the most common commissural orientation for the bicuspid aortic valve. *LA* left atrium, *LV* left ventricle

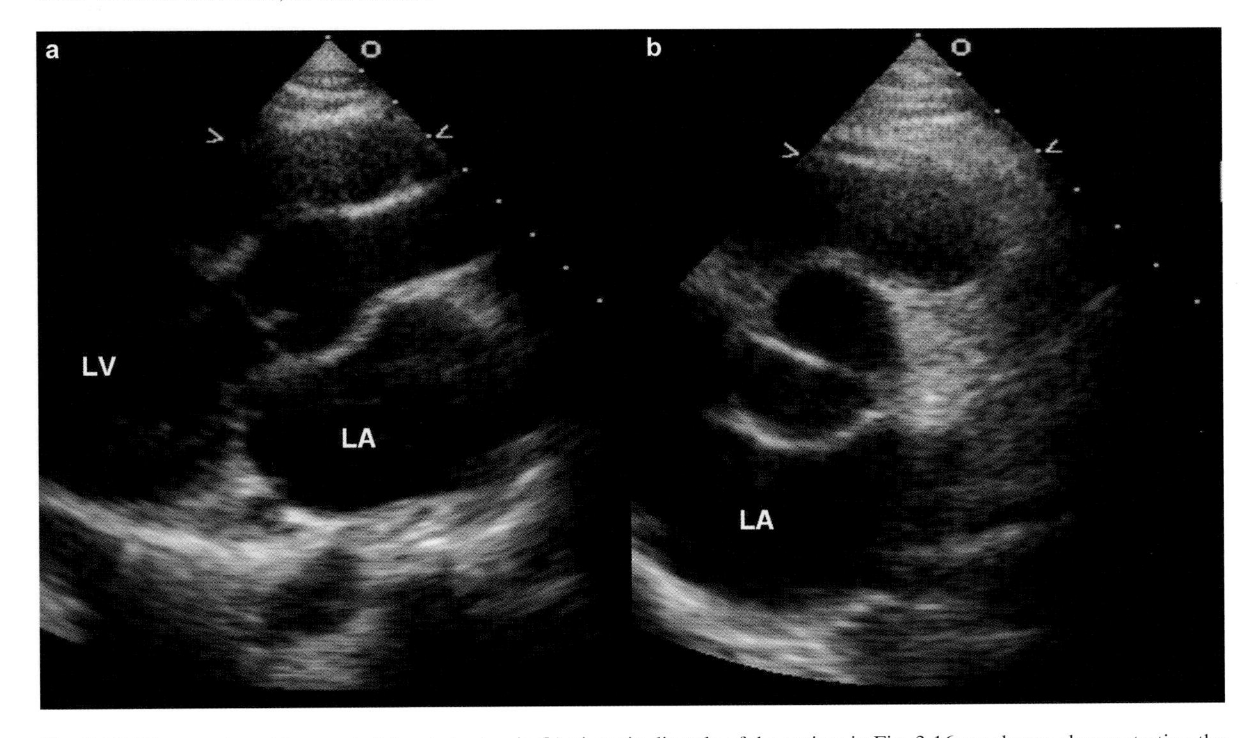

Fig. 3.17 The parasternal long-axis (**a**) and short-axis (**b**) views in diastole of the patient in Fig. 3.16 are shown, demonstrating the commissural orientation of the bicuspid aortic valve. *LA* left atrium, *LV* left ventricle

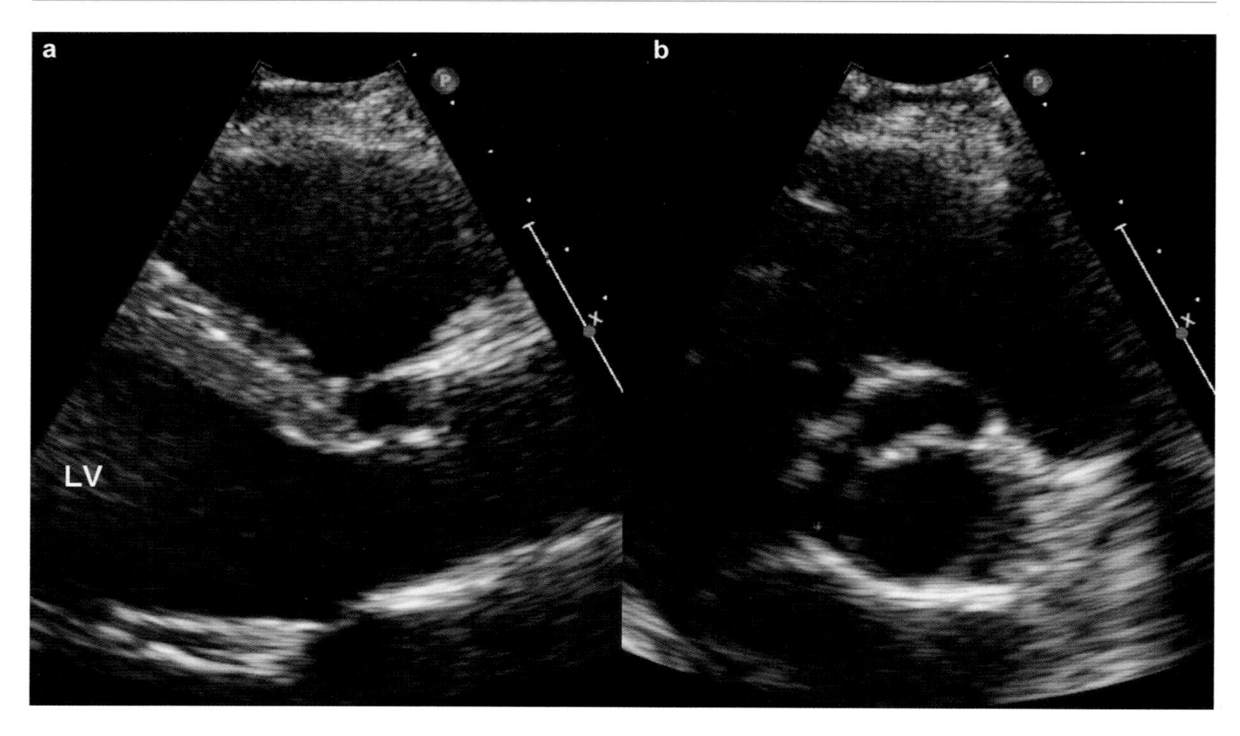

Fig. 3.18 The next common commissural orientation for the bicuspid aortic valve is shown in the long-axis (**a**) and short-axis (**b**) views in systole. There is mild doming and the commissure runs from 2 o'clock to 6 o'clock. This can be referred to as fusion of the right and non-coronary cusps. *LV* left ventricle

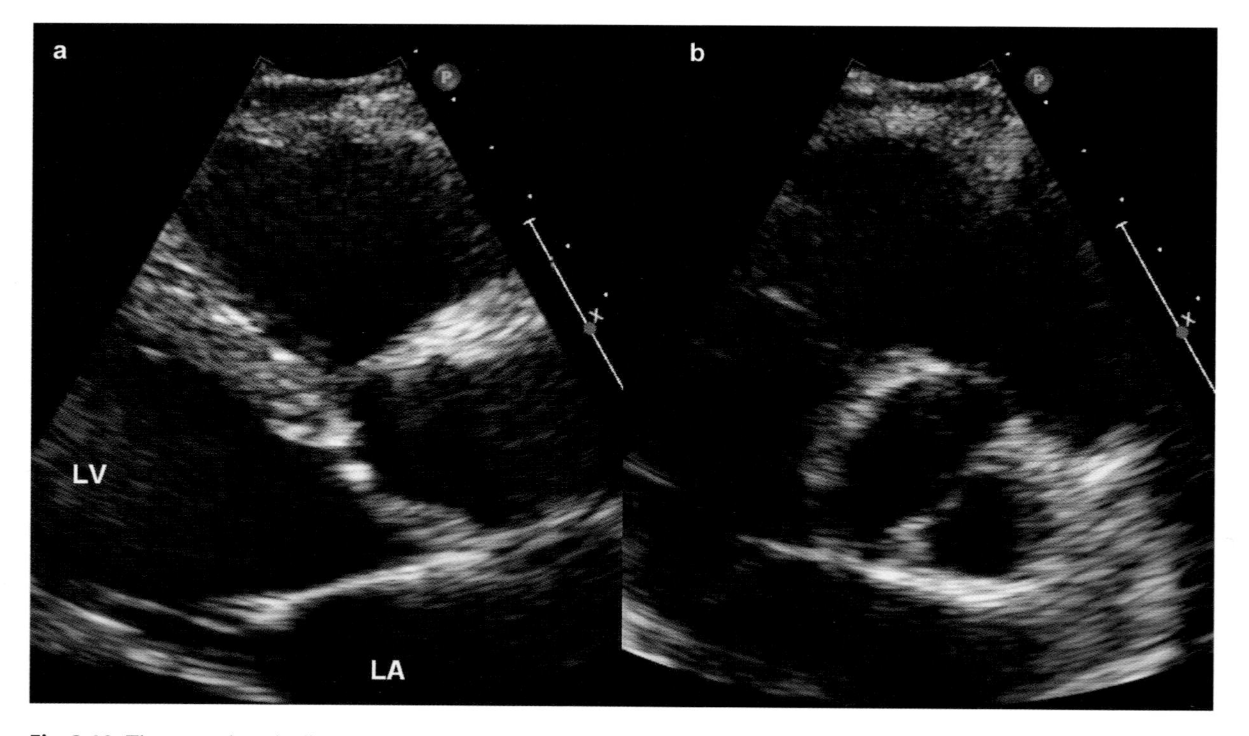

Fig. 3.19 The same views in diastole for the patient in Fig. 3.18 are shown with the long-axis view in (**a**) and short-axis view in (**b**). The commissure is clearly imaged in the short-axis view (**b**). *LA* left atrium, *LV* left ventricle

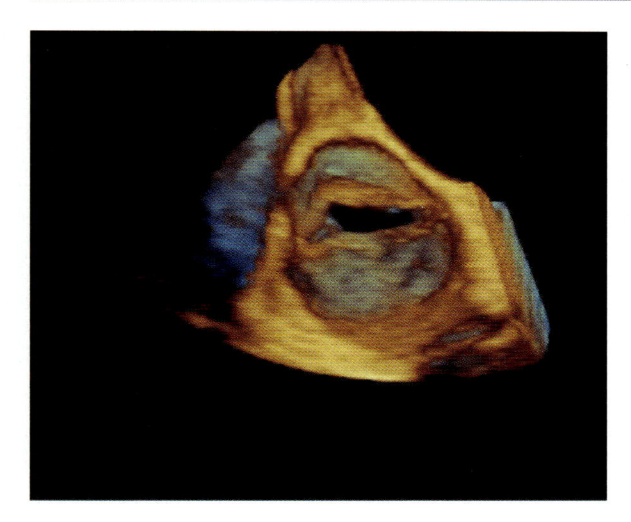

Fig. 3.20 This is a 3D view of a bicuspid aortic valve. The free edge of the cusps shows mild thickening giving a rolled up appearance

aortic valve does not extend right up to the aortic wall (Figs. 3.21, 3.22). During systole, a unicommissural unicuspid valve has an eccentric circular opening such that it gives a typical appearance of a small circle, which is the aortic valve orifice, within a larger circle, which is the aorta root, in the short axis view. Acommissural unicuspid aortic valve usually presents with severe aortic stenosis during the prenatal or the neonatal stage. This condition has not been observed in adults.

The parasternal window is preferred in the assessment of the aortic valve. Both long axis and short axis views are useful. The opening and closing motion of the aortic cusps is best appreciated with the long axis view. In aortic stenosis, restriction in aortic cusp opening is invariably present. Aortic closure abnormalities are usually present in the setting of aortic regurgitation. These are best appreciated in the parasternal long-axis view. In the long-axis view, the anterior cusp represents the right coronary cusp and the posterior cusp can be either the non-coronary cusp or the left coronary cusp depending upon the angulation of the imaging plane. If bicuspid aortic valve is suspected, it is appropriate to refer to the cusps in this view as the anterior and the posterior cusps, since the commissure orientation cannot be determined in this view and thus it is difficult to know the precise orientation of the commissure.

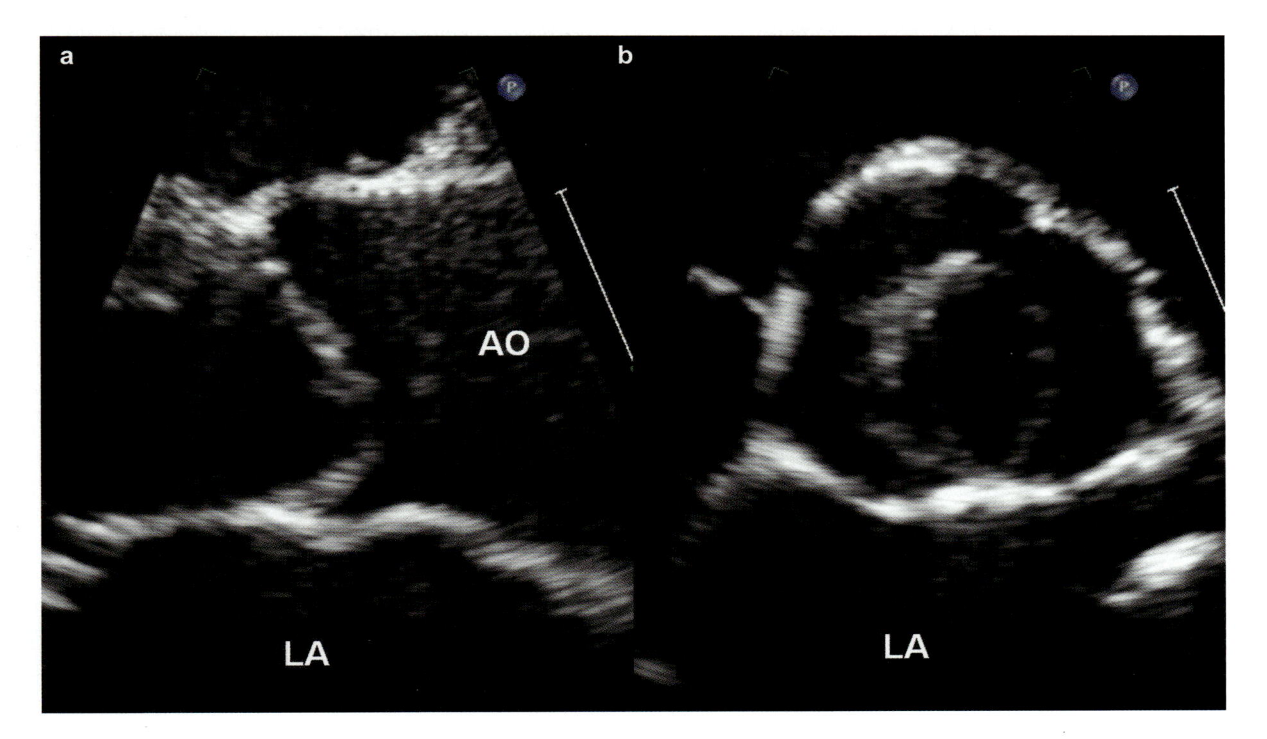

Fig. 3.21 The unicommissural unicuspid aortic valve is shown in the long-axis (**a**) and short-axis (**b**) views. The aortic valve shows marked degree of doming indicating significant restriction to cusp excursion. The short-axis view gives a typical "circle within a circle" appearance, as there is only one inferiorly located commissure

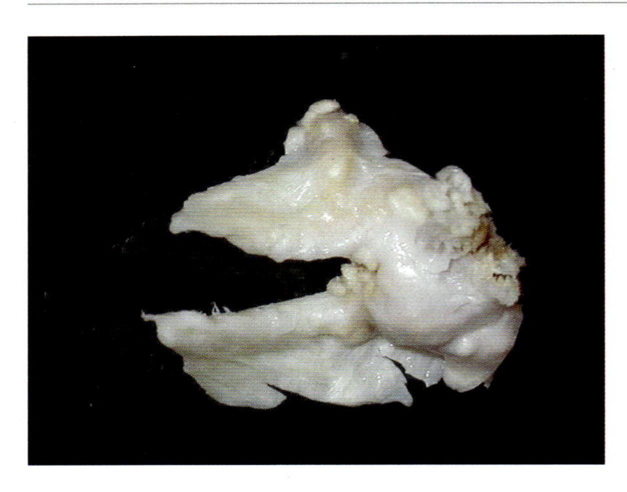

Fig. 3.22 An excised unicommissural unicuspid aortic valve with severe degenerative changes

The morphology of the aortic valve is best appreciated in the parasternal short axis view. In addition to the opening and closing motion of the aortic cusps, the number of cusps can also be determined. Care needs to be taken to sweep the imaging plane cephalic to fully appreciate the extent of the commissures, which arise slightly more cephalic than the coaptation line of the cusps. Fine adjustment by careful rotation of the imaging plane is essential to obtain a true short axis view in order to visualize the commissures cleanly (Figs. 3.17, 3.19). If this view is oblique, the commissures may not be optimally seen and a normal tricuspid aortic valve can be mistaken for a bicuspid valve or even a quadricuspid aortic valve. In our experience, it is best not to commit to the aortic valve morphology unless a true short axis view is obtained with clear visualization of the commissures extending all the way to the aortic wall. The same approach is applied when examining the aortic valve by transesophageal echocardiography, so that oblique section should not be used to determine aortic valve morphology. Freeze frame is useful for a proper appreciation of the excursion of the aortic cusps. In young healthy individuals, the aortic valve orifice assumes a circular shape during maximal excursion (Fig. 3.1). With the aging process, the free edge of the aortic cusp may become fibrotic with a slight degree of restriction to excursion, and in this situation, the aortic orifice assumes a triangular shape at maximal excursion (Fig. 3.23).

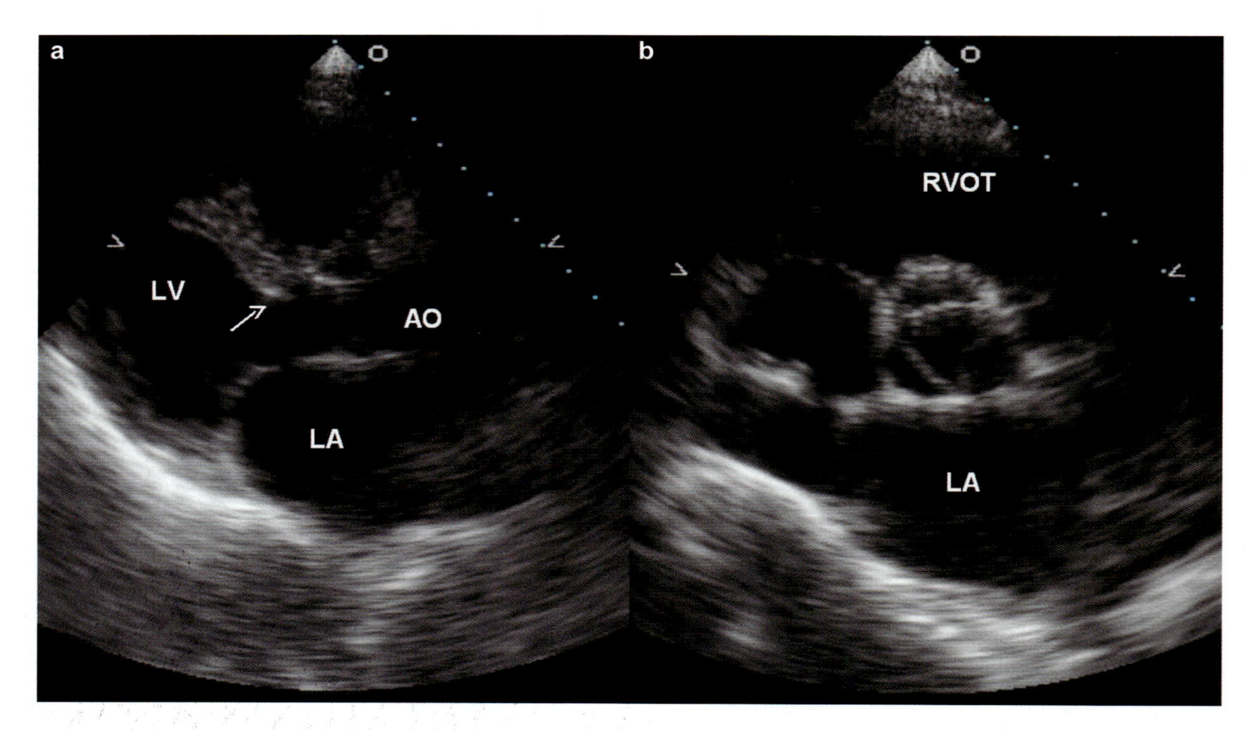

Fig. 3.23 The parasternal long-axis (**a**) and short-axis (**b**) in systole showed the typical age-related changes. In the long-axis view (a) the ventricular septum is angulated (*arrow*) and there is slight restriction to aortic cusp excursion. The left atrium is also dilated. In the short-axis view (b), the aortic valve is shown in its maximal excursion and the aortic orifice is triangular in shape indicating that there is restriction to the excursion of all three cusps, although there is no nodular thickening of any of the three cusps. *Ao* aorta, *LA* left atrium, *LV* left ventricle, *RVOT* right ventricular cutflow tract

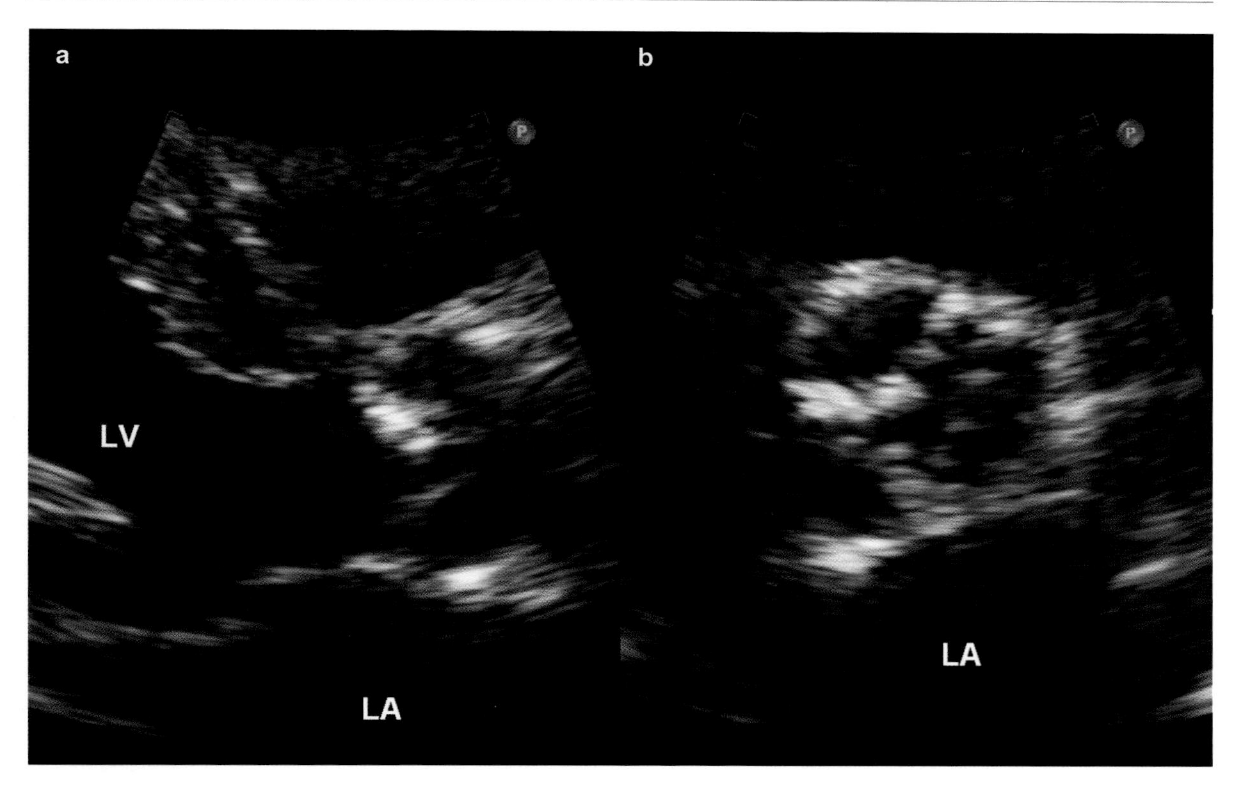

Fig. 3.24 The parasternal long-axis (**a**) and short-axis (**b**) views show that the aortic valve is tricuspid with nodular thickening involving the right coronary cusp representing a mild focal calcification. *LA* left atrium, *LV* left ventricle

Another important morphologic feature of the aortic valve is the presence of localized brightness or thickening consistent with calcification. The severity of aortic valvular calcification has been suggested to be a predictor of rapid progression of aortic stenosis [23]. The severity of calcification can be semi-quantitated by the extent of involvement of the aortic cusps (Figs. 3.24, 3.25). Patients with moderate or severe aortic valvular calcification should have more frequent follow-up to check for progression of aortic stenosis.

Assessment of Aortic Stenosis Severity

There are many indices of AS, but by far the most widely used are the transvalvular aortic velocity, peak, and mean transvalvular gradients and aortic valve area. The definition of severe AS is maximum velocity ≥4 m/s, dimensionless index which is the peak left ventricular outflow tract (LVOT) velocity divided by peak AS velocity ≤0.25, mean gradient ≥40 mmHg, aortic valve area ≤1.0 cm^2 [24, 25]. The transvalvular aortic gradient is obtained using the modified Bernoulli equation which is: pressure gradient = $4V^2$, where V is the maximum velocity across the aortic valve. The aortic valve area (AVA) is obtained using the continuity equation:

$$AVA = \frac{LVOT_{area} \times VTI_{LVOT}}{VTI_{AV}}$$

where LVOT area is the area of left ventricular outflow tract at the annulus, VTI_{LVOT} is the velocity time integral of Doppler velocity of LVOT, and VTI_{AV} is the velocity time integral of Doppler velocity at the aortic valve (Fig. 3.26). The equation can be simplified by substituting VTI_{LVOT} and VTI_{AS} with peak velocity at LVOT and peak AS velocity.

In order to avoid underestimating the severity of AS, the AS velocity should be obtained from multiple windows, particularly the apical and right sternal border windows (Fig. 3.27). Although imaging continuous wave Doppler is usually adequate, non-imaging

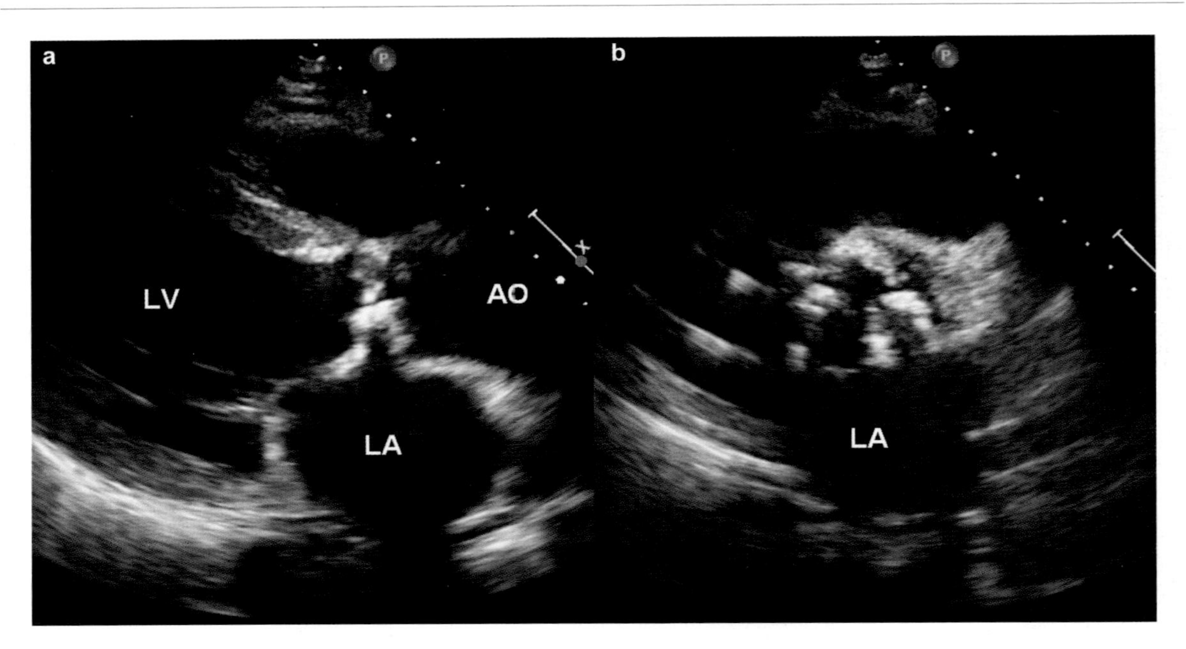

Fig. 3.25 The parasternal long-axis (**a**) and short-axis (**b**) views show that there are multiple nodular densities involving the aortic valve representing severe calcification. The number of cusps cannot be determined in this patient. *Ao* aorta, *LA* left atrium, *LV* left ventricle

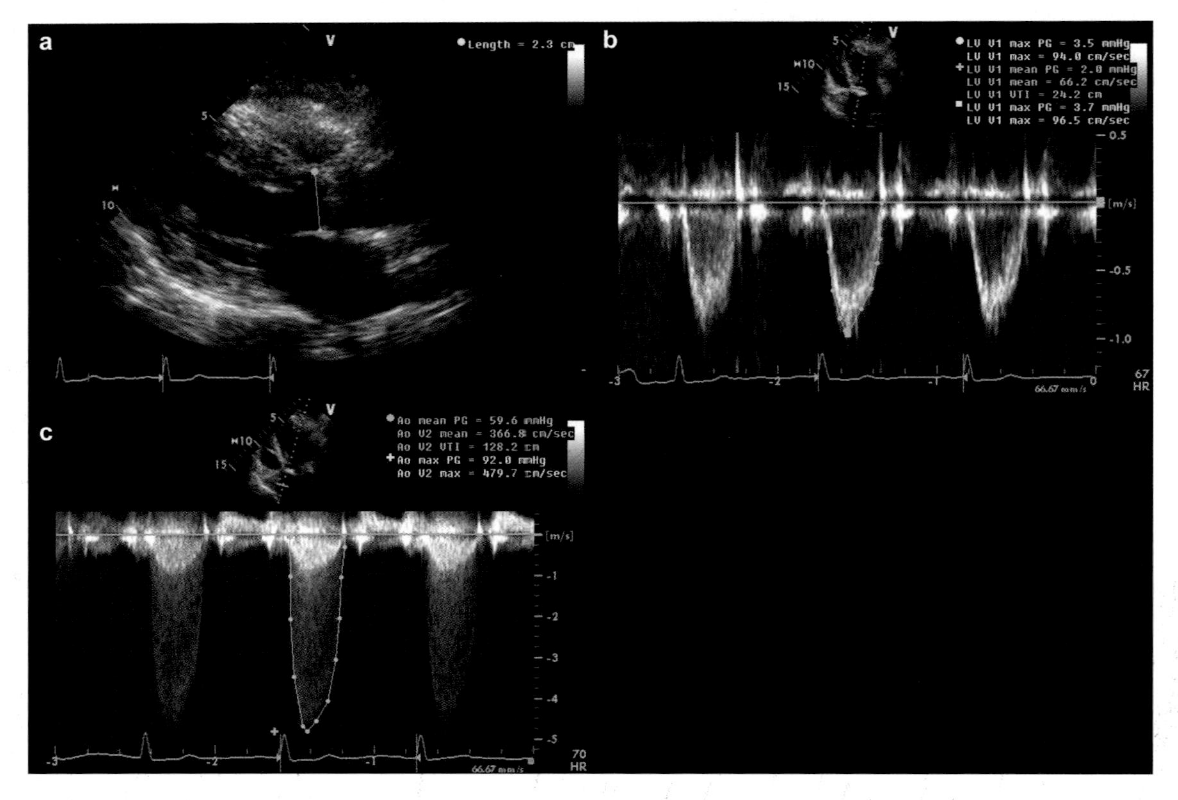

Fig. 3.26 In this patient with aortic stenosis, the aortic annulus in systole measures 2.3 cm in diameter in the long-axis view (**a**). The pulsed wave Doppler of the left ventricular outflow tract is shown in (**b**), and the continuous wave Doppler of the aortic stenosis velocity is shown in (**c**). Using the continuity equation, the aortic valve area is calculated to be 0.78 cm^2 indicating severe aortic stenosis

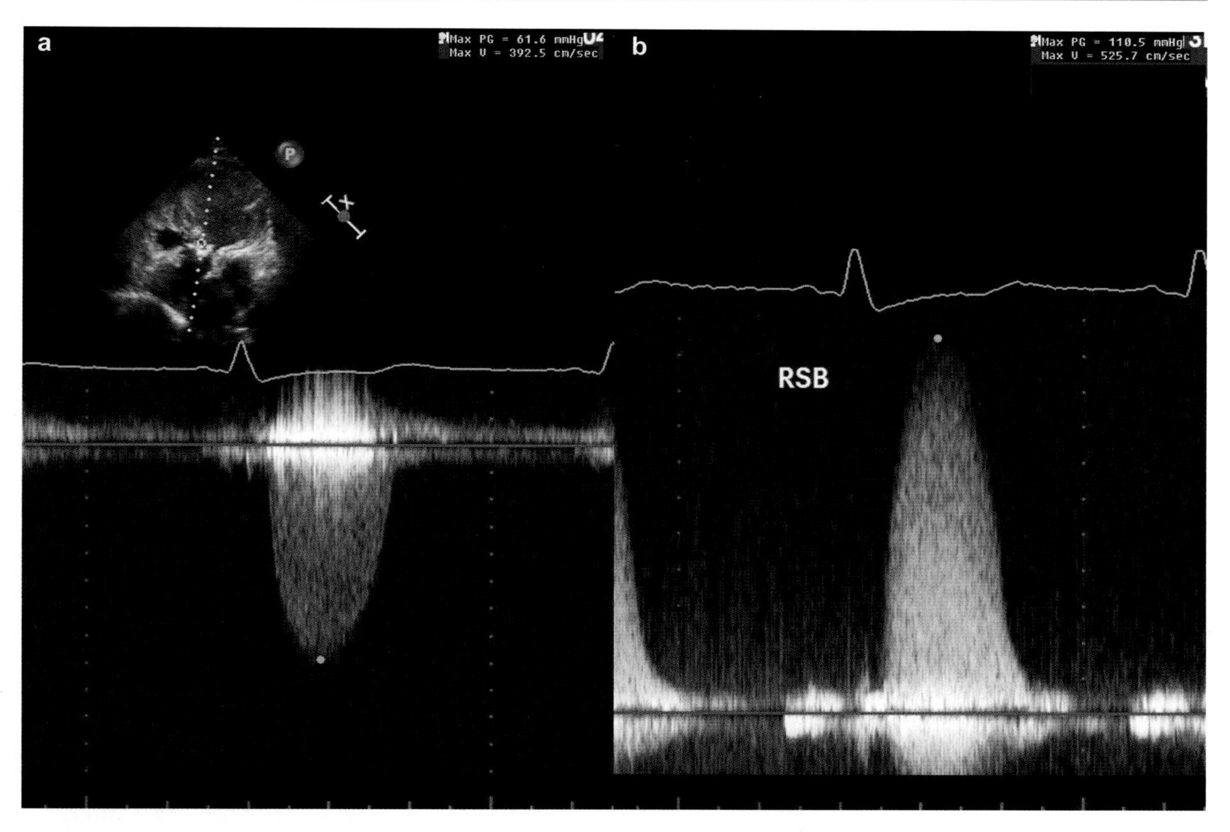

Fig. 3.27 In assessing the severity of aortic stenosis, multiple acoustic windows should be attempted. In our experience the two most useful windows are the apical window and the right suprasternal (*RSB*) window. In this patient with aortic stenosis, complete Doppler signals can be obtained from the apex (**a**) and from the right sternal border (**b**). The peak velocity from the right sternal border is 5.2 m/s, which is considerably higher than that from the apex, which is 3.9 m/s, underscoring the importance of interrogating multiple acoustic windows even after apparently optimal aortic stenosis velocity has been obtained from one particular window

continuous wave transducer should be used to optimize alignment of the AS signal so as to achieve the highest velocity. When dealing with severe AS, the highest wall filter should be used to enhance the signal to noise ratio. Avoidance of excessive Doppler gain is useful to obtain clean envelopes in order to avoid obscuring the envelope and overestimating the maximum velocity. Other ways to enhance a weaker AS signal include decreasing the sweep speed from 100 to 50 mm/s and the use of echo contrast agents.

It is not uncommon that a patient may have one or two indices suggesting severe AS and the remaining indices suggesting less than severe AS. Indeed among patients with AS, aortic valve area is the most likely measure to indicate severe AS, while the other measures may indicate otherwise. When this situation arises, it is useful to examine the aortic annulus dimension which should be 1.9–2.6 cm in diameter in most patients. Underestimating the diameter of the aortic annulus is a common reason for an underestimation of the aortic valve area. We prefer using the aortic annulus to the left ventricular outflow tract diameter in the calculation of aortic valve area as the landmarks for aortic annulus are clearly defined, while the determination of left ventricular outflow tract diameter is subjective as the left ventricular outflow tract is more of a functional entity than an anatomic structure [25]. It is also useful to calculate the stroke volume at the left ventricular outflow tract which is $LVOT_{area} x VTI_{LVOT}$ and to compare with the stroke volume calculated from the left ventricular volumes. If the former is substantially less than the latter, the aortic annulus is likely underestimated. On the other hand, if the former is substantially greater than the latter, the sample volume may have been too close to the aortic annulus.

An important entity is low gradient severe AS. In this clinical setting aortic valve area indicates severe AS and yet both maximal velocity and transvalvular gradients are not very elevated and the aortic annulus diameter appears appropriate. In these patients the dimensional index also indicates AS. Two groups of patients have been identified to manifest this phenomenon [26, 27]. The first group of patients is those with left ventricular systolic dysfunction resulting in reduced stroke volume to account for the reduced transvalvular gradients. Dobutamine stress-echo has been shown to be useful in these patients to differentiate those with true severe AS from those with pseudo-severe AS (Fig. 3.28). Patients with pseudo-severe AS are those with aortic valves that demonstrate improved excursion with improvement in left ventricular systolic function during dobutamine infusion. The second group of patients has a normal left ventricular systolic function with paradoxic low gradients due to reduced stroke volume as a result of decreased left ventricular volumes. These are more likely to be elderly women with concentric left ventricular hypertrophy leading to reduced left ventricular volumes (Fig. 3.29). Thus, interpretation of severity of aortic stenosis should not be based upon a single measure alone but should be

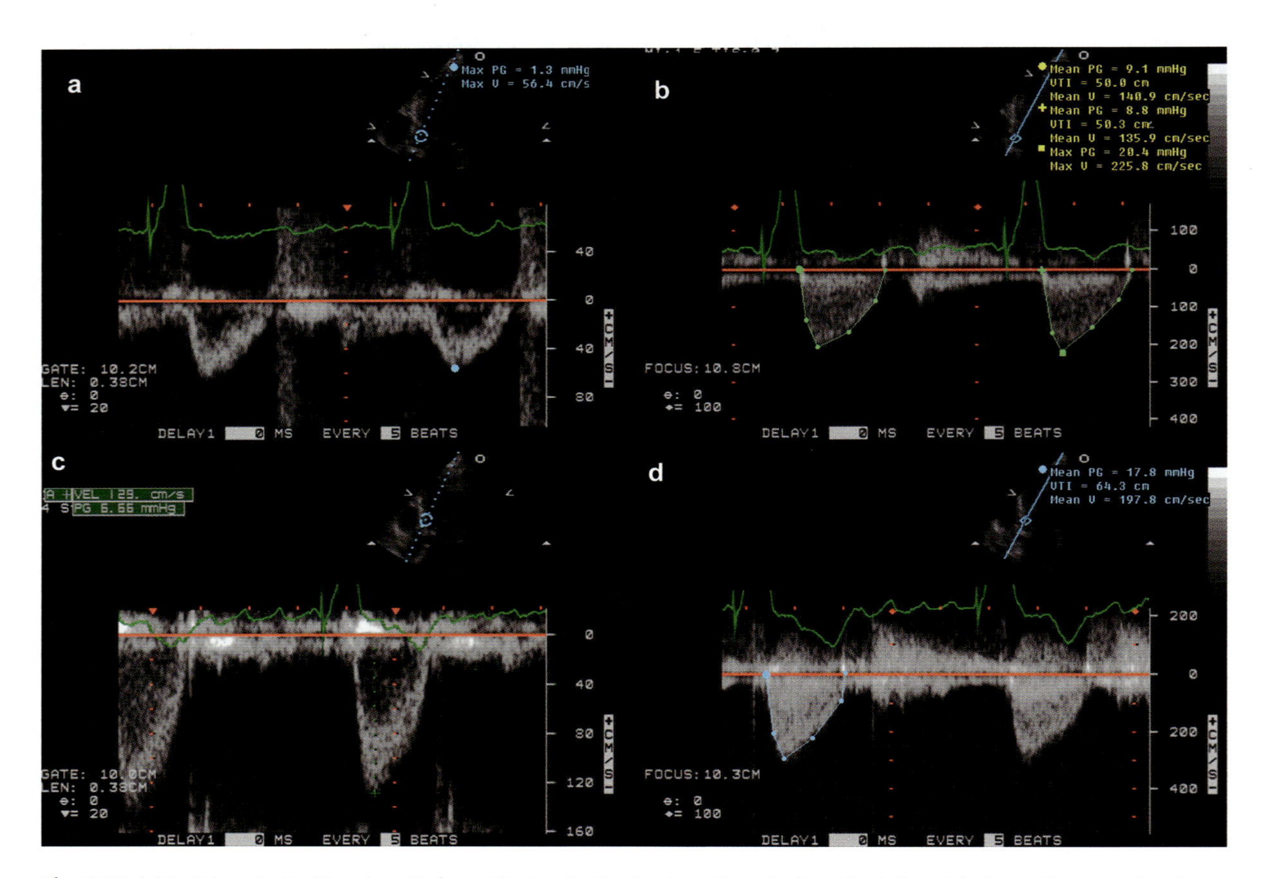

Fig. 3.28 (**a**) In this patient with reduced left ventricular ejection fraction, the velocity at the left ventricular outflow tract is reduced at 0.56 m/s. (**b**) The peak aortic stenosis velocity is 2.26 m/s giving a peak gradient of 20 mmHg and a mean gradient of 9 mmHg. The calculated aortic valve area based on the continuity equation is 0.78 cm^2 indicating severe aortic stenosis. (**c**) During dobutamine infusion, there is improvement in left ventricular systolic function with a corresponding increase in the velocity at the left ventricular outflow tract at 1.29 m/s. (**d**) The peak aortic stenosis velocity is 3 m/s giving a peak gradient of 36 mmHg and a mean gradient of 18 mmHg. By the continuity equation, the aortic valve area is calculated to be 1.35 cm^2 (annulus diameter 2 cm). This substantial increase in aortic valve area indicates that this patient has pseudo-severe AS and the small calculated aortic valve area at rest is due to low cardiac output

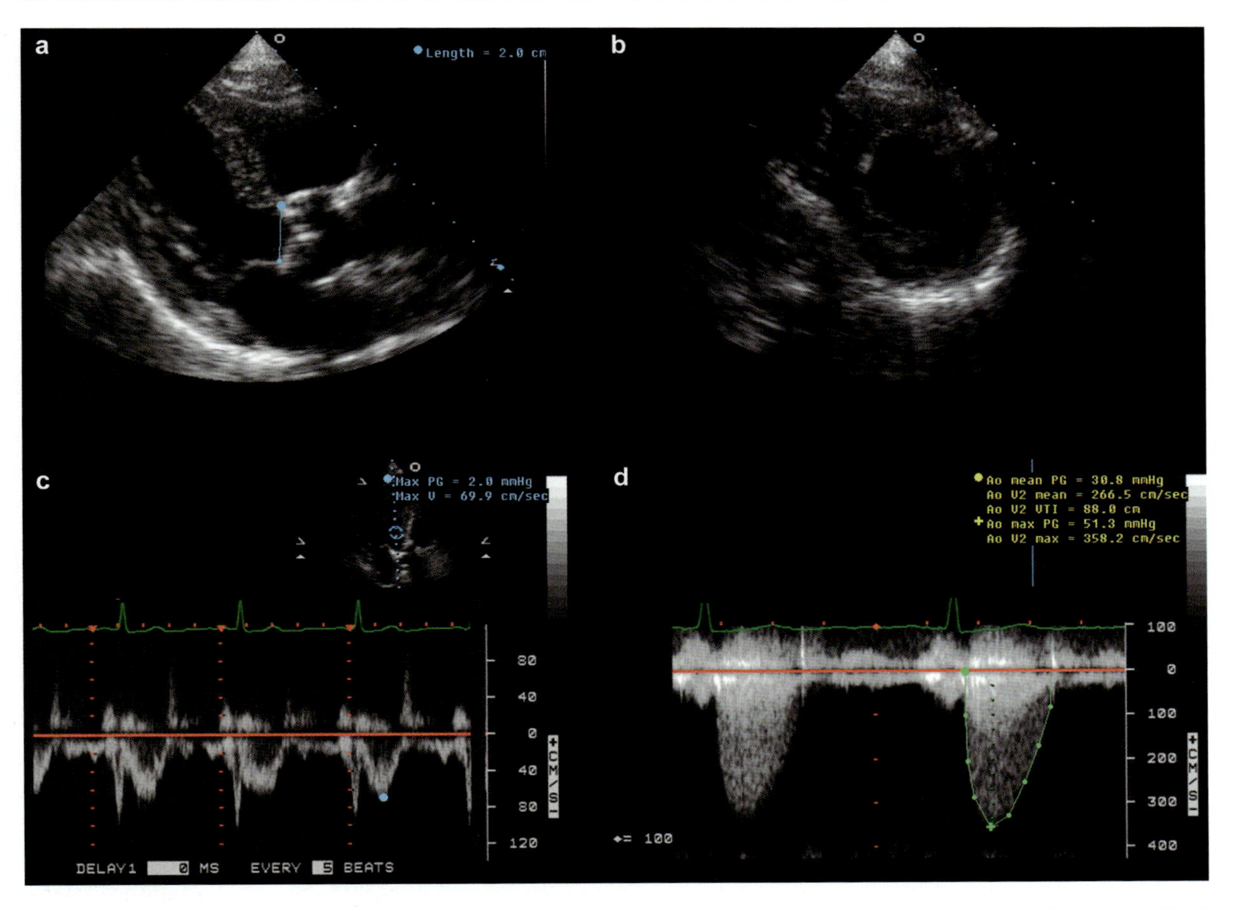

Fig. 3.29 In this patient with aortic stenosis, the aortic annulus measures 2 cm (**a**). The left ventricular cavity is relatively small and the ejection fraction is normal (**b**). The Doppler velocity at the left ventricular outflow tract is shown in (**c**) and the aortic stenosis velocity shown in (**d**). The calculated aortic valve area is 0.61 cm^2 based on the continuity equation, although the peak and mean aortic stenosis gradients are modest at 51 and 31 mmHg, respectively. Patients such as this one are expected to benefit from aortic valve replacement

based upon a careful consideration of different measures, including aortic annulus diameter and stroke volume. Measurements such as maximal velocity, transvalvular gradients and aortic valve area are flow dependent and thus may be misleading in low flow conditions such as those discussed above. Other measures such as valve resistance and stroke work loss have been proposed to be relatively flow independent; however they have been shown to be affected by flow and have not gained wide acceptance.

As structure and function go hand in hand in AS, assessment of the degree of thickening or calcification of the aortic cusps, the excursion of the aortic cusps, and the planimetry of the aortic orifice area are very helpful when there is discordance among the different indices of AS severity. Transesophageal echocardiography provides high quality images and should be used in this setting (Figs. 3.30, 3.31).

Left Ventricular Adaptation to Aortic Stenosis

Development of left ventricular hypertrophy can be quite variable among patients with AS. Patients with left ventricular hypertrophy and presence of intracavitary obstruction appeared to have a more complicated perioperative course following aortic valve replacement [28] (Fig. 3.32). Mitral annular velocities are reduced in

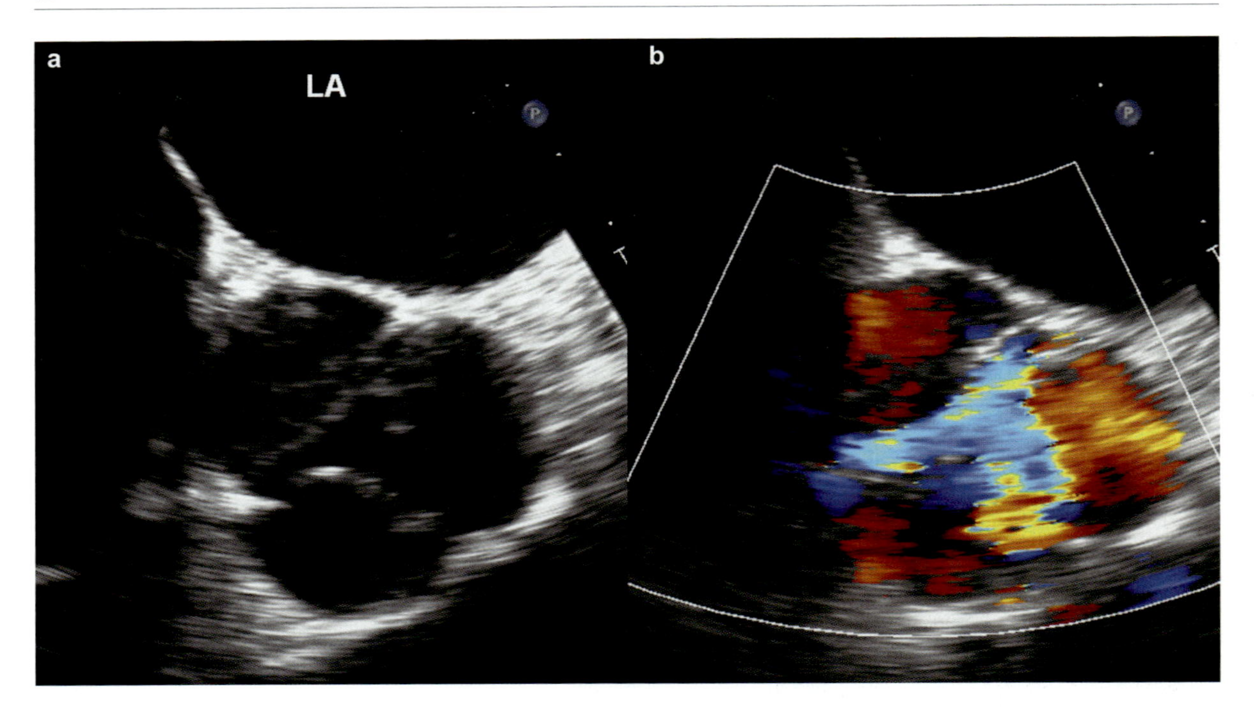

Fig. 3.30 This is a transesophageal echocardiogram (**a**, **b**) of the aortic valve in a patient with low gradient severe aortic stenosis. The aortic valve is tricuspid. Other than focal nodular calcification at the commissure between the right and non-coronary cusp, the aortic cusps appear quite normal, suggesting that the patient has pseudo-severe aortic stenosis. *LA* left atrium

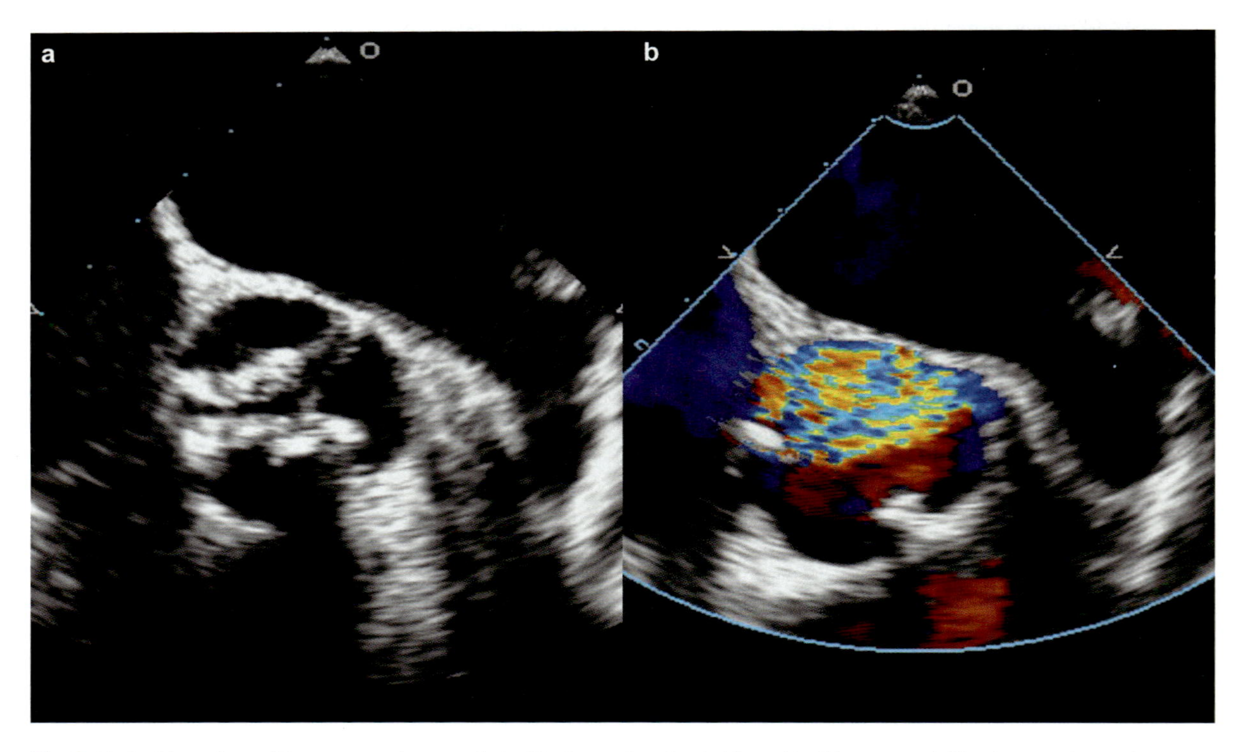

Fig. 3.31 In this patient with severe aortic stenosis (**a**, **b**), the aortic valve is bicuspid with severe calcification restricting the excursion of both cusps. The findings are in keeping with true severe aortic stenosis

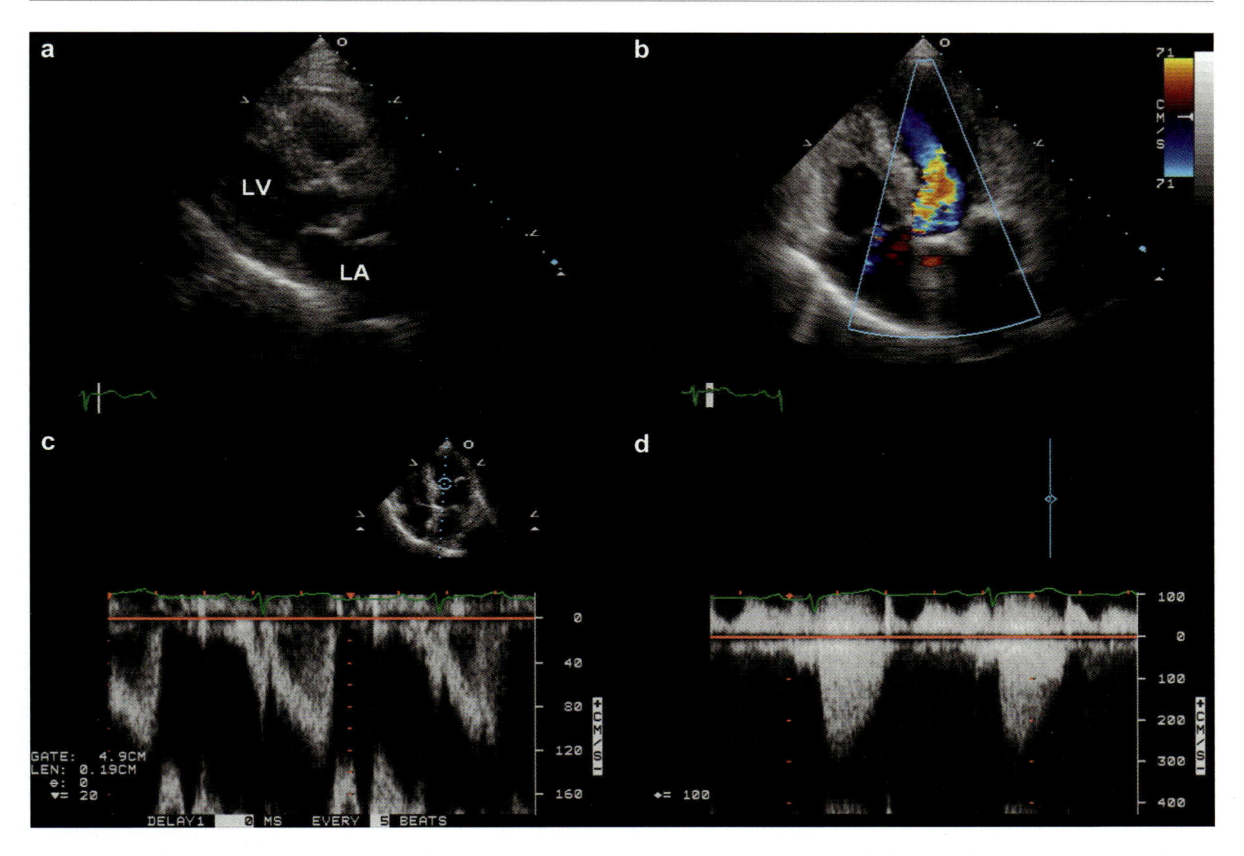

Fig. 3.32 In this patient with aortic stenosis, the parasternal long-axis view is shown in (**a**), the apical five chamber view in (**b**), pulse wave Doppler of the left ventricular outflow tract (**c**) and the aortic stenosis velocity by continuous wave Doppler in (**d**). The left ventricular cavity is relatively small with an angulated ventricular septum. Pulse wave Doppler of the left ventricular outflow tract indicates that there is an increased intracavitary velocity at this region. Myectomy of the basal ventricular septum may be indicated at the time of aortic valve replacement in these patients. *LA* left atrium, *LV* left ventricle

patients with aortic stenosis and the degree of reduction appears to be related to the severity of aortic stenosis (Fig. 3.33). It remains unclear whether these measures have predictive value in identifying patients who will develop early symptoms during follow-up [29].

Aortic Valve Regurgitation

Aortic valve regurgitation may be due to abnormalities of the aortic valve cusps or the adjacent aortic root. The most common mechanisms that cause valve regurgitation are aortic annular dilatation, valve cusp prolapse, scar retraction of the cusps, and cusp perforation [30]. The most common valve cusp causes of aortic regurgitation include: (a) rheumatic – post-inflammatory changes, (b) infective endocarditis, (c) congenitally bicuspid valve, (d) iatrogenic causes including balloon valvotomy, and (e) cusp prolapse – such as prolapse into an adjacent ventricular septal defect (VSD).

Congenitally Bicuspid Valve

Congenitally bicuspid aortic valves are not uncommon, being found in 1–2% of the population. A variant type, termed the "atypical" variant, has been described to account for up to 3–24% of these. This variant has a fenestrated raphe on the conjoined cusp so that there is continuity between the conjoined cusp sinuses. The resulting raphal chord is often only a few mm in thickness and may be calcified (Fig. 3.34) [31]. Rarely such

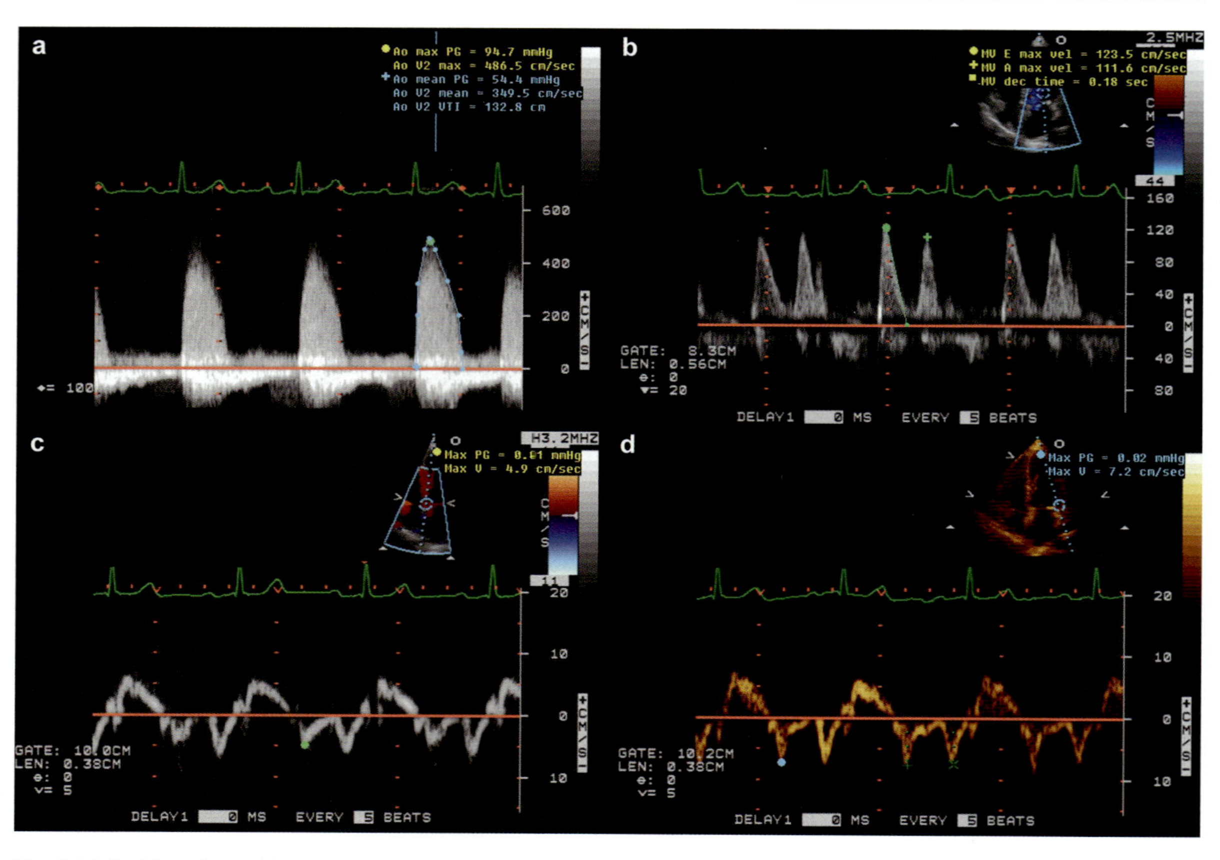

Fig. 3.33 In this patient with severe aortic stenosis, the peak and mean aortic gradients are 95 and 54 mmHg, respectively (**a**). The mitral inflow velocities are shown in (**b**), and the septal and lateral annular velocities are shown in (**c**) and (**d**) respectively. With increasing severity of aortic stenosis, the annular tissue velocities are generally reduced. Whether these velocities have prognostic value remains to be investigated

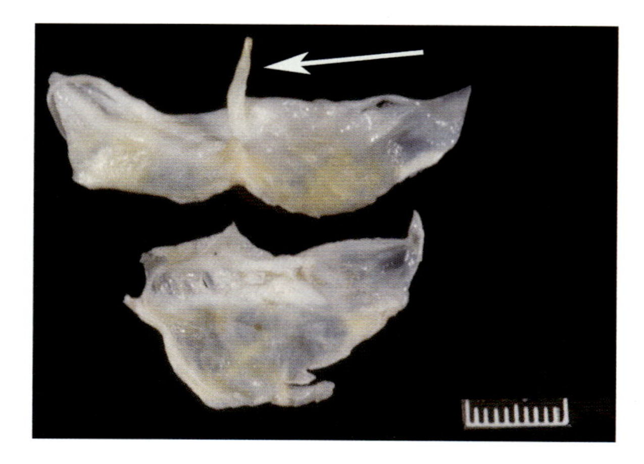

Fig. 3.34 Congenitally bicuspid aortic valve with atypical raphe. The conjoined upper cusp has a thin fibrous chord like raphe (*arrow*). The valve cusps are also thin and probably myxomatous

chords may rupture giving rise to acute aortic regurgitation (Figs. 3.35–3.37). In such cases, there may be raphal remnants on the cusp, attached to the aortic wall, or both. These remnants must be distinguished from the residua of cusp perforations secondary to healed infective endocarditis, and from valve fenestrations which are in different locations on the cusps and generally not associated with aortic regurgitation. The raphe remnant may also be misinterpreted as a valve vegetation or thrombus since the clinical situation is acute aortic insufficiency with a mobile valve mass.

Post-inflammatory Changes

Post-inflammatory cusp disease produces fibrosis, calcification, and commissural fusion of the cusps, similar to

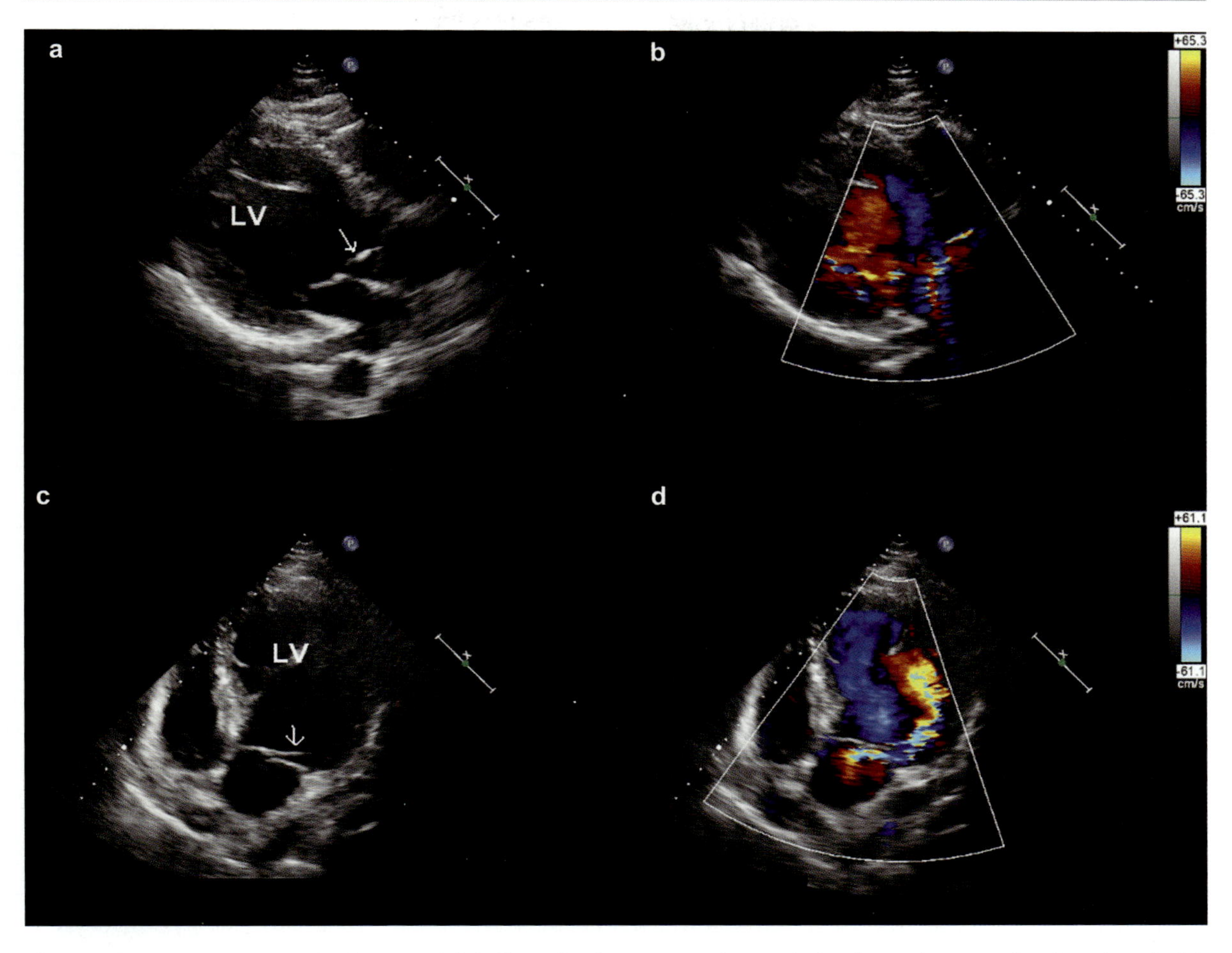

Fig. 3.35 In parasternal long-axis view (**a**), a bright linear density appears to be attached to the aortic cusp and prolapse into the left ventricular outflow tract during diastole. The corresponding color flow images shown in (**b**) demonstrates the presence of posteriorly directed aortic regurgitation. This bright linear structure is better seen in the apical long-axis view in (**c**) and the corresponding color flow image in (**d**) clearly demonstrates the presence of aortic regurgitation which is posteriorly directed

the pathology seen in stenotic rheumatic valves. However, in these cases, the fusion and cusp immobility fix the valve orifice open, rather than hold it closed. It should be apparent that rheumatic disease may give a valve that is mixed in its hemodynamics (Figs. 3.10, 3.38). However, usually either the regurgitation or the stenosis predominates in any one case. Radiation may produce significant cusp fibrosis and retraction of the cusps [32]. Systemic lupus erythematous (SLE) may scar the cusps with cusp retraction, poor opposition, and regurgitation. Aortitis may cause root dilation and regurgitation but some types of aortitis, such as that seen in syphilis and ankylosing spondylitis, may cause the cusps to scar and cause valvular aortic insufficiency.

Other Valvular Causes of Aortic Regurgitation

Infective endocarditis may cause destruction of the cusps. The infected thrombi, known as vegetations, destroy the cusps leading to defects, erosions, and acquired aneurysms that may eventually perforate and leave a hole in the cusp (Fig. 3.39). After the acute episode, healed infective endocarditis may leave large defects or valve irregularities causing poor valve closure.

Balloon valvotomy of the aortic valve is not done because of its limited effectiveness when it is performed. By the destructive nature of the procedure, the

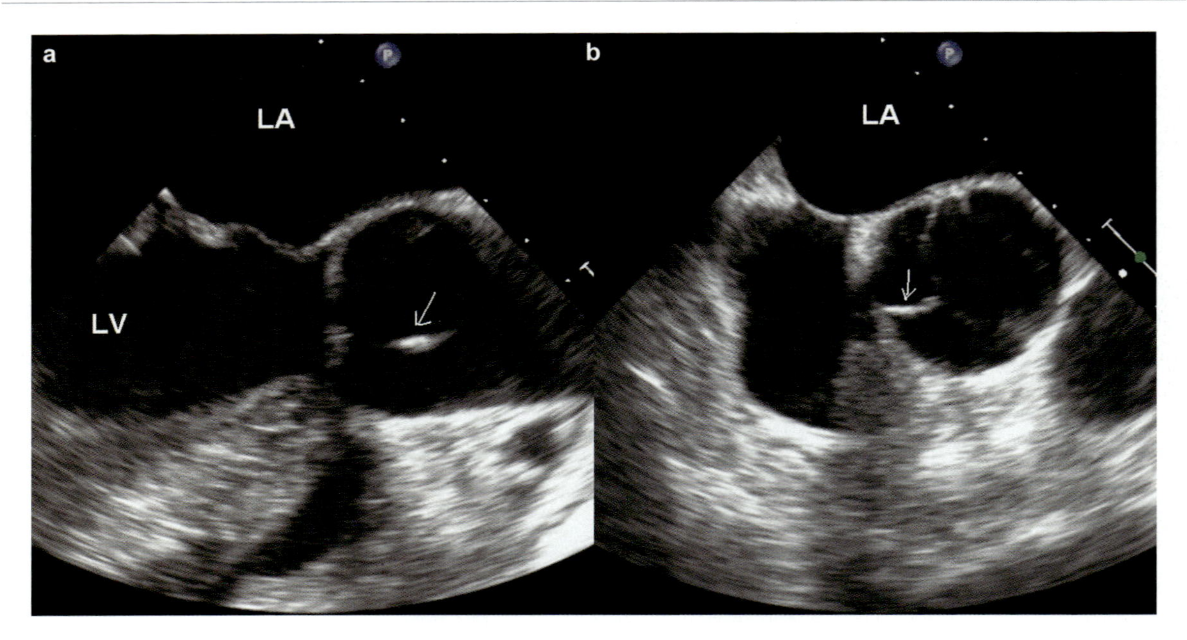

Fig. 3.36 The ruptured raphe of the bicuspid valve is demonstrated in the long-axis (**a**) and short-axis views of the aortic valve (**b**) by transesophageal echocardiography. The ruptured raphe (*L*) is shown to attach to the right cusp. This is the same patient as in Fig. 3.35. *LA* left atrium, *LV* left ventricle

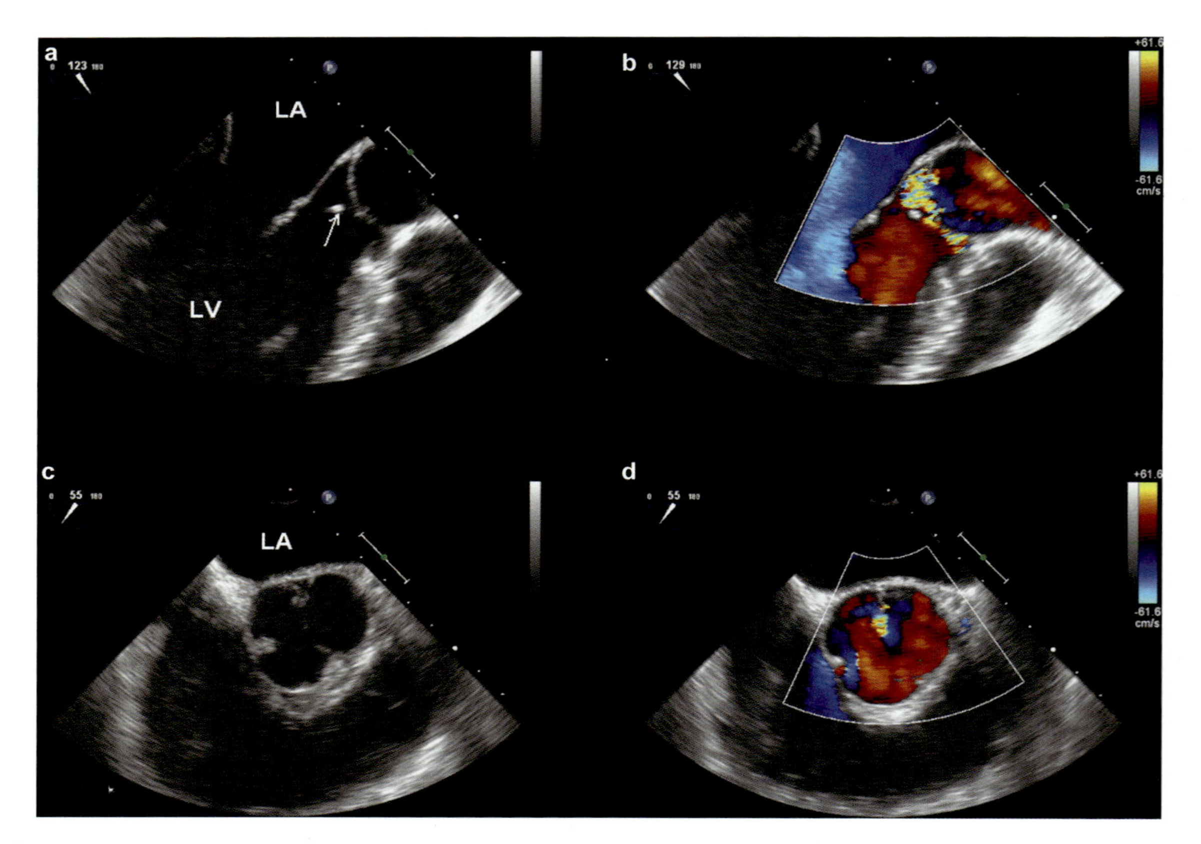

Fig. 3.37 The location and functional consequence of the torn raphe are demonstrated in the long-axis (**a**, **b**) and short-axis (**c**, **d**) transesophageal views of the aortic valve. The posteriorly directed aortic regurgitant jet is clearly demonstrated by color-flow imaging in (**b**) and (**d**). *LA* atrium, *LV* left ventricle

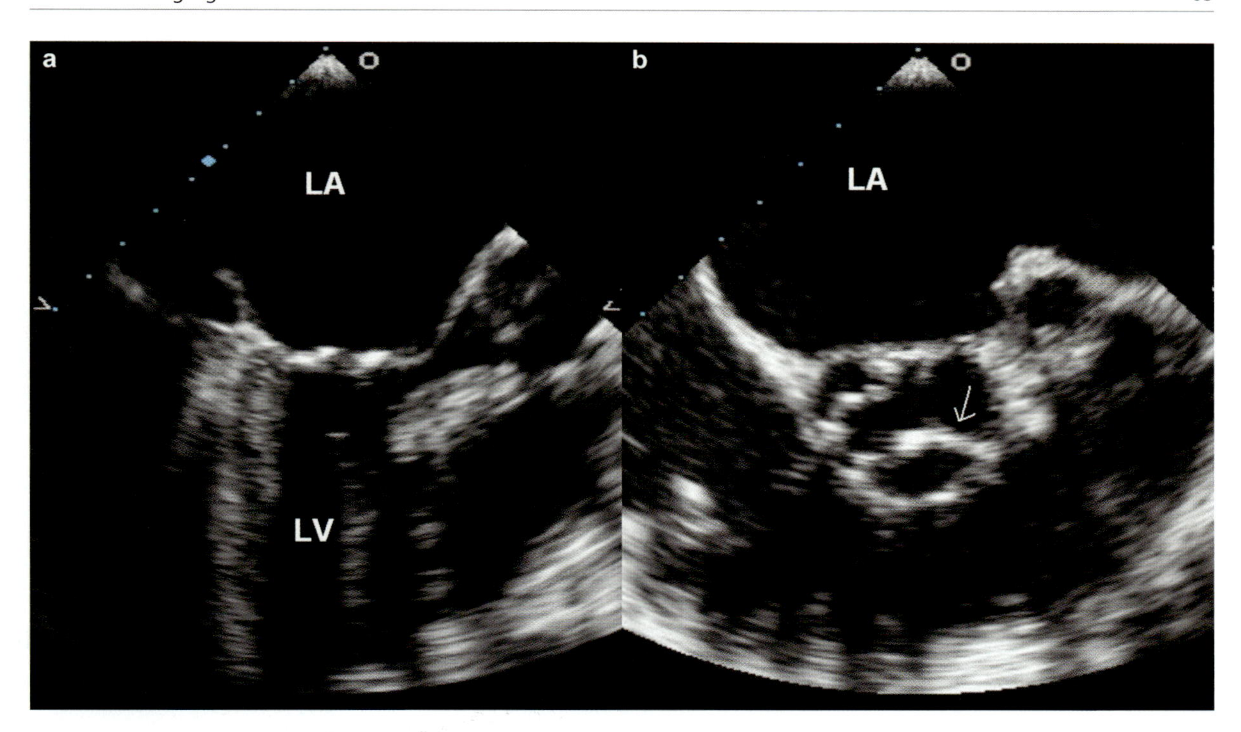

Fig. 3.38 The mitral valve demonstrates thickening and restriction of the tips of both the anterior and posterior mitral leaflets which are typical changes of rheumatic mitral stenosis (**a**). The aortic valve of the same patient is shown in (**b**). There is fusion of the commissure (*arrow*) between the right and left coronary cusps with the diffuse nodular thickening, representing typical rheumatic changes. Rheumatic involvement of the aortic valve is usually associated with rheumatic changes of the mitral valve. *LA* left atrium, *LV* left ventricle

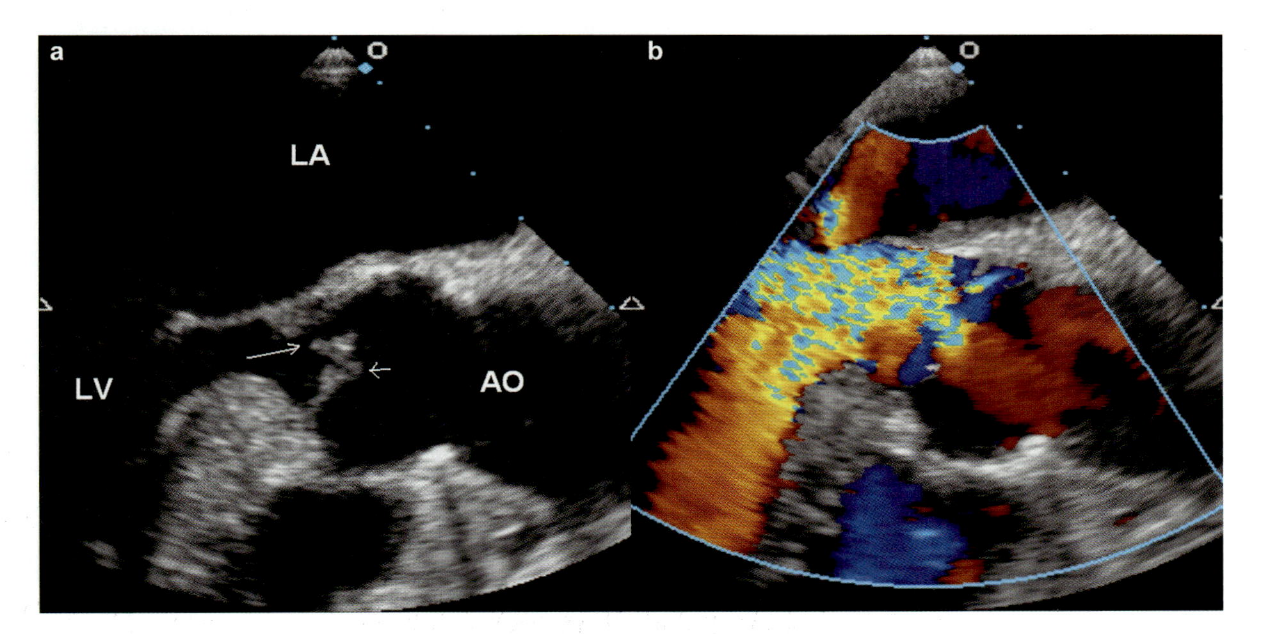

Fig. 3.39 In this patient with infective endocarditis (**a**), there are vegetations on the aortic cusps. Despite adequate cusp coarctation (*short arrow*) a perforation is seen at the base of the posterior cusp (*long arrow*). The corresponding color flow image (**b**) shows the presence of severe aortic regurgitation mainly arising from the perforation. *Ao* aorta, *LA* left atrium, *LV* left ventricle

valve cusps may tear and dehisce from the aortic root. The treatment may lead to a severely regurgitant valve. A normal aortic valve may prolapse into an adjacent membranous ventricular septal defect (VSD). This is treated by re-suspension of the valve and patch of the hole (Trusler plication and VSD repair).

Aortic Causes of Aortic Valve Regurgitation

The other category of conditions commonly leading to aortic valve regurgitation has normal valve cusps to begin with, and the chief pathology is in the aortic root where they are attached (Fig. 3.40). These aortic diseases include: (a) age-related and systemic arterial hypertension related aortic medial degeneration, (b) connective tissue disorders such as Marfan's and Ehlers Danlos, (c) aortic dissection, and (d) aortitis. Diseases that produce annular dilatation include aortic cystic medial necrosis (medial degenerative changes), forms of congenital heart disease, and aortitis. Aortic medial degenerative changes may be an age-related change, or may be related to connective tissue diseases including Marfan's syndrome. The aorta progressively dilates due to loss of its normal collagenous and elastic framework. Both systemic arterial hypertension and connective tissue disorders are observed in patient with aortic dissection, which can acutely cause valve regurgitation.

Aortic root disorders and dilatation are becoming more common. This probably has to do with improved survival of patients with systemic arterial hypertension,

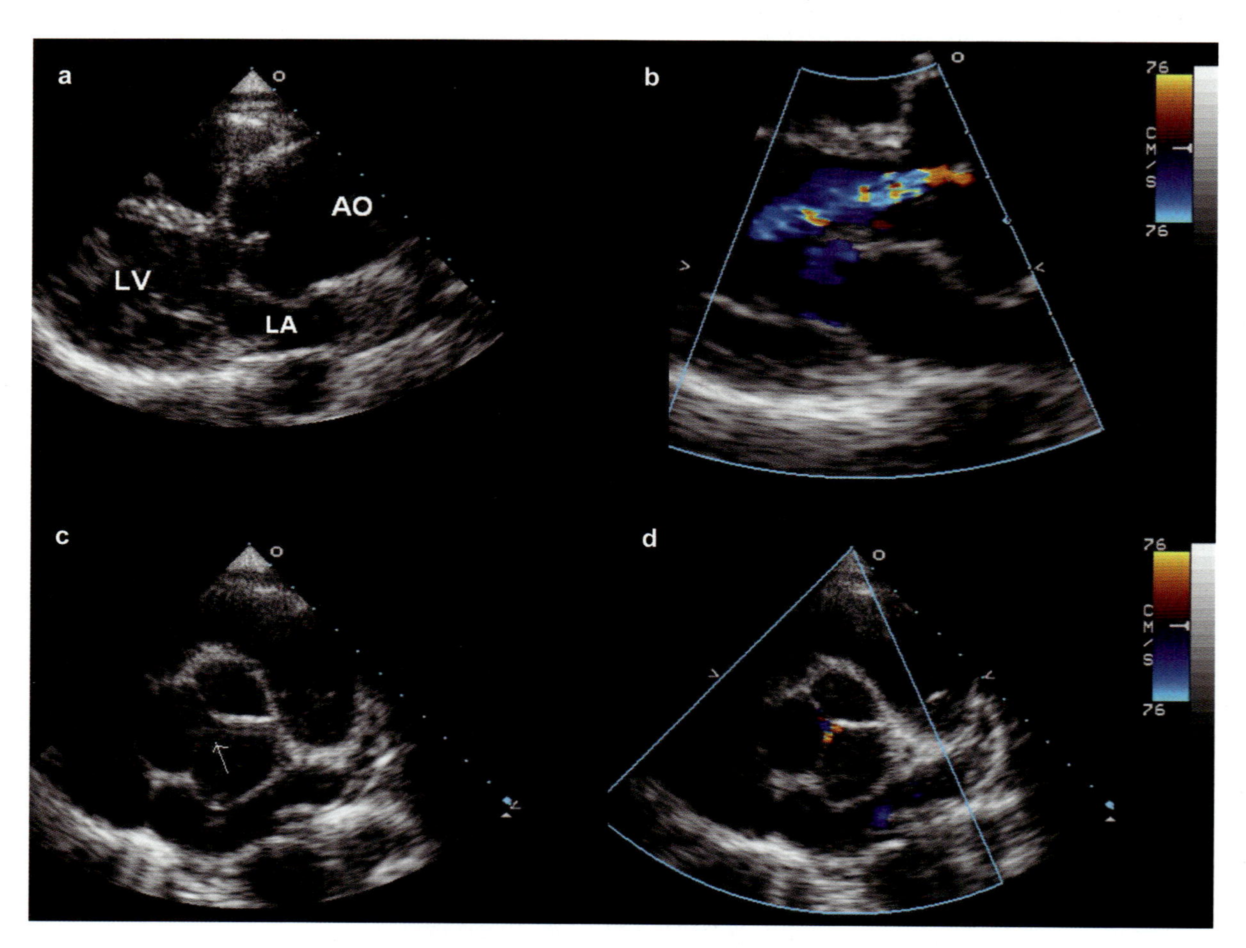

Fig. 3.40 In this patient with dilated aortic root as shown in (**a**), the aortic valve is tricuspid and quite normal, shown in (**c**). The presence of aortic regurgitation is illustrated in (**b**) and (**d**). There is a small central regurgitant area (*arrow*) due to the dilatation of the aortic annulus associated with the root enlargement. *Ao* aorta, *LA* left atrium, *LV* left ventricle

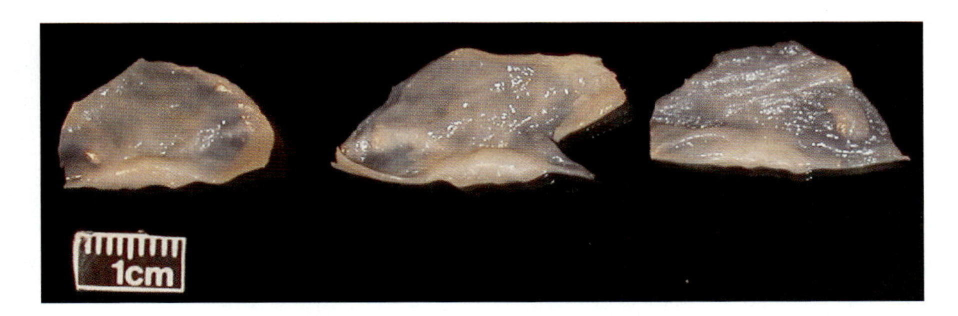

Fig. 3.41 Excised aortic valve from a patient with a dilated aortic root and chronic valve regurgitation. The valve cusps are thin and myxomatous and the free edges are rolled and thickened from the chronic regurgitation

increasing population age, and improving survival of adult congenital heart disease patients. In the latter group, as the patients get older, we continue to discover new complications of their congenital heart disorders and aortic root dilatation is a common complication in these patients.

The valve often stretches as the aorta and the aortic root dilates. This is manifest grossly as thin or myxomatous cusps with rolled free edges due to chronic hemodynamic stress (Fig. 3.41). In some aortitis conditions such as ankylosing spondylitis and syphilis, the cusp may fibrose and scar. Acute aortic dissection may extend back to the valve area. In a type A dissection, the aortic valve may be dehisced from the aortic root either by the dissection or the thrombus in the false lumen.

Echocardiographic Consideration in Aortic Regurgitation

Color Doppler imaging is a very sensitive tool in the detection of aortic regurgitation [33]. In many patients with mild aortic regurgitation detected by color flow Doppler, aortic regurgitation murmur may not be detectable. Trivial aortic regurgitation may be a normal finding, detectable in about 5% of patients with no obvious aortic valvular abnormality. A careful examination of the aortic valve is indicated whenever aortic regurgitation is present.

As many diseases may affect the aortic valve leading to aortic regurgitation, the underlying mechanism leading to aortic regurgitation is more important. A good understanding of the mechanism may allow the selection of candidates for valve repair. Aortic valve repair in patients with aortic regurgitation is gaining popularity as the short to medium term results have steadily improved. The best imaging planes to determine the mechanism of aortic regurgitation are the parasternal long and short axis views. Transesophageal echocardiogram should be used to assess the mechanism of regurgitation if the transthoracic images are suboptimal.

Proper coaptation of the aortic valve requires adequate coaptation along the entire area of the commissures. Incomplete coaptation is present when there is insufficient coaptation between the aortic cusps frequently resulting in a central regurgitation orifice which can be imaged (Fig. 3.42). When the regurgitant orifice can be imaged by transthoracic echocardiography, at least moderate aortic regurgitation is present. Fibrosis and retraction of the aortic cusps and dilatation of the aortic root, particularly at the level of the sinotubular junction, are two common reasons for this type of coaptation abnormality.

Aortic cusp prolapse is best detected by using the long axis view showing excessive protrusion of the aortic cusps into the left ventricular outflow tract beyond the aortic annulus during diastole, interfering with proper coaptation (Fig. 3.43). The common cause for this type of coaptation abnormality is myxomatous changes of the aortic valve in patients with connective tissue disease such as Marfan syndrome and bicuspid aortic valve. In some patients with bicuspid aortic valve, one of the aortic cusps, usually the conjoined cusp, can be quite large and redundant resulting in prolapse.

Flail of the aortic cusp is present when the cusp demonstrates excessive motion with the tip pointing to the left ventricular outflow tract instead of the aorta during diastole. This is caused by one or more tears of the aortic cusp extending beyond the coaptation zone (Fig. 3.44). Endocarditis is the most common cause. Closed chest trauma can also result in this abnormality.

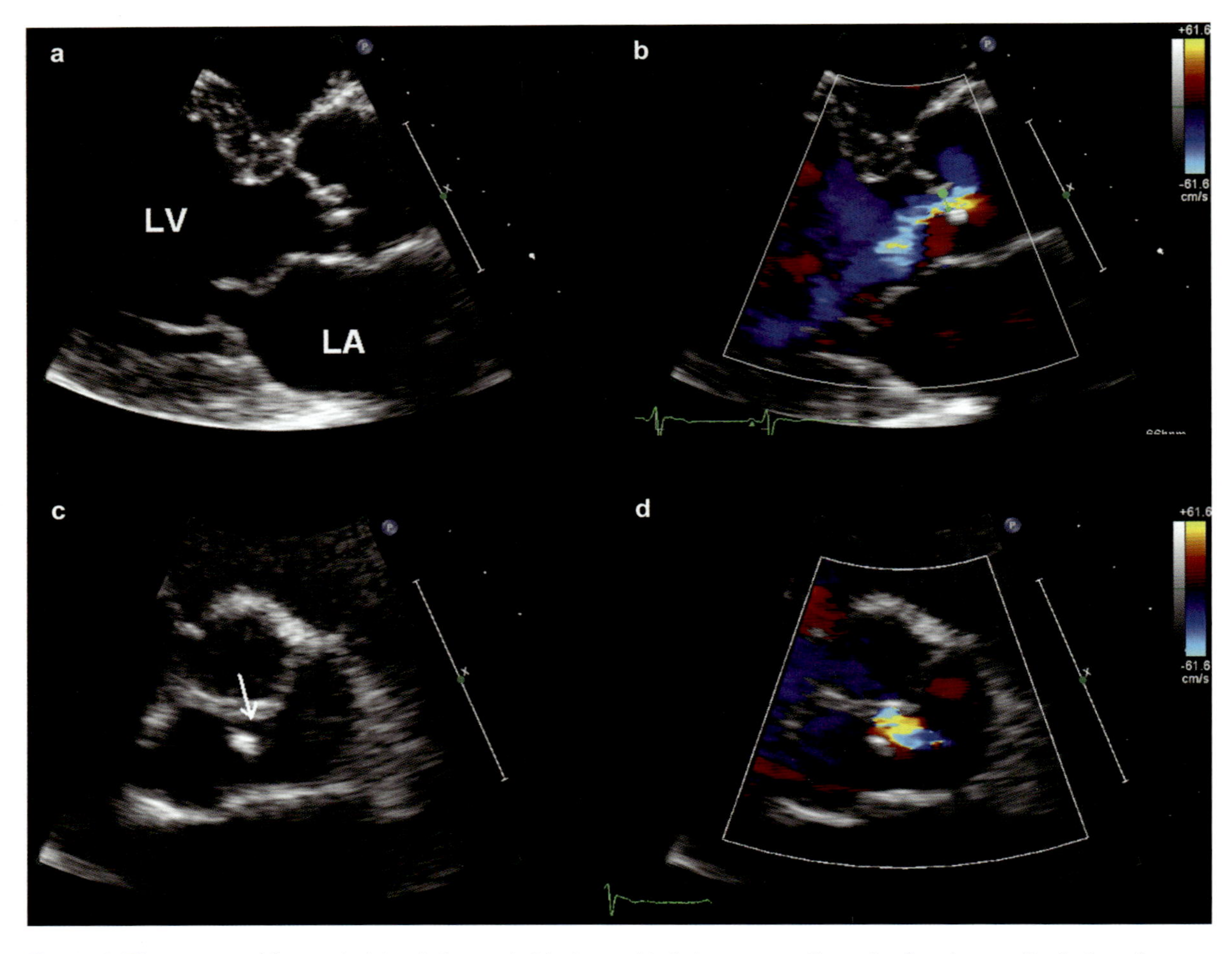

Fig. 3.42 The parasternal long-axis (**a**) and short-axis (**c**) views with their corresponding color-flow images (**b**, **d**) show the presence of aortic regurgitation and the underlying mechanism for the regurgitation. There is nodular thickening involving the closing edge of the right and non-coronary cusps. The tip of the non-coronary cusp is retracted creating a regurgitant orifice (*arrow*) which is demonstrated by color-flow imaging in (b) and (d). *LA* left atrium, *LV* left ventricle

Perforation of the aortic cusp should be suspected whenever the aortic regurgitant jet appears to arise from the base of the cusp rather than from the site of cusp coaptation. The actual defect can frequently be imaged using the transesophageal window (Fig. 3.39). This abnormality is almost exclusively due to endocarditis, and frequently the perforation coexists with a diverticulum or aneurysm. These abnormalities are further discussed in the chapter on infective endocarditis.

Careful examination of the aortic regurgitant jet can help identify the specific type of coaptation abnormalities. Particular attention should be paid to the location of the flow convergence within the aortic root during diastole. Perforation is likely if the flow convergence is not located at the coaptation site, but rather at the base of the cusp. Eccentricity of the aortic regurgitant jet indicates one specific aortic cusp may be primarily involved. A posterior directed aortic regurgitant jet suggests that the anterior cusp plays the dominant role, whereas an anteriorly directed aortic regurgitant jet suggests that the abnormality of the posterior cusp is responsible for the aortic regurgitation. In some patients, particularly in those with endocarditis, multiple coaptation abnormalities may coexist. Elucidation of the mechanism of aortic regurgitation helps the planning of surgical repair. For instance, if the mechanism is incomplete coaptation, reconfiguration of the aortic annulus and the sinotubular junction may eliminate aortic regurgitation and obviate the need for aortic valve replacement. In patients with small perforation of the aortic cusp, pericardial patch repair of the perforation is frequently feasible.

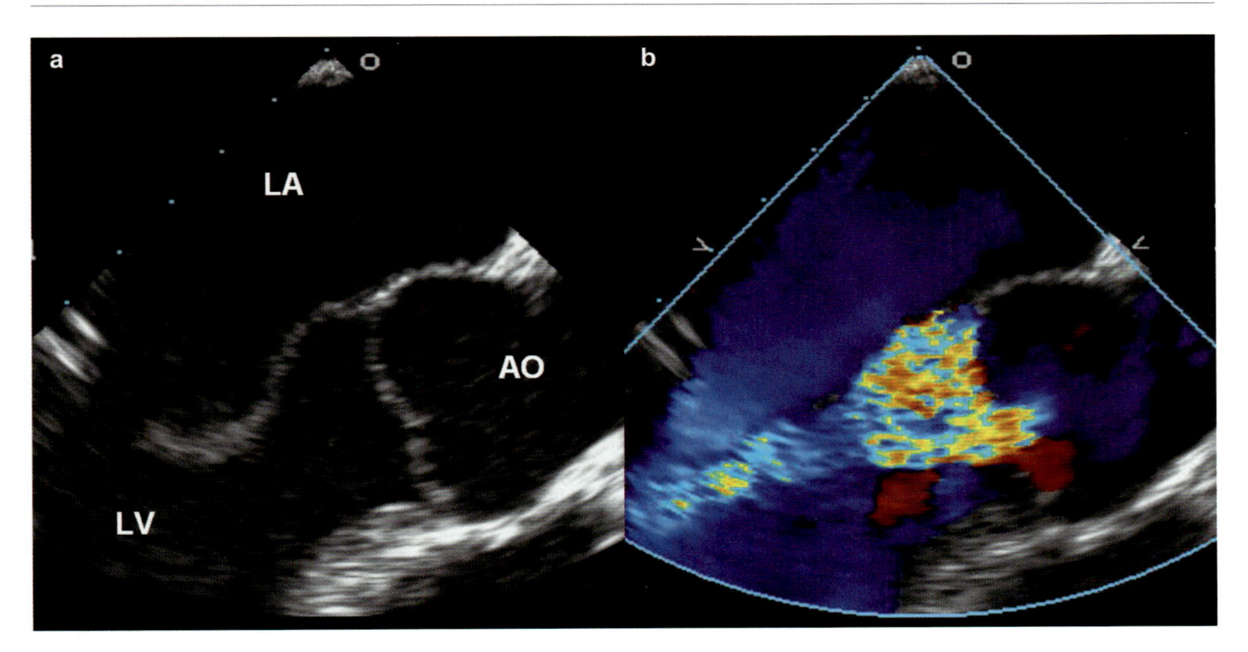

Fig. 3.43 In this patient with bicuspid aortic valve, aortic valve prolapse is demonstrated in (**a**) and the presence of severe aortic regurgitation is shown in (**b**). *Ao* aorta, *LA* left atrium, *LV* left ventricle

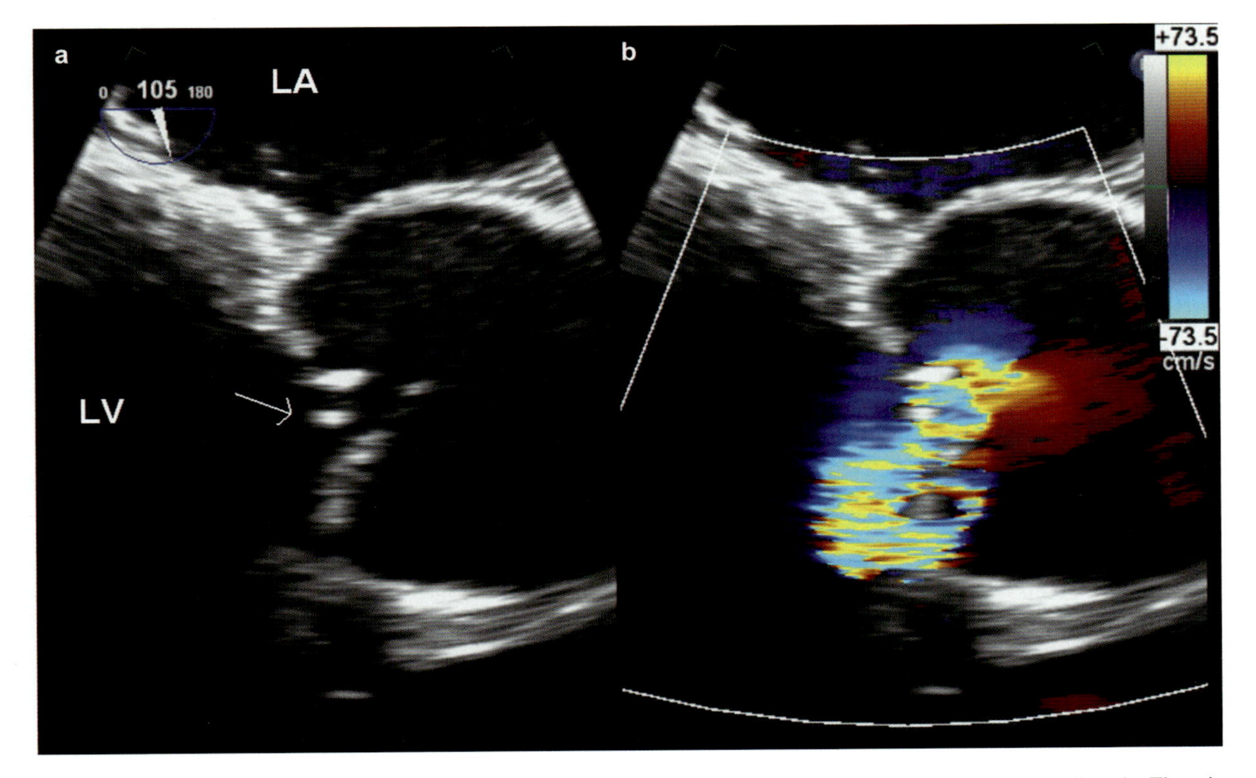

Fig. 3.44 In (**a**), the posterior aortic cusp is flail with the tip pointing into the left ventricular outflow tract during diastole. There is severe aortic regurgitation which is directed anteriorly and is shown in (**b**). *LA* left atrium, *LV* left ventricle

Assessment of Aortic Regurgitation Severity

Multiple measures of aortic regurgitant severities are available [32] (Table 3.1). Many of the measures are non-specific and the best approach is to incorporate multiple measures. We pay particular attention to the jet width, which is less gain dependent and more reproducible than other measures of the aortic regurgitant jets such as intrusion distance and jet area (Figs. 3.45, 3.46) (Table 3.2). Flow convergence can be difficult to assess in aortic regurgitation, but if present, generally indicates greater than moderate aortic regurgitation (Fig. 3.47). A very short aortic regurgitant half-time (<200 ms) indicates the presence of severe aortic regurgitation (Figs. 3.48, 3.49). There is significant variability of the aortic half-time from study to study and thus it is not a good measure for assessing the change in severity. The presence of an A-dip in the aortic regurgitant signal has recently been suggested to indicate severe aortic regurgitation and in our experience has proven to be a useful sign when it is present. Unfortunately, it is detected only in a minority of patients with severe aortic regurgitation. Detection of retrograde flow in diastole in the descending thoracic aorta and abdominal aorta should be routinely performed, although in many patients optimal images may not be obtainable (Fig. 3.50).

When assessing patients with aortic regurgitation, it needs to be underscored that there is a good correlation

Table 3.1 Qualitative and quantitative measures in the assessment of severity of aortic regurgitation

	Mild	Moderate		Severe
Structural parameters				
LV size	Normal*	Normal or dilated		Usually dilated**
Aortic leaflets	Normal or abnormal	Normal or abnormal		Abnormal/flail, or wide coaptation defect
Doppler parameters				
Jet width in LVOT – Color flow[ξ]	Small in central jets	Intermediate		Large in central jets; variable in eccentric jets
Jet density – CW	Incomplete or faint	Dense		Dense
Jet deceleration rate – CW (PHT, ms)[ψ]	Slow > 500	Medium 500–200		Steep < 200
Diastolic flow reversal in descending aorta –PW	Brief, early diastolic reversal	Intermediate		Prominent holodiastolic reversal
Quantitative parameters[φ]				
VC width (cm)[ξ]	<0.3	0.3–0.60		>0.6
Jet width/LVOT width (%)[ξ]	<25	25–45	46–64	≥65
Jet CSA/LVOT CSA (%)[ξ]	<5	5–20	21–59	≥60
R Vol (mL/beat)	<30	30–44	45–59	≥60
RF (%)	<30	30–39	40–49	≥50
EROA (cm^2)	<0.10	0.10–0.19	0.20–0.29	≥0.30

Source: Reproduced from Zoghbi et al. [33]. With permission

*Unless there are other causes for LV dilatation

**Except in acute AR

[ξ]At a Nyguist limit of 50–60 cm/s

[ψ]Pressure half-time (PHT) is shortened with increasing LV diastolic pressure and may be lengthened in chronic adaptation to severe AR

[φ]Quantitative measures can sub-classify moderate AR into mild-to-moderate and moderate-to-severe AR

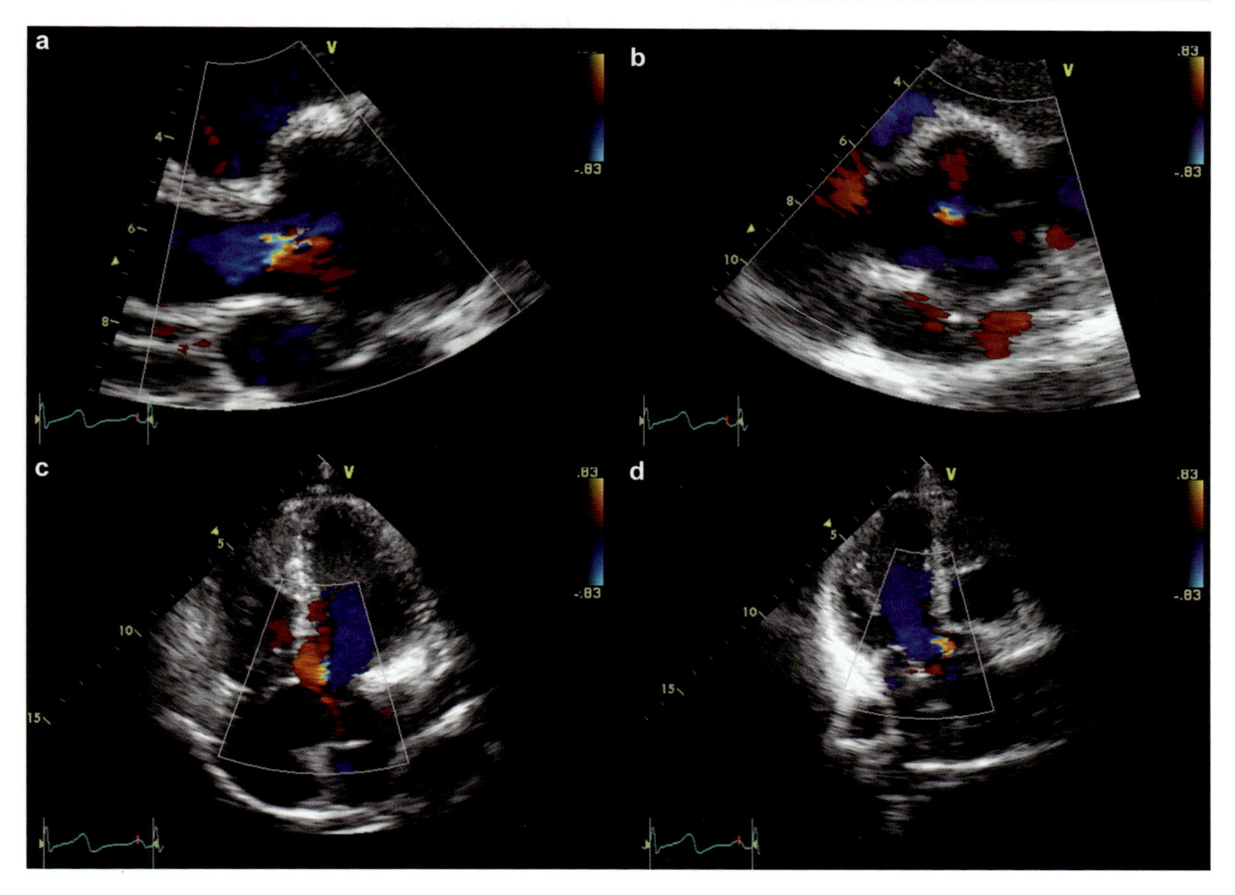

Fig. 3.45 Mild aortic regurgitation is demonstrated in multiple views including the parasternal long-axis (**a**), short axis (**b**), apical five chamber (**c**), and apical long-axis (**d**) views. The width of the aortic regurgitant jet is narrowed with a short protruding distance

between morphology and function. Careful assessment of the mechanism for aortic regurgitation is paramount. If coaptation abnormality is present, significant aortic regurgitation is likely. Useful features of the aortic regurgitant jet such as flow convergence and jet width need to be carefully assessed. Finally, the impact of aortic regurgitation on left ventricular size and function should be an integral part of the assessment of patients with aortic regurgitation (Fig. 3.51).

Summary

Aortic stenosis is a common valvular disease and its prevalence increases with age. Mild to moderate aortic stenosis is generally well tolerated, but severe aortic stenosis is associated with a high risk of cardiovascular events. Severe aortic stenosis is usually due to calcified and rigid aortic cusps. On the other hand, aortic regurgitation can be a result of several different mechanisms.

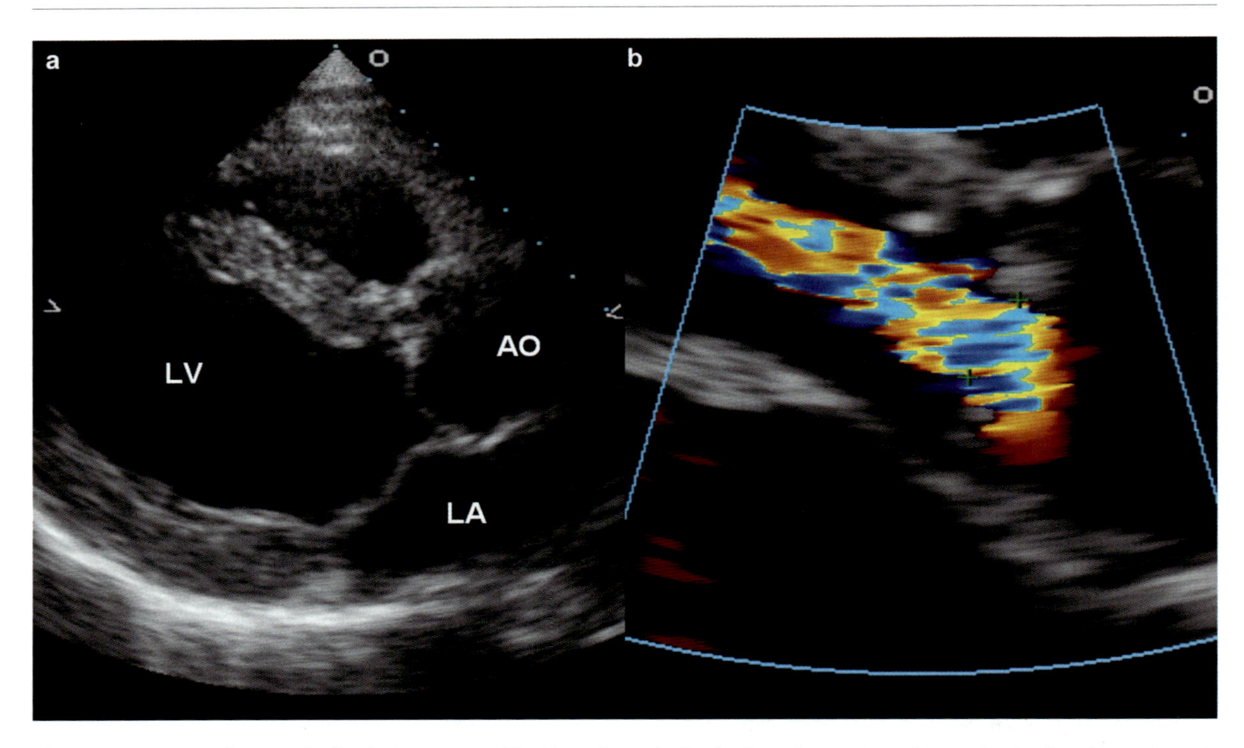

Fig. 3.46 Severe aortic regurgitation is demonstrated in this patient who has had previous aortic valve repair. Aortic valve prolapse is seen in (**a**) and color-flow imaging shows a regurgitant jet with a large width shown in (**b**). *Ao* aorta, *LA* left atrium, *LV* left ventricle

Table 3.2 Advantages and limitations of echo and Doppler measures in the assessment of aortic regurgitation severity

	Utility/advantages	Limitations
Structural parameters		
LV size	Enlargement sensitive for chronic significant AR, important for outcomes. Normal size virtually excludes significant chronic AR	Enlargement seen in other conditions. May be normal in acute significant AR
Aortic cusps alterations	Simple, usually abnormal in severe AR, Flail valve denotes severe AR	Poor accuracy, may grossly underestimate or overestimate the defect
Doppler parameters		
Jets width or jet cross-sectional area in LVOT –color flow	Simple, very sensitive, quick screen for AR	Expands unpredictably below the orifice. Inaccurate for eccentric jets
Vena contracta width	Simple, quantitative, good at identifying mild or severe AR	Not useful for multiple AR jets. Small values; thus small error leads to large % error
PISA method	Quantitative. Provides both lesion severity (EROA) and volume overload (R Vol)	Feasibility is limited by aortic valve calcifications. Not valid for multiple jets, less accurate in eccentric jets. Provides peak flow and maximal EROA. Underestimation is possible with aortic aneurysms. Limited experience
Flow quantitation – PW	Quantitative, valid with multiple jets and eccentric jets. Provides both lesion severity (EROA, RF) and volume overload (R Vol)	Not valid for combined MR and AR, unless pulmonic site is used
Jet density – CW	Simple. Faint or incomplete jet compatible with mild AR	Qualitative. Overlap between moderate and severe AR. Complementary data only
Jet deceleration rate (PHT) – CW	Simple	Qualitative; affected by changes in LV and aortic diastolic pressures
Diastolic flow reversal in descending aorta – PW	Simple	Depends on rigidity of aorta. Brief velocity reversal is normal

Source: Reproduced from Zoghbi et al. [33]. With permission

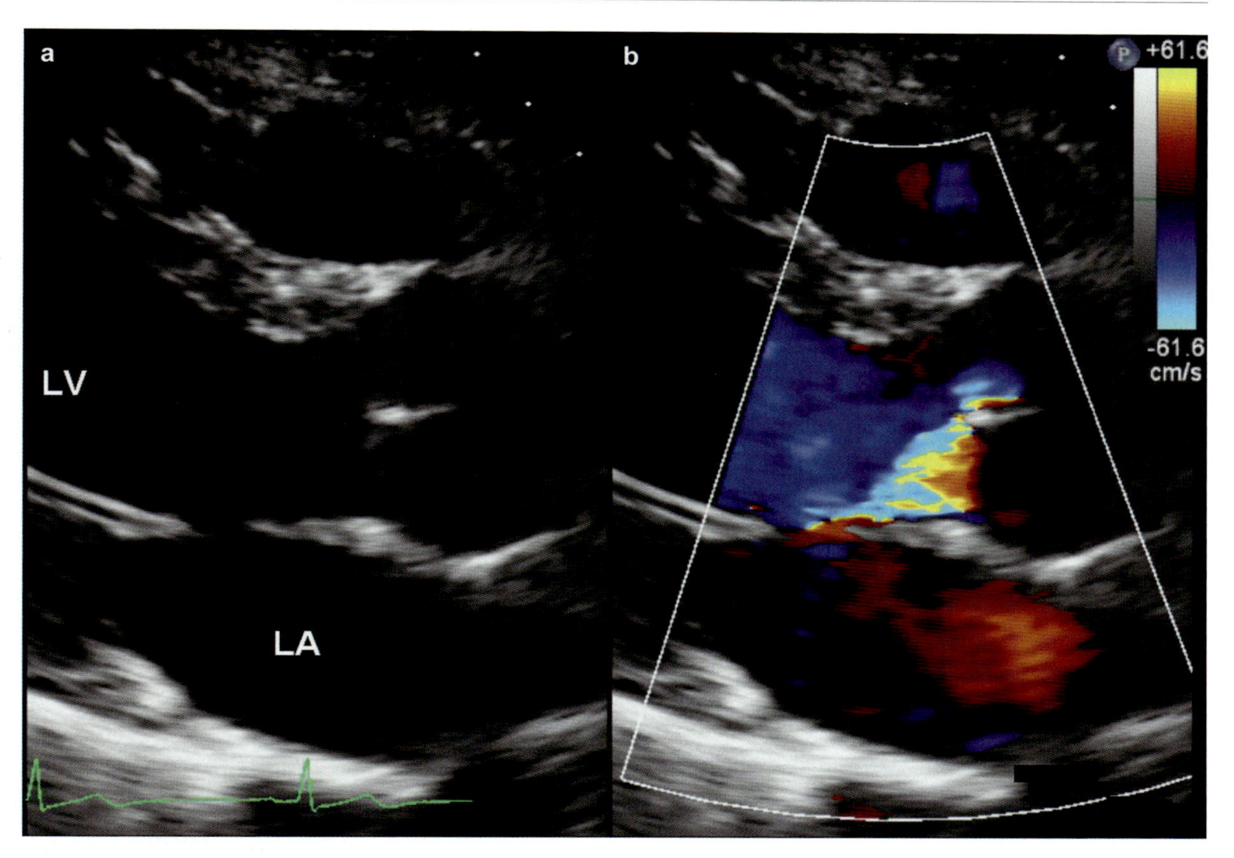

Fig. 3.47 Although the aortic coaptation appears normal as shown in the long-axis view in (**a**), there is an eccentric aortic regurgitant jet directed posteriorly shown in the color image in (**b**). A flow convergence area can be clearly seen indicating that the aortic regurgitant is at least moderate in severity. *LA* atrium, *LV* left ventricle

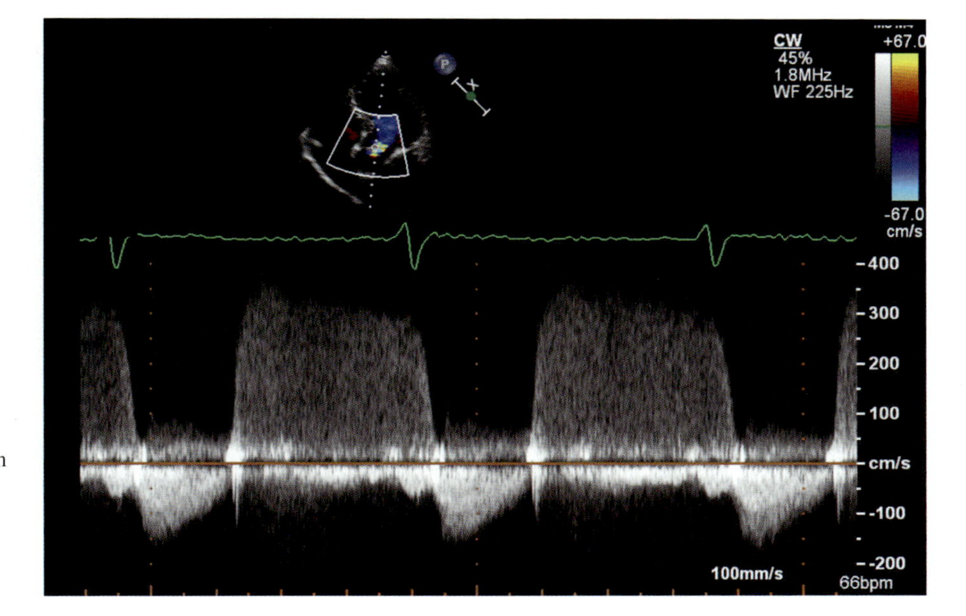

Fig. 3.48 Continuous wave Doppler tracing of a patient with mild aortic regurgitation is shown. The aortic regurgitation decay slope is gentle indicating that the aortic regurgitation is not severe

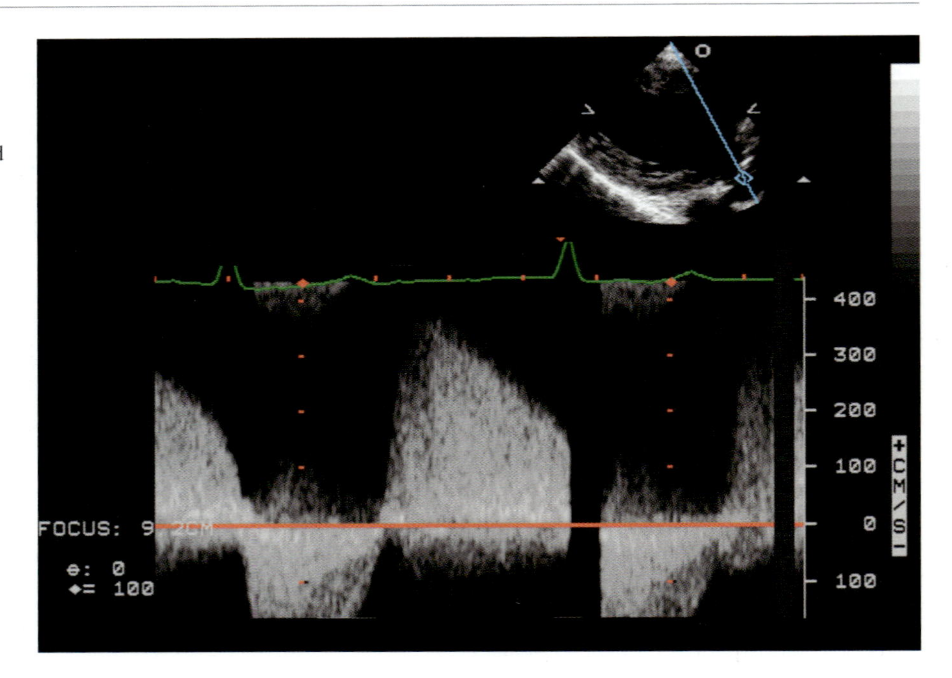

Fig. 3.49 This is a continuous wave Doppler tracing of a patient with combined aortic stenosis and aortic regurgitation. There is a rapid decay slope of aortic regurgitation velocity indicating a short pressure half time consistent with severe aortic regurgitation

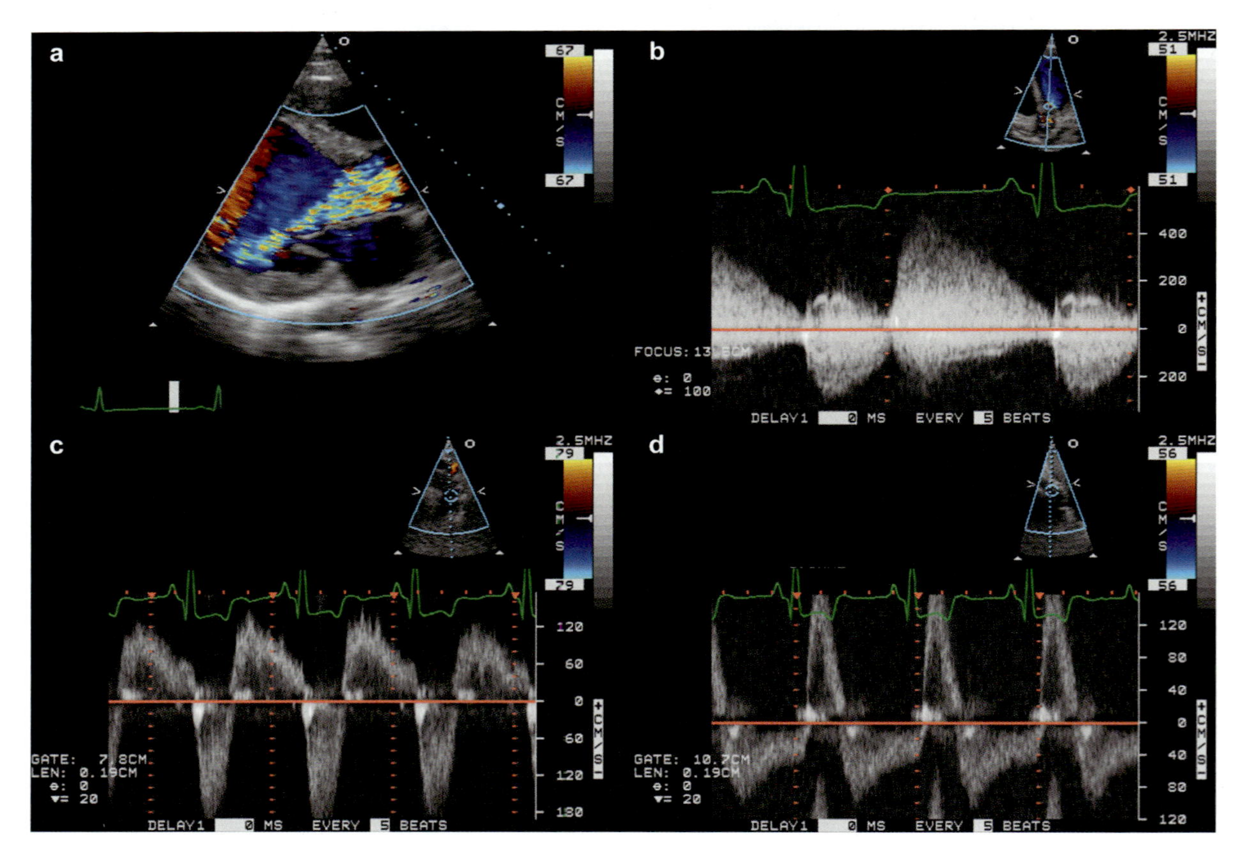

Fig. 3.50 Multiple indices of severe aortic regurgitation are shown in this patient. There is a large jet filling the entire left ventricular outflow tract shown in (**a**). A short pressure half-time is demonstrated in (**b**). A large retrograde diastolic flow is detected in the descending thoracic aorta in (**c**) and in the abdominal aorta in (**d**)

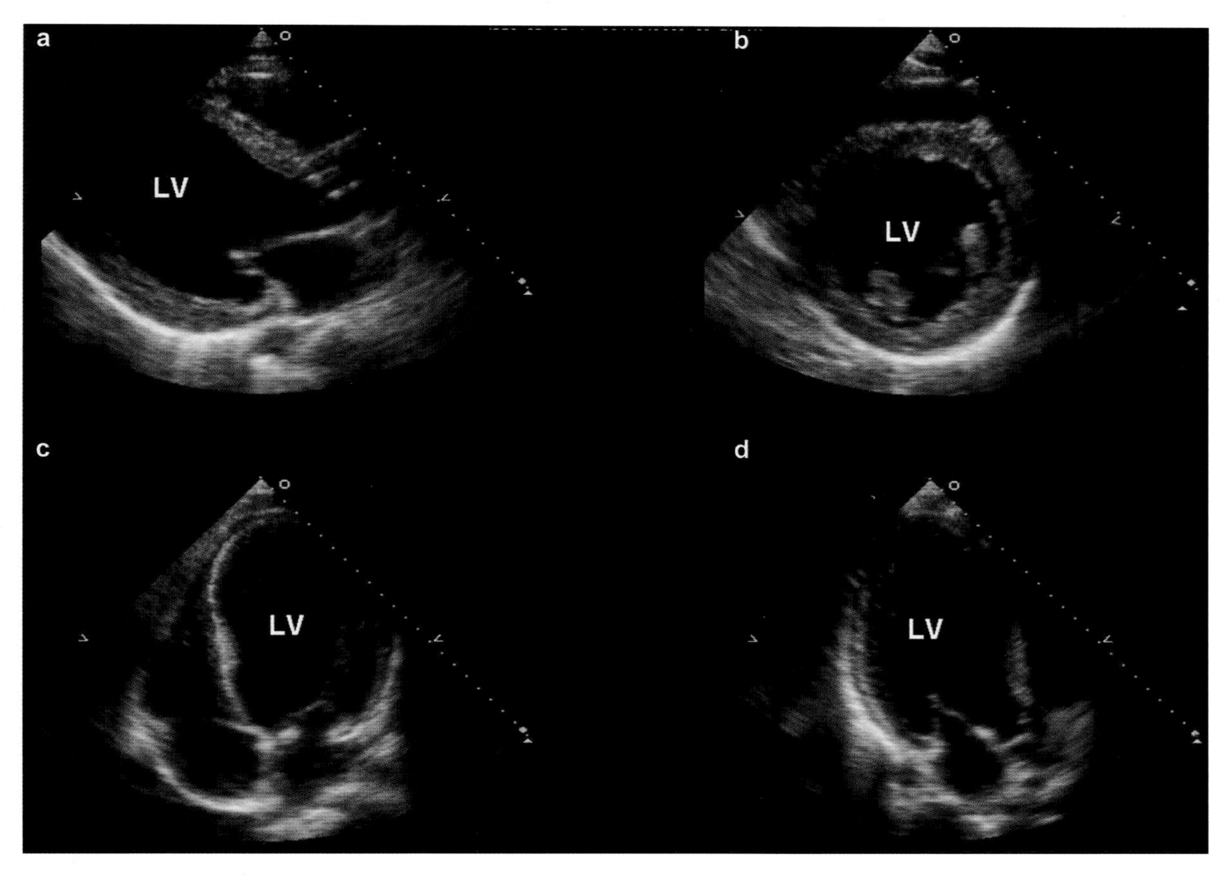

Fig. 3.51 In this patient with chronic severe aortic regurgitation, the severely increased left ventricular volume is demonstrated in multiple views including the parasternal long-axis (**a**), parasternal short-axis (**b**), apical four chamber (**c**), and apical long-axis (**d**) views. The left ventricle in this setting not only increases in size but also assumes a more globular shape. In the absence of significant increase in left ventricular volume, chronic severe aortic regurgitation is unlikely to be present. *LV* left ventricle

In aortic stenosis, accurate assessment of the severity and the adaptive changes of the left ventricle is important to the management. In aortic regurgitation, the feasibility of valve repair is based on the knowledge of the mechanism in addition to the severity or regurgitation.

References

1. Veinot JP. Pathology of inflammatory native valvular heart disease. *Cardiovasc Pathol*. 2006 Sept;15(5):243-251.
2. Dare AJ, Veinot JP, Edwards WD, Tazelaar HD, Schaff HV. New observations on the etiology of aortic valve disease: a surgical pathologic study of 236 cases from 1990. *Hum Pathol*. 1993;24(12):1330-1338.
3. Mohler ER III. Mechanisms of aortic valve calcification. *Am J Cardiol*. 2004 Dec 1;94(11):1396-1402.
4. Rajamannan NM, Subramaniam M, Rickard D, et al. Human aortic valve calcification is associated with an osteoblast phenotype. *Circulation*. 2003 May 6;107(17):2181-2184.
5. Wallby L, Janerot-Sjoberg B, Steffensen T, Broqvist M. T lymphocyte infiltration in non-rheumatic aortic stenosis: a comparative descriptive study between tricuspid and bicuspid aortic valves. *Heart*. 2002 Oct;88(4):348-351.
6. Mohler ER III, Gannon F, Reynolds C, Zimmerman R, Keane MG, Kaplan FS. Bone formation and inflammation in cardiac valves. *Circulation*. 2001 Mar 20;103(11): 1522-1528.
7. Wierzbicki A, Shetty C. Aortic stenosis: an atherosclerotic disease? *J Heart Valve Dis*. 1999 July;8(4):416-423.
8. Palta S, Pai AM, Gill KS, Pai RG. New insights into the progression of aortic stenosis: implications for secondary prevention. *Circulation*. 2000 May 30;101(21):2497-2502.

9. Aronow WS, Ahn C, Kronzon I, Goldman ME. Association of coronary risk factors and use of statins with progression of mild valvular aortic stenosis in older persons. *Am J Cardiol*. 2001 Sept 15;88(6):693-695.
10. Srivatsa SS, Harrity PJ, Maercklein PB, et al. Increased cellular expression of matrix proteins that regulate mineralization is associated with calcification of native human and porcine xenograft bioprosthetic heart valves. *J Clin Invest*. 1997 Mar 1;99(5):996-1009.
11. Davies MR, Hruska KA. Pathophysiological mechanisms of vascular calcification in end-stage renal disease. *Kidney Int*. 2001 Aug;60(2):472-479.
12. Kajbaf S, Veinot JP, Ha A, Zimmerman D. Comparison of surgically removed cardiac valves of patients with ESRD with those of the general population. *Am J Kidney Dis*. 2005 July;46(1):86-93.
13. Veinot JP, Elstein D, Hanania D, Abrahamov A, Srivatsa S, Zimran A. Gaucher's disease with valve calcification: possible role of Gaucher cells, bone matrix proteins and integrins. *Can J Cardiol*. 1999 Feb;15(2):211-216.
14. de Sa M, Moshkovitz Y, Butany J, David TE. Histologic abnormalities of the ascending aorta and pulmonary trunk in patients with bicuspid aortic valve disease: clinical relevance to the ross procedure. *J Thorac Cardiovasc Surg*. 1999 Oct;118(4):588-594.
15. Roberto S, Kosanke S, Dunn ST, Jankelow D, Duran CMG, Cunningham MW. Pathogenic mechanisms in rheumatic carditis: focus on valvular endothelium. *J Infect Dis*. 2001;183:507-511.
16. Oliver JM, Gonzalez A, Gallego P, Sanchez-Recalde A, Benito F, Mesa JM. Discrete subaortic stenosis in adults: increased prevalence and slow rate of progression of the obstruction and aortic regurgitation. *J Am Coll Cardiol*. 2001 Sept;38(3):835-842.
17. Stassano P, Di TL, Contaldo A, et al. Discrete subaortic stenosis: long-term prognosis on the progression of the obstruction and of the aortic insufficiency. *Thorac Cardiovasc Surg*. 2005 Feb;53(1):23-27.
18. Haley JH, Sinak LJ, Tajik AJ, Ommen SR, Oh JK. Dynamic left ventricular outflow tract obstruction in acute coronary syndromes: an important cause of new systolic murmur and cardiogenic shock. *Mayo Clin Proc*. 1999 Sept;74(9):901-906.
19. Spooner PH, Perry MP, Brandenburg RO, Pennock GD. Increased intraventricular velocities: an unrecognized cause of systolic murmur in adults. *J Am Coll Cardiol*. 1998 Nov 15;32(6):1589-1595.
20. Pober BR. Williams-Beuren syndrome. *N Engl J Med*. 2010 Jan 21;362(3):239-252.
21. Davies MJ, Treasure T, Parker DJ. Demographic characteristics of patients undergoing aortic valve replacement for stenosis: relation to valve morphology. *Heart*. 1996 Feb;75(2): 174-178.
22. Roberts WC, Ko JM, Hamilton C. Comparison of valve structure, valve weight, and severity of the valve obstruction in 1849 patients having isolated aortic valve replacement for aortic valve stenosis (with or without associated aortic regurgitation) studied at 3 different medical centers in 2 different time periods. *Circulation*. 2005 Dec 20;112(25):3919-3929.
23. Chan KL, Teo K, Dumesnil JG, Ni A, Tam J. Effect of Lipid lowering with rosuvastatin on progression of aortic stenosis: results of the aortic stenosis progression observation: measuring effects of rosuvastatin (ASTRONOMER) trial. *Circulation*. 2010 Jan 19;121(2):306-314.
24. Bonow RO, Carabello BA, Chatterjee K, et al. ACC/AHA 2006 guidelines for the management of patients with valvular heart disease: a report of the American College of Cardiology/American Heart Association Task Force on Practice Guidelines (writing Committee to Revise the 1998 guidelines for the management of patients with valvular heart disease) developed in collaboration with the Society of Cardiovascular Anesthesiologists endorsed by the Society for Cardiovascular Angiography and Interventions and the Society of Thoracic Surgeons. *J Am Coll Cardiol*. 2006 Aug 1;48(3):e1-148.
25. Quinones MA, Otto CM, Stoddard M, Waggoner A, Zoghbi WA. Recommendations for quantification of Doppler echocardiography: a report from the Doppler Quantification Task Force of the Nomenclature and Standards Committee of the American Society of Echocardiography. *J Am Soc Echocardiogr*. 2002 Feb;15(2):167-184.
26. Clavel MA, Fuchs C, Burwash IG, et al. Predictors of outcomes in low-flow, low-gradient aortic stenosis: results of the multicenter TOPAS Study. *Circulation*. 2008 Sept 30;118(14 Suppl):S234-S242.
27. Hachicha Z, Dumesnil JG, Bogaty P, Pibarot P. Paradoxical low-flow, low-gradient severe aortic stenosis despite preserved ejection fraction is associated with higher afterload and reduced survival. *Circulation*. 2007 June 5;115(22): 2856-2864.
28. Aurigemma G, Battista S, Orsinelli D, Sweeney A, Pape L, Cuenoud H. Abnormal left ventricular intracavitary flow acceleration in patients undergoing aortic valve replacement for aortic stenosis. A marker for high postoperative morbidity and mortality. *Circulation*. 1992 Sept;86(3):926-936.
29. Jassal DS, Tam JW, Dumesnil JG, et al. Clinical usefulness of tissue Doppler imaging in patients with mild to moderate aortic stenosis: a substudy of the aortic stenosis progression observation measuring effects of rosuvastatin study. *J Am Soc Echocardiogr*. 2008 Sept;21(9):1023-1027.
30. Olson LJ, Subramanian R, Edwards WD. Surgical pathology of pure aortic insufficiency: a study of 225 cases. *Mayo Clin Proc*. 1984;59:835-841.
31. Walley VM, Antecol DH, Kyrollos AG, Chan K-L. Congenitally bicuspid aortic valves: study of a variant with fenestrated raphe. *Can J Cardiol*. 1994;10:535-542.
32. Veinot JP, Edwards WD. Pathology of radiation-induced heart disease: a surgical and autopsy study of 27 cases. *Hum Pathol*. 1996 Aug;27(8):766-773.
33. Zoghbi WA, Enriquez-Sarano M, Foster E, et al. Recommendations for evaluation of the severity of native valvular regurgitation with two-dimensional and Doppler echocardiography. *J Am Soc Echocardiogr*. 2003 July;16(7): 777-802.

4 Mitral Valve

To understand mitral valve dysfunction the anatomy of the valve must be understood. The mitral valve is an atrioventricular valve with leaflets and chordae that attach to papillary muscles. There are two leaflets: the anterior and the posterior (Fig. 4.1). On either side of the leaflets there are commissures. The mitral valve has no septal chordal attachments. The anterior leaflet is in fibrous continuity with the aortic valve (Fig. 4.2). The leaflets have free edges and closing margins, approximately a few mm from the edge. The mitral valve annulus is better defined than the right sided annulus, and a fibrous annular band can be grossly seen. The posterior leaflet has three scallops that are discernible and formed to varying degrees. These small indentations allow redundancy to the valve, which is important for leaflet overlap and competency.

The chordae are complex and are classified differently by different investigator groups: first order chords (attached to free edge of leaflet), second-order chords (attached mid leaflet), and third order chords (attached to papillary muscle); or strut, commissural, basal chords, and rough zone chords (Fig. 4.3). Only the posterior leaflet has basal chords, which run between the leaflet and the adjacent posterior left ventricle wall. Only the anterior leaflet has strut chords – these are two

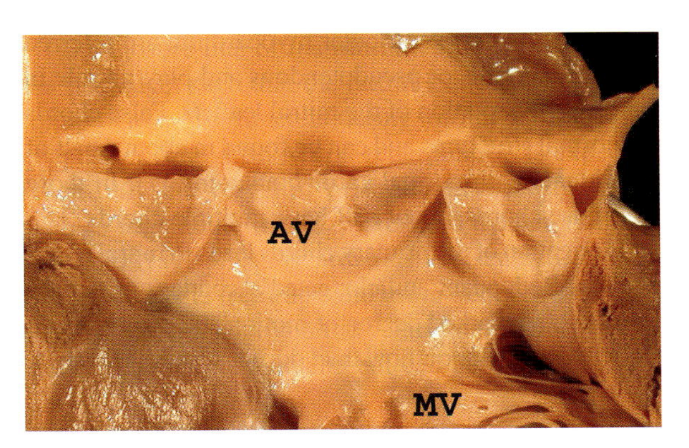

Fig. 4.2 The left ventricle outflow tract opened to show the continuity between the aortic valve (*AV*) and the anterior mitral leaflet (*MV*)

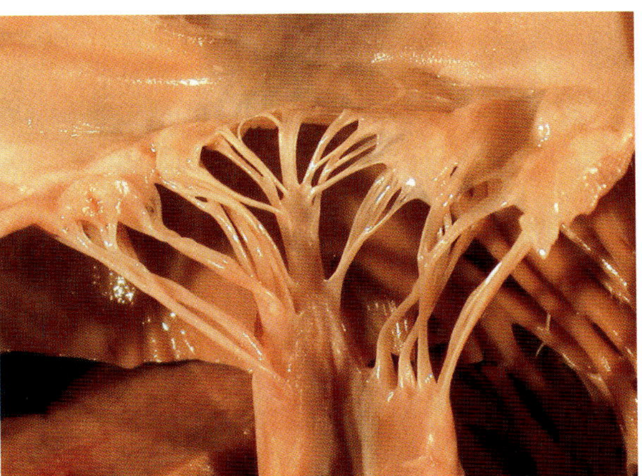

Fig. 4.3 Mitral valve opened with commissural chordae noted

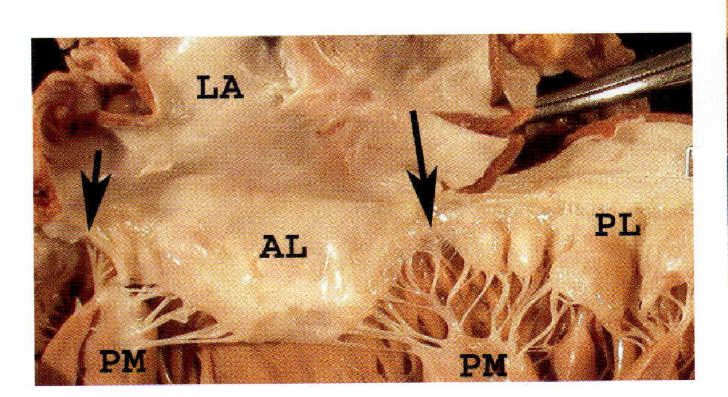

Fig. 4.1 Mitral valve with anterior leaflet (*AL*) and the posterior leaflet (*PL*), which has been cut through with heart opening. Two commissures are present on either side of the leaflets (*arrows*). Left atrium is above (*LA*) the valve and the left ventricle papillary muscles are below (*PM*), connected by the chordae tendonae

K.-L. Chan and J.P. Veinot, *Anatomic Basis of Echocardiographic Diagnosis*,
DOI: 10.1007/978-1-84996-387-9_4,

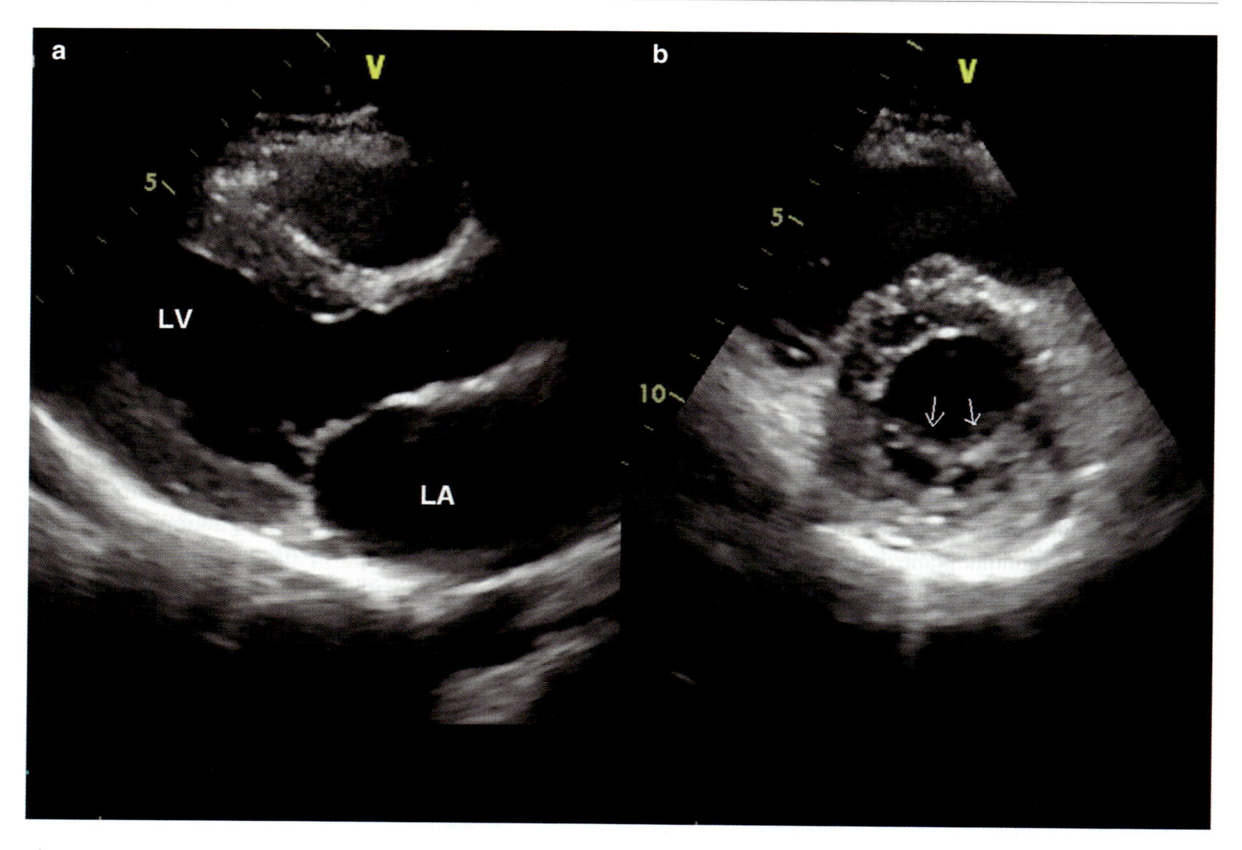

Fig. 4.6 The parasternal long-axis (**a**) and short-axis (**b**) views of the mitral valve in systole show proper coaptation of the anterior and posterior mitral leaflet (*arrows*). In the short-axis view (**b**), multiple folding along the entire coaptation can be seen. *LA* left atrium, *LV* left ventricle

the parasternal and apical windows (Figs. 4.10, 4.11). In evaluating the thickness of the mitral leaflet, it is important to recognize that the rough zone will appear thicker due to the insertion of the chords. The papillary muscles can be readily imaged using the parasternal short-axis and apical views (Figs. 4.11, 4.12). The number of papillary muscles and their individual heads should be routinely assessed. The anterolateral papillary muscle is usually imaged in the apical four-chamber view, while the posteromedial papillary muscle is seen in the apical long-axis view (Fig. 4.11).

Mitral Stenosis

Mitral stenosis is usually due to leaflet fibrosis, commissural fusion and calcification. Almost all cases are post-inflammatory, rheumatic in etiology. Commonly, rheumatic valve stenosis is also associated with some degree of valve regurgitation. Rheumatic fever is a late inflammatory non-suppurative complication of pharyngitis caused by Group A beta-hemolytic Streptococci. This multi-system disease is characterized by involvement of the heart, joints, central nervous system, subcutaneous tissues and skin [2].

Rheumatic carditis is an important and frequent acquired cardiovascular disease in children and adolescents and an important cause of death from cardiac disease in young people in developing countries. The pathoetiology of the disease is complex and the incidence and prevalence vary among countries. Environmental conditions may play a factor with some climates having an increased frequency of rheumatic fever. Genetic determination also plays a role. Important antigenic structures of the Streptococcus include M, R and T proteins. Streptococcal M-protein, which determines the serotype, extends from the cell surface as an alpha-helix with structural homology to

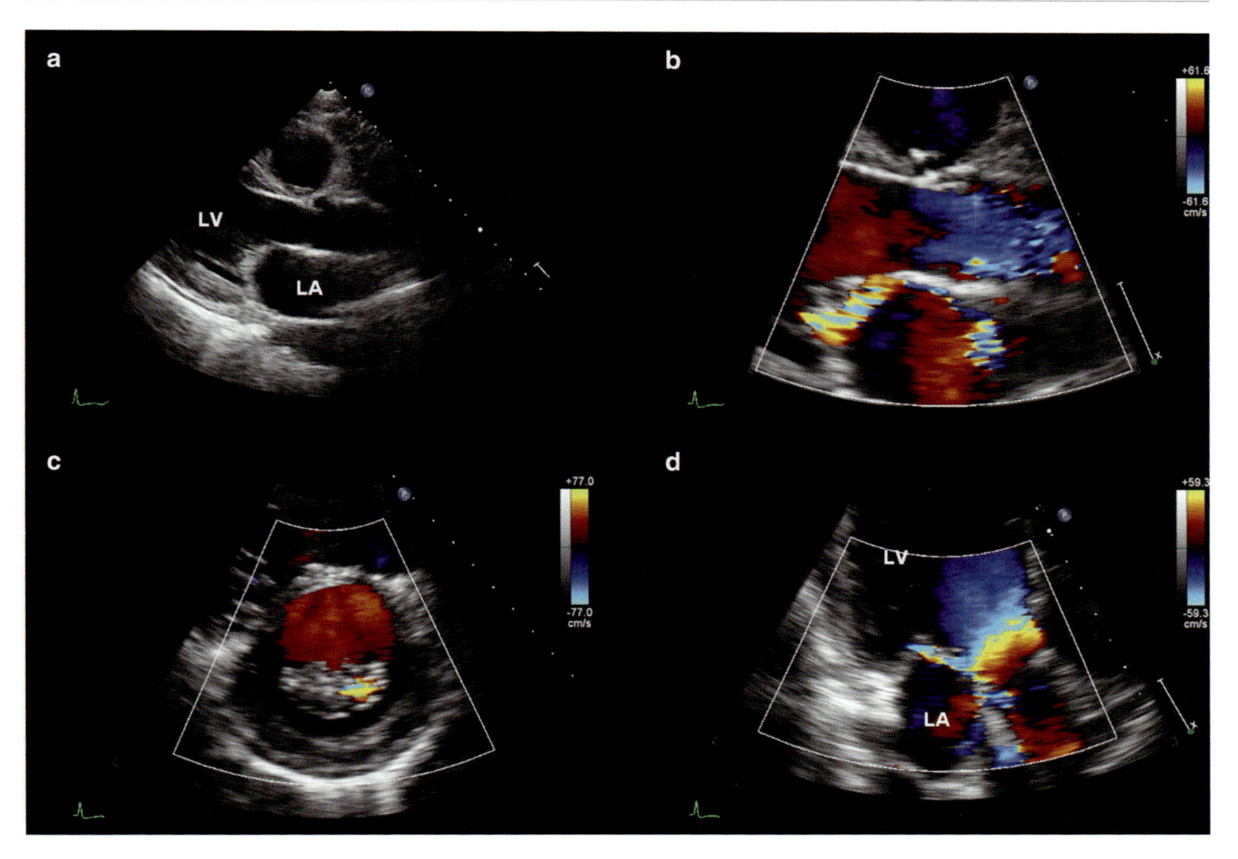

Fig. 4.7 This patient has localized prolapse of the lateral scallop of the posterior mitral leaflet (P1). In the parasternal long-axis view (**a**) the prolapsed scallop is not visualized as the mid scallops of the anterior and posterior mitral leaflets, but not the other scallops, are visualized in this view. The color-flow imaging (**b–d**) shows a localized mitral regurgitant jet arising from the lateral aspect of mitral leaflet coaptation and directed anteriorly consistent with prolapse of the lateral scallop of the posterior mitral leaflet. *LA* left atrium, *LV* left ventricle

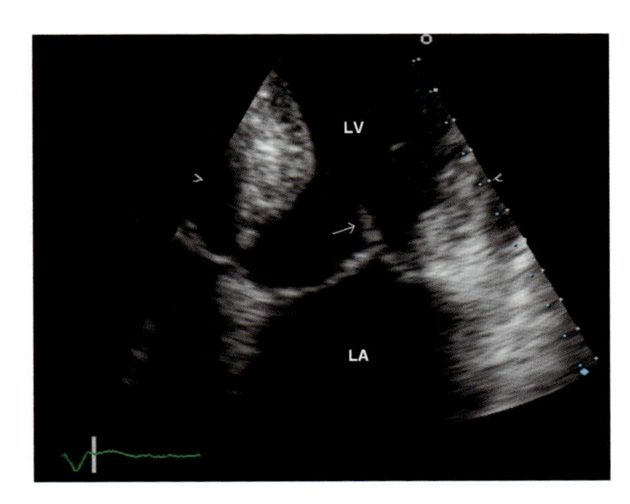

Fig. 4.8 This is a zoomed apical four chamber view showing the proper coaptation between the anterior and posterior mitral leaflets in systole (*arrow*). The two leaflets are opposed for several millimeters in this case. *LA* left atrium, *LV* left ventricle

myosin and other alpha-helix coiled molecules [3]. The M-protein is a virulence factor with potent anti-phagocytic activity [4]. In outbreaks, bacterial colonies isolated from those with rheumatic fever tend to have a mucoid morphology with thick capsules and certain M-proteins are more common [5, 6].

The pathogenesis of rheumatic fever relates to humoral and cellular mediated immune responses with development of autoimmunity [7]. The clinical manifestations of acute rheumatic fever occur 1–3 weeks after the onset of Streptococcal infection. After an apparent convalescence of the pharyngitis, products of the Streptococcus have "molecular mimicry" to human tissue and are recognized by the immune system, thus initiating an autoimmune response. Individuals develop antibodies to the carbohydrate and the M protein of the Streptococcal organism. The anti-carbohydrate antibodies cross react with the valvular endothelium. This

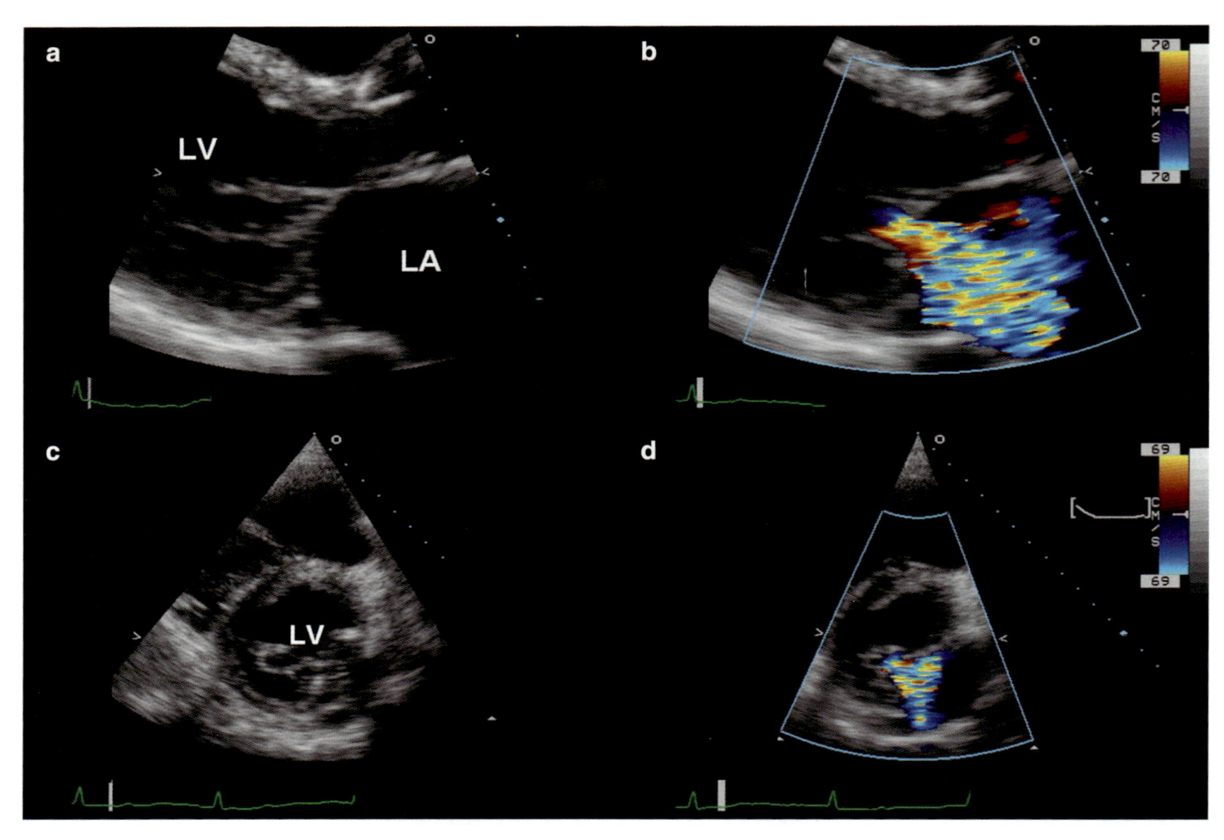

Fig. 4.9 This patient has dilated cardiomyopathy and the mitral leaflets are not properly opposed (**a**, **c**), resulting in severe mitral regurgitation (**b**, **d**). *LA* left atrium, *LV* left ventricle

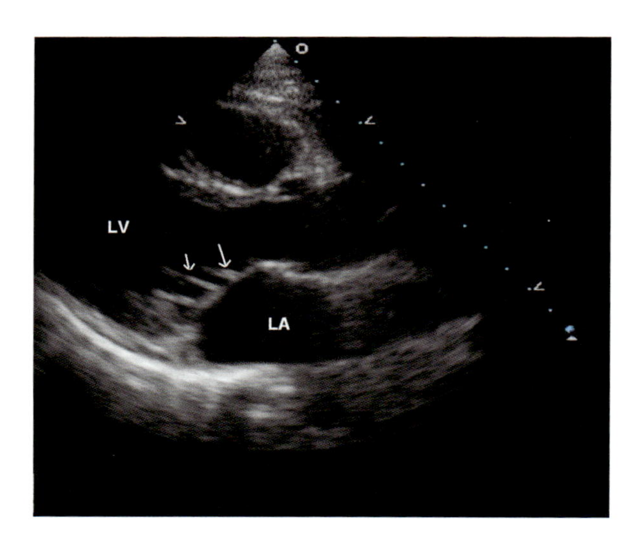

Fig. 4.10 This parasternal long-axis view shows chordal attachment on the ventricular surface of the anterior mitral leaflet beyond the free edge (*arrows*). *LA* left atrium, *LV* left ventricle

produces valve injury or dysfunction with up regulation of cell adhesion molecules facilitating lymphocyte infiltration into the valve. The M-protein antibodies contribute to the valve disease via molecular mimicry with myosin. Cardiac myosin is not present in the valve, but laminin links myosin in the valve. The anti-myosin antibody recognizes laminin, an extracellular matrix alpha helix coiled protein, part of the valve basement membrane structure [3, 7].

T-cells responsive to the Streptococcal M-protein infiltrate the valve through the valvular endothelium activated by the binding of anti-Streptococcal carbohydrate antibodies cross reactive to the endothelium. Within the valve tissue the inflammatory cells are responsible for local cytokine release, and interstitial cell damage with neovascularization and chronic inflammation [7]. The T cells produce cytokines including tumor necrosis factor and interleukins. Macrophages are activated and attract T cells [8].

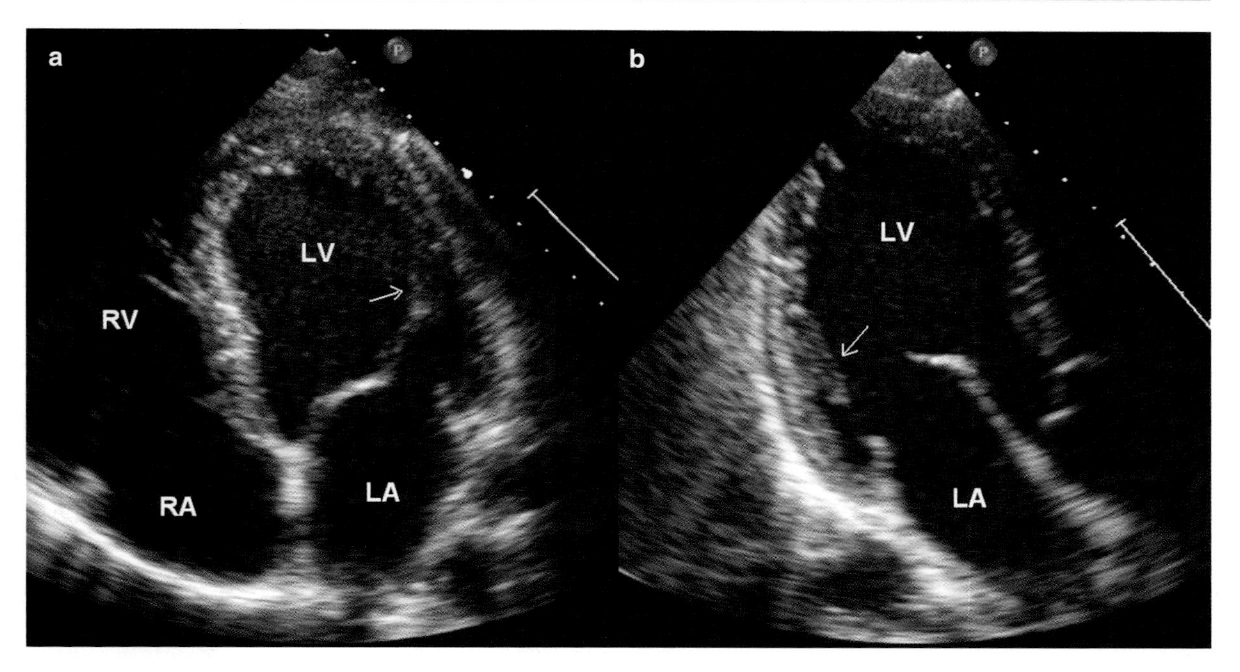

Fig. 4.11 The anterolateral papillary muscle (*arrow*), with its chordal attachment to the anterior mitral leaflet, is shown in the apical four chamber view (**a**). The posteromedial papillary muscle (*arrow*) is imaged using the apical long-axis view (**b**). *LA* left atrium, *LV* left ventricle, *RA* right atrium, *RV* right ventricle

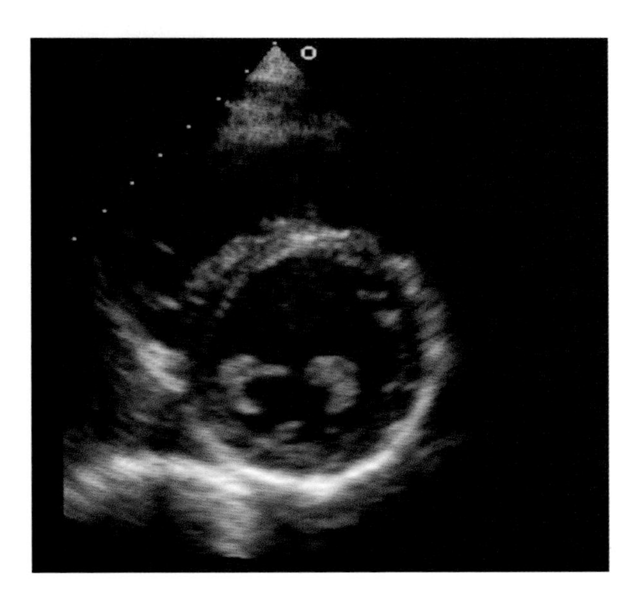

Fig. 4.12 The parasternal short-axis view is preferred in the assessment of the papillary muscles. Both the location and the number of heads of the papillary muscles can be assessed using this view

The acute involvement of the heart in rheumatic fever is pancarditis with inflammation of the myocardium, pericardium and endocardium. Endocarditis and acute valve disease may be asymptomatic or present with a new murmur. In the acute phase, murmurs do not indicate a permanent valve defect and the murmur may be transient. The valves most affected by rheumatic fever are the mitral, aortic, tricuspid and pulmonary, in that order. In acute disease, thrombi form along the lines of valve closure. These small thrombi have been termed "verrucous" endocarditis and do not produce valve destruction. The leaflets may have associated edema and inflammatory cell infiltration [4, 9]. Such acute disease is rarely recognized by ante-mortem investigations.

The chronically scarred, inflamed and neovascularized valve is most commonly encountered by the pathologist and the cardiac clinician. The mechanism of stenosis is due to leaflet fibrosis, calcification, commissural fusion, chordal fusion and shortening. Chronic rheumatic fever leads to neovascularization, chronic inflammation, commissural fusion, valve thickening and calcification. Once the valve is inflamed and there is neovascularization, lymphocytes can infiltrate the valve both through the valve surface as well as through the new vessels. Even in old calcified rheumatic valves, lymphocytes and neovascularization are still present, indicating progression or persistence of disease in the valve.

Grossly chronic rheumatic valves have fibrosis, with or without calcification (Figs. 4.13–4.15). The commissures are often fused. Valve leaflets may be thickened and show scar retraction. The chordae are often thick and shortened. The subvalvular chordal space may seem to disappear with short thick chords attached almost directly to the papillary muscles. The subvalvular apparatus pathology can be graded by echocardiography and the results used to plan valve surgery or interventional procedures [10]. At the commissures of mitral valves there is often loss of surface endothelium with erosion and overlying thrombus material (Fig. 4.16). This does not seem to be as common in the aortic position. Histology shows neovascularization, chronic inflammation and fibrosis with alteration and damage of the underlying valve architecture. Large fibrous endocardial onlays are present on microscopic examination. These thicken the leaflets and encase the chordae.

Other rare causes of mitral stenosis include storage diseases and medication – related pathology especially ergot and migraine medications. Ergotamine associated valve disease chiefly affects the mitral valve and produces a carcinoid like gross appearance that may be severe. Mitral stenosis and regurgitation have been seen. Valve leaflets are typically very thick with chordal fusion and shortening and commissural fusion. Large "myxoid collagenous" myofibroblast rich plaques are stuck on the underlying valve proper without underlying valve leaflet destruction [11, 12].

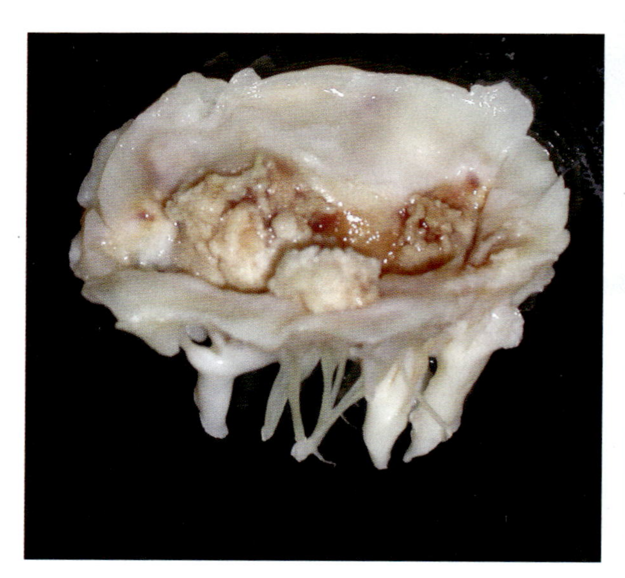

Fig. 4.13 Excised mitral valve with severe fibrosis of leaflets, chordal thickening and extensive calcific deposits. Commissures are fused

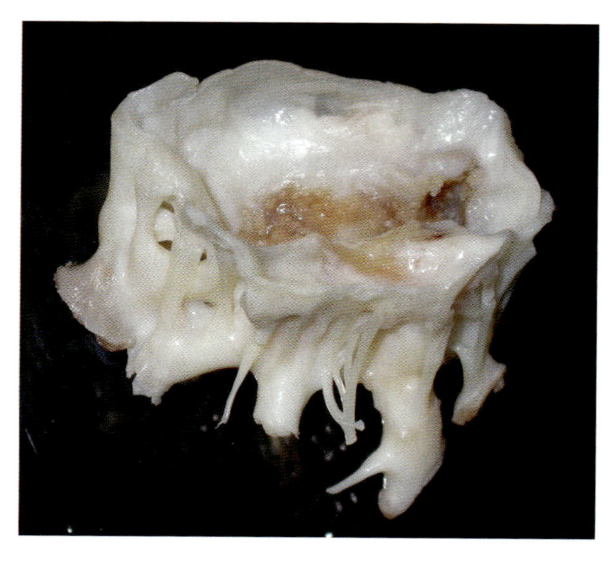

Fig. 4.14 Another excided rheumatic mitral valve with severe fibrosis and marked chordal thickening

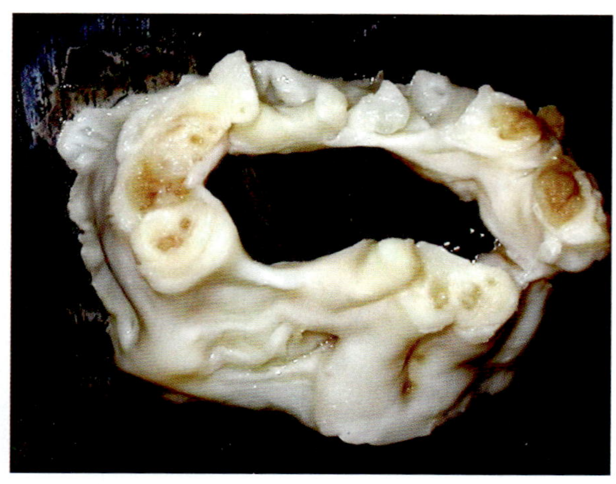

Fig. 4.15 Rheumatic valve chordae seen on end show marked fibrous thickening

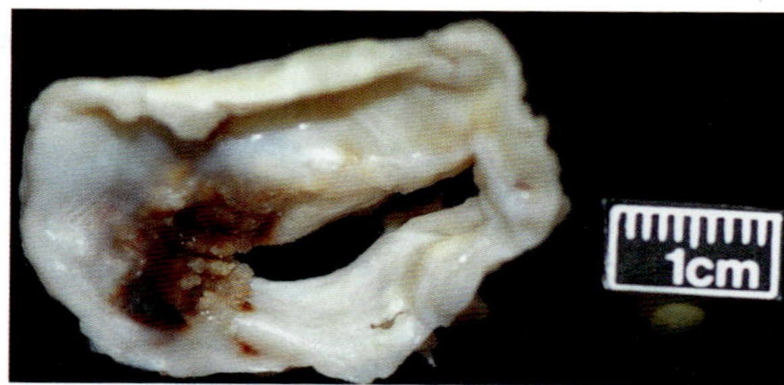

Fig. 4.16 Rheumatic mitral valve with leaflet fibrosis and commissural fusion. At one commissure there is erosion and thrombus deposit

The secondary effects of mitral valve stenosis upon the heart involve the left atrium and the right heart. Chronically the left atrium enlarges. With enlargement and stretching the interatrial septum may open its foramen ovale leading to Lutembacher syndrome (an acquired secundum atrial septal defect) and shunting. The cardiomyocytes undergo degenerative changes and the atrium is prone to fibrillation. Paroxysmal fibrillation may eventually lead to permanent fibrillation. The large atrial size and arrhythmia lead to stasis and thrombi with risk of embolism. The left atrial enlargement may also manifest in unusual ways – dysphagia as it presses against the esophagus, cough as it irritates the bronchi, and hoarseness as the recurrent laryngeal nerve is displaced (Ortner's syndrome). The most common manifestation of mitral valve stenosis is left heart failure with orthopnea, paroxysmal nocturnal dyspnea and dyspnea. Pleural effusions may occur. The left heart failure may cause hemoptysis. The left heart failure may lead to right heart failure with peripheral edema, ascites, organomegaly and weight gain.

Echocardiography Considerations

Mitral stenosis is described as the condition where there is obstruction to blood flow from the left atrium into the left ventricle during diastole. Although obstruction is most frequently at the mitral leaflet level, obstruction at other levels can occur. Despite the decrease in incidence of rheumatic fever, the most common cause remains rheumatic mitral stenosis. In the Western world, pure rheumatic mitral regurgitation is extremely rare, as a certain degree of mitral stenosis is invariably present. This is not the case in the developing world where repeated early infection can result in pure rheumatic mitral regurgitation at a young age.

The rheumatic pathological changes are not restricted to the mitral leaflets, although the leaflet changes are more readily identified by echocardiography (Figs. 4.17, 4.18). The mitral leaflets are slightly thickened particularly at the closing edge resulting in the typical doming or "hockey stick" appearance. This limitation in excursion is more pronounced in the posterior mitral leaflet, which is considerably shorter than the anterior mitral

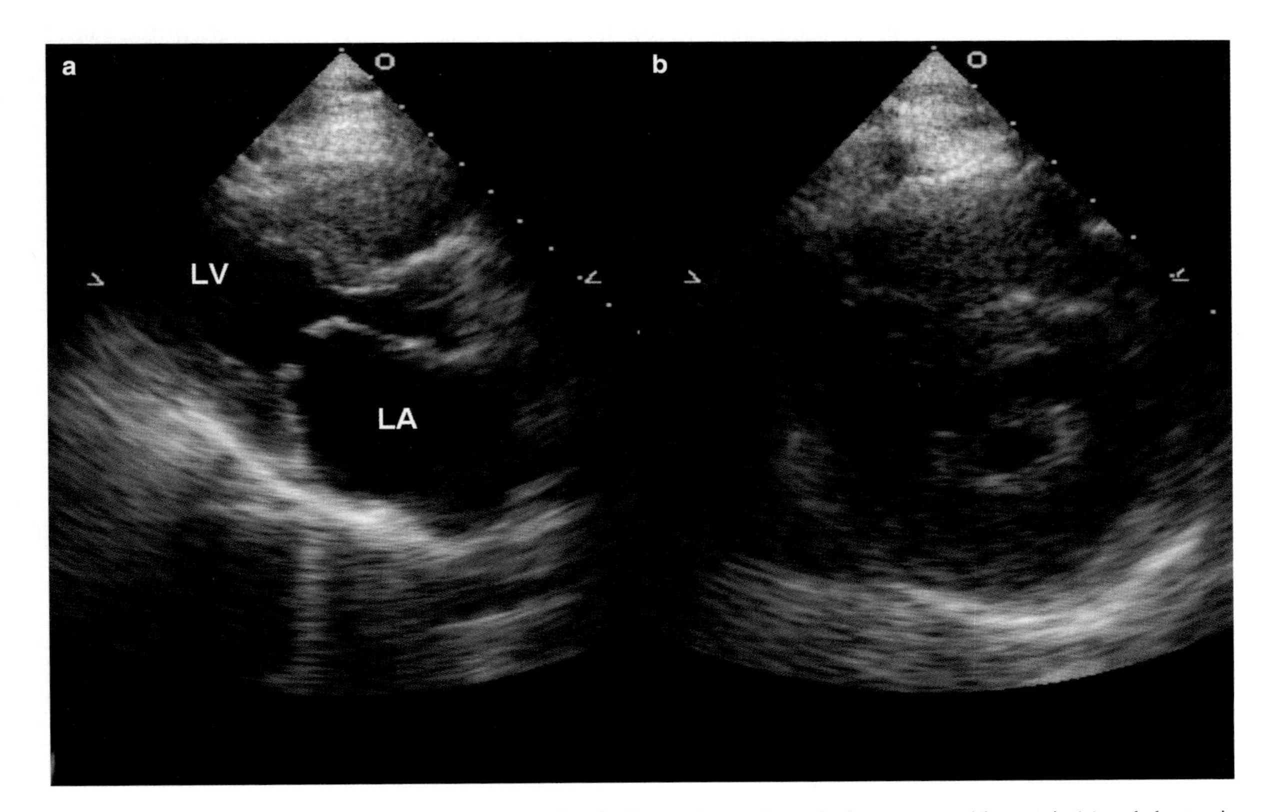

Fig. 4.17 The typical morphologic features of rheumatic mitral stenosis are shown in the parasternal long-axis (**a**) and short-axis (**b**) views. The tips of the mitral leaflets are thickened and tethered but the bellies of the leaflets remain mobile producing a "hockey stick" appearance. In the short-axis view (**b**) fusion at both commissures is present producing a fish-mouth appearance. *LA* left atrium, *LV* left ventricle

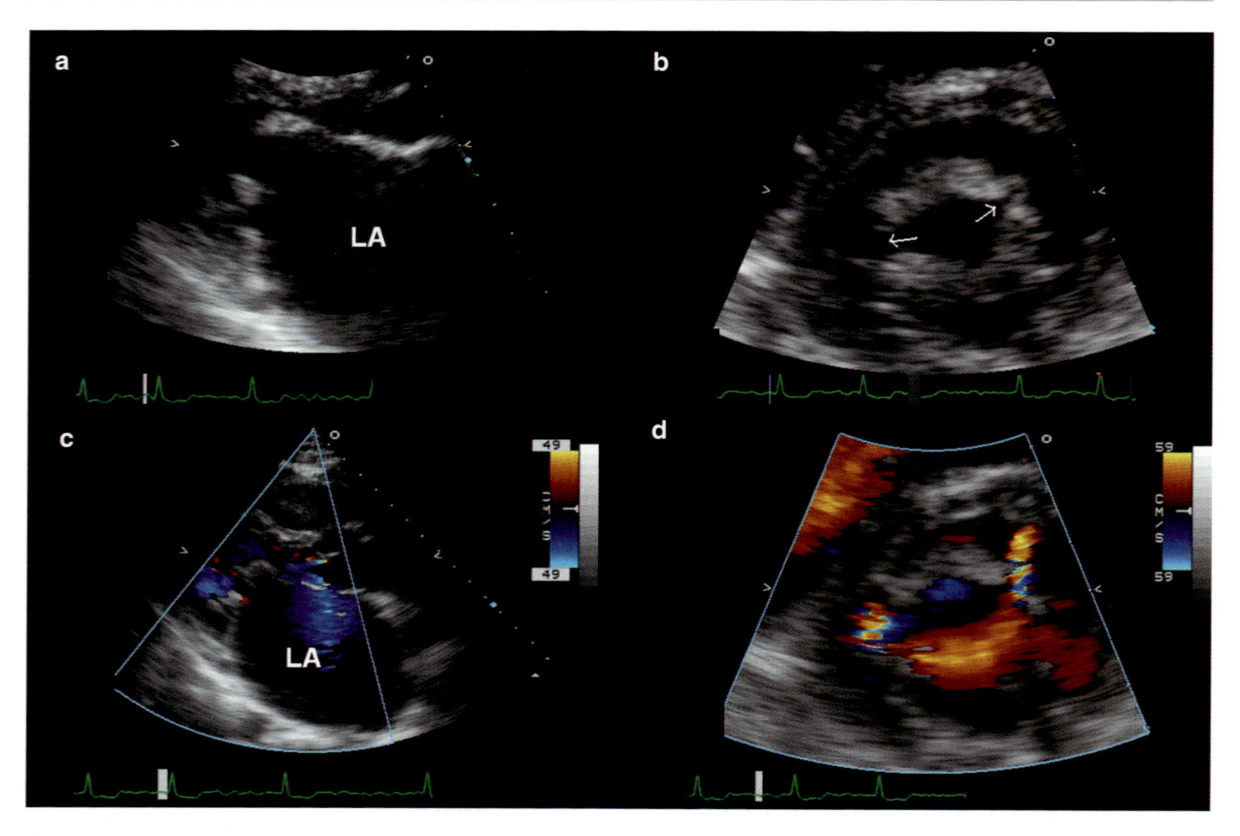

Fig. 4.18 This patient has rheumatic mitral stenosis and has had previous surgical commissurotomy. The mitral leaflets demonstrate mild restriction in excursion involving the tips of both mitral leaflets (**a**). In the short-axis view (**b**), splits at both the medial and lateral commissures are shown (*arrows*). Color-flow images (**c**, **d**) shows no significant flow acceleration during diastole, suggesting that there is no significant residual mitral stenosis. Diastolic antegrade flow across the split commissures is present. *LA* left atrium

leaflet. The rheumatic process results in fusion of the commissures, a pathognomonic finding. In the short-axis view, the mitral orifice has a "fish-mouth" appearance which is a result of commissural fusion fibrosis and restricted excursion of the leaflets (Figs. 4.13, 4.15, 4.16, 4.19). Calcification of the mitral leaflet, particularly at the tips of the leaflets, and at both commissures, is common. This is recognized as localized echo-dense nodules. Thickening, retraction and fusion of the subvalvular chords should be assessed. Scoring systems assessing different aspects of the mitral valve have been proposed to select patients for balloon valvotomy [10, 13]. These scoring systems, such as the one proposed by Wilkins et al. should be used in all patients with mitral stenosis, even in those who have mild disease and not being considered for valvotomy. The routine use of these scoring systems ensures that the mitral valve morphology is comprehensively assessed. The scoring system proposed by Wilkins provides a semi-quantitative assessment of mitral leaflet thickness, leaflet mobility, leaflet calcification and subvalvular involvement [13]. A low score (<8) suggests that the patient is more likely to have a good result from balloon valvotomy. However, this scoring system does not assess the degree of commissural fusion and does not differentiate fibrosis from calcification. The assessment of leaflet thickness was based on echocardiographic systems in the 1980s, so that the grading based on the suggested thickness is certainly incorrect using current imaging systems.

Mitral annular calcification (MAC) is sometimes included as a cause for mitral stenosis, although most patients with mitral annular calcification do not have mitral stenosis. In general, mitral stenosis is present only when the anterior mitral leaflet is also involved by the sclerotic change (Fig. 4.20). The tip of the anterior mitral leaflet is mobile, but the base of the anterior mitral

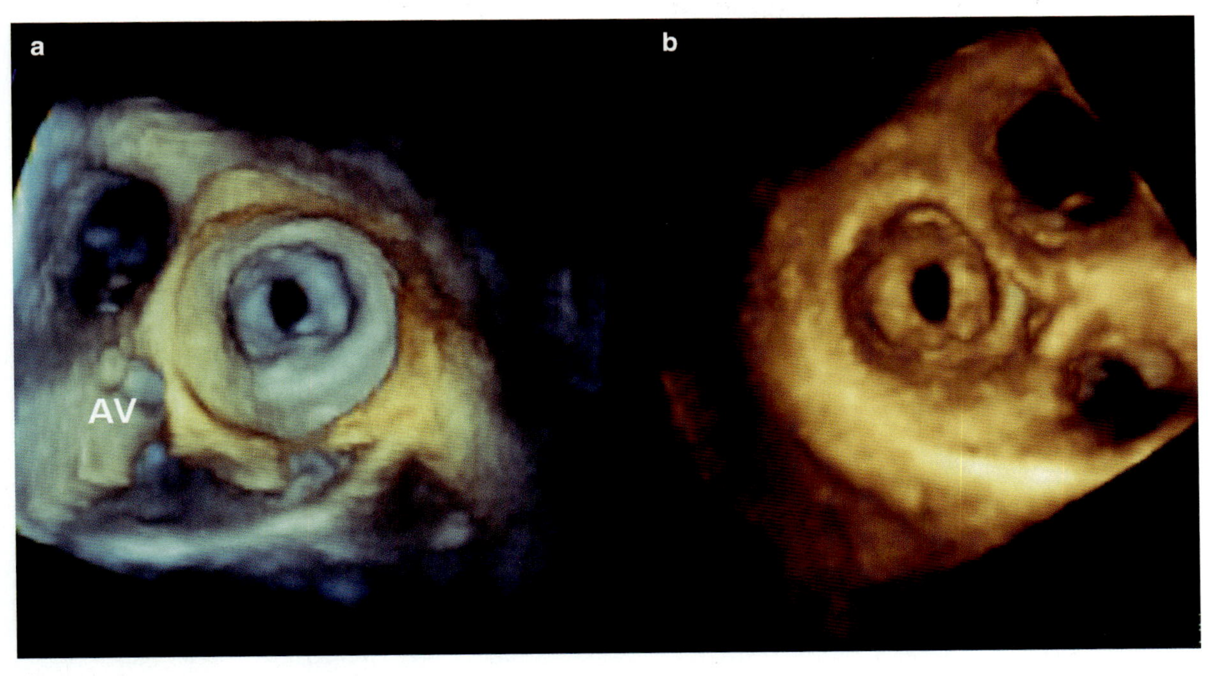

Fig. 4.19 This is a three-dimensional view of the mitral orifice from the perspective of the left atrium (**a**) and from the perspective of the left ventricle (**b**). The typical fish mouth appearance of the mitral orifice is evident. *AV* aortic valve

leaflet is rigid and immobile. There is no commissural fusion which differentiates it from rheumatic mitral stenosis. Management of these patients is problematic as they are elderly and there is extensive calcification involving the entire fibrous skeleton of the heart.

Non-valvular causes of mitral stenosis include obstruction of the mitral orifice by obstructing masses caused by endocarditis, particularly fungal endocarditis, or tumor mass such as a prolapsing myxoma, obstruction above the mitral valve level such as cor triatriatum and supramitral valvular ring (Fig. 4.21) and subvalvular obstruction related to papillary muscle abnormalities such as a parachute mitral valve (Fig. 4.22).

Assessment of Severity of Mitral Stenosis

The severity of mitral stenosis can be evaluated by several related measurements which are mitral valve area (MVA), transmitral peak and mean gradients, and the right ventricular systolic pressure. Among these measures, mitral valve area is least affected by loading conditions, concomitant mitral regurgitation and alteration in left ventricular function. There are different methods to obtain the mitral area (Table 4.1) [14]. The orifice of the mitral valve is best visualized in the parasternal short-axis view. Fine adjustment is required to image the mitral valve orifice just at the leaflet tip level where it demonstrates the typical "fish-mouth" appearance. When adequate images of the mitral valve orifice are obtained, mitral valve area by planimetry has been shown to be better than measurements by other methods. Three-dimensional (3D) echocardiography appears to be even better by virtue of its ability to obtain proper orthogonal view of the mitral orifice, but 3D is more time consuming (Fig. 4.23). The strength and limitations of these methods are listed in Table 4.1.

Management of patients with mitral stenosis is dependent on the inter-play between symptom, valve morphology and intracardiac hemodynamics. The common symptoms are fatigue and dyspnea, both of which are non-specific and can be seen in many diseases. Mild mitral stenosis is well tolerated and generally does not produce symptoms. Even in patients with severe mitral stenosis, they often delay in seeking medical attention because the symptoms are insidious and non-specific. Thus, objective testing is required to

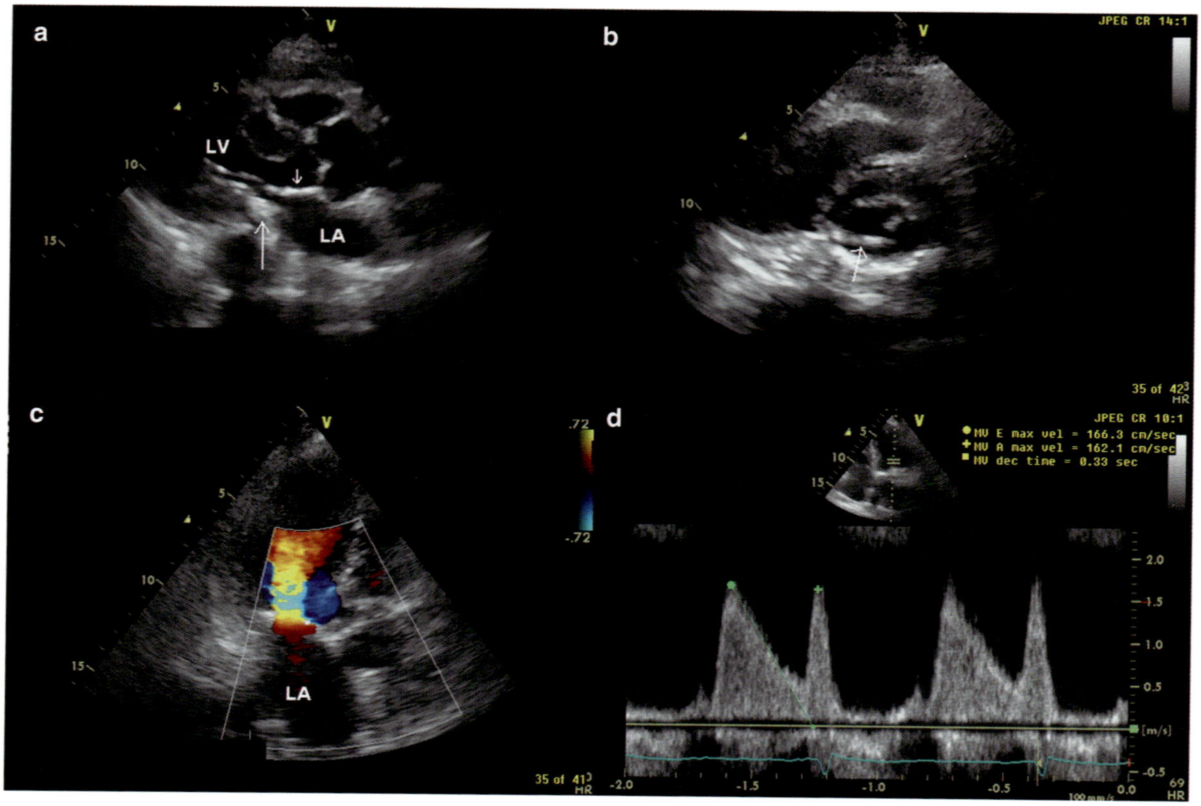

Fig. 4.20 This 80-year-old woman has mitral annular calcification (*long arrow*) and thickening and restriction of the base of the anterior mitral leaflet (*short arrow*) on the parasternal long-axis view shown in (**a**). In the parasternal short-axis view (**b**), the extent of mitral annular calcification is well seen and involves the medial half of the posterior annulus (*arrow*). Color-flow examination using the apical long-axis view (**c**) shows that there is increased flow velocity across the mitral valve which is confirmed on the continuous wave Doppler shown in (**d**). The mean transmitral valvular gradient is calculated to be 6 mmHg. *LA* left atrium, *LV* left ventricle

assess the degree of functional limitation in these patients. The intracardiac hemodynamics in mitral stenosis can be reliably assessed by Doppler echocardiography. A comprehensive assessment should include transmitral gradients, both peak and mean, mitral valve area and pulmonary artery pressure. The presence of a transmitral gradient is the hemodynamic hallmark of mitral stenosis, although it is flow dependent. Mitral valve area, on the other hand, has the advantage of being independent of flow and is the preferred index of severity in most instances. Pulmonary artery pressure determination should be included in the assessment as it may be a better predictor of functional limitation.

Among the several different methods to measure mitral valve area, planimetry is the most simple and reliable method, provided that the mitral orifice is optimally visualized (Fig. 4.24; Table 4.1). This may be difficult in mitral valves that are heavily calcified or have had prior commissurotomy. Excellent correlation between this method and measurements by pathologic examination has been demonstrated. The stenotic mitral valve is funnel shaped and it is crucial that planimetry be done at the tip of the funnel to avoid over-estimation of the valve area. Excessive gain can lead to under-estimation of the mitral valve area while non-orthogonal imaging plane may lead to over-estimation. This method is unaffected by the presence of co-existing mitral regurgitation or aortic regurgitation. The mitral pressure half-time method is based on the observation that the pressure decay between the left atrium and left ventricle is related to the severity of mitral stenosis. The more severe the disease, the slower the decay of the pressure difference, and the longer the half-time. The mitral valve area (MVA) can be calculated using the empiric formula:

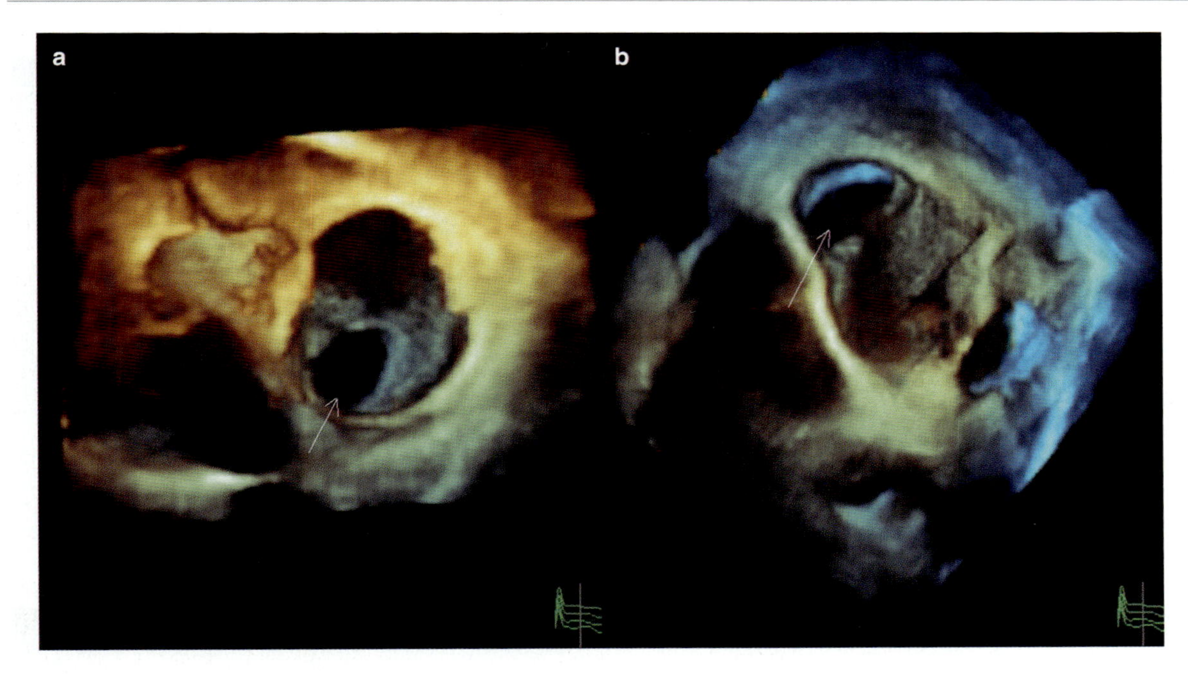

Fig. 4.21 This is a 3D image from the perspective of the mitral valve (**a**) and the posterior left atrium (**b**), showing a large membrane partitioning the left atrium into a posterior and an anterior chambers. There is a communication between the two chambers which is located medially and posteriorly (*arrow*). This is a cor triatriatum, since it is located posterior to the left atrial appendage (not shown)

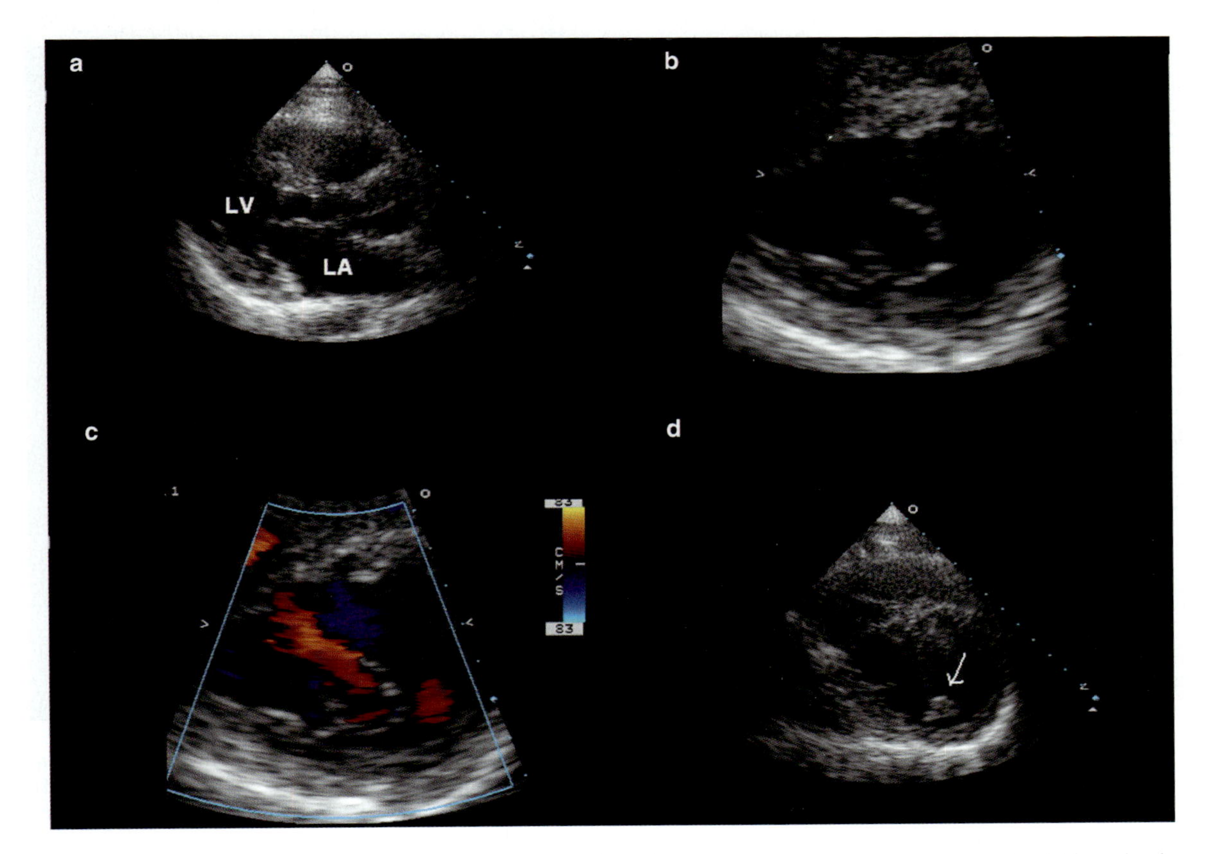

Fig. 4.22 The parasternal long-axis (**a**) and short-axis (**b–d**) views showing a parachute mitral valve with chordal insertion into a solitary papillary muscle (*arrow*)

Table 4.1 Advantages and limitations of the echocardiographic methods in assessing severity of mitral stenosis

Method	Strengths	Limitations
Planimetry	Simple, reliable	May be difficult in calcified valves or valve post-commissurotomy
Pressure half-time	Simple, not effected by orifice morphology	Variability from beat to beat, non-linear deceleration slope, and may be unreliable post-commissurotomy
Diameters of stenotic jet	Functional orifice, not effected by MR	Unusual orifice shape, contamination by AR
Flow convergence	Gain independent, not effected by MR	Non-hemispheric shape, time consuming, cumulative error
Pulse Doppler quantitative method	Not effected by orifice morphology	Not applicable if there is MR or AR, time consuming, cumulative errors
3D planimetry	Allows proper alignment	Requires dedicated equipment, time consuming, needs more validation

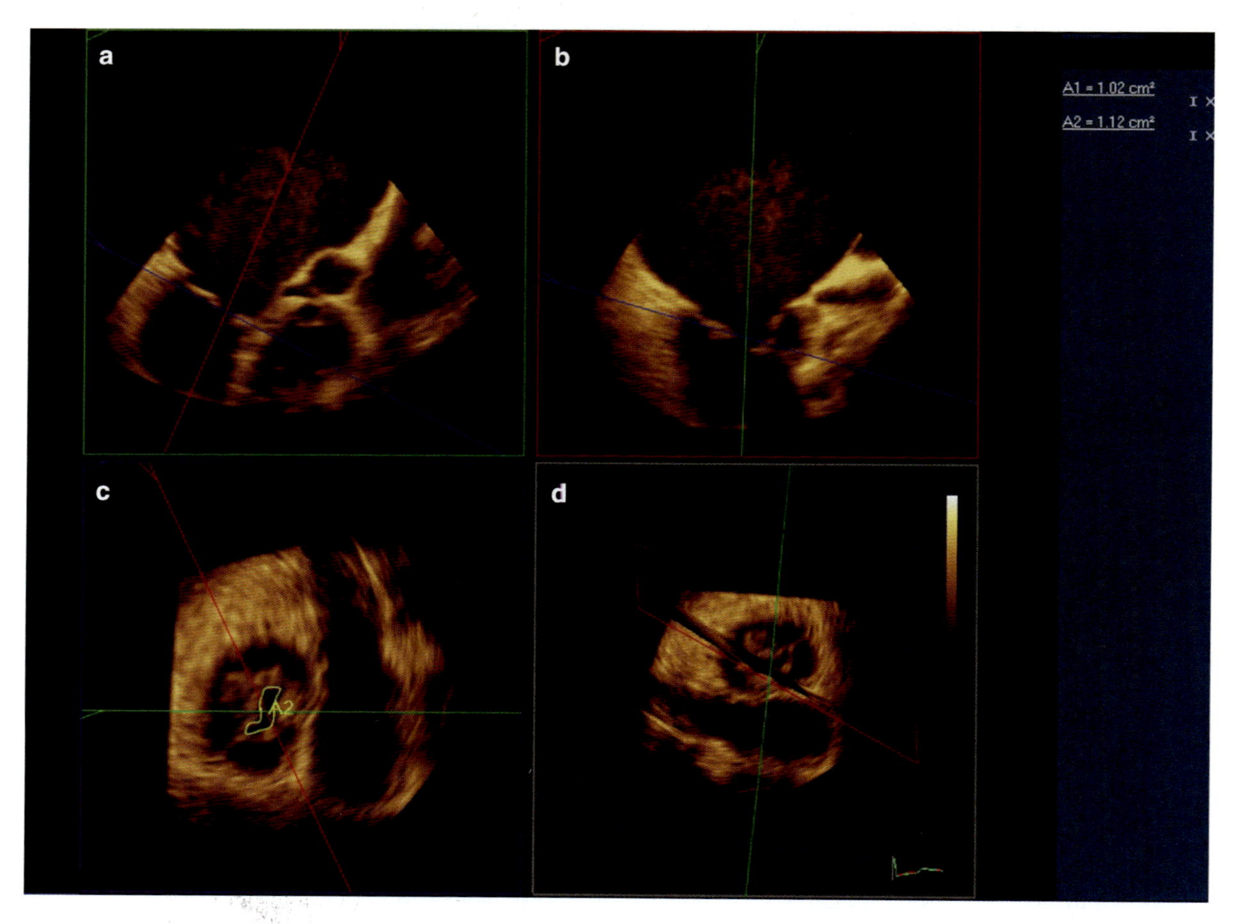

Fig. 4.23 The 3D echocardiography can be used to provide proper alignment of the imaging plane to the mitral orifice as demonstrated in (**a**) and (**b**). This allows the visualization of the mitral orifice at the tip of the mitral leaflets as show in (**c**) and (**d**). Planimetry of the mitral valve area using this approach may provide a more accurate measurement, although more validation data are required

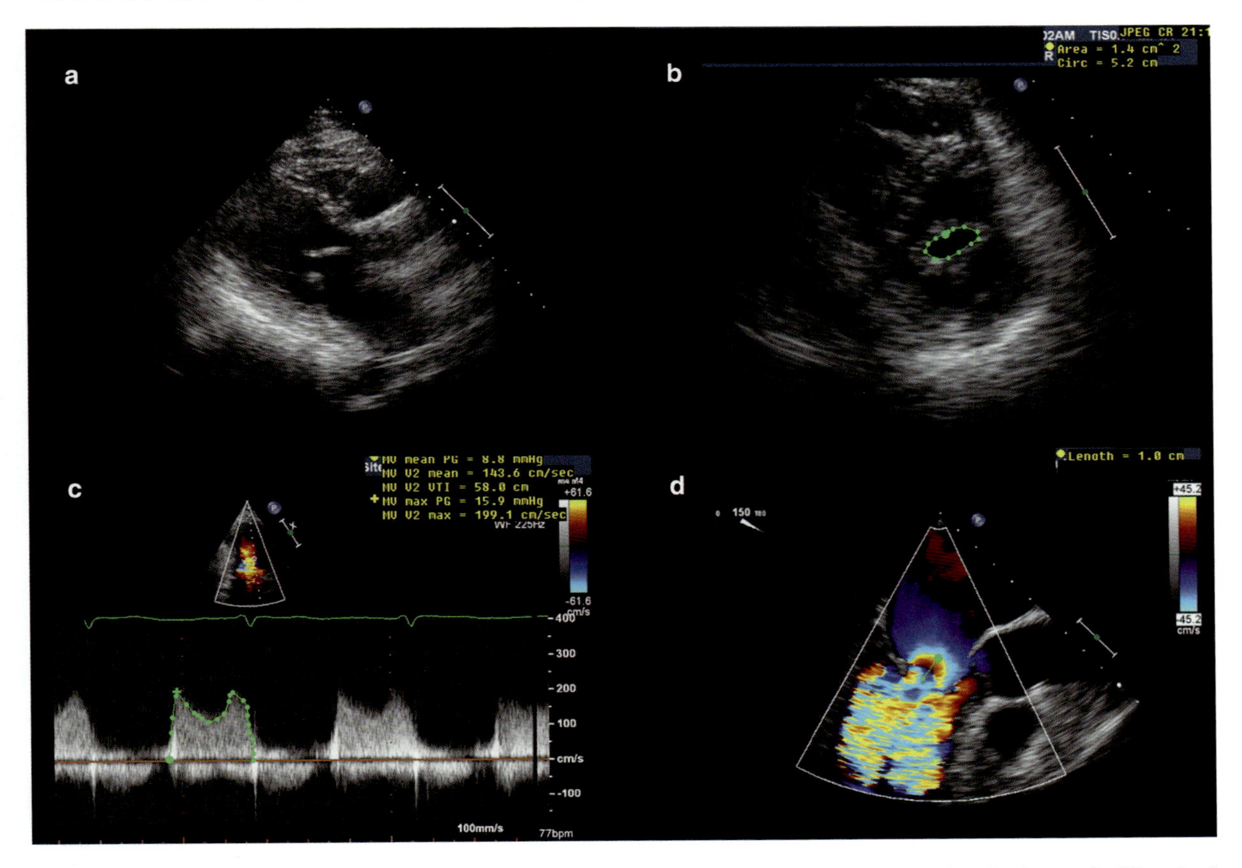

Fig. 4.24 The parasternal long-axis (**a**) and short-axis (**b**) views show typical features of rheumatic mitral stenosis. The mitral valve area by planimetry is performed using the short-axis view (**b**) and is 1.4 cm². The transmitral valvular gradients are assessed by continuous wave Doppler (**c**). The peak and mean gradients are 15.9 and 8.8 mmHg, respectively. The radius of flow convergence is 1 cm with an aliasing velocity of 45.2 cm/s (**d**). Continuous wave Doppler shows a maximum mitral stenosis velocity of 199.1 cm/s (**c**), and the calculated mitral valve area is 1.43 cm² which is similar to the mitral valve area by planimetry

$$\text{MVA cm}^2 = \frac{220}{\text{pressure half time}},$$

or

$$= \frac{220}{\text{deceleration time } \times 0.29}$$

This is the most popular method to obtain mitral valve area due to of its ease of use. It is also relatively independent of the angle of interrogation and not effected by the orifice morphology. On the other hand the slope of the signal may not be linear making determination difficult. There can be significant variability from beat to beat. In patients shortly following balloon mitral valvotomy, mitral valve area determined by the half-time method has been shown to be unreliable. Variability of this measurement is particularly problematic in the setting of atrial fibrillation (Fig. 4.25). Measurement of multiple sequential beats is required. The so-called "ski slope" phenomenon describes a rapid slope at the beginning of diastole followed by a gentler slope. In this situation it is advisable to use the mean slope, rather than the initial slope, to determine the half-time. The mitral jet area, which is approximated by the jet area, can be calculated by obtaining orthogonal diameters of the mitral inflow jet. The jet area is calculated by: $\pi/4 \times$ the product of the two diameters. This measurement assesses the functional mitral orifice and is unaffected by coexisting mitral regurgitation. The flow convergence or the proximal isovelocity surface method is based on the phenomenon of accelerating flow exceeding the aliasing velocity and creating multiple hemispheric isovelocity shells as it

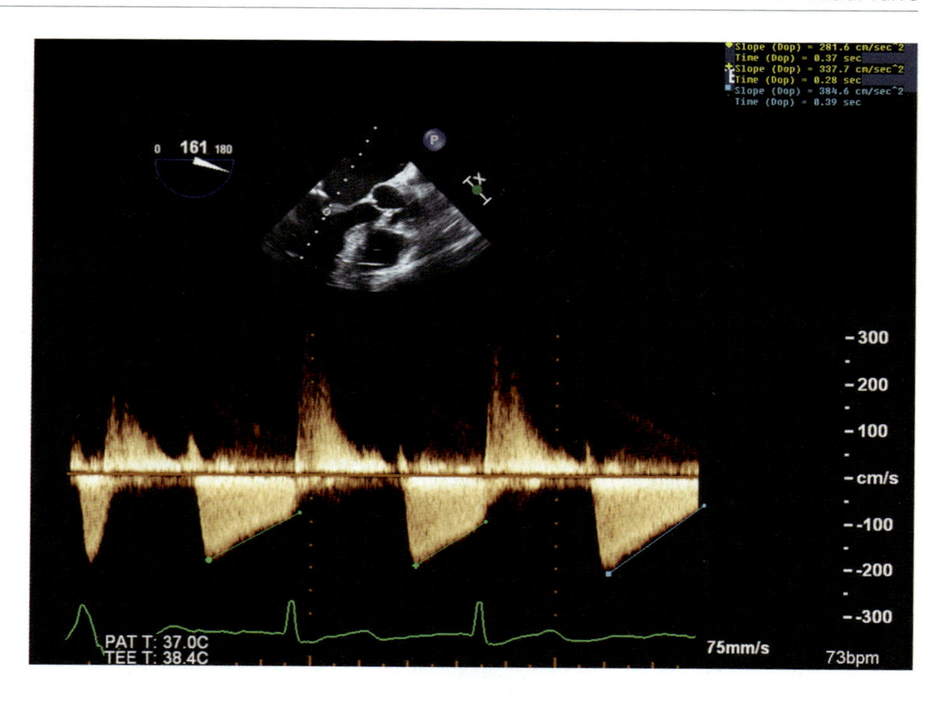

Fig. 4.25 The continuous wave Doppler of the mitral velocity from the transesophageal window shows beat to beat variability as the patient is in atrial fibrillation

approaches an obstructing orifice. The instantaneous flow rate at any given iso-velocity shell is the product of the specific aliasing velocity times the surface area of the shell, and should equal the instantaneous flow rate at the obstructing orifice.

Thus,

$$\text{MVA} \times \text{V}_{\text{MS}} = 2\pi r_{\text{A}}^{\;2} \times \text{V}_{\text{A}},$$

and

$$\text{MVA} = \frac{2\pi r^2 \times \text{V}_{\text{A}}}{\text{V}_{\text{MS}}},$$

where V_{MS} is the maximal mitral stenosis velocity, r_A is the radius and V_A is the velocity of the isovelocity shell. Correction for the angle should be made if the flow convergence is not a perfect hemisphere (Fig. 4.26). The advantages of this method include gain independence, not being affected by concomitant mitral regurgitation, and relative independence of the 2D image quality. The disadvantages are that it is time consuming and requires multiple calculations.

The continuity equation is also applied in the pulsed Doppler quantitative method which requires calculating the stroke volumes at the aortic valve and the mitral valve.

$$\text{MVA} = \frac{\text{AVA} \times \text{VTI}_{\text{AV}}}{\text{VTI}_{\text{MV}}}$$

where AVA= aortic valve area or area of left ventricular outflow tract, VTI_{AV} = velocity time integral at the aortic valve and VTI_{MV} = velocity time integral at the mitral valve. This method has the advantage that it is not affected by the orifice shape. It is however not applicable when there is concomitant significant aortic regurgitation or mitral regurgitation. It is also time consuming with multiple calculations, and the errors in the measurements may compound themselves. Three-dimensional (3D) appears to be a very promising method in measuring MVA, but more validation data are needed (Figs. 4.19, 4.23). In patients in whom multiple methods can be applied, measurements by planimetry appears to be the most reliable method and is technically the most straightforward to apply [14].

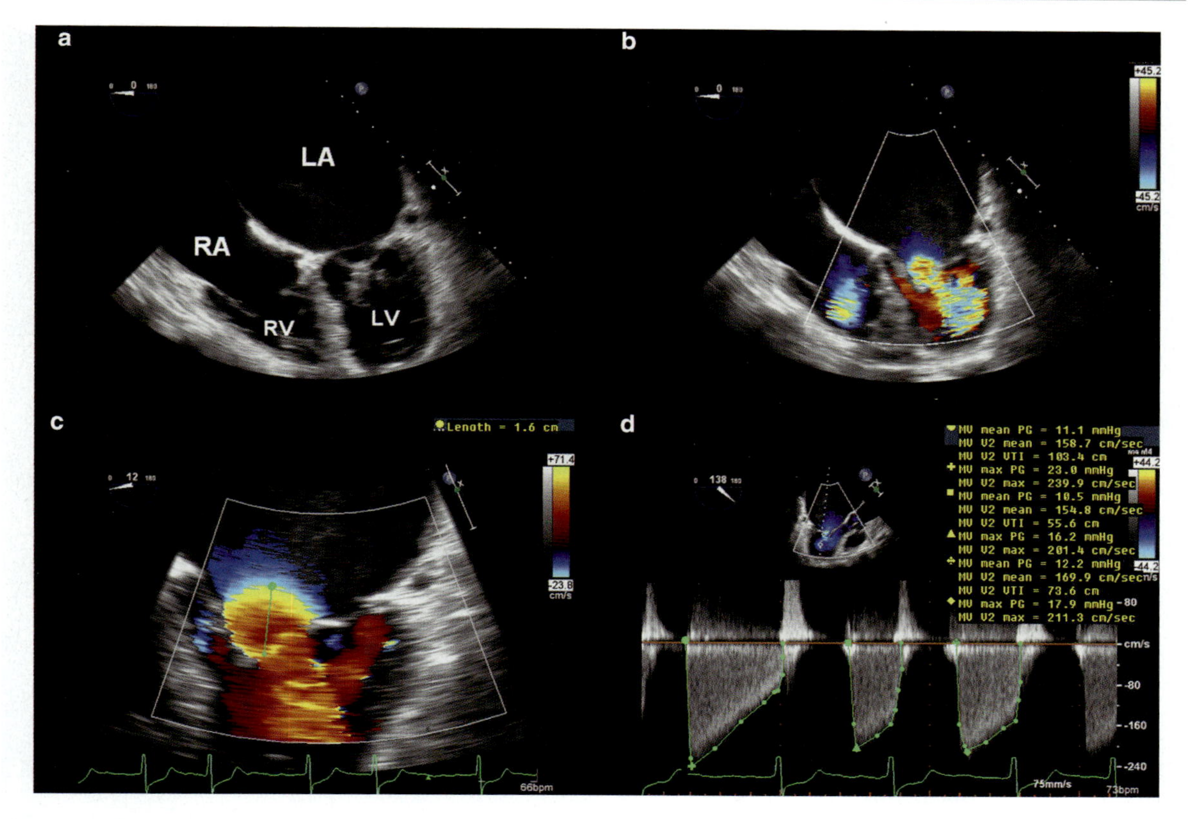

Fig. 4.26 The transesophageal four-chamber view in this patient with mitral stenosis is shown in (**a**), and the color images in (**b**) and (**c**). The flow convergence is not hemispheric in shape but rather occupies about a 90° angle. The continuous wave Doppler of mitral velocity is shown in (**d**), and the average maximum mitral stenosis velocity is 218 cm/s. Using the continuity equation and adjusting for a 90° angle of the convergence area, the mitral valve area is calculated to be 0.88 cm^2

Exercise is useful in the evaluation of patients with mitral stenosis (Fig. 4.27). When doing the exercise study, it is important to obtain a comprehensive assessment. The mitral gradients and the pulmonary artery pressure should be obtained at multiple stages of exercise. However, mitral pressure half-time is of limited usefulness. A marked increase in transvalvular mitral gradients and pulmonary systolic pressure indicates that mitral stenosis is functionally significant.

Mitral Insufficiency

Anatomical Considerations

The mitral valve apparatus is a complicated structure with numerous components, all of which must function to ensure valve competence. The leaflets, annulus, chordae, papillary muscles and even the left ventricle all must work together to ensure normal valve function. Different diseases may affect multiple parts of the valve. An organized method of categorizing causes of mitral insufficiency is to consider each anatomical structure separately— leaflet, annulus, chordae, papillary muscles and left ventricle.

Leaflet Causes of Mitral Regurgitation

Abnormalities of the leaflet causing regurgitation include: perforation (postinfective endocarditis), scar retraction (post-inflammatory causes, often rheumatic), medications (anorectic drugs), and importantly the degenerative floppy mitral valve (myxomatous degeneration).

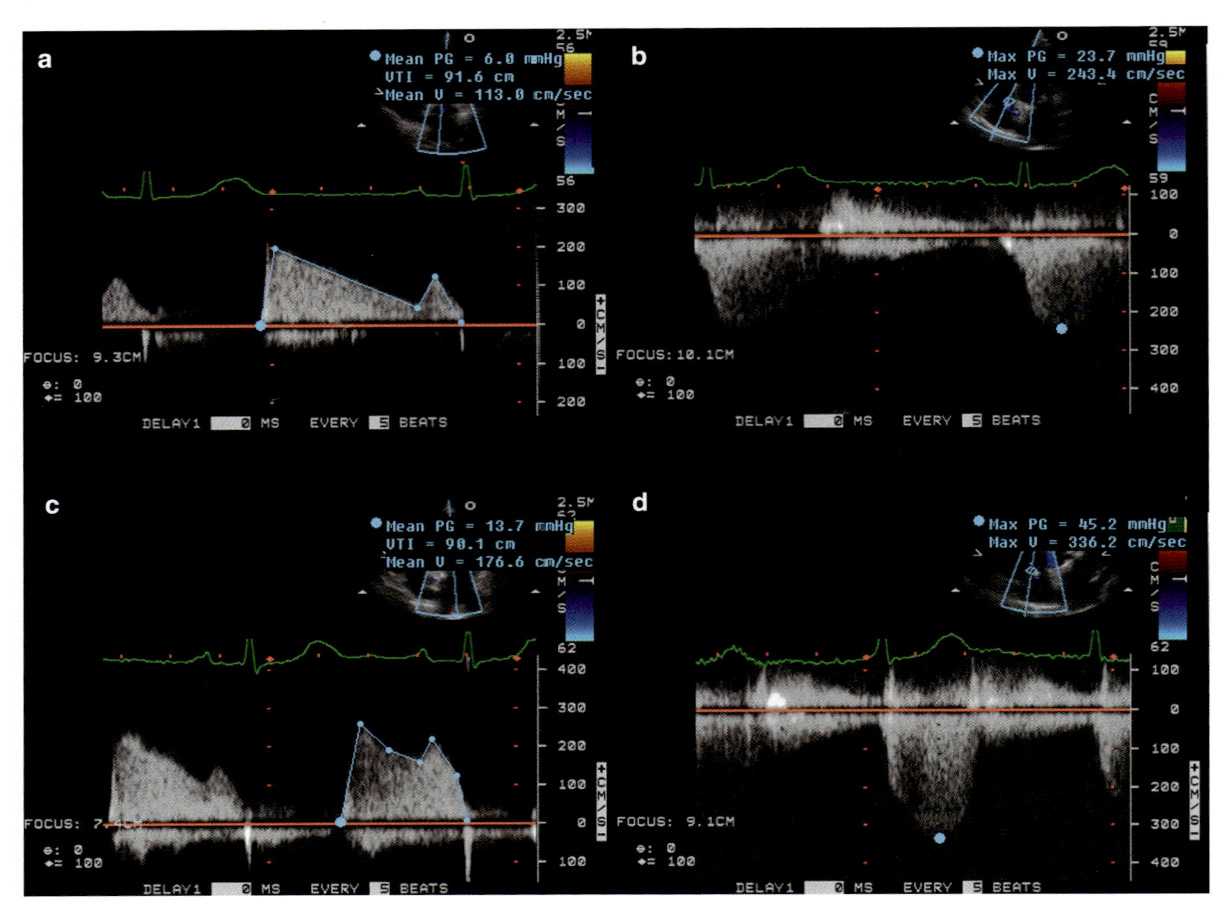

Fig. 4.27 This is an exercise study to assess the hemodynamic changes in a 77-year-old woman with mitral stenosis and previous mitral valve repair. The resting peak and mean mitral gradients at a heart rate of 46 beats/min are 16 and 6 mmHg, respectively (**a**), and the right ventricular systolic pressure is 34 mmHg with an estimated right atrial pressure of 10 mmHg (**b**). At a peak heart rate of 70 beats/min, the peak and mean mitral gradients are 25 and 14 mmHg, respectively (**c**), and the right ventricular systolic pressure is 55 mmHg (**d**)

Myxomatous Valve Disease

Mitral valve prolapse may be seen with myxomatous valve degeneration as a degenerative age related change or in association with syndromes such as Marfan's, Ehlers Danlos or osteogenesis imperfecta. These are the classic large redundant, thickened, "floppy" valves with endocardial fibrous thickening and accumulation of ground substances (glycosaminoglycans) in the valve spongiosa layer. Mitral valve prolapse may also be seen with Turner's syndrome, hypertrophic cardiomyopathy, atrial septal defect, ischemic heart disease and chest trauma. The myxomatous change is most common in the posterior leaflet and the process may be very marked in just one scallop (Figs. 4.28–4.30). Anterior leaflet degeneration occurs less commonly. The entire valve may be severely involved with large thick redundant leaflets— some have termed this Barlow's syndrome (in fact Barlow actually described mitral valve prolapse of many types not just from myxomatous degeneration). Most myxomatous degeneration is age related in nature and thus the incidence of this abnormality seems to be increasing.

Myxomatous changes of the mitral valve can be recognized by redundant or thick mitral leaflets, with multiple folding particularly along the coaptation margin best recognized in the short-axis view. The rough zone of the mitral leaflet, particularly the anterior mitral leaflet, may appear thickened during diastole as the secondary chords located in this area can make the leaflet

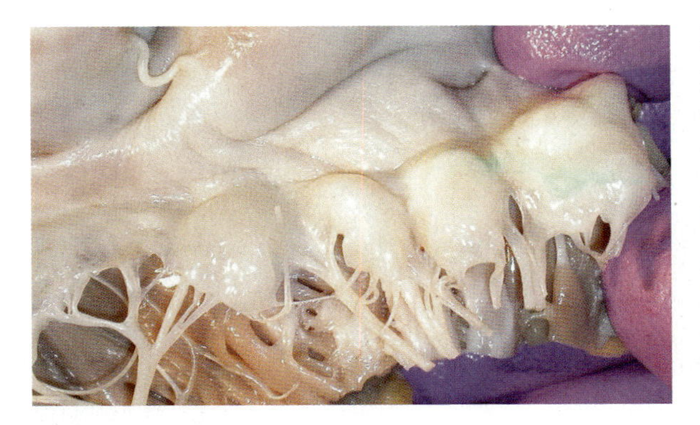

Fig. 4.28 Floppy myxomatous mitral valve with severe degeneration of the posterior leaflet tissue. The scallops of the leaflet are exaggerated and the leaflet tissue is thickened, although soft

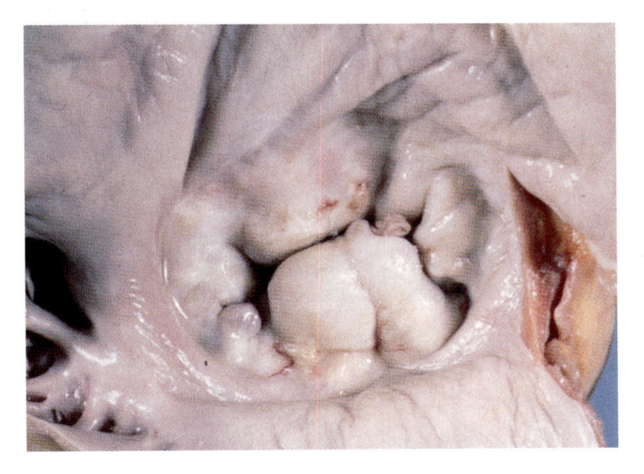

Fig. 4.29 Myxomatous mitral valve prolapse, as seen through the opened left atrium. The leaflets are thickened and redundant, especial the mid posterior leaflet

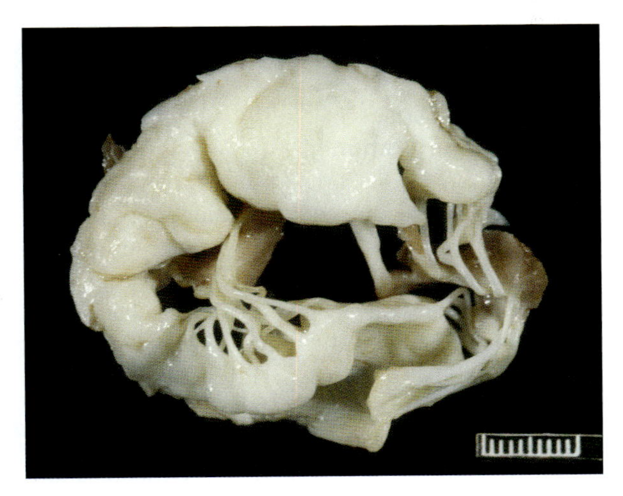

Fig. 4.30 Excised myxomatous valve which appears thickened and redundant. A surgically excised entire valve like this is now rare. With valve repair less tissue is excised, if any

look thicker than normal. Frame to frame analysis during diastole can provide a ready differentiation between chords and actual leaflets. The redundancy of the leaflet can give a doming appearance of the anterior mitral leaflet (Figs. 4.31, 4.32). Again frame-to-frame analysis in both the long- and short-axis view should dispel any notion of restriction to excursion. Commissural fusion, best seen in the short-axis view, is absent. Another common cause for mitral valve prolapse is fibroelastic deficiency. In this setting, the mitral leaflets are less redundant and on the short-axis view show far less folding compared to the myxomatous mitral valves (Fig. 4.33). Regardless of the etiology of mitral valve prolapse, ruptured chords leading to flail of one or more scallops of the mitral leaflets is a common complication.

When severe prolapse is present, a flail segment should be suspected. In our experience, a small flail segment due to the rupture of a few chords can easily be missed by trans-thoracic imaging, and thus transesophageal imaging should be considered in this setting. The sign of a flail segment is the presence of erratic chords protruding in the left atrium during systole (the snake tongue deformity) (Figs. 4.34, 4.35). Color flow imaging is helpful to identify the leaflets involved. If the mitral regurgitation jet is directed anteriorly, the posterior mitral leaflet is the culprit. A posterior directed mitral regurgitant jet suggests that an abnormality is located on the anterior mitral leaflet. As indicated previously, the mitral regurgitation can be eccentric making it difficult to determine the origin and the direction of the jet. One example is prolapse or flail localized to either the lateral or medial commissural areas of the leaflet. If the medial scallops leaflet area is affected, the origin of the mitral regurgitant jet is located at the medial commissure and directed laterally. The opposite is true when the lateral commissural leaflet is flail (Fig. 4.36). It is important to assess the commissural leaflet area, since isolated involvement of this area can be readily repaired with good result. When imaging the mitral valve in the short-axis view, it is clear that the mitral orifice area is dynamic in nature with a maximal opening in early diastole and the mitral opening was circular in shape approximating the area of the mitral annulus. The anterior mitral leaflet is continuous with the posterior mitral leaflet forming essentially a continuous curtain draping from the mitral annulus. Between the anterior and posterior mitral leaflet are the commissural leaflets which should be included in assessing the structural integrity of the mitral valve (Fig. 4.37).

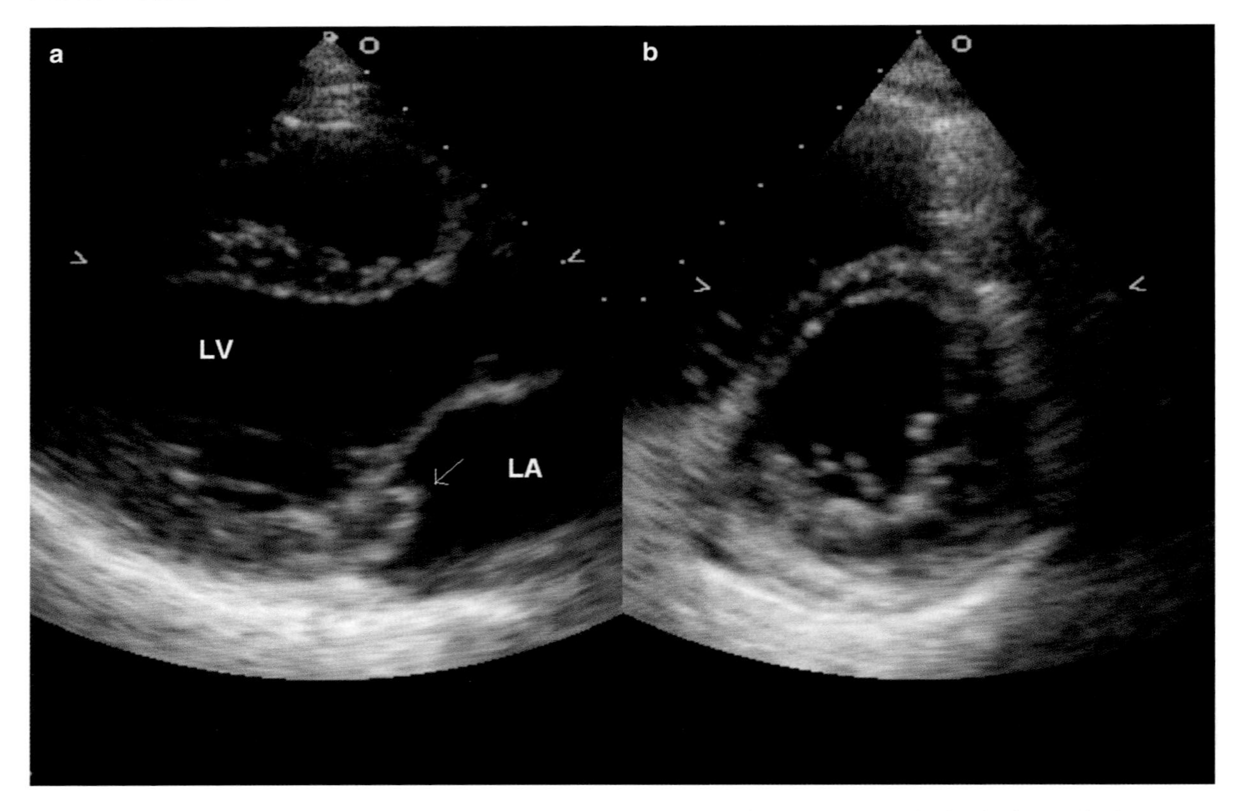

Fig. 4.31 The parasternal long-axis (**a**) and short-axis (**b**) views of a patient with myxomatous mitral valve in systole show severe prolapse of the posterior mitral leaflet (*arrow*). *LA* left atrium, *LV* left ventricle

Infective Endocarditis

Infective endocarditis may lead to leaflet and chordal destruction. Acutely, the infection may weaken the leaflet tissue leading to an acquired out-pouching or aneurysm. In the process of healing, or if the infection continues, the aneurysm may become like a sieve due to perforation (Fig. 4.38). Infected thrombi may also destroy the chords and cause them to rupture. Chronically the infections may lead to leaflet and chordal loss with valve defects and holes.

Fibrotic changes involving the mitral leaflet due to the rheumatic process or endocarditis gives rise to leaflets that are truly thickened. The leaflets may be retracted leading to incomplete coaptation and in these cases, a mitral regurgitant orifice can usually be imaged both from the long and short-axis views. Color imaging shows that the mitral regurgitation arises from the coaptation area and is generally directed centrally. This should be distinguished from leaflet perforation which is usually caused by endocarditis (Fig. 4.39). Unusual causes of mitral leaflet perforation include suture dehiscence following quadrangular resection of the posterior mitral leaflet and iatrogenic damage following ablation near the mitral annulus.

Drug Related Causes of Mitral Regurgitation

Medications, including anorexogenic drugs (fenfluramine-phentermine), ergotamine and methysergide (migraine medications) have been described as producing carcinoid-like valve disease. The mechanism of valve injury is thought to be activation or agonist activity of the 5HT-2B receptors. Ergot alkaloid drugs include methysergide and ergotamine, both used for treatment of migraine headaches. The anorectic diet medications have previously been used as monotherapy for short duration therapy for many years. The combination of fenfluramine and phentermine (Fen-Phen)

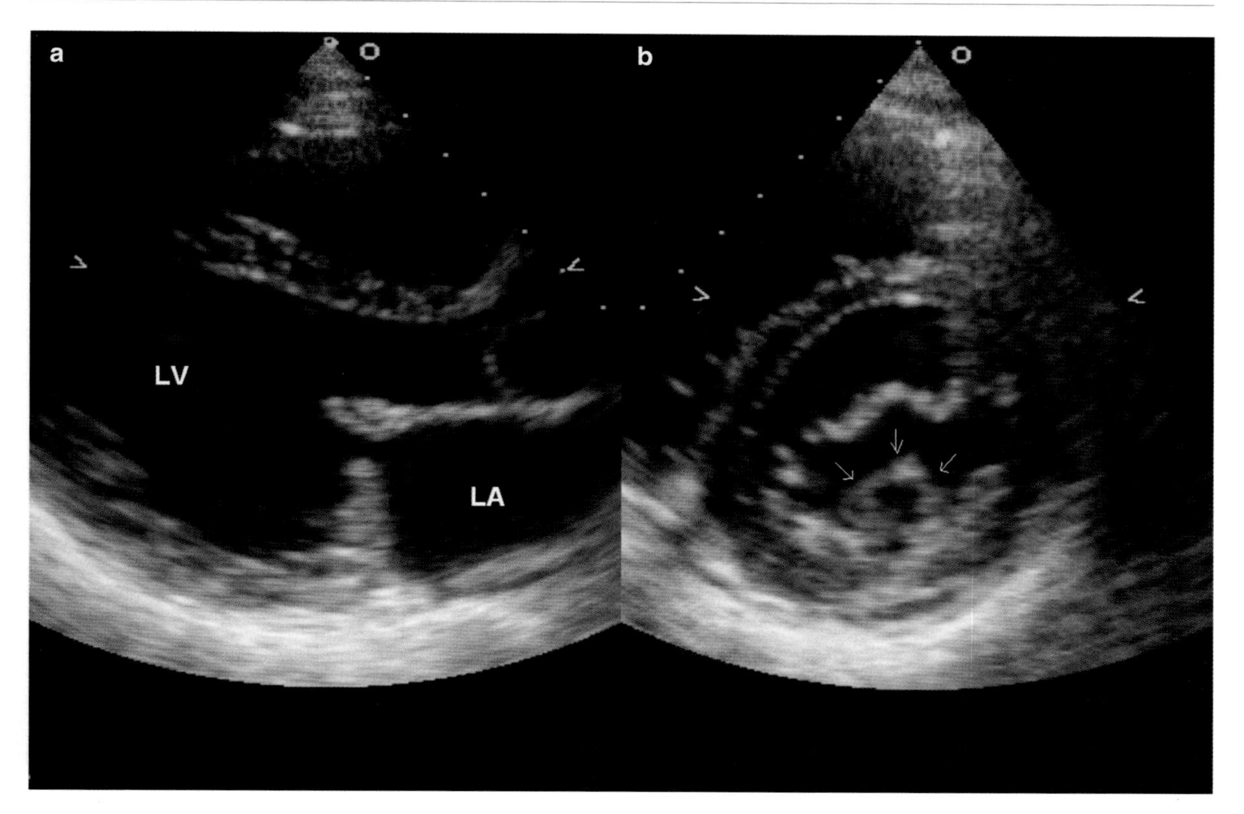

Fig. 4.32 The parasternal long-axis (**a**) and short-axis (**b**) views of the same patient as in Fig. 4.31 in diastole highlight the redundant nature of the mitral leaflets. Both leaflets appear thickened in the long-axis view (**a**). In the short-axis view the multiple foldings particularly involving the mid scallop of the posterior mitral leaflet (*arrows*) can be appreciated. *LA* left atrium, *LV* left ventricle

was introduced in North America in the mid-1990s. There was little knowledge concerning effectiveness or chronic effects. Connolly et al. reported heart valve disease shortly thereafter in 1997 [15]. There is still some debate as to the actual risk and incidence of the valvulopathy associated with anorexogenic agents, but it is probably low [16]. Susceptibility or risk may depend upon the medication dose, the duration of treatment and individual risk factors including the presence of pre-existing valve disease and concomitant medication use [17].

Grossly and microscopically, the valve disease or valvulopathy associated with anorexogenic drugs has been reported to be similar morphologically to that of carcinoid valve disease [15, 18]. The left sided valves are predominantly affected. White plaques are noted grossly and there may be chordal encasement and fusion, but not rupture. The commissures are not fused, in contrast to rheumatic disease. Doming or hooding of the mitral leaflets is not seen, in contrast to floppy valve disease. By microscopic examination, the valves have myofibroblast and glycosaminoglycan rich endocardial lesions with preservation of the underlying valve architecture. These lesions are onlays of glycosaminoglycan, collagen, and myofibroblasts that are superficial to the valve elastic membrane, but deep to the surface endothelium. The valve proper may have myxoid degeneration with accumulation of glycosaminoglycans. The onlays also may contain chronic inflammatory cells (CD3 positive lymphocytes and CD68 positive macrophages) and there is neovascularization within the onlay lesions and in the valve proper [19].

Similar carcinoid like valve disease has also been noted recently with Pergolide, an ergot derived dopamine receptor agonist used for treatment of Parkinson's disease [20, 21]. Tricuspid and mitral valve regurgitation have been reported. Pergolide is another medication that has been described to activate serotonin 5HT-2B receptors.

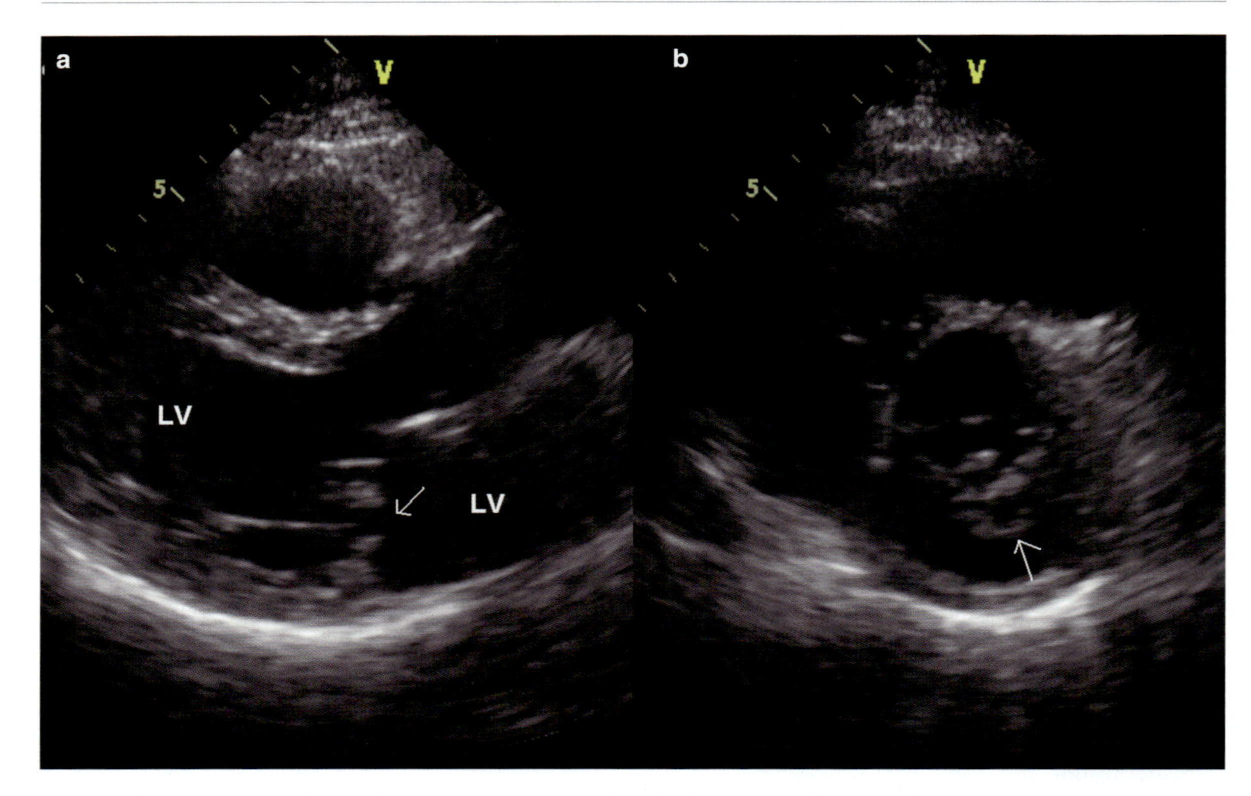

Fig. 4.33 This is a patient with mitral valve prolapse related to fibroelastic deficiency. Prolapse of the posterior mitral leaflet (*arrow*) is demonstrated in the parasternal long-axis (**a**) and short-axis (**b**) views. The prolapse largely involves the mid scallop of the posterior mitral leaflet which is shown in the short-axis view (**b**). Compared to the patient shown in Figs. 4.31 and 4.32, the mitral leaflets appear to be of normal thickness with a less degree of folding during leaflet coaptation

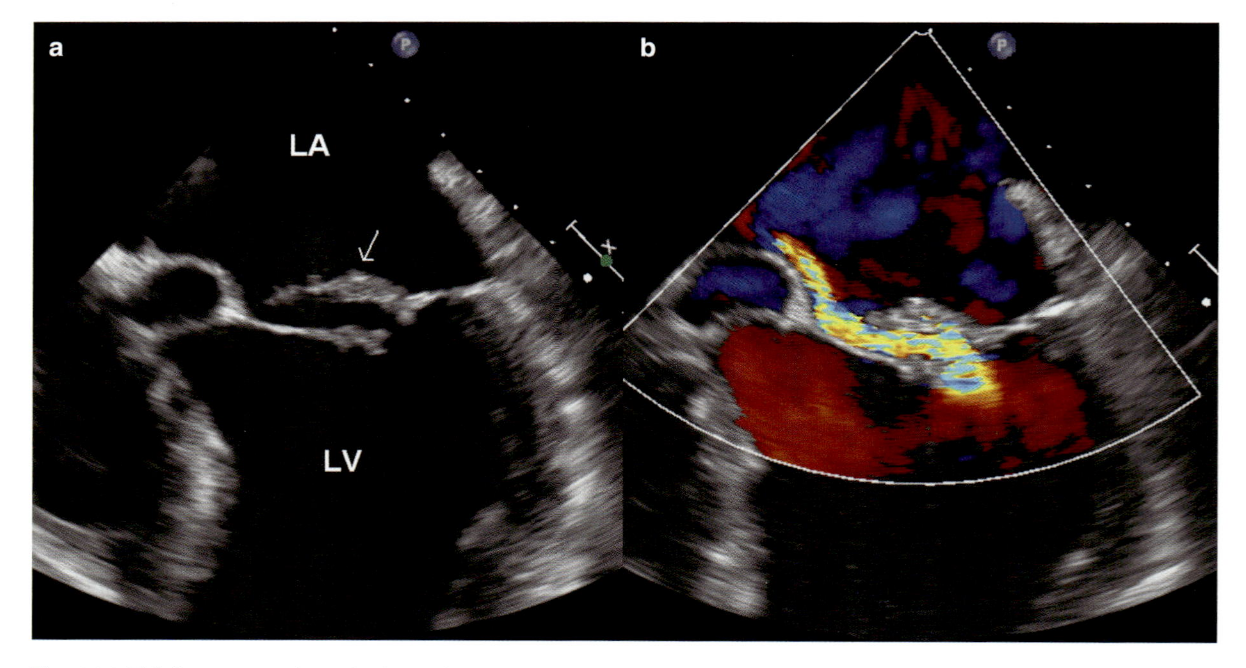

Fig. 4.34 This is a transesophageal echocardiogram in a patient with a flail mid scallop (P2) of the posterior mitral leaflet (*arrow*). The flail scallop prolapses to close behind the anterior mitral leaflet in systole (**a**) and a large anterior directed mitral regurgitant jet is present (**b**). *LA* left atrium, *LV* left ventricle

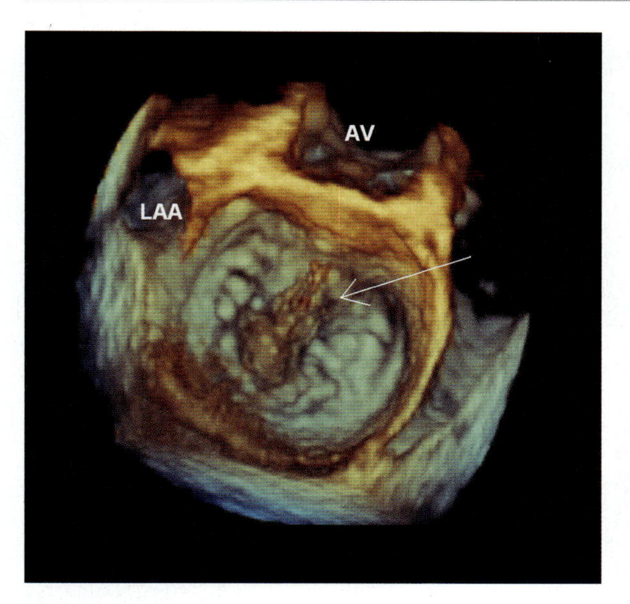

Fig. 4.35 This is a 3D transesophageal view of a patient with flail mid scallop (P2) of the posterior mitral leaflet, demonstrating the prolapsed scallop with multiple ruptured chords flailing in the left atrium (*arrow*). *AV* aortic valve, *LAA* left atrial appendage

Chordal Causes of Mitral Regurgitation

Chordal abnormalities causing regurgitation are due to chordal elongation, as observed in a myxomatous floppy valve, or actual chordal rupture from a floppy valve or after infective endocarditis. The two have vastly different consequences. In elongation and myxomatous change, the regurgitation is chronic leading to left ventricle dilatation and progressive heart failure. In rupture, the regurgitation is sudden leading to acute ventricle dilatation and marked left heart failure leading to dyspnea and pulmonary edema. The size of the left atrium and its ability to adapt to the volume overload are key to how the patient will present. In myxomatous valves studies have shown structural anomalies in not only the leaflets but also the chordae. These are of abnormal composition and are weak and prone to elongation and rupture.

The presence of an elongated chord is detected by displacement of the subservient mitral leaflet into the left atrium during leaflet coaptation. The tip of the

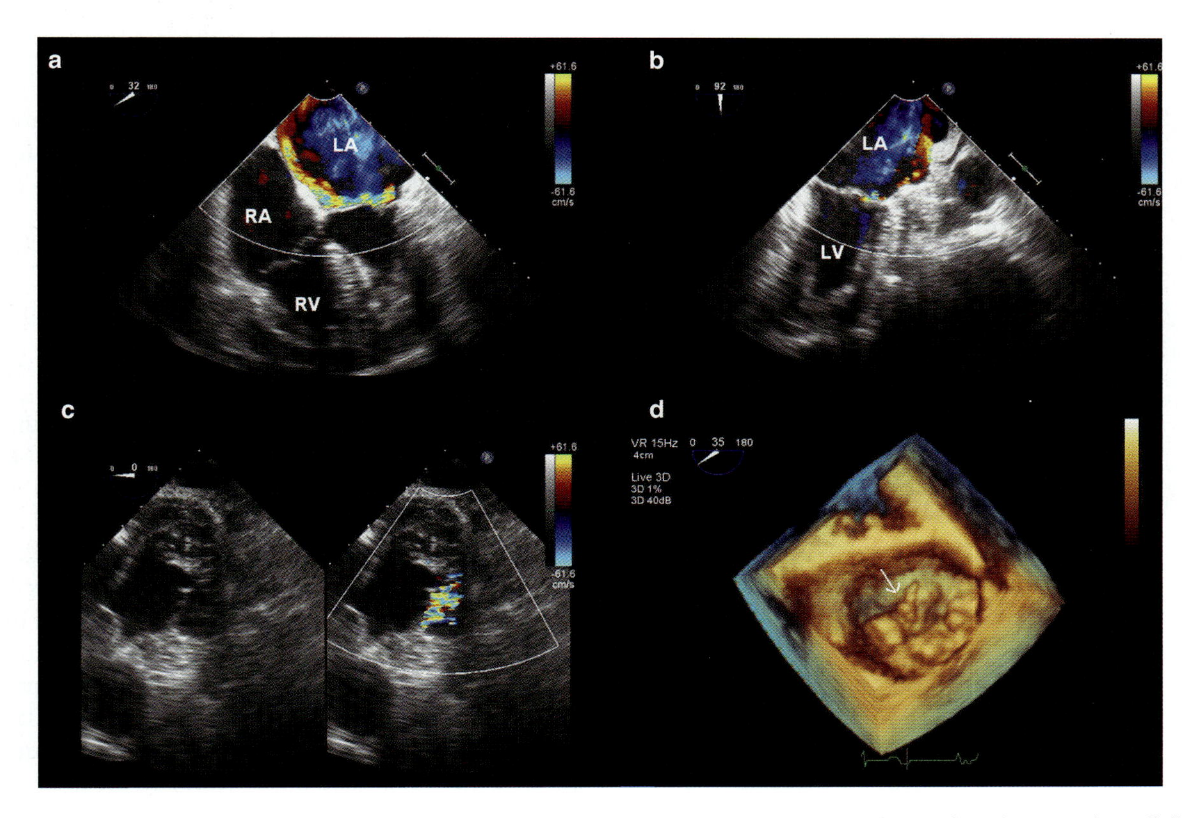

Fig. 4.36 This is a patient with localized flail involving the lateral scallop (P1) of the posterior mitral leaflet. The eccentric medially directed mitral regurgitant jet is demonstrated in the transesophageal four-chamber view (**a**) and not in the two-chamber view (**b**). The trans-gastric view (**c**) of the mitral valve shows that the mitral regurgitation originates from the lateral aspect of the leaflet coaptation. Transesophageal 3D image (**d**) is a very good way to assess mitral valve morphology and shows that there is diffuse prolapse involving the posterior mitral leaflet but the flail segment is localized to the lateral scallop (*arrow*)

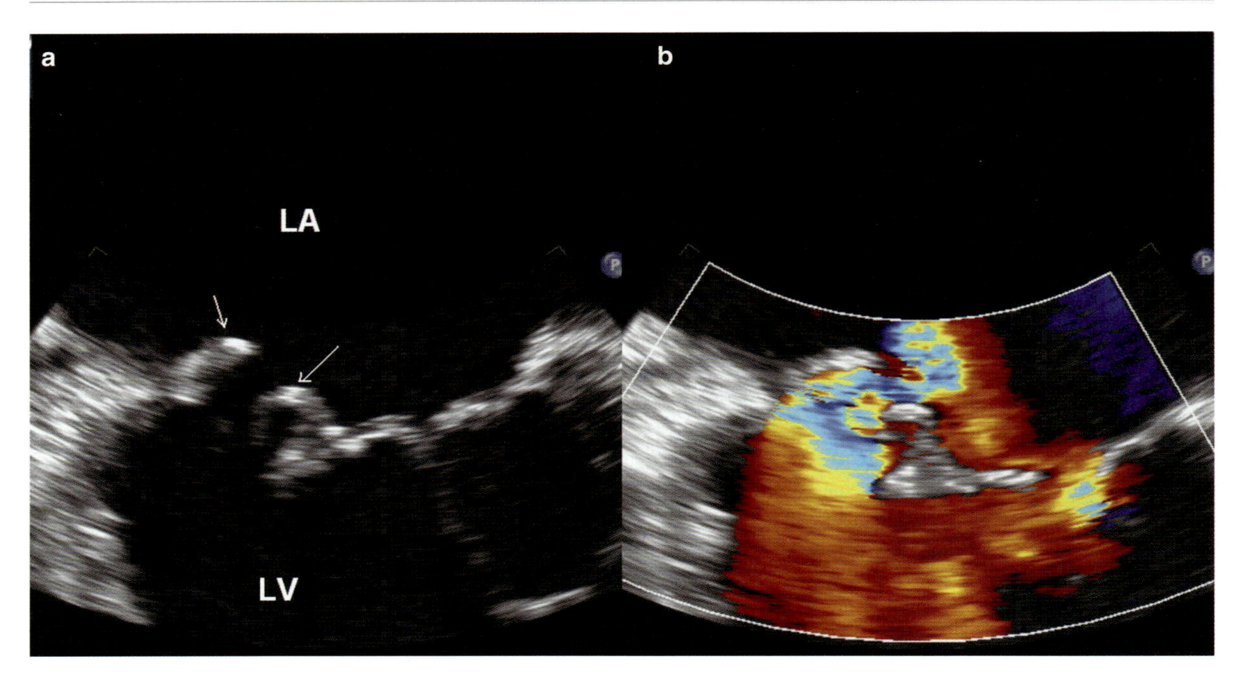

Fig. 4.37 Transesophageal longitudinal view (**a**) of the mitral valve shows that the commissure leaflet (*short arrow*) is severely involved in the myxomatous process and demonstrates marked prolapse. Severe mitral regurgitation is confirmed by color flow imaging (**b**). *LA* left atrium, *LV* left ventricle

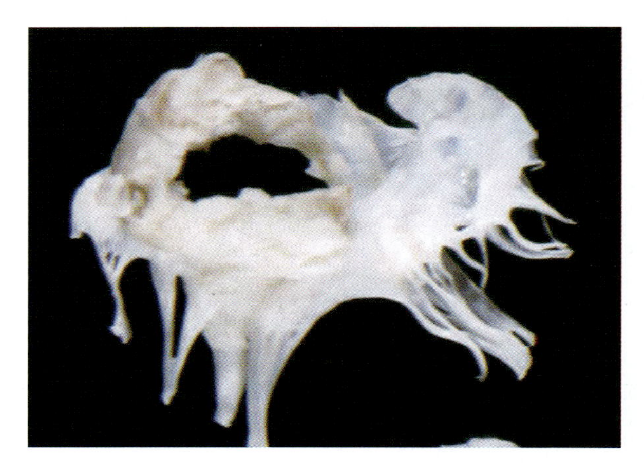

Fig. 4.38 Surgically excised anterior mitral leaflet with large defect from destruction by bacterial infective endocarditis. Endocarditis may cause mitral regurgitation in many ways: endocarditis may destroy the leaflet, the chords and cause ring and myocardial abscesses. Emboli may cause infarct and rupture of the papillary muscle leading to a flail leaflet

involved leaflet still points into the left ventricular cavity and chaotic motion of a ruptured chord is not present. Elongated chords can be due to myxomatous changes of the chords, which are prone to rupture. Rheumatic involvement can also lead to elongation of the chords providing one reason for the development of mitral regurgitation in this setting (Fig. 4.40).

Ventricular Causes of Mitral Regurgitation

Abnormal dilatation or fibrosis and calcification of the annulus may also lead to regurgitation. A dilated mitral annulus is a result of left atrial enlargement which is invariably present in the setting atrial fibrillation and in patients with mitral regurgitation. There is truth in the saying that "mitral regurgitation begets mitral regurgitation" as progressive left atrial dilatation secondary to mitral regurgitation leads to enlargement of the mitral annulus further contributing to the failure of proper mitral leaflet coaptation. In addition, left ventricle dilation of any cause may lead to poor opposition of the mitral leaflets (Fig. 4.41). This is due to the annular dilatation and also to misalignment of the papillary muscles with leaflet "restriction" due to the geometrical distortion of the ventricle. Part of mitral valve repair

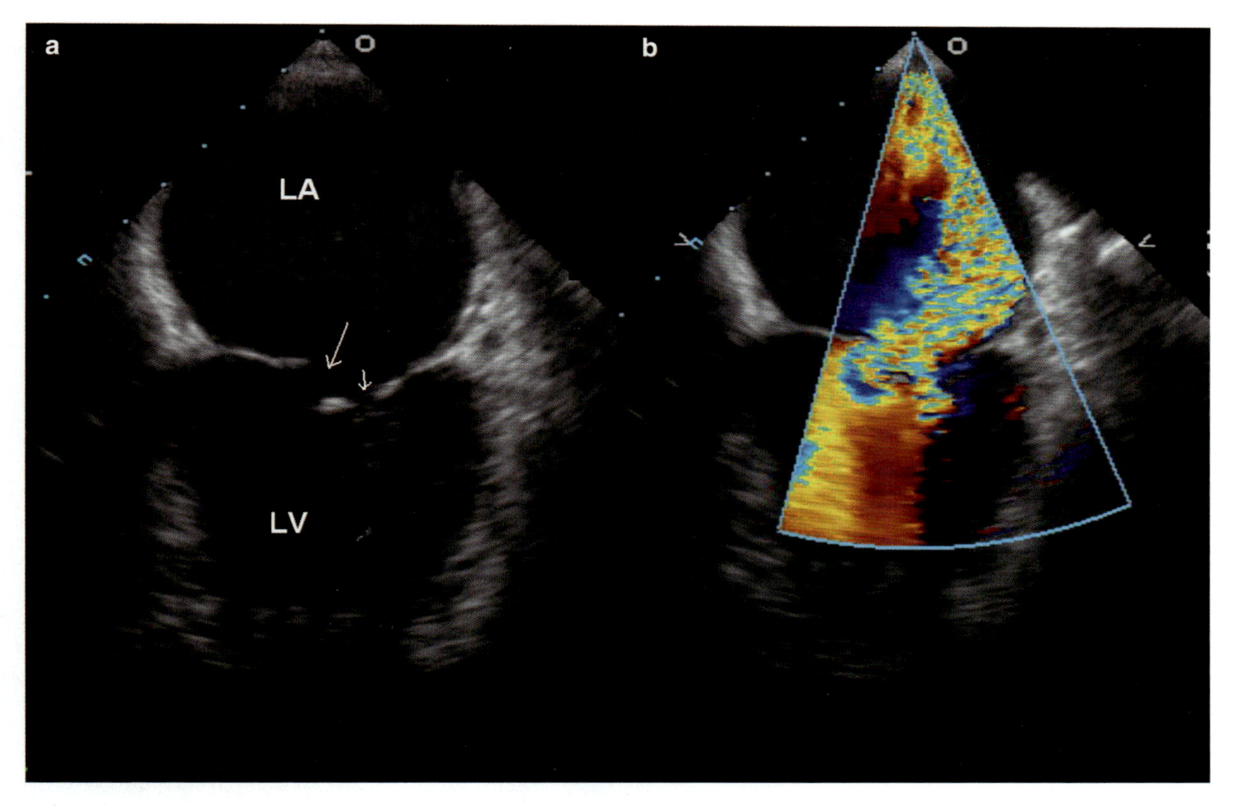

Fig. 4.39 This patient has infective endocarditis involving the mitral valve. The transesophageal view (**a**) in systole shows that the mitral leaflet coaptation (*short arrow*) appears normal but there is a large defect (*long arrow*) on the anterior mitral leaflet. The color-flow image (**b**) shows severe mitral regurgitation mainly from the perforation at the anterior mitral leaflet as evidenced by the large flow convergence. *LA* left atrium, *LV* left ventricle

is to re-establish good contact between the leaflets. Ventricular aneurysm surgery may involve ventricular remodeling in an attempt to improve leaflet contact.

Mitral Annular Calcification

Mitral annular calcification (MAC) is a common finding in the hearts of elderly patients, especially females. MAC is probably a pathological process due to degenerative changes in the mitral annulus. Its incidence is about 8–10% in those over the age of 50 years; however, the incidence of MAC increases to over 40% in those over 90 years.

Although it is frequently considered as a cause for mitral regurgitation, our experience suggests that it is an associated finding rather than a cause for mitral regurgitation. We have observed a similar prevalence and severity of mitral regurgitation in the elderly patients with or without MAC, after adjusting for age and other clinical variables such as systemic hypertension. When moderate or greater mitral regurgitation is present in a patient with MAC, it is important to look for another cause before ascribing the mitral regurgitation to the presence of mitral annular calcification.

MAC can co-exist with sclerotic changes of the mitral leaflets, which are thickened and retracted, causing mitral regurgitation (Fig. 4.42). It is often associated with myxomatous degeneration of the mitral valve leaflets and in fact some think the leaflet disorder puts stress on the annulus causing it to secondarily degenerate. The calcium is localized to the mitral ring, the most common site being the base of the posterior mitral leaflet (Fig. 4.43). Rarely the calcified mass may extend onto the leaflet, fixing it and producing leaflet immobility. It also may liquefy and form a left atrial posterior wall mass that can be confused with a granuloma or/and abscess. The annulus normally contracts

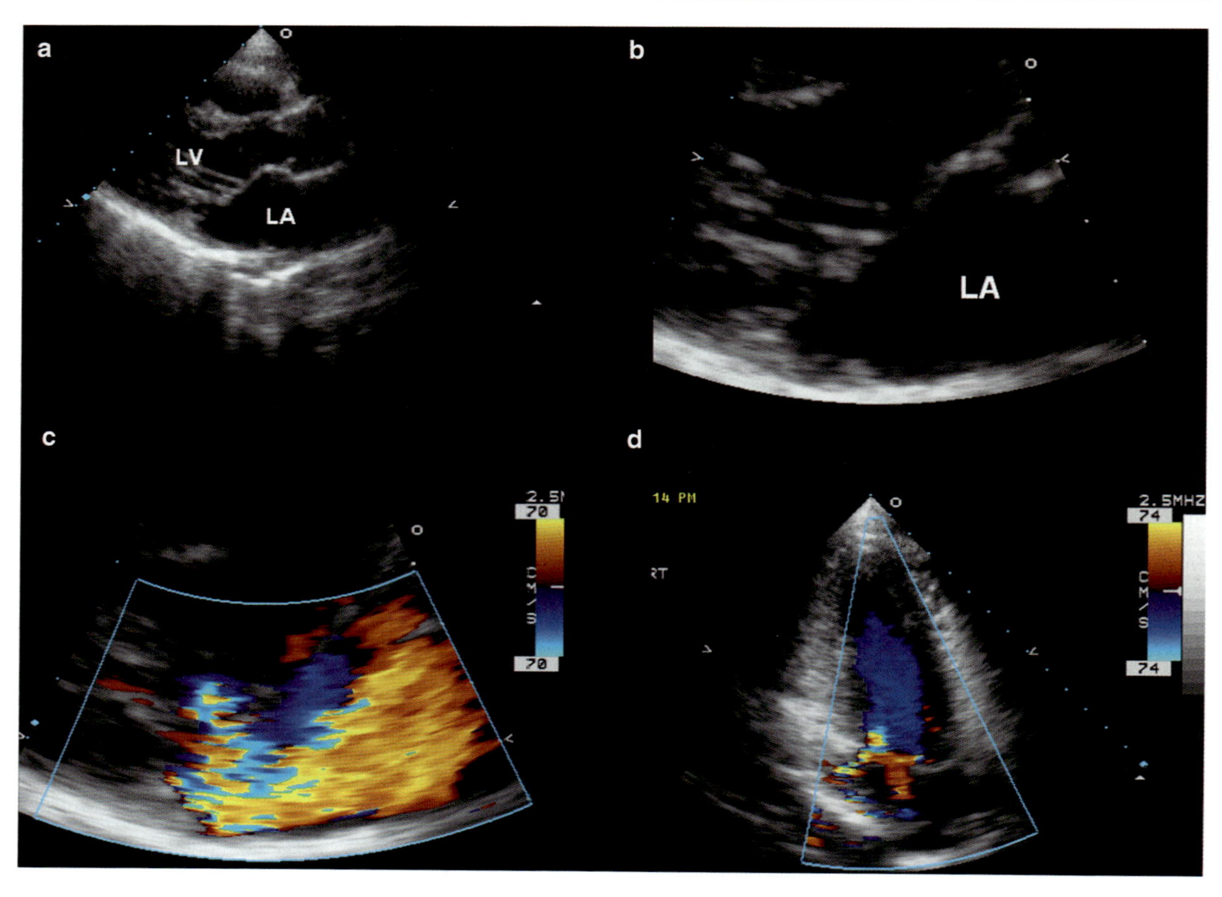

Fig. 4.40 The parasternal long-axis view (**a**, **b**) shows mitral valve prolapse with no flail segments. In addition to the redundant leaflets, the chords are also elongated such that the anterior leaflet is closing behind the posterior mitral leaflet. Color flow imaging in the parasternal long-axis and apical two-chamber views (**c**, **d**) show that mitral regurgitation is directed posteriorly. *LA* left atrium, *LV* left ventricle

with the ventricle and the ventricle squeezes and shortens with systole. If the annulus is rigid, the ring cannot contract and some of the constriction and squeezing motions of systole are lost. MAC may also ulcerate with thrombus deposition with potential for embolization (Fig. 4.44) [22].

Papillary Muscle Causes of Mitral Regurgitation

The left ventricle papillary muscles may become dysfunctional and contribute to valvular regurgitation. With myocardial ischemia the muscles may temporarily stop contracting, a process known as stunning. With chronic heart failure and chronic ischemia the myocytes may undergo degenerative myocytolysis and lose their myofilaments reverting to a more fetal or primitive phenotype for survival. This is known as hibernating myocardium. This myocardium is not contractile, but is viable and salvageable, so papillary muscle function may return.

In acute myocardial infarction, the muscles may infarct and die. This dead muscle is no longer contractile. In the most dramatic manifestation, the papillary muscle may rupture leading to acute mitral regurgitation and severe congestive heart failure. Mitral valve replacement is often necessary. Rupture of the posterior medial papillary muscle is more common as it generally has a single blood supply from the right coronary artery, whereas the anterolateral papillary muscle can

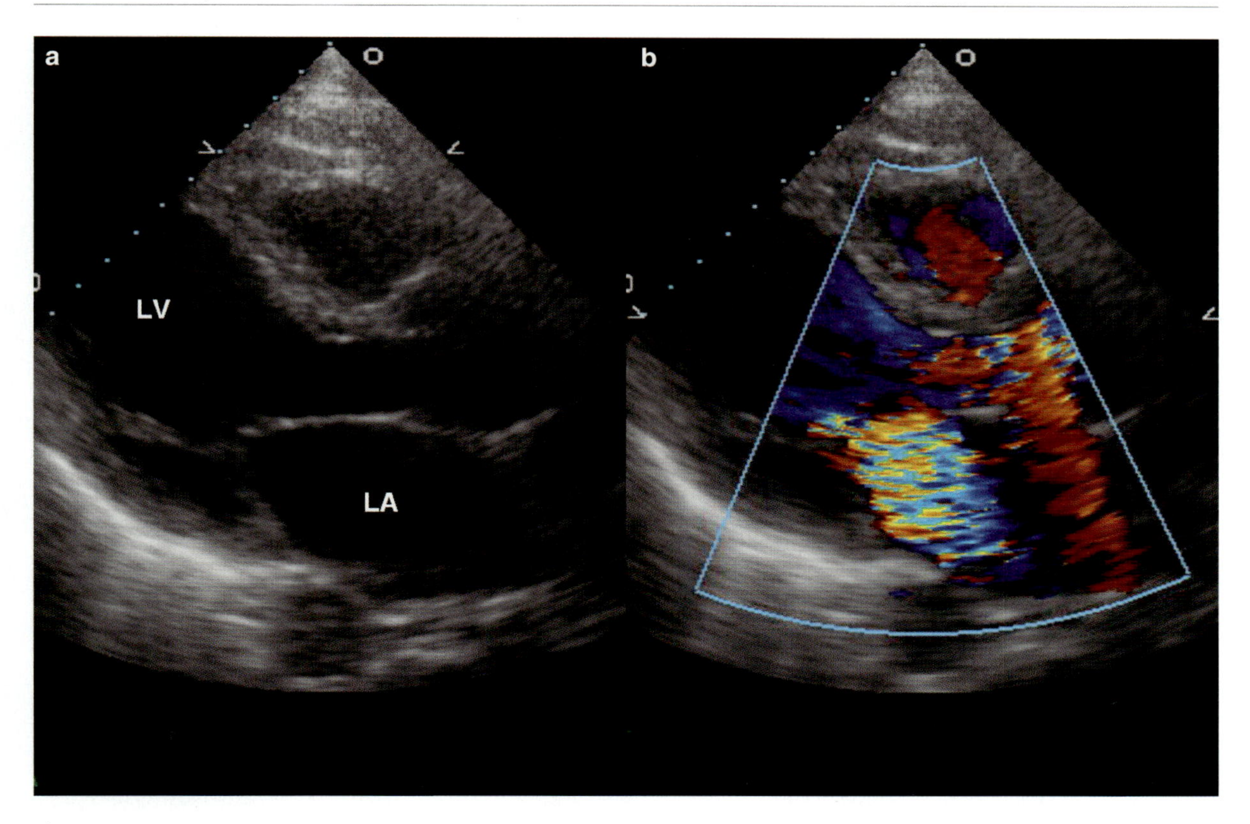

Fig. 4.41 The parasternal long-axis view in systole (**a**) shows that the left ventricle is dilated and the mitral annulus is similarly dilated. The mitral leaflet coaptation is apically displaced consistent with tethering of the leaflets due to left ventricular dilatation. The color-flow image (**b**) confirms that presence of severe mitral regurgitation. *LA* left atrium, *LV* left ventricle

have dual blood supply from both the right coronary artery and the left circumflex artery. Rupture of one head of the papillary muscle leads to severe mitral regurgitation, but rupture of the whole head of the papillary muscle results in torrential mitral regurgitation and cardiogenic shock. In the latter situation, the murmur of mitral regurgitation may not be evident, and when present it may appear to be short in duration and not the typical pan-systolic murmur associated with mitral regurgitation.

The ruptured head of the papillary muscle demonstrates excessive movement associated with a flail mitral leaflet (Figs. 4.45, 4.46). The ruptured head protrudes into the left atrium during systole and needs to be differentiated from a vegetation or the curled up end of a ruptured chord. The main differentiating feature is the presence of underlying regional wall motion abnormality and the absent head of the corresponding papillary muscle.

Partial rupture of the papillary muscle is illustrated by a break in the normal contour of the papillary muscle and underlying regional wall motion abnormality (Fig. 4.47). It leads to improper coaptation of the mitral leaflets and significant mitral regurgitation. This is an important condition to recognize, due to the high likelihood of progression to complete rupture leading to worse mitral regurgitation and severe heart failure. Patients with papillary muscle rupture usually have no prior myocardial infarction and relatively preserved left ventricular systolic function. Their prognosis is much improved with prompt surgical intervention.

When a myocardial infarct heals, the papillary muscle may fibrose and become non-contractile. Scar retraction and underlying ventricular distortion and

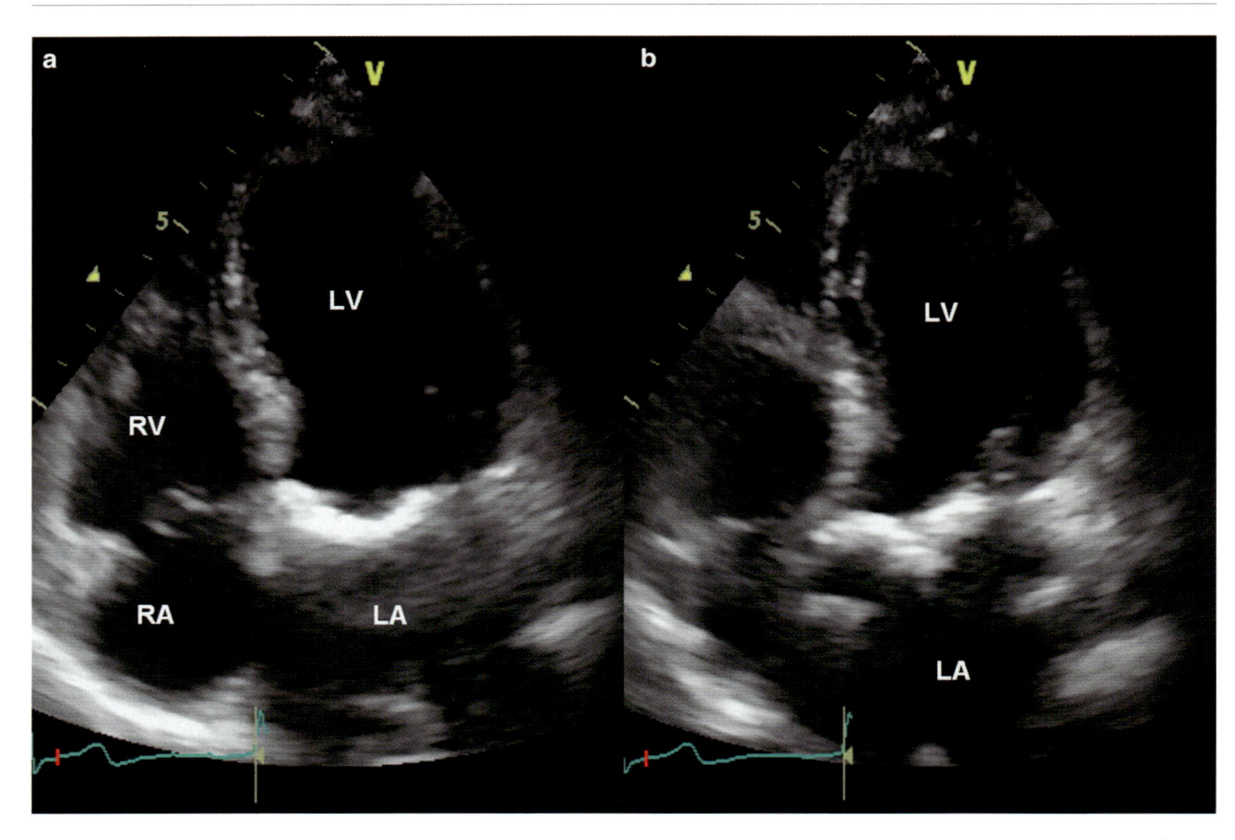

Fig. 4.42 The apical four-chamber (**a**) and five-chamber (**b**) views show that this patient has extensive calcification involving the anterior mitral leaflet in addition to the mitral annular calcification. *LA* left atrium, *LV* left ventricle, *RA* right atrium, *RV* right ventricle

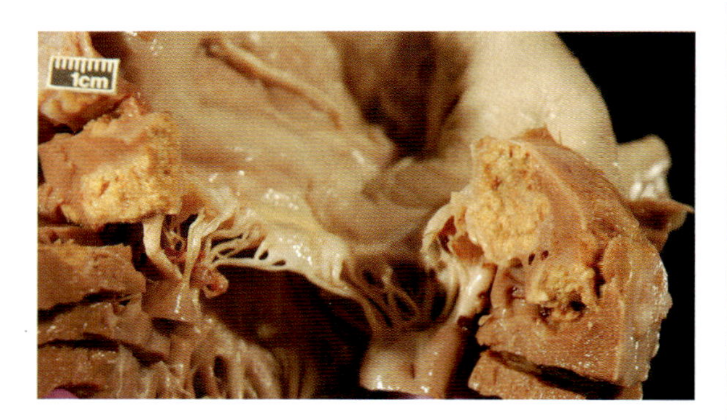

Fig. 4.43 Mitral annular calcification noted at the junction of the left atrium and the left ventricle. This involves the posterior annulus. The calcification restricts ventricular annular movement and may attach to the overlying leaflet fixing it to the ventricular wall ventricle. This involves the posterior annulus. The calcification restricts ventricular annular movement and may attach to the overlying leaflet fixing it to the ventricular wall

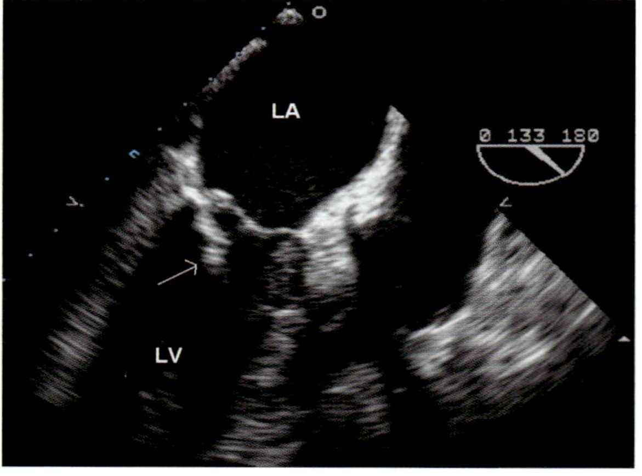

Fig. 4.44 In this transesophageal view, a mobile mass is present attaching to the ventricular surface to the ventricular surface of the mitral annulus, which is calcified. This mass is shown to be organized thrombus at the time of coronary bypass surgery

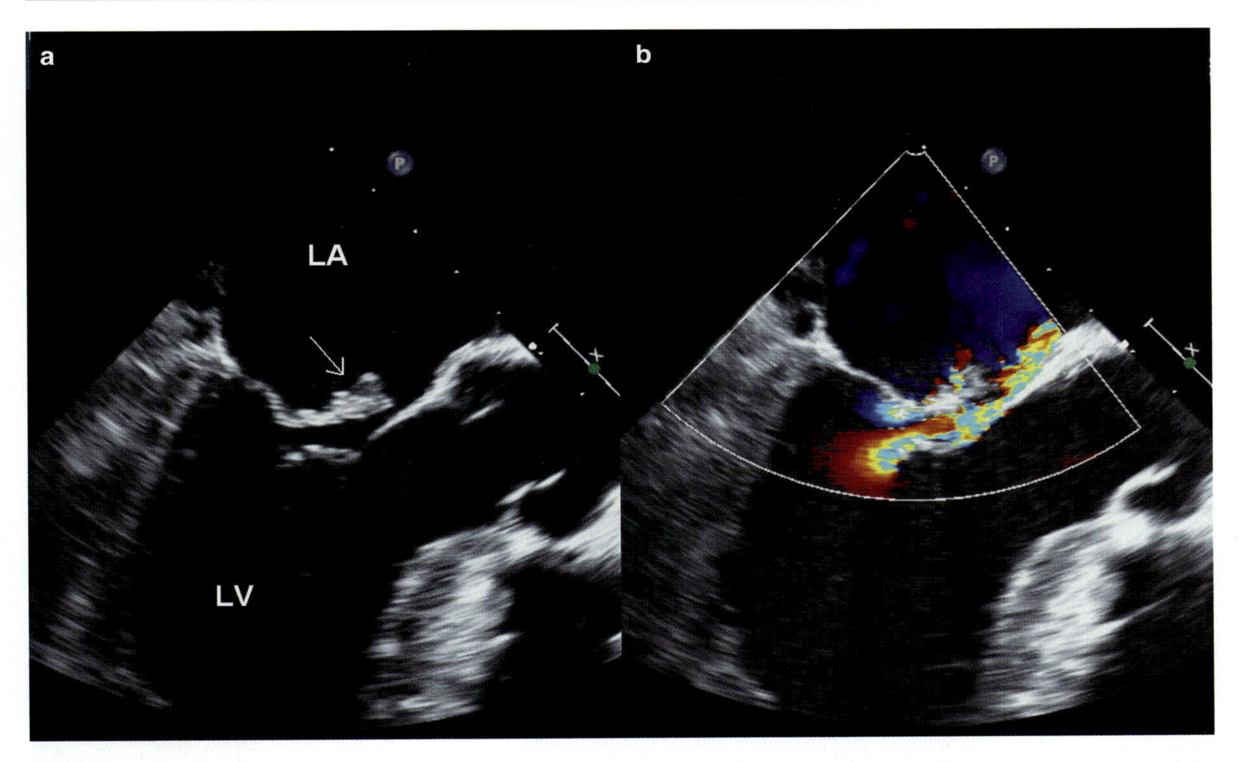

Fig. 4.45 This transesophageal echocardiogram (**a**) shows that there is a large mass which is attached to the posterior mitral leaflet with prolapse into the left atrium. This mass is a ruptured head of the posterior medial papillary muscle. The posterior wall in this view is thin and akinetic. The color-flow image (**b**) shows the presence of anteriorly directed mitral regurgitation. *LA* left atrium, *LV* left ventricle

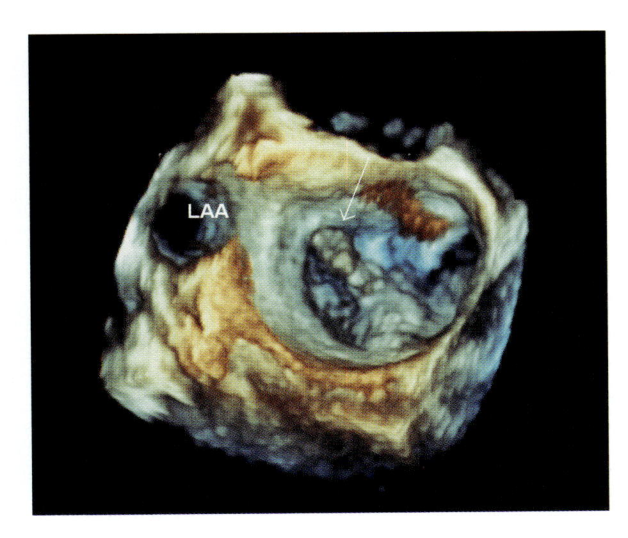

Fig. 4.46 This is a transesophageal 3D image showing the rupture of the papillary muscle head (*arrow*) prolapsing into the left atrium. This is the same patient as in Fig. 4.45. *LAA* left atrial appendage

dilatation from the infarct may distort or restrict the normal mitral valve architecture (Figs. 4.48, 4.49).

Displacement of the papillary muscles from variable causes, but usually in the setting of left ventricular dilatation such as in patients with dilated cardiomyopathy, can also cause improper mitral leaflet coaptation and mitral regurgitation (Fig. 4.41). Both mitral leaflets may have restricted motion, which has been described as tethering. This abnormality is usually more prominent with the posterior mitral leaflet. Tethering of the anterior mitral leaflet in some cases has been attributed to the presence of secondary chords restricting full excursion of the anterior mitral leaflet during systole. In some of these patients, improvement of leaflet excursion and coaptation associated with reduction in mitral regurgitation has been reported with selective cutting of these secondary chords. So far there is still little long term data about the durability of this procedure.

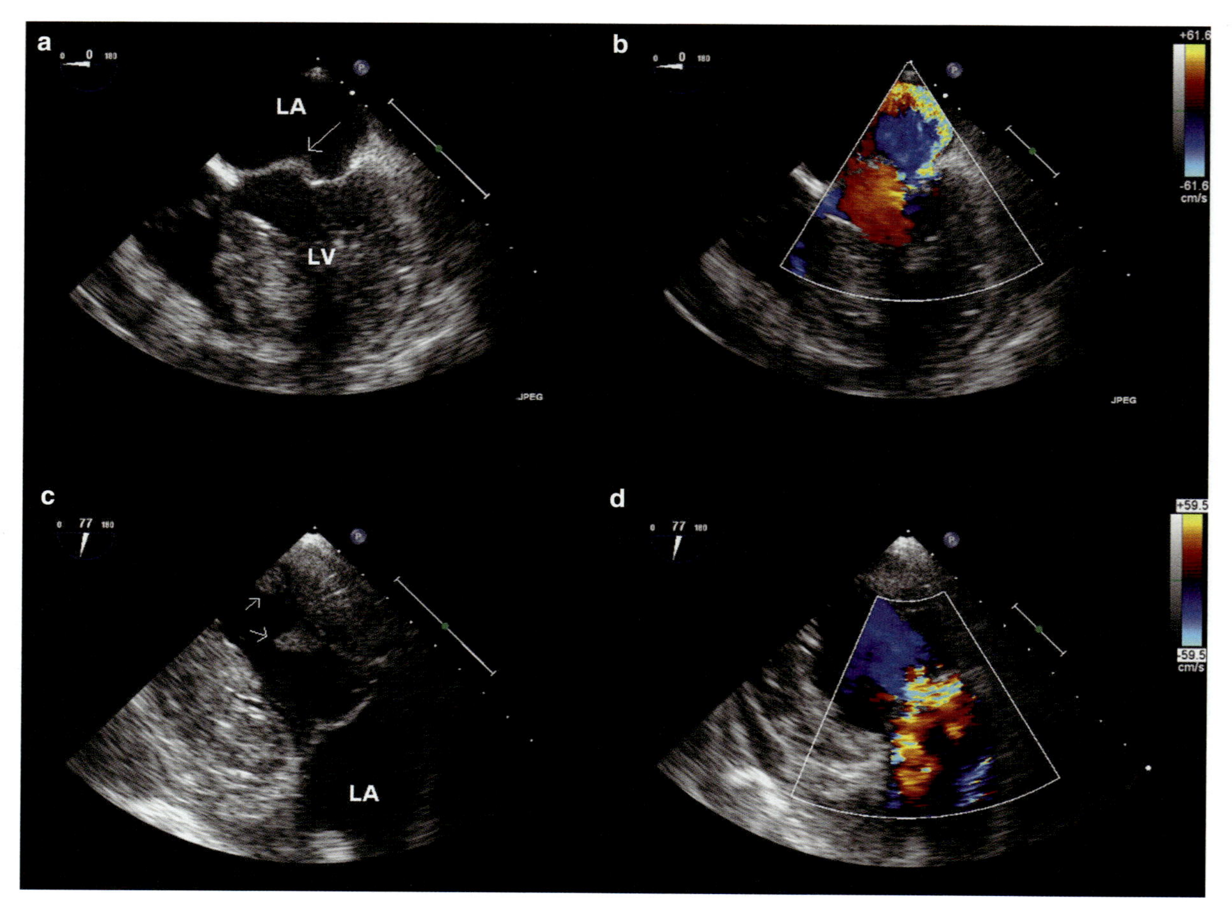

Fig. 4.47 In the transesophageal four-chamber view (**a**) the anterior mitral leaflet shows a marked degree of prolapse (*arrow*) associated with posterior directed mitral regurgitation (**b**). In the trans-gastric left ventricular long-axis view (**c**), the discontinuity of the posteromedial papillary muscle is shown (*arrows*). Part of the papillary muscle is still in continuity thus preventing the papillary muscle from prolapsing into the left atrium during systole. Color-flow image of the trans-gastric view (**d**) confirms severe mitral regurgitation. Patients with partial rupture of the papillary muscle should be considered for urgent surgery as they are at risk for developing complete rupture resulting in torrential mitral regurgitation and cardiogenic shock

Post-mitral Valve Repair

Mitral valve repair has been the procedure of choice in the surgical treatment of degenerative mitral regurgitation. Mitral valve repair usually consists of two components. The first is to correct the specific component of the mitral apparatus responsible for the abnormal coaptation leading to MR. The second is to remodel and stabilize the mitral annulus by the placement of an annular ring or band. Asymmetric leaflet prolapse as a result of redundant leaflet tissue or ruptured chords, particularly involving the posterior mitral leaflet, can be managed by resection of more than one-third of the posterior mitral leaflet. If the anterior mitral leaflet is involved, chordal reconstruction using chordal transfer or artificial chords can be performed. Some form of annuloplasty is then performed to remodel the annulus and to support the leaflet repair. A complete annular ring, be it flexible or rigid, is widely used for this purpose. Recently, the use of an incomplete ring or posterior band to remodel the mitral annulus has become popular (Fig. 4.50). In order to ensure proper coaptation of the mitral leaflets, the Alfieri procedure may be performed. This

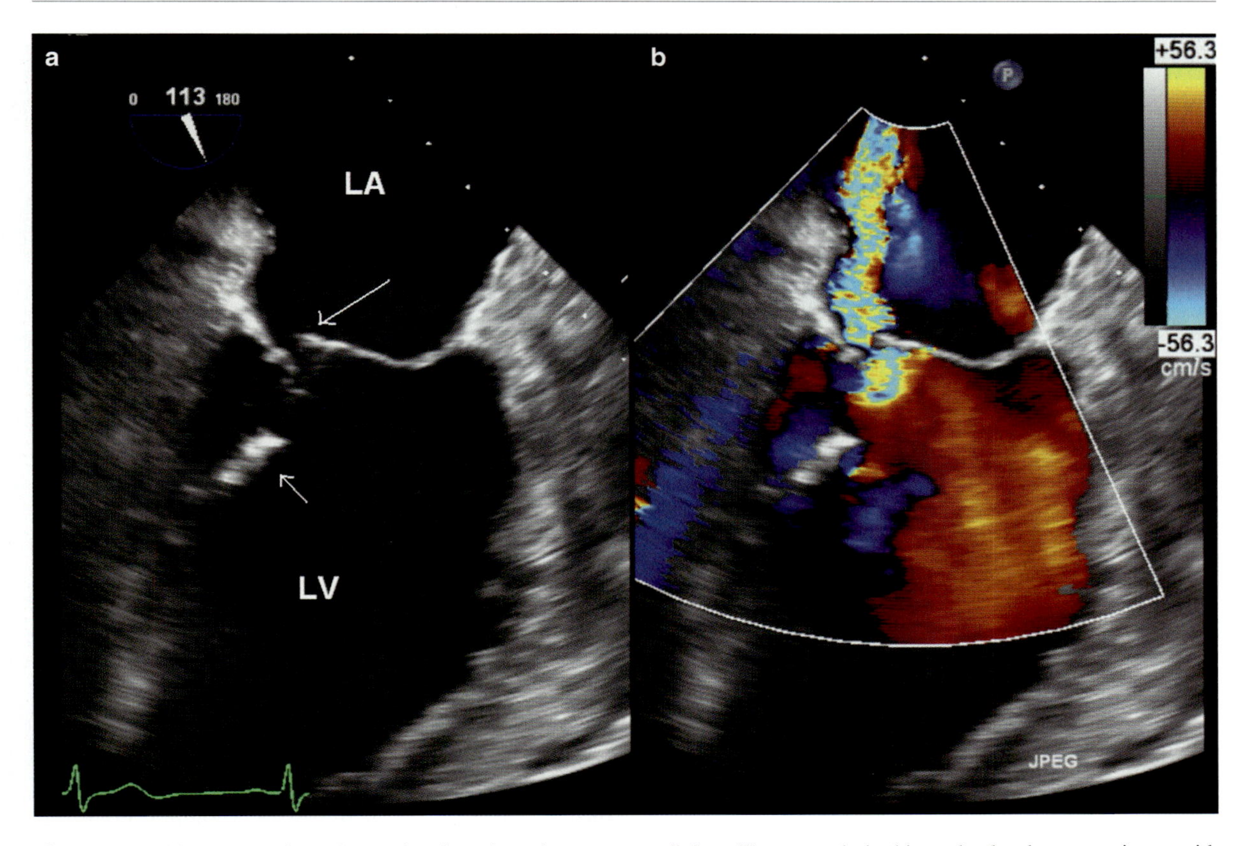

Fig. 4.48 In this transesophageal two-chamber view, the posteromedial papillary muscle is thin and echo-dense consistent with fibrosis secondary to previous infarction (**a**). The anterior mitral leaflet prolapses into the left atrium without evidence of a flail segment. Color-flow image (**b**) shows severe mitral regurgitation which is posteriorly directed. *LA* left atrium, *LV* left ventricle

involves suturing the tips of the mitral leaflets creating a double-orifice mitral valve (Fig. 4.51).

The mitral valve area is certainly reduced as a result of the procedure. The mitral annulus is reduced in size with the implantation of the annular ring or posterior band, and resection of the posterior mitral leaflet, which can be greater than one-third of the leaflet, not only reduces the area of the posterior mitral leaflet, but also frequently restricts the excursion of the posterior mitral leaflet. There may also be a tendency to use an undersized ring to increase the degree of leaflet coaptation. These anatomic changes should be considered in the echocardiographic follow-up of these patients. Proper coaptation of the mitral leaflets is the result of a successful mitral repair surgery, but excursion of the leaflets should be evaluated as well. One or both mitral leaflets may be restricted in excursion as a result of the surgery. The mid portion of the posterior leaflet following quadrangular resection frequently appears immobile, best seen in the parasternal long-axis view, and yet not associated with functional significance. On the other hand restricted excursion of the anterior mitral leaflet due to chordal transfer from the posterior mitral leaflet may be associated with some degree of mitral stenosis (Fig. 4.52). Systolic anterior mitral leaflet motion is a dreaded complication, as it may be an indication of dynamic subaortic stenosis which can have severe functional consequences. The integrity of the mitral annular ring is an essential component of the long term success of the surgery. Dehiscence of the ring can occur months to years after repair surgery and should be considered in patients who develop mitral regurgitation following mitral valve repair.

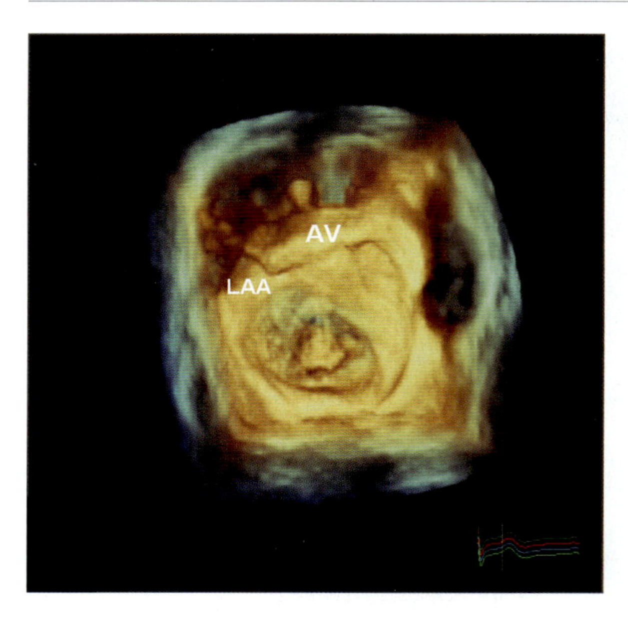

Fig. 4.49 Transesophageal 3D image of the mitral valve from the atrial perspective showing that the anterior mitral leaflet appears normal, but demonstrates marked degree of prolapse into the left atrium. This is the same patient as in Fig. 4.48. The prolapse of the anterior mitral leaflet is related to infarcted and fibrotic posteromedial papillary muscle. *AV* aortic valve, *LAA* left atrial appendage

Assessment of Severity of Mitral Regurgitation

A small degree of mitral regurgitation can frequently be seen by color flow imaging, and thus it is important to differentiate a small amount of physiological mitral regurgitation from clinically significant mitral regurgitation. Due to the sensitivity of color flow imaging in the detection of mitral regurgitation, many individuals are diagnosed to have mild mitral regurgitation which is not clinically significant and not associated with a systolic murmur. At the same time, significant mitral regurgitation can be missed since the mitral regurgitant jet is frequently eccentric and may escape detection if only the conventional views are used. Mitral leaflet coaptation is the key event in patients with suspected mitral regurgitation. If proper leaflet coaptation is present, significant mitral regurgitation is highly unlikely. Similarly abnormal leaflet coaptation is invariably associated with mitral regurgitation and the type of the coaptation abnormality predicts the direction and severity of the mitral regurgitant jet.

There are many echocardiographic findings that have been reported to be useful in assessing the severity of mitral regurgitation, but there is no one consistently reliable measure. A comprehensive approach is essential to avoid pitfalls. Such an approach includes careful assessment of the integrity of the entire mitral apparatus due to the close relationship between structure and function. Helpful guidelines have been developed and provide useful framework on how to approach mitral regurgitation from an echocardiographic viewpoint (Table 4.2) [23]. It is crucial to recognize the strengths and limitations of all the different measures of the severity of mitral regurgitation (Table 4.3).

Quantitative Approach

Recent studies suggest that quantitative measures of mitral regurgitation are preferred in the assessment of mitral regurgitation and these predict outcome. The proposed measures are the effective regurgitant orifice area and the regurgitant volume (Table 4.2). The continuity equation is the basis for the calculation of regurgitant volume. The same stroke volume that passes through the mitral valve in diastole also passes through the aortic valve in systole, if there is no mitral or aortic regurgitation. When there is mitral regurgitation, but no aortic regurgitation, the stroke volume through the mitral orifice during diastole exceeds the stroke volume through the aortic valve during systole, with the difference being the mitral regurgitant volume. Accurate assessment of the flow volumes at the mitral and aortic valves is a prerequisite for the calculation of the regurgitant volume. There are a number of technical issues involved in this calculation. The mitral orifice area shows dynamic change throughout diastole making it difficult to be quantified. Thus, the flow volume at the mitral annulus level is used instead of the flow volume at the mitral orifice. Outside of research studies, there is substantial variability in calculating the flow volume at the mitral annulus which may not necessarily be circular and its dimension can be difficult to be determined accurately.

The effective regurgitant orifice area is calculated using the flow convergence or proximal isovelocity surface area method (Fig. 4.53). This calculation is also based on the principle that the volume flow at the isovelocity shell equals the volume flow passing through the regurgitant orifice at the same instant. The instantaneous

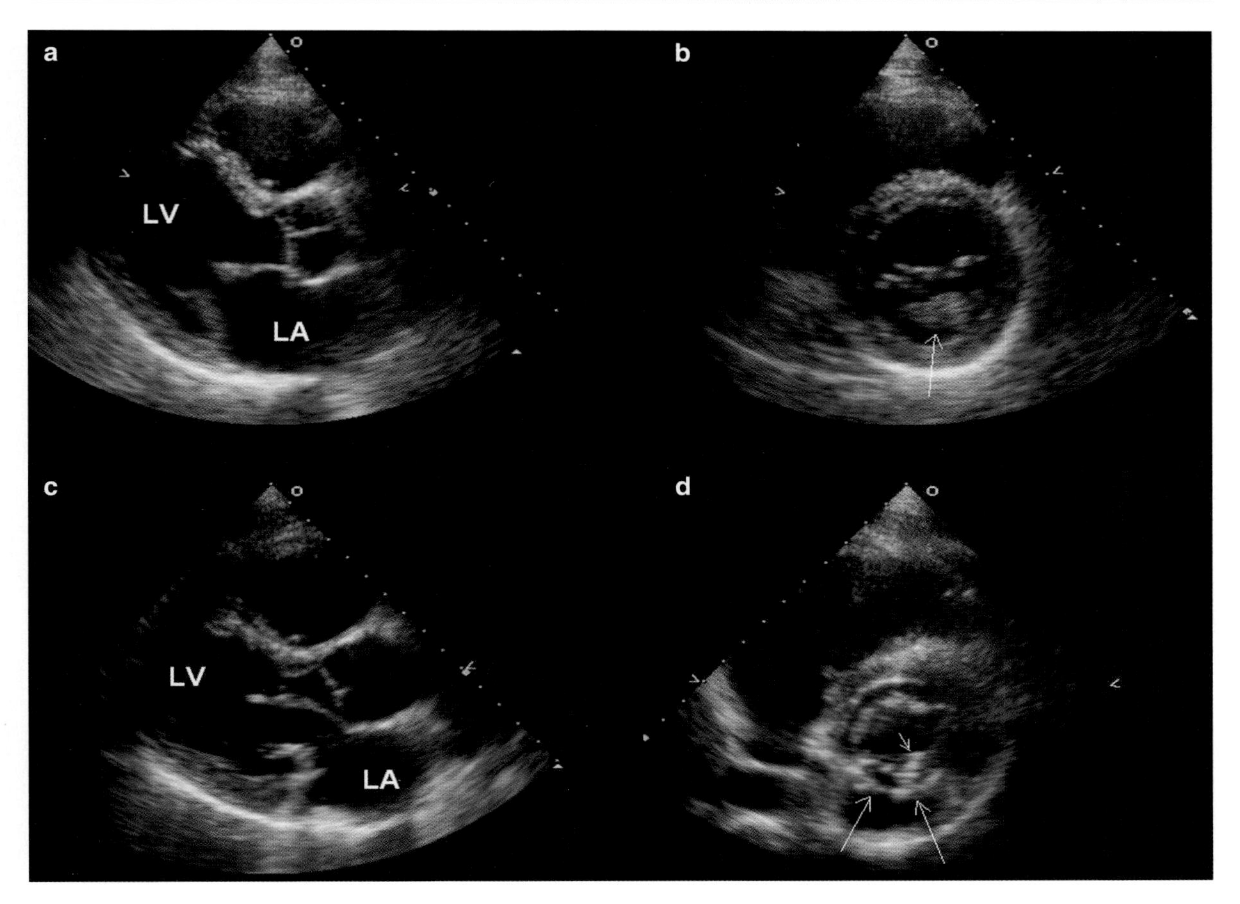

Fig. 4.50 This patient has had mitral valve repair. The pre-operative parasternal long-axis (**a**) and short-axis (**b**) views show that the posterior mitral leaflet is myxomatous best seen in the short-axis view (*arrow*). The mid scallop (P2) of the posterior mitral leaflet is predominantly involved. The postoperative parasternal long-axis (**c**) and short-axis (**d**) views show that a posterior band has been implanted (*long arrows*). There is linear brightness involving the mid portion of the posterior mitral leaflet (*short arrow*) consistent with quadrangular resection of the mid scallop of the posterior mitral leaflet

regurgitant flow at the isovelocity hemispheric shell is the product of the hemispheric area (with radius r_A) times the aliasing velocity (V_A).

Thus, $2\pi r_A^2 \times V_A$ = effective regurgitant orifice area (EROA) × maximum mitral regurgitation (MR) velocity, and

$$\text{EROA} = \frac{2\pi r_A^2 \times V_A}{V_{MR}}$$

Adjusting the color scale and baseline to achieve a hemispheric shell can be challenging. Frequently the isovelocity shell is not hemispheric in shape and it is difficult to adjust for the variation in the shape in the calculation. The largest convergence area is used but the convergence area is dynamic and may change throughout systole. The maximum mitral regurgitant velocity is used in the calculation, although the maximal velocity may not necessarily coincide in timing with convergence area chosen for this calculation. In day-to-day practice, there is substantial variability in these calculated measures. In order for this to be adopted into routine practice, there needs to be data specific to one's own laboratory to confirm that the inter- and intra-observer variabilities in these measures are within the acceptable range.

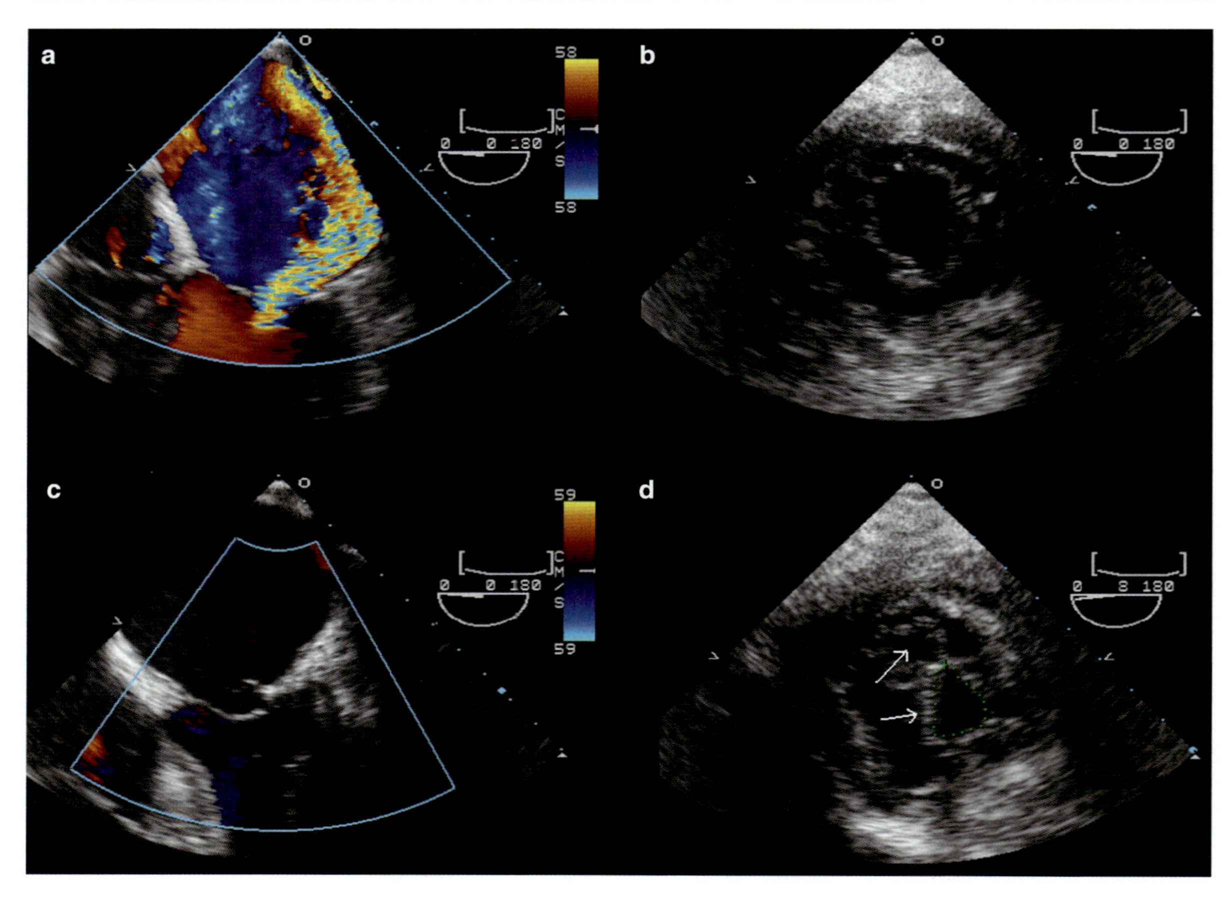

Fig. 4.51 This patient has had mitral valve repair with the Alfieri procedure. The preoperative transesophageal views (**a**, **b**) show that there is severe mitral regurgitation. The postoperative views (**c**, **d**) show that a posterior annular band is implanted. The short-axis view of the mitral valve (**d**) shows that the mitral valve assumes a double orifice appears (*arrows*) due to a suture between the anterior and posterior mitral leaflet. There is no significant residual mitral regurgitation (**c**)

Qualitative Approach

Among the qualitative or semi-quantitative measures, the jet area remains the most popular. The jet area has many pitfalls. It is gain dependent and very much influenced by loading conditions, which explains the consistent underestimation of mitral regurgitation severity in intra-operative echocardiographic studies. The jet area can also underestimate severity when the mitral regurgitant jet is eccentric or wall hugging. Multiple imaging planes need to be used to fully assess the extent of the mitral regurgitant jet (Fig. 4.36). The dimension of the flow convergence area, vena contracta and jet width provide an estimation of the regurgitant area. These measures are less gain dependent but are still affected by eccentricity of the mitral regurgitant jet. In many patients, more than one mitral regurgitant jet is present and this needs to be taken into

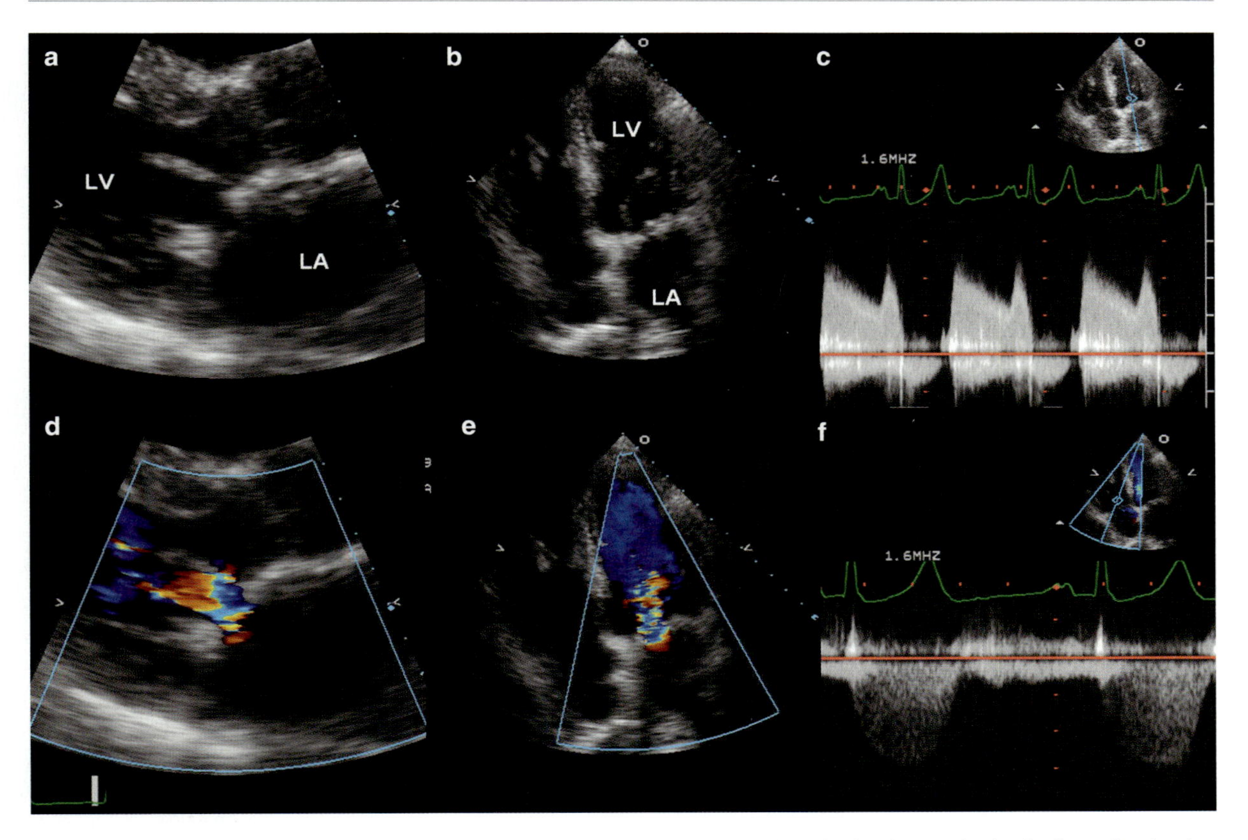

Fig. 4.52 The parasternal long-axis view (**a**) shows typical findings consistent with mitral valve repair. A mitral annular ring has been implanted and the posterior mitral leaflet is thickened and restricted in excursion. Color-flow image of the parasternal long-axis view (**b**) shows a restricted mitral inflow orifice. The apical four-chamber view (**c**) shows the presence of a complete mitral annular ring and the corresponding color-flow image (**d**) shows a narrowed mitral orifice with increased transvalvular velocity which is confirmed by continuous wave Doppler (**e**). The mean resting mitral gradient is 10 mmHg. There is also elevation in right ventricular systolic pressure as evidenced by the tricuspid regurgitation velocity (**f**)

consideration in assessing severity. Another useful qualitative indicator of severe mitral regurgitation is blunted or reverse systolic flow in the pulmonary veins (Fig. 4.54) [24]. Systolic blunting of the pulmonary venous flow can also be seen in patients with severe left ventricular dysfunction and is therefore not a specific sign for severe mitral regurgitation, whereas systolic flow reversal appears to be specific for severe mitral regurgitation. Both the pulsed wave and continuous wave spectral signals can be useful. Severe mitral regurgitation is associated with a dominant E-wave and a dense MR envelope. The MR CW signal demonstrating late systolic blunting indicates rapid rise in left atrial pressure which is seen in severe and acute mitral regurgitation (Fig. 4.55).

We believe that an integrated approach using all the structural information from 2D and hemodynamic data from Doppler provides the best way to assess the severity of mitral regurgitation. If there is clear evidence of abnormal leaflet coaptation such as the demonstration

Table 4.2 Qualitative and quantitative echocardiographic measures in the assessment of mitral regurgitation severity

	Mild	Moderate	Severe
Structural parameters			
LA size	Normal*	Normal or dilated	Usually dilated**
LV size	Normal*	Normal or dilated	Usually dilated**
Mitral leaflets or support apparatus	Normal or abnormal	Normal or abnormal	Abnormal/flail leaflet/ruptured papillary muscle
Doppler parameters			
Color flow jet area[$]	Small, central jet (usually <4 cm^2 or <20% of LA area)	Variable	Large central jet (usually >10 cm^2 or >40% of LA area) or variable size wall-impinging jet swirling in LA
Mitral inflow – PW	A wave dominant[φ]	Variable	E wave dominant[φ](E usually 1.2 m/s)
Jet density – CW	Incomplete or faint	Dense	Dense
Jet contour – CW	Parabolic	Usually parabolic	Early peaking-triangular
Pulmonary vein flow	Systolic dominance	Systolic blunting	Systolic flow reversal
Quantitative parameters[$]			
VC width (cm)	<0.3	0.3–0.69	≥0.7
R Vol (mL/beat)	<30	30–44 45–59	≥60
RF (%)	<30	30–39 40–49	≥50
EROA (cm^2)	<0.20	0.20–0.29 0.30–0.39	≥0.40

Source: Reproduced by Zoghbi et al. [23]. With permission

* unless there are other reasons for LA or LV dilatation

** except in acute mitral regurgitation

[φ] usually above 50 years of age, in the absence of mitral sterosis or causes of elevated LA pressure.

[$] quantitative paraneters can sub-classify morderate MR into mild-to-moderate and moderate-to-severe.

Table 4.3 Advantages and limitations of echocardiographic measures in the assessment of mitral regurgitation severity

	Utility/advantages	Limitations
Structural parameters		
LA and LV Size	Enlargement sensitive for chronic significant MR, important for outcomes. Normal size virtually excludes significant chronic MR	Enlargement seen in other conditions. May be normal in acute significant MR
MV leaflet/support apparatus	Flail valve and ruptured papillary muscle specific for significant MR	Other abnormalities do not imply significant MR
Doppler parameters		
Jet area – color flow	Simple, quick screen for mild or severe central MR; evaluates spatial orientation of jet	Subject to technical, hemodynamic variation; significantly underestimates severity in wall-impinging jets
Vena contracta width	Simple, quantitative, good at identifying mild or severe MR	Not useful for multiple MR jets; intermediate values require confirmation. Small values; thus small error leads to large % error
PISA method	Quantitative; presence of flow convergence at Nyquist limit of 50–60 cm/s alerts to significant MR. Provides both lesion severity (EROA) and volume overload (R Vol)	Less accurate in eccentric jets; not valid in multiple jets. Provides peak flow and maximal EROA
Flow quantitation – PW	Quantitative, valid in multiple jets and eccentric jets. Provides both lesion severity (EROA, RF) and volume overload (R Vol)	Measurement of flow at MV annulus less reliable in calcific MV and/or annulus. Not valid with concomitant significant AR unless pulmonic site is used
Jet profile – CW	Simple, readily available	Qualitative; complementary data
Peak mitral E velocity	Simple, readily available, A-wave dominance excludes severe MR	Influenced by LA pressure, LV relaxation, MV area, and atrial fibrillation. Complementary data only, does not quantify MR severity
Pulmonary vein flow	Simple, systolic flow reversal is specific for severe MR	Influenced by LA pressure, atrial fibrillation. Not accurate if MR jet directed into the sampled vein

Source: Reproduced by Zoghbi et al. [23]. With permission

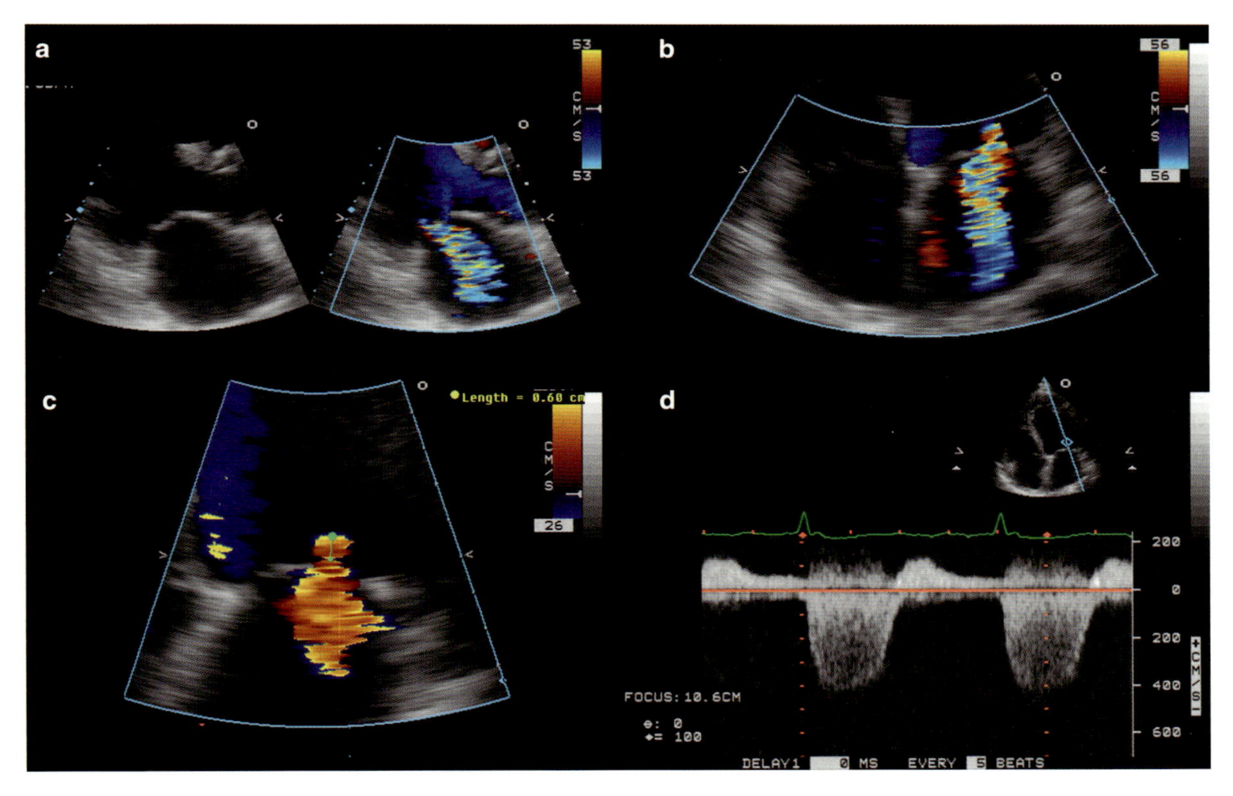

Fig. 4.53 The parasternal long-axis views (**a**) in a patient with functional mitral regurgitation show that the mitral valve is normal, but the coaptation is apically displaced resulting in a centrally directed mitral regurgitation jet, which is confirmed by the four-chamber apical view (**b**). The flow convergence becomes more apparent by down-shifting the aliasing velocity to 26 cm/s (**c**). The peak mitral regurgitation velocity is 4 m/s (**d**). The effective regurgitation orifice area is calculated to be 0.15 cm^2 which is indicative of mild mitral regurgitation

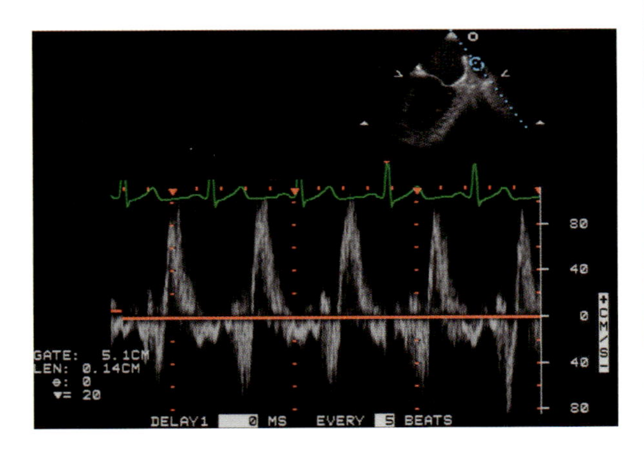

Fig. 4.54 The pulmonary venous flow obtained by transesophageal echocardiography shows systolic flow reversal, which is a specific sign for severe mitral regurgitation

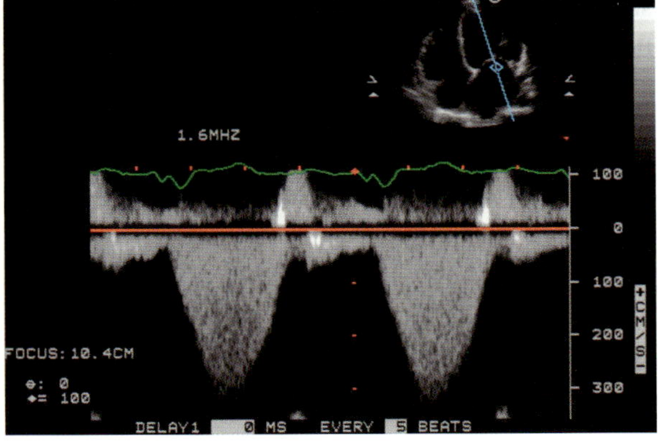

Fig. 4.55 Continuous wave Doppler is used to obtain the mitral regurgitation spectral signal in a patient with dilated cardiomyopathy. The dense, triangular appearance of the mitral regurgitation velocity is indicative of severe mitral regurgitation. The profile of the mitral regurgitation velocity during the early part of systole is consistent with severe left ventricular systolic dysfunction

5 Tricuspid and Pulmonary Valve

Anatomical Considerations

The tricuspid valve has three leaflets, the anterior, the septal and the posterior (Fig. 5.1). The anterior leaflet is the largest of the three. As with all cardiac valves there is a free edge and a line of closure, located on the atrial side of the tricuspid valve. There are three commissures separating each leaflet. Each leaflet has chordae tendonae attached to ventricular papillary muscles, which can vary in number. One of the defining characteristics of a tricuspid valve is that the septal leaflet chordae attach directly to the underlying, adjacent ventricular septum.

The anterior papillary muscle is usually the largest and has multiple heads, as is also common with the posterior muscle. The septal papillary muscle, also termed the muscle of Lancisi, may get smaller with age. There can be considerable variations in the papillary muscles. Multiple small septal papillary muscles are not uncommon. The annulus of the tricuspid valve is discontinuous and not as well formed as the mitral annulus. The tricuspid valve is different than the mitral valve as it is separate from the corresponding semilunar valve, the pulmonary valve. The separation is due to the presence of the infundibular ventricular septum of the morphological right ventricle [1].

The pulmonary valve and the aortic valve are both semilunar valves, a name derived from their shape. They both have corona shaped annulus like a crown. The pulmonary valve is separate from its atrioventricular valve, the tricuspid valve. There are normally three cusps (Fig. 5.2). These are separate from each other at three commissures. The cusps are the anterior, and the left and right cusps. The cusps have a free edge and a line of closure which is along the ventricular surface.

The right-sided cardiac valves, tricuspid and pulmonary valves, have received less attention compared to the left-sided cardiac valves, even though right-sided valvular insufficiency, particularly tricuspid regurgitation, is common in many forms of heart disease [2–4]. The tricuspid and pulmonary valves may become both stenotic

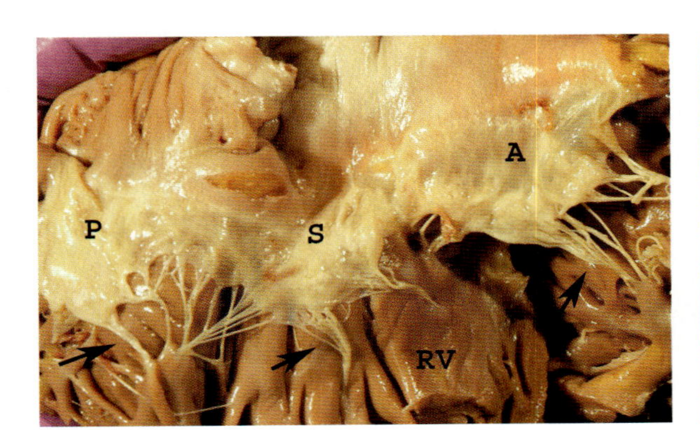

Fig. 5.1 Opened normal tricuspid valve with anterior (*A*), septal (*S*), and posterior (*P*) leaflets. Chordae (*arrows*) connect the leaflets to the papillary muscles and septum of the right ventricle (*RV*)

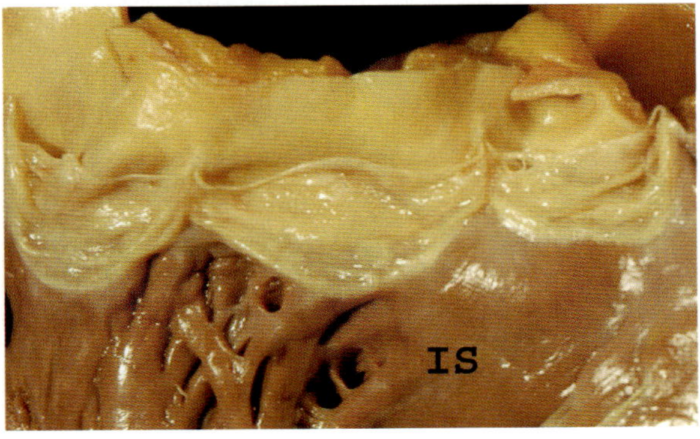

Fig. 5.2 Opened right ventricle outflow tract with pulmonary valve. This is a semilunar valve with three cusps. The infundibular septum (*IS*) separates the pulmonary valve from the tricuspid valve

K.-L. Chan and J.P. Veinot, *Anatomic Basis of Echocardiographic Diagnosis*,
DOI: 10.1007/978-1-84996-387-9_5, © Springer-Verlag London Limited 2011

or regurgitant. Tricuspid regurgitation is usually related to right ventricular dilatation and dysfunction which are frequently related to left-sided heart disease. In the cases with associated heart failure, the tricuspid valve is structurally normal but the annulus dilates and the leaflets or cusps do not oppose properly. There may be some ventricular distortion with an element of chordal restriction in the case of a dilated right ventricle.

Echocardiography Considerations

The tricuspid valve is made up of three leaflets namely anterior, posterior and septal leaflets, with the anterior leaflet being the dominant leaflet and well visualized in most imaging planes. The septal tricuspid leaflet is best seen using the four-chamber view. In the right ventricular inflow tract view, the degree of angulation of the transducer determines which leaflets are visualized. With the transducer angulated slightly rightward from the left ventricular long-axis plane such that the left ventricle can still be present posterior to the right ventricle, the tricuspid leaflets visualized are the anteriorly placed anterior leaflet and the septal leaflet posteriorly. With more extreme rightward and inferior tilt, the right ventricular posterior free wall is visualized with the disappearance of the left ventricle from the view. The two tricuspid leaflets imaged in this fashion are the anteriorly placed anterior leaflet and the posteriorly placed posterior leaflet (Fig. 5.3). All three leaflets can be seen in the same imaging plane, if a true short-axis of the tricuspid valve is obtained either from the subcostal window using a transthoracic approach or the transgastric window using the transesophageal approach (Figs. 5.4, 5.5). The number of papillary muscles is variable. There is invariably a large anterior papillary muscle with its base in proximity with the moderator band. There are two to four small papillary muscles on the septum. Thus septal attachment of the atrioventricular valve is a strong indication that the valve in question is the tricuspid valve rather than the mitral valve.

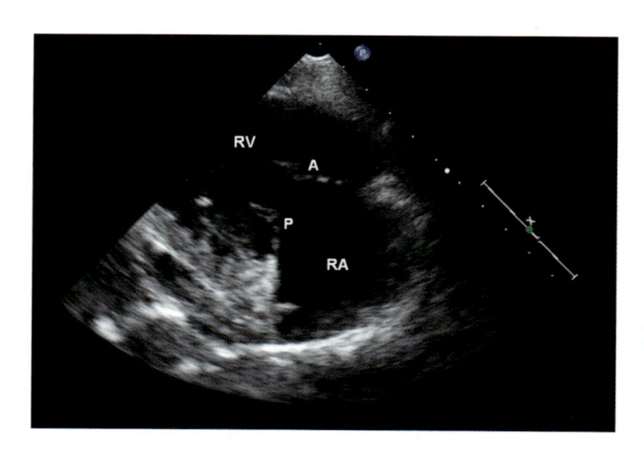

Fig. 5.3 The parasternal right ventricular inflow view shows the anterior and posterior tricuspid leaflets. *A* anterior tricuspid leaflet, *P* posterior tricuspid leaflet, *RA* right atrium, *RV* right ventricle

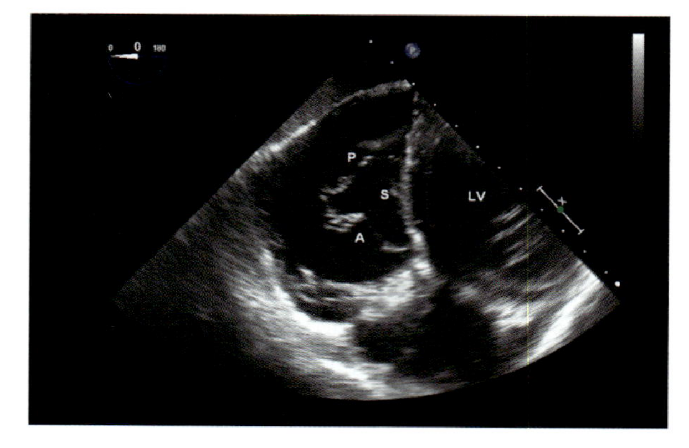

Fig. 5.4 The transesophageal transgastric view shows all three tricuspid leaflets. *A* anterior tricuspid leaflet, *LV* left ventricle, *P* posterior tricuspid leaflet, *S* septal tricuspid leaflet

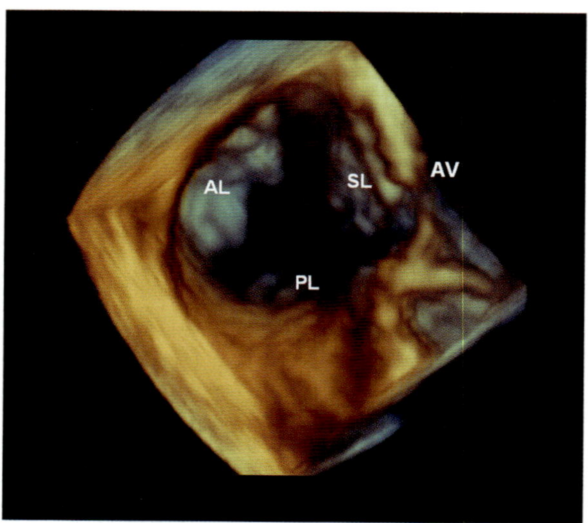

Fig. 5.5 Three-dimensional image of the tricuspid valve is obtained by transesophageal echocardiography. All three tricuspid leaflets can be seen, and the anterior tricuspid leaflet is the largest leaflet. *AV* aortic valve, *AL* anterior tricuspid leaflet, *PL* posterior tricuspid leaflet, *SL* septal tricuspid leaflet

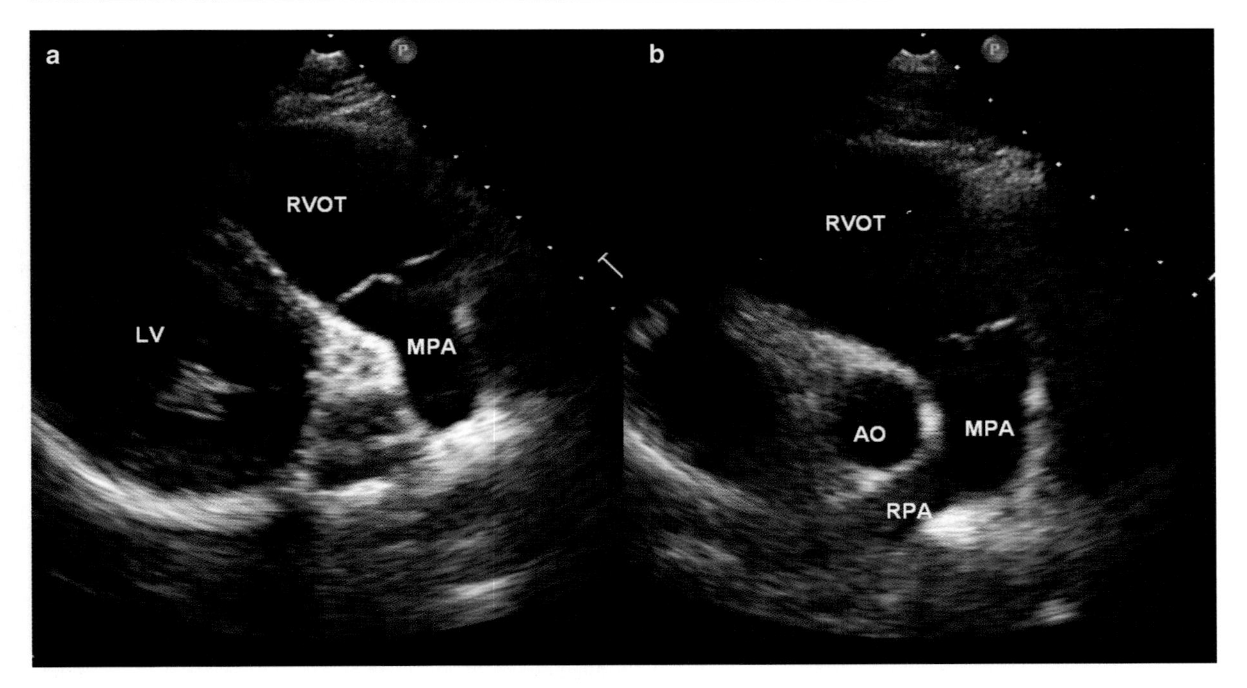

Fig. 5.6 The pulmonary valve can be well imaged using the parasternal window, although a true short-axis of the pulmonic valve usually cannot be obtained. The pulmonic valve and the right ventricular outflow tract are shown in (**a**), and the main and right pulmonary arteries in (**b**). *Ao* aorta, *MPA* main pulmonary artery, *RPA* right pulmonary artery, *RVOT* right ventricular outflow tract

The pulmonary valve is not well seen by echocardiography and its motion is difficult to assess, since it is frequently imaged obliquely. A high left parasternal view is generally best to show the motion of the pulmonic valve with the main pulmonary artery imaged in its long-axis (Fig. 5.6). Since a good short-axis view is difficult to obtain, it is difficult to be sure about which two cusps are displayed in the high left parasternal view. It is of limited clinical significance to identify the exact cusps in the imaging plane. The pulmonary valve can also be well seen using the subcostal short-axis imaging plane, particularly in patients with obstructive lung disease (Fig. 5.7).

Tricuspid Valve Regurgitation

Tricuspid regurgitation is very common and indeed a mild degree of tricuspid regurgitation is ubiquitous and is a normal finding. It is important to note that the severity of tricuspid regurgitation and increasing tricuspid regurgitation velocity do not necessarily go hand in hand (Fig. 5.8). For instance, in patients with primary pulmonary hypertension, the degree of tricuspid regurgitation may be mild or even trivial before the onset of right ventricular dysfunction and dilatation, and yet the velocity of tricuspid regurgitation is high indicative of the elevated right ventricular systolic pressure.

The most common cause for pathologic degree of tricuspid regurgitation, which is at least moderate, is the presence of left heart failure leading to pulmonary hypertension and right ventricular dysfunction and dilatation (Fig. 5.9). In this setting, the tricuspid valve is morphologically normal but the tricuspid annulus is enlarged causing incomplete leaflet coaptation. Evaluated by 3D echocardiography showed that normal tricuspid annulus is ellipsoid and non-planar with a somewhat saddle shape [5]. With progressive enlargement, the annulus of the tricuspid valve becomes more planar and circular. It is uncertain whether it is necessary to reconstitute the non-planar shape of the annulus to ensure long term success of tricuspid annuloplasty to reduce the severity of tricuspid regurgitation.

Tricuspid valve prolapse has been reported in about 20% of patients with myxomatous mitral valve

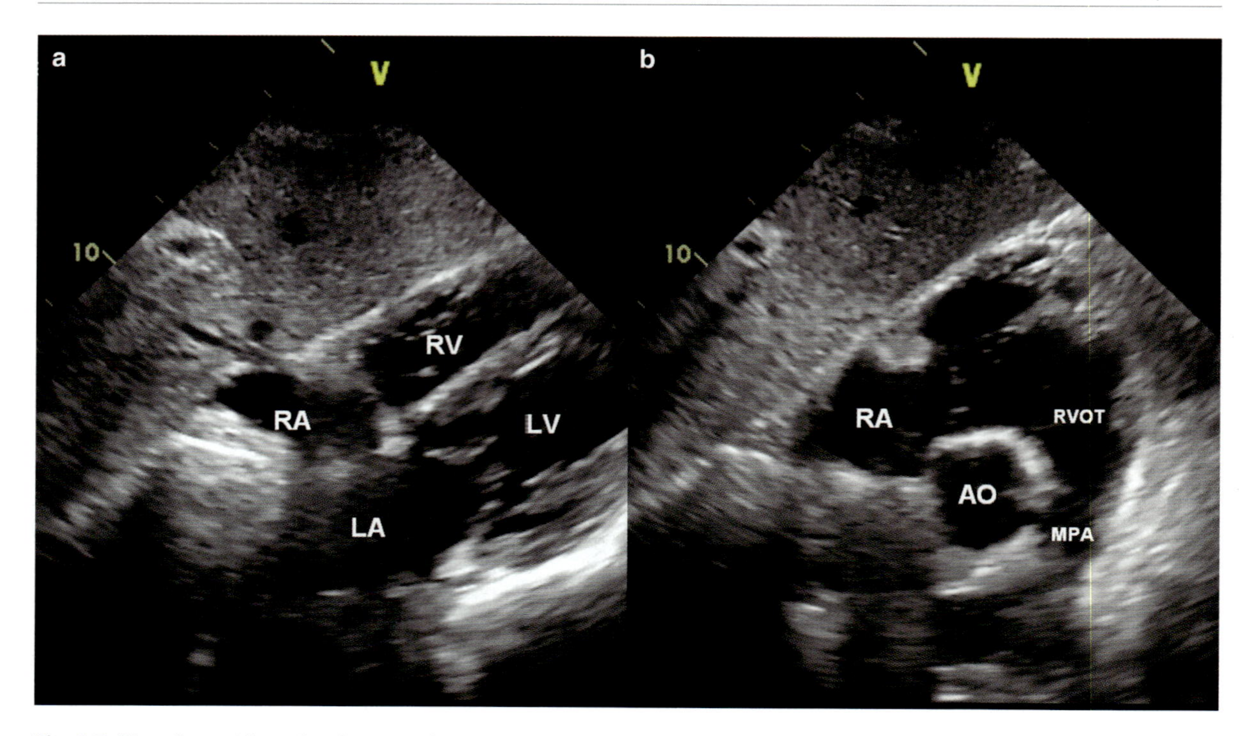

Fig. 5.7 The subcostal four-chamber (**a**) and short-axis (**b**) views can frequently be obtained particularly in patients with obstructive lung disease. The right ventricular outflow tract, pulmonary valve and main pulmonary artery can be imaged using the short-axis view (**b**). *Ao* aorta, *LA* left atrium, *LV* left ventricle, *MPA* main pulmonary artery, *RA* right atrium, *RV* right ventricle, *RVOT* right ventricular outflow tract

prolapse, but the diagnostic criteria for tricuspid valve prolapse are not well defined [6]. Some degree of systolic billowing of the tricuspid leaflets is a normal finding and tricuspid valve prolapse should only be diagnosed when there is excessive billowing associated with redundancy of the tricuspid leaflets (Fig. 5.10). Multiple views should be performed to image all the three leaflets, because prolapse may be quite focal involving only one leaflet and sparing the other two leaflets (Fig. 5.11).

With the decreased prevalence of rheumatic valvular heart disease, rheumatic involvement of tricuspid valve is a rarity in the western world [2, 3]. Nonetheless this should be suspected in patients with evidence of rheumatic mitral valve disease. The changes of the tricuspid leaflets resemble those of the mitral leaflets, namely the leaflets and/or chords are thickened with restriction in excursion and incomplete coaptation of the leaflets leading to tricuspid regurgitation.

Flail of the tricuspid leaflet is recognized by a ruptured chord or a ruptured papillary muscle with excessive motion and protrusion in to the right atrium during systole. Closed chest trauma can lead to papillary muscle rupture and flail of the tricuspid leaflet [7–10]. Another important cause is right ventricular endomyocardial biopsy which inadvertently damages the papillary muscle or valve chord resulting in flail of the tricuspid leaflet (Fig. 5.12). This is an important consideration in patients post cardiac transplant that develop severe tricuspid regurgitation during follow-up [11, 12]. Although pacemaker leads are well tolerated and not associated with tricuspid valve dysfunction in most patients, they can result in severe tricuspid regurgitation in some patients [13]. This complication may occur when the pacemaker lead interferes with tricuspid leaflet motion due to excessive looping of the pacemaker lead. Other mechanisms include leaflet adhesion, erosion or perforation. (Figs. 5.13, 5.14). In these patients, removal or reposition of the lead needs to be considered to reduce the severity of tricuspid regurgitation, but this needs to be balanced with the

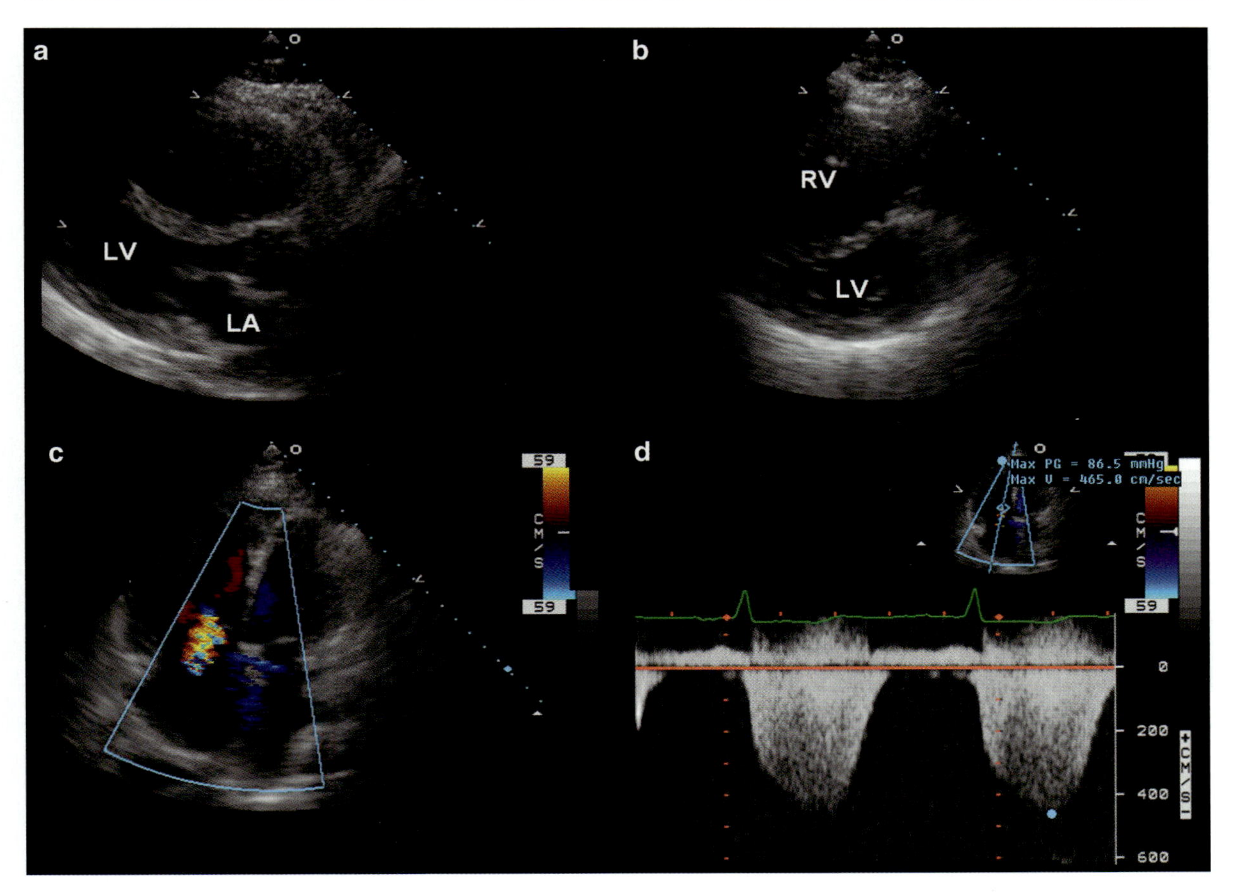

Fig. 5.8 In this patient with severe idiopathic pulmonary hypertension, the parasternal long-axis (**a**), short-axis (**b**) and apical four-chamber (**c**) views show severe dilatation of the right ventricle. There is flattened ventricular septum in keeping with pulmonary hypertension. The continuous wave Doppler (**d**) shows that tricuspid regurgitation has a very high velocity (4.7 m/s), but the severity of tricuspid regurgitation is only mild to moderate (**c**)

risk of further damage to the tricuspid leaflets during extraction of the lead. Other causes of tricuspid regurgitation are infective endocarditis and Ebstein's anomaly. Infective endocarditis can cause tricuspid regurgitation in many ways, including leaflet erosion, retraction, chordal rupture, leaflet perforation, annular dilatation and interference of leaflet coaptation by the vegetation [14–16]. These are discussed in greater detail in the chapter on endocarditis.

Ebstein's Anomaly

Ebstein's anomaly is an important cause of tricuspid regurgitation in the young and the old. Normally, the atrioventricular valves delaminate from their underlying developing ventricle. In the case of the tricuspid valve, the three leaflets delaminate from the out pouched and rotating bulbus chamber. Failure to delaminate causes the valve leaflets to become elongated and only come off the wall of the ventricle close to the apex (Figs. 5.15, 5.16). The right atrium seems huge (in reality it usually is) and the ventricle has "atrialized." Not unexpectedly the valve leaflets are not well formed and are dysplastic [17]. The posterior and septal leaflets are usually the ones that are chiefly affected by the apical displacement and the anterior leaflet often is the most dysplastic. The anterior leaflet may be large, thick, abnormally formed and with multiple orifices and defects. The chordae are often short and thick. Underneath the leaflets the right ventricle

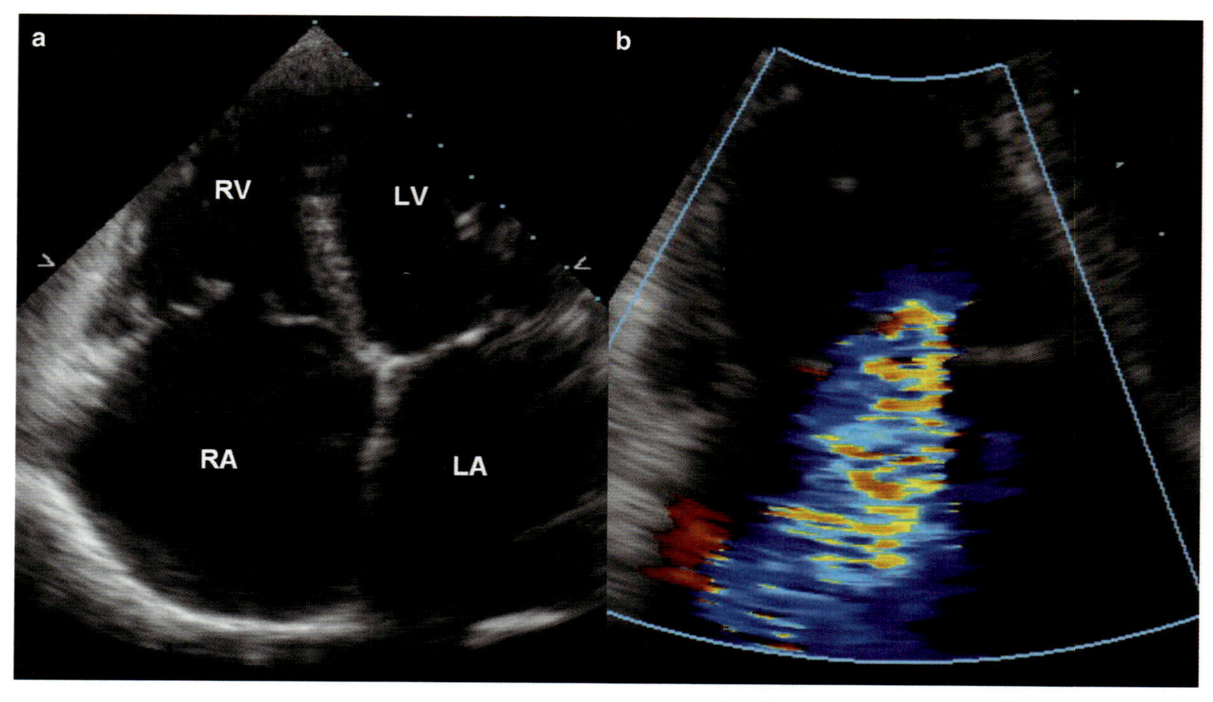

Fig. 5.9 The apical four-chamber view (**a**) in this 82-year-old woman with a history of hypertension and atrial fibrillation shows severe dilatation of the tricuspid annulus with a lack of coaptation of the tricuspid leaflets. The color-flow image (**b**) confirms severe tricuspid regurgitation. *LA* left atrium, *LV* left ventricle, *RA* right atrium, *RV* right ventricle

undergoes eccentric hypertrophy from volume overload and chronic regurgitation. The right ventricle wall may be thin or thick and the chamber may be markedly dilated. Due to the regurgitation the atrium is usually markedly dilated and an associated atrial septal defect secundum type is common.

Ebstein's anomaly is often associated with accessory atrioventricular pathways and Wolfe Parkinson White syndrome [18]. These pathways are associated with ventricular pre-excitation and may cause arrhythmias and sudden death. In Ebstein's anomaly the pathways are usually right sided, posterior on the annulus and may be multiple. Ebstein's anomaly may be left sided in the case of corrected transposition [19].

The key echocardiographic findings of Ebstein's anomaly are displacement of the tricuspid leaflet attachment, and dysplastic changes and dysfunction of the tricuspid valve and the right ventricle [20]. The diagnosis is commonly made by the apical four-chamber view, showing excessive apical displacement of the septal tricuspid leaflet. One commonly used cut-off value is 8 mm/m^2, which is the displacement of the tricuspid septal leaflet in relation to the mitral annulus indexed for the body surface area [20]. The attachment of the septal and posterior tricuspid leaflets is preferentially displaced with the maximal displacement at the commissure between these two leaflets (Fig. 5.17) [21]. Displacement of the posterior leaflet should be carefully assessed with the right ventricular inflow view, because the leaflet displacement may be localized such that the involvement of the septal leaflet may be quite mild (Fig. 5.18). In many cases, the leaflets are extensively tethered or adherent to the ventricular wall rather than truly displaced. The attachment of the anterior tricuspid leaflet is usually not displaced, but dysplastic changes are common. The anterior leaflet is large, sail-shaped and frequently protruding into the right ventricular outflow tract during diastole.

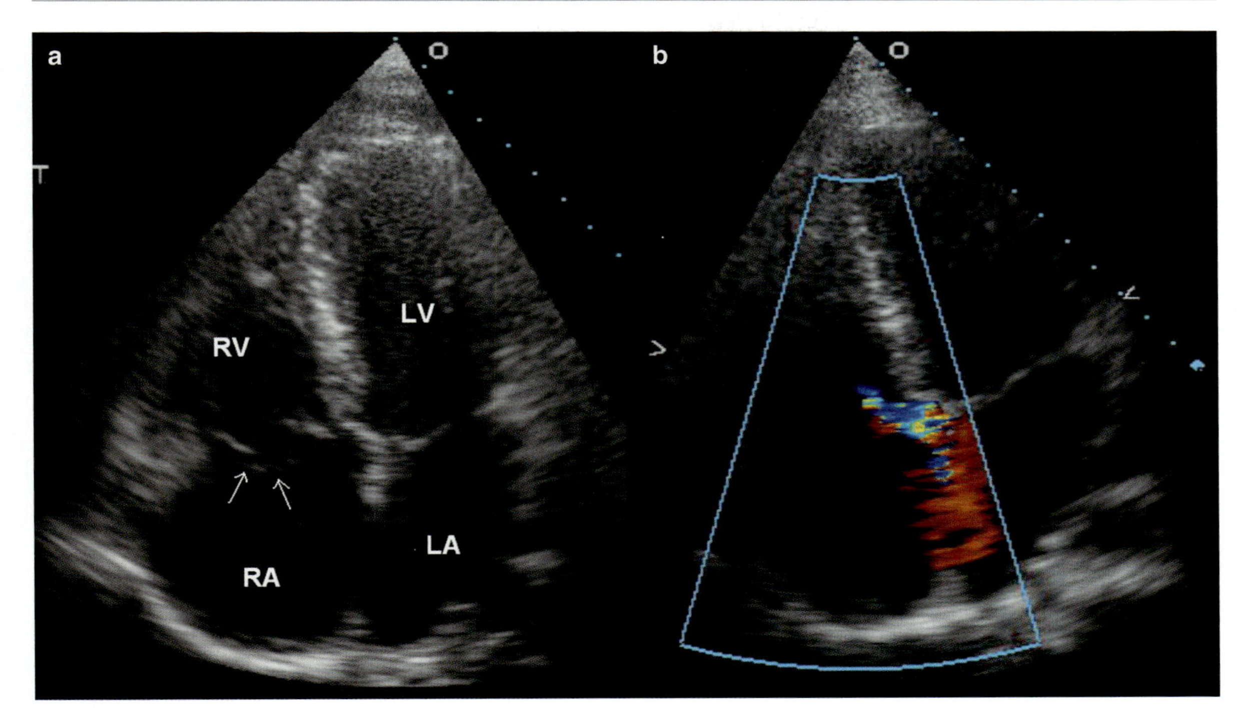

Fig. 5.10 Severe prolapse of the anterior tricuspid leaflet (*arrows*), is shown in the apical four-chamber view (**a**). Color-flow image (**b**) shows eccentric tricuspid regurgitation directed to the atrial septum consistent with prolapse of the anterior tricuspid leaflet. *LA* left atrium, *LV* left ventricle, *RA* right atrium, *RV* right ventricle

Other dysplastic changes include tethering by large fibrous bands or abnormal chordae to the septum or right ventricular free wall (Fig. 5.19) [22]. If the dysplastic changes of the anterior tricuspid leaflet are mild, tricuspid valve repair rather than replacement may be feasible [22]. Varying degree of tricuspid regurgitation is invariably present due to the dysplastic changes of the leaflets. The tricuspid orifice and the tricuspid regurgitant jet are apically displaced. The tricuspid regurgitation jet can frequently be eccentric and typically has a low velocity (Fig. 5.20). Tricuspid stenosis can occur but is rare in adults with this condition [21].

Dilated right atrium is expected due to the presence of tricuspid regurgitation and the inclusion of the atrialized right ventricle. The wall of the atrialized right ventricle is thin and fibrotic. The functional right ventricle may be small or dilated. In fact the functional right ventricle is dilated in over half of the patients, and right ventricular dysfunction is common [21]. Atrial septal defect can be detected in about 25% of the cases and the prevalence of patent foramen ovale may be even higher. Pulmonary stenosis has also been reported [21].

Severe tricuspid regurgitation can result from dysplastic changes affecting the tricuspid leaflets without significant displacement (Figs. 5.21, 5.22) [23]. These patients should not be diagnosed to have Ebstein's anomaly, since in our experience these patients seldom have dysplastic changes of their right ventricle and respond favorably to valve repair.

Carcinoid Valve Disease

Carcinoid valve disease most commonly affects the tricuspid and the pulmonary valves. The disease is commonly related to metastatic carcinoid tumor in the liver usually from a metastatic primary in the gastrointestinal

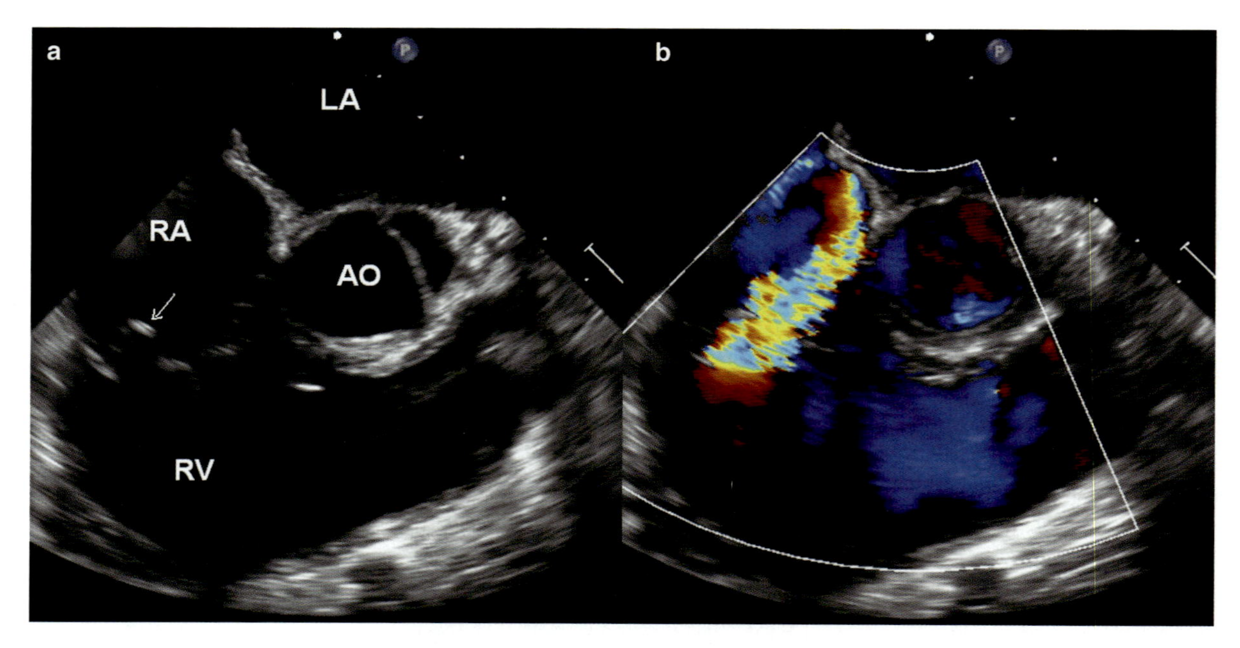

Fig. 5.11 (**a**) The transesophageal longitudinal view shows focal prolapse involving the posterior tricuspid leaflet (*arrow*). The prolapse is not seen in other views. Colur-flow image (**b**) shows severe tricuspid regurgitation. *Ao* aorta, *LA* left atrium, *RA* right atrium, *RV* right ventricle

tract. Carcinoid heart disease is seen in approximately 50% of patients with carcinoid syndrome [24]. Left-sided disease may occur rarely if there is a patent foramen ovale. The valves are white and thickened by gross examination (Figs. 5.23–5.25). The thickening is due to fibromuscular plaques or endocardial onlays. The plaques involve the cusps of the semilunar valves and the leaflets, chords and papillary muscles of the atrioventricular valves. The endocardial plaques cause valve thickening and retraction leading to valvular regurgitation and stenosis. Regurgitant valves are most common, with mixed pulmonary stenosis and pulmonary insufficiency and tricuspid insufficiency.

The valve thickening is due to cellular proliferation of myofibroblast like cells and accumulation of extracellular matrix in the endocardial onlay plaque valvular lesions. These onlays or plaques tend to occur on the arterial surface of the pulmonary valve and both surfaces of the tricuspid valve, but predominantly the ventricular side. Carcinoid plaques do not destroy the underlying valve architecture. The plaque matrix is rich in collagen and ground substances and some studies have found small amounts of elastin. Autopsy studies have noted a high degree of neovascularization and the presence of chronic inflammation. Mast cells are variable in number. Mast cells tend to be in areas of neovascularization and they may also be in adjacent valve tissue and not actually in the endocardial plaque.

Carcinoid valve disease is classified with other serotonin associated valve disorders. These include carcinoid valve disease and disease associated with serotonin agonists such as migraine and diet medications (Fen-Phen). The valvulopathy associated with these agents is hyperplastic in nature with hyperplastic endocardial lesions [25]. Carcinoid valve disease is postulated to relate to increased serum levels of serotonin which induces transforming growth factor (TGF) beta expression in the valve via serotonin 5HT-2A and 5HT-2B receptors [25–27]. In vitro, the addition of serotonin to cultured valve interstitial cells increases TGF beta expression and increased extracellular matrix probably through this serotonin receptor mechanism [26, 28]. TGF beta can induce valvular endothelial cells and interstitial cells to trans-differentiate into myofibroblasts which produce the plaques [28, 29].

Typical echocardiographic findings are diffusely thickened tricuspid valve leaflets with restricted

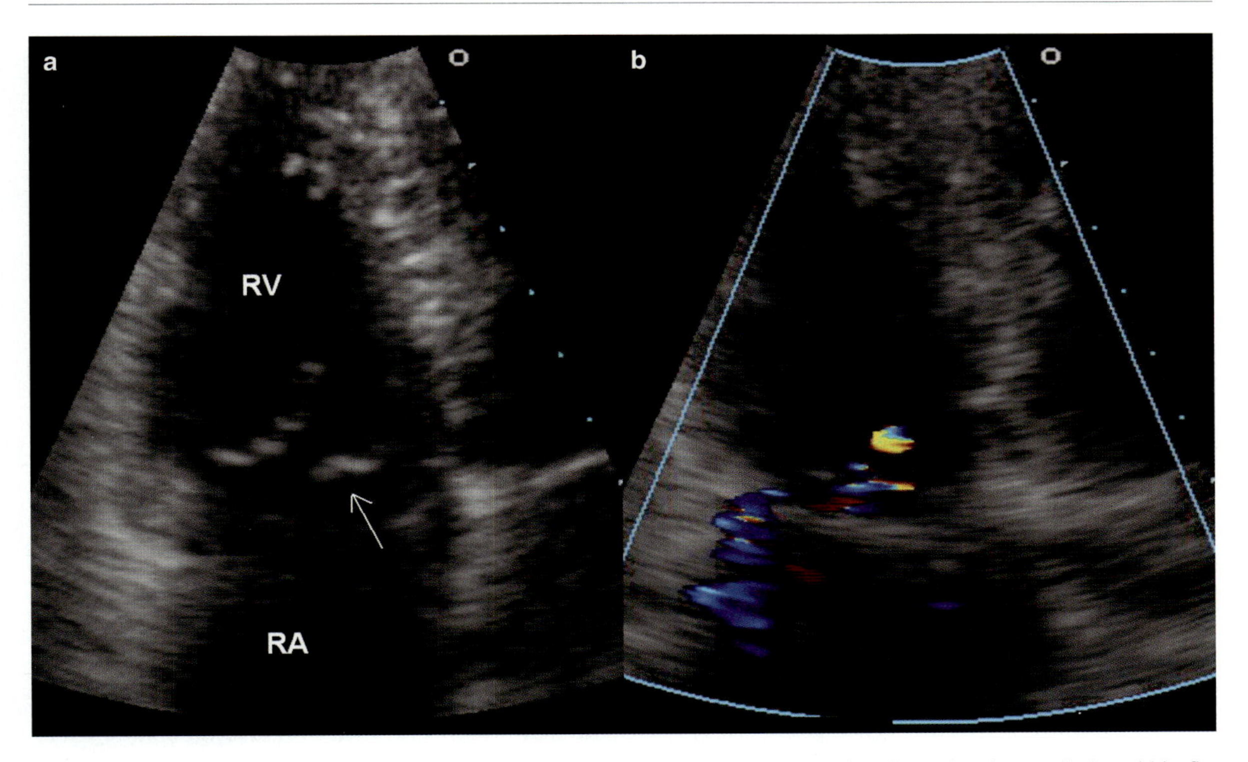

Fig. 5.12 The apical four-chamber view (**a**) in a patient who has had cardiac transplantation shows that the septal tricuspid leaflet is flailed with the tip of the leaflet pointing into the right atrium during systole. The color-flow image (**b**) confirms eccentric tricuspid regurgitation. The tricuspid valve abnormality is likely due to inadvertent damage of the tricuspid valve during endomyocardial biopsy. *RA* right atrium, *RV* right ventricle

motion which is best described as "frozen in space." During systole, there is no coaptation of the leaflets resulting in a large regurgitant orifice and torrential tricuspid regurgitation (Figs. 5.26, 5.27). Similar changes involving the pulmonic valve are frequently present. There may also be diffuse thickening and brightness of the right ventricular endocardium due to endothelial fibrosis [30].

Severity of Tricuspid Regurgitation

Like the other heart valves, coaptation of the tricuspid leaflets is the key to normal valve function and needs to be carefully assessed. Proper leaflet coaptation excludes severe tricuspid regurgitation, and conversely lack of leaflet coaptation indicates the presence of severe tricuspid regurgitation. Determination of the severity of tricuspid regurgitation follows the same principles used in assessing the severity of mitral regurgitation.(Table 5.1) [31] Commonly used for this purpose are measures of the tricuspid regurgitation color flow jet, particularly the color jet area and jet width. The presence of an easily detectable flow convergence indicates at least moderate severity for the tricuspid regurgitation (Fig. 5.28). Systolic flow reversal in the hepatic vein can be detected by color flow imaging or pulsed-wave Doppler (Fig. 5.29). Its presence indicates severe tricuspid regurgitation [32]. Confirmatory findings such as right atrial and right ventricular enlargement should be present. The advantages and limitations of these measures are summarized in Table 5.1.

We use a semi-quantitative approach as recommended by the American Society of Echocardiography to classify tricuspid regurgitation into mild, moderate and severe (Table 5.2) [31]. This determination takes into consideration all the different measures that we have discussed.

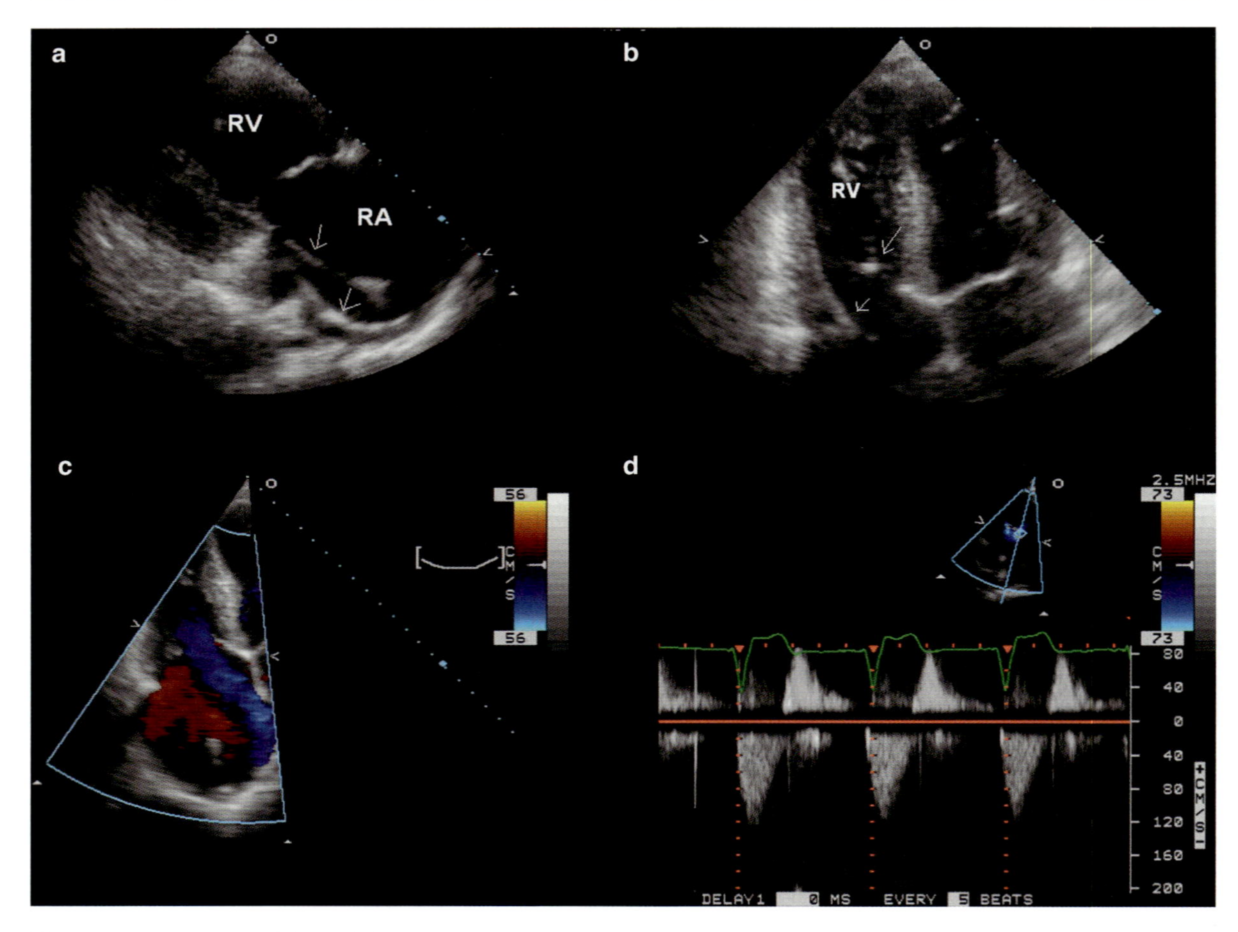

Fig. 5.13 In this patient with two right ventricular pacemaker leads (*arrows*), there is lack of tricuspid leaflet coaptation shown in the parasternal right ventricular inflow (**a**) and four-chamber (**b**) views, far in excess of the mild degree of tricuspid annular dilatation. The color-flow image (**c**) shows severe tricuspid regurgitation of a lower velocity. This is confirmed by the continuous wave Doppler (**d**). The tricuspid velocity is triangular in contour with early peaking, indicative of severe regurgitation

Tricuspid Valve Stenotic Lesions

These are uncommon valve disorders. Tricuspid stenosis may be due to a dysplastic valve which may be associated with Ebstein's anomaly [21]. Acquired stenosis is usually rheumatic and is invariably associated with concomitant left sided valve disease. Fungal endocarditis or large vegetations from intravenous drug use may cause valve stenosis due to the large size of the vegetations. Indwelling catheters, shunt lines, pacemaker leads and defibrillator leads may incorporate into the valve leaflets or chords, but unless associated with thrombus they do not usually cause significant valve destruction or stenosis. Some lines are associated with calcific masses termed calcified amorphous tumors [33]. These pseudotumors probably represent calcified thrombus and are also associated with coagulation disorders such as lupus anticoagulant [34].

Tricuspid valve repair is increasingly performed in association with other valve surgeries to reduce or eliminate tricuspid regurgitation [35], and may emerge as an important cause of tricuspid stenosis (Fig. 5.30). This may be related to over-reduction of the tricuspid annulus associated with additional procedures such as bicuspidalization and Alfieri repair. Thus in these patients, Doppler assessment for tricuspid stenosis should be performed in addition to the evaluation of the severity of residual tricuspid regurgitation.

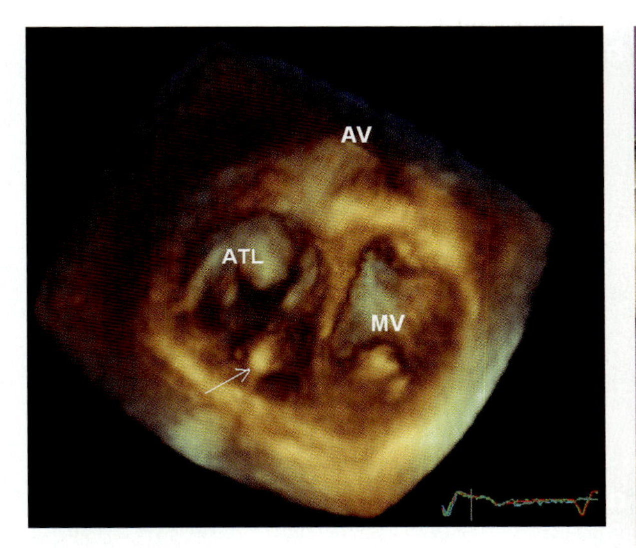

Fig. 5.14 The transthoracic 3D view near the crux of the heart shows that the septal tricuspid leaflet is restricted in excursion such that there is a large tricuspid regurgitation orifice. The restricted excursion appears to be related to the pacemaker lead (*arrow*) traversing the tricuspid valve. *ATL* anterior tricuspid leaflet, *AV* aortic valve, *MV* mitral valve

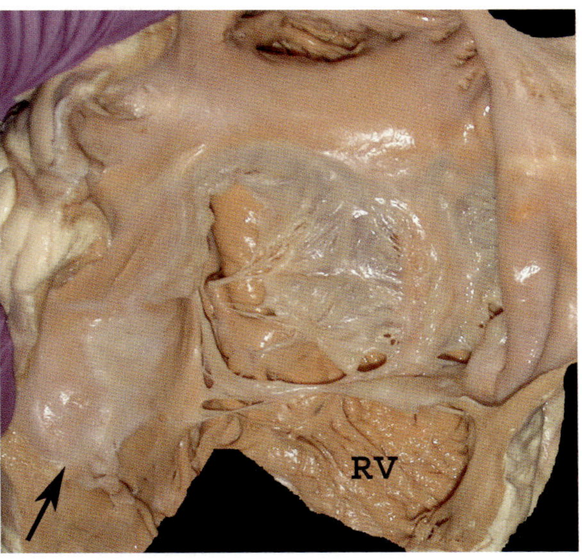

Fig. 5.16 Another individual with Ebstein's anomaly of the tricuspid valve. There are abnormally formed valve leaflets which also appear to be adherent (*arrow*) to the underlying right ventricle (*RV*)

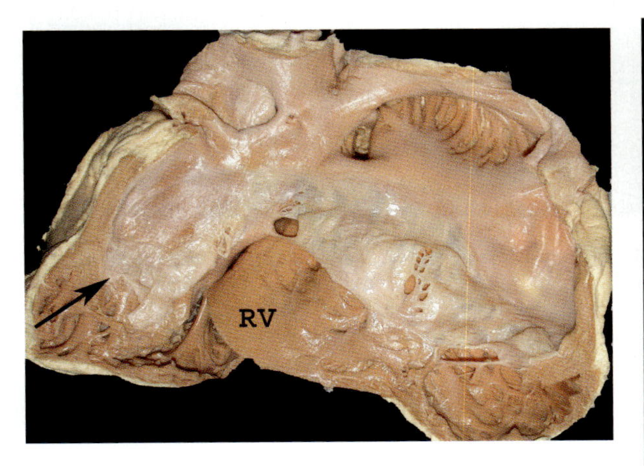

Fig. 5.15 Ebstein's anomaly of the tricuspid valve. The leaflets are elongated and abnormally attached to the underlying ventricular wall (*arrow*). The leaflets are also malformed. The right ventricle is thin under the leaflets (*RV*)

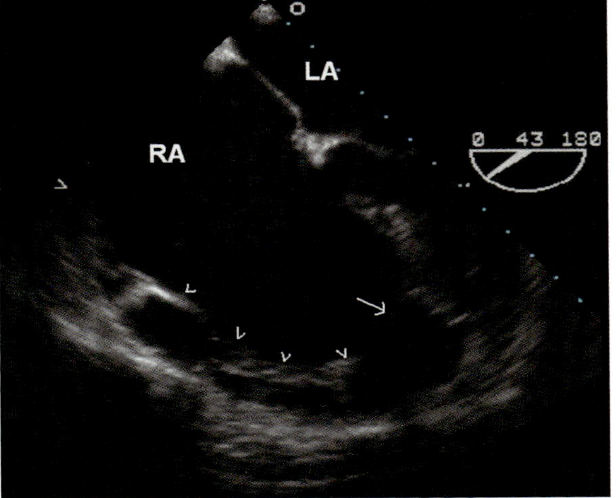

Fig. 5.17 The transesophageal four-chamber view shows the severe apical displacement of the septal tricuspid leaflet (*arrow*). The anterior leaflet is elongated and demonstrates tethering to the ventricular wall by multiple fibrous bands (*arrowheads*). *LA* left atrium, *RA* right atrium

Pulmonary Stenosis

Unicuspid and bicuspid pulmonary valves may be isolated or associated with syndromes including tetralogy of Fallot and Noonan's syndrome (usually with an atrial or ventricular septal defect). Unicuspid valves are acommissural dome shaped or unicommissural teardrop shaped, analogous to their aortic counterparts

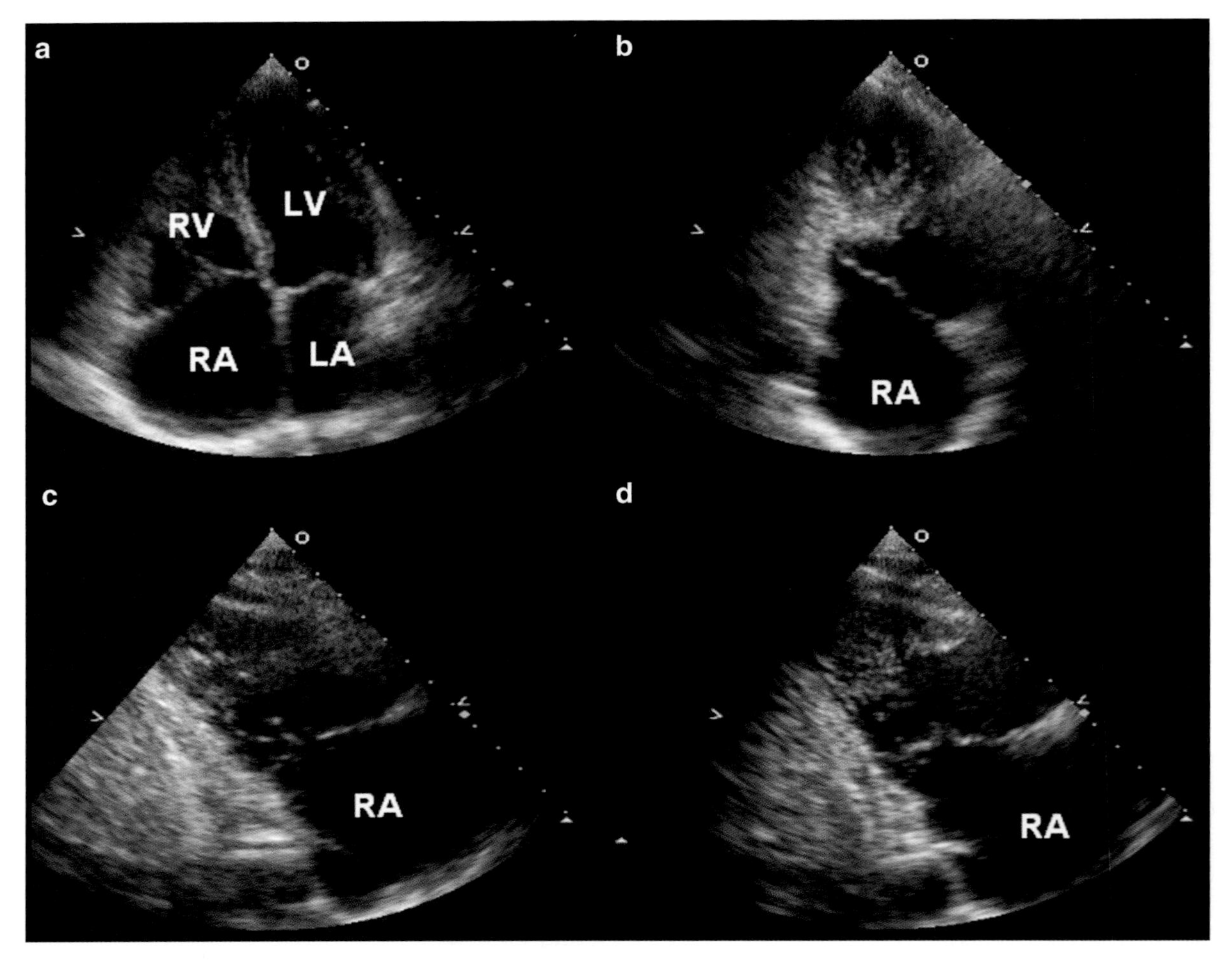

Fig. 5.18 In this patient with Ebstein's anomaly, the apical displacement of the tricuspid leaflet is localized to the posterior leaflet which is best shown in the apical two-chamber (**b**) and right ventricular inflow (**d**) views. In the apical four-chamber view (**a**), the attachment of the septal tricuspid leaflet is normal. In the right ventricular inflow view (**c**) the apical displacement of the posterior tricuspid leaflet is less severe compared to (**d**), highlighting the localized nature of the leaflet displacement. *LA* left atrium, *LV* left ventricle, *RA* right atrium, *RV* right ventricle

(Fig. 5.31). Raphes may be present in both variants. These valves are stenotic and usually symptomatic after a time. Traditionally they were replaced, but now are repaired with valvuloplasty or stented (including percutaneous stenting) with reasonable results. Bicuspid pulmonary valves may be asymptomatic and may be regurgitant or stenotic. These are more common than unicuspid valves.

In most adult patients, the pulmonary valve is not well visualized by echocardiography. Pulmonary stenosis usually due to congenital bicuspid pulmonary valve is generally well tolerated in the adult population (Fig. 5.32). The pulmonary valve demonstrates doming which is a sign of restricted excursion of the cusps (Fig. 5.33). There is post stenotic dilation of the main pulmonary artery and the proximal right and left pulmonary arteries (Fig. 5.34). Typically, the left pulmonary artery is more dilated than the right pulmonary artery. Percutaneous pulmonary valvotomy can be considered in symptomatic patients or patients with severe pulmonary stenosis. Mild to moderate pulmonary stenosis seldom progresses and is usually benign.

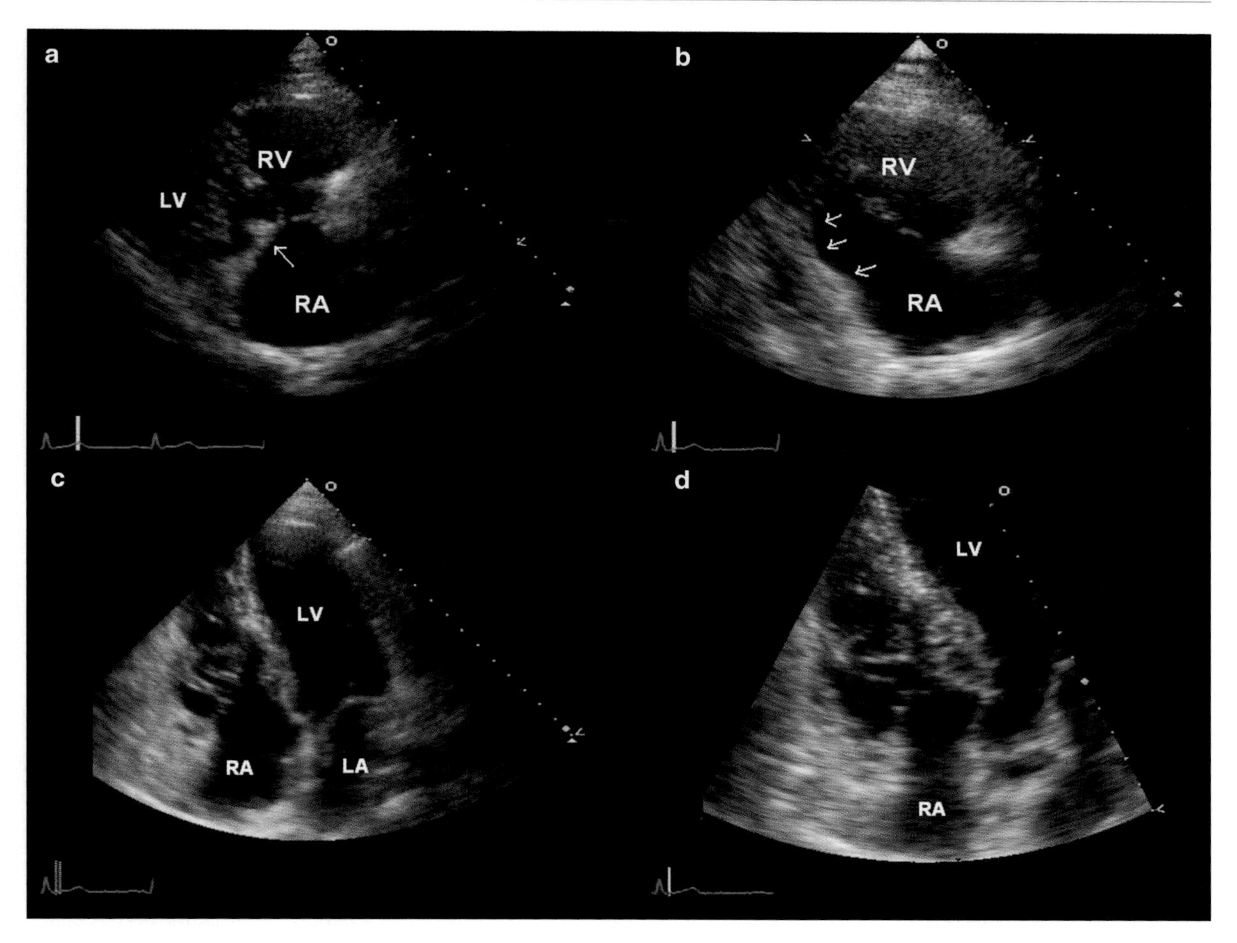

Fig. 5.19 In this patients with Ebstein's anomaly, part of the posterior tricuspid leaflet (*arrows*) is severely apically displaced (**b**), while other portions of the posterior leaflet (*arrow*) has normal attachment (**a**). The anterior tricuspid leaflet is dysplastic and tethered to the ventricular wall by multiple fibrous bands and abnormal chordae (**c**, **d**)

Pulmonary Regurgitation

Once again leaflet coaptation is the key finding and should be assessed from multiple imaging windows. Similar to tricuspid regurgitation, a slight degree of pulmonic regurgitation is ubiquitous and is a normal finding (Fig. 5.35). The presence of "A dip" in the pulmonary regurgitation spectral sign is a common and normal finding, unlike the situation in aortic regurgitation (Fig. 5.36). Pathologic pulmonary regurgitation may be caused by endocarditis, prior pulmonic valvotomy for pulmonary stenosis and transannular patch of the right ventricular outflow tract. Measures of the color jet size are useful in estimating the severity although complete visualization of the pulmonary regurgitation jet may be difficult because of the orientation of the infundibulum (Fig. 5.37). The Doppler spectral signal of severe pulmonary regurgitation is dense compared to the antegrade flow and demonstrates rapid deceleration to the baseline (Fig. 5.38) [36]. In this setting right ventricular dilatation is invariably present. The advantages and limitations of these measures are summarized in Table 5.3 [31].

In tetralogy of Fallot, the right ventricle outflow tract stenosis may be valvular due to a dysplastic, a unicuspid or a bicuspid pulmonary valve. However, an infundibular tract muscular stenosis may co-exist and may require resection of subvalvular ventricular muscle at surgical repair for tetralogy.

There are also quadricuspid pulmonary valves which are usually competent and not associated with symptoms.

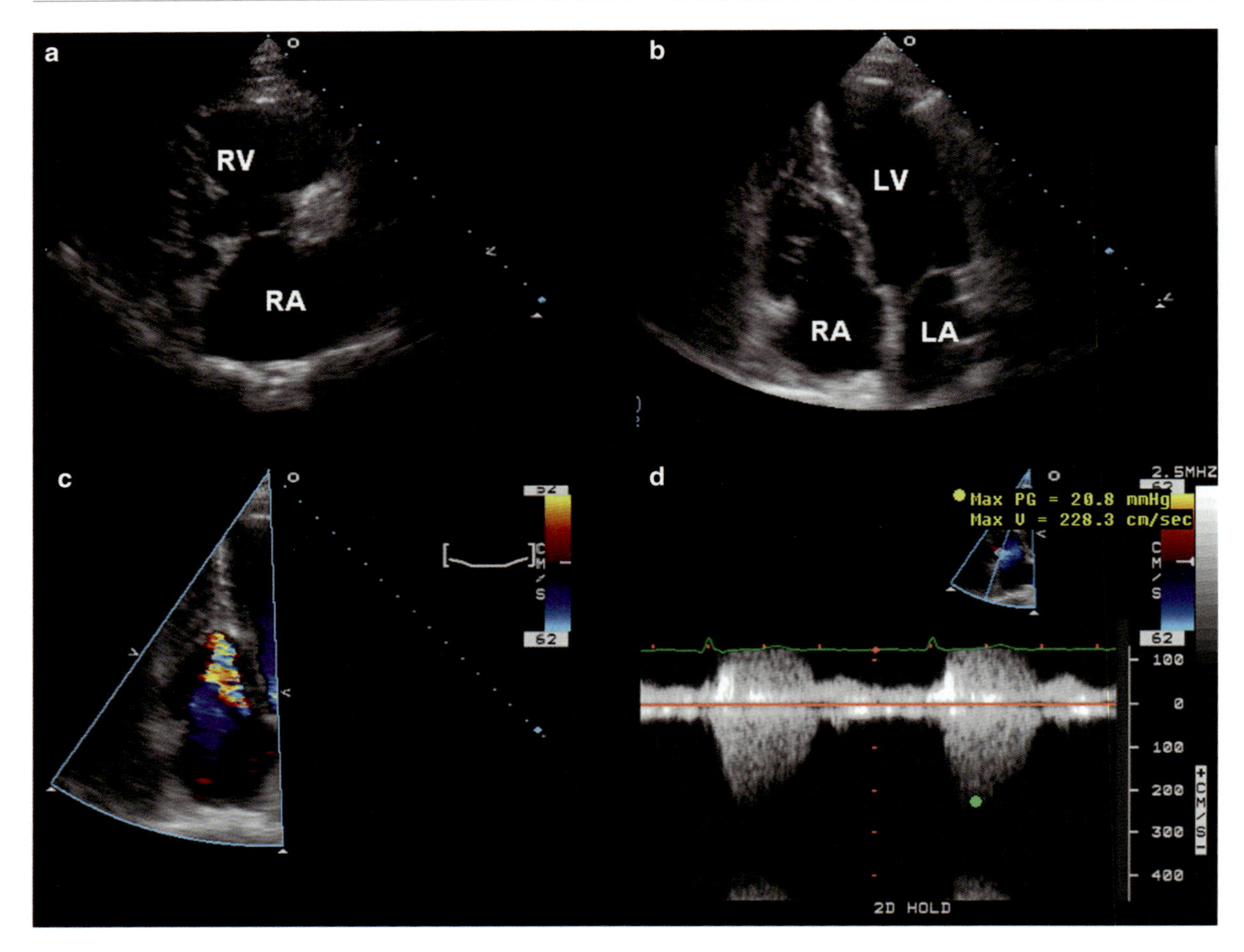

Fig. 5.20 In this patient with Ebstein's anomaly, the attachment of the septal tricuspid leaflet is severely displaced shown in the apical four-chamber view (**b**), while the posterior leaflet has normal attachment shown in the parasternal right ventricular inflow view (**a**). Moderate tricuspid regurgitation is present (**c**). The continuous wave Doppler (**d**) shows that the velocity of the tricuspid is not high indicating normal pulmonary artery systolic pressure

Tricuspid and Pulmonary Valve Infective Endocarditis

Right sided tricuspid or pulmonary valve infective endocarditis may be associated with indwelling lines or catheters, pacemakers or defibrillator lead infections, or intravenous drug use. The valve destruction is more likely to be clinically silent than left sided valve disease, with the development of progressive right heart failure and pulmonary manifestations including pulmonary emboli, pulmonary infarcts, pulmonary abscesses, empyema, pleuritis and effusions (Figs. 5.39, 5.40)

Summary

A mild degree of regurgitation of the tricuspid or pulmonary valve is common and certainly can be physiological. A more severe degree of regurgitation is abnormal and can lead to right ventricular volume overload. The underlying mechanism responsible for the valvular regurgitation should be understood, in order to determine the feasibility of valve repair and the type of surgical approach, since early invasive intervention to eliminate regurgitation has been shown to improve long-term outcome.

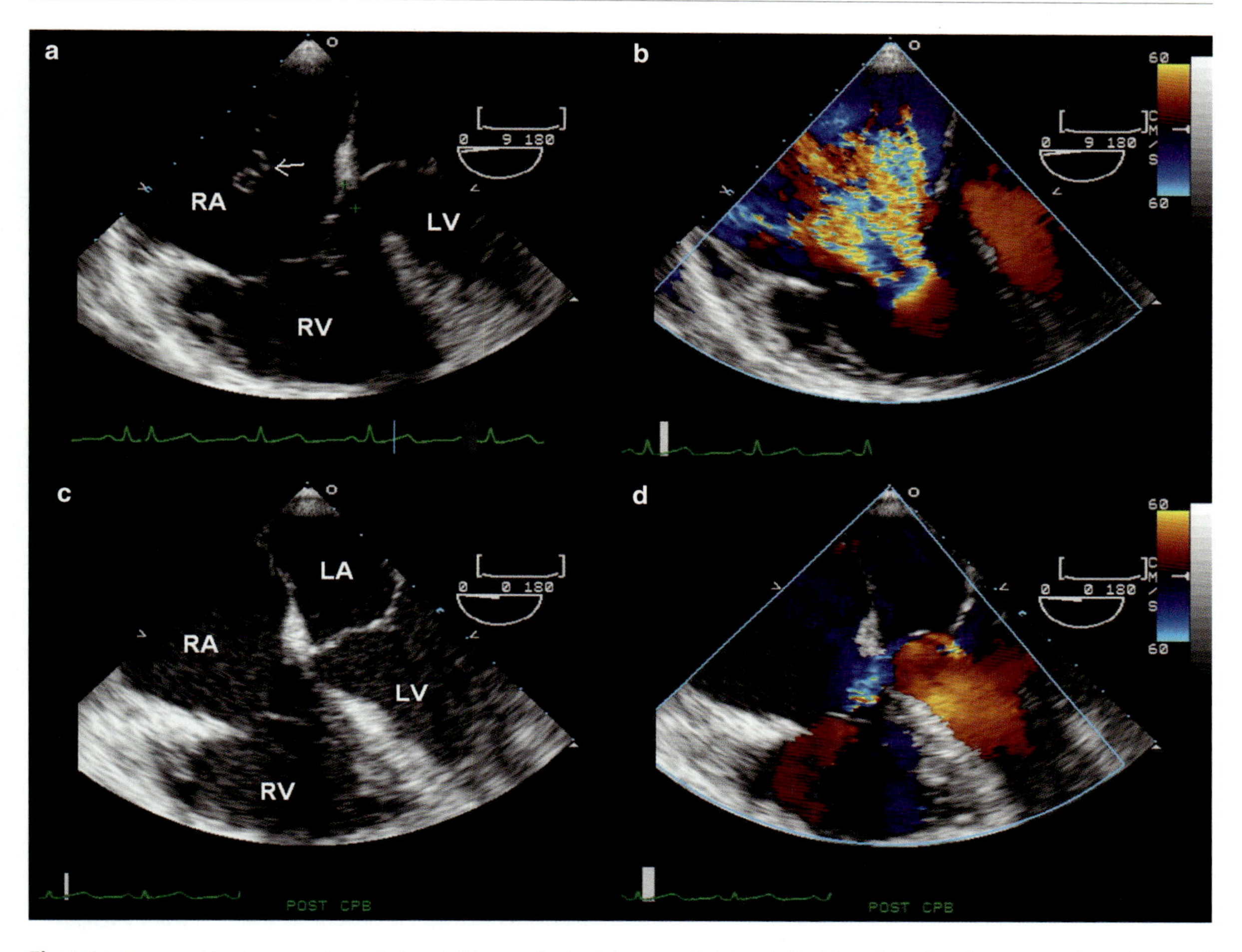

Fig. 5.21 Preoperative transesophageal view (**a**) in a patient with congenital dysplastic tricuspid valve shows normal attachment of the tricuspid leaflets and color flow image (**b**) shows severe tricuspid regurgitation. A prominent Eustachian valve (*arrow*) is present. Post-operative images (**c**, **d**) show smaller tricuspid annulus, proper leaflet coaptation and trivial regurgitation. *LA* left atrium, *LV* left ventricle, *RA* right atrium, *RV* right ventricle

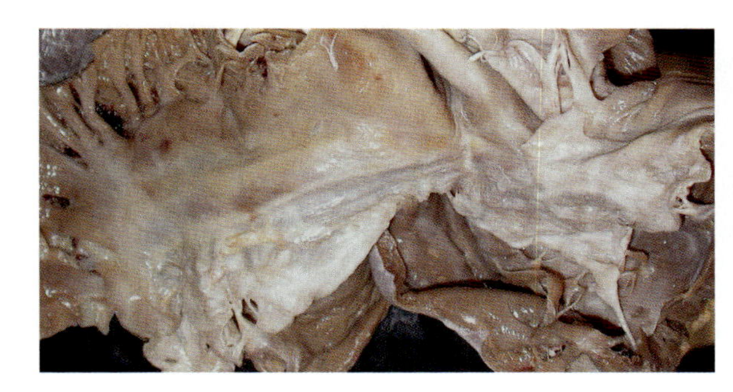

Fig. 5.22 Tricuspid valve dysplasia with abnormally formed valve leaflets, but no displacement

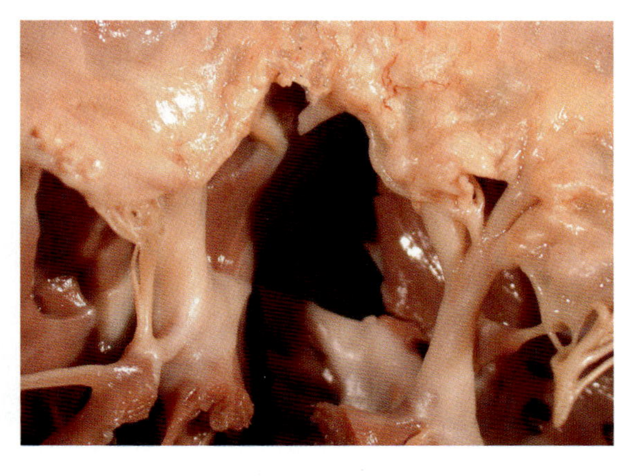

Fig. 5.23 Carcinoid disease involving the tricuspid valve causes leaflet and chordal thickening with white fibromuscular endocardial plaques. The valve structure is normal underneath, and the plaques deposit on the valve tissue and distort it. Such valves are usually predominantly regurgitant

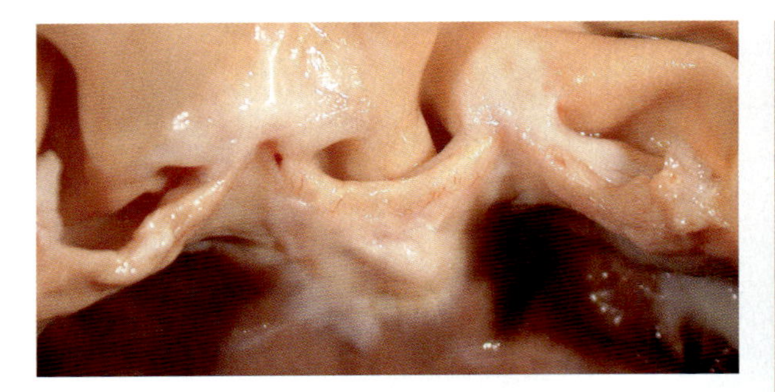

Fig. 5.24 Carcinoid disease involving the pulmonary valve with white discoloration and cusp thickening. The fibromuscular onlays deposit on the valve and thicken it. Such valves are usually mixed stenotic and regurgitant

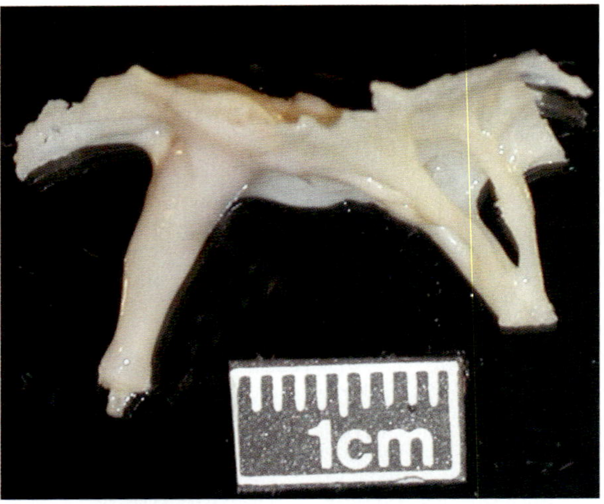

Fig. 5.25 Surgically excised tricuspid valve tissue with thickened leaflet and chords

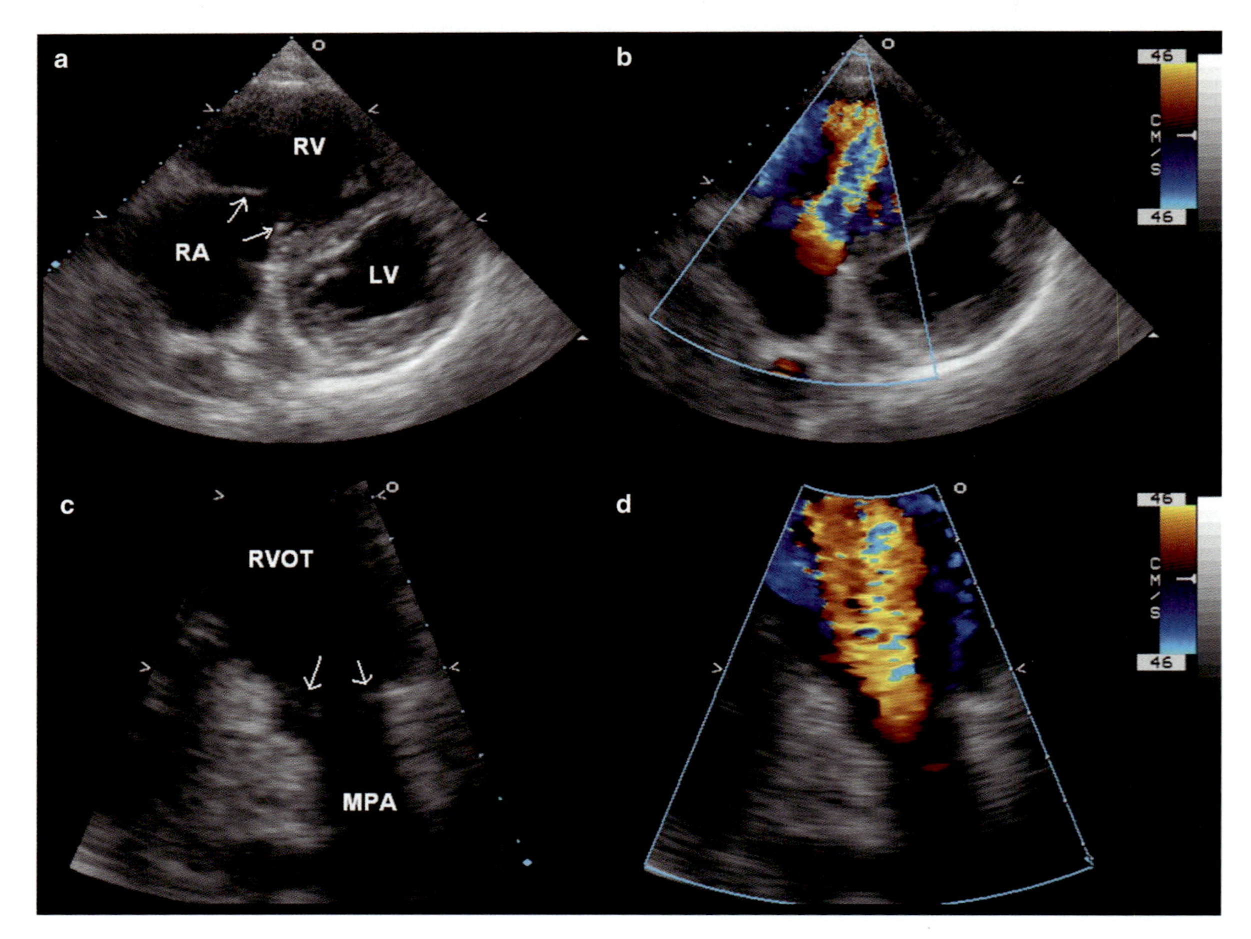

Fig. 5.26 The diastolic images of the tricuspid valve (**a**) and the pulmonary valve (**c**) shows diffuse thickening and restriction in excursion of both valves (*arrows*). Color-flow images shows a mild degree of tricuspid stenosis (**b**) and the presence of severe pulmonic regurgitation (**d**) due to a lack of coaptation of the pulmonary cusps. *LV* left ventricle, *RA* right atrium, *RV* right ventricle, *RVOT* right ventricular outflow tract

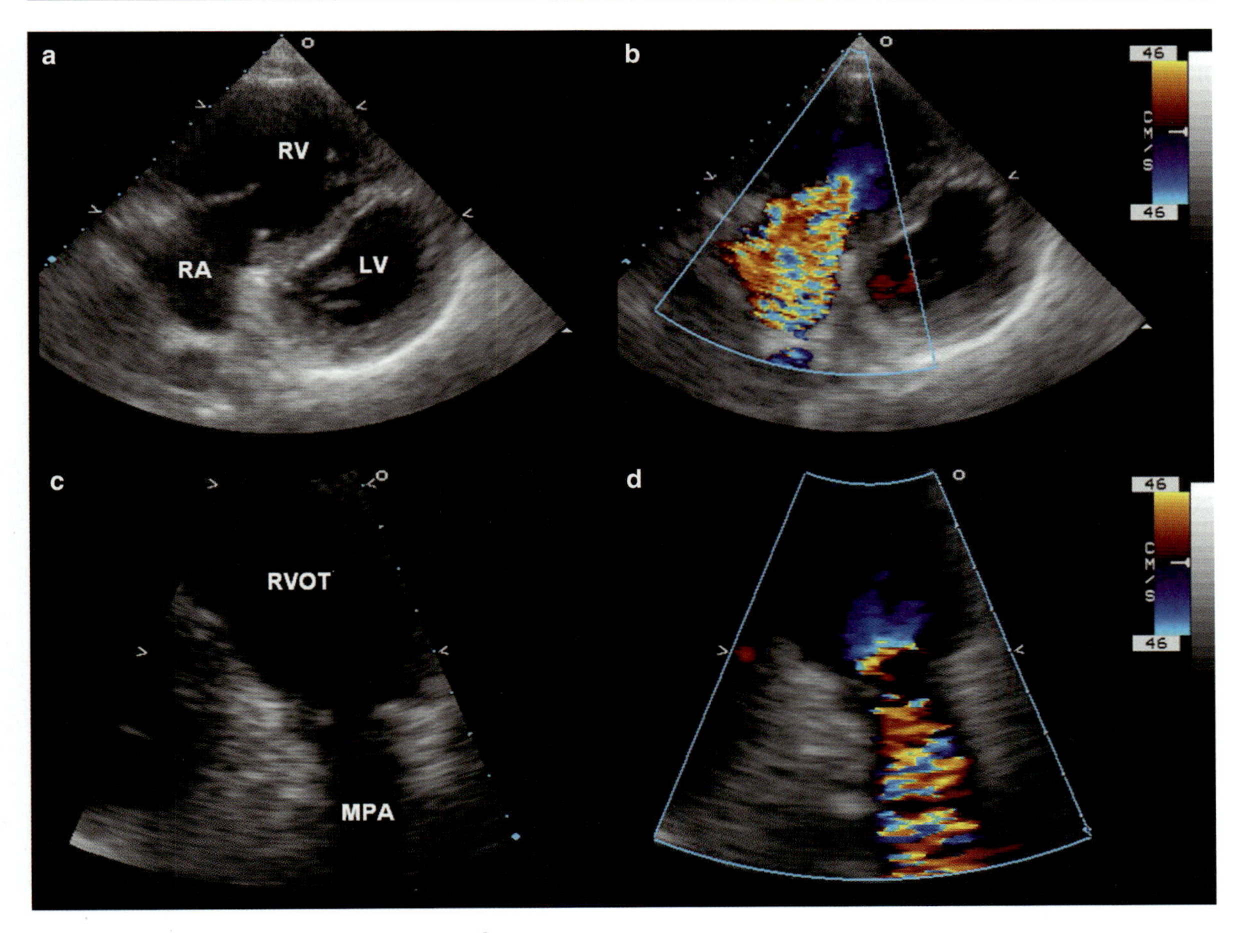

Fig. 5.27 These are the systolic images of the tricuspid valve (**a**, **b**) and the pulmonary valve (**c**, **d**) of the same patient in Fig. 5.21. The tricuspid and pulmonary valves are diffusely thickened and restricted in excursion. Color-flow image shows severe tricuspid regurgitation due to a lack of coaptation of the tricuspid leaflets (**b**). There is also flow acceleration at the pulmonary valve due to restricted systolic excursion of the pulmonary cusps (**d**). *LV* left ventricle, *MPA* main pulmonary artery, *RA* right atrium, *RV* right ventricle, *RVOT* right ventricular outflow tract

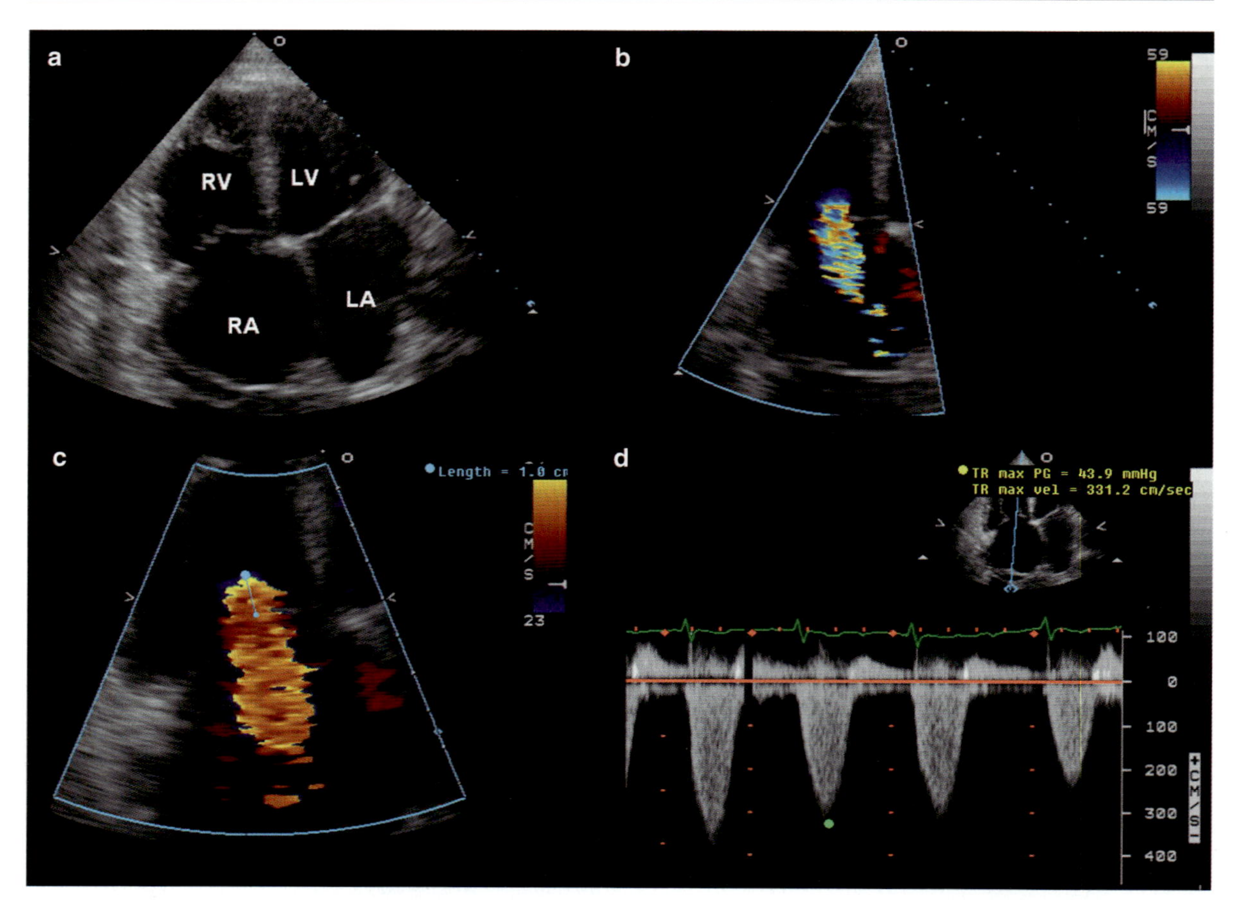

Fig. 5.28 The apical four-chamber view (**a**) shows severe dilatation of the right ventricle and right atrium. Color-flow image (**b**) shows a large tricuspid regurgitant jet with a prominent flow convergence and a jet width of 0.8 cm in diameter. At a Nyquist limit of 23 cm/s, the radius of the flow convergence is 1 cm (**c**). The tricuspid regurgitation spectral signal is shown in (**d**). The tricuspid regurgitant orifice area is calculated to be 0.44 cm^2. These parameters are consistent with severe tricuspid regurgitation. *LA* left atrium, *LV* left ventricle, *RA* right atrium, *RV* right ventricle

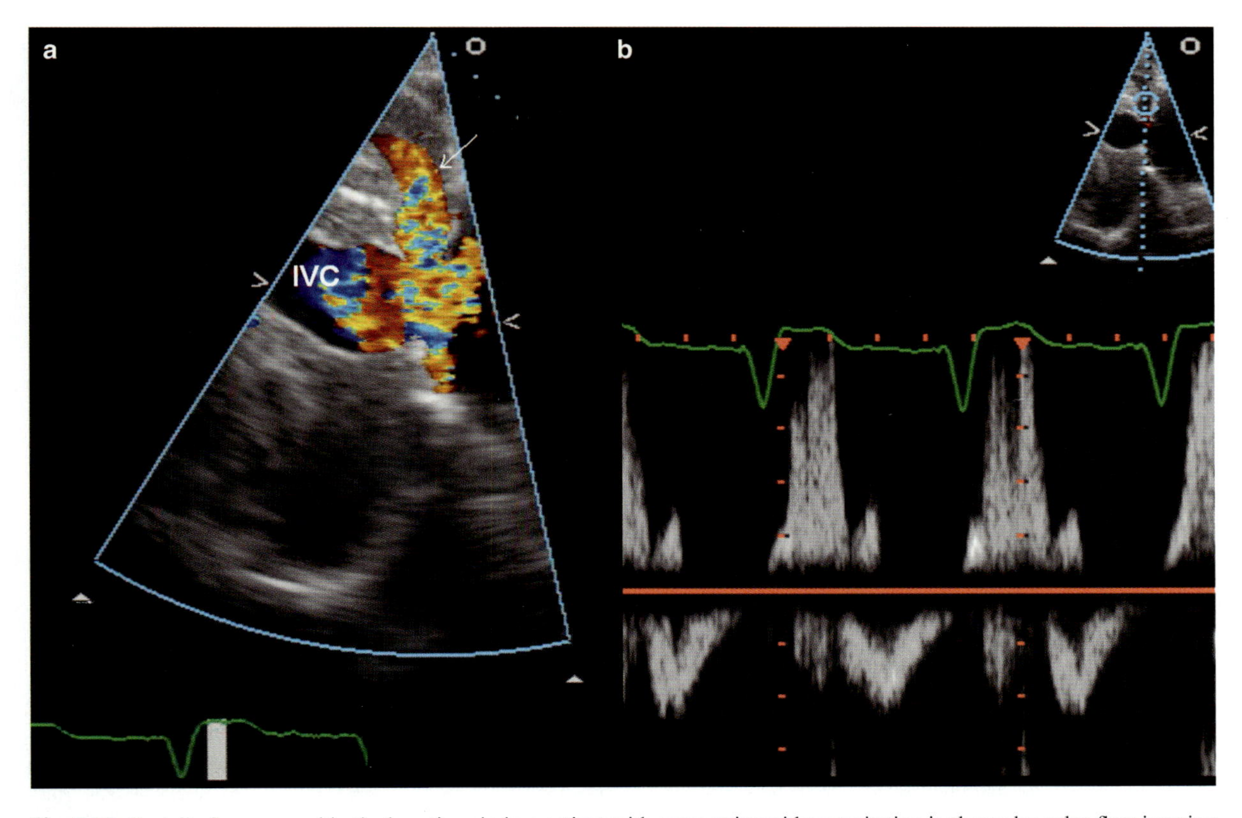

Fig. 5.29 Systolic flow reversal in the hepatic vein in a patient with severe tricuspid regurgitation is shown by color-flow imaging (*arrow*) (**a**) and pulsed wave Doppler examination (**b**). *IVC* inferior vena cava

Table 5.1 Strengths and limitations of echocardiographic and Doppler parameters in the assessment of tricuspid regurgitation

Parameter	Utility/advantages	Limitations
RV/RA/IVC size	Enlargement sensitive for chronic significant TR. Normal size virtually excludes significant chronic TR	Enlargement seen in other conditions. May be normal in acute significant TR
TV leaflet alterations	Flail valve specific for significant TR	Other abnormalities do not imply significant TR
Paradoxical septal motion (volume overload pattern)	Simple sign of severe TR	Not specific for TR
Jet area – color flow	Simple, quick screen for TR	Subject to technical and hemodynamic factors. Underestimates severity in eccentric jets
Vena contracta width	Simple, quantitative, separates mild from severe TR	Intermediate values require further confirmation
PISA method	Quantitative	Validated in only a few studies
Flow quantitation – PW	Quantitative	Not validated for determining TR regurgitant fraction
Jet profile – CW	Simple, readily available	Qualitative, complementary data
Peak tricuspid E velocity	Simple, usually increased in severe TR	Depends on RA pressure and RV relaxation, TV area, and atrial fibrillation; complementary data only
Hepatic vein flow	Simple; systolic flow reversal is sensitive for severe TR	Influenced by RA pressure, atrial fibrillation

CW continuous wave Doppler, *EROA* effective orifice regurgitant area, *IVC* inferior vena cava, *PISA* proximal isovelocity surface area, *PW* pulsed wave Doppler, *RA* right atrium, *RV* right ventricle; *TV* tricuspid valve, *TR* tricuspid regurgitation
Source: Reproduced from Zoghbi et al. [31]. With permission

Table 5.2 Semi-quantitation of severity of tricuspid regurgitation based on echocardiographic and Doppler parameters

Parameter	Mild	Moderate	Severe
Tricuspid valve	Usually normal	Normal or abnormal	Abnormal/flail leaflet/poor coaptation
RV/RA/IVC size	Normal[a]	Normal or dilated	Usually dilated[b]
Jet area-central jets (cm^2)[c]	<5	5–10	>10
VC width (cm)[d]	Not defined	Not defined, but <0.7	>07
PISA radius (cm)[e]	<0.5	0.6–0.9	>0.9
Jet density and contour – CW	Soft and parabolic	Dense, variable contour	Dense, triangular with early peaking
Hepatic vein flow[f]	Systolic dominance	Systolic blunting	Systolic reversal

CW continuous wave Doppler, *IVC* inferior vena cava, *RA* right atrium, *RV* right ventricle, *VC* vena contracts width
[a]Unless there are other reasons for RA or RV dilation. Normal 2D measurements from the apical four-chamber view: RV medio-lateral end-diastolic dimension ≤ 4.3 cm, RV end-diastolic area ≤ 35.5 cm^2, maximal RA medio-lateral and supero-inferior dimensions ≤ 4.6 and 4.9 cm, respectively, maximal RA volume ≤ 33 mL/m^2 (35;89)
[b]Exception: acute TR
[c]At a Nyquist limit of 50–60 cm/s. Not valid in eccentric jets. Jet area is not recommended as the sole parameter of TR severity due to its dependence on hemodynamic and technical factors
[d]At a Nyquist limit of 50–60 cm/s
[e]Baseline shift with Nyquist limit of 28 cm/s
[f]Other conditions may cause systolic blunting (e.g., atrial fibrillation, elevated RA pressure)
Source: Reproduced from Zoghbi et al. [31]. With permission

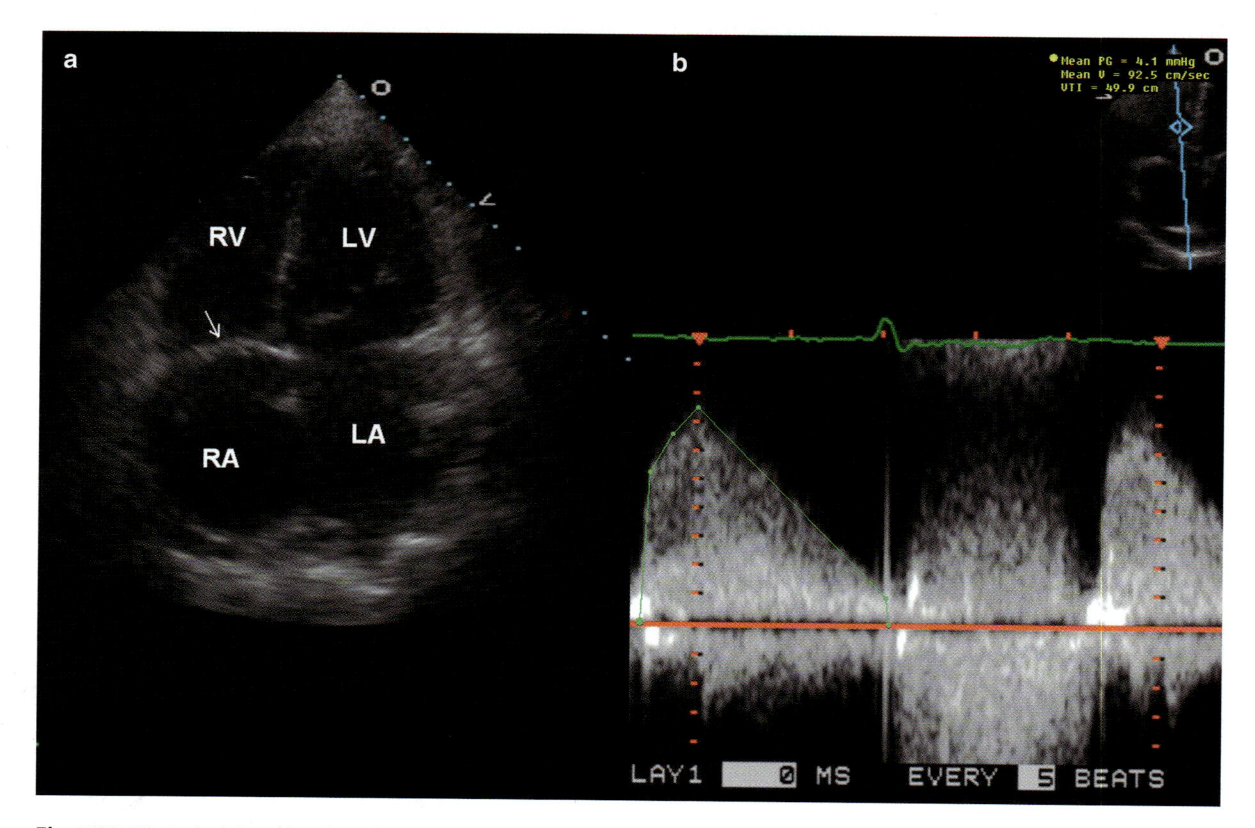

Fig. 5.30 The apical four-chamber view (**a**) in a patient who had tricuspid valve repair for tricuspid regurgitation shows restriction in excursion of the tricuspid leaflet (*arrow*). Tricuspid stenosis is confirmed by the continuous wave Doppler (**b**). The mean tricuspid gradient is 4.1 mmHg. *LA* left atrium, *LV* left ventricle, *RA* right atrium, *RV* right ventricle

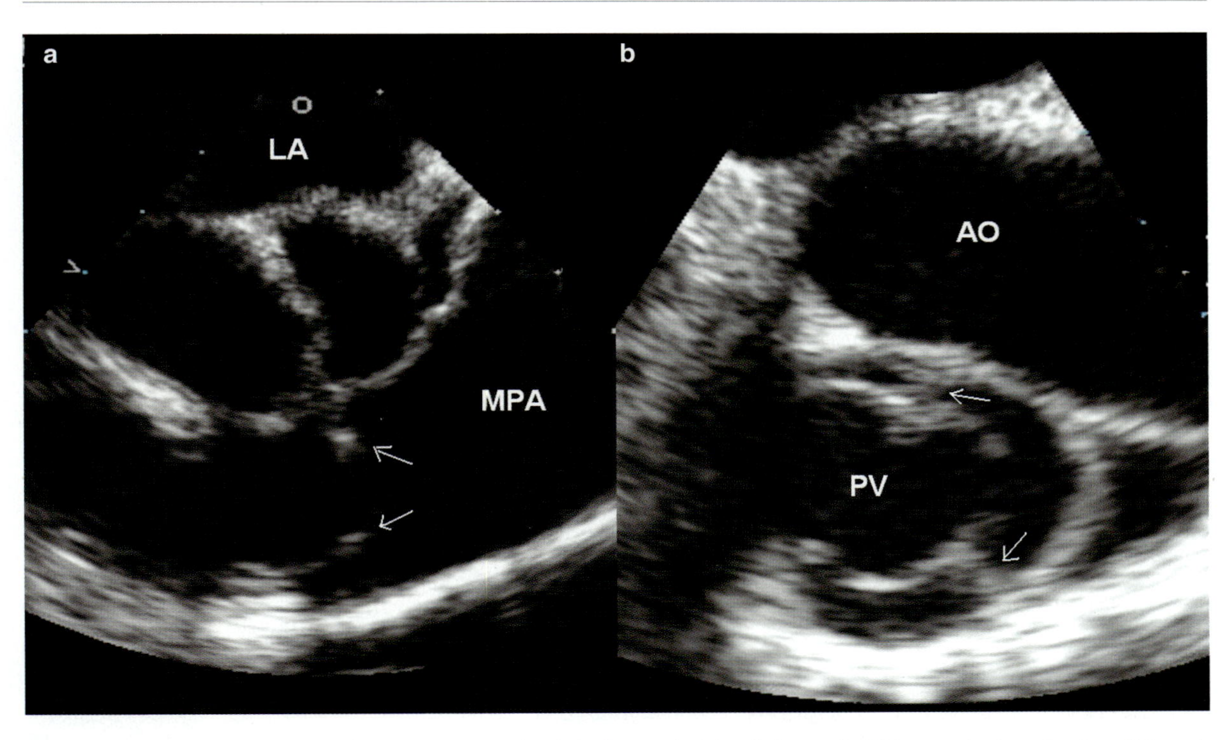

Fig. 5.31 Transesophageal views of the pulmonary valve in its long-axis (**a**) and short-axis (**b**) in systole show doming of the pulmonary valve consistent with mild pulmonary stenosis and the presence of two raphes (*arrows*) (**b**) suggesting this may be a unicuspid pulmonary valve. *Ao* aorta, *LA* left atrium, *MPA* main pulmonary artery, *PV* pulmonary valve

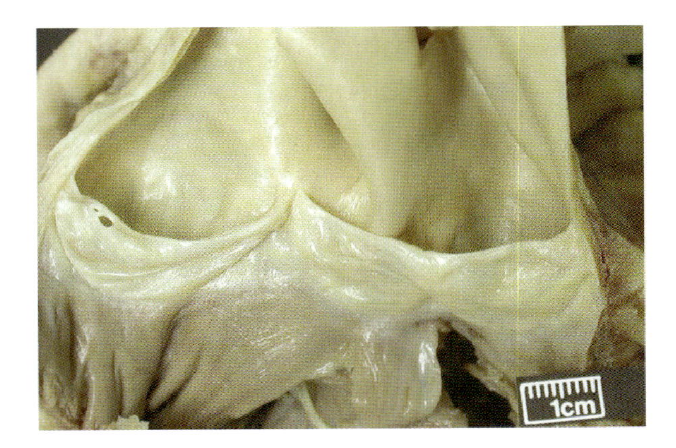

Fig. 5.32 Congenitally bicuspid pulmonary valve. Only two cusps are present. This was clinically not apparent. Interestingly this is the same patient as shown in Fig. 5.22, the individual with tricuspid valve dysplasia

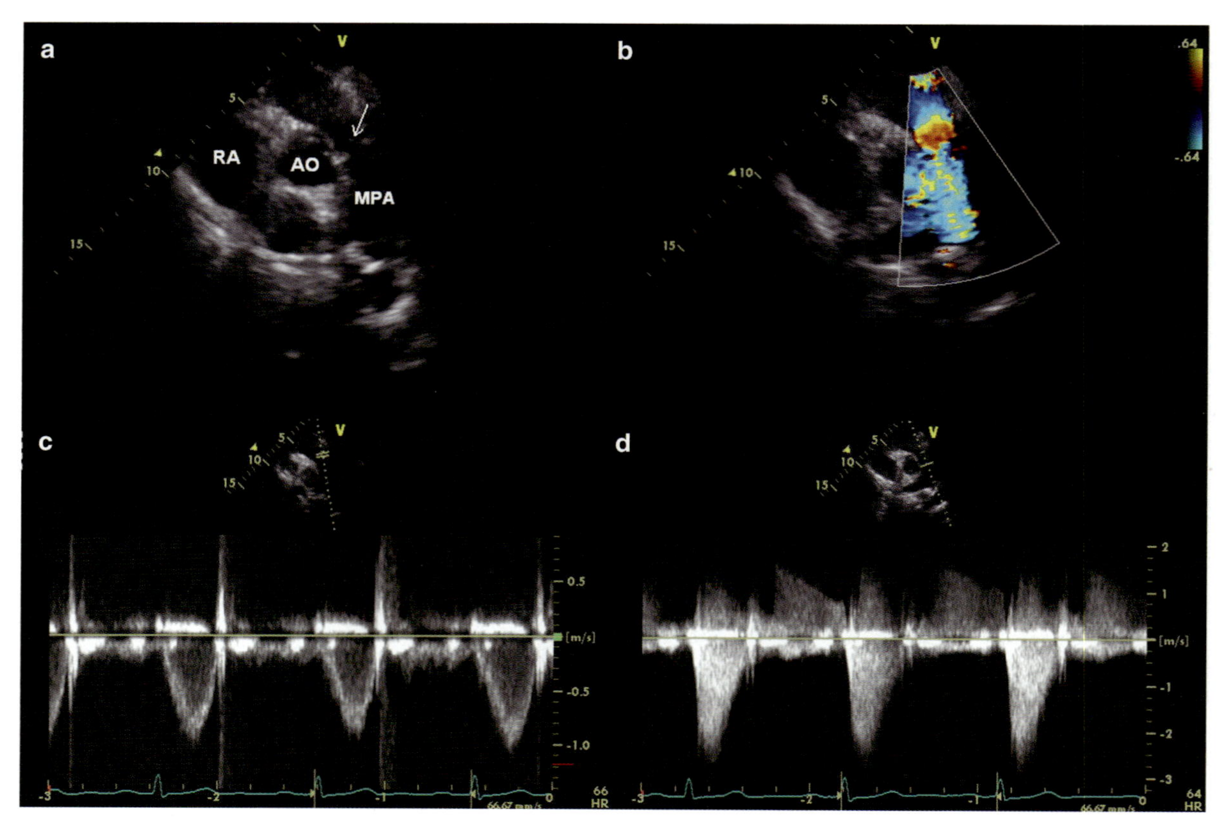

Fig. 5.33 In this patient with mild pulmonary valvular stenosis, the pulmonary valve (*arrow*) is not well seen in the parasternal short-axis view (**a**). Color-flow image (**b**) shows flow acceleration at the pulmonary valve consistent with pulmonary stenosis. Pulsed wave Doppler examination (**c**) shows normal systolic velocity in the right ventricular outflow tract, and continuous wave Doppler (**d**) shows a peak gradient of 28 mmHg with a mean gradient of 13 mmHg across the pulmonary valve consistent with mild pulmonary stenosis. *Ao* aorta, *MPA* main pulmonary artery, *RA* right atrium

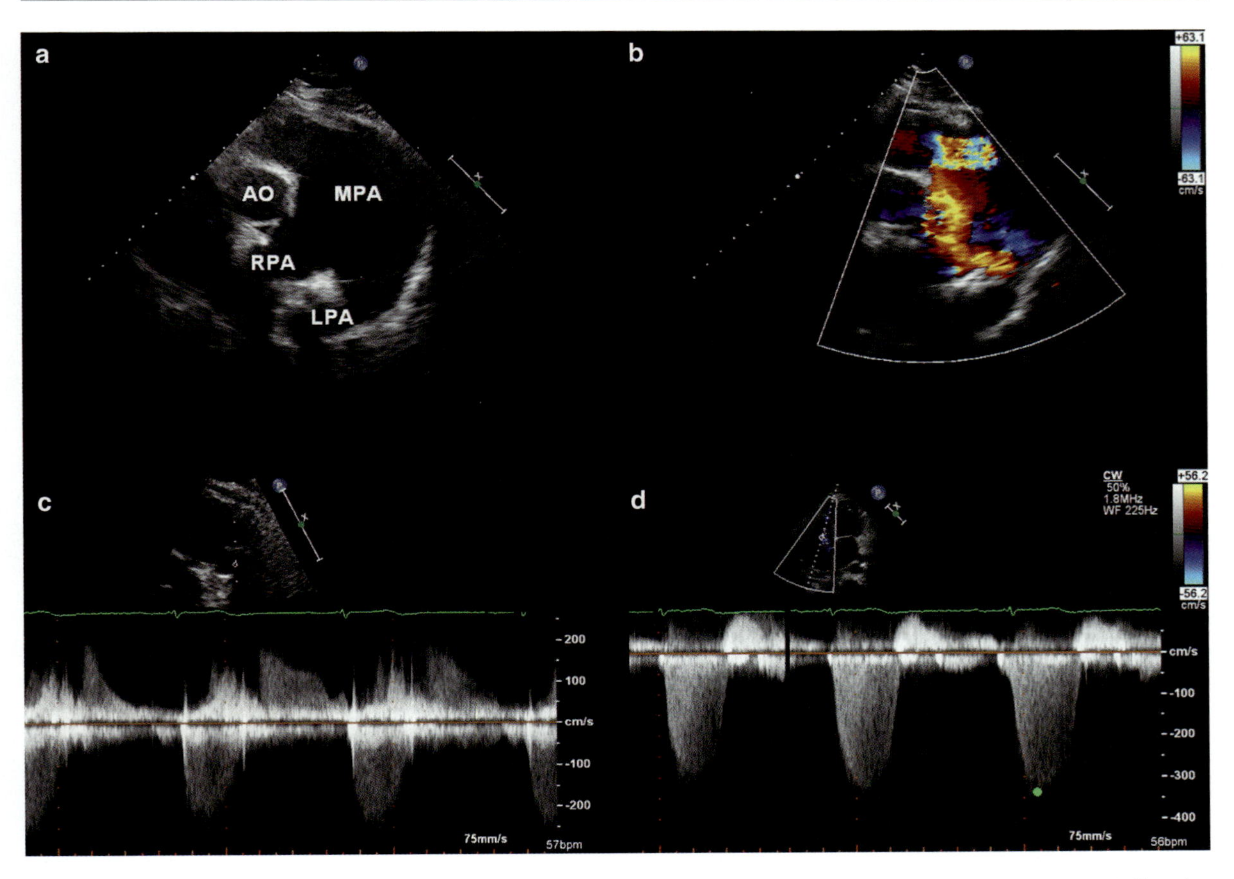

Fig. 5.34 This patient with moderate pulmonary stenosis shows severe dilatation of the main pulmonary artery and mild dilatation involving the proximal right and left pulmonary arteries (**a**). Color-flow image shows flow acceleration at the pulmonary valve confirming valvular pulmonary stenosis (**b**). Doppler examination (**c**, **d**) confirms moderate pulmonary stenosis with a peak gradient of 50 mmHg and a mean gradient of 24 mmHg. *Ao* aorta, *LPA* left pulmonary artery, *MPA* main pulmonary artery, *RPA* right pulmonary artery

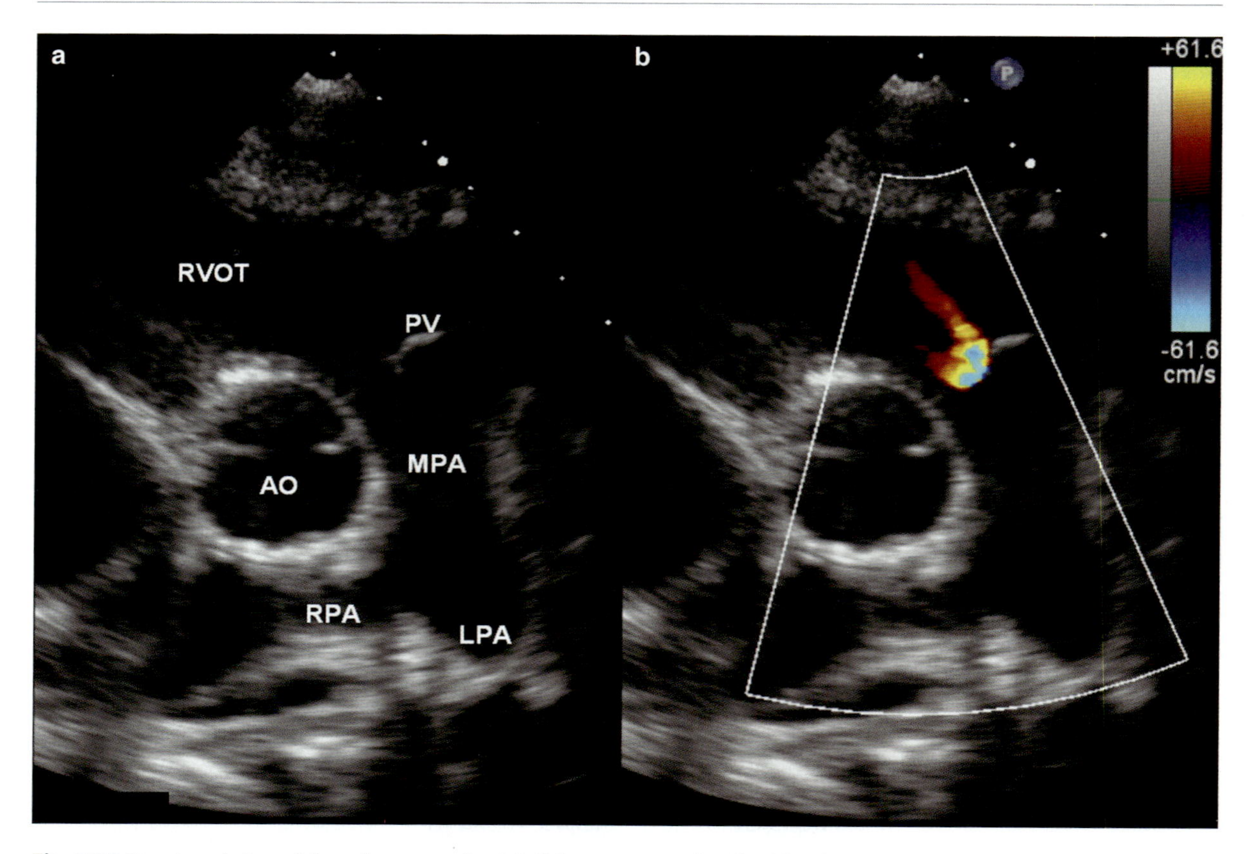

Fig. 5.35 Parasternal view of the pulmonary valve (**a**). Other structures visualized in this view include the right ventricular outflow tract and the pulmonary arteries. Color-flow image (**b**) shows mild pulmonary regurgitation which is physiological and not an abnormal finding. *Ao* aorta, *LPA* left pulmonary artery, *MPA* main pulmonary artery, *PV* pulmonic valve, *RPA* right pulmonary artery, *RVOT* right ventricular outflow tract

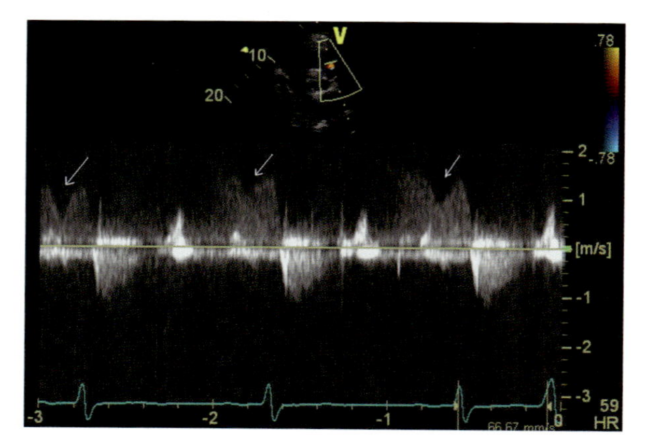

Fig. 5.36 Continuous wave Doppler across the pulmonary valve showing prominent A-dip *arrows*) in the pulmonary regurgitation velocity profile, which is a normal finding

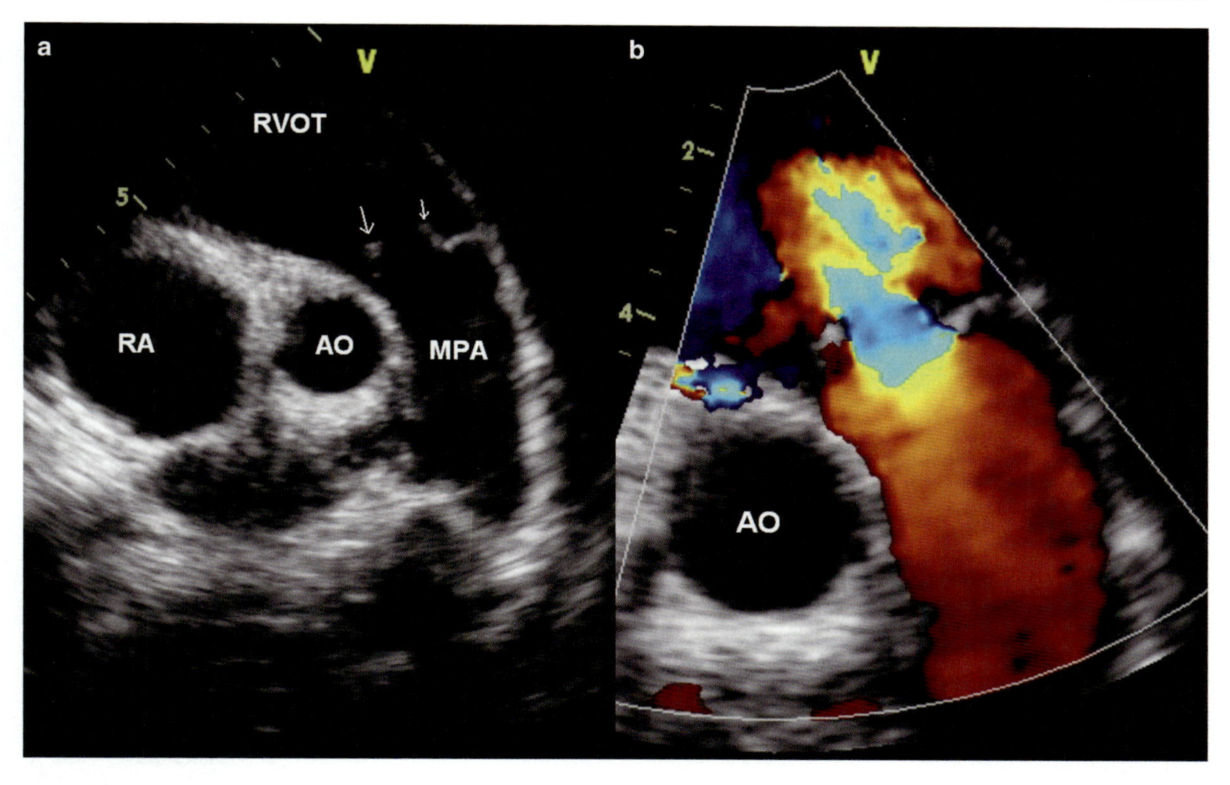

Fig. 5.37 The parasternal short-axis view shows that the pulmonary valve is flailed (*arrows*) in a patient who had pulmonary valvotomy for pulmonary stenosis. Color-flow image (**b**) shows a large pulmonary regurgitant jet consistent with severe pulmonary regurgitation. *Ao* aorta, *MPA* main pulmonary artery, *RA* right atrium, *RVOT* right ventricular outflow tract

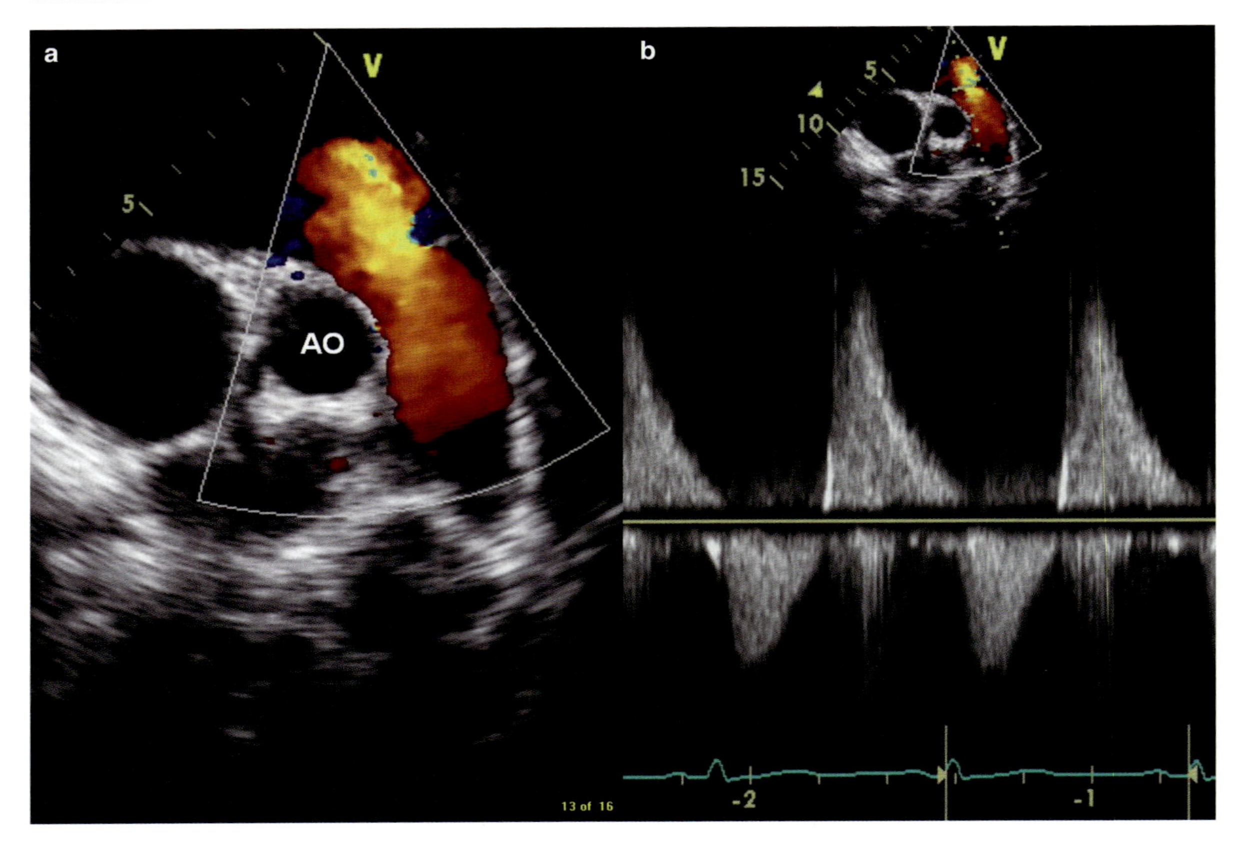

Fig. 5.38 The parasternal short-axis view (**a**) and the continuous wave Doppler (**b**) of the same patient in Fig. 5.26. There is a typical pulmonary regurgitation velocity profile of severe pulmonary regurgitation. (**b**) The regurgitation velocity is dense with a rapid deceleration to the baseline. *Ao* aorta

Table 5.3 Strengths and limitations of echocardiographic and Doppler parameter in the assessment of pulmonary regurgitation

Parameter	Utility/advantages	Disadvantages
RV size	RV enlargement sensitive for chronic significant PR. Normal size virtually excludes significant PR	Enlargement seen in other conditions
Paradoxical septal motion (volume overload pattern)	Simple sign of severe PR	Not specific for PR
Jet length – color flow	Simple	Poor correlation with severity of PR
Vena contracta width	Simple quantitative method that works well for other valves	More difficult to perform; requires good images of pulmonary valve; lacks published validation
Jet deceleration rate – CW	Simple	Steep deceleration not specific for severe PR
Flow quantitation – PW	Quantitates regurgitant flow and fraction	Subject to significant errors due to difficulties of measurement of pulmonic annulus and a dynamic RVOT; not well validated

CW continuous wave, *RV* right ventricle, *PR* pulmonic regurgitation, *RVOT* right ventricular outflow tract
Source: Reproduced from Zoghbi et al. [31]. With permission

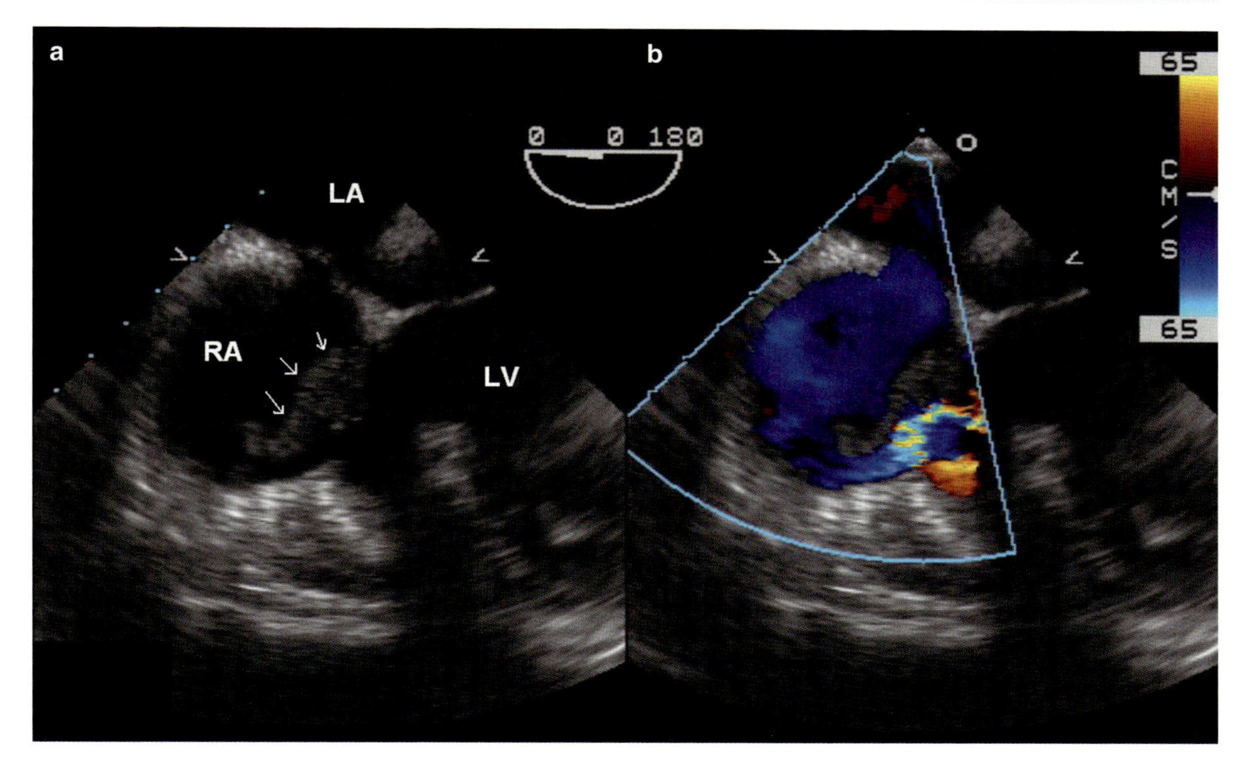

Fig. 5.39 (**a**) Transesophageal echocardiogram in a patient with right-sided endocarditis shows a large vegetation (*arrows*) on the tricuspid leaflet prolapsing into the right atrium during systole. The color-flow image (**b**) shows mild tricuspid regurgitation

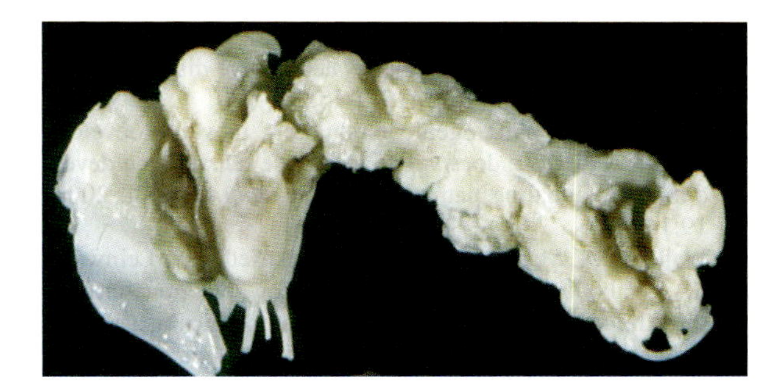

Fig. 5.40 Tricuspid valve infective endocarditis. Excised piece of tricuspid valve. Large vegetations are typical, especially with fungal infections, Right side infections are often culture negative. Presentations with emboli, including pulmonary emboli occur. Empyema, effusions, pulmonary infarcts and abscesses may complicate right-sided infection

6 Cardiomyopathies

Cardiomyopathies are cardiac disorders characterized by predominant myocardial dysfunction – expressed as diastolic or systolic ventricular dysfunction. Before the advent of molecular biology, cardiomyopathies were considered heart muscle disease of unknown etiology. The most recently accepted definition of a cardiomyopathy is a heterogeneous group of diseases of the myocardium associated with mechanical or electrical dysfunction that usually (but not invariably) exhibit inappropriate ventricular hypertrophy or dilation and are due to a variety of causes that frequently are genetic [1]. Cardiomyopathies are either confined to the heart (primary cardiomyopathies) or are part of generalized systemic disorders (secondary cardiomyopathies). Within the group of primary cardiomyopathies, some are thought to be genetic (hypertrophic cardiomyopathy), some acquired (post-myocarditis), and some mixed (dilated cardiomyopathy) in pathoetiology [1]. Traditionally, three general cardiomyopathy groups are widely recognized – dilated, hypertrophic, and restrictive cardiomyopathies [2, 3]. It is expected that these cardiomyopathy classifications will evolve and change especially in view of the increasing knowledge of genetic mutations and their relationship to diseases. In the future we may classify cardiomyopathies according to categories of mutations of cytoskeleton elements, sarcomeric proteins, and components of the intercalated disk or ion channels [4].

Symptoms related to cardiomyopathy can be quite variable. At the early stage of the disease, patients are generally asymptomatic. Although there are some differences in the pattern of symptoms among the different cardiomyopathies, as the disease progresses, typical symptoms of heart failure will develop, irrespective of the type of cardiomyopathy. The common symptoms are dyspnea, palpitations, fatigue, and peripheral edema. The onset of heart failure predicts a poor prognosis with a mortality rate of 20% at 1 year and 70–80% at 6 years [5]. Sudden death can occur in all cardiomyopathies, but may be particularly important in specific subsets of patients with hypertrophic cardiomyopathy and patients with arrhythmogenic right ventricular cardiomyopathy.

Dilated Cardiomyopathy (DCM)

Dilated cardiomyopathy (DCM) is a disease of the myocardium characterized by dilatation and impaired systolic contraction of one or both ventricles [6]. Dilated cardiomyopathy is the most common cardiomyopathy, and may affect patients of any age. DCM is characterized by dilatation of all four cardiac chambers and biventricular hypertrophy (Figs. 6.1–6.3) [2]. The weight of the heart may be severely increased predominantly from eccentric ventricular hypertrophy (ventricular dilatation and hypertrophy together). The ventricle wall thickness may be thin, due to stretching of the myocytes as the ventricle dilates. This is sometimes confusing; a dilated heart may be severely hypertrophied in terms of increased ventricular mass, despite having thin walls due to failure and dilatation of the chambers. There may be atrial or ventricular thrombus in all chambers, including both atrial appendages. Myocardial scars may be noted grossly in the wall of either ventricle. It is important that there be no significant coronary disease, large myocardial infarcts, congenital heart disease, or valve disease that might otherwise explain the myocardial damage.

The common microscopic findings include myocyte nuclear hypertrophy, fibrosis which can be endocardial, interstitial, perivascular and pericellular, and often myocyte sarcoplasmic degenerative changes with myocyte clearing or vacuolization. Myofiber attenuation

K.-L. Chan and J.P. Veinot, *Anatomic Basis of Echocardiographic Diagnosis*,
DOI: 10.1007/978-1-84996-387-9_6,

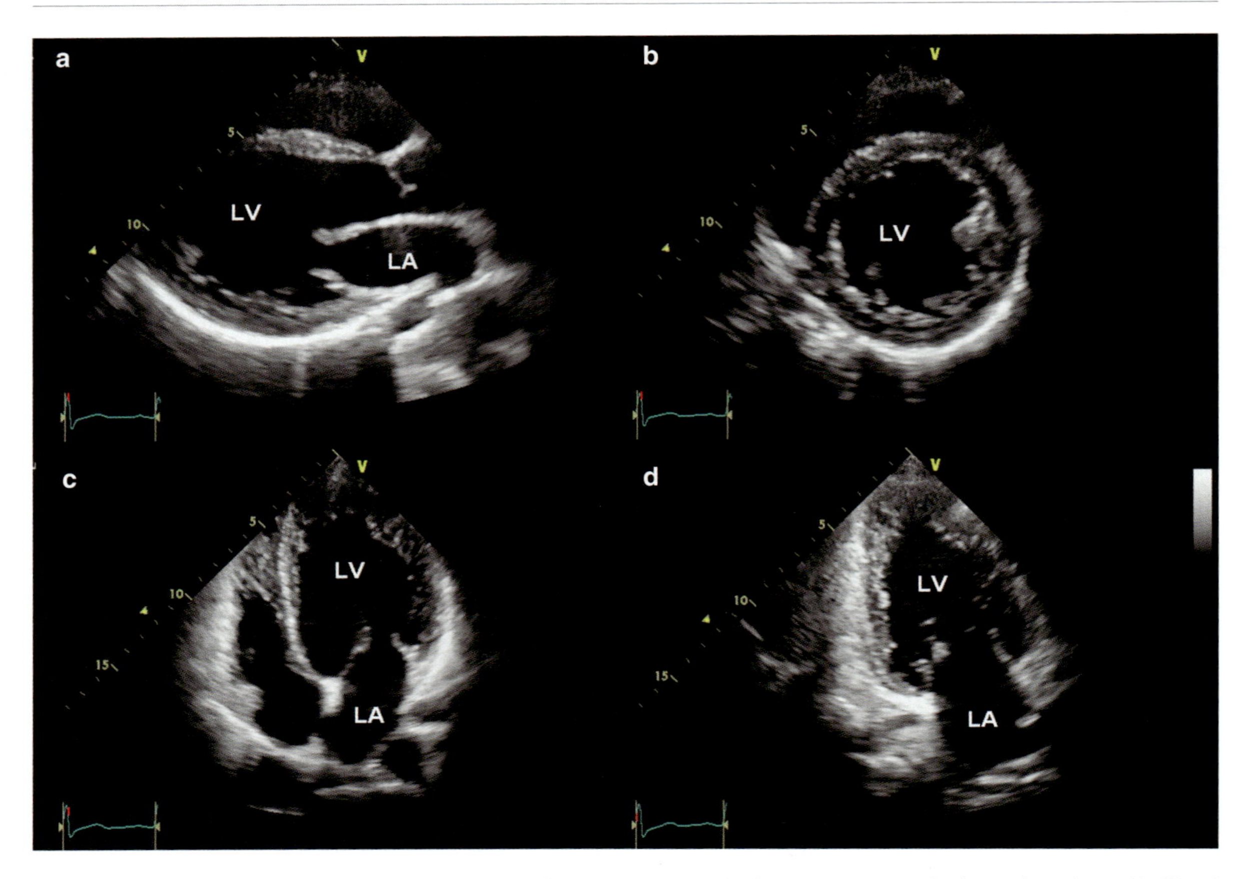

Fig. 6.1 Parasternal long-axis (**a**), short-axis (**b**), apical four-chamber (**c**) and apical two-chamber (**d**) views of a patient with dilated cardiomyopathy in diastole showing a dilated and globular left ventricle. *LA* left atrium, *LV* left ventricle

and stretching may be marked. Nuclei may be irregular in shape and hyperchromatic. Interstitial fibrosis is mostly pericellular and endocardial, but may also be perivascular in location. Interstitial cells should not be confused with inflammatory cells and misinterpreted as evidence for myocarditis. However, true myocarditis is not uncommon either as an underlying etiology or as a result of treatment (catecholaminergic and hypersensitivity myocarditis from pressor agents and other medications).

Dilated cardiomyopathy may be complicated by biventricular congestive heart failure, supraventricular and ventricular arrhythmias, thromboemboli, and sudden death. It is common to have some degree of tricuspid and mitral valve regurgitation with DCM as the ventricular dilatation and annular stretching cause poor apposition of the valve leaflets.

To accurately diagnose primary dilated cardiomyopathy, the clinical information of the individual must be known, including knowledge of other illnesses, toxin and drug exposures, and systemic diseases. The correct clinical context includes the absence of significant valvular heart disease, coronary artery disease, and long-standing hypertension.

Myocarditis is found histologically in about 10% of cases of DCM, hence its classification as a mixed pathoetiology within the primary cardiomyopathy group (Fig. 6.4) [1, 7, 8]. Myocarditis may lead to DCM as the initial viral infection may lead to myocyte destruction, followed by a chronic immunological attack of the myocytes with autoantibodies and also involvement of the cellular immune system. Viral proteases may cleave and disrupt the normal dystrophin protein relationship it has with the sarcolemmal membrane. Interestingly, dystrophin mutations and other cytoskeleton protein mutations are the ones commonly associated with genetic DCM and cardiomyopathy associated with Duchenne and Becker muscular dystrophy.

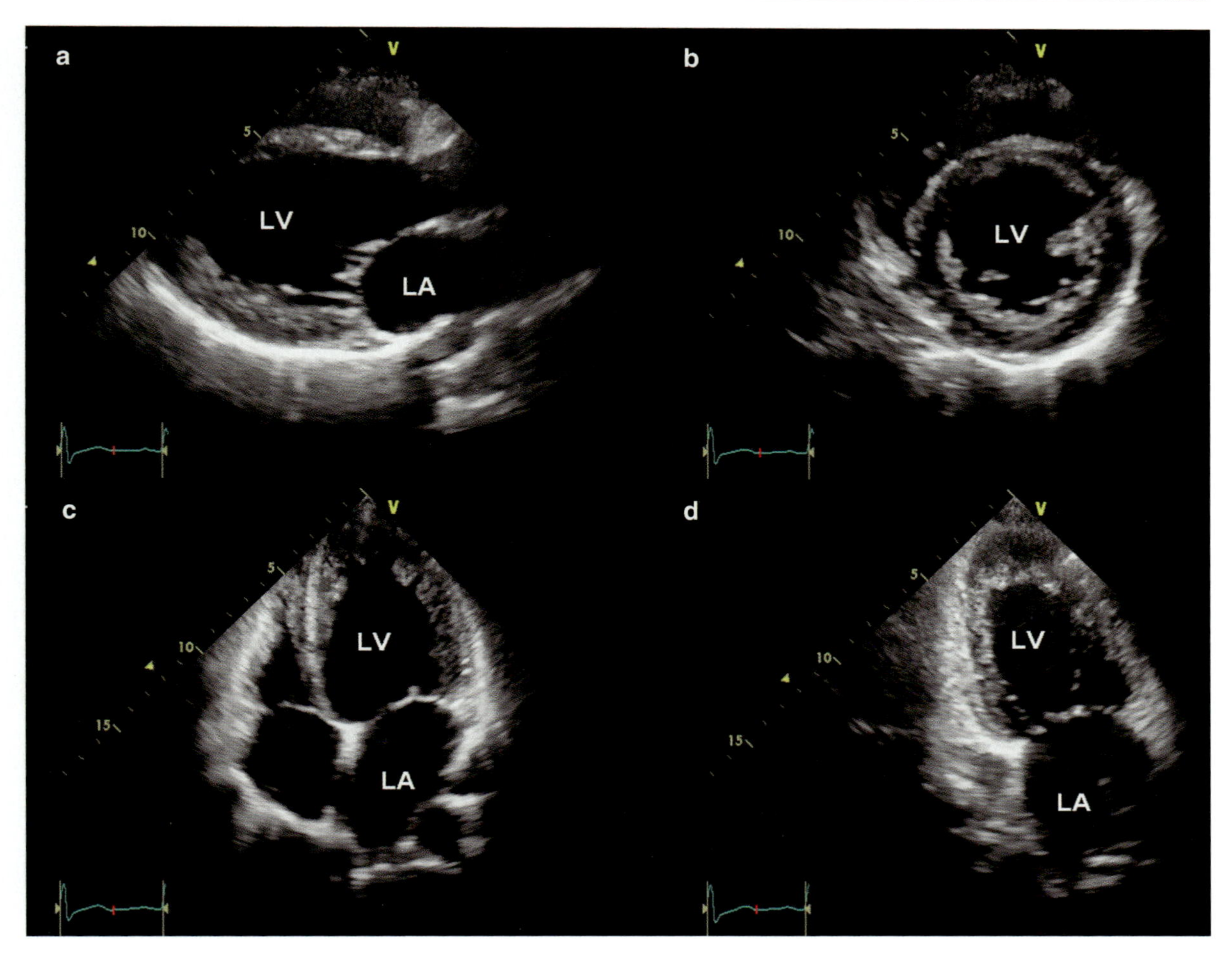

Fig. 6.2 Parasternal long-axis (**a**), short-axis (**b**), apical four-chamber (**c**) and apical two-chamber (**d**) views in systole in the same patient as in Fig. 6.1 show that the left ventricle remains globular in shape with global hypokinesia. *LA* left atrium, *LV* left ventricle

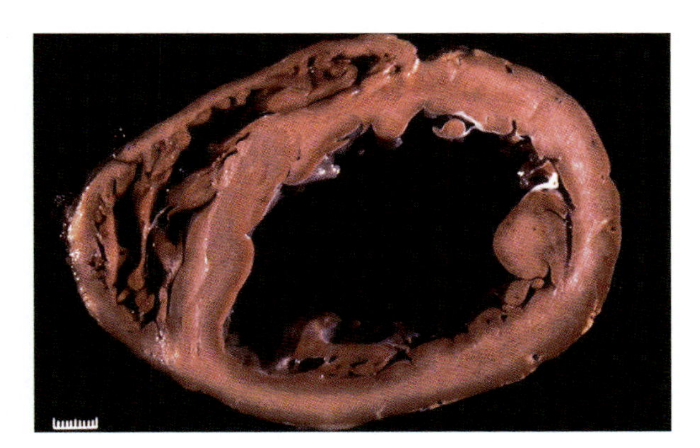

Fig. 6.3 Primary dilated cardiomyopathy. The patient has biventricular hypertrophy and dilatation. Congestive heart failure was present

Causes of secondary DCM include myopathies that also involve the skeletal muscles, radiation, adriamycin exposure, nutritional deficiencies, alcohol, diabetes, human immunodeficiency virus (HIV) infection, hepatitis C infection, and the peripartum state [9-12]. Thought should be given to the investigation of skeletal muscle if there is clinical fatigue. Many forms of generalized myopathy can have myocardial involvement and the diagnosis may be more easily obtained by biopsying an involved peripheral muscle (Fig. 6.5).

Familial DCM represents approximately 20% of cases of DCM [11, 13, 14]. The nonfamilial and familial forms of DCM cannot be distinguished by routine histology or imaging [15].

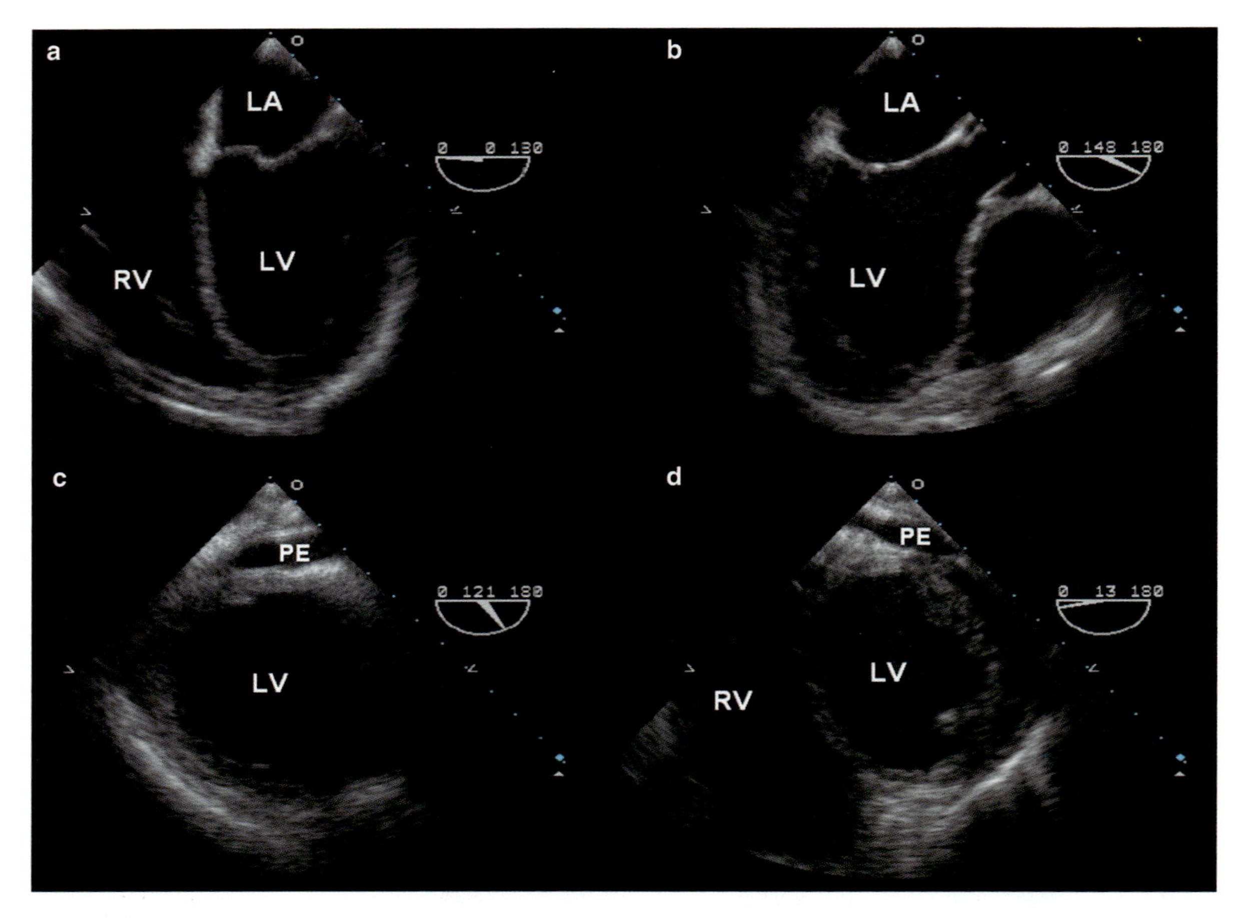

Fig. 6.4 Transesophageal views (**a**, **b**, **c**, **d**) in a patient with giant cell myocarditis show that the left ventricle is severely dilated with global hypokinesia. The right ventricle is also dilated and hypokinetic. A small pericardial effusion is present. *LA* left atrium, *LV* left ventricle, *PE* pericardial effusion, *RV* right ventricle

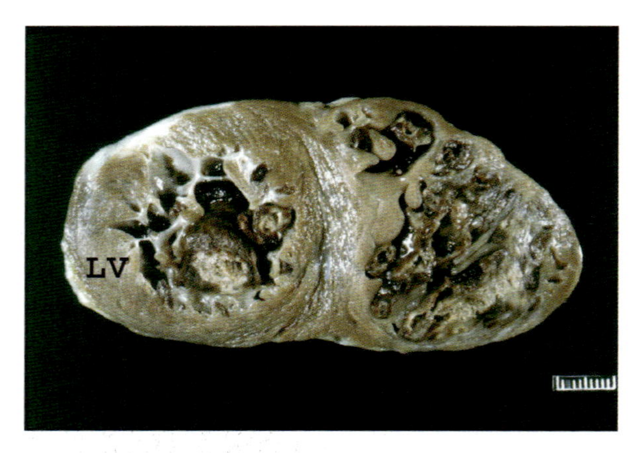

Fig. 6.5 Becker's muscular dystrophy related cardiomyopathy. This patient had congestive heart failure. Bilateral ventricular thrombi are noted. Skeletal muscle involvement was also clinically present. *LV* left ventricle

As the name DCM implies, the typical echocardiographic finding is a dilated left ventricle with global hypokinesia resulting in reduced stroke volume [16]. The left ventricular wall is generally of normal thickness or thin. With the increased left ventricular size, the left ventricular mass is also increased despite the normal left ventricular wall thickness (eccentric hypertrophy). Although global hypokinesia is the norm, some degree of regional differences can be observed. The basal walls and the septum are usually severely hypokinetic, as compared to the anterior and lateral free walls. Myocardial scar, evidenced by a thin echodense ventricular wall, is uncommon, and when it is present, coronary artery disease should be suspected.

The degree of left ventricular dysfunction can run the whole gamut from very mild to severe systolic dysfunction. The increase in left ventricular volume may be subtle at the beginning of the disease. As the dilatation becomes more apparent, the heart assumes a more globular shape [17, 18]. With moderate or severe left ventricular dysfunction, spontaneous contrast within the left ventricular cavity can be seen, especially when a high frequency transducer is used. In this setting, spontaneous contrast can be differentiated from artifact by its typical swirling motion pattern.

In dilated cardiomyopathy, the myopathic process affects both ventricles and right ventricular function should be carefully assessed. Indeed, the presence of right ventricular dysfunction in the setting of left ventricular dysfunction is an indication that the etiology of left ventricular disease is more likely to be cardiomyopathy than ischemic heart disease. Right ventricular function is more sensitive to loading conditions than the left ventricle. While the left ventricle can maintain normal output over a wide range of after load, right ventricular output may decrease markedly even with a relatively small increase in after load [19]. The increase in after load due to the increase in back pressure in a failing left ventricle is another important reason for the presence of right ventricular dysfunction. It is not surprising that right ventricular dysfunction provides incremental prognostic value in determining outcome, including exercise capacity and survival in patients with heart failure [20].

Left ventricular thrombus is an uncommon complication in dilated cardiomyopathy, and anticoagulation treatment is not routinely used in patients who remain in sinus rhythm. The location of thrombus is most common at the left ventricular apex (Fig. 6.6). The differentiating

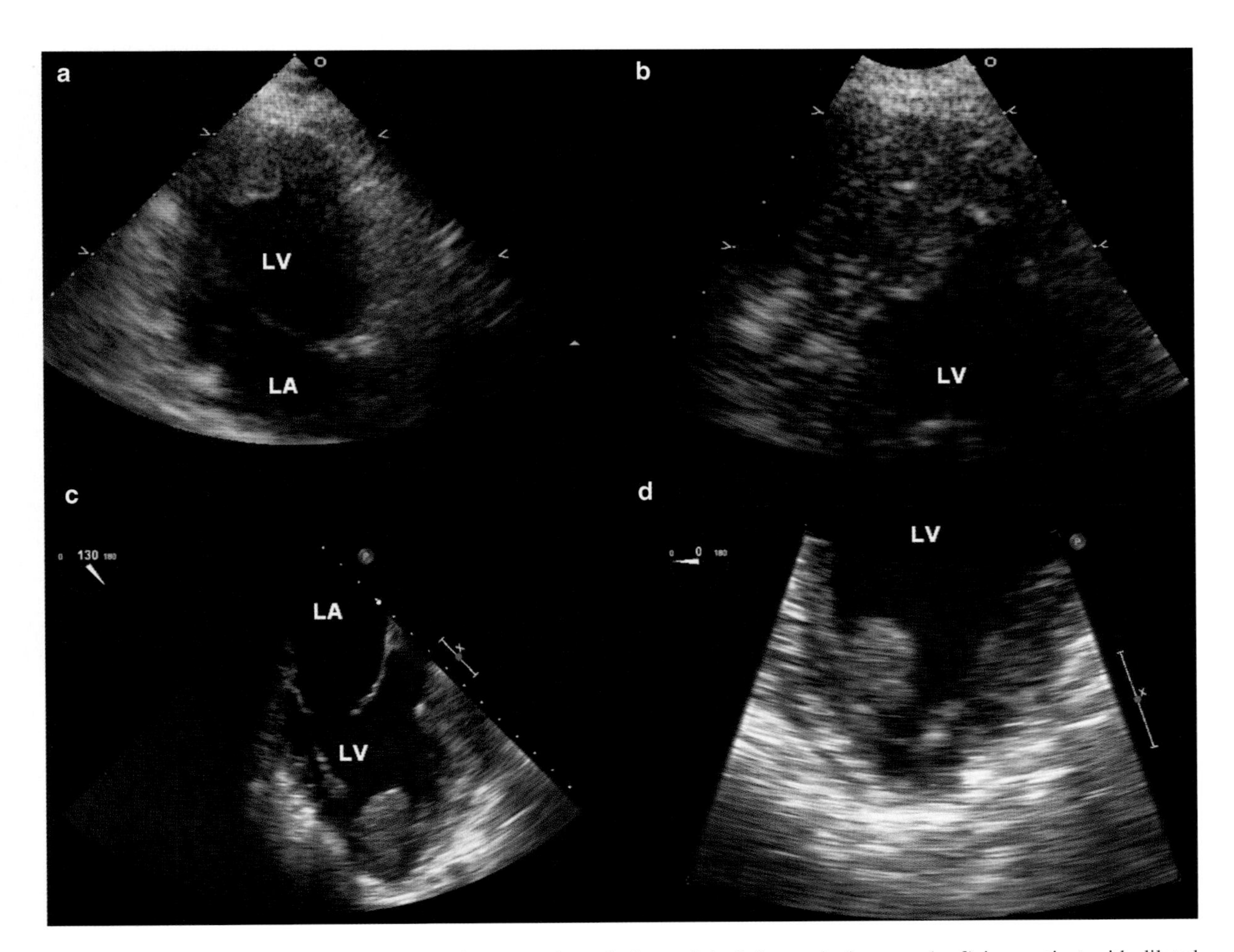

Fig. 6.6 Transthoracic apical views (**a, b**) and transesophageal views of the left ventricular apex (**c, d**) in a patient with dilated cardiomyopathy show a large apical thrombus. The left ventricular apex is trabeculated and it can be difficult to differentiate thrombus from trabeculations, as demonstrated in the transthoracic image in (**b**). *LA* left atrium, *LV* left ventricle

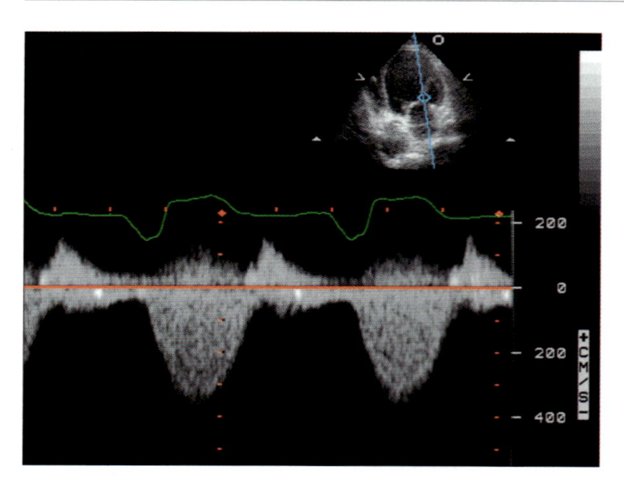

Fig. 6.7 Mitral regurgitation is common in patients with dilated cardiomyopathy. The continuous wave Doppler signal is intense and triangular in contour consistent with severe mitral regurgitation. The delay in reaching peak flow velocity indicates severe left ventricular dysfunction

features between left ventricular thrombus and near gain artifact are discussed in Chap. 7. The ventricular apex in dilated cardiomyopathy can be quite trabeculated and the appearance may suggest noncompaction, but ventricular walls are thin and do not have a two-layered myocardium [21]. Small laminated thrombi may be difficult to identify among the trabeculations. Mitral regurgitation is common as a result of mitral annular dilatation and systolic tethering of the mitral leaflets, leading to passive pulmonary hypertension and right ventricular dysfunction (Fig. 6.7).

Diastolic dysfunction generally coexists with systolic dysfunction, and can be the dominant abnormality so that patients can have severe heart failure symptoms despite only mildly reduced systolic function. Many of the diastolic echocardiographic measurements are abnormal in these patients. Diastolic filling period is usually reduced in DCM, and this is worse in the presence of heart block. Pacing with optimization of the atrioventricular interval can be helpful [22]. Restrictive filling pattern with a short mitral deceleration time is indicative of high left ventricular filling pressure and predicts a poor prognosis (Fig. 6.8) [23]. The Doppler indices can also be used to follow the response to treatment (Fig. 6.9). A detailed approach for the assessment of diastolic function is described in Chap. 16.

Noncompaction of the Ventricle

Isolated noncompaction of the ventricle is grouped with dilated cardiomyopathy. Ventricular noncompaction can be familial in nature [24]. In this disorder, the inner left ventricle has marked trabeculations giving it a two-layered appearance. The left ventricle demonstrates heavy trabeculations with deep crevices, an appearance akin to the right ventricle rather than the usually smooth endocardial surface of the left ventricle. The trabeculations are most prominent in the inferolateral wall and the apex, and a meshwork of trabeculation is frequently present in the apex (Fig. 6.10) [21]. This disorder has systolic dysfunction, arrhythmias, and propensity for endocardial thrombus formation with embolization. The latter propensity may be due to the increased endocardial trabecular surface area of the ventricle and stasis as a result of ventricular dysfunction. Color flow imaging and the use of contrast can illustrate the differences between the compact and noncompacted layers by highlighting the deep crevices. Small laminated thrombus is difficult to detect in this condition.

The echocardiographic features are listed in Table 6.1 (Figs. 6.10, 6.11). The most diagnostic feature of isolated ventricular noncompaction is the ratio (>2:1) of the trabeculated ventricular wall component to the non-trabeculated compact ventricular wall component in systole [21]. Excessive ventricular trabeculation may also be seen with ventricular outflow tract obstruction and congenital heart disease, including pulmonary atresia. Although noncompacted ventricles, they are not isolated. While one or more of the features may be present in other disease conditions including dilated cardiomyopathy and hypertensive heart disease, only isolated noncompaction has most, if not all, of these findings [21]. Increased wall thickness of the noncompacted wall is a good differentiating feature to exclude dilated cardiomyopathy, and the two-layered appearance of myocardium is generally not seen in hypertensive heart disease. Isolated noncompaction has been associated with some systemic neuromuscular myopathies or muscular dystrophies. In view of the propensity for the development of arrhythmias and thrombi, defibrillator and anticoagulation may be considered.

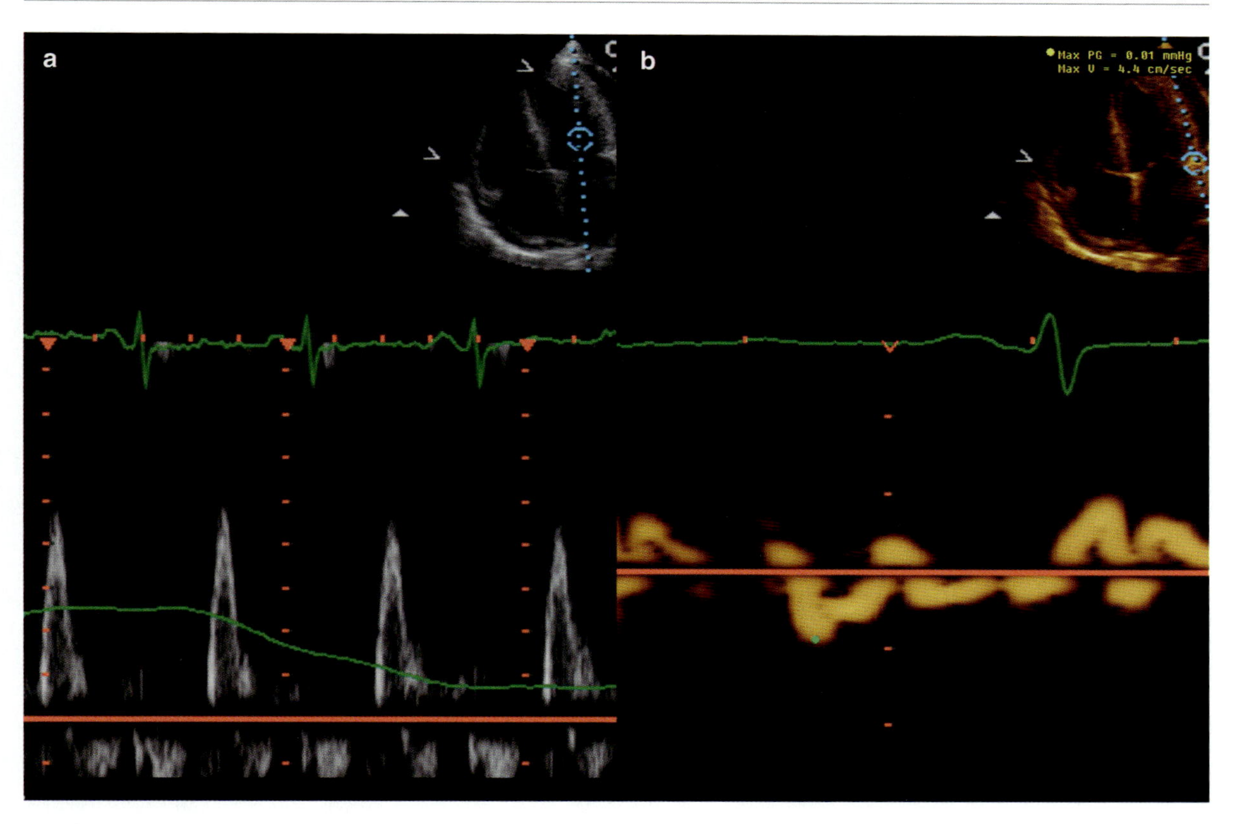

Fig. 6.8 The mitral inflow signal (**a**) shows an increased early diastolic velocity with very low late diastolic velocity. The deceleration time is very short consistent with severe elevation in left ventricular filling pressure and predicts a poor prognosis. Tissue Doppler imaging at the lateral annulus shows a severely reduced early diastolic velocity

Hypertrophic Cardiomyopathy (HCM)

Hypertrophic cardiomyopathy (HCM) is an important clinical entity that may have both systolic and diastolic dysfunction. It is an inherited cardiomyopathy and is responsible for many sudden deaths, especially under the age of 35. [25, 26]. Hypertrophic cardiomyopathy has many synonyms including idiopathic hypertrophic subaortic stenosis and hypertrophic obstructive cardiomyopathy, but no single name fully captures the wide clinical and pathological variation seen in the disorder [27]. There may be asymmetrical septal hypertrophy, or this may be absent. Hypertrophy itself may be absent or only minimal. Obstruction of the ventricular outflow tract and ischemia may be major problems [28].

The diagnostic features of HCM have been described for pathology, echocardiography, electrocardiology, clinical examination, and hemodynamic studies [27, 29-31]. These features include diastolic dysfunction, ventricular hypertrophy, and systolic motion of the anterior mitral leaflet. Many of these features are not unique to HCM. For instance, age-related angulation of the ventricular septum or severe hypertension-related left hypertrophy may give rise to systolic anterior motion of the anterior mitral leaflet particularly when the patients become hypovolemic. Genetic studies to detect typical mutations in the myosin gene have become increasingly important in the diagnosis and prognosis of patients with this condition.

It should also be remembered that many variants of HCM exist, and not all are asymmetrical septal hypertrophy in phenotype. Many patients have symmetrical left ventricular hypertrophy mimicking changes seen with systemic arterial hypertension. An apical variant

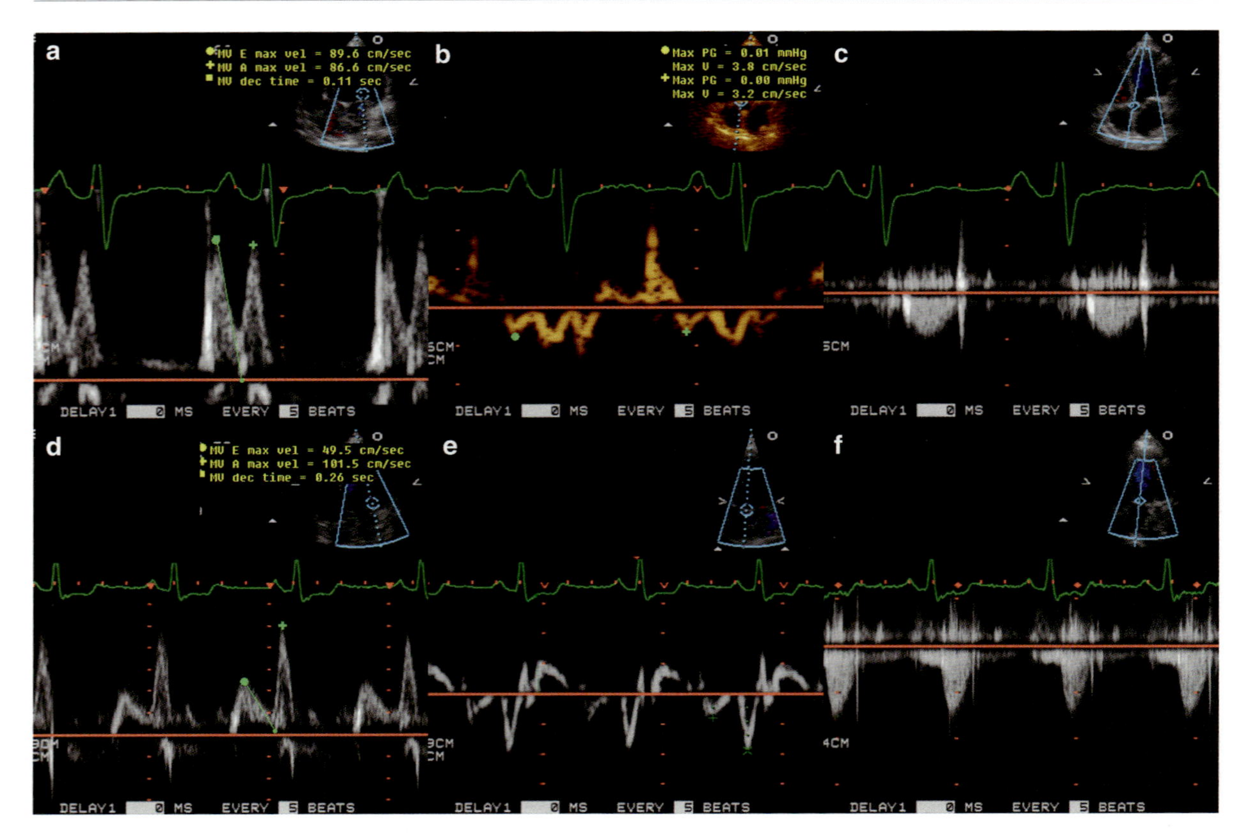

Fig. 6.9 The response to treatment in a patient with dilated cardiomyopathy and heart failure can be assessed by the Doppler assessment. Before treatment, elevated left ventricular filling pressure is indicated by the mitral inflow velocities (**a**) and the septal tissue annular velocities (**b**). The low stroke volume is evidenced by the continuous wave Doppler at the left ventricular outflow tract (**c**). After treatment, there is reduction in left ventricular filling pressure such that the mitral inflow velocities (**d**) demonstrate an impaired relaxation pattern. The diastolic annular tissue velocities remain unchanged (**e**). The stroke volume as determined by continuous wave Doppler at the left ventricular outflow tract shows a slight improvement (**f**). These findings indicate a positive response to heart failure therapy

has been described, in which the gross hypertrophy and histological disarray of the myocytes is centered at the LV apex. With this variant there is no outflow tract obstruction, although obstruction at the apex can be present.

Grossly these hearts are often severely hypertrophied, although the hypertrophy may not be apparent at an early age (Fig. 6.12). This is important for childhood screening as a child with no hypertrophy on imaging must be longitudinally followed in case hypertrophy subsequently develops. The hypertrophy is usually apparent when the child reaches physical maturity, although recent studies suggest that in some patients with HCM cardiac hypertrophy may develop much later in life [25]. The left atrium is usually dilated and the mitral valve is thickened, a problem that increases with systolic anterior motion of the anterior leaflet with trauma against the ventricular septum (Fig. 6.13). Chronic congestive heart failure, which may occur in some of these patients, may cause the right-sided chambers to dilate or become hypertrophic.

Explanted or autopsy hearts characteristically show myocyte hypertrophy, interstitial fibrosis, myocyte disarray, and thick intramyocardial arterioles. Disarray is actually normal in the heart and thus is not specific for HCM. Disarray of myocytes may also be found if a prior biopsy site is re-biopsied and in tetralogy of Fallot, pulmonary atresia, aortic atresia, and regressed papillary muscles after atrioventricular valve resection. The difference with the disarray between these entities and HCM is quantitative rather than qualitative [32].

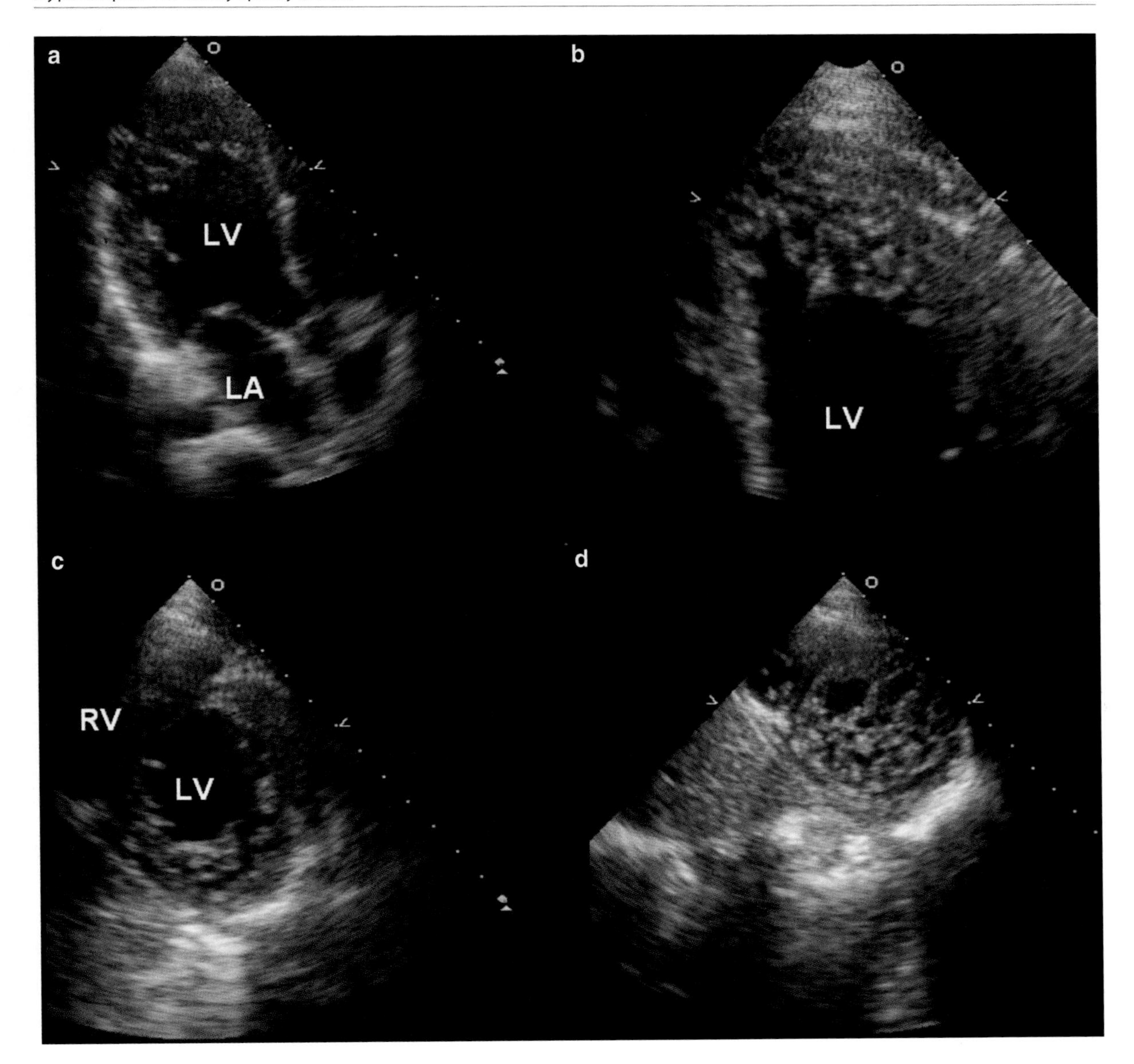

Fig. 6.10 There are heavy trabeculations with deep recesses in the mid-segments and apical segments of the left ventricle which are seen in the apical long-axis (**a, b**) and short-axis (**c, d**) views. These features are consistent with left ventricular noncompaction. *LA* left atrium, *LV* left ventricle, *RV* right ventricle

Table 6.1 Diagnostic features of left ventricular noncompaction

• Thickened ventricular segments
• Two-layered myocardium
• Non-compacted layer to compacted layer at end systole ≥ 2:1
• Deeply perfused recesses
• Prominent meshwork in mid-segments or apical segments
• Hypokinesia of affected segments

Source: Modified from Frischknecht et al. [21]

Microinfarcts with replacement type fibrosis are not uncommon. Large scars mimicking old myocardial infarcts may occur in the "dilated" phase of the disease where the diastolic failure is succeeded by systolic congestive heart failure (Fig. 6.14). Only about 10% of individuals with HCM develop this complication. These "burnt out" cases still have pathological myocardial findings characteristic of HCM and extensive scars are usually present, but the cause is uncertain.

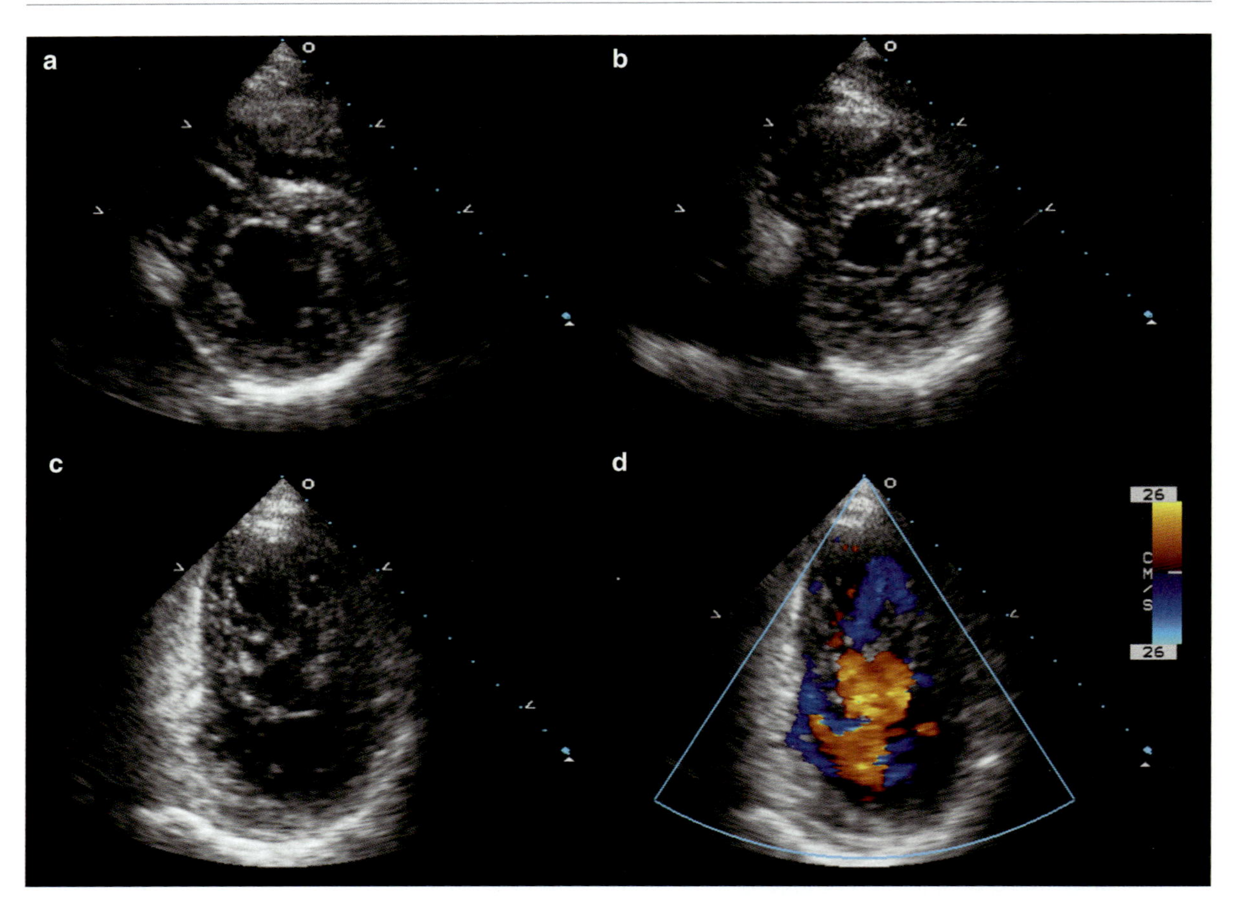

Fig. 6.11 Parasternal short-axis views of mid-left ventricle and apical left ventricle (**a, b, c**) show prominent meshwork in mid-segments and apical segments with deep perfused recesses demonstrated by color-flow imaging (**d**)

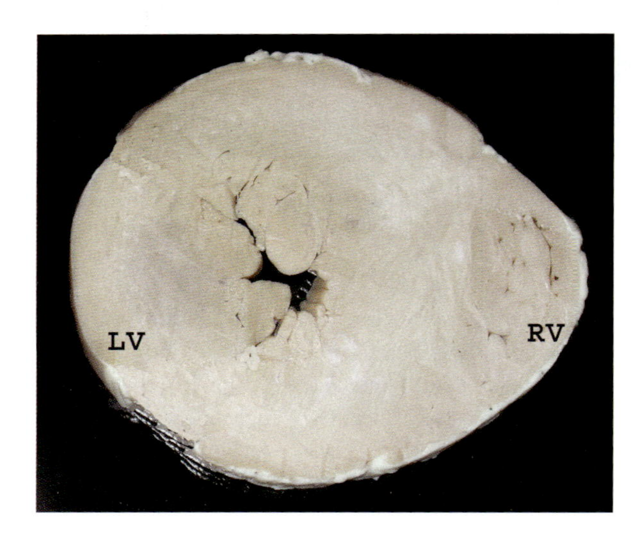

Fig. 6.12 Cross section of a heart from a young person who died suddenly from hypertrophic cardiomyopathy (HCM). Marked left ventricle hypertrophy that is symmetrical. Myocyte disarray was abundant. *LV* left ventricle, *RV* right ventricle

When comparing usual HCM cases with "burnt out" HCM ones, the major morphological difference is the degree of scarring [33].

HCM has many mimics including amyloid, Fabry disease, and other glycogen storage disorders [30]. Amyloid stains such as Congo red, sulfated alcian blue, or methyl violet should be routinely performed on heart biopsy specimens, especially if HCM is a clinical consideration. Storage diseases such as Fabry disease or glycogen storage disease may be detected. Mutations of the gene encoding gamma-2 regulatory subunit of the AMP-activated protein kinase (PRKAG) have been described in patients with atrial fibrillation and a cardiac phenotype that mimics primary hypertrophic cardiomyopathy (Fig. 6.15) [34].

Molecular biology may change the diagnosis of HCM, as the mutations become known. The most common abnormalities include sarcomeric mutations in the beta-myosin heavy chain, troponin T, and alpha-tropomyosin

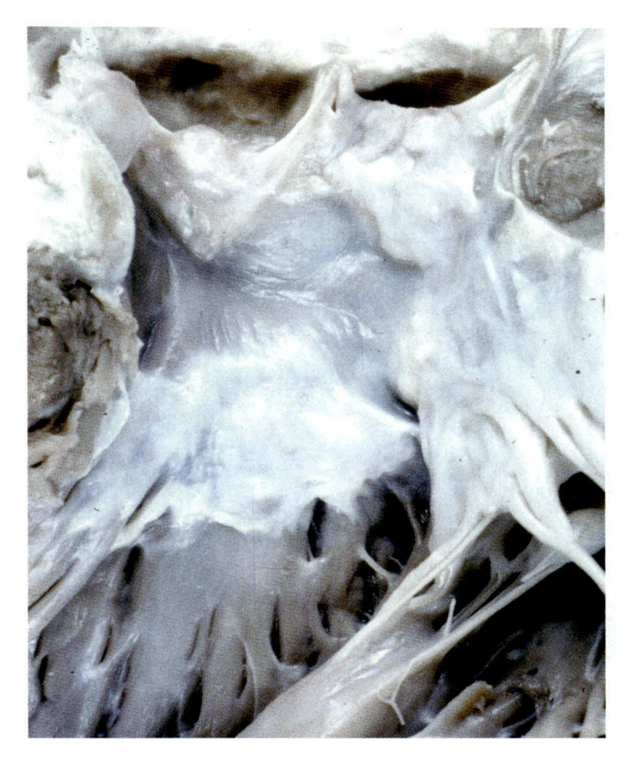

Fig. 6.13 Individual with hypertrophic cardiomyopathy (HCM) with outflow tract obstruction. The mitral valve impact on the ventricular septum has produced a ridge of fibrous endocardial thickening – the septal contact lesion. Such lesions are seen in HCM, but are not specific for this diagnosis

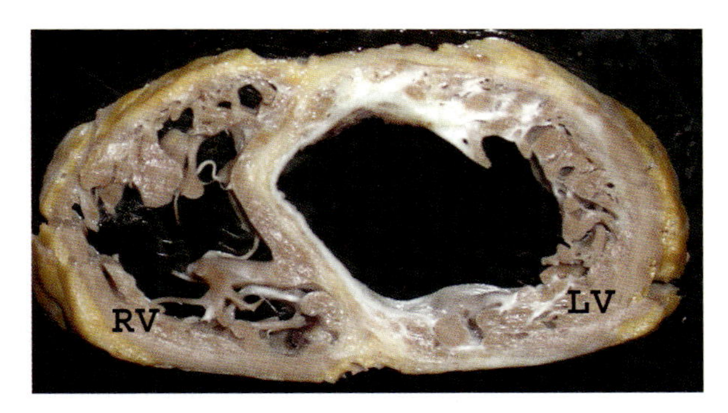

Fig. 6.14 "Burnt out" hypertrophic cardiomyopathy. This patient had congestive heart failure. His heart had biventricular dilatation and hypertrophy with myocardial scarring. Despite this the characteristic myocyte disarray and small vascular disease diagnostic of hypertrophic cardiomyopathy (HCM) were present. *LV* left ventricle, *RV* right ventricle

regions [35-37]. With the use of short tandem repeat polymorphic (STRP) markers that are highly informative, and the polymerase chain reaction (PCR), the mutations can now be rapidly detected [37, 38]. These tests do not require myocardium for diagnosis but these techniques are still largely research techniques and not yet widely used. The phenotypic expression can be highly variable even within families, and coexisting disease modifiers may play a role in the phenotypic expression of certain mutations [39].

HCM is a heterogeneous disease in terms of genotypes, phenotypes, and natural history. The disease is familial in about 50% of the cases and in these cases the hereditary pattern is autosomal dominant related to sarcomere protein mutations [40]. In up to 10% of patients with HCM phenotype, the mutations may not reside in the genes encoding the sarcomeric proteins, and genetic analysis is the best way to identify these mutations. In HCM patients with sarcomeric protein mutations, the presentation can be quite variable. Phenotypic expression may be absent in about 10–15% of adult patients. Some of these patients may develop the phenotype late in life at 50–60 years of age; and some may stay phenotypically negative throughout their lives [41].

Echocardiography plays an essential role in the assessment of patients with hypertrophic cardiomyopathy, as unexplained focal or diffuse hypertrophy is the classic feature of this condition. The common echocardiographic findings are presented in Table 6.2. Some of these findings are only pertinent to specific morphologic types. Different morphologic types, based on the pattern and location of hypertrophy, have been described. There is no single generally accepted index of the extent and severity of hypertrophy. The presence of extreme hypertrophy (≥30 mm wall thickness) in one or more myocardial segments may be a risk factor for sudden death, particularly if it is associated with other risk factors such as family history of sudden death, presentation at a young age, and unexplained syncope (Fig. 6.16) [42, 43]. Abnormal blood pressure response to exercise and non-sustained ventricular tachycardia also may increase the risk of sudden death [44]. It is thus important to measure the maximal wall thickness, in addition to a comprehensive assessment, for hypertrophy of all the myocardial segments.

The classic phenotype has prominent hypertrophy of the basal septum with relative sparing of the basal posterior and inferior walls. There is an association with dynamic subaortic obstruction (Fig. 6.17). The pattern of "eject, obstruct and leak" is a good description of the intracavitary left ventricular hemodynamics in these patients [45]. During the early part of left ventricular ejection, there is rapid anterior motion of the

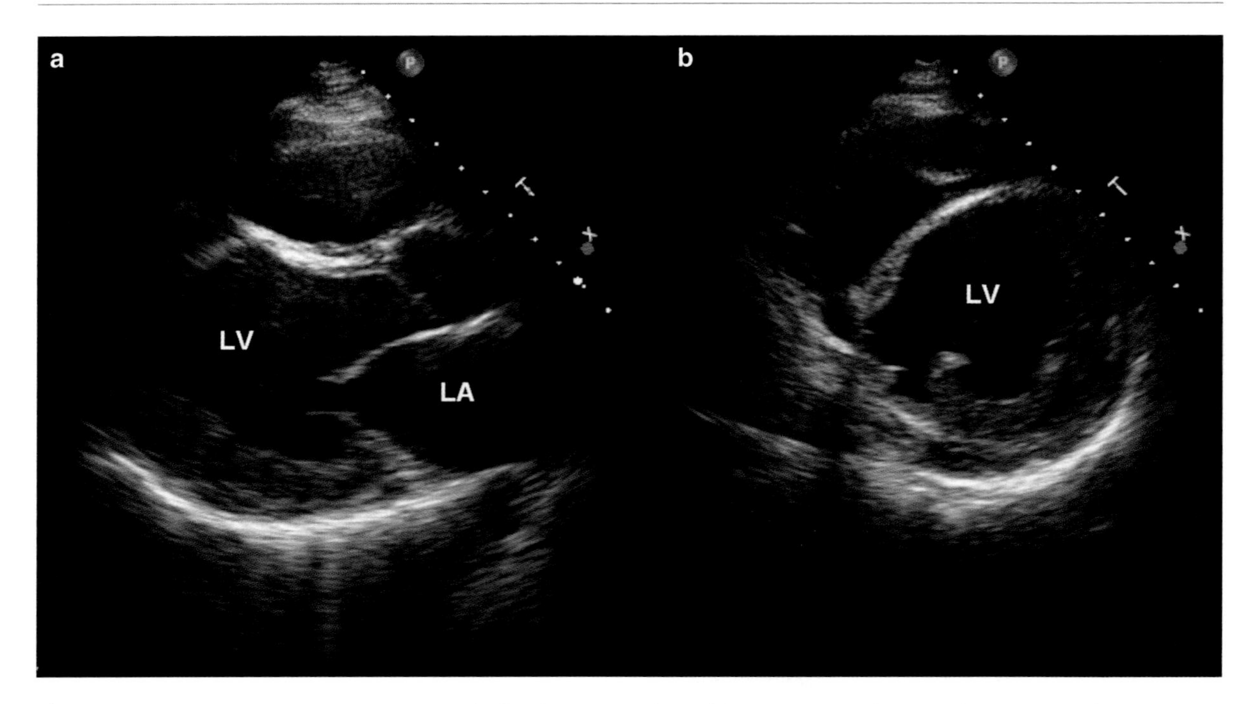

Fig. 6.15 Parasternal long-axis (**a**) and short-axis (**b**) views in a patient with PRKAG mutation show hypertrophy of the anterolateral, posterolateral, and inferior walls. The ventricular septum is thin and akinetic. The patient was diagnosed to have hypertrophic cardiomyopathy before he underwent genetic testing. *LA* left atrium, *LV* left ventricle

Table 6.2 Echocardiographic findings in hypertrophic cardiomyopathy

• LV hypertrophy (focal or diffuse)
• Increase septal to posterior wall thickness ratio (>1.3)
• Small LV cavity
• Hyperdynamic LV contraction
• RV hypertrophy
• Increased LA size
• Systolic anterior mutation (SAM) of mitral leaflet
• Ventricular septal brightness at SAM contact
• Abnormal papillary muscles
• Posteriorly directed mitral regurgitation
• Mid-systolic closure of aortic valve
• Subaortic systolic dynamic gradient (dagger shape CW signal)
• Mid-systolic or apical systolic dynamic gradient
• Relaxation asynchrony (prominent flow during IVRT)

IVRT isovolumic relaxation time, *LV* left ventricle, *RV* right ventricle, *LA* left atrium

tips of the mitral leaflets (SAM) near the coaptation site. This may be due to a narrow outflow tract, abnormal mitral leaflet orientation, and the Venturi effect. The mitral leaflets may make contact with the ventricular septum at mid-systole to late systole resulting in a subaortic gradient. At the same time, the mitral leaflets lose their proper coaptation as they turn sharply into the outflow tract leading to the development of mitral regurgitation, which is posteriorly directed and increases in severity as ejection progresses (Fig. 6.18).

A complete description of the location and severity of hypertrophy is essential for the management of these patients, as this information is crucial to the consideration of surgical septal myectomy or alcohol septal ablation (Fig. 6.19). These procedures can be considered in symptomatic HCM patients, with basal septal hypertrophy (≥15 mm) and a resting subaortic gradient (>30 mmHg) or provocable gradient (>50 mmHg) [46]. When resting subaortic obstruction is absent, manipulation of the left ventricular loading conditions with the Valsalva maneuver or amyl nitrite inhalation may bring out a provocable subaortic gradient (Fig. 6.20). Systolic

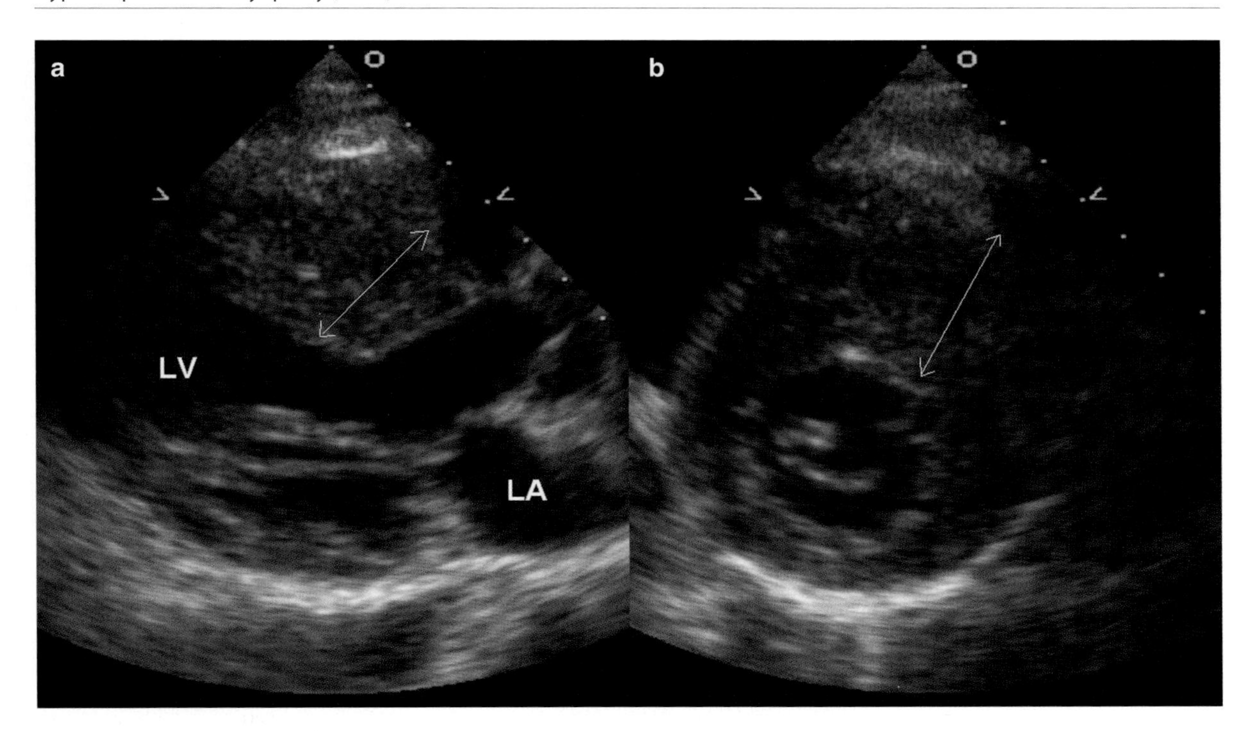

Fig. 6.16 Parasternal long-axis (**a**) and short-axis (**b**) views of a patient with hypertrophic cardiomyopathy showing very severe hypertrophy of the ventricular septum and anterior wall up to 33 mm in thickness. *LA* left atrium, *LV* left ventricle

anterior motion of the mitral leaflet indicates the presence of a subaortic gradient. In contrast, chordal systolic anterior motion can be present in patients without hypertrophic cardiomyopathy and does not necessarily indicate the presence of an intracavitary gradient. It is present in patients with redundant chords and normal left ventricular size and systolic function. Mid-systolic closure of the aortic valve is also an indication of the presence of a subaortic gradient and its presence is best appreciated on M-mode recording of the aortic valve. In association with SAM, mitral regurgitation is frequently detected and its severity increases in late systole (Fig. 6.18). The mitral regurgitation is posteriorly directed [45]. Minor variation of the papillary muscle location can be seen in this condition and may predispose to the development of subaortic obstruction [47].

Symmetrical or diffuse ventricular hypertrophy is an uncommon form of HCM (Fig. 6.21) [48]. It can be difficult to differentiate it from left ventricular hypertrophy related to long-standing, poorly controlled systemic arterial hypertension. The presence of a family history or molecular analysis showing a known sarcomere protein mutation for HCM is helpful to make the diagnosis in this situation. In this morphologic type, subaortic dynamic obstruction is uncommon but mid-intracavitary gradient may be present.

Apical HCM is another uncommon morphologic type; it was first described in the Japanese population, but has now been reported in all ethnic groups [49, 50]. Although the apical four-chamber view is apt to show this condition with its typical "spade shaped" left ventricular cavity, the apical hypertrophy may be difficult to visualize (Fig. 6.22). Indeed the left ventricular apex may appear akinetic and be confused for apical infarct (Fig. 6.23). When this condition is suspected, the use of an echo contrast agent is useful to detect this condition (Fig. 6.24). An apical systolic gradient may be present and can be demonstrated by color-flow imaging and pulse wave interrogation of the left ventricular apex. A better view to assess the hypertrophy of the left ventricular apex is the short axis view of the apex with the transducer at the fourth or fifth intercostal space near the mid-clavicular line (Fig. 6.24). It may be helpful with the patient at a slight left decubitus close to a supine position instead of the standard left lateral decubitus position. Apical infarct is a known complication

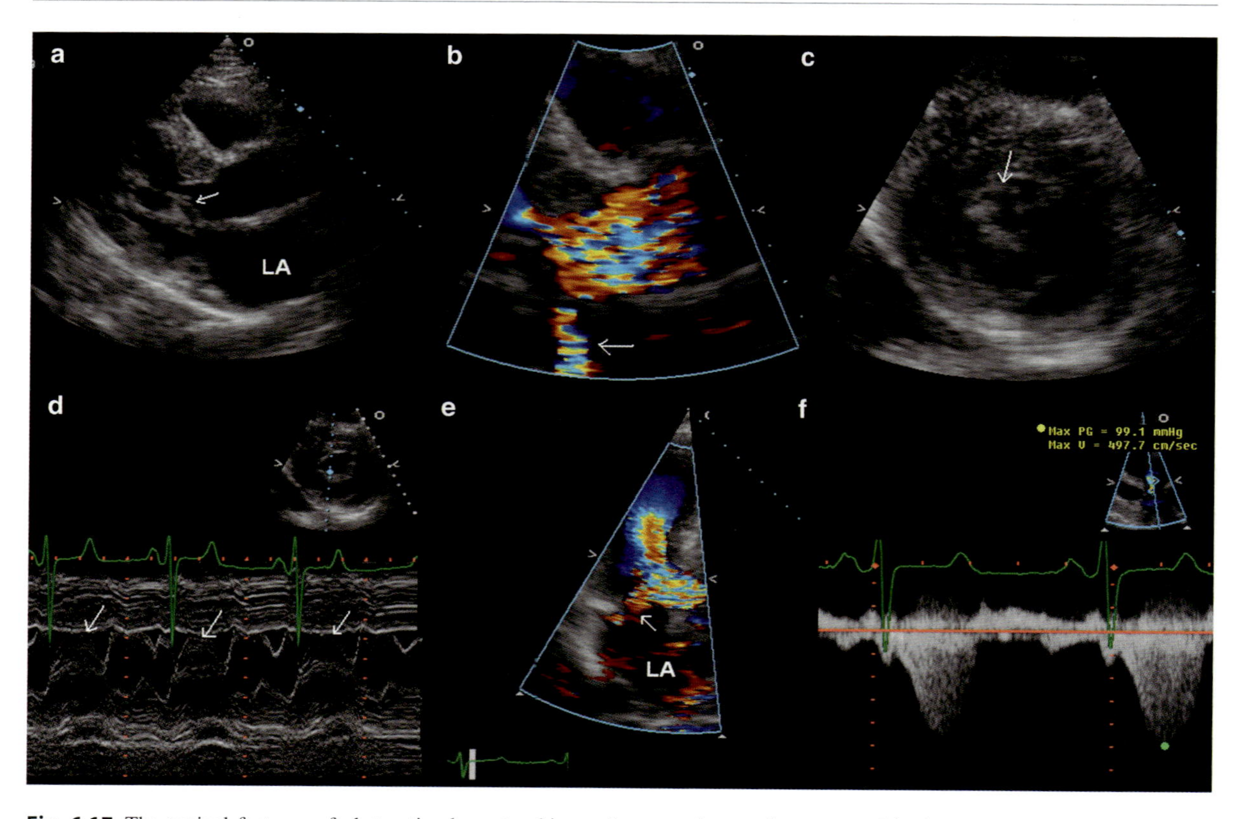

Fig. 6.17 The typical features of obstructive hypertrophic cardiomyopathy are demonstrated in the parasternal long-axis (**a, b**), short-axis (**c**), M-mode of the mitral valve (**d**), color-flow imaging (**b, e**) and continuous wave Doppler across the left ventricular outflow tract (**f**). Systolic anterior motion of the mitral leaflet is present in both the long- and short-axis views (**a, c**). This is clearly demonstrated by M-mode (*arrows*, **d**). Color-flow imaging shows flow acceleration in the left ventricular outflow tract and the presence of mitral regurgitation (*arrow*). The left ventricular outflow tract obstruction is confirmed by the continuous wave Doppler (**f**). *LA* left atrium

in patients with apical hypertrophic cardiomyopathy (Fig. 6.25a, b) [51]. Left ventricular thrombus needs to be considered and the injection of the echo contrast agent should be an integral part of the evaluation of patients with apical hypertrophic cardiomyopathy suspected to have apical aneurysm or thrombus.

Unusual morphological types of hypertrophic cardiomyopathy can be seen. In some patients, the hypertrophy may be quite mild (Fig. 6.26). Affected family members with a familial hypertrophic cardiomyopathy may have different morphologic types. Extreme hypertrophy (≥30 mm) is less common in the older than in the younger HCM patients, suggesting a natural attrition in the young HCM patients with this finding, probably due to sudden death [42, 43].

The degree of hypertrophy varies during the first 2 decades of life, and rapid changes in left ventricular morphology and hypertrophy can occur during adolescence. After physical maturity there is generally little further increase in wall thickness. However, recent studies suggest that in a subset of HCM patients, particularly those with myosin-binding protein C mutations, hypertrophy may appear late in life in the fifth or sixth decade [41]. This has an important implication in family screening. In families with a known mutation for HCM, negative genetic studies can definitely exclude the diagnosis. When no known mutation for HCM is identified in the index case, echo to detect hypertrophy should be performed annually in the young family members and every 3–5 years in adult family members.

Right ventricular involvement can be quite common in HCM. A recent study showed that the majority of HCM patients have RV hypertrophy on cardiac magnetic resonance imaging [52]. The clinical significance of this finding remains unclear.

Systolic function is normal or supranormal in HCM. Left ventricular dysfunction can occur in about 10% of HCM patients. This has been described as end-stage or

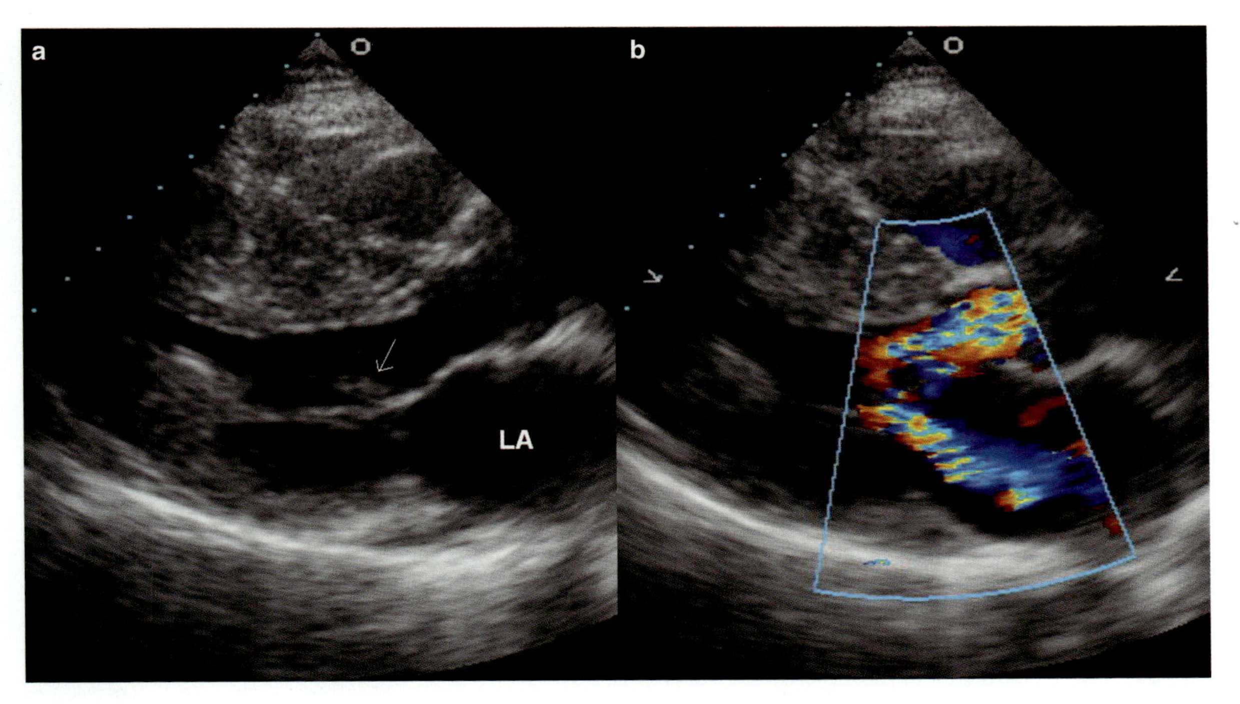

Fig. 6.18 Parasternal long-axis view (**a**) shows systolic anterior motion of the mitral leaflet (*arrow*). Color-flow imaging (**b**) shows flow acceleration in the left ventricular outflow tract consistent with obstruction and the presence of posteriorly directed mitral regurgitation. *LA* left atrium

"burnt-out HCM" because it predicts a poor prognosis with a high risk of sudden death [53]. Although wall thinning and cavity enlargement can occur, persistent hypertrophy with non-dilated left ventricular cavity may persist.

Diastolic abnormalities are common in patients with hypertrophic cardiomyopathy. Measures such as E/E′ and deceleration time that are predictive of left ventricular filling pressure in other cardiac diseases are not good predictors of filling pressure in hypertrophic cardiomyopathy [54]. Determination of left ventricular filling pressure should not be based on one or two measures, but should take in all available echo and Doppler findings [55]. It has been reported that reduced diastolic annular velocity is present in patients carrying known mutations for the disease but are phenotypically negative for hypertrophy, and a low early diastolic annular velocity may be used to identify these patients (Fig. 6.26) [56, 57]. This interesting observation requires further validation.

Asynchrony in left ventricular relaxation is common and can give rise to a prominent antegrade flow from the base of the left ventricular cavity to the apex during the isovolumic relaxation phase. This may be mistaken for a prominent mitral E velocity if careful attention is not paid to the timing of this flow velocity (Fig. 6.27). The relaxation asynchrony can extend into the diastolic filling phase such that the diastolic gradient may exist between the basal portion of the left ventricular cavity and the left ventricular apex (Fig. 6.28). If an apical aneurysm is present, intriguing multiphasic flow velocity can be detected communicating between the left ventricular aneurysm and the main cavity of the left ventricle. To illustrate the complexity of intracavitary flow dynamics in these patients, frame by frame assessment of the color flow images and careful sequential interrogation of different locations within the left ventricular cavity using pulsed wave Doppler is essential. M-mode of the intracardiac color flow can be very useful for timing and location of these intracardiac flows.

Restrictive Cardiomyopathy

Restrictive cardiomyopathy, the least common type of cardiomyopathy, is characterized by a heterogeneous group of disorders with restricted diastolic ventricular

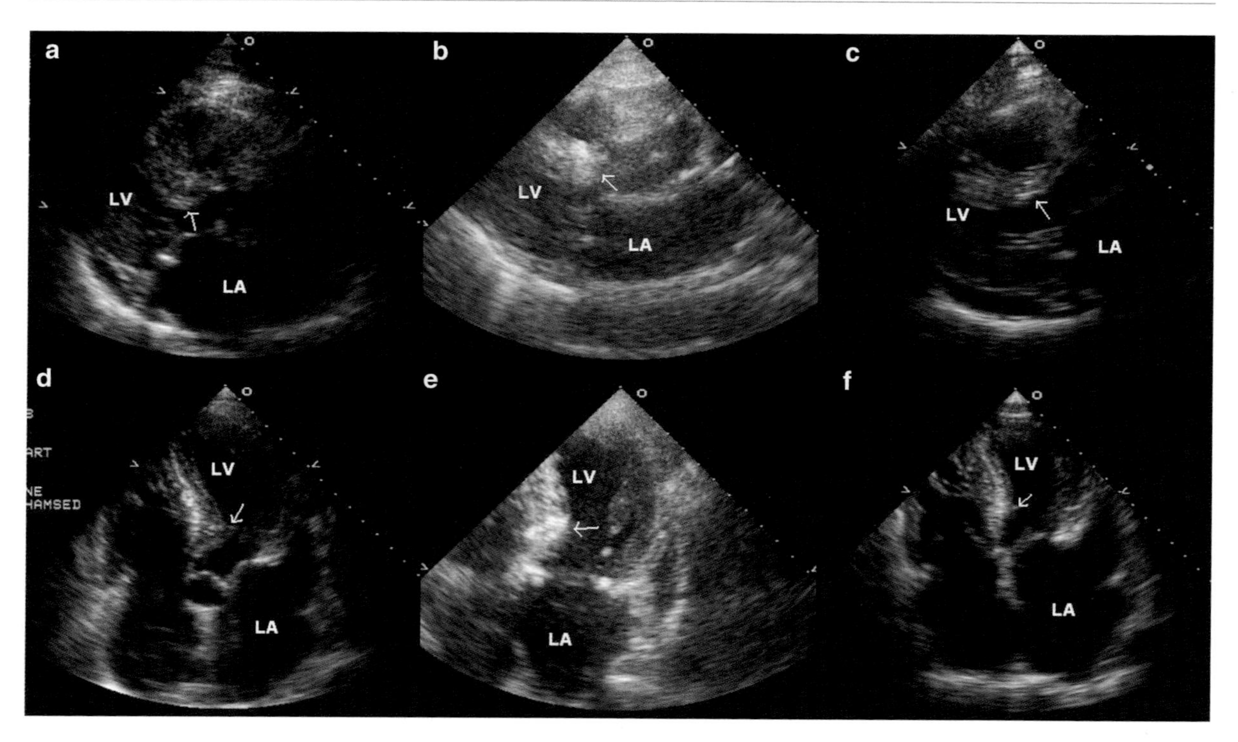

Fig. 6.19 This patient with hypertrophic cardiomyopathy has undergone alcohol septal ablation. The parasternal long-axis (**a**) and apical five-chamber (**d**) views before the procedure show prominent hypertrophy of the basal septum (*arrow*). During the alcohol septal ablation procedure, the perfusion pattern of the septum is assessed by injection of echo contrast into the selected septal branch. The parasternal long-axis (**b**) and apical four-chamber (**e**) views show echo enhancement of the basal anterior septum indicating the appropriateness of using this septal branch for alcohol infusion. A month post-procedure, the parasternal long-axis (**c**) and apical four-chamber (**f**) views show a reduction in thickness of the basal anterior septum as a result of the procedure. *LA* left atrium, *LV* left ventricle

filling and varying degree of systolic dysfunction. In some of these patients, systolic function may be preserved [58]. Included in this group are primary restrictive cardiomyopathy, Loffler's fibroplastic parietal endocarditis, endocardial fibrosis, and hypereosinophilic syndrome. There are numerous secondary causes of diastolic failure including common diseases such as acute and chronic ischemia and systemic arterial hypertension.

In restrictive cardiomyopathy the ventricular size is normal, or nearly normal, and there is increased ventricular filling pressure, decreased ventricular compliance, normal or near normal ventricular systolic function, and atrial dilatation [59]. The largest chambers are the atria, as they are the ones that have to empty into a noncompliant ventricle. There is usually no significant ventricular hypertrophy. Pericardial constriction needs to be excluded as the clinical presentation may be similar and patients with constriction benefit from pericardiectomy.

The two major primary restrictive cardiomyopathies are the eosinophilic endomyocardial type and the non-eosinophilic type [2]. The eosinophilic type may be associated with hypereosinophilia, eosinophilic myocarditis, and endomyocardial fibrosis. The eosinophils are thought to be toxic to the microvasculature and the myocytes. The disease initially starts with a necrotic eosinophilic myocarditis stage, progresses to a thrombotic stage, and results in fibrosis of the endomyocardium. In the acute phase of the eosinophilic type, eosinophilic cationic protein and major basic protein, lead to myocyte and microvasculature damage [60]. As the disease progresses, the endocardial thrombus organizes causing a fibrotic rind in the endocardium that gradually obliterates the ventricular cavities. Mitral and tricuspid valves become tethered to the endocardium

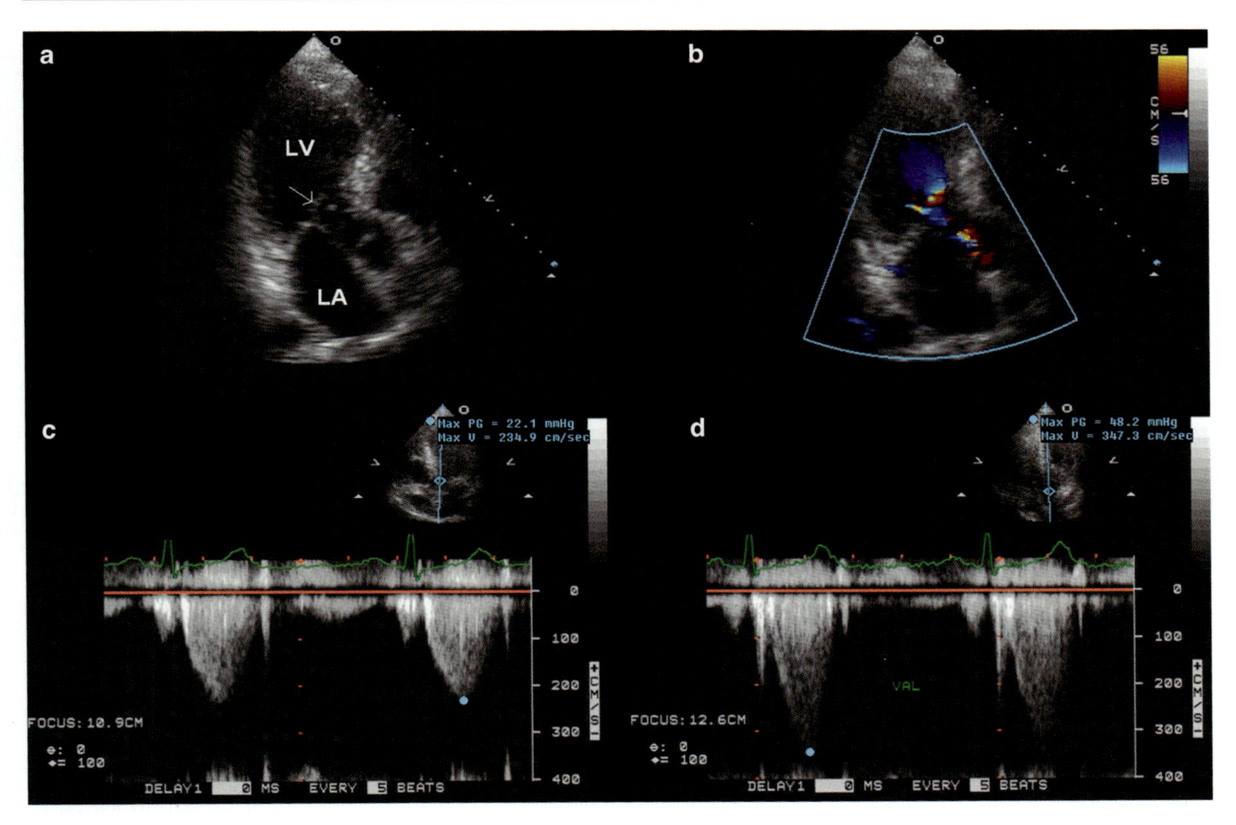

Fig. 6.20 The Valsalva maneuver can be used to increase the subvalvular gradient in a patient with hypertrophic cardiomyopathy. The apical long-axis view (**a**) shows systolic anterior motion of the anterior mitral leaflet and the hypertrophy involving the basal anterior septum. Color-flow imaging (**b**) shows flow acceleration in the left ventricular outflow tract. Doppler examination at rest (**c**) shows a small subaortic gradient which increases during the strain phase of the Valsalva maneuver (**d**). *LA* left atrium, *LV* left ventricle

and dysfunctional. The atria markedly enlarge and heart failure ensues. At the later fibrotic stage, an endomyocardial biopsy material yields only fibrous tissue, if the ventricles can be biopsied at all.

The non-eosinophilic type of primary restrictive cardiomyopathy pathologically has nonspecific myocyte hypertrophy and interstitial fibrosis, similar to most other cardiomyopathies [58]. There may be sampling error when performing endomyocardial biopsy as the disease tends to involve primarily the ventricular inflow tracts where it may have major effects on valve mobility [61].

Endomyocardial biopsy is often useful to determine the cause of restrictive cardiac dysfunction. In the early phase of eosinophilic restrictive cardiomyopathy, the results may be diagnostic. Thrombus, eosinophils, myocyte necrosis, and granulation-like tissue rich in eosinophils will be present. Other causes of secondary cardiomyopathies causing restriction may also be detected by heart biopsy. These include storage disease, hemochromatosis, and amyloidosis. Amyloid may cause restrictive hemodynamics, and thus an amyloid stain must be done. Hypertrophic cardiomyopathy may also present with restrictive findings but usually does not require endomyocardial biopsy to distinguish from restrictive cardiomyopathy. Desmin myopathy, which may be associated with skeletal myopathy and restrictive cardiomyopathy, could be diagnosed by endomyocardial biopsy examination [62, 63].

It is essential to differentiate restrictive cardiomyopathy from constrictive pericarditis. The pericardium should be visualized by magnetic resonance imaging (MRI) or computerized tomography (CT) to detect calcification or thickening. Hemodynamic study and echocardiography are also useful in making the distinction between restriction and constriction. Myocardial

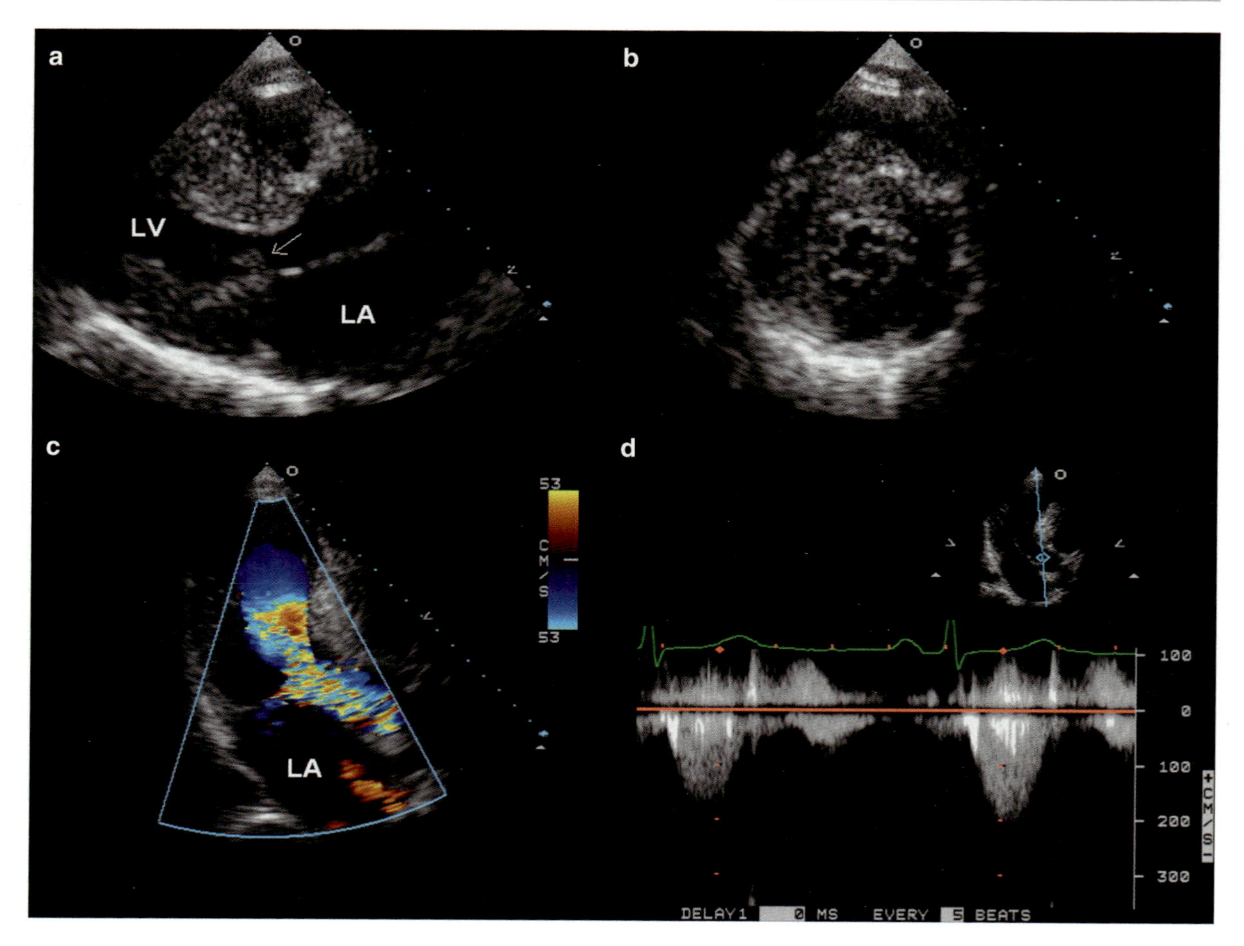

Fig. 6.21 In this patient with hypertrophic cardiomyopathy the hypertrophy is quite diffuse and symmetrical as shown in the parasternal long-axis (**a**) and short-axis (**b**) views. Systolic anterior motion of the mitral leaflets (*arrow*) is shown in (**a**). The presence of subaortic obstruction is demonstrated by color-flow imaging (**c**) and continuous wave Doppler (**d**)

biopsy in patients with constrictive pericarditis shows that the myocytes are normal sized or slightly atrophic. In contrast, the biopsy in primary restrictive cardiomyopathy will demonstrate interstitial fibrosis and myocyte hypertrophy. This is true of both the late fibrotic phase of the eosinophilic type and of the non-eosinophilic type [30].

The typical echocardiographic findings of restrictive cardiomyopathy are normal or slightly reduced left ventricular cavity size with normal or slightly increased left ventricular wall thickness (Fig. 6.29). The left ventricular systolic function may be normal or reduced. Restrictive cardiomyopathy can be reliably differentiated from constrictive pericarditis by assessing the annular velocities which are severely reduced in restrictive cardiomyopathy but are generally normal in patients with constriction [64]. The differentiating features are discussed in Chap. 10.

Arrhythmogenic Right Ventricular Dysplasia – Arrhythmogenic Cardiomyopathy

Arrhythmogenic right ventricular dysplasia or arrhythmogenic cardiomyopathy (ARVC) was first described under this name in 1978 [65]. It is a frequent cause of sudden death in young people and may cause arrhythmias and congestive heart failure. ARVC is characterized by fibrofatty atrophy of the right ventricular myocardium with resultant electrical

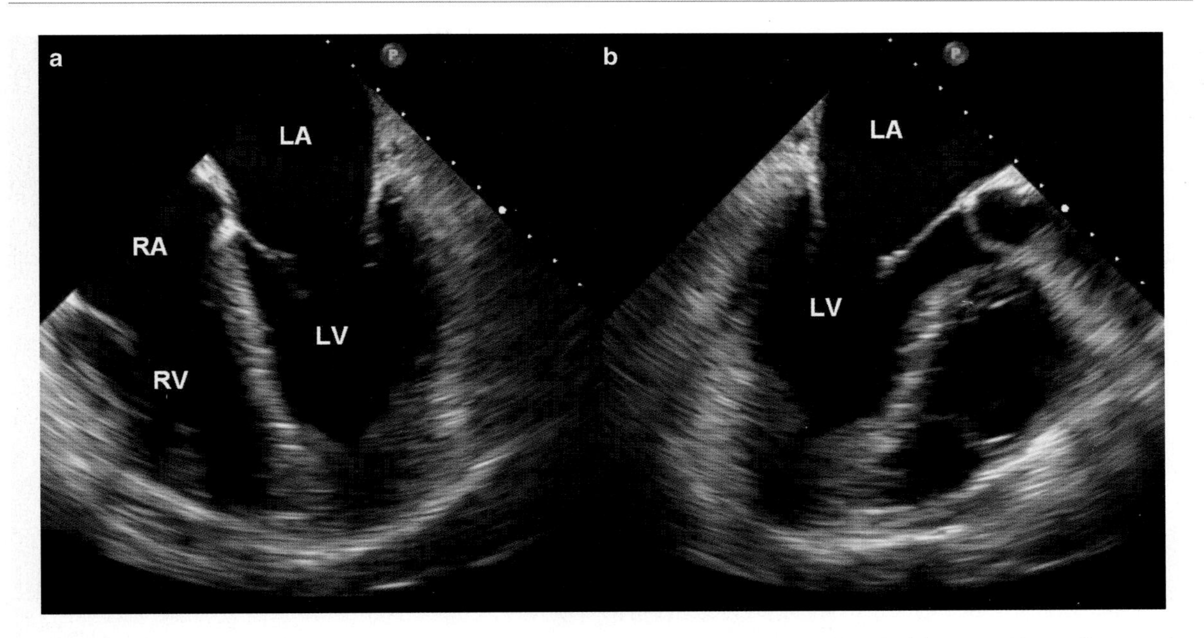

Fig. 6.22 Transesophageal views showing the typical apical involvement in a patient with apical hypertrophic cardiomyopathy. *LA* left atrium, *LV* left ventricle, *RA* right atrium, *RV* right ventricle

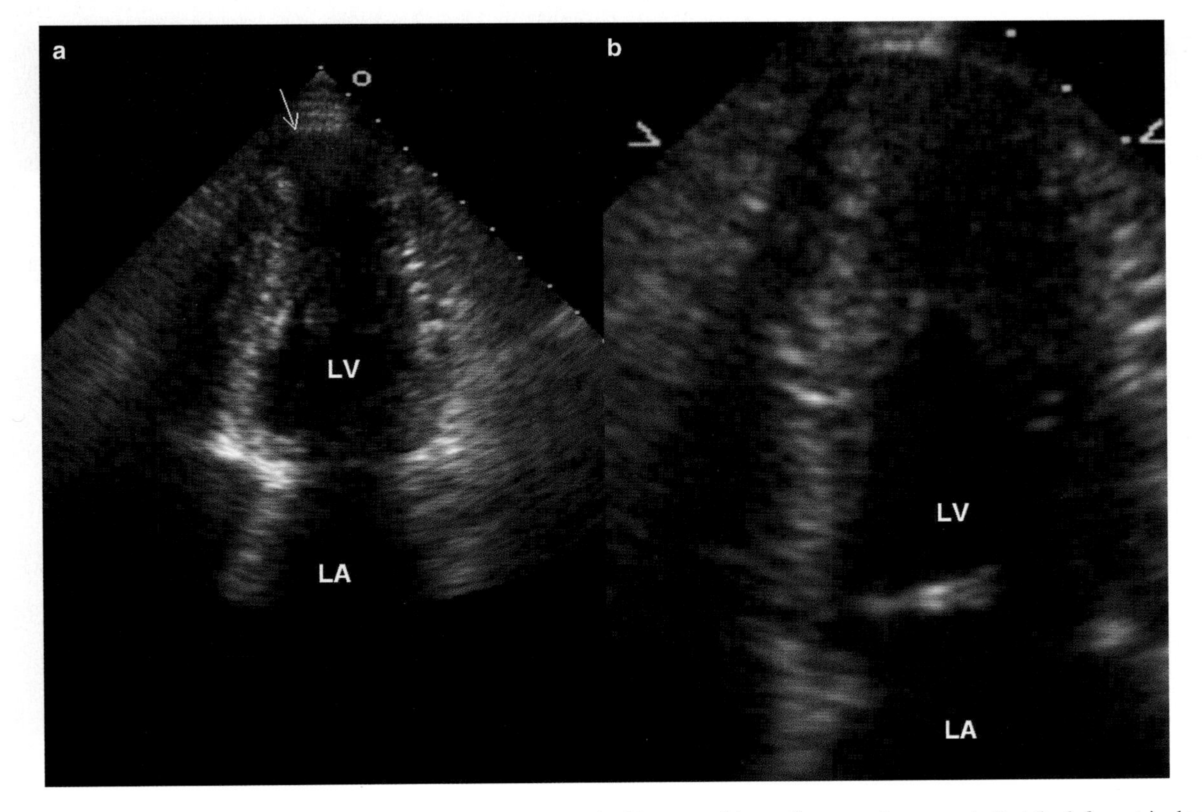

Fig. 6.23 (**a**) The apical four-chamber view in a patient with apical hypertrophic cardiomyopathy suggests that the left ventricular apex may be dyskinetic (*arrow*) consistent with left ventricular apical aneurysm. (**b**) The focus view with careful adjustment of the near gain clearly shows severe apical hypertrophy. *LA* left atrium, *LV* left ventricle

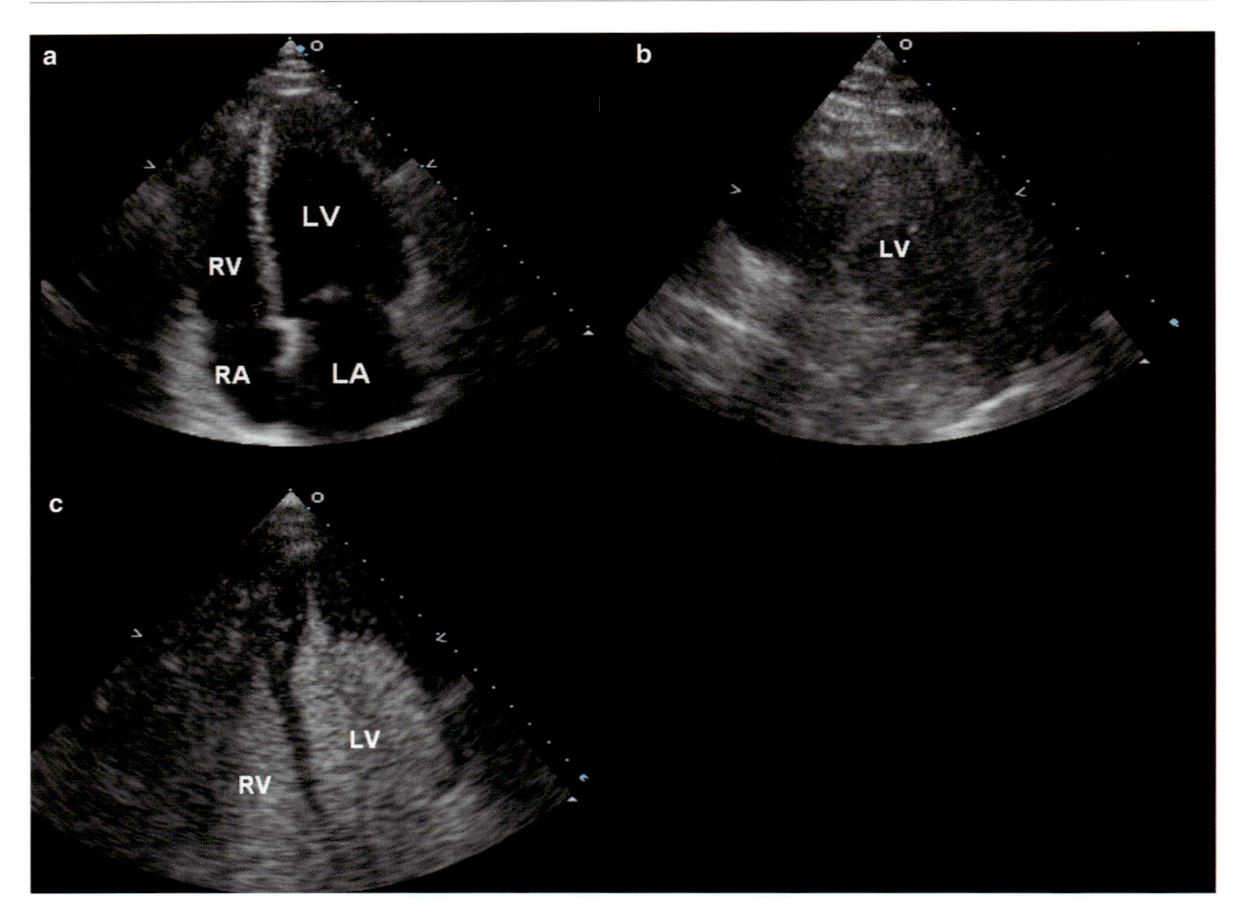

Fig. 6.24 The apical four-chamber view (**a**) is unable to demonstrate the apical hypertrophy, which can be better seen using the apical short-axis view (**b**) with careful adjustment of the near gain. The apical hypertrophy can be demonstrated using an echo contrast agent (**c**). The suspicion of an apical pathology such as apical aneurysm, thrombus or hypertrophy is a good indication for the use of an echo contrast agent. *LA* left atrium; *LV* left ventricle, *RA* right atrium, *RV* right ventricle

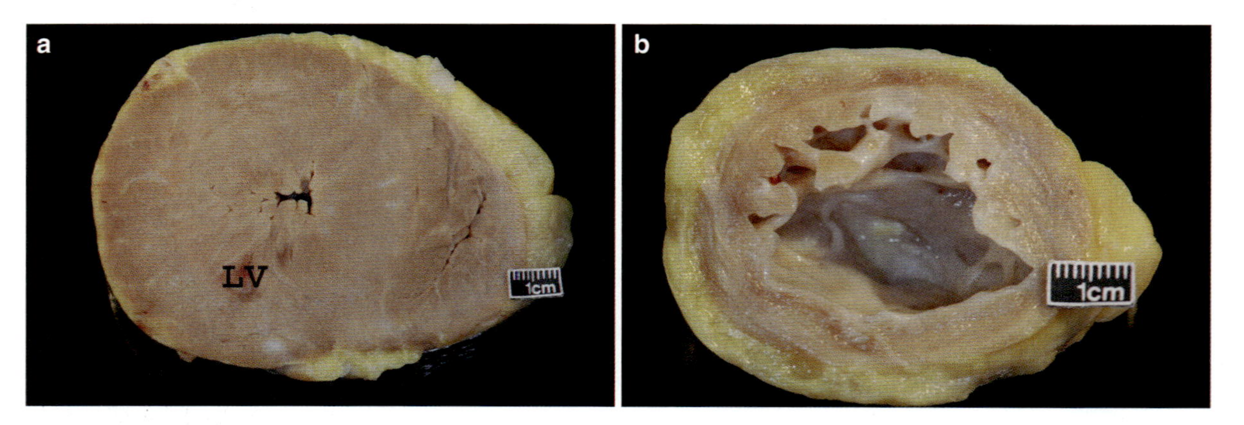

Fig. 6.25 (**a**) Cross section of the heart showing severe concentric symmetrical hypertrophy. The patient had ventricular arrhythmias refractory to medical therapy and had undergone ablations. Her heart weighed over 700 g and had the characteristic myocyte disarray. (**b**) The left ventricular apex in this patient shows severe interstitial fibrosis and thinning, consistent with apical aneurysm due to prior infarction

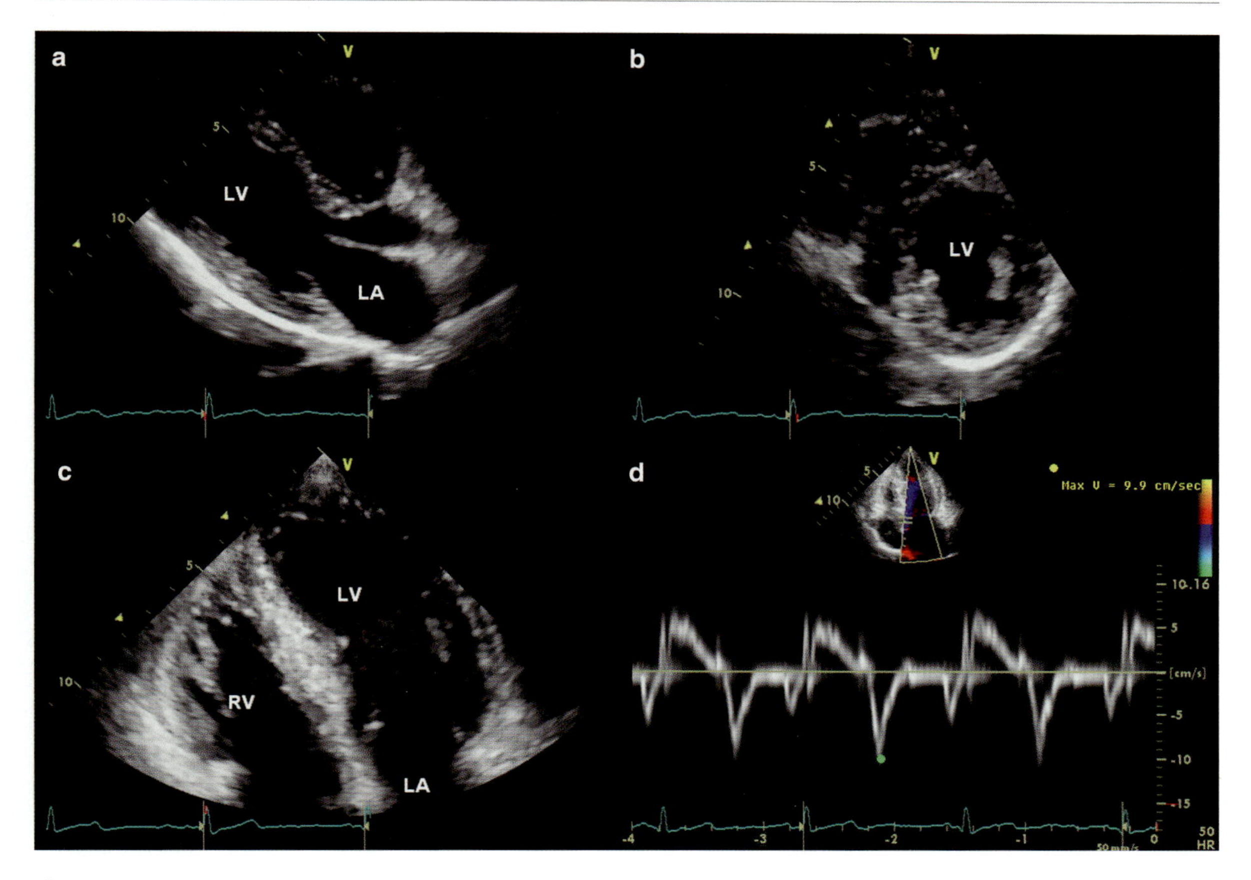

Fig. 6.26 In this 24-year-old woman with a proven mutation for hypertrophic cardiomyopathy, the left ventricular hypertrophy is quite mild and localized as seen in the parasternal long-axis (**a**), short-axis (**b**) and apical four-chamber (**c**) views. The hypertrophy is most pronounced in the mid-inferior wall (**b**). Tissue Doppler imaging (**d**) shows that the septal early diastolic velocity is mildly reduced for her age

instability or myocardial dysfunction [66, 67]. Its etiology is still under debate with theories of a developmental abnormality, a degenerative change, apoptotic cell death or an end result of myocarditis. Mutations in proteins of the intercalated disk, including desmoplakin, desmoglobin, and plakophillin, have been described [68]. Familial cases exist, and the disease has been mapped to a genetic abnormality at chromosome 14q 23-q24 [66].

The clinical presentation consists of ventricular arrhythmias (often recurrent and sometimes refractory), right heart failure, murmur, complete heart block, and sudden death [69, 70]. ARVC is an important cause of sudden unexpected death, especially in some geographic locations. The diagnosis is often suspected clinically, but the proof of the diagnosis lies with the demonstration of transmural replacement of the right ventricular myocardium by fibrofatty tissue and cardiomyopathic changes in the myocardium. This is usually possible at autopsy or surgery, although imaging may detect abnormalities useful for the diagnosis. Magnet resonance imaging (MRI) is frequently used for this purpose due to its ability to characterize the abnormal tissue, although a recent report suggests that the diagnostic accuracy of MRI is low [71].

The echo findings are summarized in Table 6.3. Echocardiography has a reasonable sensitivity in the diagnosis of this condition, with one finding present in 62% and two or more findings in 38% of the proven cases (Fig. 6.30) [72]. Recent modification of the diagnostic criteria has introduced quantitative measures in addition to the qualitative findings listed in Table 6.3. To fulfill the major criterion based on echo, the right ventricular outflow tract in diastole needs to be ≥ 32 mm

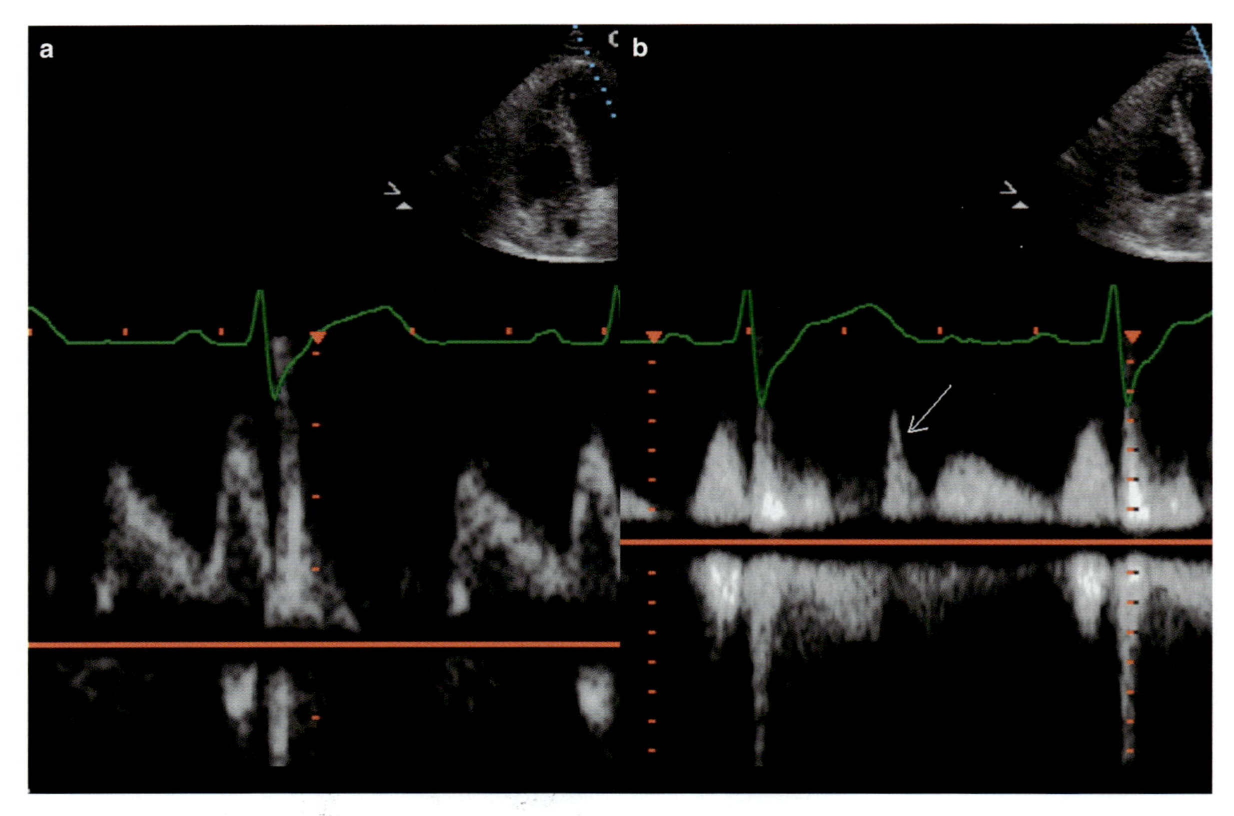

Fig. 6.27 The mitral inflow velocities by pulse-wave Doppler (**a**) and by continuous-wave Doppler (**b**) show a prominent early velocity (*arrow*) detected by continuous wave Doppler but not by pulse-wave Doppler, resulting from asynchrony in left ventricular relaxation such that there is antegrade flow from the left ventricular cavity into the left ventricular apex during the isovolumic relaxation phase. This phenomenon is common in patients with hypertrophic cardiomyopathy as well as patients with long-standing hypertension

in the parasternal long-axis view and≥36 mm in the short-axis view, in addition to severe right ventricular regional abnormalities [73].

Grossly the right ventricle may be dilated and aneurysmal bulging may be noted. The wall is thinned and gross fat infiltration may be noted (Figs. 6.31, 6.32). Anatomically, the most involved areas form the "triangle of dysplasia," extending between the right ventricular infundibulum, the apex, and the diaphragmatic surface of the right ventricle [70, 74]. The septum is not commonly involved. Left ventricular involvement is well described in up to 47% of cases, with typical pathologic changes manifested as fibrofatty scarring in the left ventricle (Fig. 6.33) [66, 75-79]. The individual with prominent left ventricle disease may have severe left ventricle systolic dysfunction with a clinical picture of a dilated cardiomyopathy. Since both DCM and ARVC have heart failure and arrhythmias, imaging becomes important in making this distinction. Directed endomyocardial biopsy of the free wall has been proposed by some. If this is performed, surgical backup is necessary due to the risk of perforation. Imaging and electrophysiological (EP) study guided biopsy has been proposed to aid in biopsying the areas that are abnormal.

By microscopic examination, the areas of involvement show severe infiltration of the right ventricular wall by mature fat cells (Fig. 6.34). These are invariably associated with changes of cardiomyopathy including interstitial fibrosis (pericellular and microscopic microinfarct

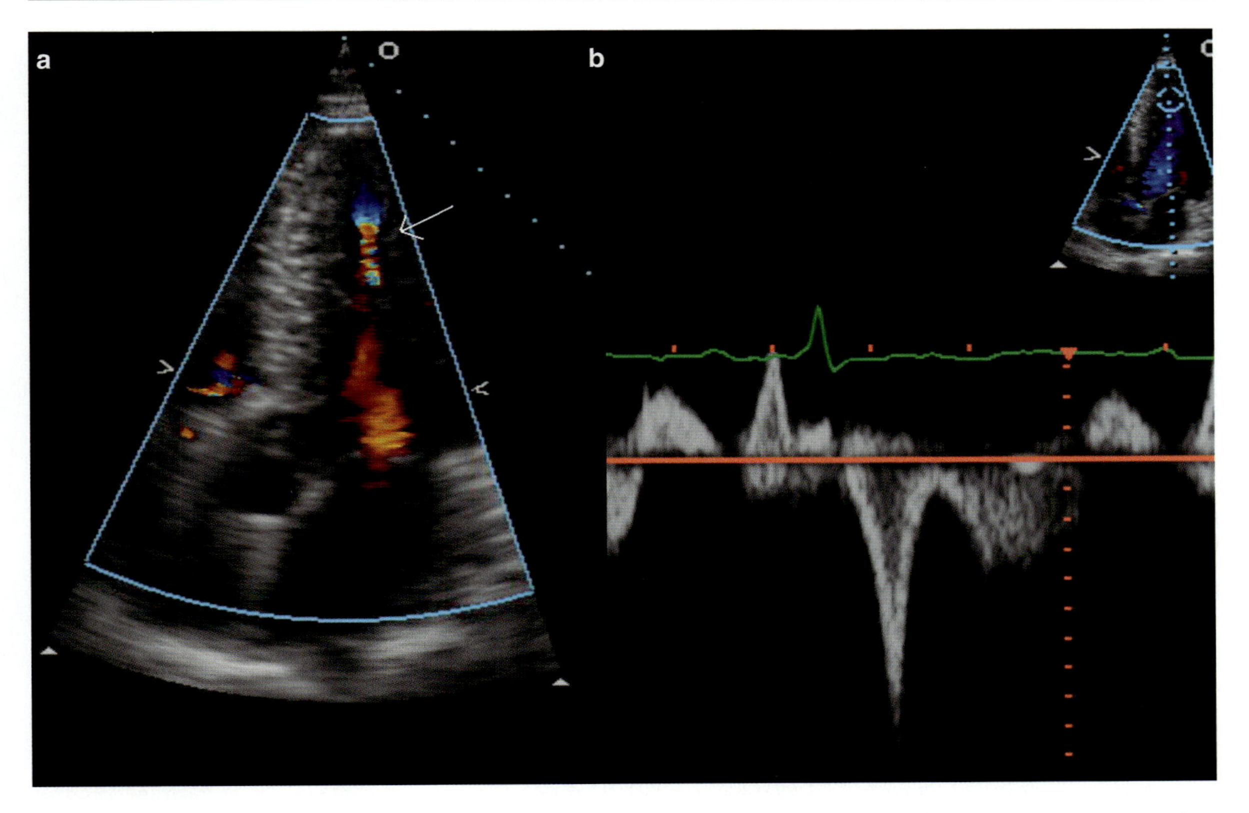

Fig. 6.28 The color-flow image (**a**) in a patient with hypertrophic cardiomyopathy and severe hypertrophy of the apex shows flow from the apex into left ventricular cavity, simultaneous with early diastolic flow from the left atrium into the left ventricular cavity. The complex intracardiac flow dynamics are illustrated by the pulsed-wave Doppler with the sample volume near the left ventricular apex (**b**). Flow from the left ventricular apex to the left ventricular cavity is present both in systolic and early diastole. These intracardiac velocities are caused by asynchrony in relaxation and contraction which is common in hypertrophic cardiomyopathy

replacement types), myocyte degeneration, and myocyte nuclear hypertrophy. Active and borderline myocarditis may also be noted [78]. Myocyte atrophy is also found [69, 74]. Characteristically, the disease begins in the subepicardial myocardium with preservation of the inner trabeculae until late. This may be noted on imaging and can be helpful for diagnosis.

Fat is normal in the epicardium of the heart and some infiltration along the vessels and into the myocardium invariably occurs. Endocardial fat is also present normally in small amounts. Fat is thought to increase with age, and fat may contribute up to 52% of the heart weight [80]. The difference between normal and ARVC may be quantitative rather than qualitative. Studies have quantitated the amount of fat present in biopsies and attempted to determine what percentage is abnormal, and over 20–50% fat in the biopsy area is considered to be strongly suggestive of ARVC [81, 82].

In the correct clinical situation, the presence of adipose tissue and cardiomyopathic changes is strongly suggestive or supportive of the diagnosis. However, correlation of the clinical situation with the imaging findings is a necessity in all cases. The usual course of diagnosis would involve correlation of a combination of the patient's findings on echocardiography, angiography, hemodynamic study, electrocardiographic findings,

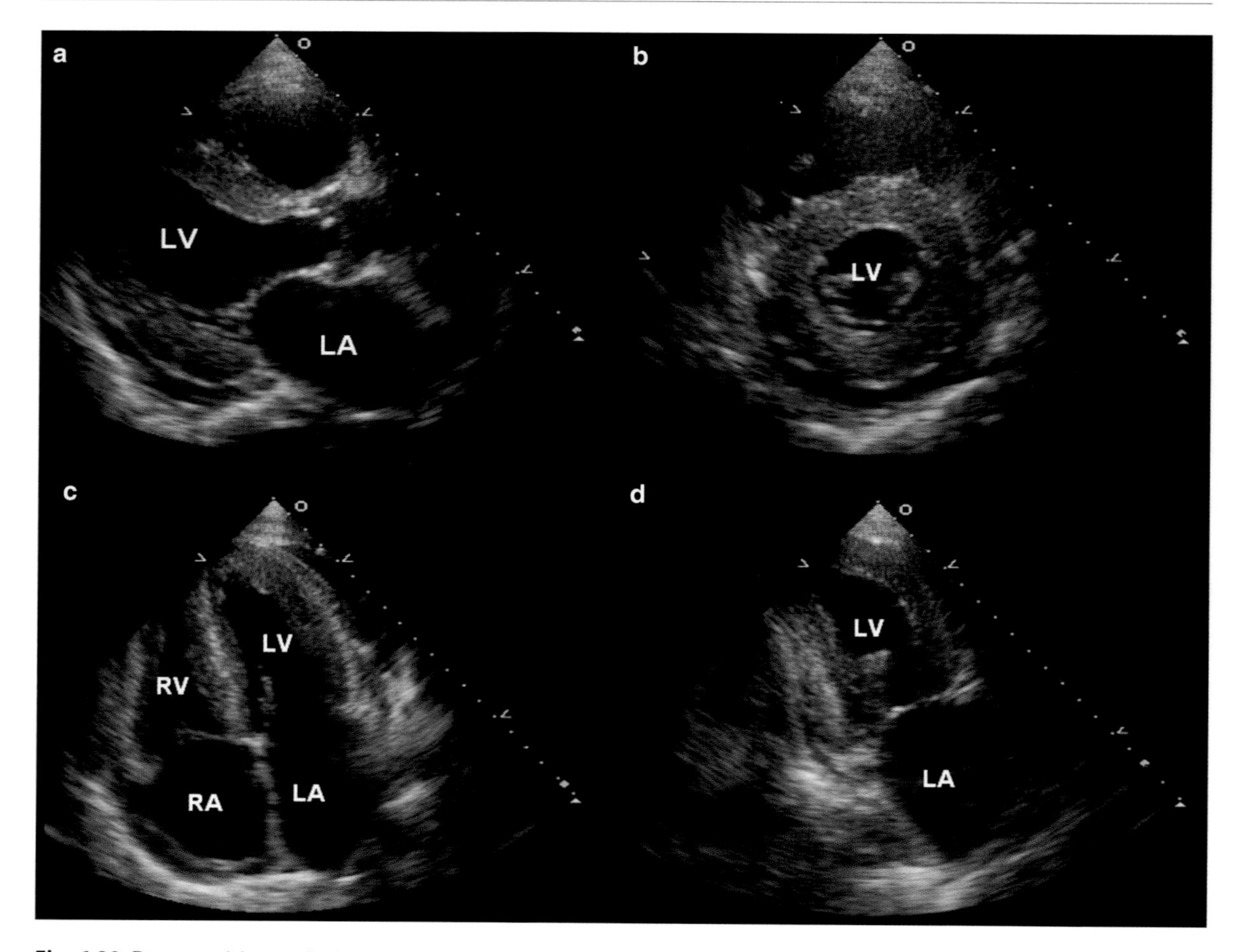

Fig. 6.29 Parasternal long-axis (**a**), short-axis (**b**), apical four-chamber (**c**) and apical two-chamber (**d**) views in a patient with amyloid heart disease show diffuse increase in wall thickness, non-dilated left ventricular cavity and mild global hypokinesia. A small circumferential pericardial effusion is present. *LA* left atrium, *LV* left ventricle, *RA* right atrium, *RV* right ventricle

Table 6.3 Echocardiographic findings of arrhythmogenic right ventricular cardiomyopathy

• Severe RV dilatation with reduced function
• Regional RV akinesia, dyskinesia or aneurysm
• Hyper-reflective moderator band
• Excessive trabeculations
• Sacculations

RV right ventricle
Source: Modified from Yoerger et al. [72]

clinical history, and results of an endomyocardial biopsy. Major and minor criteria for diagnosis have been established and incorporate the findings of the endomyocardial biopsy [83].

Diagnosis of this disease is of importance in counseling families of sudden death patients, and for prognosis of survivors of ventricular fibrillation [84]. Transplantation or implantable defibrillators are therapeutic options. In a clinically normal patient with a high probability of ARVC, the correct treatment is uncertain.

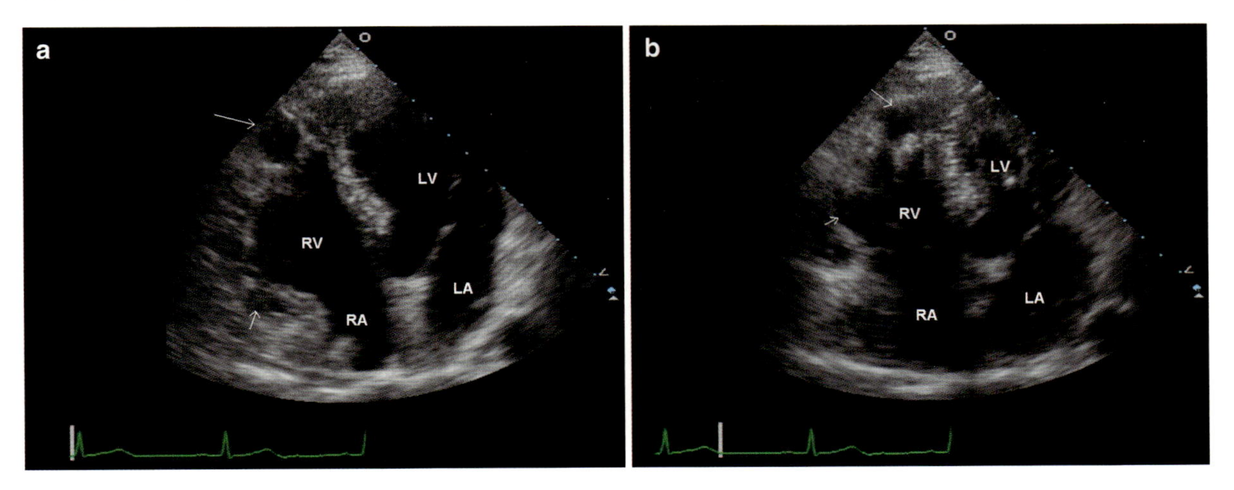

Fig. 6.30 (**a**) Four-chamber view in diastole in a patient with arrhythmogenic right ventricular cardiomyopathy shows dilated right ventricle with two focal areas of wall thinning. (**b**) Apical four-chamber view in systole confirms severe right ventricular dysfunction and systolic outpouchings at the areas of wall thinning. *LA* left atrium, *LV* left ventricle, *RA* right atrium, *LV* left ventricle

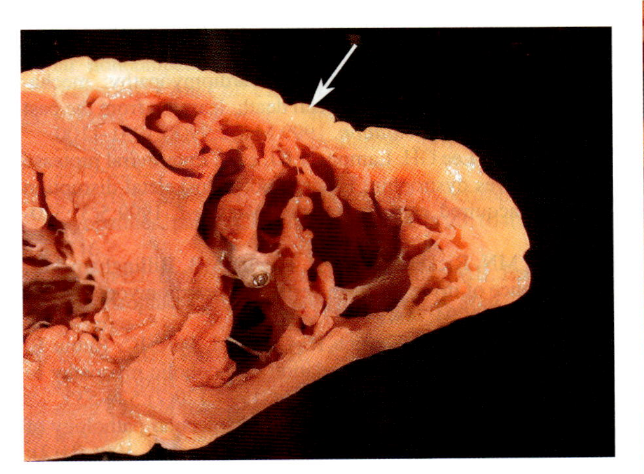

Fig. 6.31 Right ventricle cross section in an individual with arrhythmogenic right ventricular cardiomyopathy. The anterior (*arrow*) and lateral walls show severe fatty replacement. The right ventricle is dilated. There is an implantable defibrillator lead

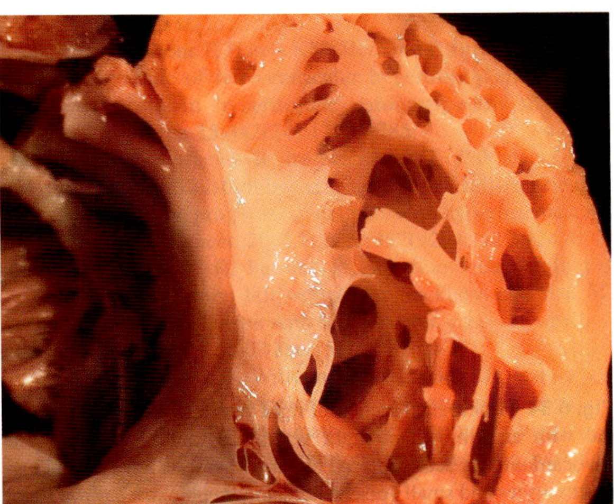

Fig. 6.32 Right ventricle free wall in an individual with arrhythmogenic right ventricular cardiomyopathy. The wall shows thinning and fatty replacement

Table 7.1 Non-atherosclerotic causes of myocardial ischemia

Coronary artery spasm
Dissection • Primary coronary artery dissection • Dissection related to aortic dissection
Coronary Embolism • Endocarditis, paradoxic embolism, cardiac tumors
Trauma • Blunt chest trauma • Iatrogenic coronary arterial trauma during angiography
Coronary Arterial thrombosis due to pro-thrombotic state • Polycythemia vera • Thrombocytosis • Erythrocytosis
Metabolic disease leading to abnormal coronary arteries • Mucopolysaccharidosis • Fabry disease
Increased demand-supply relationship • Left ventricular hypertrophy • Hypotension, severe anemia • Aortic regurgitation
Congenital coronary artery anomalies Coronary ostial stenosis • Calcification of the sinotubular junction • Vasculitis – syphilis, Takayasu disease Cocaine

band necrosis and coagulative necrosis [7]. In the absence of collaterals, irreversible myocardial injury occurs after 20 min of coronary occlusion. With necrotic myocyte death, there is reactive inflammation to the necrotic fibers. The myocardial wall becomes non-contractive and may not move during contraction or it may paradoxically bulge out during systole. These changes are manifest on imaging as akinesia, dyskinesia or aneurysmal wall motion abnormalities. There is also diastolic dysfunction which is invariably present when there is significant systolic dysfunction.

Grossly infarcted myocardium may be dark and hemorrhagic if significant reperfusion occurs (Fig. 7.1). Otherwise there is pallor, edema and peripheral congestion of the infarcted area. Over a few days, the infarct edema lessens, the infarct becomes mottled and tanned, and the wall thins (Figs. 7.2–7.4). Ventricular wall thinning is seen early in the time course of an infarction, but it becomes most marked after about 5 days [9].

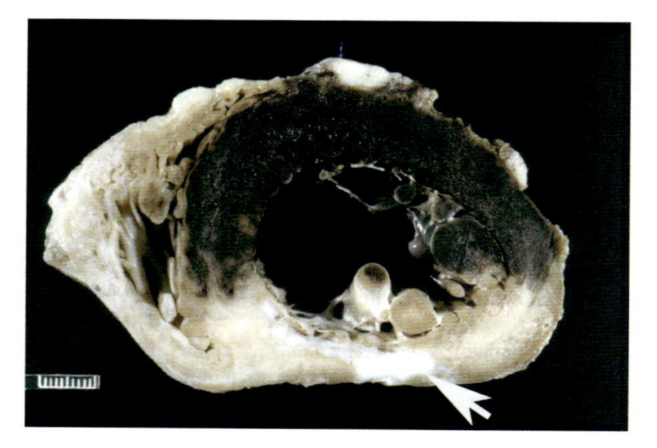

Fig. 7.1 Cross section of a heart with a large reperfused transmural hemorrhagic anteroseptal wall myocardial infarct. There is also a smaller old transmural infarct seen as a transmural white scar (*arrow*)

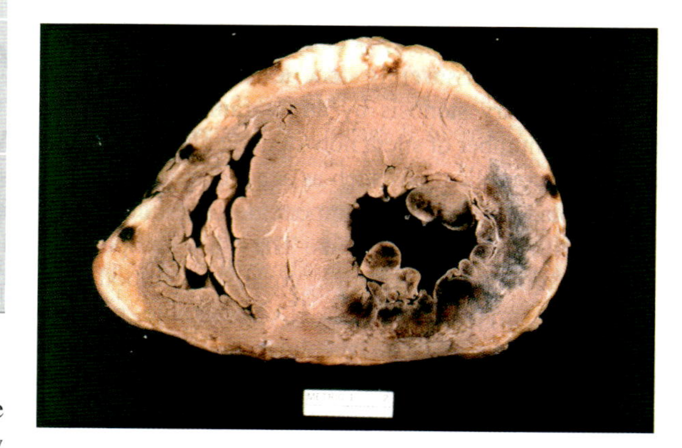

Fig. 7.2 Cross section of a heart with a recent subendocardial myocardial infarct involving the lateral and inferior left ventricle walls. The infarct is still mostly in the inner third of the ventricle wall. Mild reperfusion has occurred

Global and Regional Function

The coronary arteries can be directly visualized using current echo equipment both from the chest wall and from the esophagus, although only the proximal arterial segments are usually imaged (Figs. 7.5–7.7). From the chest wall, color-flow imaging is an essential aid to locate the coronaries. The imaging of coronary arteries has not gained wide acceptance as it is time consuming and requires operator experience [10].

The foundation of echocardiography in patients with coronary artery disease is the assessment of global

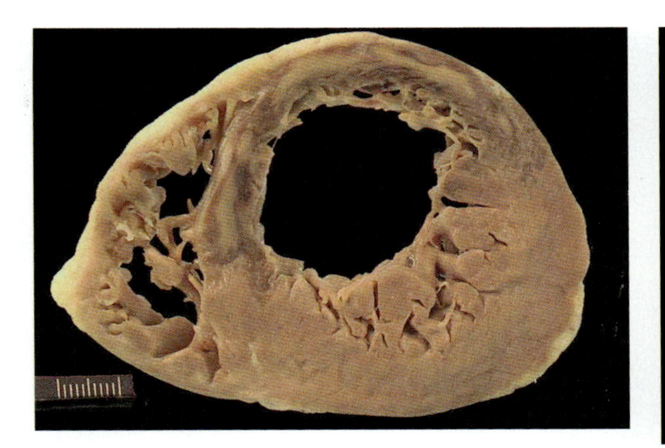

Fig. 7.3 Cross section of heart with a recent anterior anteroseptal transmural myocardial infarct. The infarct is healing with mottling and peripheral congestion. Note the wall thinning of the infarct

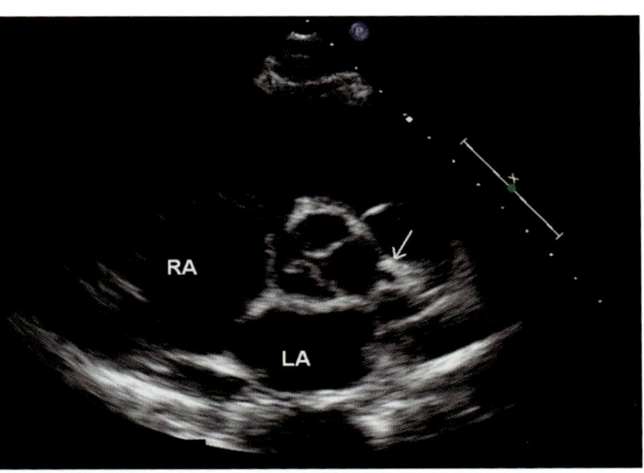

Fig. 7.5 Parasternal short-axis view showing the origin of the left main coronary artery (*arrow*) which can usually be imaged by the transthoracic approach. *LA* left atrium, *RA* right atrium

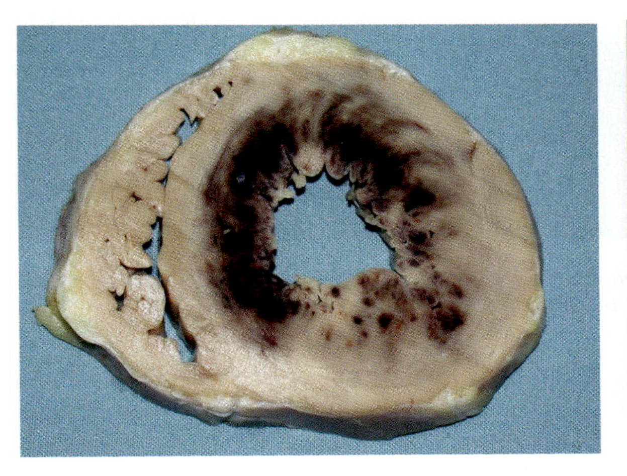

Fig. 7.4 Cross section of a heart in a patient with a large reperfused circumferential left ventricular myocardial infarct. There was significant multivessel coronary artery disease

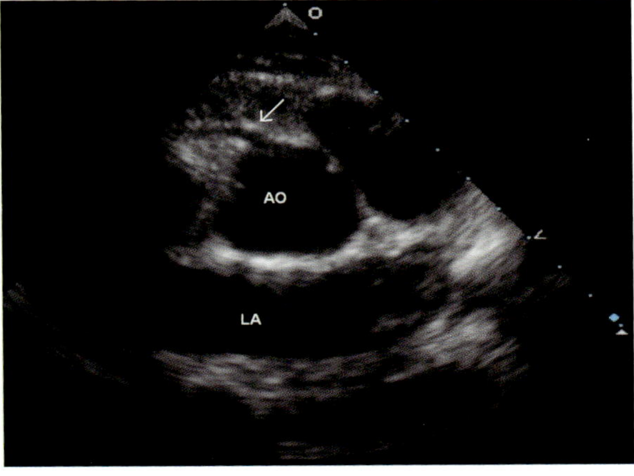

Fig. 7.6 Parasternal short-axis view showing the proximal right coronary artery (*arrow*). The imaging plane needs to be angled more superiorly from the plane used to image the left main coronary artery. *Ao* aorta, *LA* left atrium

ventricular function and the detection of regional wall motion abnormalities. There are multiple measures of left ventricular global function, but ejection fraction (EF) remains the most widely used despite being preload and after load dependent. It has been shown to be a strong predictor of mortality during follow-up [11, 12]. It has incremental prognostic value beyond symptoms, extent of coronary artery narrowing and perfusion defect [13, 14]. There are multiple methods to calculate EF. Visual estimate is widely used and has been shown to have good correlation with the measured EF [15]. Nonetheless we believe that EF should be routinely measured to allow for easy comparison during follow-up and routine practice should help to reduce the study to study variability. Our preference is to use the modified Simpson method when there is adequate endocardial visualization of the left ventricle in the apical views, and the combined echo-Doppler method when the endocardial visualization is suboptimal. The latter method is based upon calculating the stroke volume at the left ventricular outflow tract and the left ventricular diastolic volume by the Teicholz method,

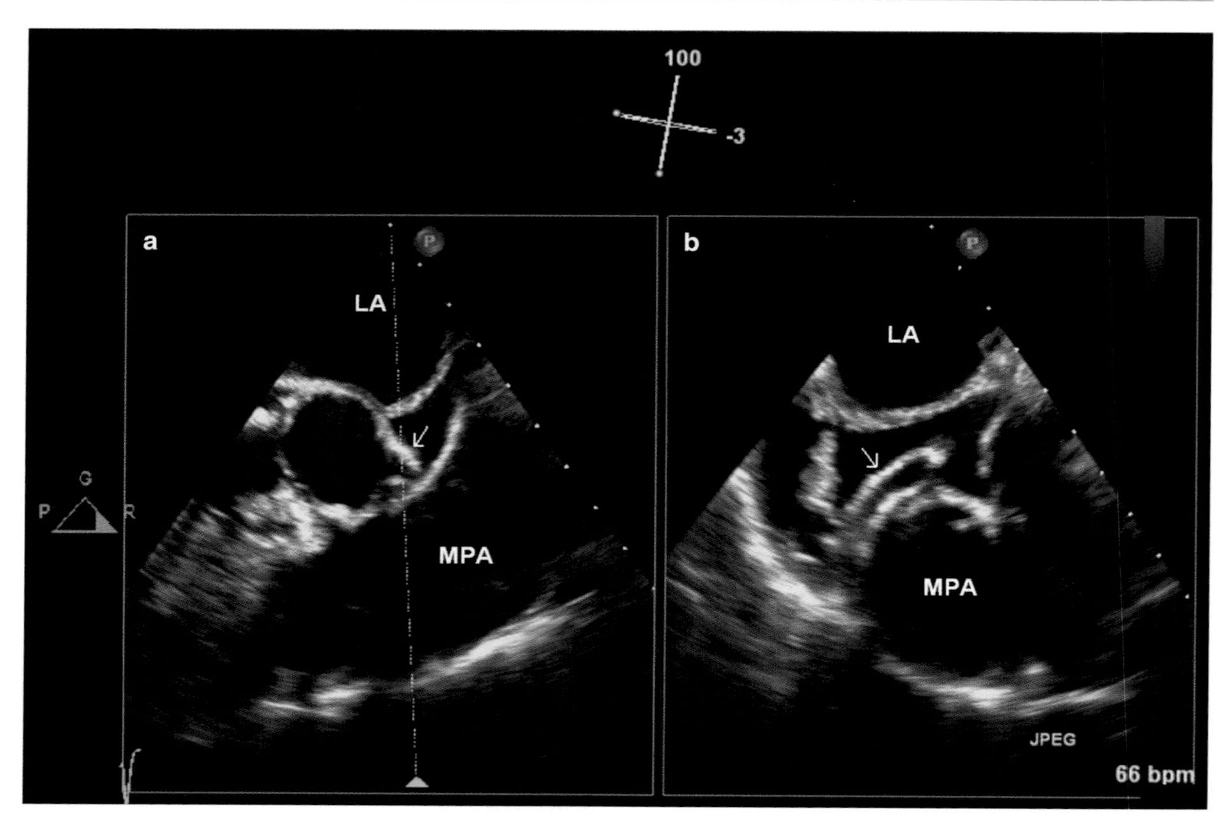

Fig. 7.7 Biplane transesophageal views showing the left main coronary artery (*arrow*) in the transverse plane (**a**) and the proximal left anterior descending artery (*arrow*) in the longitudinal plane (**b**). *LA* left atrium, *MPA* main pulmonary artery

provided that there is no concomitant moderate to severe mitral regurgitation. EF obtained by this method has been shown to have good correlations with EF obtained by radionuclide imaging [16]. The calculated EF should be compared with the EF estimate based upon wall motion score index (see below) and the visual estimate. If a substantial discrepancy is present, EF measurement by other means such as radionuclear imaging should be considered.

Tissue Doppler imaging is a new and easy method to assess systolic and diastolic function. The systolic velocity (S wave) appears to correlate with systolic function and indeed may be a more sensitive measure as it may be able to detect occult systolic dysfunction. More validation data are needed [17].

Although there are many different ways to detect wall motion using echo, the two most practical approaches are endocardial excursion and wall thickening. Endocardial excursion refers to the motion of the endocardium from end diastole to end systole. When the endocardium is poorly visualized, epicardial motion is frequently used as a substitute. Although there are quantitative methods utilizing off-line endocardial tracing with either a fixed centroid or a floating centroid model, visual assessment is widely used in the clinical setting. In general, assessment of endocardial motion is more sensitive, but less specific, in the detection of coronary artery disease as compared to wall thickening, since wall motion can be passive and easily affected by the translational motion of the heart.

Wall thickening is a better measure of regional systolic function than endocardial excursion as the increase in thickness of the myocardium from end diastole to end systole is a more specific measure of myocardial contraction [18, 19]. Although quantitative measures dividing the left ventricular myocardium into multiple regions have been proposed to assess regional function, visual assessment remains the most clinically relevant approach. There is heterogeneity in wall thickening among myocardial segments with the basal inferior wall and posterior wall showing less systolic thickening as compared to the other walls. Furthermore, the mid and apical segments in general demonstrate more wall thickening as compared to the basal walls. The exception is in the patient with an apical cleft in whom the apical wall thickening is less compared to the other segments. The normal range for wall thickening is quite wide but in general an increase in ≥ 30% in wall thickness from end diastole to end systole is considered normal.

When there is an absence of wall thickening from end diastole to end systole, the wall is considered akinetic. From 0% to 30% thickening, the wall is judged to be hypokinetic. Hyperkinesia refers to thickening more than 30%, usually associated with increased endocardial excursion. When there is paradoxic excursion (that is the wall moves away from the centroid during systole) associated with no thickening, the wall is considered dyskinetic, and an aneurysmal wall is one that demonstrates obvious diastolic bulging with further expansion during systole. A scoring system has been proposed and widely used to assess the severity of wall motion abnormalities (Table 7.2) [20, 21].

Since wall motion abnormalities form the basis of echocardiographic diagnosis of myocardial ischemia or infarction, it is not surprising that transmural myocardial infarcts can be detected by echocardiography in over 90% of the cases, while 50% of the non-transmural myocardial infarcts may escape detection [22, 23]. The location and extent of wall motion abnormality are good predictors of the involvement of specific coronary arteries. Wall motion abnormalities restricted to the anterior wall and apex are likely related to disease involving the left anterior descending artery. Similarly wall motion abnormalities of the inferior wall and inferior septum indicate that the right coronary artery is likely the culprit.

Table 7.2 Wall motion score to assess regional myocardial contraction abnormalities

Score	Description	Wall thickening	Endocardial excursion
1	Normal	≥30%	Normal
2	Hypokinetic	<30%	Normal or reduced
3	Akinetic	0%	Reduced or absent
4	Dyskinetic	0%	Paradoxic motion
5	Dyskinetic associated with diastolic bulge	0%	Paradoxic motion

The basal inferior wall often appears hypokinetic, and this is a normal finding. In some patients, the basal and mid inferior or posterior walls may appear dyskinetic simulating an inferior wall infarction (Figs. 7.8, 7.9). Yet, wall thickening remains normal and can be recognized by frame-to-frame analysis. This "pseudodyskinesis" may be due to an elevated diaphragm and should not be mistaken for inferior wall infarction [19].

To quantitate the extent of left ventricular involvement, the left ventricle may be divided into 16 or 17 segments with the wall motion of each segment graded from normal to aneurysmal, as previously described (Fig. 7.10). An overall wall motion score can be obtained by dividing the total score of all segments visualized by the number of visualized segments to arrive at a wall motion score index, which is an indicator of the overall involvement of the left ventricle [20, 21]. The wall motion score index has been shown to predict short and medium term outcomes, including death and re-hospitalization [24, 25]. The higher the score, the more is the severity and extent of myocardial ischemia and the worse is the outcome. Furthermore there is a relationship between left ventricular global function, such as ejection fraction, and the wall motion score index [26, 27]. In general a wall motion score index less than 1.5 is unlikely to be associated with significant left ventricular systolic dysfunction. At the same time a patient with a wall motion score index greater than 2 is highly likely to have an abnormal EF; and a score index > 2.5 indicates severely depressed systolic function with EF ≤ 30% [27].

Strain and strain rate imaging are new methods to assess global and regional functions. It is easy to use and quite reproducible. Both strain and strain rate assess the deformation of the myocardium during systole (Fig. 7.11). They are less affected by cardiac motion or tethering [28]. The strain and strain rate can be displayed in a format that allows comparison between myocardial segments to promptly detect

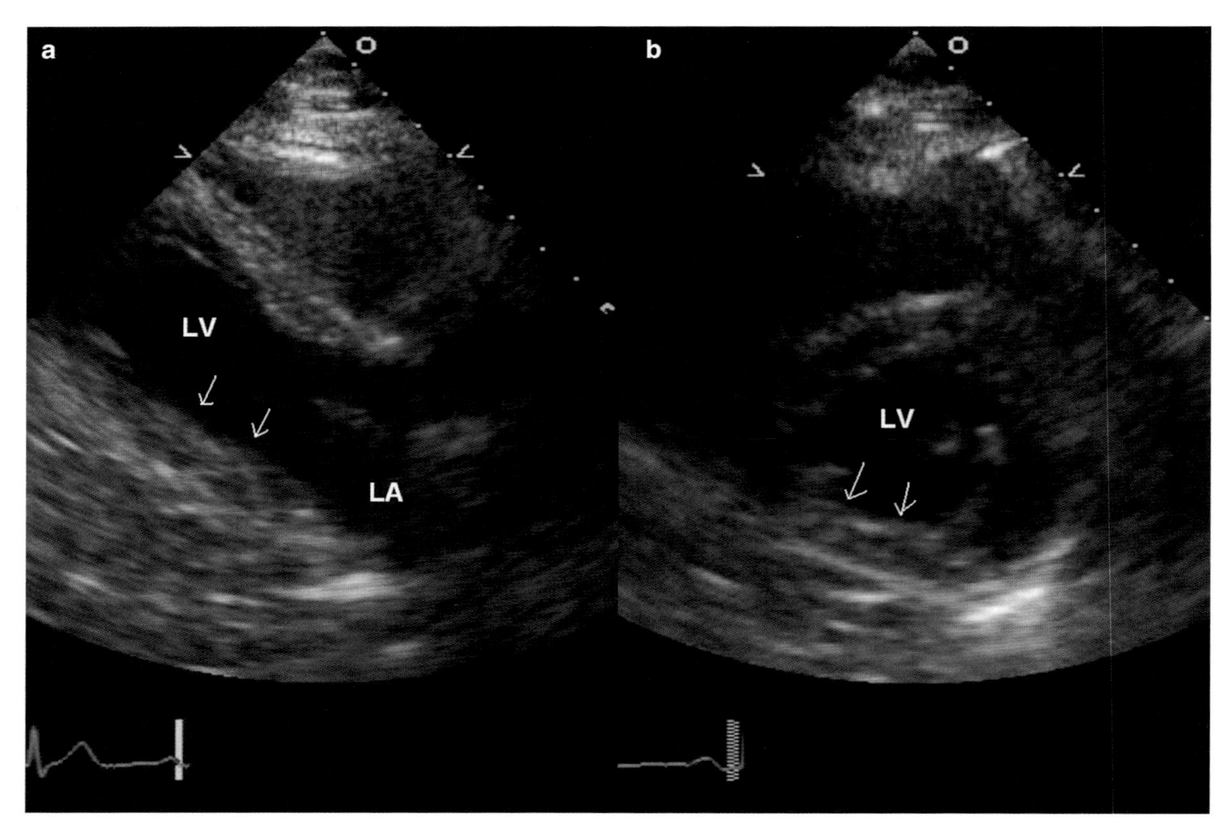

Fig. 7.8 Parasternal long-axis (**a**) and short-axix (**b**) views in diastole show that the posteroinferior wall (*arrows*) appears to be flattened. *LA* left atrium, *LV* left ventricle

abnormal walls (Fig. 7.12). In a study of 222 consecutive patients with myocardial infarction or ischemic cardiomyopathy, Delgado et al. compared global longitudinal strain in these patients with that of 20 age matched normal controls [29]. Global longitudinal strain was obtained in all patients and controls with an inter-observer variability of $0.3 \pm 0.6\%$. They reported a good correlation between EF and global longitudinal strain (Fig. 7.13). Strain and strain rate are very promising measures in the assessment of global and regional function in patients with ischemic heart disease, and more validation studies are forth-coming.

Chest Pain Assessment

Echocardiography has proven useful in the assessment of patients presenting with chest pain at the Emergency Room. The detection of regional wall motion abnormality in patients without a prior history of myocardial infarction indicates that there is a high likelihood of coronary artery disease and that the chest pain is due to myocardial ischemia. In patients with no wall motion abnormalities, the prognosis is good, although the possibility of a myocardial infarction is not completely excluded. In these patients, echo is much more useful in excluding serious conditions that mimic myocardial infarction.

Acute pulmonary embolism, particularly of massive or submassive nature, can be identified by the presence of right ventricular enlargement and dysfunction. In rare cases, the actual pulmonary embolus can be visualized in the proximal pulmonary arteries.

Aortic dissection is another critically important diagnosis to consider, since prompt surgical intervention is frequently necessary to ensure survival (Fig. 7.14). The echocardiographic features of aortic dissections are discussed in Chap. 9. This is an important and sometimes confusing diagnosis, since the

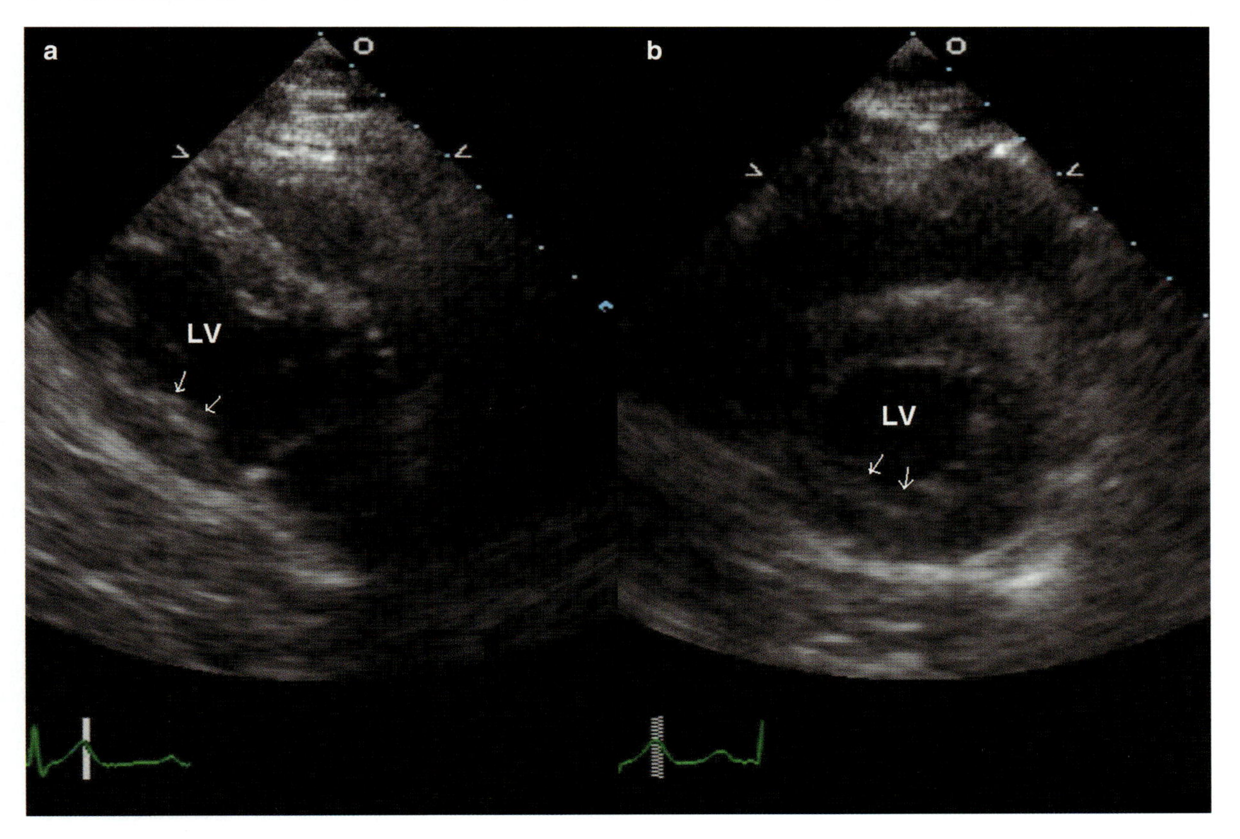

Fig. 7.9 Parasternal long-axis (**a**) and short-axis (**b**) views in systole in the same patient as in Fig. 7.7.7 show that the posteroinferior wall has a paradoxic outward movement during systole but the endocardial thickening (*arrows*) is normal. This finding has been termed pseudodyskinesia which may be related to an elevated left hemidiaphragm and should not be confused with myocardial infarction involving the posteroinferior wall. *LV* left ventricle

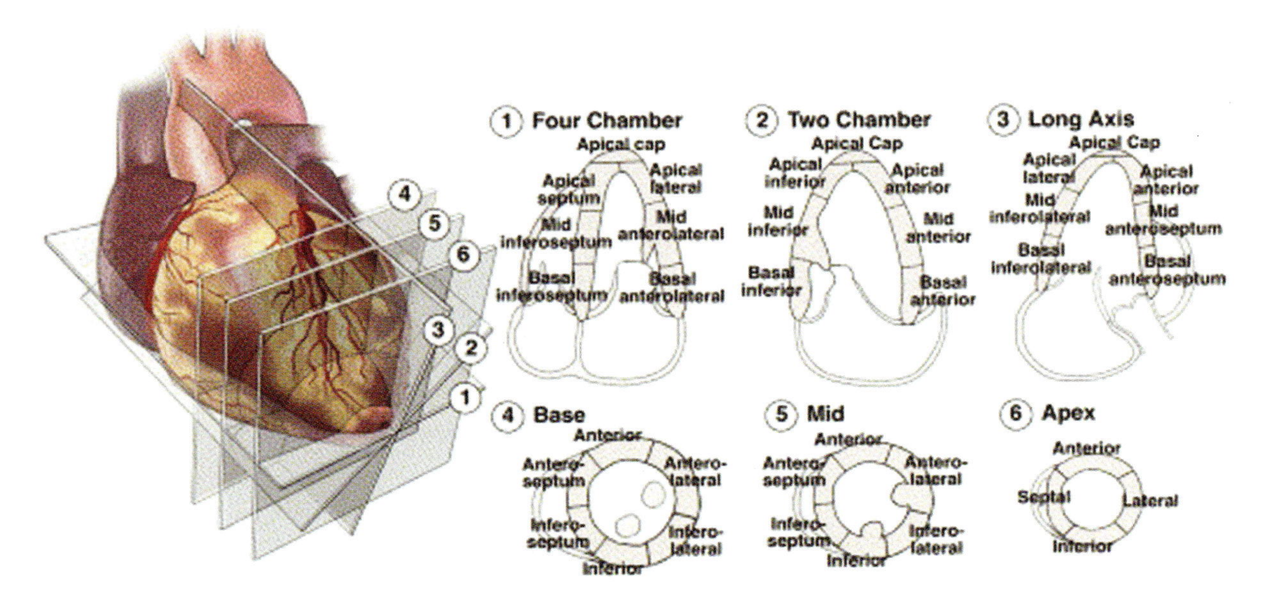

Fig. 7.10 Schematic diagram showing the 17 segment model to assess left ventricular regional wall motion abnormalities (Reproduced with permission from Lang et al. [21])

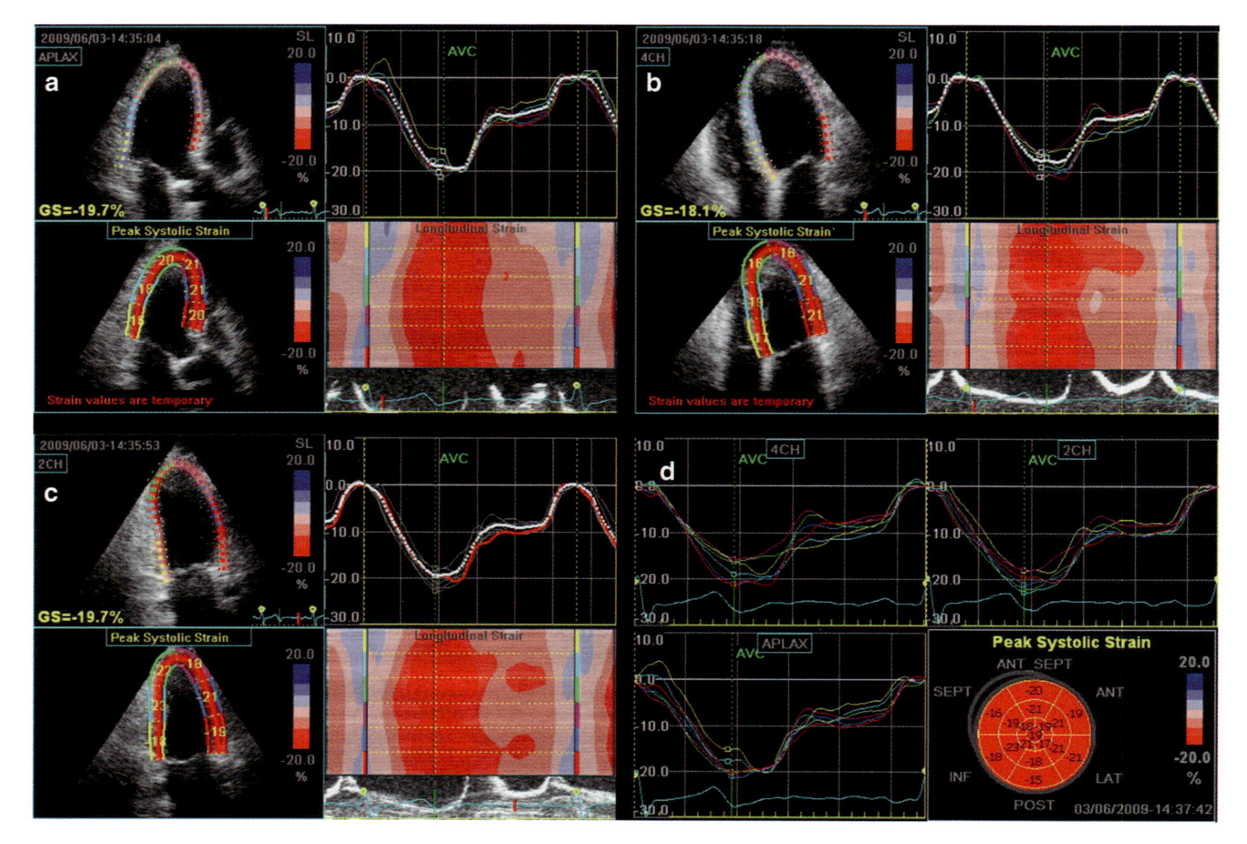

Fig. 7.11 Global and regional longitudinal strain measurements in the apical long-axis (**a**), four-chamber (**b**) and two-chamber (**c**) view are shown in a patient with no coronary artery disease. The summary strain data is shown in (**d**)

aortic dissection flap can occlude one of the coronary ostia, particularly the right coronary ostium, resulting in electrocardiographic changes of acute inferior wall myocardial infarction. Infarct and acute dissection can thus co-exist.

In patients with intermittent chest pain and no resting wall motion abnormalities, the diagnosis of coronary artery disease can be supported by the demonstration of stress induced regional wall motion abnormality. In the diagnosis of coronary artery disease, the use of echocardiographic imaging to detect wall motion increases the sensitivity of the stress test to 70–80% and specificity to 80–90%, which are similar to radionuclide stress test [30–33].

Exercise is the preferred stress modality in patients who can exercise. There are two main modalities in exercise stress echo, namely treadmill exercise and supine bicycle exercise tests, with similar sensitivity and specificity for the diagnosis of coronary artery disease [33]. The latter has the advantage of assessing wall motion at different stages of exercise. In patients who are unable to exercise, pharmacologic agents such as dobutamine, arbutamine and dipyridamole have been used to bring out reversible wall motion abnormalities. In stress echocardiography, the echo images during stress are more likely to be suboptimal due to increased respiration and body movement during stress. Echo contrast agents have been successfully used to improve the image quality and thus the diagnostic confidence in the assessment of stress induced wall motion abnormalities (Fig. 7.15).

Myocardial Infarction

In patients with prolonged chest pain consistent with myocardial ischemia, the presence of regional wall motion abnormalities is diagnostic of acute myocardial infarction in those with no history of prior myocardial

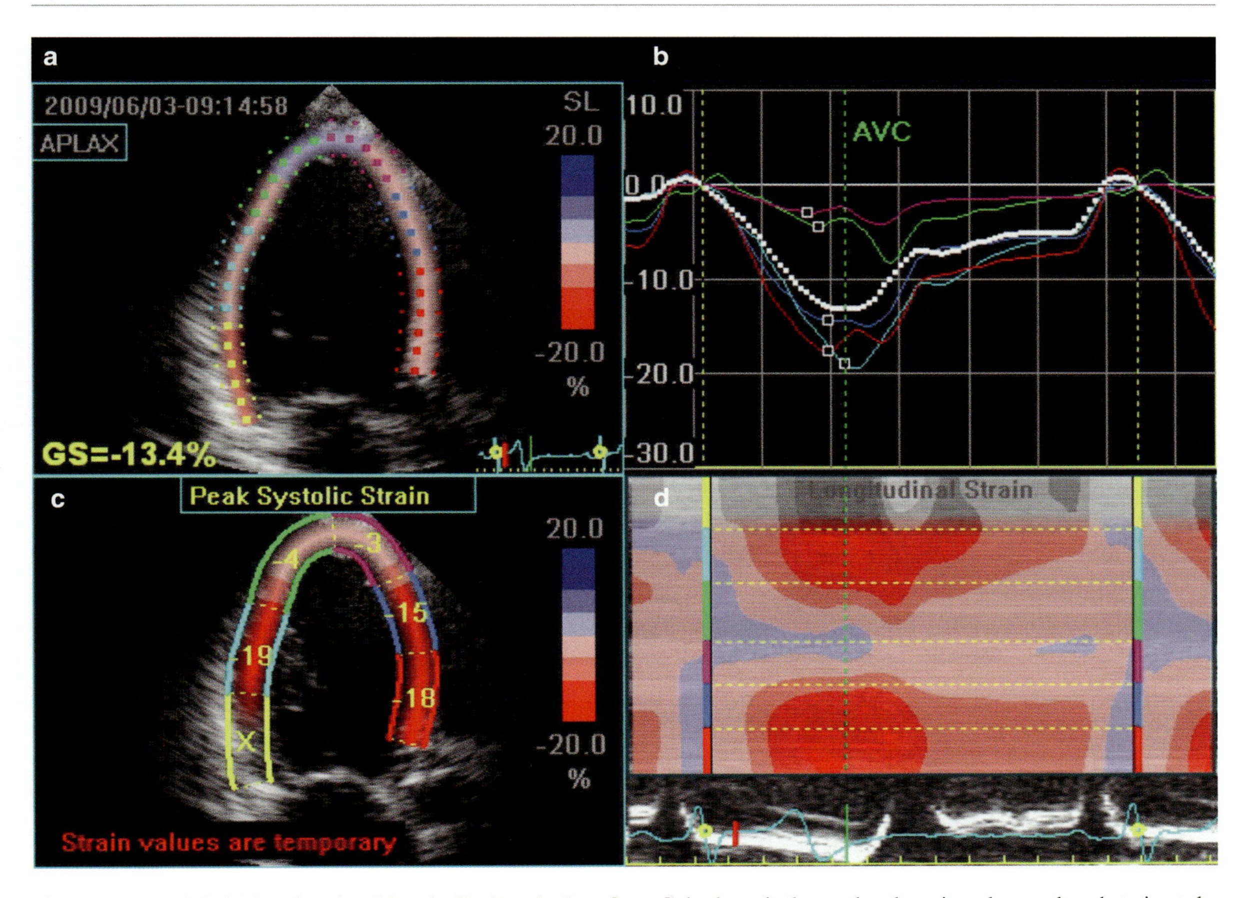

Fig. 7.12 The global (**a**) and regional longitudinal strain data (**b**, **c**, **d**) in the apical two-chamber view show reduced strain at the apex consistent with apical myocardial infarction. The global strain is reduced as a result of reduced strain at the apex

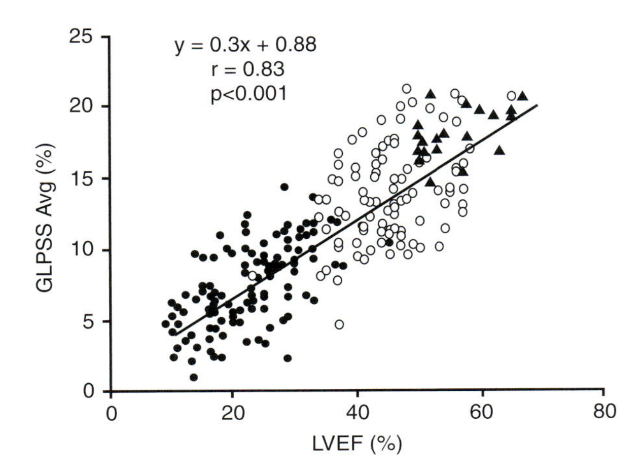

Fig. 7.13 Correlation between global longitudinal strain and left ventricular ejection fraction showing a close relationship between these two values (Reproduced with permission from Delgado et al. [29])

infarction. The location of regional wall motion abnormalities is a good indicator of the culprit coronary lesion (Figs. 7.16–7.18). As previously discussed wall motion abnormalities involving the anterior wall are indicative of obstructive lesion of in the left anterior descending artery. Conversely, wall motion abnormalities in the inferior wall indicate the presence of right coronary artery disease.

The extent of the wall motion abnormalities is a good reflection of the extent of the affected myocardium and can help to identify patients with multivessel disease from those with single vessel disease (Figs. 7.4, 7.19). In patients with single vessel disease, such as obstructive lesions of the left anterior descending artery, there is hypokinesia or akinesia of the anterior wall but also hyperkinesia of the inferior wall. The absence of hyperkinesia in the inferior wall in these

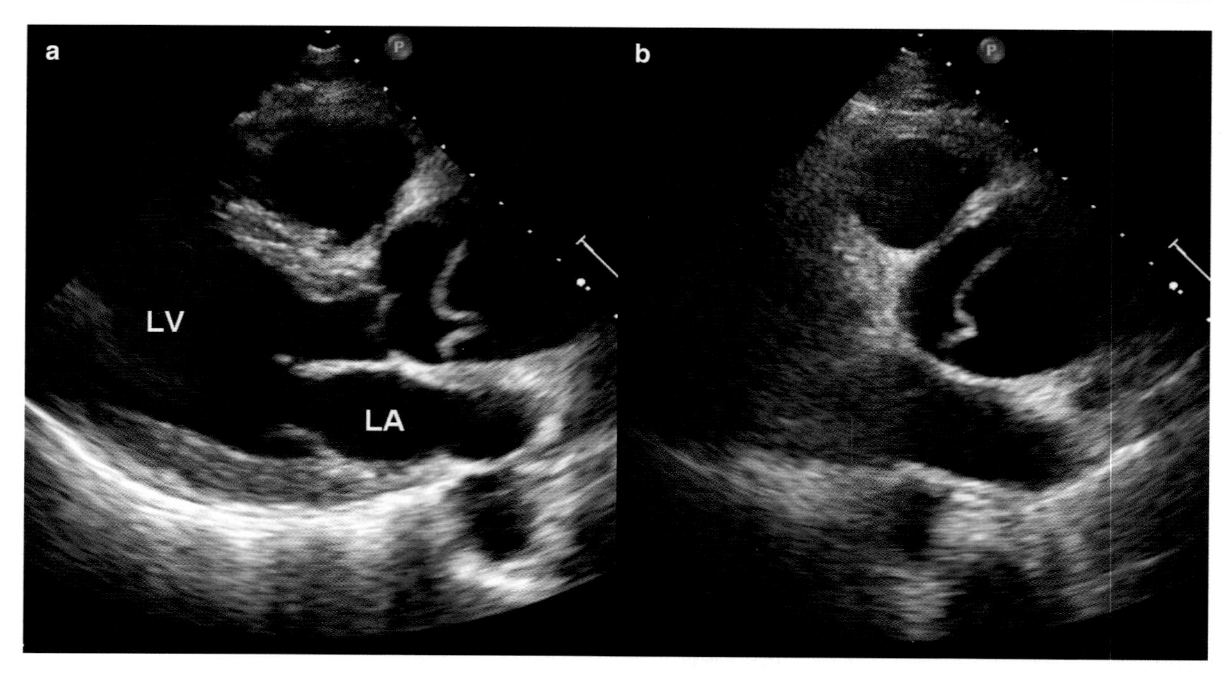

Fig. 7.14 Parasternal long-axis (**a**) and short-axis (**b**) views show a large intimal flap in the aortic root diagnostic of type A aortic dissection. *LA* left atrium, *LV* left ventricle

patients suggests that there is concomitant right coronary artery disease. In patients with suboptimal echo images, echo contrast agent can be used to diagnose the wall motion abnormalities (Fig. 7.20).

The absence of wall motion abnormality in patients with prolonged chest pain lowers the likelihood of myocardial infarction, although small non-transmural myocardial injury can be present with no significant wall motion abnormalities. Therefore in patients with equivocal history and non-diagnostic electrocardiographic findings, echocardiography can be very useful in the diagnosis or exclusion of acute myocardial infarction.

Acute infarct complications may be mechanical or non- mechanical [34]. Some of the non- mechanical ones are quite common including diastolic dysfunction, congestive heart failure, atrial and ventricular arrhythmias, deep venous thrombosis and depression. Fibrinous pericarditis is common immediately after myocardial infarction and this may be complicated by a pericardial effusion. After several weeks post- infarct, Dressler's phenomenon, an autoimmune pericarditis, may develop and may be associated with a pericardial effusion.

The role of echocardiography is particularly important in dealing with patients with acute myocardial infarction complicated by shock (Table 7.3). Shock complicating myocardial infarction carries a high mortality and needs to be aggressively managed to improve the prognosis. Echocardiography provides prompt and accurate diagnosis in these critically ill patients.

The conditions giving rise to shock in this setting can be divided into those associated with or without a new cardiac murmur. A word of caution is that the murmur in this setting may be soft and difficult to detect with certainty in view of the hypotension and tachycardia in these patients. Acute mechanical complications include ventricular free wall rupture and hemopericardium, papillary muscle rupture and ventricular septal rupture. These can occur in any combination, even all three complications in the same individual. These mechanical complications can be accurately assessed by echocardiography.

Papillary Muscle Rupture

The ventricular papillary muscles may be ischemic or infarcted and become immobile and stunned [35]. This may lead to transient mitral valve regurgitation. If the

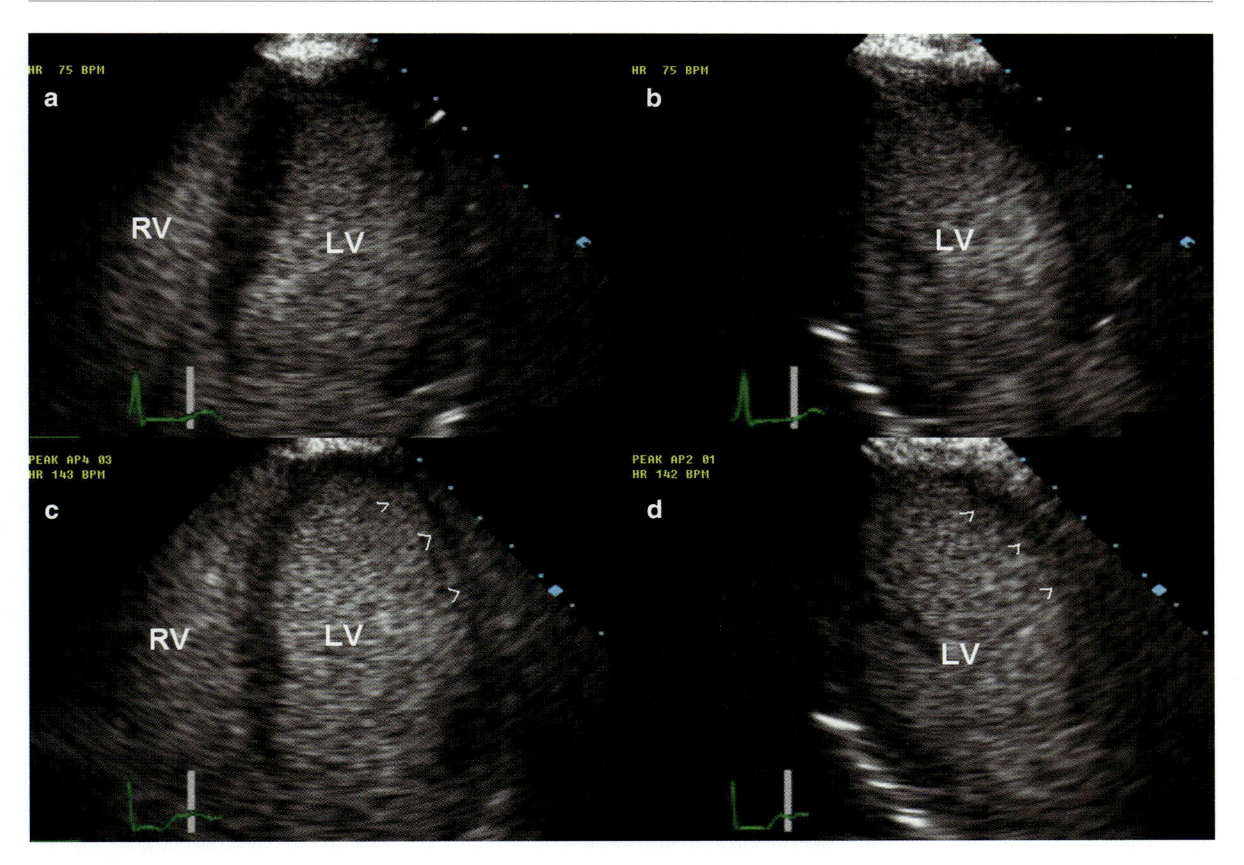

Fig. 7.15 Contrast stress-echocardiograms comparing the resting apical four-chamber (**a**) and apical two-chamber (**b**) views with the peak stress apical four-chamber (**c**) and two-chamber (**d**) views show that the anterolateral walls (arrowheads) become akinetic at peak exercise, consistent with diseases in the left anterior descending and left circumflex arteries. The use of an echo contrast agent has been shown to increase the diagnostic confidence of stress echocardiography. *LV* left ventricle, *RV* right ventricle

papillary muscles rupture, this usually occurs at 4–5 days post infarct when the affected myocardium is maximally necrotic and inflamed. Rupture of a part of the muscle or the entire muscle may occur leading to severe mitral regurgitation and heart failure (Figs. 7.21–7.23) [9]. Echocardiography is an accurate means to diagnose this complication [36]. Papillary muscle rupture can occur with either subendocardial or transmural infarction. All the other mechanical complications require transmural infarction. Rupture or partial rupture of the papillary muscle can lead to severe mitral regurgitation. This usually occurs in the setting of inferior wall infarction when the posteromedial papillary muscle is involved. The posteromedial papillary muscle is generally supplied by the right coronary artery, while the anterolateral papillary muscle has a dual blood supply from both the right coronary artery and left circumflex artery and therefore rupture of the anterior papillary muscle is less common. The typical setting of this complication is an elderly patient with first myocardial infarction and a history of systemic hypertension.

The overall systolic function may be preserved or only mildly reduced with focal regional wall motion abnormalities involving the inferior wall. If this condition is suspected, close examination of the papillary muscle is required to ensure that both heads are intact. In complete rupture of the papillary muscle, the affected mitral leaflet demonstrates a flail portion with the papillary muscle protruding into the left atrium during systole. In partial rupture, obvious flail is not seen, but there would be a marked degree of prolapse of the affected mitral leaflet, and partial disruption of the base of the affected papillary muscle (Figs. 7.24, 7.25). This

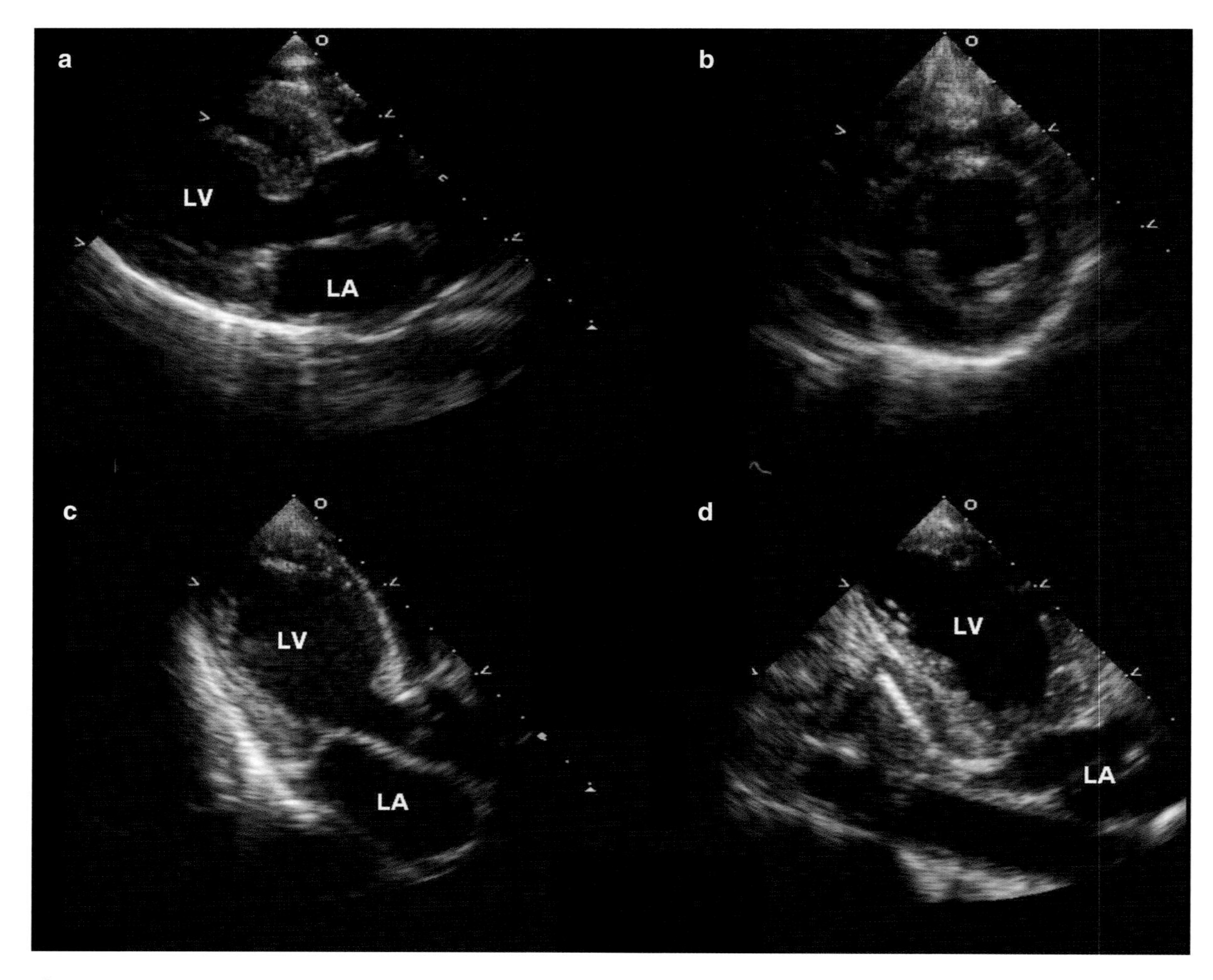

Fig. 7.16 Parasternal long-axis (**a**), short-axis (**b**), apical long-axis (**c**) and apical two-chamber (**d**) views show that the mid and apical anterior wall and anterior septum are thinned out and akinetic consistent with anterior wall myocardial infarction. *LA* left atrium, *LV* left ventricle

condition requires prompt attention as it is a prelude to complete rupture resulting in more severe mitral regurgitation. When the entire papillary muscle is ruptured, there is usually torrential mitral regurgitation accompanied by shock. Emergent surgery is generally indicated as these patients do not respond to medical treatment alone. A systolic murmur is generally detected, although the murmur may appear to be systolic ejection in nature due to its decrescendo nature from the rapid equalization of pressures between the left atrium and left ventricle during the later part of systole.

Ventricular Septal Rupture

Ventricular septal rupture is another condition that is associated with the presence of a systolic murmur which is typically located at the lower left sternal border. There are two clinically distinct septal defects associated with myocardial infarction [9, 37]. In patients with large inferior wall myocardial infarction, ventricular septal rupture can occur involving the basal inferior septum (Figs. 7.26, 7.27). The defect in this situation is usually quite large and may be associated with right ventricular dysfunction. Because of the location and size of the

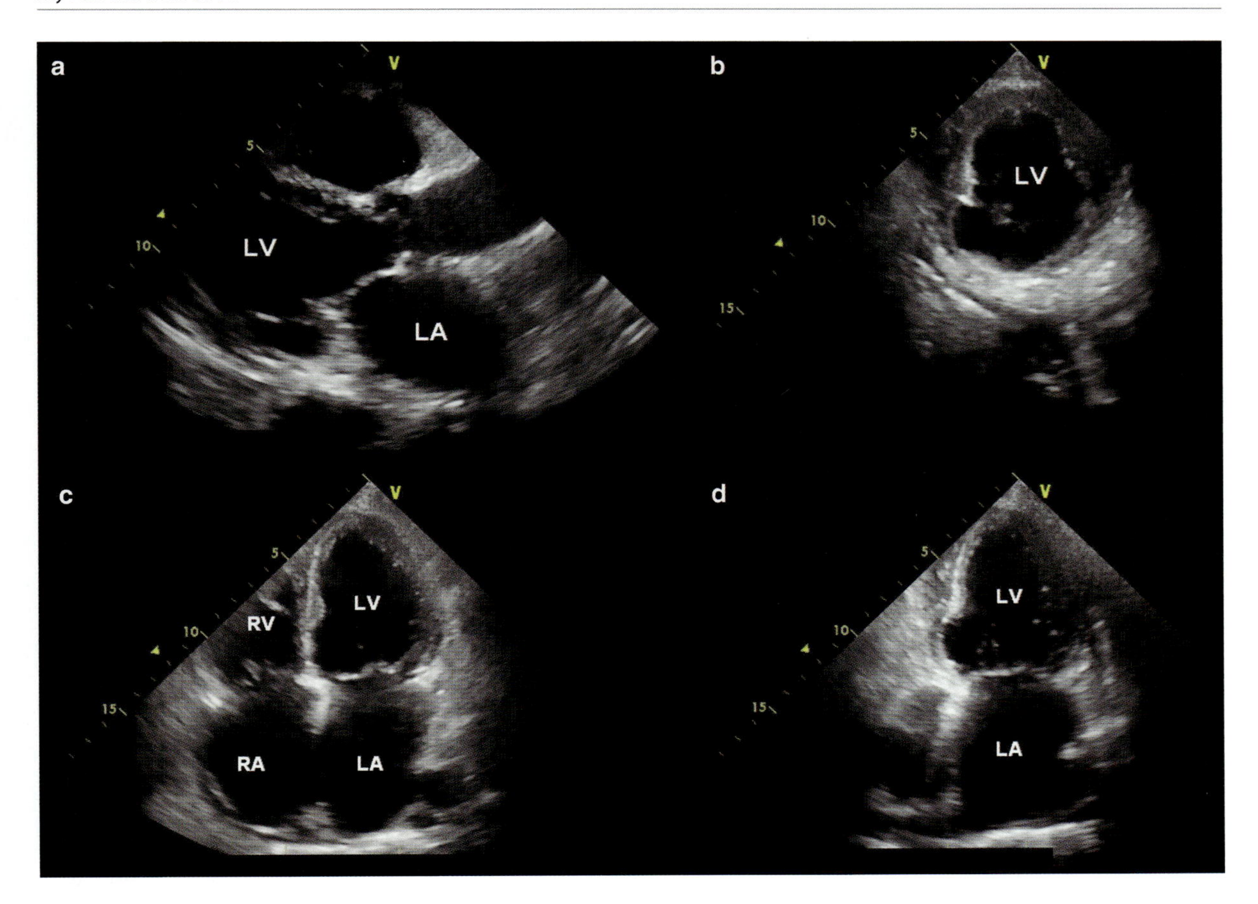

Fig. 7.17 Parasternal long-axis (**a**), short-axis (**b**), apical four-chamber (**c**) and apical two-chamber (**d**) views show localized thinning and akinesia consistent with old infarction involving the basal and mid inferior and posterior walls. *LA* left atrium; *LV* left ventricle, *RA* right atrium, *RV* right ventricle

defect, these defects are generally difficult to repair surgically and the prognosis of these patients is poor. The other type of ventricular septal rupture involves the apical septum in the setting of anterior wall infarction (Fig. 7.28). These defects generally have a serpiginous tract and the degree of left to right shunting may not be severe. These defects are more amenable to surgery particularly if the surgery can be delayed for several weeks to allow resolution of inflammation and development of some degree of fibrosis.

Dynamic Subaortic Stenosis

The development of subaortic obstruction in the setting of anterior myocardial infarction is an uncommon cause of cardiogenic shock, but this is an important condition to recognize since it may respond to treatment with beta-blocker therapy and it may worsen with inotropic agent therapy [38]. This usually occurs in patients with anterior wall myocardial infarction with sparing of the basal septum. The basal septum in these patients becomes hyperkinetic leading to the development of systolic anterior motion of the mitral leaflets and a subaortic gradient (Fig. 7.29). Treatment with inotropes accentuates the gradient and worsens the systemic hypotension. The proper management includes optimal fluid replacement and the use of a beta-blocker to relieve the subaortic gradient. After the acute phase of myocardial infarction, patients with this condition generally do quite well as they tend to have reasonably preserved left ventricular function.

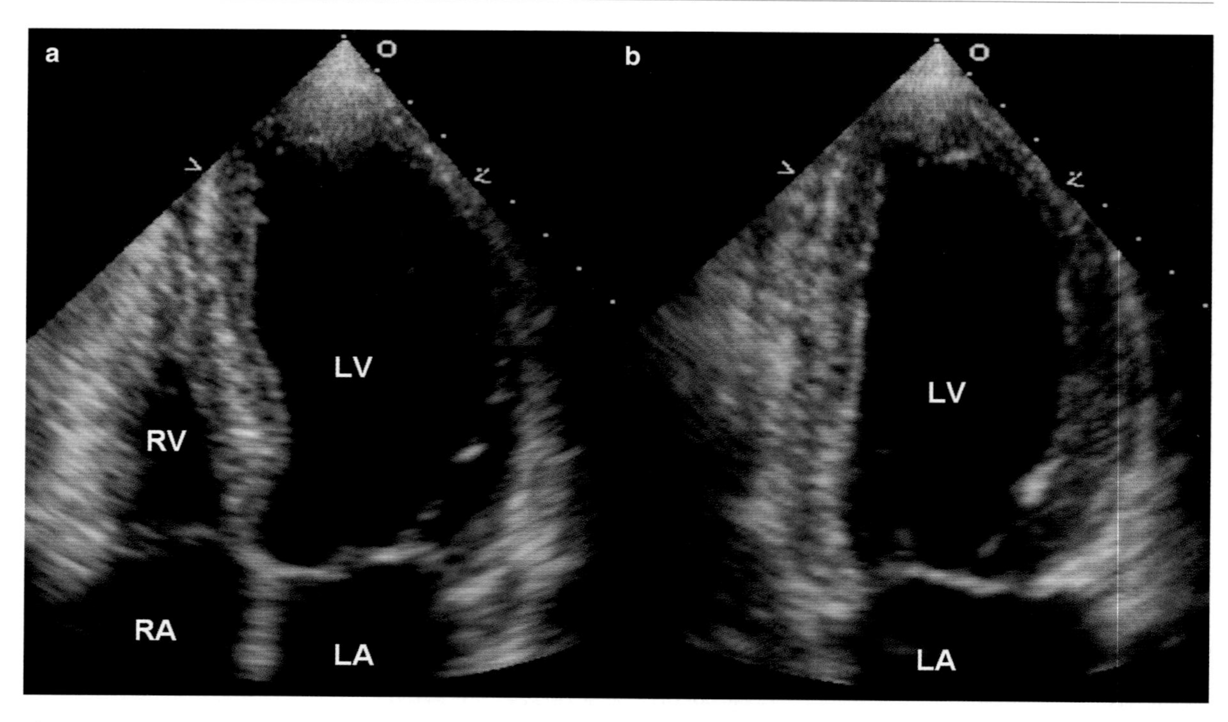

Fig. 7.18 Apical four-chamber (**a**) and two-chamber (**b**) views show thinning and akinesia of the lateral wall. The anterior wall and inferior wall showed normal thickness. *LA* left atrium, *LV* left ventricle, *RA* right atrium, *RV* right ventricle

Free Wall Rupture

Free-wall rupture should always be considered in patients in shock complicating myocardial infarction. Free wall rupture may occur in the first 24 h after the infarct or at 4–5 days [9, 39]. Most individuals with this condition are female, have post-infarct hypertension, and of course have suffered a transmural infarct. This is usually the individual's first myocardial infarct, as a previous older infarct would leave scar which would be protective against rupture. The early rupture is due to a so called "dissecting hematoma" that cleaves the myocardium and causes rupture. This type of complication may have become more common with thrombolytic therapy, but this is debatable, since thrombolytic therapy has likely decreased free wall rupture overall as the therapy leads to limitation of infarct size resulting in smaller infarcts that are less transmural and less prone to this complication.

At 4–5 days post infarct the affected myocardium has extensive necrosis and the infiltrating neutrophils have degranulated. No fibroblasts have entered the infarct yet, so this is the time of maximal wall weakness. Rupture commonly occurs near the base of the papillary muscles or between them, or at the anterior apex (Fig. 7.30) [39]. These are areas where the muscle fibers are undergoing extensive changes in direction leading to potential areas of ventricular weakness. Free wall rupture may be gradual and associated with fibrinous pericarditis (Fig. 7.31).

With free-wall rupture the pericardium fills with blood such that an effusion may be visualized by imaging (Fig. 7.32) [40]. The pericardium is a fibrous structure and is not acutely distensible, thus even a small fluid accumulation (> 100 mL) leads to a rapid increase in intrapericardial pressure resulting in cardiac tamponade. The pathognomonic sign is the detection of blood in the pericardium which on echocardiography appears as an echo-dense pericardial effusion. Localized thinning of the left ventricular free wall associated with excessive motion in the adjacent myocardium is a frequent associated finding. A high index of suspicion is crucial in making this diagnosis, since some of these patients may stabilize for some time due to sealing off of the free-wall rupture by the pericardial hematoma. The use of an echo contrast agent may

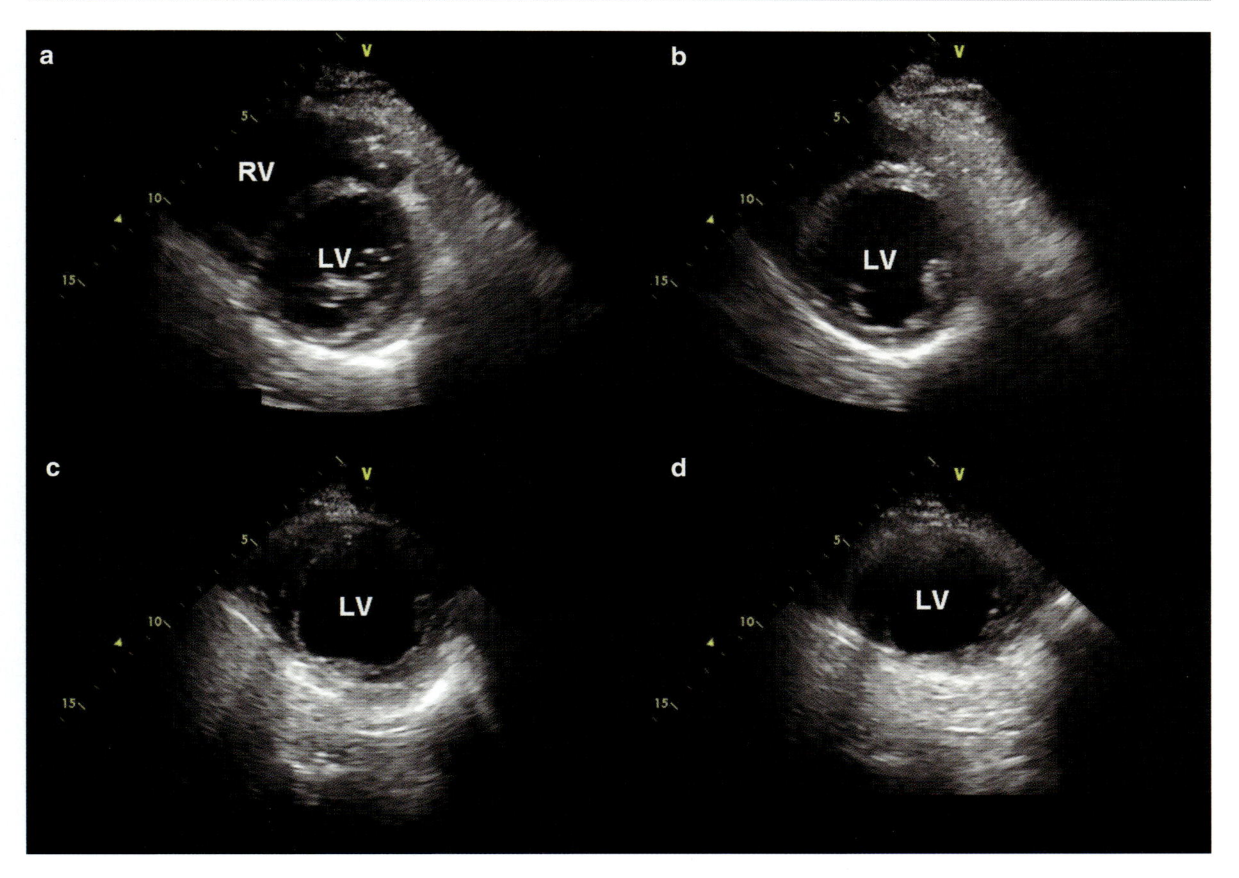

Fig. 7.19 Parasternal short-axis views from base to apex (**a–d**) in this patient with multiple myocardial infarctions show thinning of multiple myocardial segments including the inferior wall, anterior wall and apex. *LV* left ventricle, *RV* right ventricle

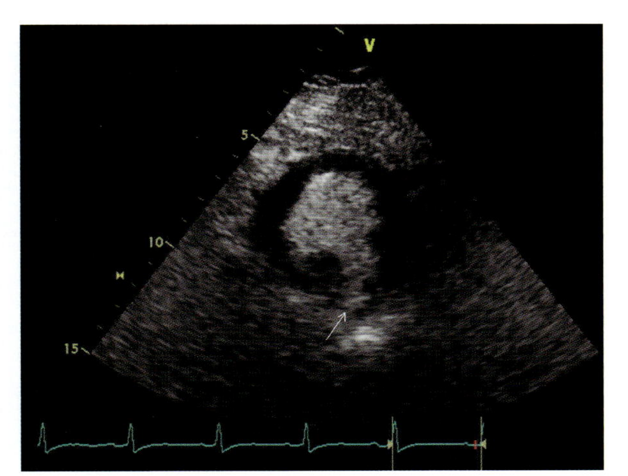

Fig. 7.20 Parasternal short-axis view with injection of echo contrast identifies local thinning and akinesia involving the inferior wall (*arrow*)

Table 7.3 Causes of shock following acute myocardial infarction

Associated with new murmur
Ruptured papillary muscle
Ventricular septal rupture
Dynamic subaortic stenosis
Not associated with new murmur
Free wall rupture
Takotsubo cardiomyopathy
Extensive myocardial necrosis
Right ventricular infarction

demonstrate the localized thinning of the myocardium more effectively, but it remains unclear whether it can help make a firm diagnosis particularly in those whose defect has been sealed off temporarily by the pericardial hematoma.

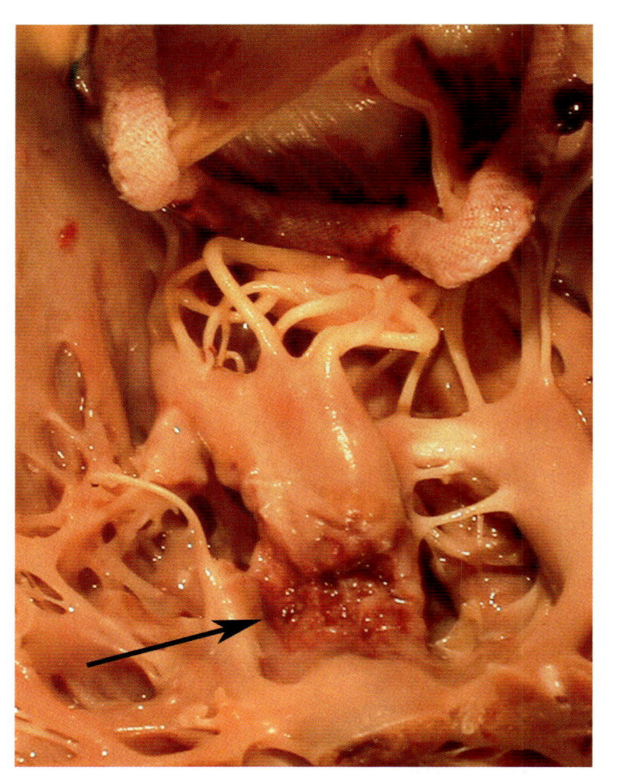

Fig. 7.21 Papillary muscle rupture post MI. This patient ruptured part of their papillary muscle and had valve replacement for mitral insufficiency. At autopsy the residual papillary muscle tissues show the area of prior rupture (*arrow*). Superior to this the valve prosthesis can be seen

Takotsubo Cardiomyopathy

An unusual myocardial infarction is one that is brought on by excessive mental stress. It commonly occurs in elderly post-menopausal women. This condition is termed "Takotsubo cardiomyopathy", as the left ventricle takes on the shape of a Japanese pot vessel used to catch octopus [41]. The shape is a result of preservation of basal function with akinesia to dyskinesia of all the mid and apical segments. Angiography shows no culprit coronary lesions and pathologic myocardial findings are consistent with catecholamine induced myocarditis. After the acute phase of this disease, these patients generally have a good prognosis as they usually have good recovery of left ventricular function (Fig. 7.33). The typical appearance of the left ventricle during the acute phase can be reliably detected by echocardiography.

Right Ventricular Infarction

Right ventricular infarction can cause cardiogenic shock as the right ventricle does not provide adequate preload for the left ventricle, leading to low cardiac output and hypotension. Right ventricle infarction may be isolated, but is much more commonly associated with an adjacent acute inferior left ventricle infarct (Figs. 7.34, 7.35). Right ventricular dysfunction is common in the setting of inferior wall myocardial infarction but severe right ventricular dysfunction leading to shock is uncommon. Echocardiographic detection of right ventricular inferior wall motion abnormalities is a relatively common finding and detectable in about half of the patients with inferior wall myocardial infarction, but in less than 10% of these patients, right ventricular dysfunction can be severe resulting in hemodynamic decompensation. The optimal management of these patients remains uncertain although both fluid loading and pacing have been proposed.

Chronic Complications of Myocardial Infarction

Following acute myocardial infarction, particularly if the extent of infarction is substantial, the left ventricle undergoes remodeling with thinning of the infarct area, increase in the minor axis diameter more than the left ventricular length, leading to a more globular shaped ventricle, and increased left ventricular volume (Figs. 7.36, 7.37) [42]. This remodeling process can take place from days to months. Due to loss of myocardium the ventricle increases its volume and enlarges in an attempt to maintain the stroke volume. With chamber enlargement the wall tension increases and there is a compensatory wall hypertrophy. The remodeled ventricle thus is hypertrophied and dilated, resulting in eccentric hypertrophy. Initially these changes are compensatory and beneficial, but eventually they become counter-productive and pathological with cell death, myocyte degeneration and heart failure.

The increased left ventricular volume (end diastolic or end systolic) is one of the strongest predictors of long-term adverse effects such as the development of heart failure and death. Prevention of remodeling is essential

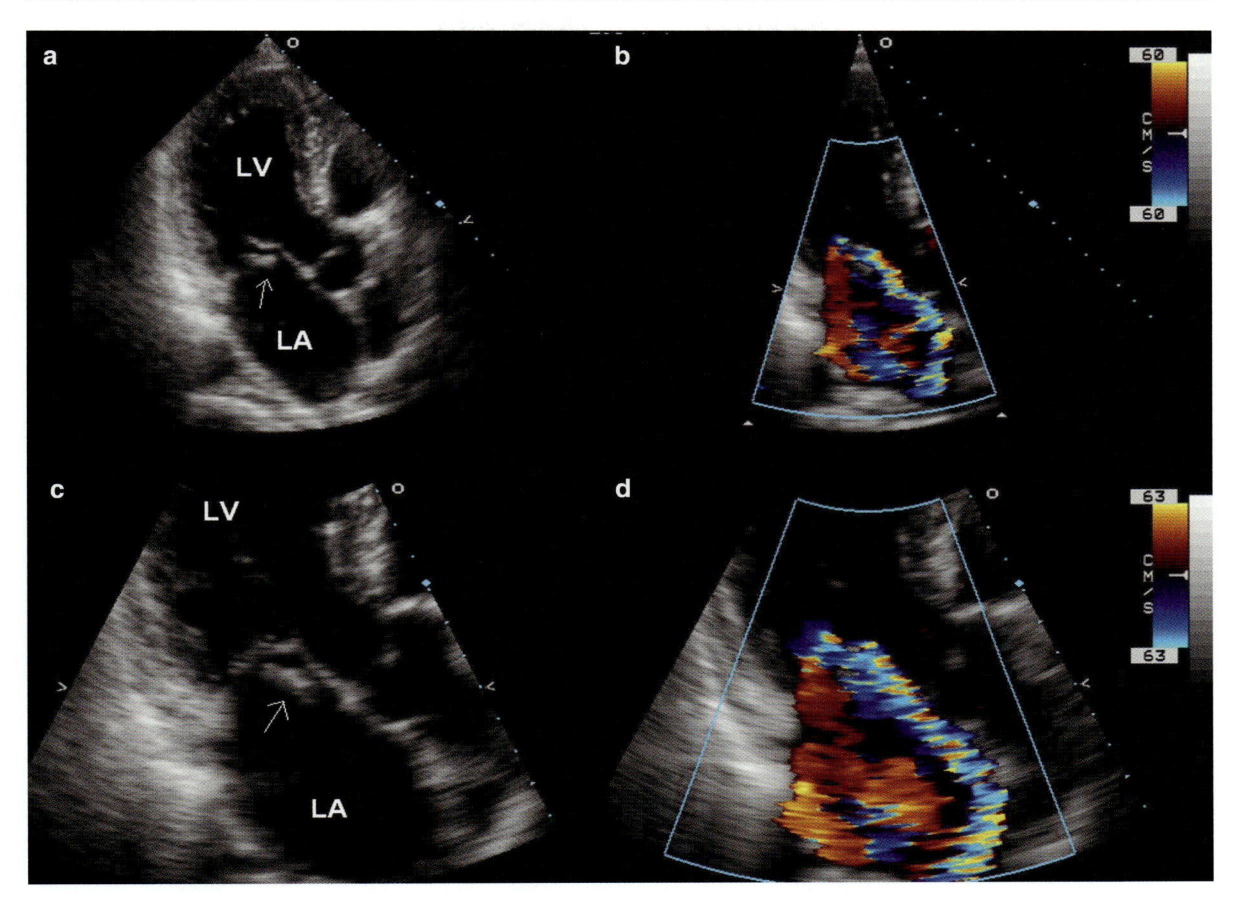

Fig. 7.22 Apical long-axis views (**a, c**) show a large mass prolapsing into the left atrium during systole. Color-flow images (**b, d**) show severe mitral regurgitation which is anteriorly directed. The large prolapsing mass represents the ruptured head of the posteromedial papillary muscle. *LA* left atrium, *LV* left ventricle

to improve the prognosis. Prompt and early revascularization limits myocardial damage and is an effective way to minimize remodeling. Treatment with a beta-blocker and/or an angiotensin converting enzyme inhibitor has been shown to limit or prevent remodeling.

The left ventricular shape should be assessed, as it is an independent predictor of outcome in median to long term follow-up of patients following myocardial infarction [43, 44]. The sphericity index, which is the ratio of short-axis to long-axis of the ventricle, is one measure of the shape change after myocardial infarction when the left ventricle becomes more spherical, as opposed to the normal ellipsoid shape (Figs. 7.36, 7.37). The spherical shape puts the ventricle at a mechanical disadvantage such that there is an increase in wall stress and abnormal distribution of the afterload. This can result in mal-alignment of the mitral subvalvular apparatus leading to mitral regurgitation. In the echocardiographic sub study of 373 patients in the SAVE study, sphericity index predicted development of heart failure and cardiac mortality during follow-up [44].

After acute myocardial infarction, varying degree of fibrosis will be present in the myocardium. This may be subendocardial, involve the papillary muscles, or be transmural. Scars involving the papillary muscles may lead to chronic mitral regurgitation due to loss of contractility or by restriction of the leaflet motion (a problem exacerbated by ventricular dilatation and distortion). If the muscle is fibrotic and the underlying ventricle has undergone enlargement and alteration of its normal shape, the leaflets may not coapt appropriately. Ischemic mitral regurgitation can occur from derangement of any components of the mitral valve apparatus. The mitral annulus can be dilated or the papillary muscles may be

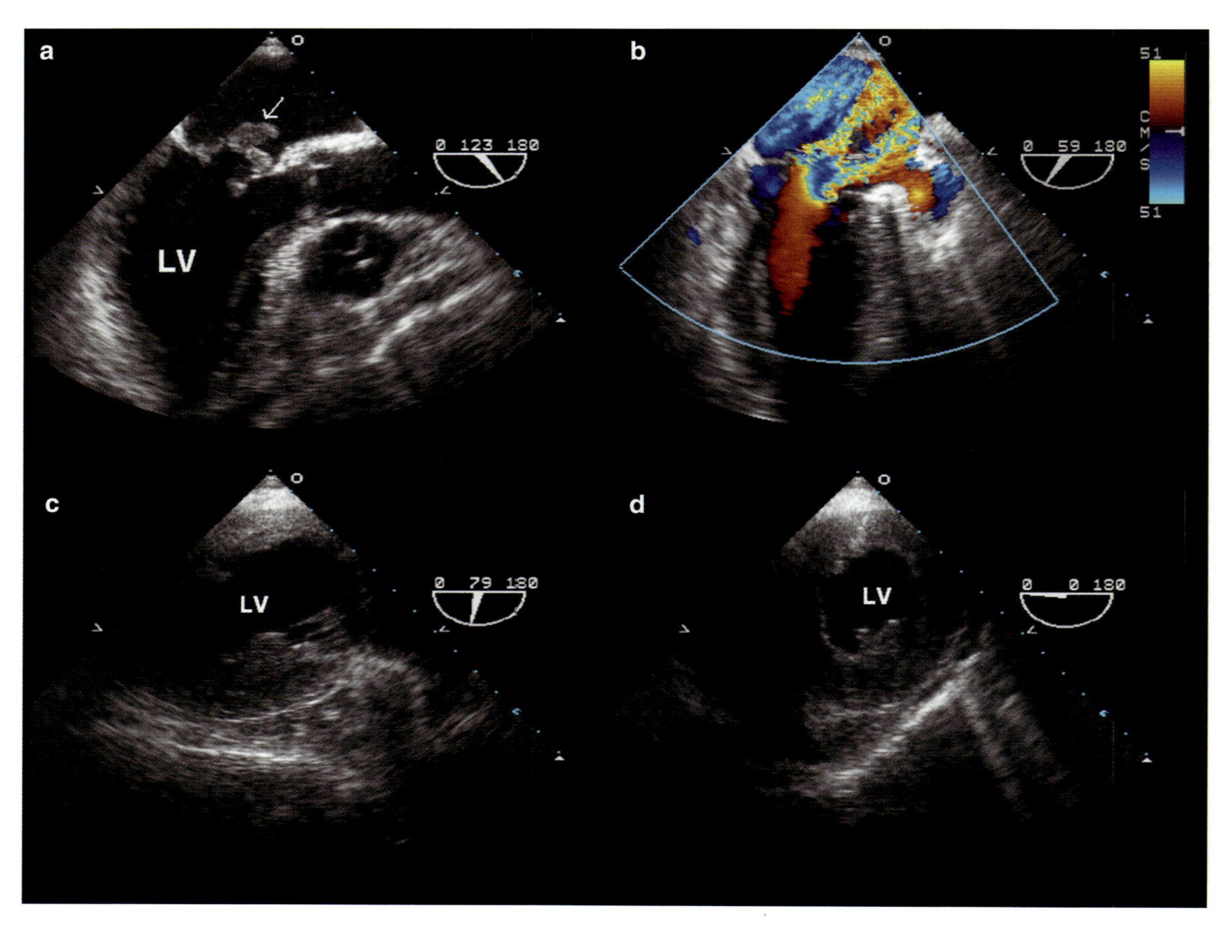

Fig. 7.23 (**a**) Transesophageal view in a patient with a ruptured papillary muscle head prolapsing in to the left atrium (*arrow*). (**b**) Color-flow imaging confirms severe mitral regurgitation. (**c, d**) The posteromedial papillary muscle is not seen in its usual location because of the complete rupture. *LV* left ventricle

scarred, pulled laterally and become misaligned due to the underlying enlarged left ventricle. Chronic mitral regurgitation is a common finding in patients with ischemic heart disease, due to the many ways that the mitral valve apparatus can be affected.

Left Ventricular True and False Aneurysm

Left ventricular aneurysm is a well recognized complication of myocardial infarction [9, 45]. It is more common in patients with anterior wall myocardial infarction, and indeed over 90% of the left ventricular aneurysms involve the left ventricular apex with the remaining 5–10% involving the inferior wall (Fig. 7.38). The incidence of aneurysm may vary partly related to variability in the definition of an aneurysm. Obviously the more restrictive the definition, the lower is the incidence. In our Laboratory, left ventricular aneurysm is defined as a localized segmental wall motion abnormality manifested by diastolic bulging with systolic expansion and a clearly defined hinge point.(Figs. 7.39–7.41). Optimal imaging of the left ventricular apex is essential to differentiate left ventricular apical aneurysm from other apical abnormalities, particularly apical hypertrophy. Patients with left ventricular aneurysm are at a higher risk of complications including left ventricular thrombus formation, arrhythmia, and heart failure [46]. It is no surprise that it confers a higher rate of short-term and long-term mortality.

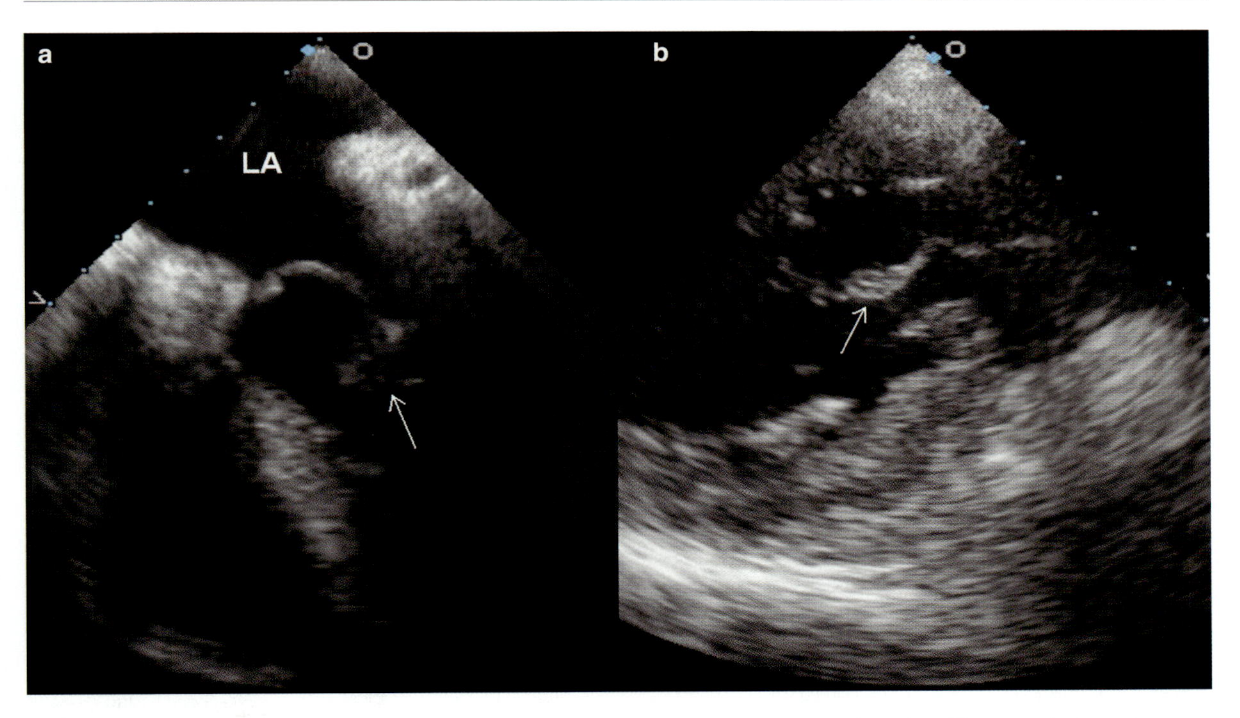

Fig. 7.24 Transesophageal (**a**) and transgastric (**b**) views show partial rupture of the anterolateral papillary muscle (*arrow*)

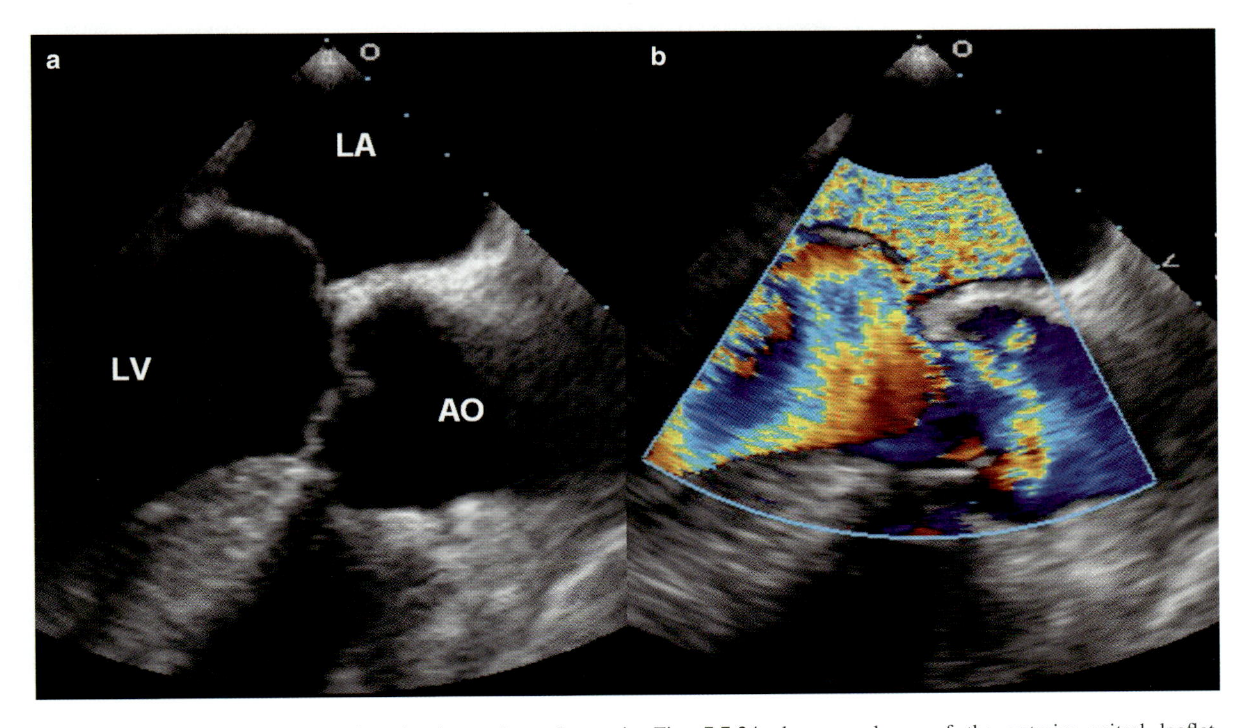

Fig. 7.25 (**a**) Transesophageal view in the patient shown in Fig. 7.7.24 shows prolapse of the anterior mitral leaflet. (**b**) Color imaging shows severe mitral regurgitation. The mitral leaflets are not flail because the papillary muscle rupture is only partial. *Ao* aorta, *LA* left atrium, *LV* left ventricle

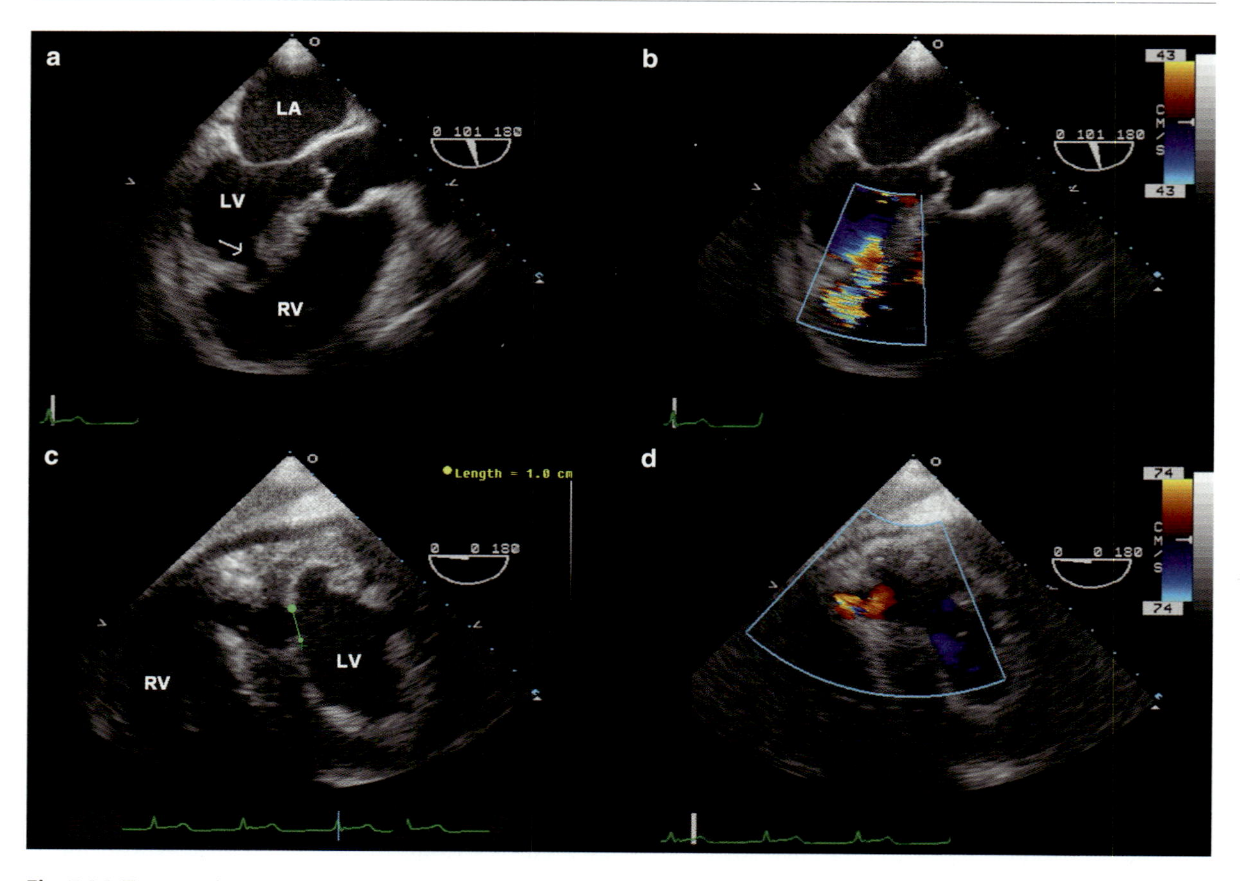

Fig. 7.26 Transesophageal views (**a, d**) in a patient with inferior wall myocardial infarction showing a large defect (*arrows*) involving the mid inferior wall. Color-flow images (**b**, **d**) confirm left to right shunting at the defect. *LA* left atrium; *LV* left ventricle, *RV* right ventricle

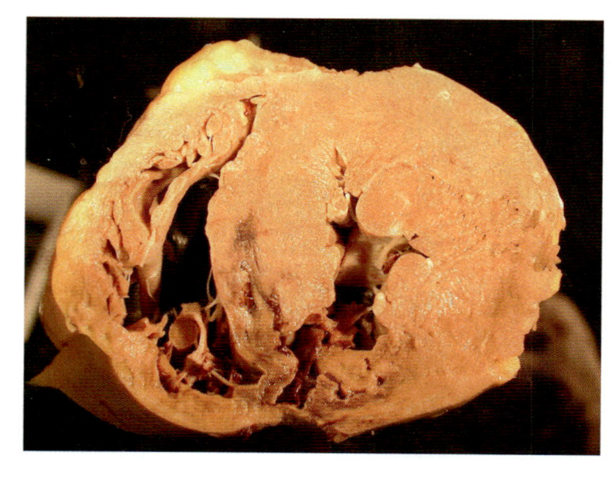

Fig. 7.27 Large complicated inferior ventricular septal defect associated with infarct of the inferior left and right ventricles. The VSD eventually ruptured externally thus making this infarct a double rupture (free wall and VSD)

The post-infarct aneurysm is commonly a true ventricular aneurysm, meaning that the aneurysm wall contains all three layers of the ventricle- the endocardium, the myocardium and the epicardium. True ventricular aneurysms have thin walls that often calcify. Aneurysms do not contract and thus are an area of stasis and may contain endocardial thrombus. True aneurysms contribute to congestive heart failure through loss of ventricular contractile function, dyskinesia, and inadvertent systolic filling with loss of forward cardiac output. They are a potential source of thrombus for systemic embolism including stroke (Figs. 7.38, 7.42) [46]. The entrapped residual myocardial fibers and the scar tissue may lead to ventricular arrhythmias.

In contrast, a false aneurysm or pseudoaneurysm is a consequence of localized ventricular free wall rupture and containment of the blood by fibrosis and adherent

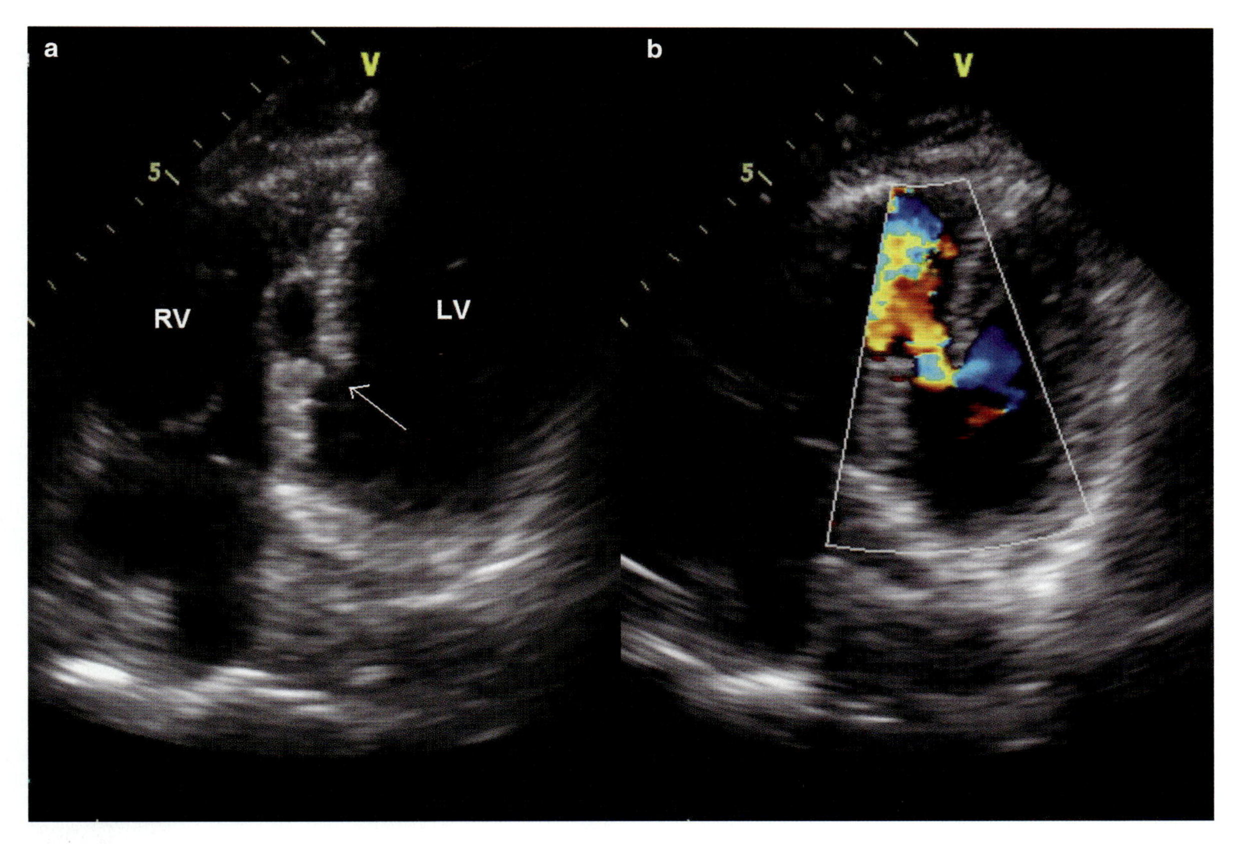

Fig. 7.28 (**a**) Apical four-chamber view in this patient with anterior wall myocardial infarction shows a ventricular septal defect involving the mid septum. (**b**) Color-flow imaging confirms shunting at the defect. *LV* left ventricle; *RV* right ventricle

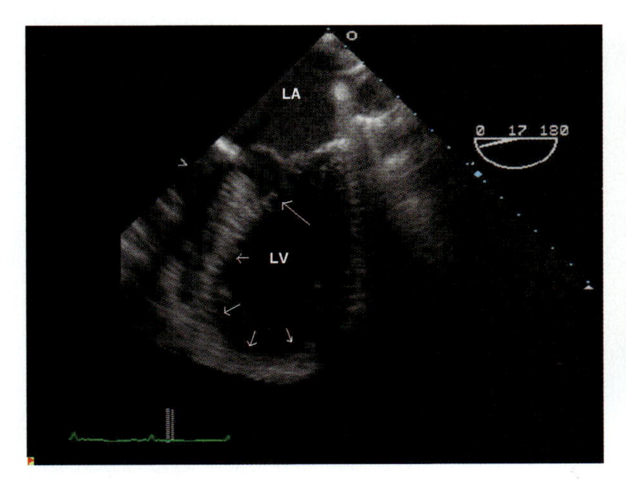

Fig. 7.29 Apical four-chamber view in a patient with anterior wall myocardial infarction shows akinesia involving the left ventricular apex (*short arrows*). The basal anterior septum is hypercontractile and there is systolic anterior motion of the mitral leaflets (*long arrow*) indicating the presence of subaortic obstruction. *LA* left atrium, *LV* left ventricle

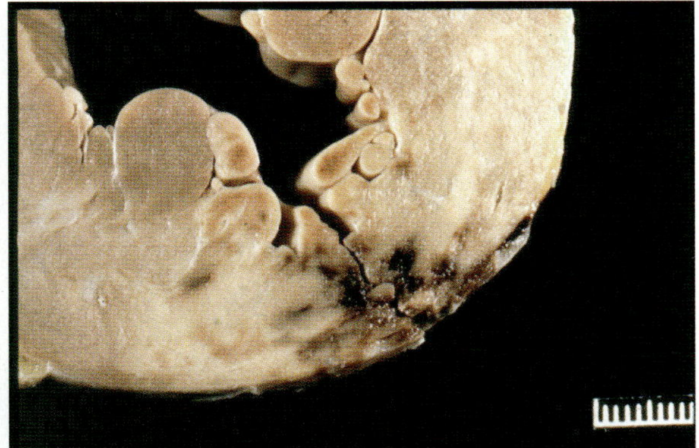

Fig. 7.30 Left ventricle free wall rupture post transmural MI. The rupture has occurred near the base of one of the papillary muscles

pericardium. There is only thrombus and fibrous tissue present in this type of aneurysm [46]. False aneurysms are less commonly seen than true aneurysms, since most free wall ruptures result in hemopericardium and

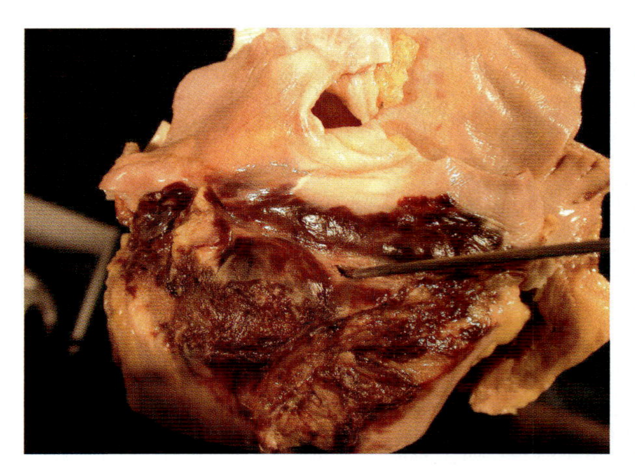

Fig. 7.31 External surface of a heart with free wall rupture post infract. There is severe fibrinous pericarditis associated with the gradual rupture process. A probe has been placed in the actual rupture tract

death, not in false aneurysms. False aneurysms may present as a chronic finding. Although the natural history is not well defined, the generally tendency is to consider surgical repair in patients who do not have severe co-morbidities that substantially increase their operative risks. The pseudoaneurysm is recognized by its characteristic narrow neck although in many circumstances, echocardiography may not be able to differentiate true aneurysm from pseudoaneurysm (Fig. 7.40).

Left Ventricular Thrombus

Anterior wall myocardial infarcts may become complicated by adherent endocardial thrombus with a risk for embolization [9, 47, 48]. This is less common with

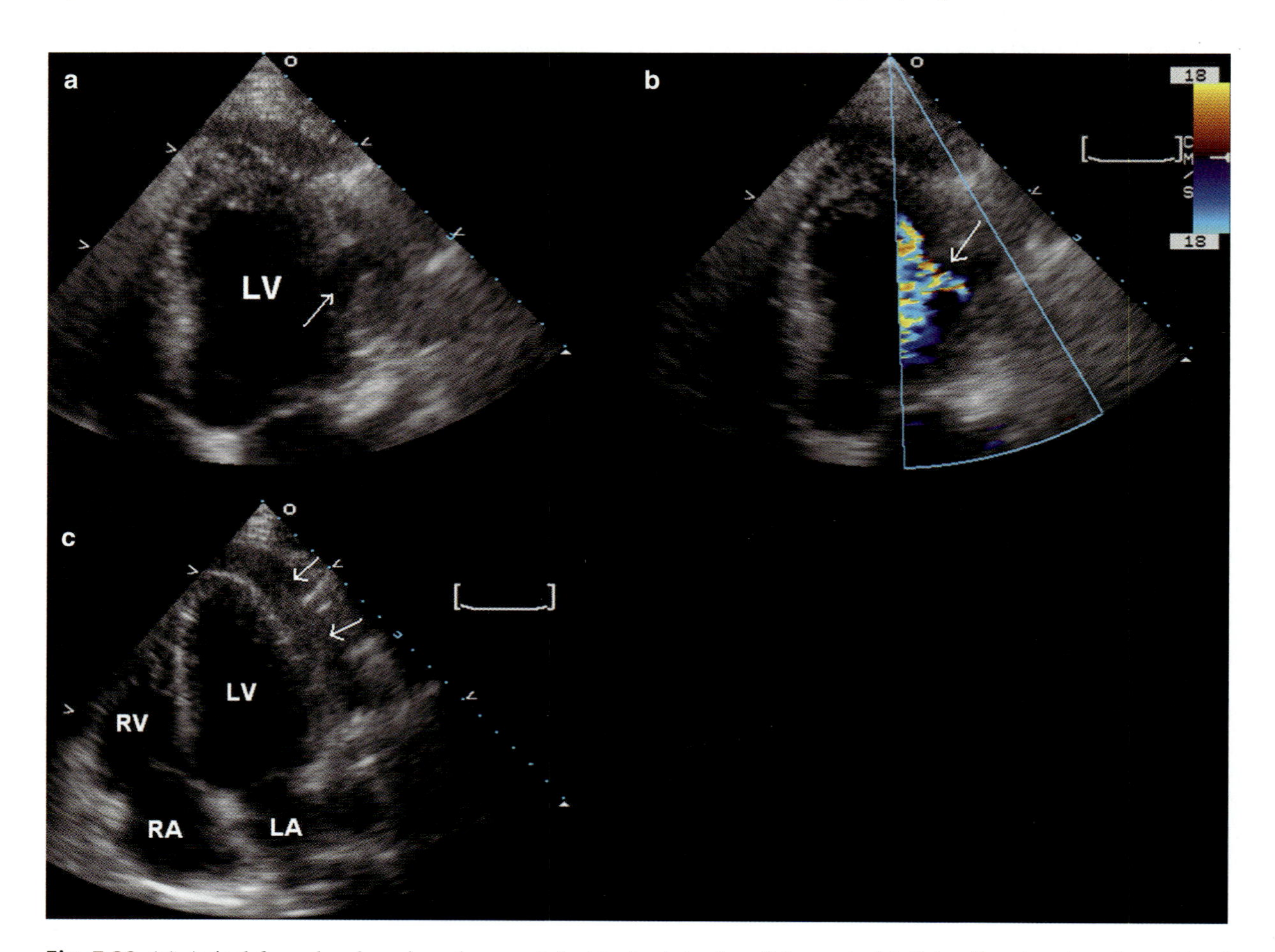

Fig. 7.32 (a) Apical four-chamber view shows a defect in the lateral wall (*arrow*). (b) Color-flow imaging shows blood flow into this defect (*arrow*). (c) A localized pericardial effusion is present (*arrows*). The pericardial effusion appears to be echo-dense consistent with hematoma which is a specific sign for left ventricular free wall rupture. *LA* left atrium, *LV* left ventricle, *RA* right atrium, *RV* right ventricle

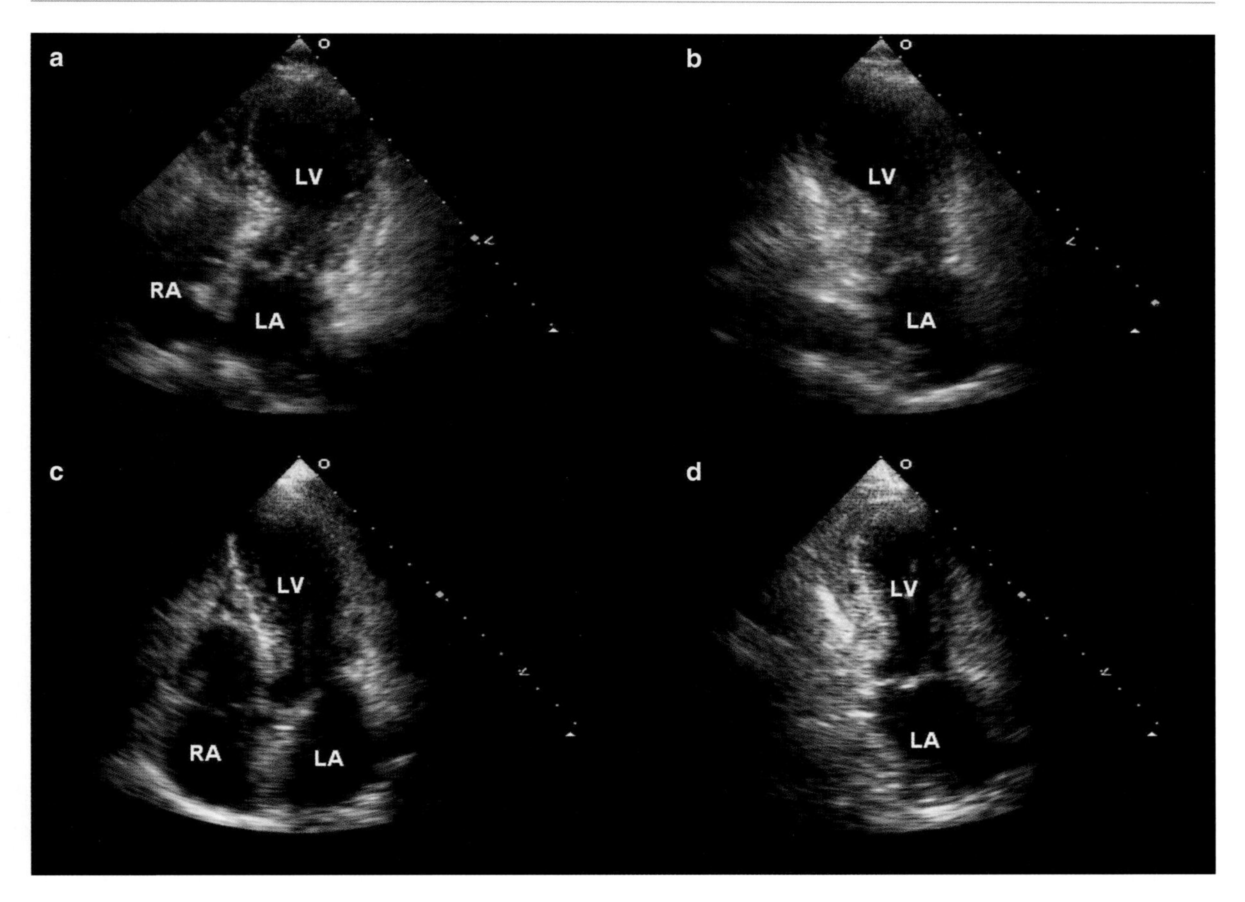

Fig. 7.33 Apical four-chamber (**a**) and two-chamber (**b**) views shows the typical apical ballooning in a 69-year-old woman with Takotsubo cardiomyopathy. There is a marked improvement in left ventricular function in the follow-up study (**c, d**). *LA* left atrium, *LV* left ventricle, *RA* right atrium

modern thrombolytic and anti-platelet agent therapy. Left ventricular thrombus is a common feature in patients with left ventricular aneurysm (Figs. 7.38, 7.42, 7.43). It is generally located at the apex, as most left ventricular aneurysms are apically located. In the apical views near gain artifact is common and may mimic a thrombus within the left ventricular apex. It is important to carefully assess the features of the presumed apical mass in order to differentiate a true thrombus from near gain artifact (Table 7.4).

In the absence of underlying regional wall motion abnormalities (usually akinesia or dyskinesia), presence of left ventricular thrombus is highly unlikely and other etiologies such as tumor are more likely. One rare exception is the hypereosinophilic syndrome in which thrombus in the left or right ventricular apices can occur in the absence of an apical wall motion abnormality (Fig. 7.44).

Intraventricular thrombus has a different acoustic property from the underlying myocardium. New thrombi are echo lucent and may be difficult to distinguish from blood, while old thrombi become more echo dense and may be very echo dense if calcification is present. If apical thrombus is suspected, the imaging depth should be reduced, the focus be set at the near field and the near field gain reduced. Intraventricular thrombus has a defined interface with the blood pool, whereas near gain artifact does not (Fig. 7.45). The short-axis view of the left ventricular apex is particularly useful to image the apex. This can be obtained with the patient close to a supine position and the transducer located more laterally than the usual apical location. In our experience, thrombus should have all the major features listed in the Table 7.4. If the left ventricular mass has some, but not all the major features,

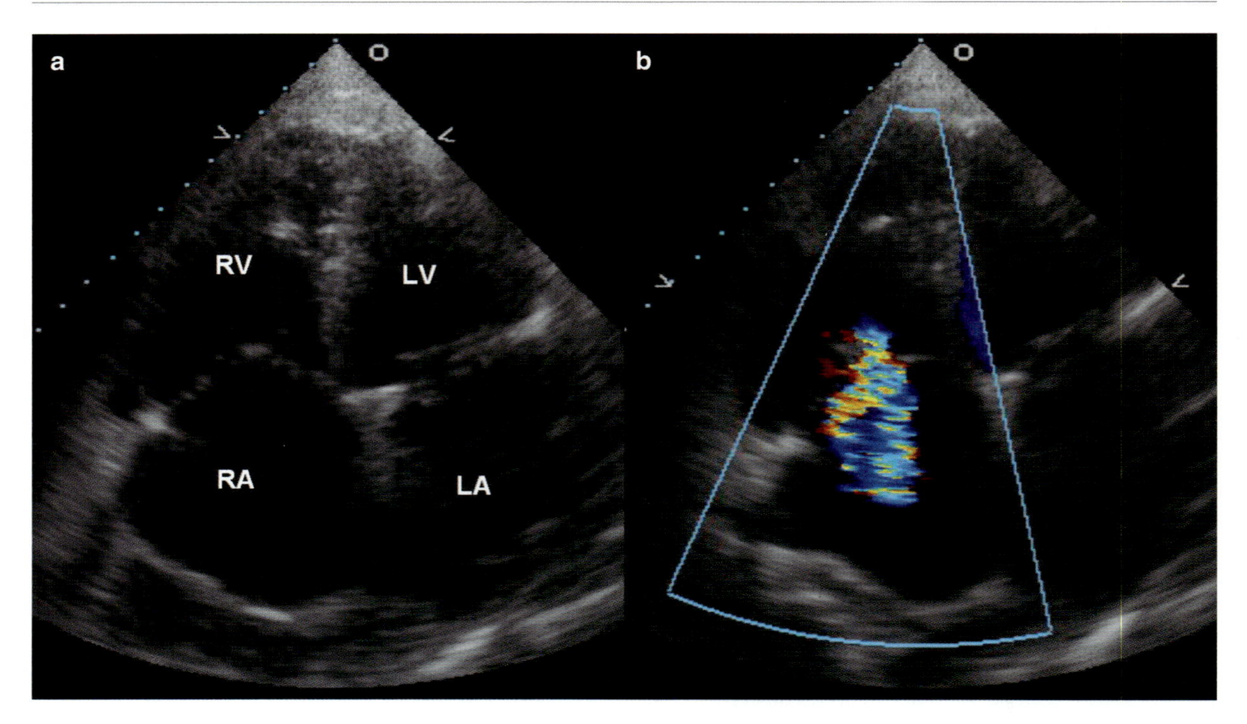

Fig. 7.34 (**a**) Apical four-chamber view in a patient with ischemic heart disease shows dilated and dysfunctional right ventricle. The right atrium is also dilated. The presence of tricuspid regurgitation is confirmed by color-flow imaging (**b**). *LA* left atrium, *LV* left ventricle, *RA* right atrium, *RV* right ventricle

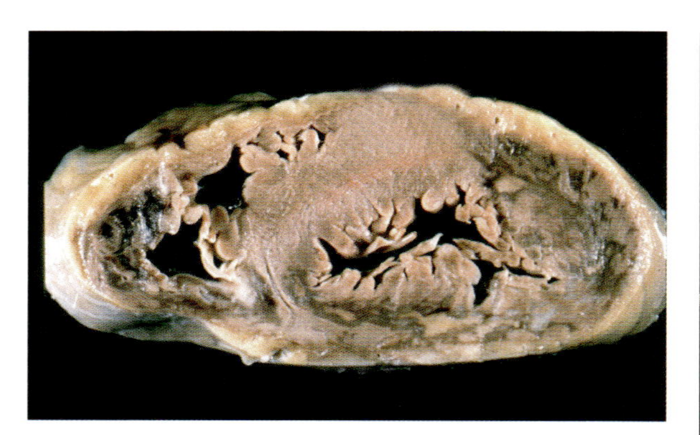

Fig. 7.35 Large healing recent transmural myocardial infarct involving the lateral wall, inferoseptum and inferior wall of the left ventricle. The right ventricle is also infarcted. This commonly occurs with inferior left ventricle infarction

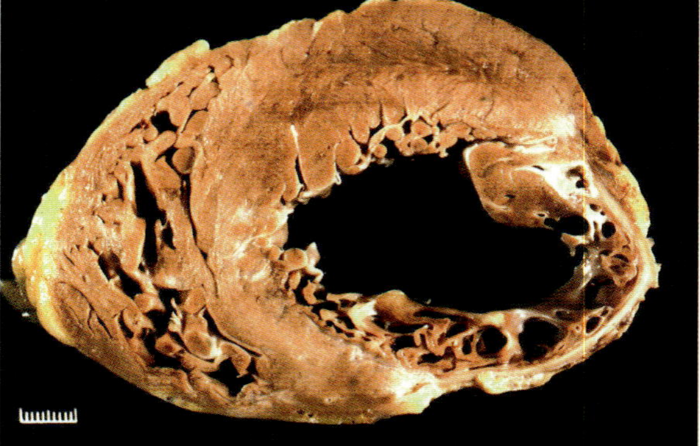

Fig. 7.36 Old inferolateral left ventricle myocardial infract. The infarct has fibrosis and severe wall thinning. The left ventricle is dilated

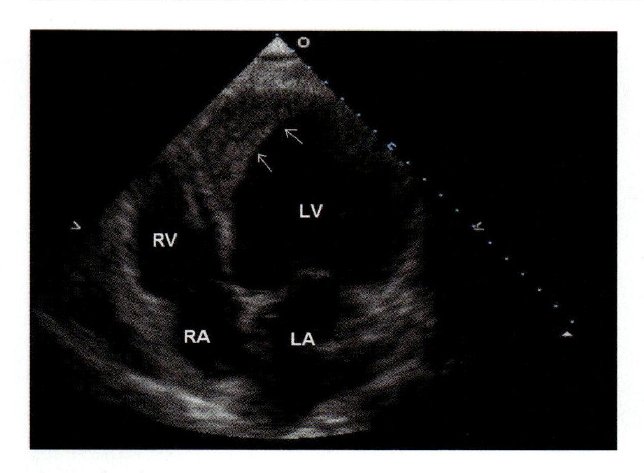

Fig. 7.37 Apical four-chamber view shows a dilated and globular left ventricle. A large laminated thrombus (*arrows*) is present at the apex. *LA* left atrium, *LV* left ventricle, *RA* right atrium, *RV* right ventricle

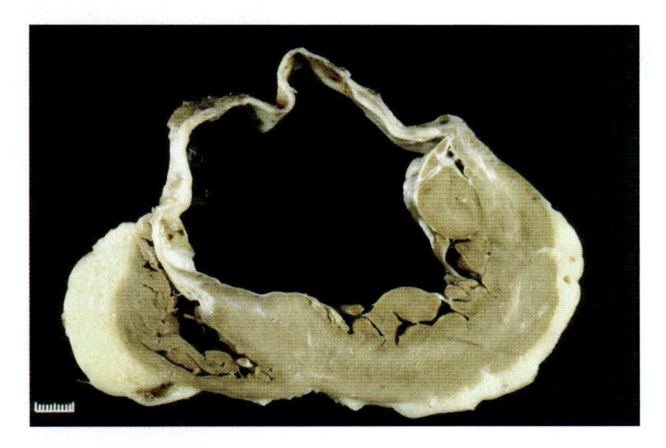

Fig. 7.38 Cross section of heart with a large anterior left ventricle aneurysm. The myocardial wall is thin and fibrotic. In addition it bulges out. There was associated endocardial thrombus more apically. Such aneurysms are now not common probably due to the success of thrombolysis and coronary interventions

our approach is to say that the diagnosis of thrombus is equivocal. The addition of echo contrast has been a welcome addition to our ability to differentiate left ventricular thrombus from artifact (Figs. 7.46, 7.47). It also helps to diagnose other types of apical abnormalities such as apical hypertrophic cardiomyopathy.

Atrial Infarction

Atrial infarction is not usually clinically evident or significant, but it can occur, usually with an adjacent ventricular infarct [49]. Both right and left atria may be affected. Atrial infarction leads to atrial arrhythmias including atria fibrillation, poor atrial contraction, stasis and thrombus, and even to atrial free wall rupture and tamponade [50]. Loss of the atrial component of ventricular filling may lead to heart failure exacerbation.

Viability

Left ventricular dysfunction following myocardial infarction can have multiple causes. It may be due to the presence of myocardial necrosis and fibrosis, but it may be more extensive than the extent of myocardial necrosis. In the setting of a patent infarct related coronary artery, the myocardial dysfunction may be transient and recovers spontaneously with time, which has been termed stunned myocardium [8]. Alternatively, myocardial dysfunction may be related to chronic myocardial ischemia with limited scar in the setting of a stenosed infarct related artery, such that improvement in myocardial function can occur after revascularization. This phenomenon is called hibernation, indicative of the presence of viable myocardium [8]. The presence and extent of viable myocardium can be assessed by positron emission tomography, nuclear imaging and pharmacological echocardiography.

Although both dobutamine and dipyridamole have been used for this indication, low dose dobutamine is more widely used and better validated. The protocol involves the intravenous infusion of dobutamine starting at 5 ug/kg/min and increases in 3–5-min intervals

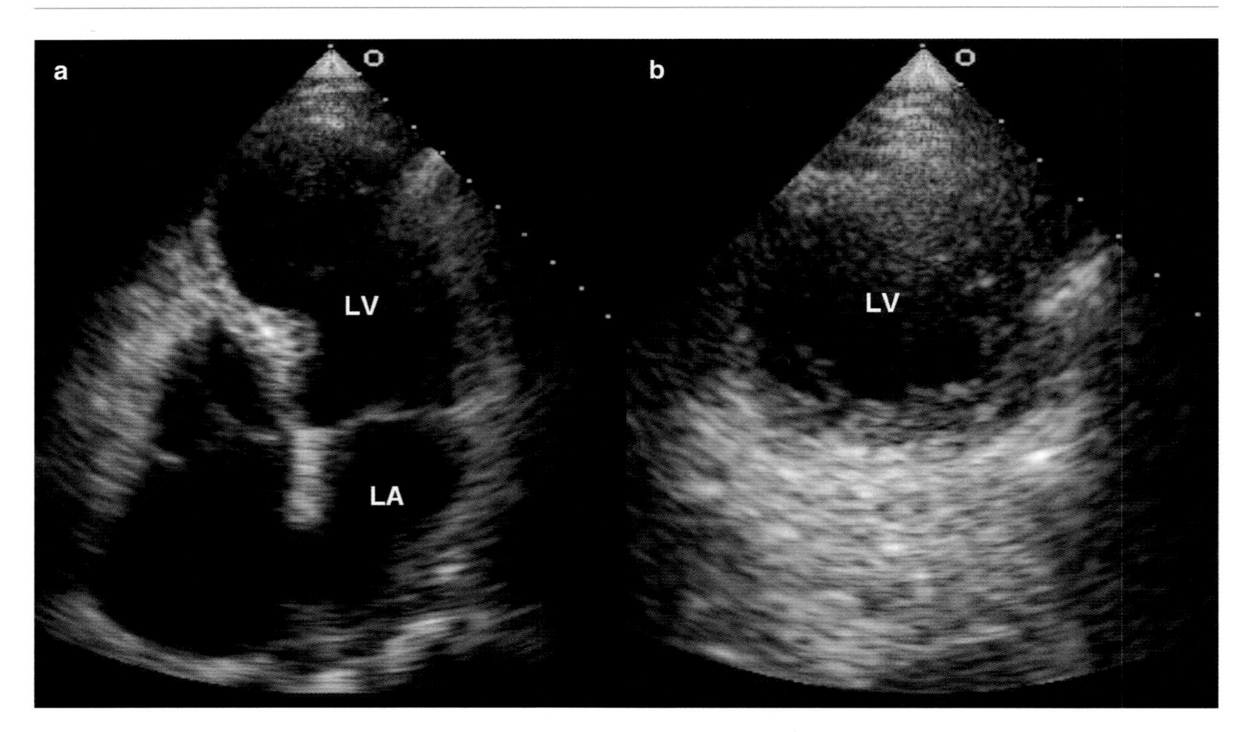

Fig. 7.39 A large apical aneurysm is shown in the apical four-chamber (**a**) and apical short-axis (**b**) views. *LA* left atrium, *LV* left ventricle

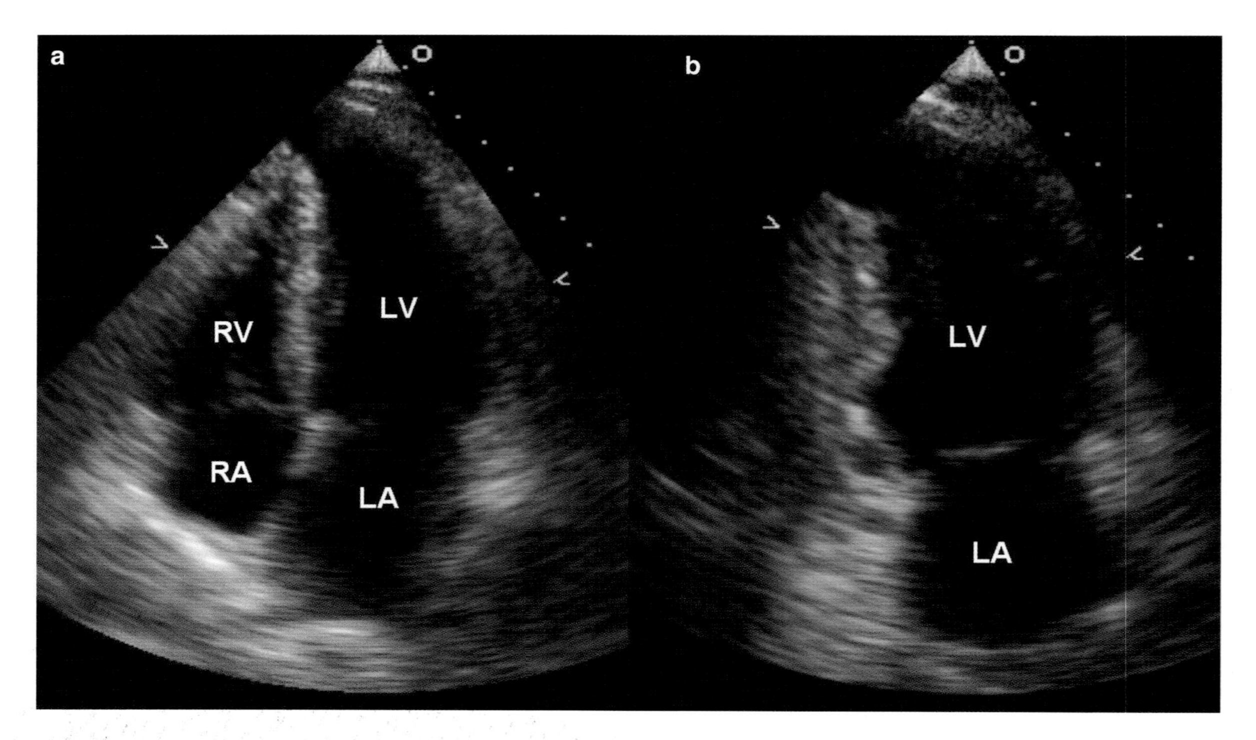

Fig. 7.40 A small apical aneurysm is shown in the apical four-chamber (**a**) and apical two- (**b**) views. A narrow neck in this case raises the possibility of a false aneurysm, although it can be very difficult to distinguish a true aneurysm from a false aneurysm based on echo findings alone. *LA* left atrium, *LV* left ventricle, *RA* right atrium, *RV* right ventricle

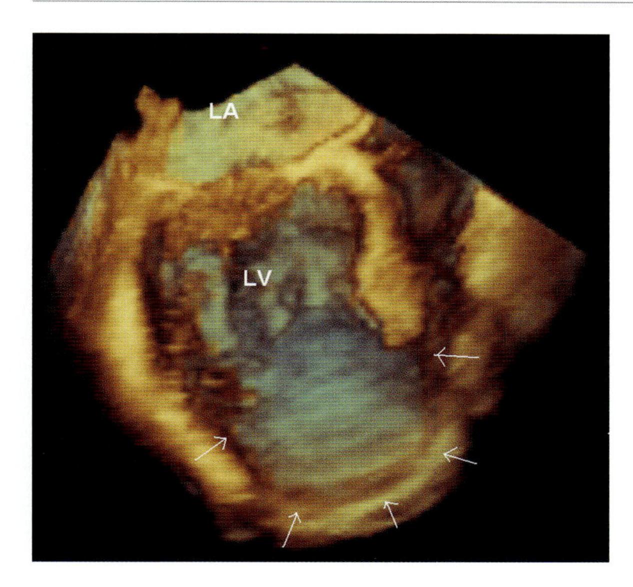

Fig. 7.41 Transthoracic 3D view of a large apical aneurysm (*arrows*). The transition from normal myocardium to the thin scar of the left ventricular aneurysm is well illustrated. *LA* left atrium, *LV* left ventricle

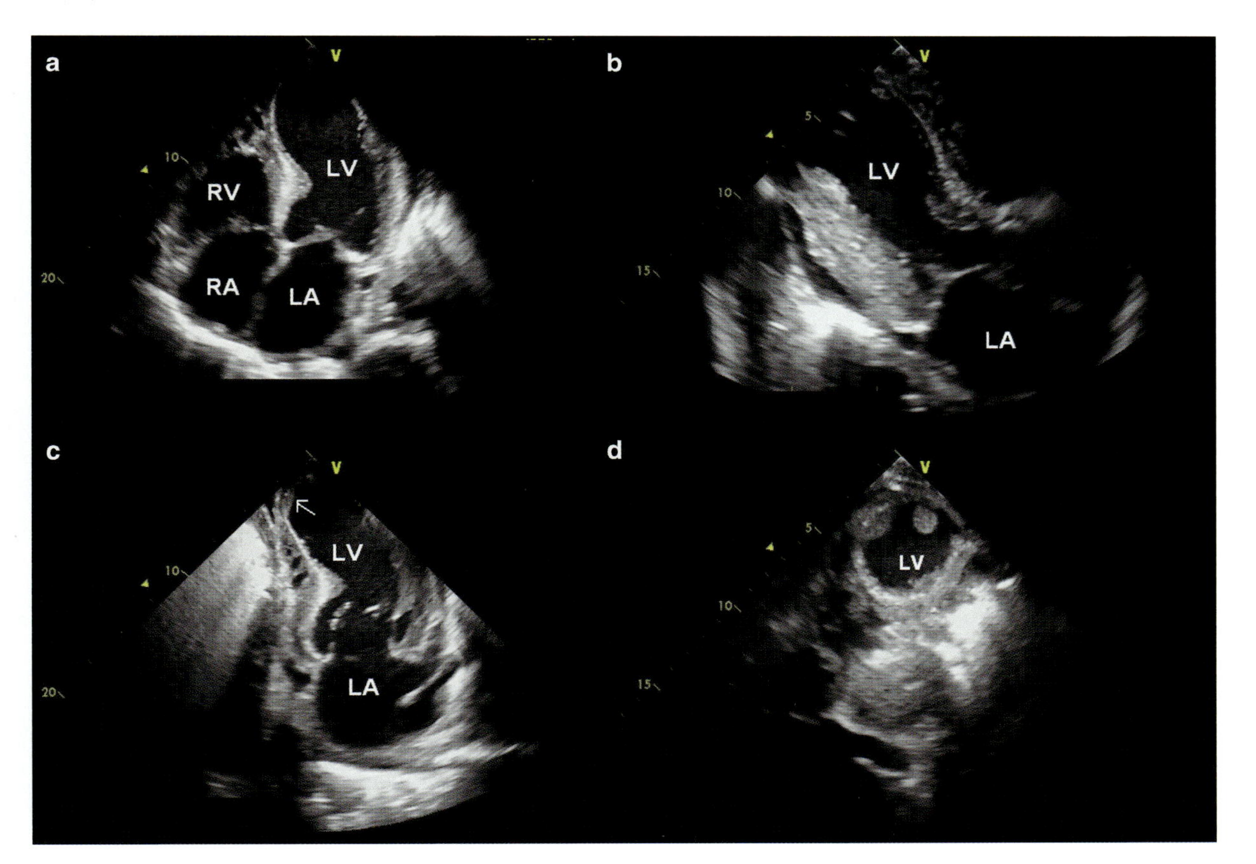

Fig. 7.42 Apical four-chamber (**a**), long-axis (**b**), two-chamber (**c**) and apical short-axis (**d**) views show an apical aneurysm with two small thrombi which are best seen (*arrow*) in the apical two-chamber and apical short-axis views. *LA* left atrium, *LV* left ventricle, *RA* right atrium, *RV* right ventricle

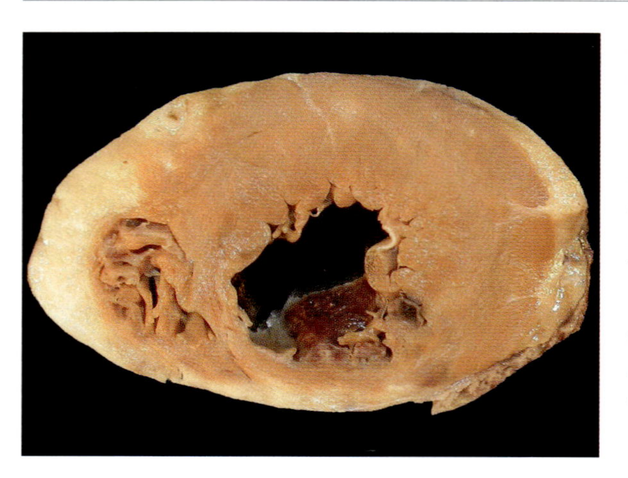

Fig. 7.43 Old inferior wall myocardial infarct with associated endocardial thrombus

Table 7.4 Echocardiographic features of left ventricular thrombus

Major features
Underlying regional wall motion abnormality
Discrete mass-blood interface
Different acoustic appearance from adjacent myocarcium
Minor Features
Apically located
Present in multiple views from multiple windows
Mobile component
Variability with time or treatment

to a peak dose of 20–40 ug/kg/min in order to assess for contractile reserve. Viable myocardium is present if one or more myocardial segments demonstrate biphasic response which is an increase in myocardial contraction at low dose followed by a decreased contraction at high dose of dobutamine infusion as compared to baseline. The biphasic response is more specific for viable myocardium, and the sensitivity and specificity (both about 80%) compare quite favorably with positron emission tomography and nuclear imaging in studies where viability is defined as recovery of contractile function following adequate revascularization [51]. Another useful and simple sign of viability is the wall thickness. If the wall thickness is well preserved (>6 mm), the wall is likely viable. Conversely if the wall is clearly thinned out (<6 mm) and echo-dense, it is highly likely to be non-viable (Fig. 7.48) [52].

Summary

In ischemic heart disease, left ventricular function is a strong predictor of outcome and can be reliably assessed by echocardiography. In patients presenting with chest pain, echocardiography can be used to diagnose the cause of chest pain, and in patients with acute myocardial ischemia echocardiography can assess the location and extent of myocardial ischemia. When shock complicates an acute infarct, a comprehensive approach is important to the management and should include a goal directed echo examination. The long term complications of myocardial infarction including ventricular remodeling, aneurysm and thrombus can be readily assessed by echocardiography. The determination of myocardial viability by dobutamine echocardiography can identify patients with left ventricular dysfunction who would benefit from revascularization.

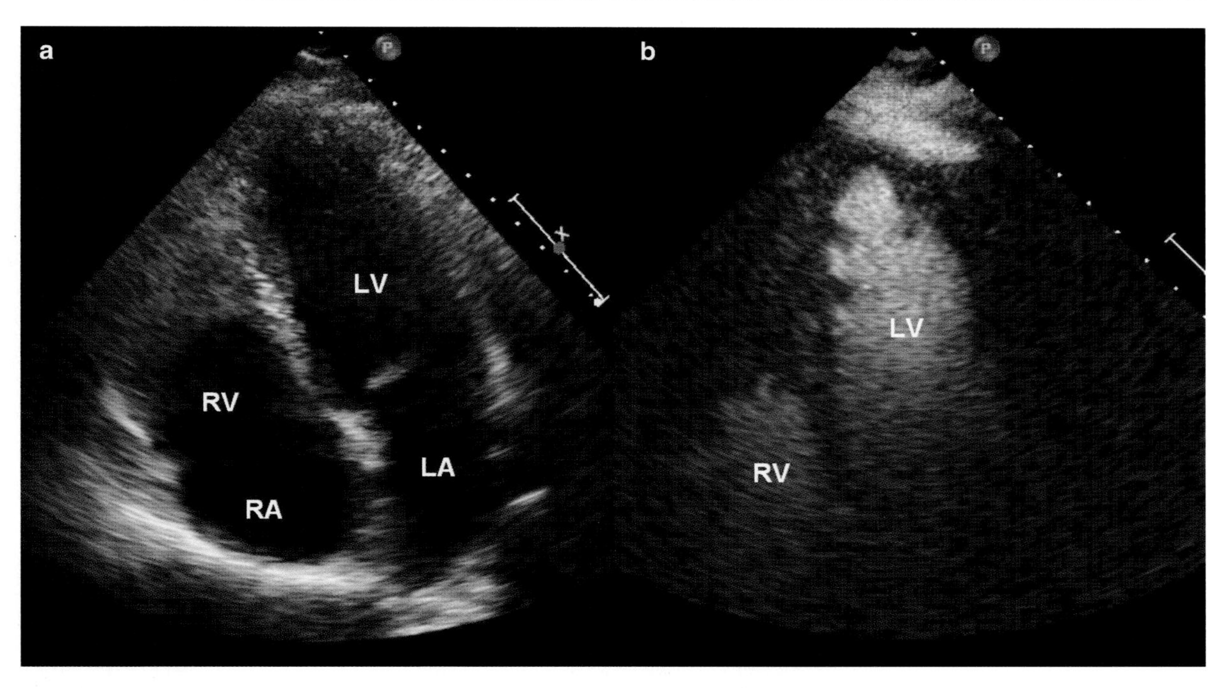

Fig. 7.44 Apical four-chamber view (**a**) in a patient with hyperesosinophilic syndrome shows the presence of thrombus within the right ventricular apex. Eosinophilic thrombus can be present in both ventricular apices, but LV thrombus is not detected by contract injection in this patient (**b**). *LA* left atrium, *LV* left ventricle, *RA* right atrium, *RV* right ventricle

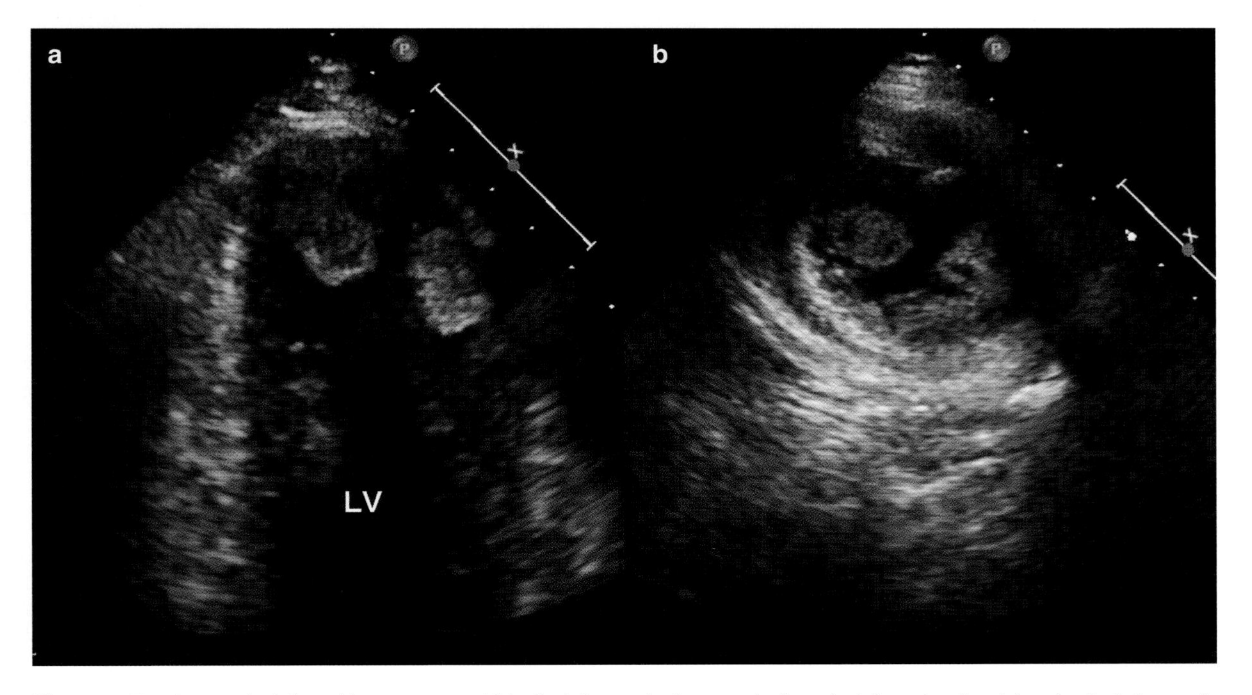

Fig. 7.45 Two large apical thrombi are present within the left ventricular apex in the apical four-chamber (**a**) and apical short-axis (**b**) views. Care needs to be taken to reduce the near gain in order not to obscure the apical thrombi. *LV* left ventricle

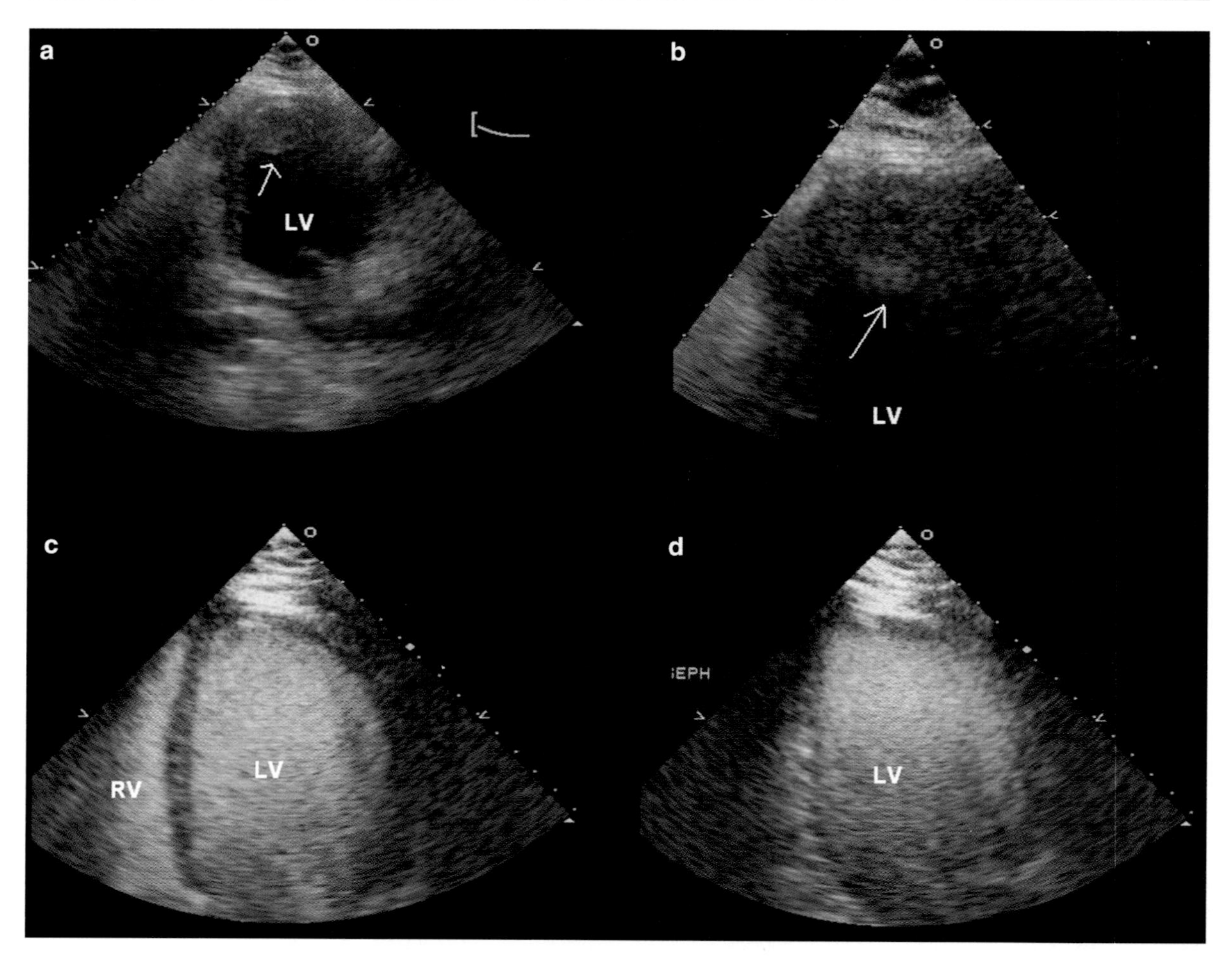

Fig. 7.46 The apical views (**a, b**) in a patient with left ventricular dysfunction show an ill defined mass (*arrow*) in the left ventricular apex suggestive of left ventricular thrombus. Contrast enhancement of the left ventricular cavity (**c, d**) shows no left ventricular thrombus indicating that the apparent left ventricular thrombus is likely near gain artifact. *LV* left ventricle, *RV* right ventricle

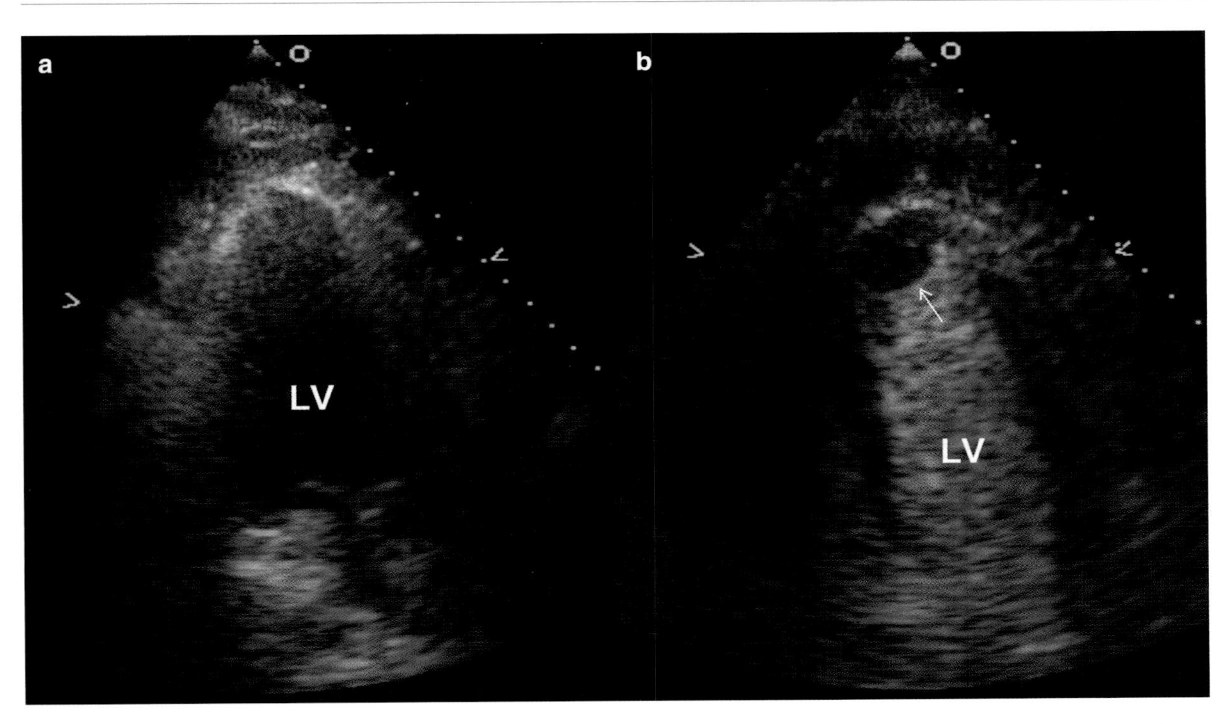

Fig. 7.47 (**a**) Apical two chamber view in a patient with anterior wall myocardial infarction cannot clearly visual the left ventricular apex. (**b**) Following injection of an echo contrast agent, the left ventricular apex is clearly imaged with detection of an apical thrombus (*arrow*). *LV* left ventricle

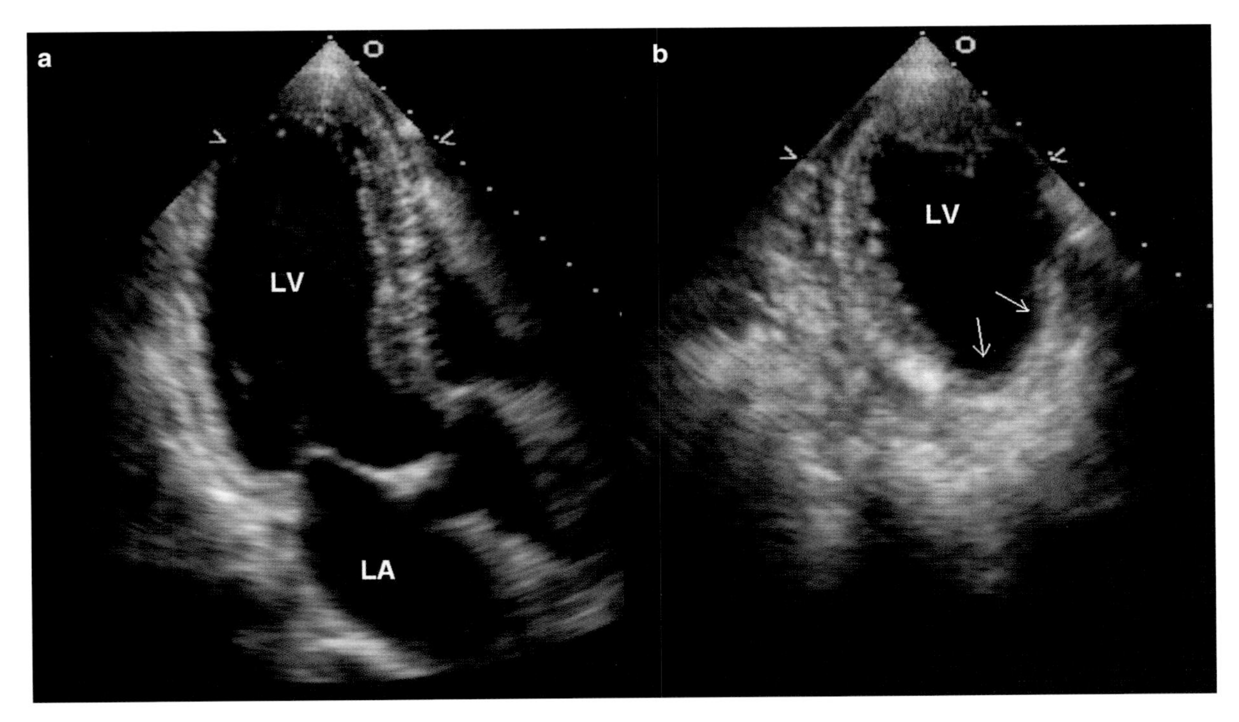

Fig. 7.48 In this patient with a posterolateral wall myocardial infarction, the affected myocardial wall (*arrows*) is severely thinned out in both the apical long-axis (**a**) and apical short-axis (**b**) views, indicating that this wall is not viable. *LA* left atrium, *LV* left ventricle

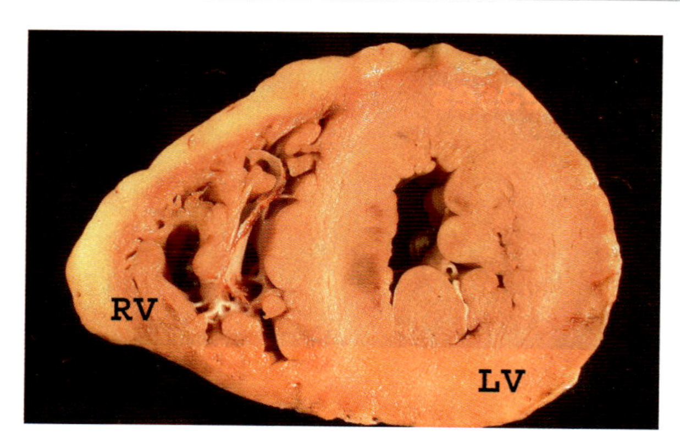

Fig. 8.3 Cross section, short axis cut, of the heart showing a normal "D" shaped right ventricle (*RV*) and a round left ventricle (*LV*)

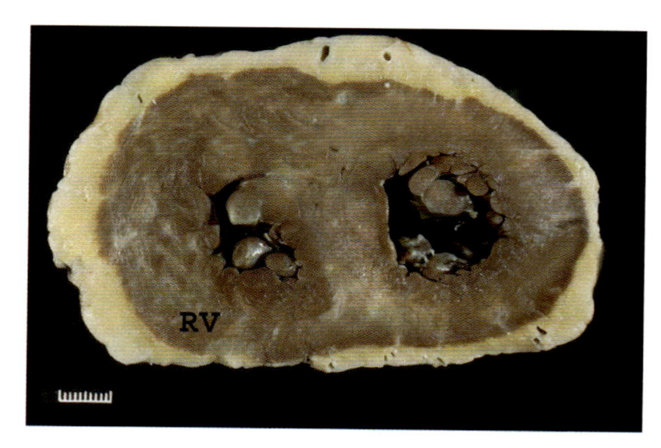

Fig. 8.4 Cross section, short axis cut of the heart with cor pulmonale from pulmonary hypertension. The interventricular septum is flat and the ventricles are almost of the same thickness due to right ventricle (*RV*) hypertrophy

[2–4]. The thin-walled RV is quite resilient, particularly in relation to volume overload. Under normal circumstances, the RV ejects into the low resistance highly compliant pulmonary circulation, and the forward flow is mainly driven by contraction of the free wall toward the septum [5]. During acute volume overload, there is dilatation of RV volume with preservation of the ejection fraction and an increase in RV stroke volume. This increase in stroke volume occurs as a result of an increase in radial function with no change in longitudinal contractility [6]. This is consistent with the clinical observation that RV systolic function remains normal in patients with long-standing volume overload due to an atrial septal defect [2]. On the other hand, the RV is much more sensitive to afterload changes than the LV, such that RV stroke volume can decrease with a modest increase in pulmonary vascular resistance [7, 8]. Thus,

Table 8.1 Causes of right ventricular failure

Intrinsic myocardial disease
• RV ischemia or infarction • Cardiomyopathies – ARVC, dilated, hypertrophic, infiltrative • RV dysplasia
Pressure overload • LV failure • Mitral valve disease • Pulmonary veno-occlusive disease • Pulmonary artery hypertension • Pulmonary hypertension due to pulmonary diseases • Pulmonary stenosis • Pulmonary arterial stenosis
Volume overload • Atrial septal defect • Anomalous pulmonary venous return • Pulmonary regurgitation • Tricuspid regurgitation
Limitation to RV filling • Tricuspid stenosis • Tamponade • Pericardial constriction

ARVC arrhythmogenic right ventricular cardiomyopathy, *LV* left ventricle, *RV* right ventricle
Source: Modified from Walker and Buttrick [9]

even modest acute increase in pulmonary vascular resistance due to pulmonary embolism can lead to a drop in RV stroke volume, and chronic RV pressure overload is likely to result in RV dilatation and failure.

There are many conditions that can affect the RV. Table 8.1 lists the major categories of pathophysiologic conditions resulting in RV failure [9]. More than one of these conditions may be present in the same patient. The most common cause is LV failure leading to increased back pressure and elevated pulmonary pressures. RV systolic function is less affected in patients with ischemic heart disease and LV failure than in those with dilated cardiomyopathy and similar LV ejection fraction, suggesting that the latter is a more diffuse process with a high likelihood of biventricular involvement [10]. In patients with heart failure, RV function and pulmonary artery pressure may be better predictors of outcome than LV ejection fraction, underscoring the importance of assessing RV function and pulmonary pressure in these patients [11]. Indeed, any diseases that can result in increased RV afterload can cause RV failure, including pulmonary embolism and chronic obstructive pulmonary disease. Although RV can tolerate volume overload, chronic and excessive volume load can lead to RV failure when the septal shift and pericardial constraint lead to reduction in LV stroke volume and compliance, which then results in increased RV afterload [12]. In addition, longstanding hyperdynamic circulation of the pulmonary vasculature may lead to fixed pulmonary hypertension further increasing the RV afterload [2].

Isolated RV infarction is rare, but some degree of RV involvement is common in the setting of inferior myocardial infarction (Fig. 8.5). In most forms of cardiomyopathies, the RV is frequently involved, although the clinical manifestations are frequently dominated by LV involvement. For instance, a large proportion of patients with hypertrophic cardiomyopathy have RV hypertrophy [13]. Arrhythmogenic right ventricular cardiomyopathy is the best known condition of cardiomyopathy with the dominant findings in the RV (Fig. 8.6). Recent modifications of the diagnostic criteria may allow a more consistent diagnosis of this condition [14]. Other forms of congenital RV dysplasia can cause RV failure and the best example is Ebstein's anomaly which is discussed in Chap. 5.

Echocardiographic Assessment of Right Ventricle

The complex RV anatomy dictates that multiple views should be performed to provide a comprehensive assessment of RV size and function [15–17]. In particular, views of the RV inflow and outflow tracts should be individually assessed since it is difficult to assess both in the same echo view. Reliance on any single linear measurement should be avoided as linear measurements are simplistic and misleading in the face of the complex RV geometry. Variability of these measurements can occur as a result of different patient positions and transducer locations. The RV area and

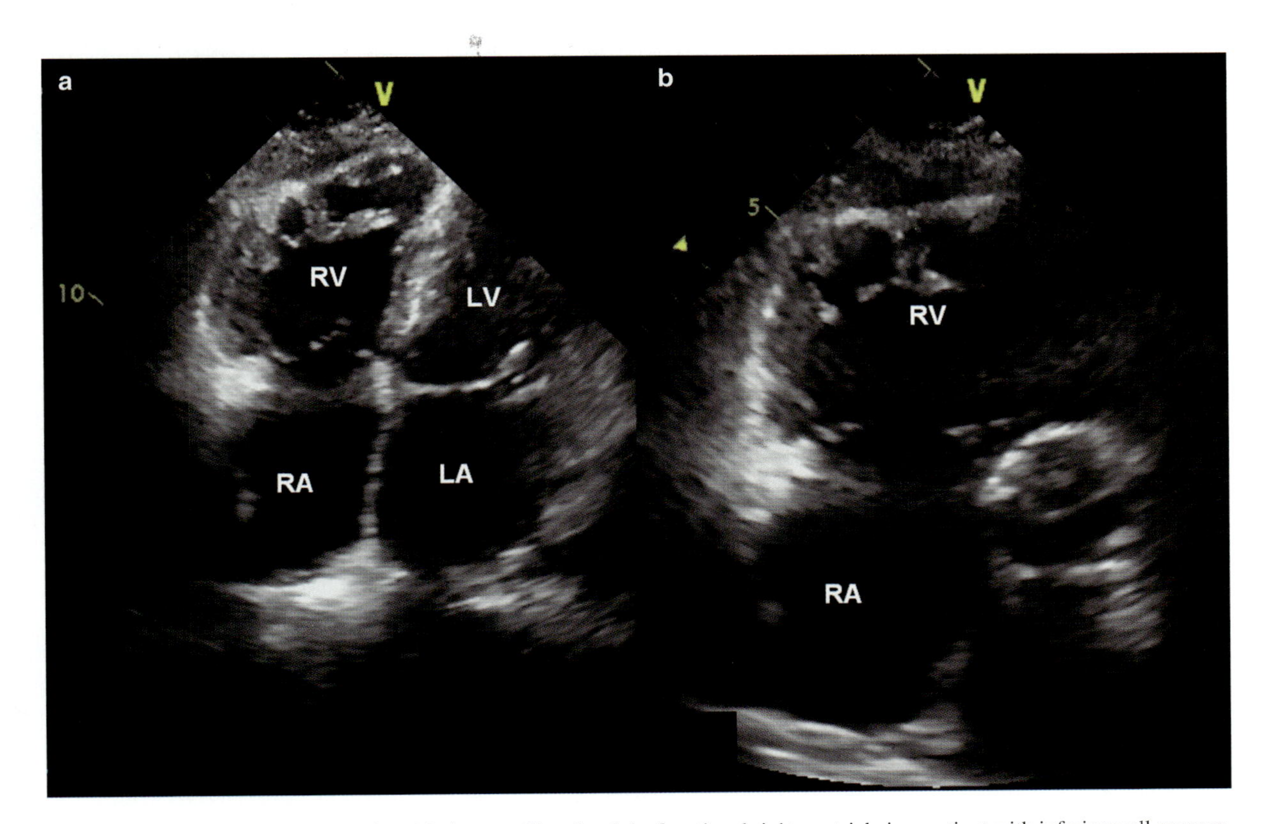

Fig. 8.5 The apical four-chamber view (**a**) shows a dilated and dysfunctional right ventricle in a patient with inferior wall myocardial infarction. The zoomed view of the right ventricular free wall (**b**) shows that the apical half of the right ventricular free wall is thinned with no thickening consistent with right ventricular infarction. *LA* left atrium, *LV* left ventricle, *RA* right atrium, *RV* right ventricle

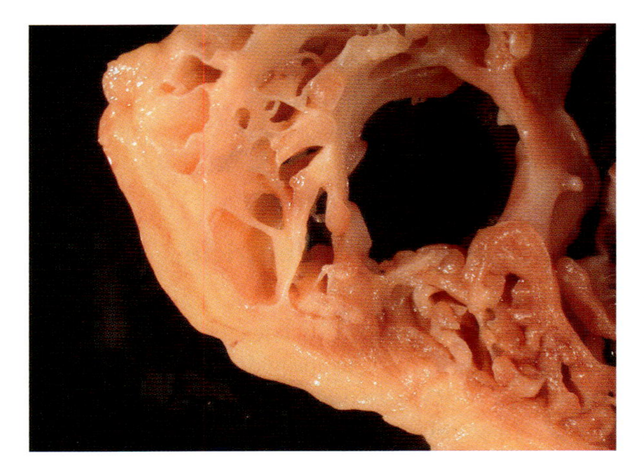

Fig. 8.6 Right ventricle wall cross section from an individual with arrhythmogenic cardiomyopathy. The right ventricle wall is replaced by fat and the right ventricle is thin and dilated

volume measurements are also fraught with uncertainties due to the lack of anatomic landmarks to ensure optimal display of the RV and the difficulty in tracing the heavily trabeculated RV endocardial surface.

The parasternal short-axis views with the transducer angled rightward to image the RV can avoid the pitfall of foreshortening the RV. Multiple short-axis views, from the base to the apex of the RV can be obtained, to assess RV global and regional function (Fig. 8.7). They can also be used to measure RV volume, although off-line analysis and spatial orientation are required and the process is time-consuming. The advent of real-time 3D echo is a promising means to assess RV volume, as 3D echo is ideally suited to assess the anatomic complexity of the RV [18–21]. However, the image quality of real-time 3D is still limited so that endocardial

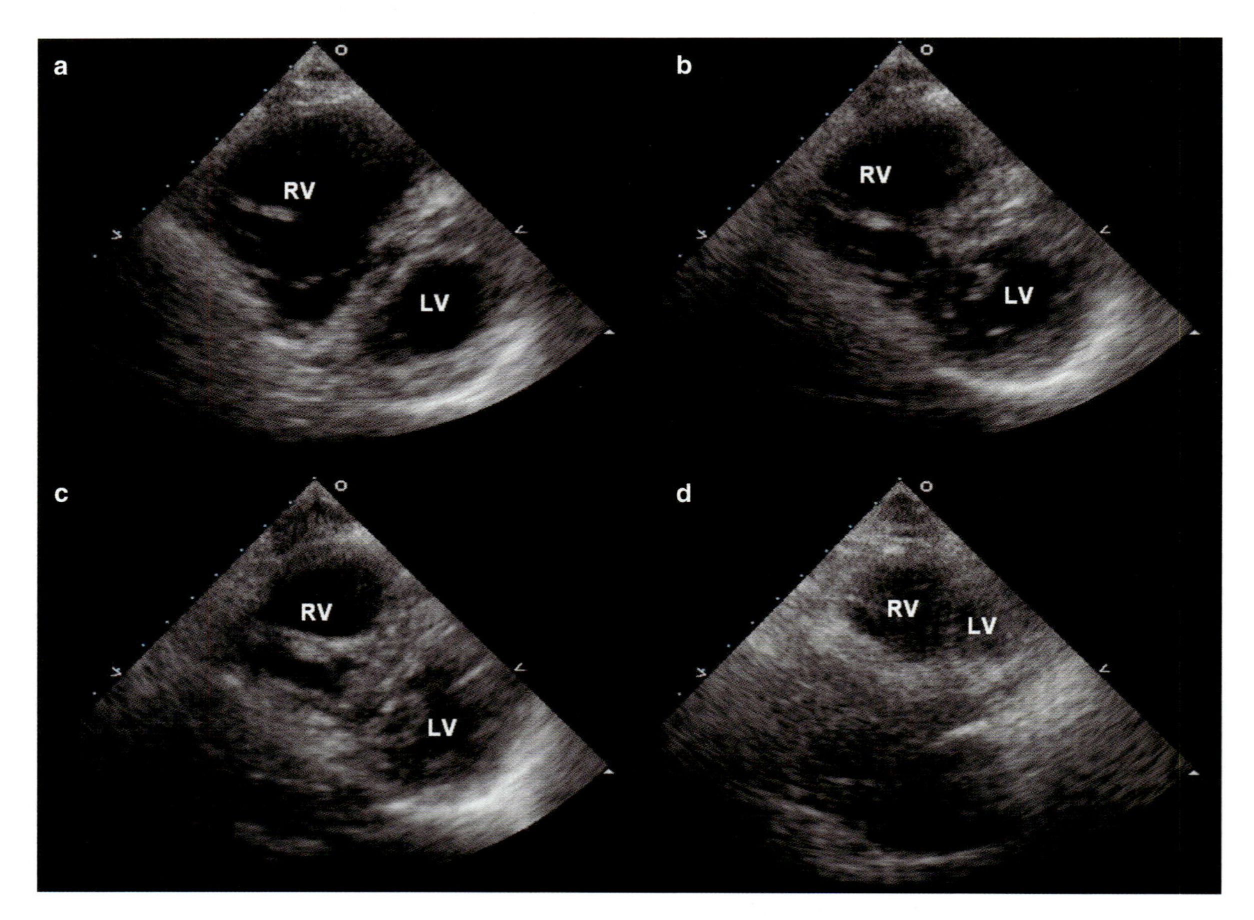

Fig. 8.7 In a patient with dilated and dysfunctional right ventricle, multiple short-axis views from base to apex (**a–d**) can be obtained from the parasternal window with the transducer tilted rightward. It is possible to obtain right ventricular volume by off-line analysis using this multiple slice approach. *LV* left ventricle, *RV* right ventricle

delineation continues to pose a challenge, such that RV volumes by 3D echo are consistently underestimated when compared to similar volumes obtained by cardiac magnetic resonance imaging (CMR) [18–21].

Thus it is not surprising that visual estimation remains the most widely used method in assessing RV size and function. The most popular echo view for this purpose is the apical four-chamber view. The RV size is assessed in relation to the LV size. In general, the RV is about two thirds the size of the LV in this view [22]. If the RV approaches the size of the LV, the RV is considered to be mildly enlarged; when it is equal in size compared to the LV, it is considered moderately enlarged; and when it exceeds the size of the LV, it is severely dilated (Fig. 8.8). It is important to avoid imaging the RV obliquely as it may overestimate RV volume in relation to the left ventricle. If the LV is dilated, allowance should be given in assessing the RV size in comparison with the LV size in this view.

In Table 8.2, we list the echo views of the RV and the useful measurements from these views [16]. The normal values of these measurements are presented in Table 8.3 [15, 16]. Our own view is that the quantitative approach to assess RV with any of these measurements requires caution. Assessment of RV size and function should take into consideration multiple echo findings and different measurements. Further refinement in real-time 3D resolution and on-line volume analysis software is required before we can routinely use RV volumes and ejection fraction in clinical practice.

Right Ventricular Areas and Fractional Area Change

The right ventricle is a thin-walled structure and systolic thickening of the right ventricular wall is difficult

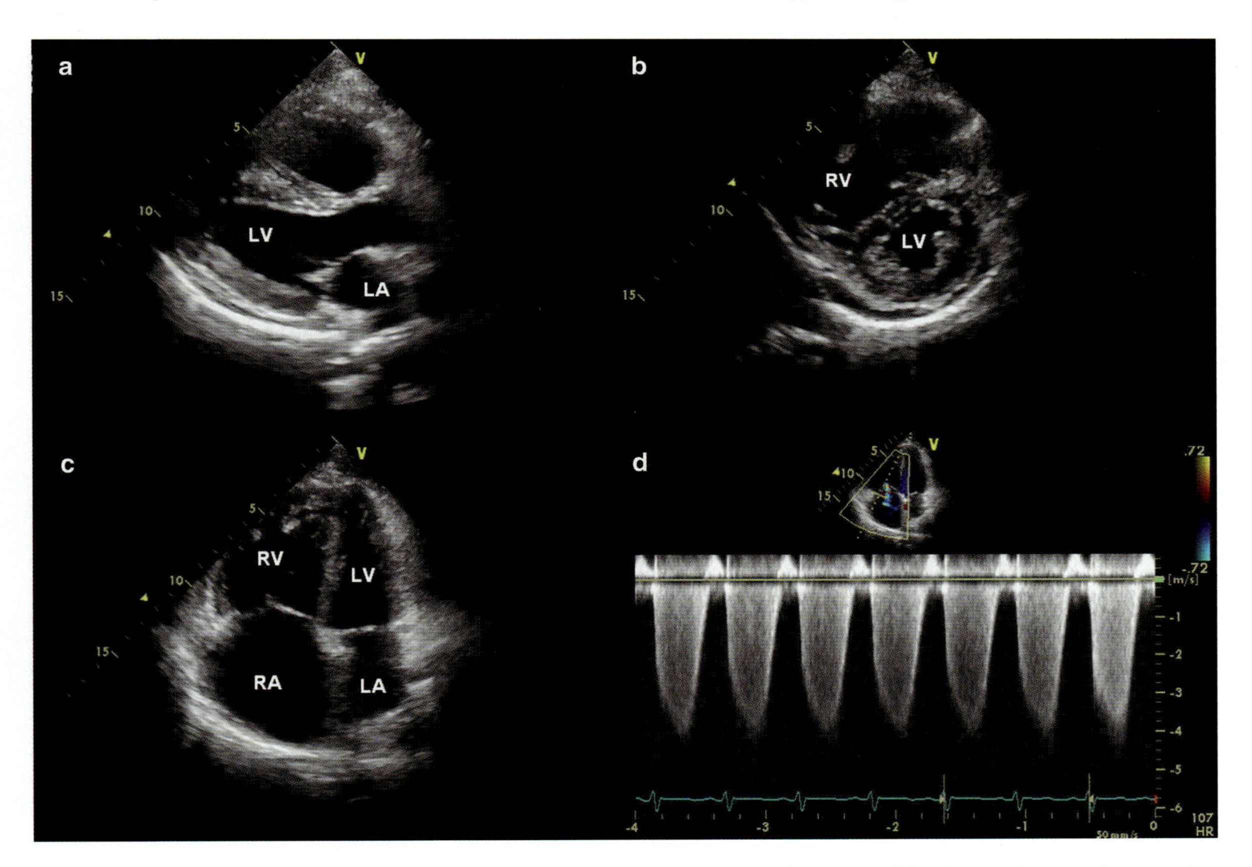

Fig. 8.8 Parasternal long-axis (**a**), short-axis (**b**) and apical four-chamber views in this patient with primary pulmonary hypertension show a severely dilated right ventricle best appreciated in the apical four-chamber view (**c**) with the right ventricle much larger than the left ventricle. Continuous wave Doppler (**d**) confirms severe elevation in right ventricular systolic pressure. *LA* left atrium, *LV* left ventricle, *RA* right atrium, *RV* right ventricle

Table 8.2 Echocardiographic assessment of the right ventricle

Imaging views
Specific measurements Parasternal long-axis • End-diastolic RVOT diameter
RV inflow view • Anatomy and function of tricuspid valve
RV outflow view • Anatomy and function of pulmonary valve
Parasternal RV short-axis views • End-diastolic and end-systolic diameters of RVOT • RVOT shortening fraction • RV size and function • RV volume by off-line reconstruction
Parasternal LV short-axis views • LV eccentricity index
Apical four-chamber view • RV size and function • RV long- and short-axis diameters • RV fractional area change • RV annular TDI • RV strain and strain rate • RV myocardial performance index • Anatomy and function of tricuspid valve • 3D RV volume and ejection fraction
Subcostal view • RVOT size and obstruction • RV free wall thickness

Source: Modified from Jurcut et al. [16]
LV left ventricle, *RV* right ventricle, *RVOT* right ventricular outflow tract, *TDI* tissue Doppler imaging

to assess. Right ventricular wall motion is largely determined by the excursion of the right ventricular free walls in the form of fractional area change (FAC). The apical four-chamber view is used to planimeter the RV area in diastole and systole. The RV FAC is the change of RV area from diastole to systole divided by the RV area in diastole, and is a measure of RV systolic function (Figs. 8.9, 8.10) [15, 16]. These measurements are limited by the technical issues including foreshortening of the RV and endocardial delineation. The RV outflow tract is not included in these measurements which are affected by both preload and afterload. Although RV area correlates with RV volume, significant overlap of RV area between normal and volume overloaded RV has been reported [23]. There is acceptable correlation between RV FAC and RV ejection fraction by CMR [24].

Right Ventricular Volumes and Ejection Fraction

The RV volumes can be obtained by 2D echo which either assumes a geometric shape which is problematic for the RV or requires time-consuming offline analysis. There is enthusiasm with the use of real-time 3D echo to measure RV volumes and ejection fraction [18–21]. Currently, this is still time-consuming as it requires offline analysis with a dedicated software package (Fig. 8.11). Excellent correlations with similar measurements by CMR have been reported. For instance, in 100 adult patients, Leibundgut et al. reported mean differences of 10.2 ± 21.2 mL in RV end-diastolic volume and $0.4 \pm 7.5\%$ in RV ejection fraction between 3D echo and CMR [19]. Compared to CMR, there is an overall underestimation of RV volume by 3D echo, which may be related to difficulty with endocardial tracing as the image quality is still not consistently optimal [18–21].

Eccentricity Index

Eccentricity index is a simple measure of LV morphology that can be used to differentiate RV volume overload from RV pressure overload [25]. It is the ratio of LV antero-posterior to septo-lateral diameters in the parasternal short-axis view. The value is 1 in both systole and diastole in normal people. In RV volume overload, there is flattening of the septum in diastole and recovery in systole, resulting in an eccentricity index > 1 in diastole (Fig. 8.12). In RV pressure overload, the septal flattening persists and may even worsen during systole, such that the eccentricity index is > 1 in diastole and systole (Fig. 8.13). A diastolic eccentricity index > 1 is a predictor of mortality in patients with pulmonary hypertension [26]. The degree of septal curvature in relation to the LV free wall reflects transeptal pressure and provides a qualitative assessment of the RV systolic pressure [27].

Tricuspid Annular Plane Systolic Excursion

Tricuspid annular plane systolic excursion (TAPSE) can be readily obtained by M-mode tracing of the lateral tricuspid annulus in the apical four-chamber view.

Table 8.3 Normal values and significance of right ventricular morphology and function

RV variable	Normal value (mean ± SD)	Significance
RVOT	22 ± 1.5	Diagnosis of AVRC
PLAX dimension (mm) PSAX dimension (mm)	27 ± 1	Diagnosis of ARVC
RVOT FS (%)	61 ± 13	Evaluation of RV failure
LV eccentricity index	1	RV volume overload versus pressure overload
RV wall thickness (mm)	3–5	RVH, good correlation with pulmonary artery pressure
RV end diastolic area (cm^2)	18 ± 5	Diagnosis of RV dilatation
RV FAC (%)	56 ± 13	RV systolic function
TAPSE (mm)	>15	Good correlation with RV systolic function
RV myocardial performance index	0.28 ± 0.04	Global assessment of RV systolic and diastolic function
RV TDI basal systolic (S) velocity (cm/s)	>12	RV systolic function
Strain (%) Basal Mid Apical	19 ± 6 27 ± 6 32 ± 6	Regional function and correlates with systolic function
RV 3D volume EDV (mL/m^2) ESV (mL/m^2) SV (mL/m^2) EF (%)	42–98 13–54 18–46 33–63	RV size and systolic function

ARVC arrhythmogenic right ventricular cardiomyopathy, *EF* ejection fraction, *EDV* end diastolic volume, *ESV* end systolic volume, *FAC* fractional area change, *FS* fractional shortening, *LV* left ventricle, *RV* right ventricle, *RVH* right ventricular hypertrophy, *RVOT* right ventricular outflow tract, *TAPSE* tricuspid annular peak systolic excursion, *TDI* tissue Doppler imaging
Source: Modified from Jurcut et al. [16] and Horten et al. [15]

Longitudinal displacement of the base of the RV during systole accounts for a greater proportion of RV volume changes than radial excursion. TAPSE has been shown to correlate with RV ejection fraction, and is a predictor of adverse events in patients with pulmonary hypertension or myocardial infarction (Figs. 8.14, 8.15) [28, 29]. Since it measures the motion of the tricuspid annulus in relation to the chest wall, TAPSE is load dependent and measures the overall cardiac motion and not just the excursion of the base of the RV. Furthermore, LV function can also affect TAPSE, due to ventricular independence [30].

Myocardial Performance Index

Myocardial performance index (MPI) is a global measure of systolic and diastolic function. It is the ratio of the sum of RV isovolumic relaxation time and isovolumic contraction time divided by the RV ejection time (Fig. 8.16) [31]. In RV failure, there is prolongation of the isovolumic times and shortened ejection time, so that MPI will be prolonged. The advantages of MPI are that it does not assume RV geometry and is relatively load independent. MPI has been shown to have prognostic value in patients with pulmonary hypertension [32]. Pseudonormalization of the MPI has been reported in patients with elevated RA pressure which leads to a shortening of isovolumic relaxation time [33]. Care needs to be taken to ensure that identical cycle lengths are used to obtain this measurement.

Tissue Doppler Imaging

Tissue Doppler imaging provides a quick and easy means to assess the tricuspid annular velocities. RV annular systolic (S) velocity has been shown to correlate with RV systolic function (Figs. 8.14, 8.15) [34, 35]. It is worth remembering that annular velocities by pulsed

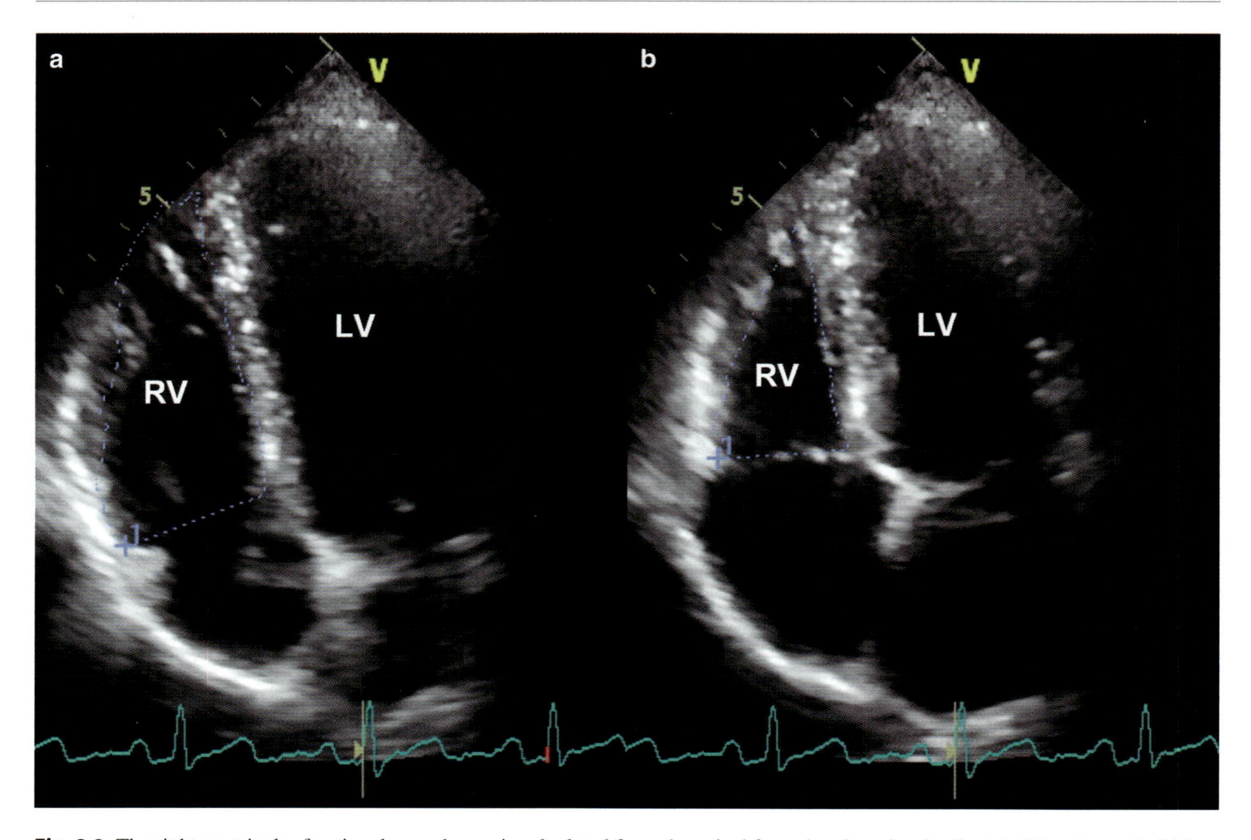

Fig. 8.9 The right ventricular fractional area change is calculated from the apical four-chamber view in diastole (**a**) and systole (**b**) in a patient with normal right ventricular function. The fractional area change is 55% which is normal. *LV* left ventricle, *RV* right ventricle

wave tissue Doppler are not the same as those measured by color tissue Doppler, as the former measures the peak myocardial velocities and the latter measures the mean myocardial velocities which are about 20% lower [36].

Strain and Strain Rate

Longitudinal RV myocardial deformation can be measured by tissue Doppler imaging or speckle tracking. Myocardial strain is the percentage of myocardial shortening during systole and a measure of myocardial systolic function. Strain can provide assessment of RV global and regional function (Fig. 8.17). Both strain and strain rate have been shown to be reduced in pulmonary hypertension, and may be useful in detecting early RV dysfunction in this clinical setting [37, 38]. They may also be a more reliable marker in the detection of arrhythmogenic right ventricular cardiomyopathy [39]. Reliable strain and strain rate measurements are dependent on good image quality. Other limitations include low temporal resolution, angle dependency, and measurement variability.

Right Ventricular Failure and Pulmonary Hypertension

There are diverse causes of RV failure (Table 8.1) [9]. Intrinsic RV myocardial diseases are rare. Arrhythmogenic right ventricular cardiomyopathy can be hereditary and is an important cause of sudden death in the young (Fig. 8.6). It is discussed in detail in Chap. 6. By far RV dysfunction is much more likely to be a secondary event in response to, or as a result of, another disease. In patients with coronary artery disease, particularly those with inferior wall infarction, RV dysfunction can be a result of RV wall infarct or passive pulmonary hypertension due to LV dysfunction. It is important to recognize that the development of RV dysfunction worsens the

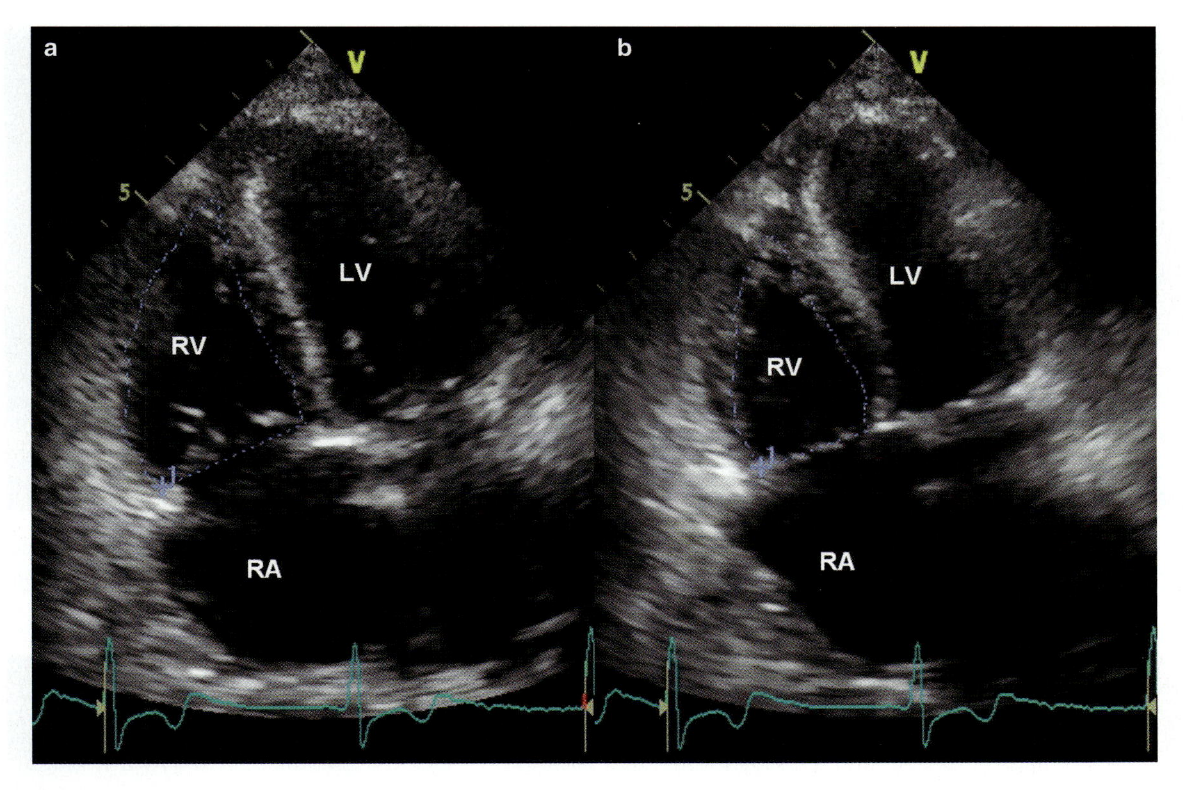

Fig. 8.10 The right ventricular fractional area change is calculated from the diastolic (**a**) and systolic (**b**) apical views a patient with right ventricular dysfunction showing an abnormal fractional area change of 33%. *LV* left ventricle, *RA* right atrium, *RV* right ventricle

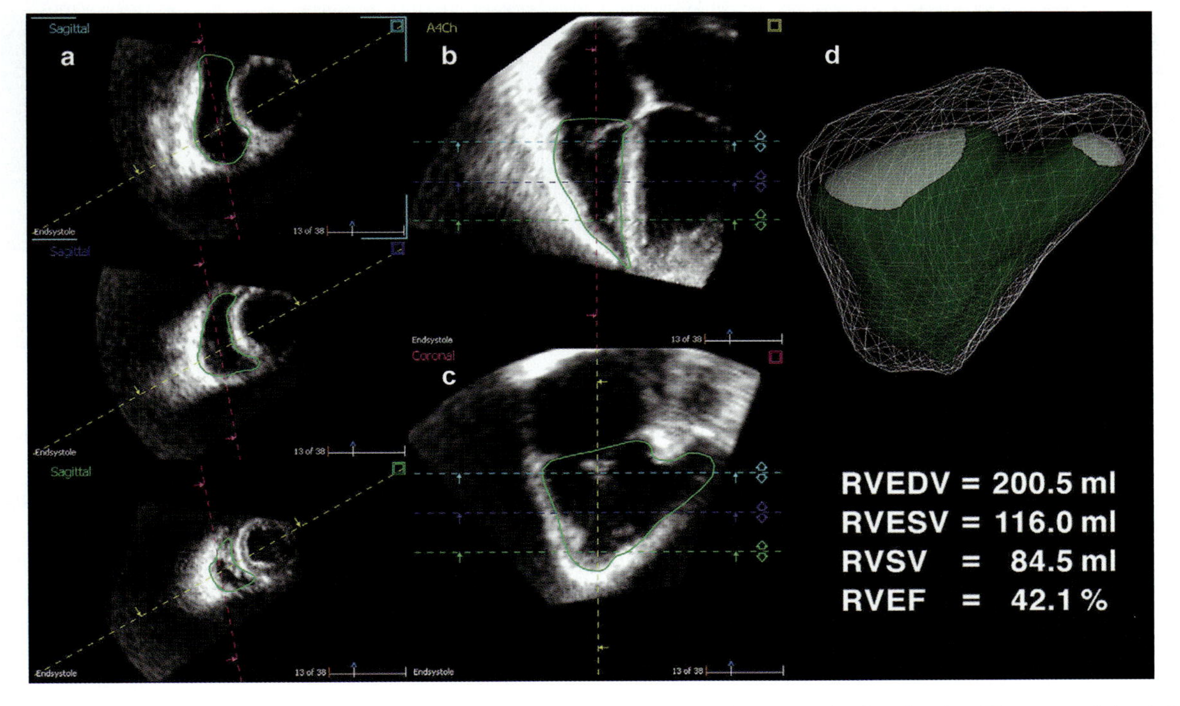

Fig. 8.11 An off-line analysis package is used to calculate right ventricular volume and ejection fraction. The areas of the right ventricle from 5 cut-planes (**a, b, c**) are automatically traced in order to produce a moving 3D model (**d**) and the volume measurements (Reproduced from Leibundgut et al. [19]. With permission)

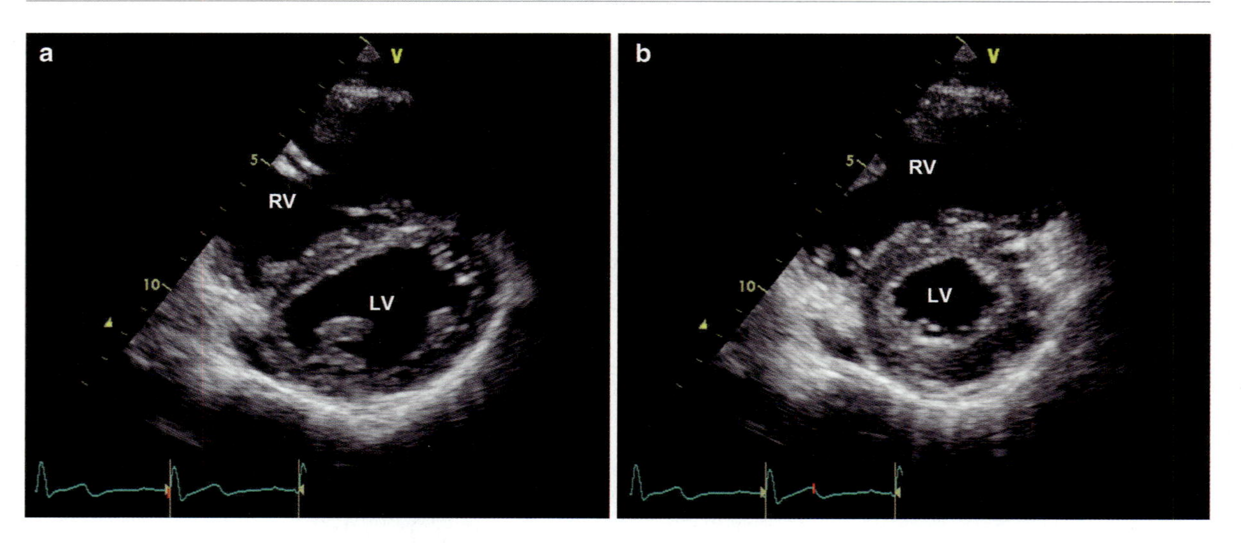

Fig. 8.12 (**a**) Parasternal short-axis view of the left ventricle in diastole in a patient with atrial septal defect shows flattening of the ventricular septum. (**b**) Parasternal short-axis view of the left ventricle in systole shows normalization of the septal curvature consistent with right ventricular volume overload. *LV* left ventricle, *RV* right ventricle

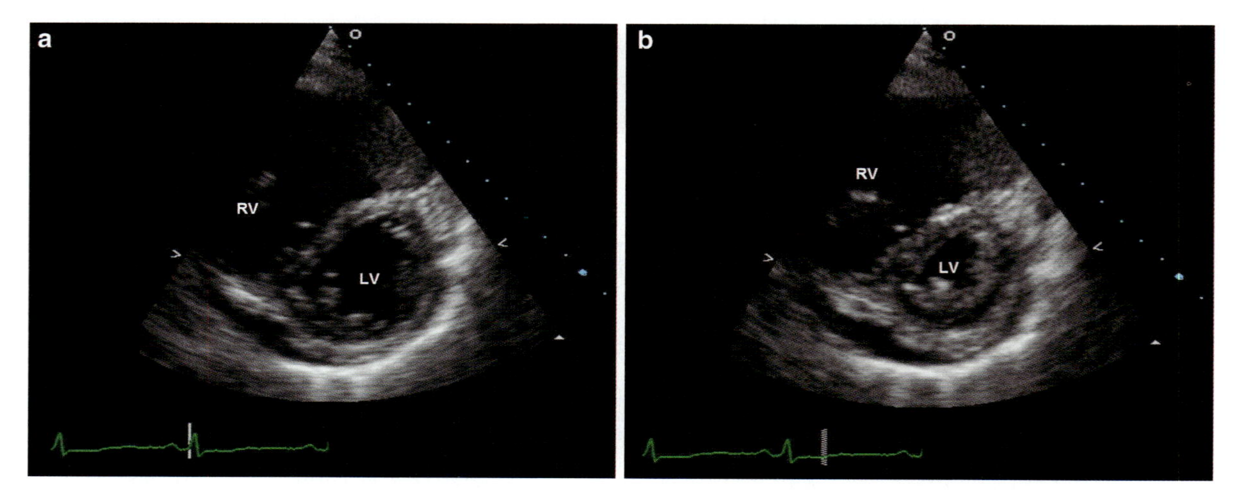

Fig. 8.13 (**a**) Parasternal short-axis view of the left ventricle in diastole in a patient with pulmonary hypertension shows flattening of the ventricular septum. A small pericardial effusion is present. (**b**) Parasternal short-axis view of the left ventricle in systole shows that the ventricular septum remains flat during systole consistent with severe pulmonary hypertension. *LV* left ventricle, *RV* right ventricle

prognosis of patients with left heart disease and should prompt consideration of early invasive interventions to improve left-sided conditions such as ischemic heart disease or mitral valve disease [29, 40].

Right ventricular dysfunction is a common end result of pulmonary hypertension which causes hypertrophy and thickening of the ventricular free wall, and the condition is termed "cor pulmonale". The RV wall may become thicker than the corresponding LV wall, thus ventricular thickness alone is not a good indicator of ventricular identity (Fig. 8.4) The RV chamber becomes distorted and may become more spherical with protrusion of the interventricular septum into the LV resulting in reduced LV end-diastolic volume and decreased LV compliance. The trabeculae carnae become even more prominent. Eventually, if the ventricle fails, the chamber dilates and tricuspid valve and pulmonary valve regurgitation occurs (Fig. 8.18) [28, 41].

In addition to chronic cor pulmonale, there are also acute cor pulmonale and subacute cor pulmonale

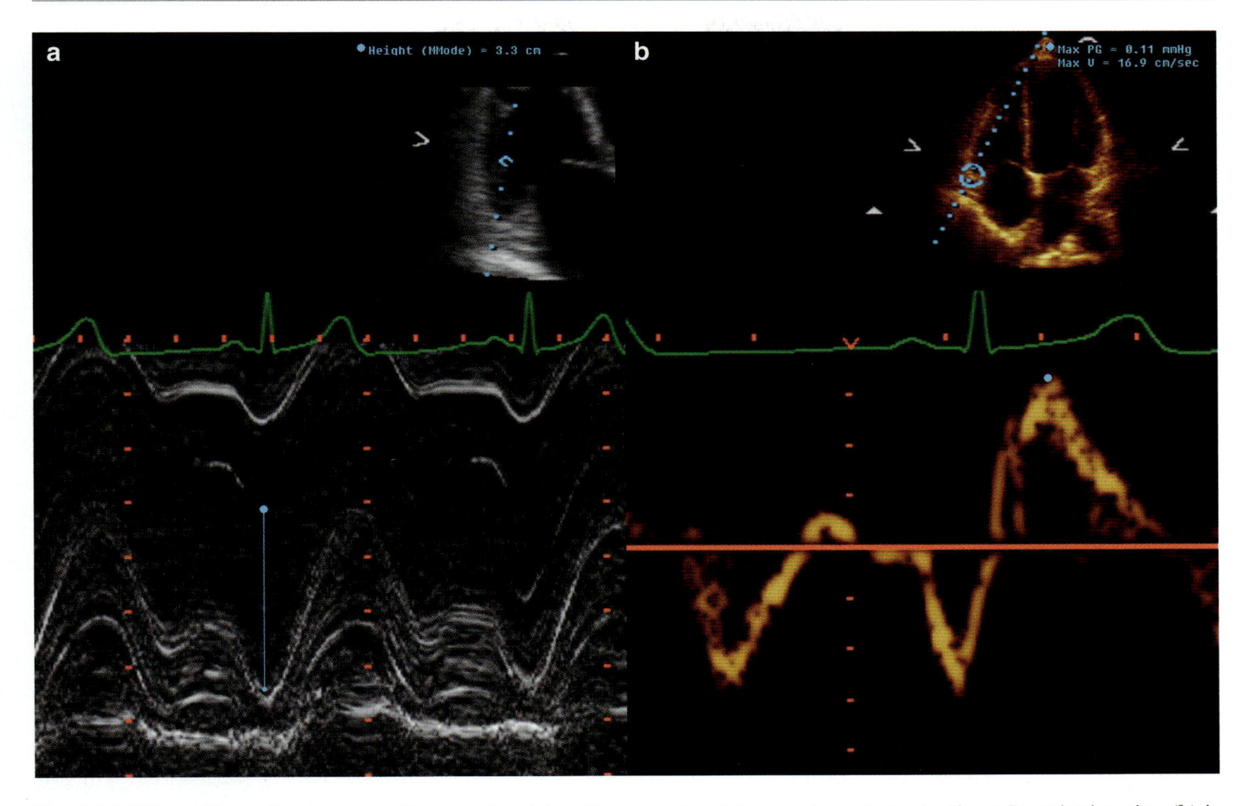

Fig. 8.14 Tricuspid annular plane systolic excursion (**a**) is 33 mm and systolic annular velocity by tissue Doppler imaging (**b**) is 16.9 cm/s in a patient with normal right ventricular size and function

situations. In acute cor pulmonale, there is severe and rapid RV pressure overload leading to a corresponding decrease in RV stroke volume due to RV failure. In this setting, the RV systolic pressure may not be very high [42]. The most common cause of acute cor pulmonale is pulmonary embolism, usually thromboembolism from deep leg veins or pelvic veins (Figs. 8.19–8.21). Combined RV pressure and volume overload may occur after a myocardial infarct complicated by an infarct-related ventricular septal defect or a papillary muscle rupture.

In subacute cor pulmonale, the RV failure develops over a few weeks and is associated with dyspnea and peripheral edema. Infections such as Schistosomiasis can cause this and is an important cause of pulmonary hypertension in the world. One other cause is tumor embolism to the pulmonary arteries and lymphatics [43]. Breast and gastric carcinomas have a propensity for this lymphangitic spread, which is usually fatal (Figs. 8.22, 8.23). The RV shows pressure overload and is dilated.

In the setting of chronic pulmonary hypertension, the RV can maintain normal volume and function for a long time. However, RV dilatation and dysfunction invariably set in. Irrespective of the reasons for pulmonary hypertension, the end result of RV response is one of dilatation and global hypokinesia. In the setting of pulmonary hypertension with a dilated and dysfunctional RV, preservation of RV apical function indicates that pulmonary thromboembolic disease is likely the underlying disease [44].

Determination of pulmonary artery pressure is an important component of the echo Doppler assessment of patients suspected to have pulmonary hypertension and can be measured by several methods. The most direct, well-validated, and widely used method is based on obtaining tricuspid regurgitation velocity (V) by continuous wave Doppler [45]. The systolic pulmonary artery pressure (PAP systolic):

$$\text{PAP systolic} = 4V^2 + \text{RAP}$$

where RAP is the right atrial pressure.

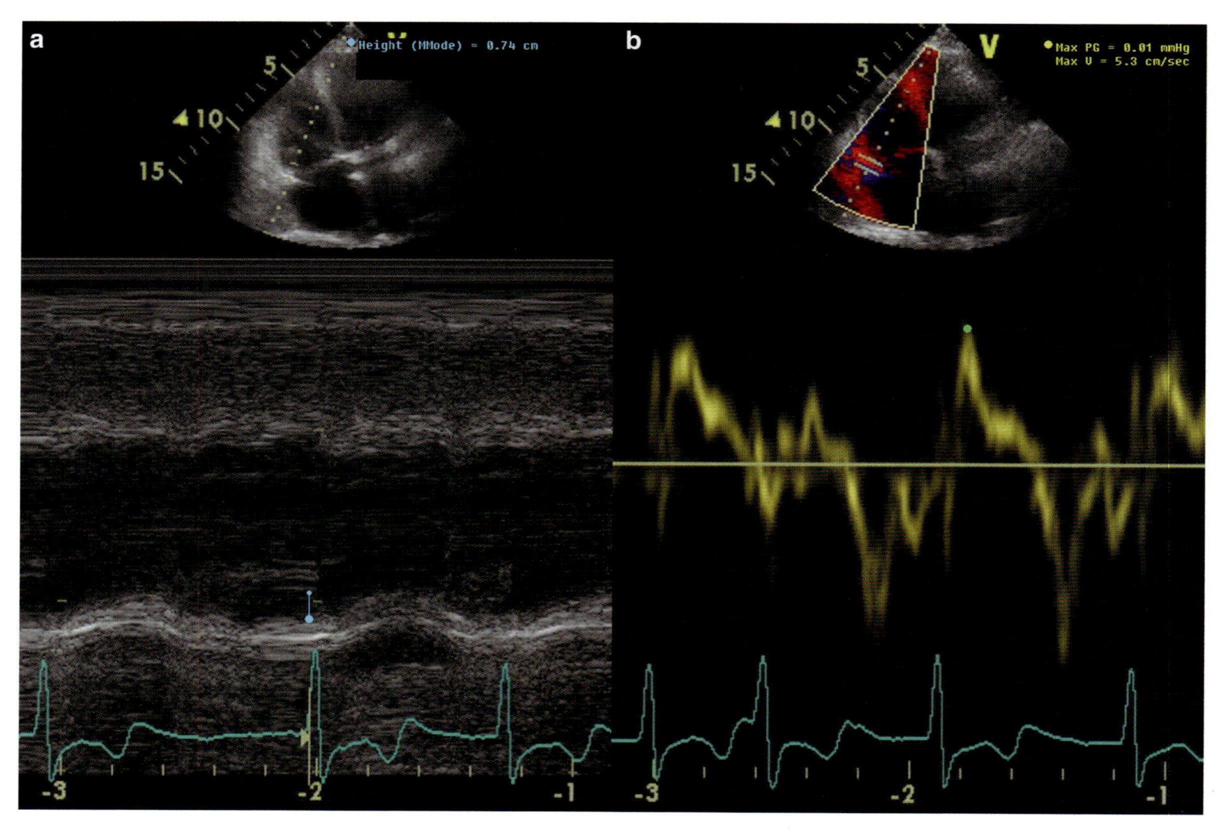

Fig. 8.15 The tricuspid annular plane systolic excursion (**a**) is 7.4 mm and systolic annular velocity by tissue Doppler imaging (**b**) is 5.3 cm/s in a patient with right ventricular dysfunction

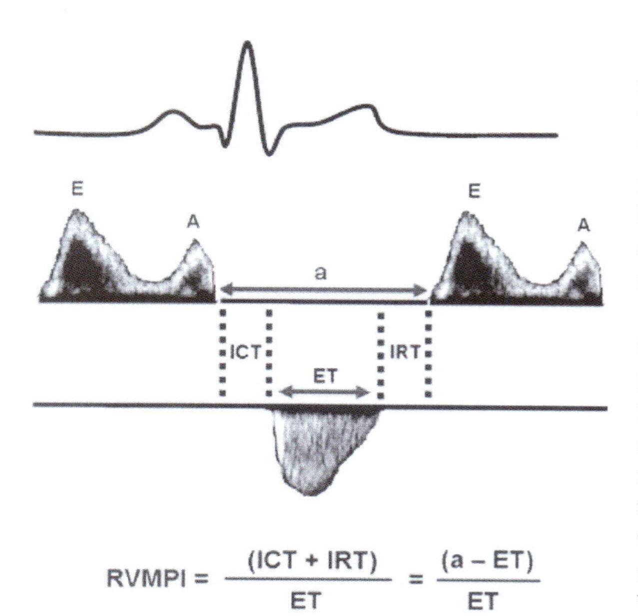

Fig. 8.16 A schematic diagram shows the measurements required to calculate the right ventricular myocardial performance index. *ET* ejection time, *ICT* isovolumic contraction time, *IRT* isovolumic relaxation time (Reproduced from Horton et al. [15]. With permission)

An adequate tricuspid regurgitation velocity signal for the calculation of PAP systolic can be obtained in up to 90% of patients [45]. It is important to emphasize that the severity of tricuspid regurgitation does not necessarily go hand in hand with that of pulmonary hypertension (Fig. 8.24). The corollary is that the lack of significant tricuspid regurgitation does not rule out severe pulmonary hypertension (Fig. 8.25).

In chronic pulmonary hypertension, the septal curvature can be a useful sign in estimating pulmonary artery pressure [27]. Diastolic flattening of the ventricular septum can be an indication of RV pressure or volume overload. In pure volume overload with normal pulmonary pressures, there is complete normalization of ventricular septal shape during systole (Fig. 8.12). If the ventricular septum remains somewhat flattened during systole, pulmonary hypertension is invariably present. When there is no improvement in the flattened septum during systole, severe pulmonary hypertension is likely, and if septal flattening worsens during systole, suprasystemic pulmonary hypertension should be suspected (Fig. 8.13).

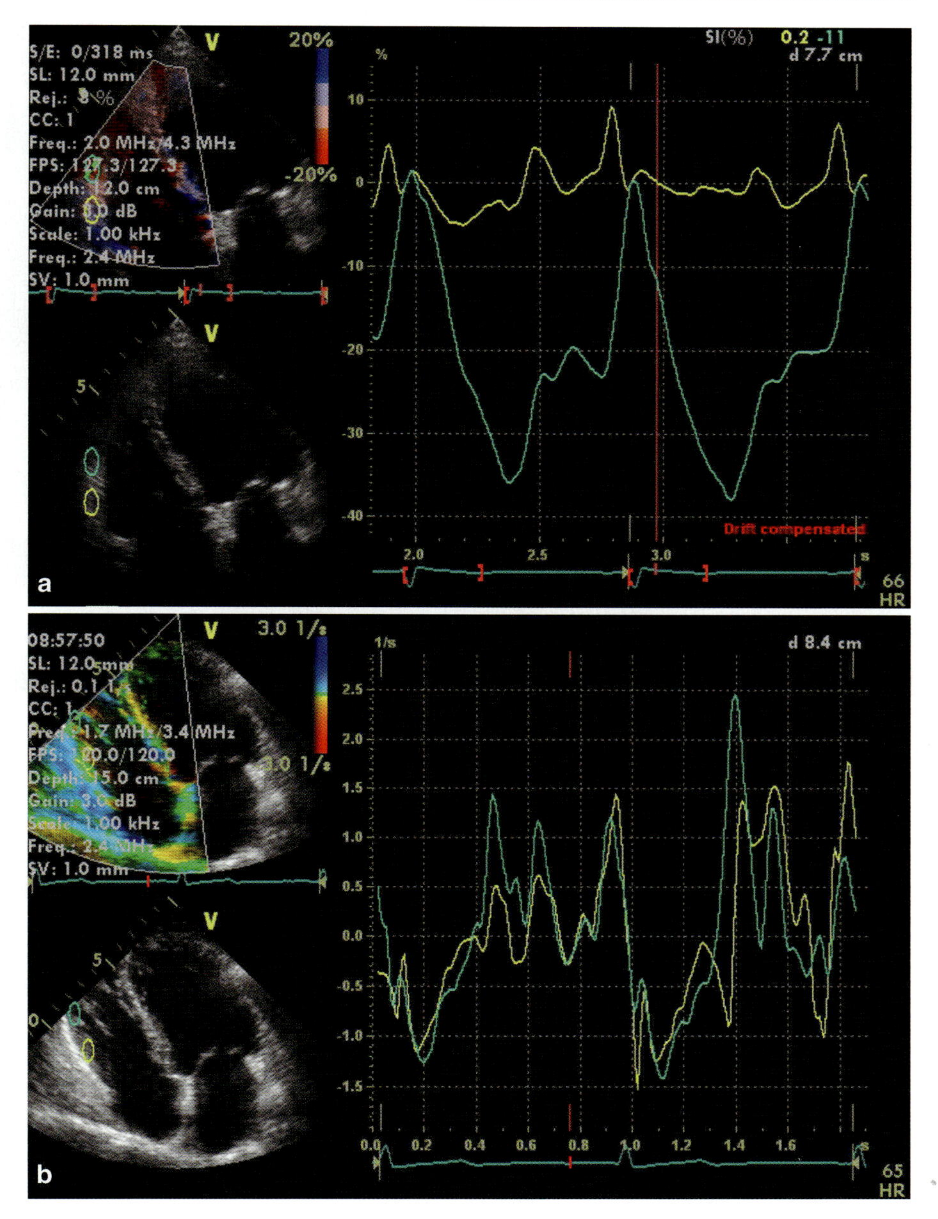

Fig. 8.17 (**a**) Right ventricular longitudinal myocardial strain by color tissue Doppler imaging at the basal and mid segments in a patient with normal right ventricular function shows that strain is higher at the mid segment. (**b**) Right ventricular longitudinal myocardial strain rate by color tissue Doppler imaging at the basal and mid segments in a patient with normal right ventricular function shows similar values at the two segments

The pulmonary arteries are usually dilated and should be examined carefully, particularly if transesophageal echocardiography is employed, to look for intraluminal thrombus which may be a result of pulmonary thromboembolism or in situ thrombus developed due to the dilated pulmonary arteries (Figs. 8.26, 8.27) [46]. When the pulmonary arteries are severely enlarged, they can protrude into neighboring cardiac structures, particularly the left atrium, simulating a left atrial mass (Fig.). Thus, in the setting of dilated pulmonary arteries, the main pulmonary and the proximal right and left pulmonary arteries need to be assessed carefully.8.28

Trauma

The anterior location of the RV under the sternum makes it vulnerable to closed chest trauma and iatrogenic trauma at surgery. Blunt closed chest injury can

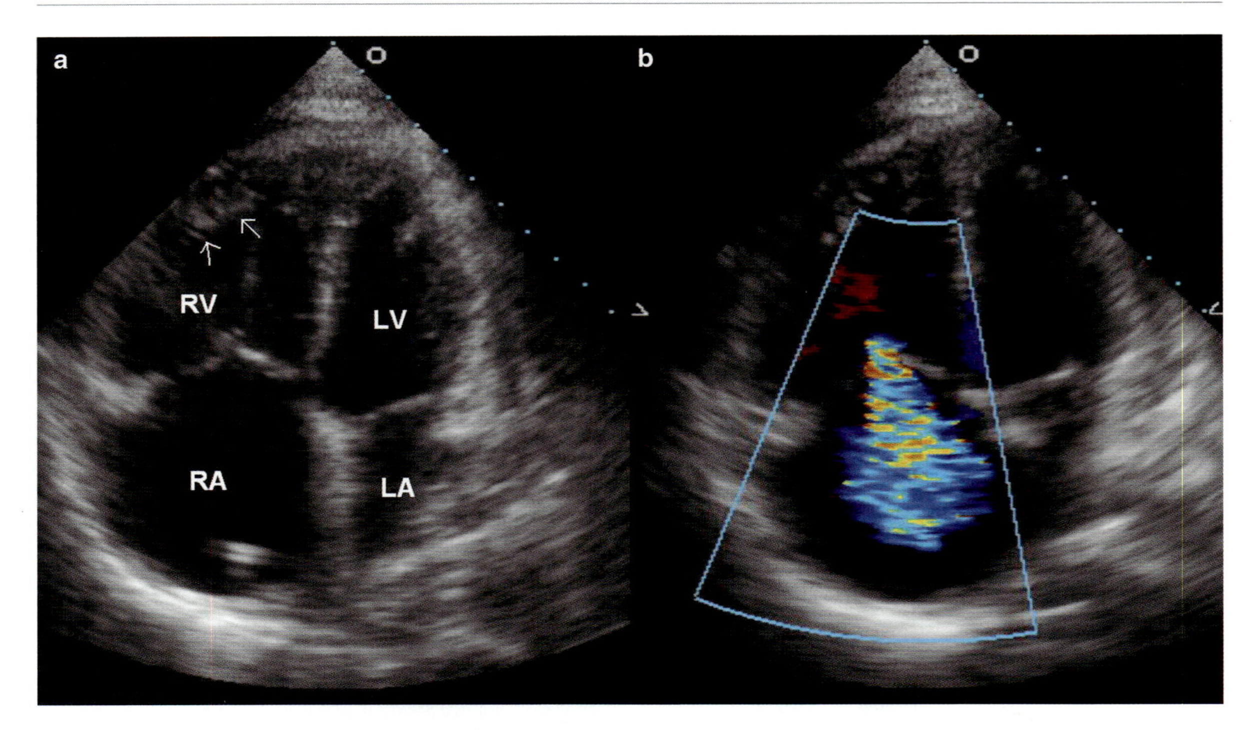

Fig. 8.18 Apical four-chamber view (**a**) in a patient with severe pulmonary hypertension shows a dilated and hypertrophied right ventricle with prominent trabeculae (*arrows*). Color-flow imaging (**b**) shows severe tricuspid regurgitation. *LA* left atrium, *LV* left ventricle, *RA* right atrium, *RV* right ventricle

occur as a result of a body deceleration (motor vehicle accident), deforming injury to chest (cardiopulmonary resuscitation, car crash, athletic injury, ungulate blow), abrupt acceleration (explosion or blast), or barotrauma (crush injury) [47–49]. In blunt chest trauma such as a car accident, the heart may move forward and hit the sternum causing a myocardial contusion. If severe, the ventricle may rupture. Papillary muscle rupture of the tricuspid valve may also occur due to blunt trauma. After sternotomy, the heart may be firmly adhered to the under surface of the sternum. At re-do surgery, the RV may be inadvertently opened and injured. It is a common practice to use preoperative imaging for patients with prior heart surgery to visualize the location of the RV and the bypass grafts so that they may be avoided during sternotomy.

Lines, Catheters, and Iatrogenic Disorders

Insertions of catheters, pacemakers, and cannulas are routine procedures for resuscitation, feeding, hemodynamic monitoring, and therapy. Local soft tissue and vascular complications have been found directly relating to these devices. Lines or catheters may contuse, tear, penetrate, perforate, tangle, or thrombose the intracardiac structures. Therapeutic valvuloplasty for treatment of valvular stenosis may also lacerate a leaflet or cusp giving rise to focal lesions and valvular regurgitation.

The most common iatrogenic catheter or line-related lesions are right-sided with endocardial lesions of the right atrium and RV, and lesions of the pulmonary and tricuspid valves [50]. These lesions are not uncommon, but are rarely of clinical significance and many, such as localized valve hemorrhages, are probably not detected by imaging (Fig. 8.29). When they are clinically significant, they are so as a result of thrombus or emboli, with or without infection.

Tricuspid valve regurgitation, as a complication of RV endomyocardial biopsy for transplant rejection monitoring, has been described. The flail leaflet is usually the septal one, almost certainly related to the practice of biopsying the septal myocardium [51]. Perforation of the right ventricle may occur with endomyocardial biopsy. The tricuspid valve and RV endomyocardium may also be torn if a line or pacemaker that has been in place chronically is removed after it has incorporated itself into the valvular apparatus.

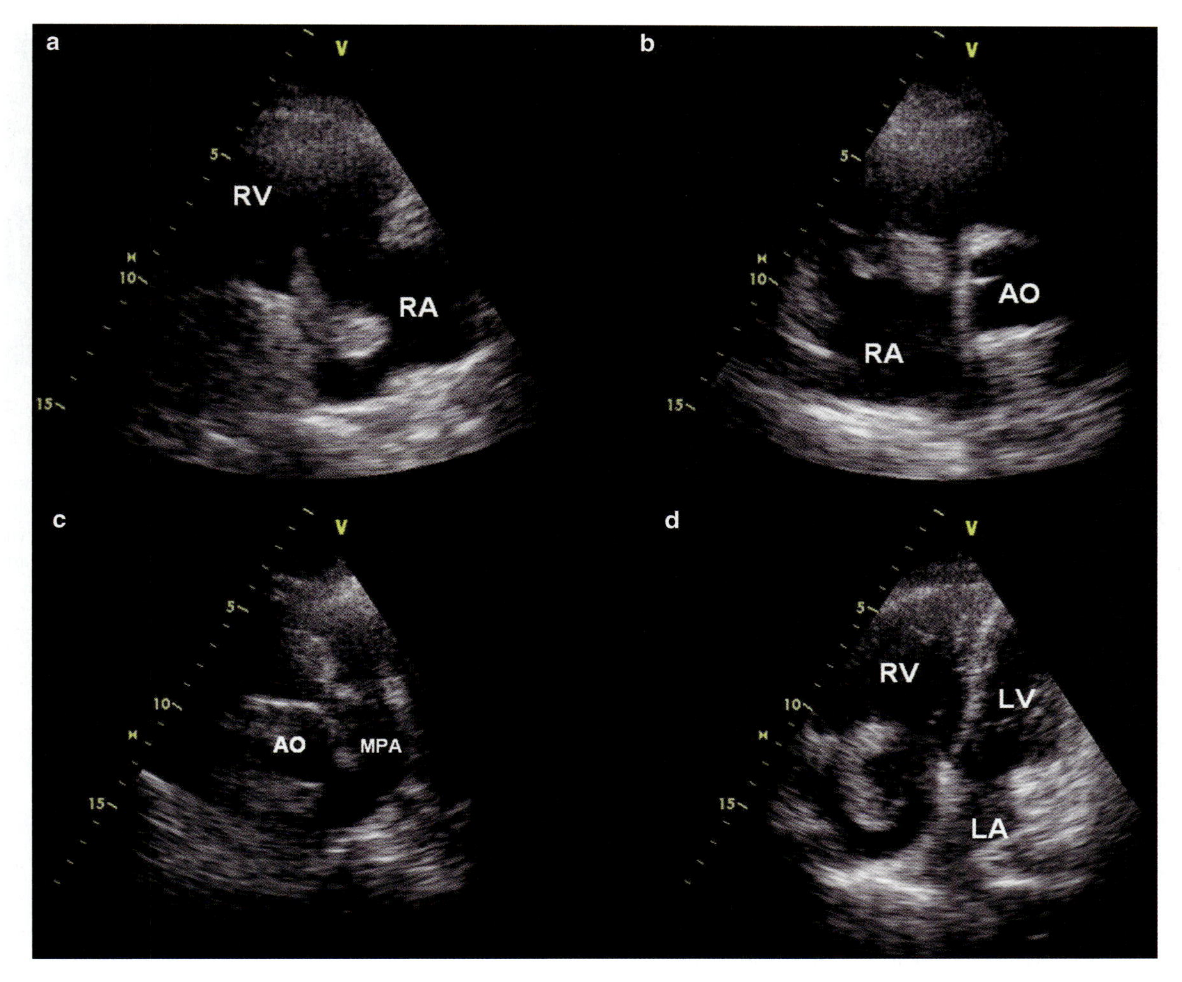

Fig. 8.19 In this patient with pulmonary embolism, a large sausage-like deep vein thrombus has embolized into the right atrium and ventricle. This large mobile thrombus can be seen in the right ventricular inflow (**a**) parasternal short-axis (**b, c**) and apical four-chamber (**d**) views. In (**c**), the thrombus prolapses into the main pulmonary artery. *Ao* aorta, *LA* left atrium, *LV* left ventricle, *RA* right atrium, *RV* right ventricle, *MPA* main pulmonary artery

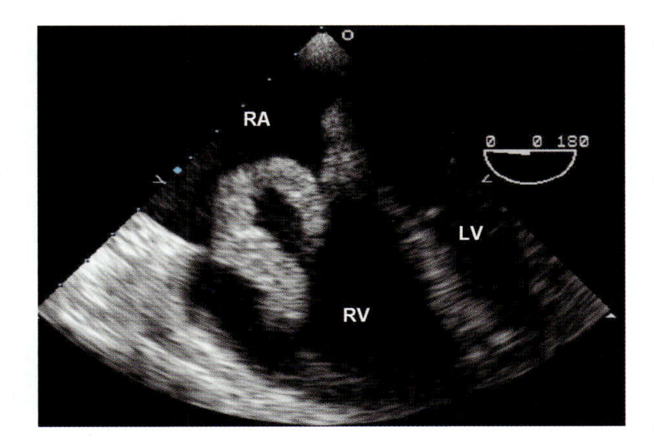

Fig. 8.20 Transesophageal transverse plane in the same patient as in Fig. 8.21 shows the large mobile sausage-like thrombus within the right atrium and right ventricle which are dilated. *LA* left atrium, *RA* right atrium, *RV* right ventricle

Summary

Right ventricular failure has diverse causes. Any condition giving rise to pulmonary hypertension can cause RV failure, as RV function is sensitive to afterload. Multiple echo views should be used to assess the RV which has a complex geometry with distinct inflow and outflow chambers. Various parameters have been used to assess RV size and function, but their usefulness is limited. Many of these parameters are based on measurements which are difficult to obtain due to the complex RV anatomy, the lack of internal landmarks to ensure proper sectioning of the RV, and the uncertainty in delineating the heavily trabeculated RV endocardial surface. Measuring RV volumes and ejection fraction by real-time 3D echo is a promising development, but

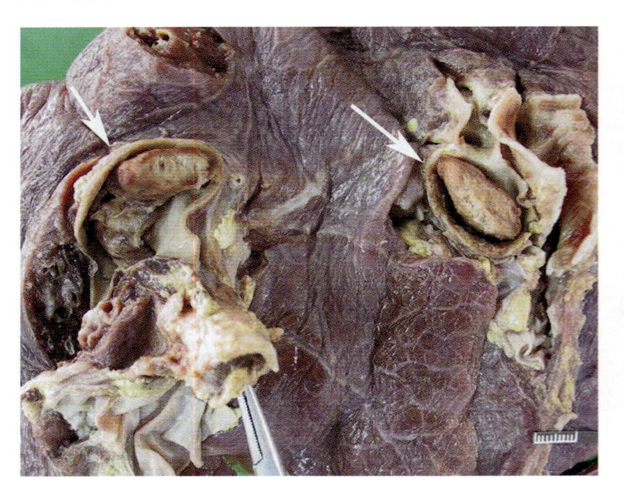

Fig. 8.21 Lungs showing pulmonary arteries containing large embolic pulmonary emboli (*arrows*). The right heart was dilated from acute obstruction

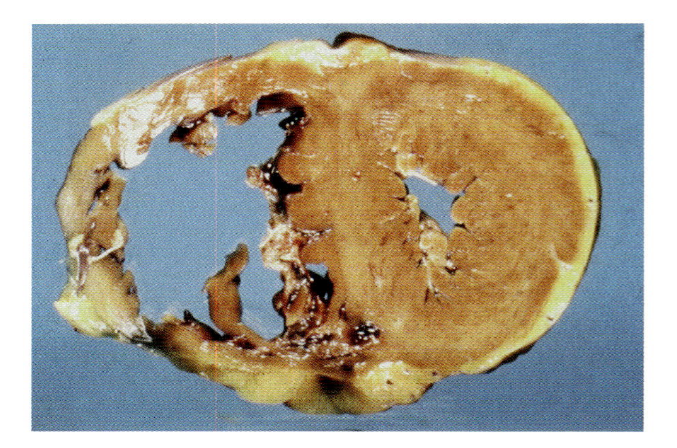

Fig. 8.22 Subacute cor pulmonale from breast cancer. The patient had severe subacute pulmonary hypertension. The breast carcinoma was discovered at autopsy. The right ventricle is severely dilated

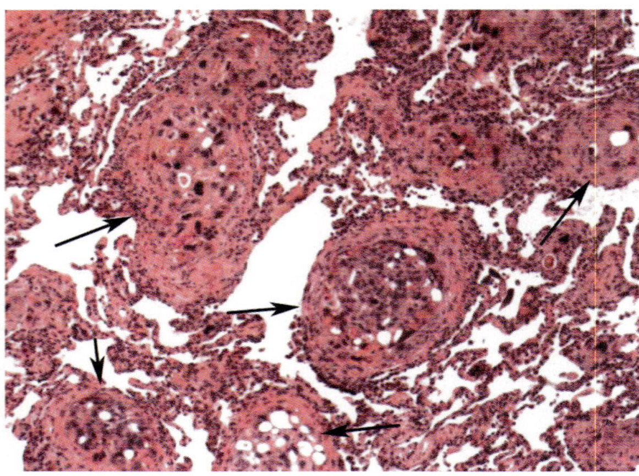

Fig. 8.23 Subacute cor pulmonale from bladder cancer tumor emboli as seen in the pulmonary arteries (*arrows*) in this histology section of the lungs. The patient had heart failure of unknown cause. This may be the first manifestation of the tumor. The heart was of normal size and weight but had a dilated right ventricle

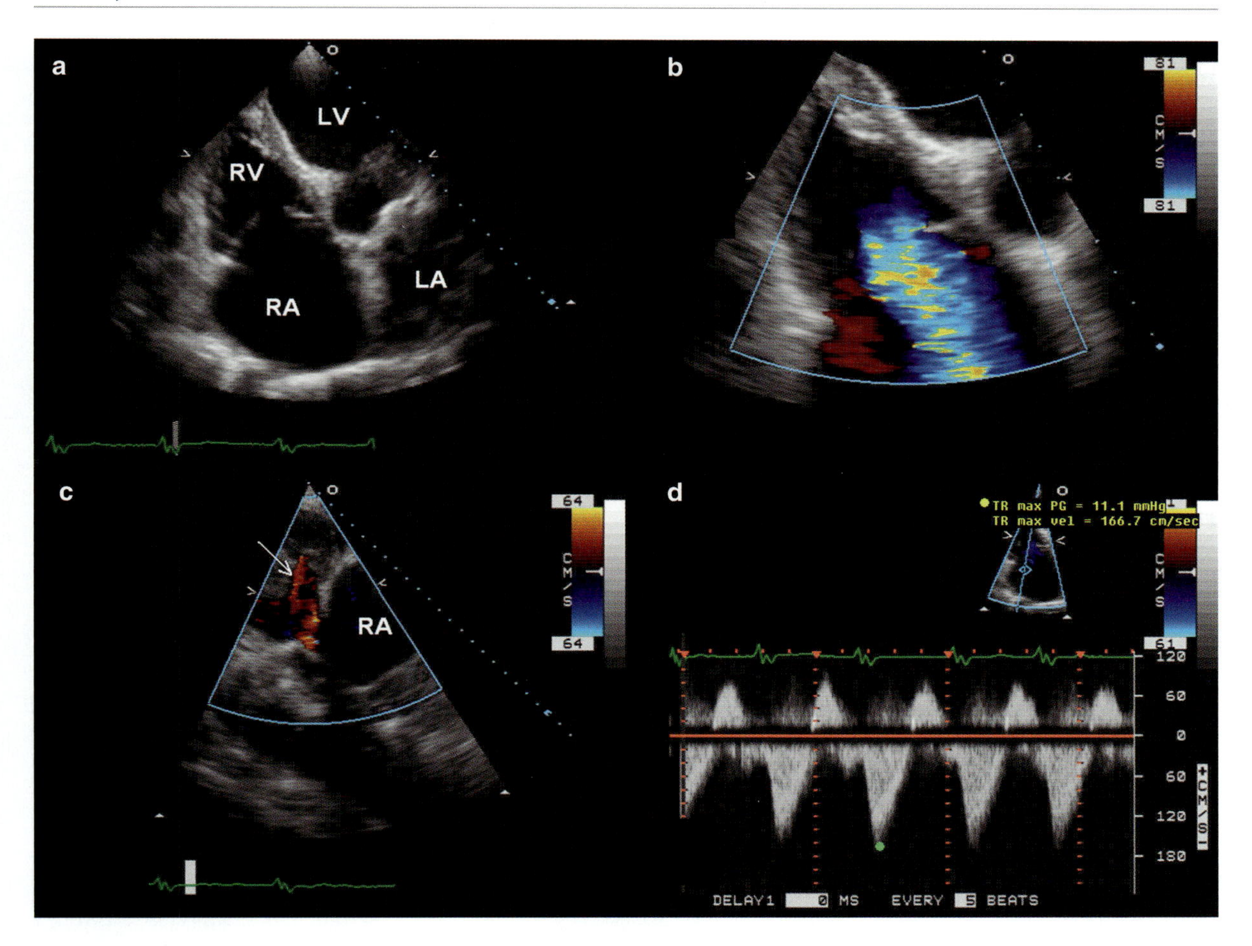

Fig. 8.24 The apical four-chamber view (**a**) shows lack of coaptation of the tricuspid leaflets due to dilated annulus in an 84-year-old woman with ischemic heart disease and longstanding atrial fibrillation, and color-flow image (**b**) shows severe tricuspid regurgitation with systolic reflux into the hepatic vein (*arrow*) shown in (**c**). Continuous wave Doppler (**d**) is in keeping with severe tricuspid regurgitation and that the right ventricular systolic pressure is not significantly elevated

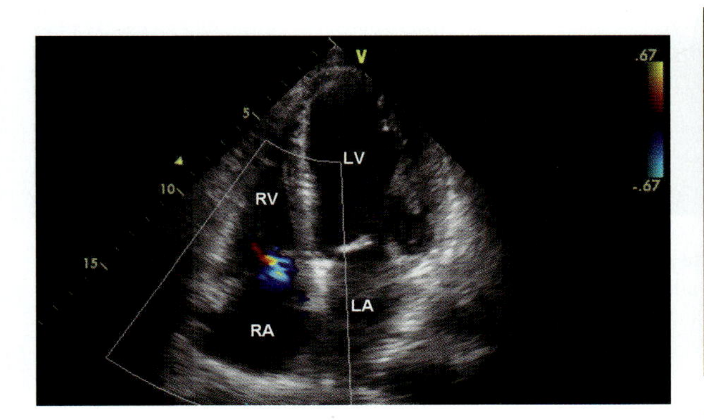

Fig. 8.25 Apical four-chamber view in a patient with coronary artery disease and severe pulmonary hypertension (pulmonary artery systolic pressure 71 mmHg) shows normal right ventricular size and only mild tricuspid regurgitation. *LA* left atrium, *LV* left ventricle, *RA* right atrium, *RV* right ventricle

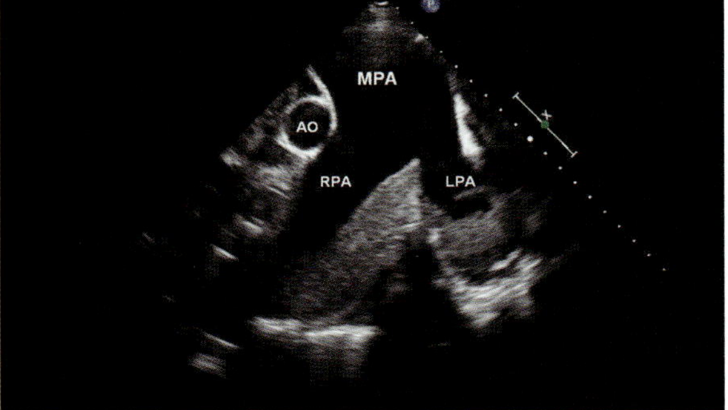

Fig. 8.26 Parasternal short-axis view shows severe dilatation of the main pulmonary artery, right pulmonary artery, and left pulmonary artery in a patient with severe primary pulmonary hypertension. A large amount of intraluminal thrombus is present in both the right and left pulmonary arteries. *Ao* aorta, *LPA* left pulmonary artery, *MPA* main pulmonary artery, *RPA* right pulmonary artery

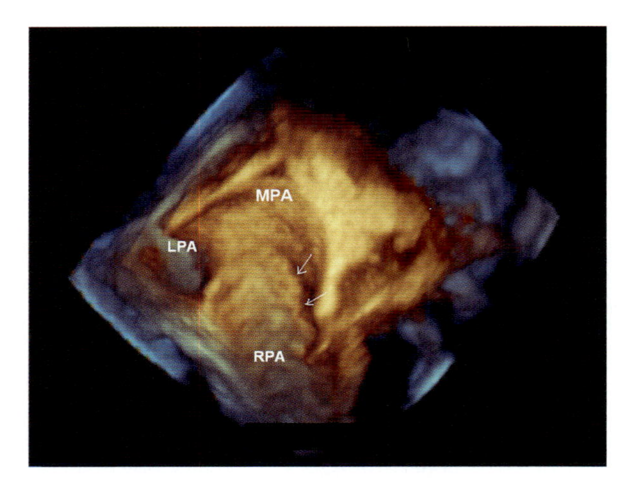

Fig. 8.27 Transthoracic 3D view of the dilated pulmonary arteries in the patient as in Fig. 8.27 shows the extensive nature of the laminated thrombus (*arrows*) within the right pulmonary artery

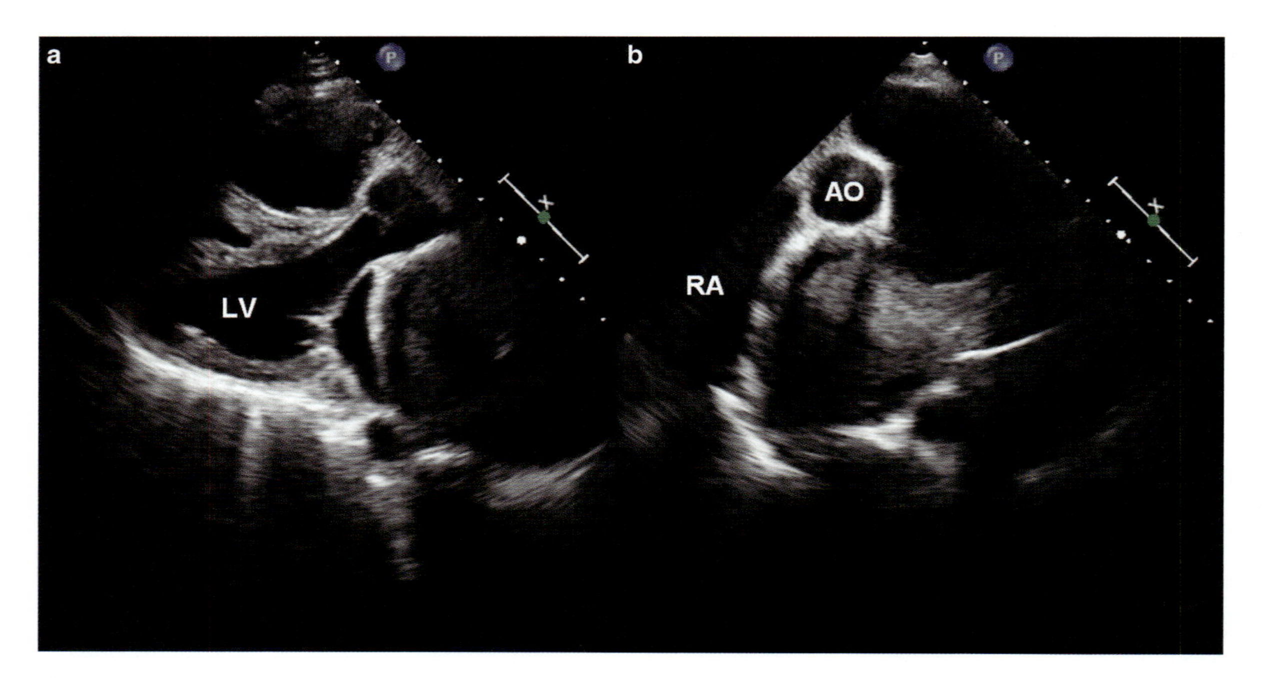

Fig. 8.28 Parasternal long-axis (**a**) and short-axis (**b**) views in the same patient as in Figs. 8.26 and 8.27 show an apparent large left atrial mass which is due to the extrinsic compression of the left atrium by the severely dilated right pulmonary artery. *Ao* aorta, *LV* left ventricle, *RA* right atrium

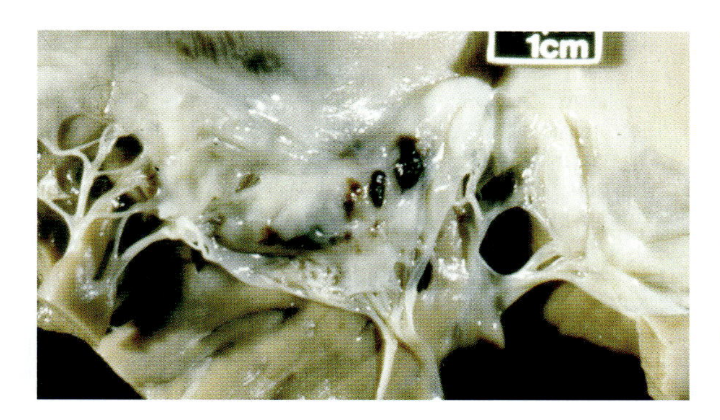

Fig. 8.29 Opened tricuspid valve with valve hemorrhages. These are not uncommon in patients with central lines and catheters. They are incidental and usually not detected by imaging

refinement of image quality and further validation are needed before 3D measurements can be used in the management of patients with RV diseases.

References

1. Ho SY, Nihoyannopoulos P. Anatomy, echocardiography, and normal right ventricular dimensions. *Heart*. 2006;92:I2-I13.
2. Webb G, Gatzoulis MA. Atrial septal defects in the adult - Recent progress and overview. *Circulation*. 2006;114(15): 1645-1653.
3. Dell'Italia LJ, Walsh RA. Application of a time varying elastance model to right ventricular performance in man. *Cardiovasc Res*. 1988 Dec;22(12):864-874.
4. Goldhaber SZ, Visani L, De RM. Acute pulmonary embolism: clinical outcomes in the International Cooperative Pulmonary Embolism Registry (ICOPER). *Lancet*. 1999 Apr 24;353(9162):1386-1389.
5. Goldstein JA. Pathophysiology and management of right heart ischemia. *J Am Coll Cardiol*. 2002;40(5):841-853.
6. Kjaergaard J, Iversen KK, Vejlstrup NG, et al. Impacts of acute severe pulmonary regurgitation on right ventricular geometry and contractility assessed by tissue-Doppler echocardiography. *Eur J Echocardiogr*. 2010 Jan;11(1):19-26.
7. Bristow MR, Zisman LS, Lowes BD, et al. The pressure-overloaded right ventricle in pulmonary hypertension. *Chest*. 1998 Jul;114(1 Suppl):101S-106S.
8. Macnee W. Pathophysiology of cor pulmonale in chronic obstructive pulmonary disease. Part One. *Am J Respir Crit Care Med*. 1994 Sep;150(3):833-852.
9. Walker LA, Buttrick PM. The right ventricle: biologic insights and response to disease. *Curr Cardiol Rev*. 2009 Jan;5(1):22-28.
10. La Vecchia L, Zanolla L, Varotto L, et al. Reduced right ventricular ejection fraction as a marker for idiopathic dilated cardiomyopathy compared with ischemic left ventricular dysfunction. *Am Heart J*. 2001 Jul;142(1):181-189.
11. Ghio S, Gavazzi A, Campana C, et al. Independent and additive prognostic value of right ventricular systolic function and pulmonary artery pressure in patients with chronic heart failure. *J Am Coll Cardiol*. 2001 Jan;37(1):183-188.
12. Louie EK, Lin SS, Reynertson SI, et al. Pressure and volume loading of the right ventricle have opposite effects on left ventricle ejection fraction. *Circulation*. 1995;92:819-824.
13. Maron MS, Hauser TH, Dubrow E, et al. Right ventricular involvement in hypertrophic cardiomyopathy. *Am J Cardiol*. 2007 Oct 15;100(8):1293-1298.
14. Marcus FI, McKenna WJ, Sherrill D, et al. Diagnosis of arrhythmogenic right ventricular cardiomyopathy/dysplasia: proposed modification of the Task Force Criteria. *Eur Heart J*. 2010 Apr;31(7):806-814.
15. Horton KD, Meece RW, Hill JC. Assessment of the right ventricle by echocardiography: a primer for cardiac sonographers. *J Am Soc Echocardiogr*. 2009 Jul;22(7):776-792.
16. Jurcut R, Giusca S, La GA, Vasile S, Ginghina C, Voigt JU. The echocardiographic assessment of the right ventricle: what to do in 2010? *Eur J Echocardiogr*. 2010 Mar;11(2):81-96.
17. Badano LP, Ginghina C, Easaw J, et al. Right ventricle in pulmonary arterial hypertension: haemodynamics, structural changes, imaging, and proposal of a study protocol aimed to assess remodelling and treatment effects. *Eur J Echocardiogr*. 2010 Jan;11(1):27-37.
18. Tamborini G, Marsan NA, Gripari P, et al. Reference values for right ventricular volumes and ejection fraction with real-time three-dimensional echocardiography: evaluation in a large series of normal subjects. *J Am Soc Echocardiogr*. 2010 Feb;23(2):109-115.
19. Leibundgut G, Rohner A, Grize L, et al. Dynamic assessment of right ventricular volumes and function by real-time three-dimensional echocardiography: a comparison study with magnetic resonance imaging in 100 adult patients. *J Am Soc Echocardiogr*. 2010 Feb;23(2):116-126.
20. Grewal J, Majdalany D, Syed I, Pellikka P, Warnes CA. Three-dimensional echocardiographic assessment of right ventricular volume and function in adult patients with congenital heart disease: comparison with magnetic resonance imaging. *J Am Soc Echocardiogr*. 2010 Feb;23(2):127-133.
21. van der Zwaan HB, Helbing WA, McGhie JS, et al. Clinical value of real-time three-dimensional echocardiography for right ventricular quantification in congenital heart disease: validation with cardiac magnetic resonance imaging. *J Am Soc Echocardiogr*. 2010 Feb;23(2):134-140.
22. Jardin F, Dubourg O, Bourdarias JP. Echocardiographic pattern of acute cor pulmonale. *Chest*. 1997 Jan;111(1):209-217.
23. Jiang L, Levine RA, Weyman AE. Echocardiographic Assessment of Right Ventricular Volume and Function. *Echocardiography*. 1997 Mar;14(2):189-206.
24. Lang RM, Bierig M, Devereux RB, et al. Recommendations for chamber quantification: a report from the American Society of Echocardiography's Guidelines and Standards Committee and the Chamber Quantification Writing Group, developed in conjunction with the European Association of Echocardiography, a branch of the European Society of Cardiology. *J Am Soc Echocardiogr*. 2005 Dec; 18(12):1440-1463.
25. Louie EK, Rich S, Levitsky S, Brundage BH. Doppler echocardiographic demonstration of the differential effects of right ventricular pressure and volume overload on left

ventricular geometry and filling. *J Am Coll Cardiol*. 1992 Jan;19(1):84-90.
26. Raymond RJ, Hinderliter AL, Willis PW, et al. Echocardiographic predictors of adverse outcomes in primary pulmonary hypertension. *J Am Coll Cardiol*. 2002 Apr 3;39(7):1214-1219.
27. King ME, Braun H, Goldblatt A, Liberthson R, Weyman AE. Interventricular septal configuration as a predictor of right ventricular systolic hypertension in children: a cross-sectional echocardiographic study. *Circulation*. 1983 Jul;68(1):68-75.
28. Forfia PR, Fisher MR, Mathai SC, et al. Tricuspid annular displacement predicts survival in pulmonary hypertension. *Am J Respir Crit Care Med*. 2006 Nov 1;174(9):1034-1041.
29. Karatasakis GT, Karagounis LA, Kalyvas PA, et al. Prognostic significance of echocardiographically estimated right ventricular shortening in advanced heart failure. *Am J Cardiol*. 1998 Aug 1;82(3):329-334.
30. Lopez-Candales A, Rajagopalan N, Saxena N, Gulyasy B, Edelman K, Bazaz R. Right ventricular systolic function is not the sole determinant of tricuspid annular motion. *Am J Cardiol*. 2006 Oct 1;98(7):973-977.
31. Tei C, Dujardin KS, Hodge DO, et al. Doppler echocardiographic index for assessment of global right ventricular function. *J Am Soc Echocardiogr*. 1996 Nov;9(6):838-847.
32. Yeo TC, Dujardin KS, Tei C, Mahoney DW, McGoon MD, Seward JB. Value of a Doppler-derived index combining systolic and diastolic time intervals in predicting outcome in primary pulmonary hypertension. *Am J Cardiol*. 1998 May 1;81(9):1157-1161.
33. Lindqvist P, Calcutteea A, Henein M. Echocardiography in the assessment of right heart function. *Eur J Echocardiogr*. 2008 Mar;9(2):225-234.
34. De Castro S, Cavarretta E, Milan A, et al. Usefulness of tricuspid annular velocity in identifying global RV dysfunction in patients with primary pulmonary hypertension: a comparison with 3D echo-derived right ventricular ejection fraction. *Echocardiography*. 2008 Mar;25(3):289-293.
35. Meluzin J, Spinarova L, Bakala J, et al. Pulsed Doppler tissue imaging of the velocity of tricuspid annular systolic motion; a new, rapid, and non-invasive method of evaluating right ventricular systolic function. *Eur Heart J*. 2001 Feb;22(4):340-348.
36. Kukulski T, Hubbert L, Arnold M, Wranne B, Hatle L, Sutherland GR. Normal regional right ventricular function and its change with age: a Doppler myocardial imaging study. *J Am Soc Echocardiogr*. 2000 Mar;13(3):194-204.
37. Borges AC, Knebel F, Eddicks S, et al. Right ventricular function assessed by two-dimensional strain and tissue Doppler echocardiography in patients with pulmonary arterial hypertension and effect of vasodilator therapy. *Am J Cardiol*. 2006 Aug 15;98(4):530-534.
38. Pirat B, McCulloch ML, Zoghbi WA. Evaluation of global and regional right ventricular systolic function in patients with pulmonary hypertension using a novel speckle tracking method. *Am J Cardiol*. 2006 Sep 1;98(5):699-704.
39. Teske AJ, Cox MG, De Boeck BW, Doevendans PA, Hauer RN, Cramer MJ. Echocardiographic tissue deformation imaging quantifies abnormal regional right ventricular function in arrhythmogenic right ventricular dysplasia/cardiomyopathy. *J Am Soc Echocardiogr*. 2009 Aug;22(8):920-927.
40. Hung J, Koelling T, Semigran MJ, Dec GW, Levine RA, Di Salvo TG. Usefulness of echocardiographic determined tricuspid regurgitation in predicting event-free survival in severe heart failure secondary to idiopathic-dilated cardiomyopathy or to ischemic cardiomyopathy. *Am J Cardiol*. 1998 Nov 15;82(10):1301-1310.
41. Chin KM, Kim NH, Rubin LJ. The right ventricle in pulmonary hypertension. *Coron Artery Dis*. 2005 Feb;16(1):13-18.
42. Schulman DS, Matthay RA. The right ventricle in pulmonary disease. *Cardiol Clin*. 1992 Feb;10(1):111-135.
43. Veinot JP, Ford SE, Price RG. Subacute cor pulmonale due to tumor embolization. *Arch Pathol Lab Med*. 1992;116:131-134.
44. McConnell MV, Solomon SD, Rayan ME, Come PC, Goldhaber SZ, Lee RT. Regional right ventricular dysfunction detected by echocardiography in acute pulmonary embolism. *Am J Cardiol*. 1996 Aug 15;78(4):469-473.
45. Currie PJ, Seward JB, Chan KL, et al. Continuous wave Doppler determination of right ventricular pressure: a simultaneous Doppler-catheterization study in 127 patients. *J Am Coll Cardiol*. 1985 Oct;6(4):750-756.
46. Moser KM, Fedullo PF, Finkbeiner WE, Golden J. Do patients with primary pulmonary hypertension develop extensive central thrombi? *Circulation*. 1995;91:741-745.
47. Bayezid O, Mete A, Turkay C, Yanat F, Deger N, Isin E. Traumatic tricuspid insufficiency following blunt chest trauma. *J Cardiovasc Surg*. 1993;34:69-71.
48. dos Santos J, de Marchi CH, Bestetti RB, Corbucci HAR, Pavarino PR. Ruptured chordae tendineae of the posterior leaflet of the tricuspid valve as a cause of tricuspid regurgitation following blunt chest trauma. *Cardiovasc Pathol*. 2001;10(2):97-98.
49. van Son JA, Danielson GK, Schaff HV, Miller FA Jr. Traumatic tricuspid valve insufficiency. Experience in thirteen patients. *Journal of Thoracic & Cardiovascular Surgery*. 1994;108:893-898.
50. Ford SE, Manley PN. Indwelling cardiac catheters: an autopsy study of associated endocardial lesions. *Arch Pathol Lab Med*. 1982;106:314-317.
51. Mielniczuk L, Haddad H, Davies RA, Veinot JP. Tricuspid valve chordal tissue in endomyocardial biopsy specimens of patients with significant tricuspid regurgitation. *J Heart Lung Transplant*. 2005 Oct;24(10):1586-1590.

9 Diseases of the Aorta

The aorta is an elastic artery that takes origin from the left ventricle. Embryologically the aorta and the pulmonary trunk derive from the truncus arteriosus in the fetus. The smooth muscle cells in variable areas of the aorta derive from different cells of origin. The ascending aorta smooth muscle cells are neural crest derived, whereas the cells in the media of the thoracic and abdominal aorta are derived from somite-derived cells and splanchnic mesoderm. The aorta is composed of an intima with endothelium, a media of elastic lamellae and smooth muscle cells, and covered by an adventitia containing collagen, nerves, and blood vessels.

The proximal few centimeters of the aorta are within the pericardial space. The ascending aorta exits the heart in a rightward direction giving rise to three arch branches – the brachiocephailc (innominate) artery, the left common carotid artery, and finally the left subclavian artery (Fig. 9.1). The ductus arteriosus is an embryological communication between the aorta and the left pulmonary artery. Its arterial origin is usually adjacent to the left subclavian artery. It closes shortly after birth in most children, but can remain patent or be kept open by medical intervention if needed. If it closes, there is usually an intimal dimple noted on both arterial sides with a fibrous connection termed the ligamentum arteriosum.

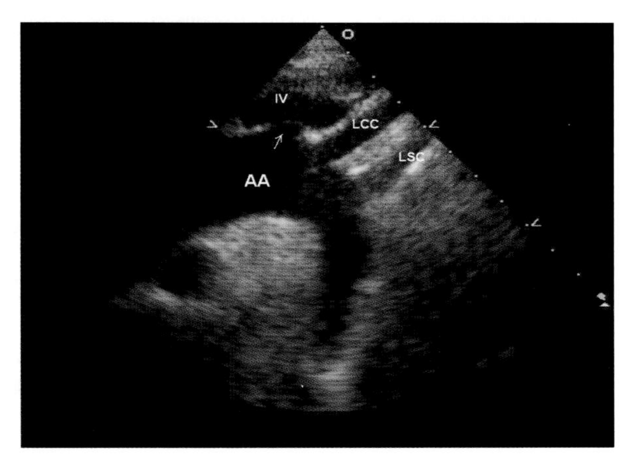

Fig. 9.1 The aortic arch is imaged from the suprasternal notch showing the three arched vessels. The origin of the innominate artery (*arrow*) can easily be seen, and the rest of the artery (not shown) can be imaged by tilting the transducer rightward. The innominate vein is present and superior to the aortic arch. *AA* aortic arch, *IV* innominate vein, *LCC* left common carotid artery, *LSC* left subclavian artery

The ascending aorta is the segment most easily seen using echocardiography (Fig. 9.2). The ascending aorta is a complex anatomical structure. It is not a simple tube with an attached aortic valve, but rather has multiple areas of curvature and protrusions or outpouchings. The aortic valve is attached to the aorta in a corona or crown-like configuration leaving areas of intercommissural fibrous trigones at each commissure (Fig. 9.3). The area of the aorta in which the aortic valve is attached is outpouched as compared to the adjacent ascending aorta. These areas are separated by a ridge – the sinotubular junction (Fig. 9.4). After the sinotubular junction, the true ascending aorta is more of a simple tube-like structure, at least until the arch vessels exit. The anatomical distinctions are important as the different areas have different behavior in native aortic disease and after valve replacement or repair. The thoracic aorta tapers progressively, with the abdominal aorta having the smallest normal diameter.

The aorta is the main conduit for the blood supply to all the major organs. It has a central location within the thorax. Important anatomic components of the intrathoracic aorta include the annulus, aortic sinus, sinotubular

K.-L. Chan and J.P. Veinot, *Anatomic Basis of Echocardiographic Diagnosis*,
DOI: 10.1007/978-1-84996-387-9_9, © Springer-Verlag London Limited 2011

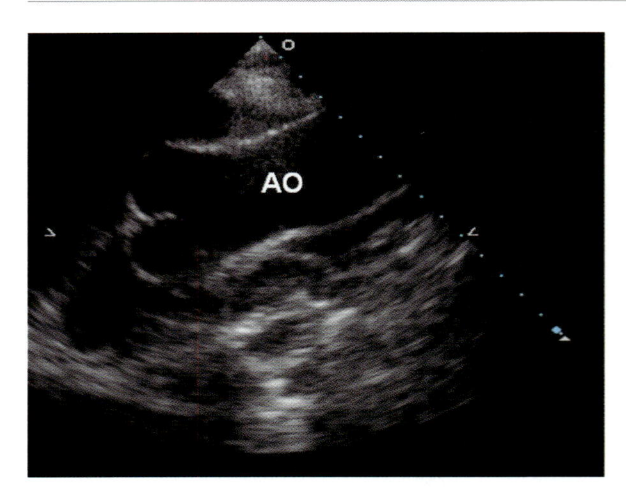

Fig. 9.2 This is a high left parasternal view of the ascending aorta showing the aortic sinus, the sinotubular junction and the ascending aorta. *Ao* aorta

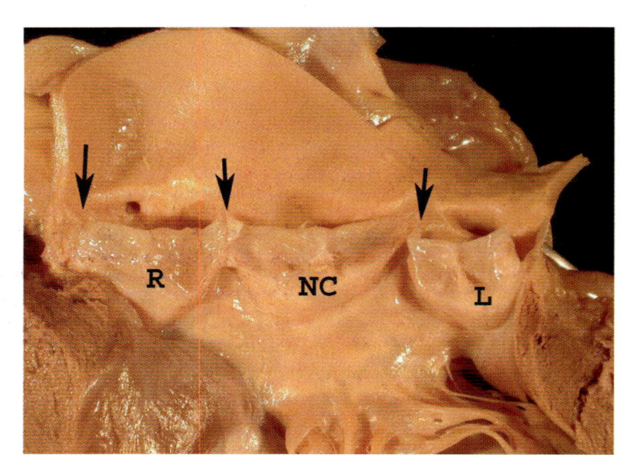

Fig. 9.3 Opened aortic valve with right (*R*), noncoronary (*NC*) and left (*L*) cusps. Commissures separate the cusps (*arrows*)

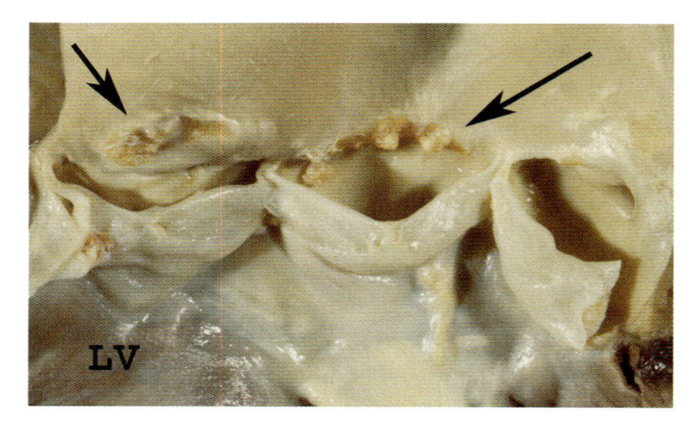

Fig. 9.4 Calcification of the sinotubular junction (*arrows*) above the aortic valve and the aortic sinuses. *LV* left ventricle

junction, tubular ascending aorta, aortic arch, and descending thoracic aorta. The sinotubular junction is usually the narrowest region of the ascending aorta. The aorta gradually tapers as it courses further distally such that the distal descending thoracic aorta is invariably smaller compared to the ascending aorta. With aging, the thoracic aorta becomes enlarged and tortuous. The proximal ascending aorta courses more anterior and rightward. The proximal descending thoracic aorta courses more posterior and leftward.

Multiple imaging modalities have been used to image the aorta (Table 9.1) [1–5]. Transthoracic echocardiography is useful to assess the aortic root and the proximal ascending aorta, but otherwise has a limited role as it produces suboptimal images of the rest of the aorta, including the aortic arch and the descending thoracic aorta [1]. On the other hand, transesophageal echocardiography (TEE) can provide an excellent evaluation of the entire thoracic aorta, although the aortic arch vessels may not be optimally seen [4].

Other imaging modalities such as computed tomography and magnetic resonance scanning can provide exquisite images of the thoracic aorta, as well as other intrathoracic abnormalities. However, both imaging modalities have limited temporal resolution compared to TEE, and they cannot be readily deployed in the assessment of critically ill patients in the intensive care unit or emergency room where transportation may be time-consuming and impose a risk to the patient. The portability of TEE allows performance at the patient's bedside and thus it is frequently the imaging modality of choice in the assessment of patients with acute aortic syndrome.

In choosing the imaging approach and management of patients with aortic disease, it is useful to divide the aortic diseases into two categories based on the acuity of the conditions (Table 9.2). Conditions in the category of acute aortic syndrome can be life threatening and need to be diagnosed promptly as surgical intervention is usually required to improve the outcome of the patients. In these patients, TEE is frequently the preferred choice due to its relative noninvasive nature and portability. The advantages and limitations of TEE in evaluating patients with aortic diseases are summarized in Table 9.3. In chronic aortic diseases, a more deliberate approach to assess the aorta can be taken and frequently computed tomography and magnetic resonance scan are preferred.

Table 9.1 Comparison of different imaging modalities for the assessment of the aorta

Diagnostic performance	Angiography	CT	MRI	TEE
Sensitivity	++	++	+++	+++
Specificity	+++	+++	+++	+++
Site of intimal tear	+/–	+/–	++	+++
Presence of thrombus	+/–	++	++	++
Pericardial effusion	–	++	++	+++
Branch vessel involvement	++	++	+++	+
Coronary artery involvement	++	+/–	–	++
No radiation exposure	–	–	+++	+++
Portability	–	–	–	+++

CT computed tomography, *MRI* magnetic resonance imaging, *TEE* transesophageal echocardiography
+++, excellent; ++, good; +, fair; –, not detected or poor
Source: Modified from Cigarroa et al. [5]

Table 9.2 Acute and chronic aortic diseases

Acute aortic syndrome
Dissection
Intramural hematoma
Rupture
Intimal tear with no hematoma
Penetrating ulcer
Aortic trauma
Chronic aortic diseases
Chronic dissection
Residual dissection post-repair
Large mobile thrombus
Aneurysm
Pseudoaneurysm
Aortitis
Atherosclerotic plaques
Aortic neoplasm

Table 9.3 Advantages and limitations of transesophageal echocardiography for the assessment of the aorta

Advantages
Portable
Rapid diagnosis
Does not interfere with resuscitation
No radiation exposure
Minimally invasive
Few complications
Limitations
Semi-invasive
Operator dependent
Blind spot in distal ascending aorta
Limited view of arch vessels
Abdominal aorta not imaged
Not applicable in patients with suspected esophageal or cervical injury

Acute Aortic Syndrome

Aortic Dissection

In acute aortic dissection, accurate and prompt diagnosis is essential as there is an increased mortality if there is a delay in making the diagnosis, with a 1% increase in mortality per hour for the first 24 h. When a clinical suspicion of aortic dissection arises, the patient should be considered for prompt investigation to rule in or rule out this diagnosis [6].

An aortic dissection is a split in the aortic media with hemorrhage between the two resulting medial layers (Figs. 9.5, 9.6). It forms part of the "acute aortic syndrome" along with penetrating aortic ulcer and intramural hematoma. An aortic dissection begins with an intimal tear which allows blood to enter and split the medial layers. An intramural hematoma is a collection of blood in the media without an apparent intimal tear. What causes the medial bleeding is unknown. By pathology many intramural hematomas are otherwise typical aortic dissections in which the intimal tear was not visible by imaging. Penetrating aortic ulcers are

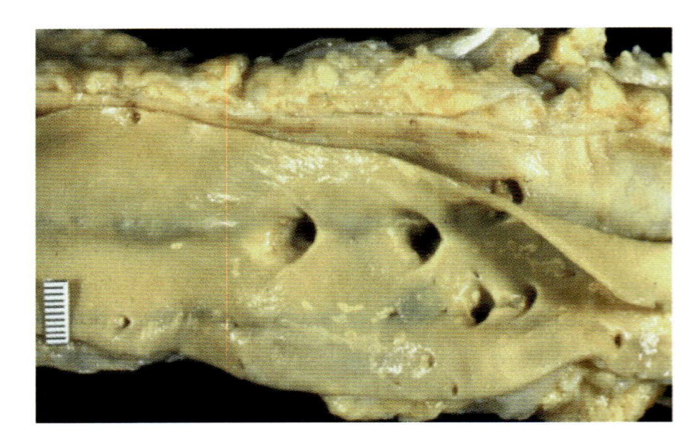

Fig. 9.5 Acute aortic dissection has resulted in split of the aorta in the medial layer

deep penetrating atheromas that extend through the vessel wall. They may rupture externally or lead to aortic dissection. They are commonly located in the proximal thoracic aorta.

Aortic dissections may be associated with many risk factors including increasing age, systemic arterial hypertension, connective tissue disease (including Marfan's, osteogenesis imperfecta, and Ehlers-Danlos), congenitally bicuspid aortic valve, aortic coarctation, aortic trauma (closed, open or iatrogenic), and hormonal-related dissection (estrogen/pregnancy) [6, 7]. The predisposing conditions of aortic dissection are summarized in Table 9.4.

Systemic arterial hypertension is the most common predisposing condition for the development of aortic dissection, but it has become increasingly recognized that familial aortopathy is an important cause. Marfan syndrome is well known for its predilection for dissection, but non-Marfan familial aortopathy is more prevalent and thus is an important consideration in patients with dissection. Dilated aorta is present in about one-third of patients with congenitally bicuspid aortic valve [8]. Patients with this condition are at risk for

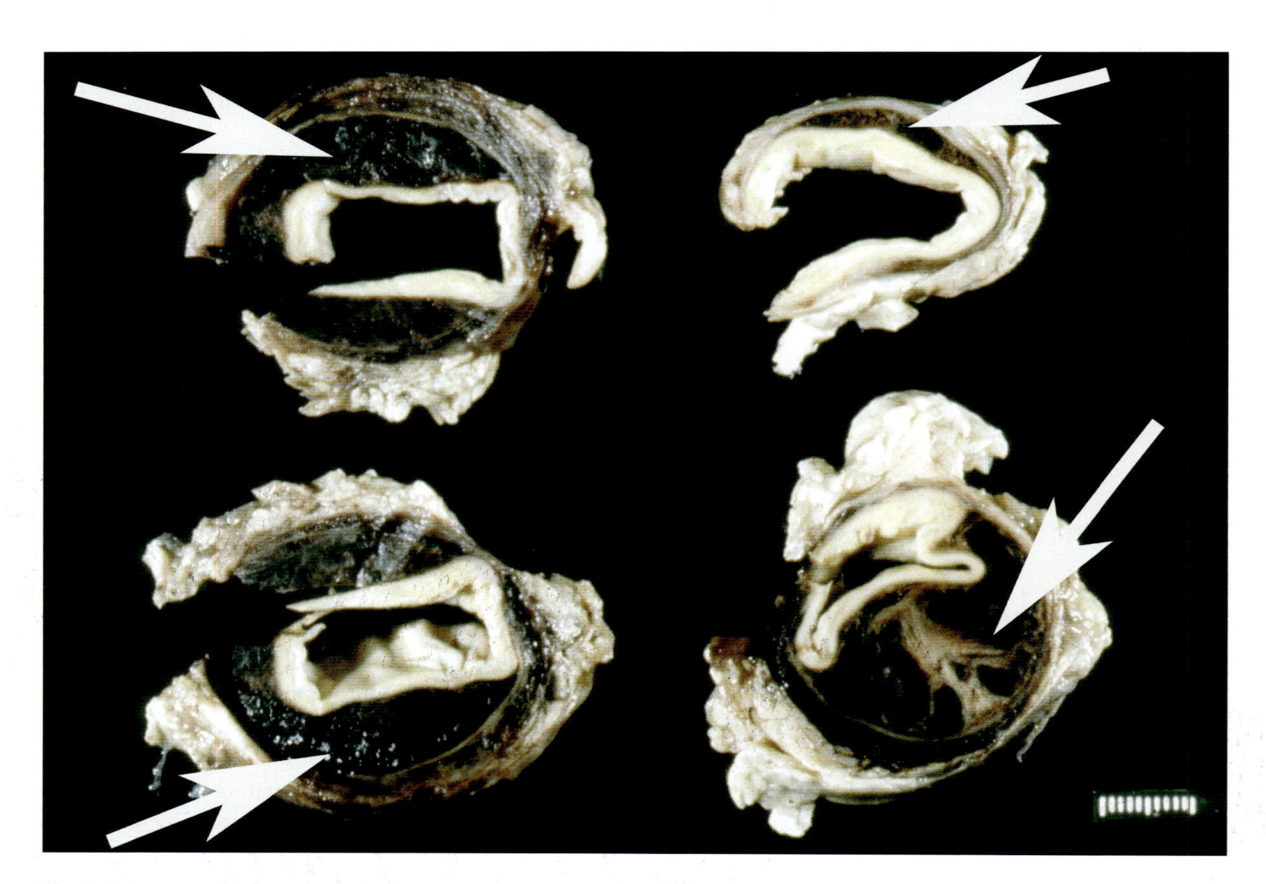

Fig. 9.6 Acute aortic dissection. The aorta has been cross sectioned demonstrating the blood clot in the false lumen (*arrows*). The true lumen of the aorta is still patent

Table 9.4 Predisposing conditions for aortic dissection

Systemic arterial hypertension
Familial aortopathy • Marfan • Non-Marfan • Others
Connective tissue disease
Congenitally bicuspid aortic valve
Coarctation of the aorta
Pregnancy
Aortitis
Aortic trauma • Cannulation, surgery • Blunt chest trauma

dissection even if the aorta is normal in size, and familial clustering has been reported. It is advisable to consider echocardiography screening of first-degree relatives for aortopathy, particularly in young patients with dissection.

Complications of aortic dissections commonly include aortic rupture, hemorrhage, vascular ostial branch compromise, and dilation of the ascending aorta with acute aortic valvular insufficiency and aneurysm formation (Fig. 9.7). Dissection is classified as type A, involving the ascending aorta, and type B, beginning after the takeoff of the right innominate artery. This dissection classification has clinical utility or meaning due to the associated complications with each type of pathology [9, 10].

Type A dissections may lead to severe complications involving the ascending aorta leading to aortic rupture in the pericardial sac with hemopericardium and tamponade, distortion and dehiscence of the aortic valve, and coronary arterial dissection with myocardial infarct. The dissection may propagate distally and involve the entire length of the aorta. Type B dissections, in contrast, usually have complications at or below the thoracic level. Although they may compromise spinal cord blood flow, cause visceral ischemia and limb loss, they are not associated with acute life-threatening emergencies such as tamponade [11]. Type A dissections should be surgically treated, whereas many type B dissections can be treated medically by reducing the force of contraction and lowering the dissection pressure.

In type A dissections the intimal tear is usually in the ascending aorta (Fig. 9.8), but rarely the intimal tear may be in the descending aorta, with the ascending aorta involved from retrograde extension of dissection. Intimal entry tears on the right side of the aorta are more commonly described. Type B dissections have tears in the descending thoracic aorta and do not involve the ascending aorta.

Underlying aortic medial degenerative changes are often observed. This pathology has been termed "cystic medial necrosis" but this is a misnomer and the term aortic medial degenerative change is preferred [12]. These degenerative medial changes consist of

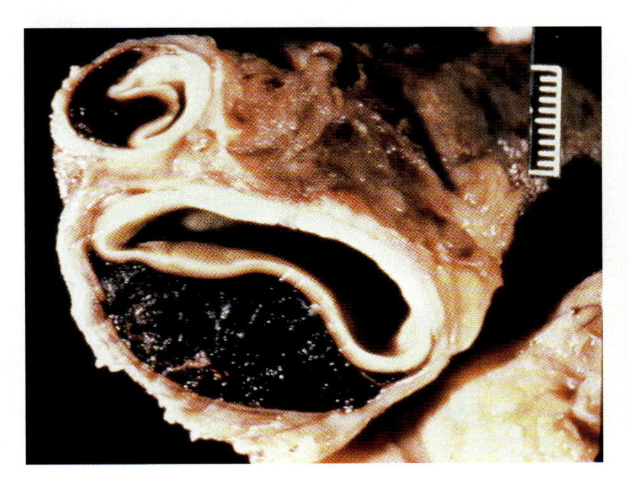

Fig. 9.7 The acute aortic dissection has split the media in the arch blood vessels. The blood clot can be seen compressing the normal lumen

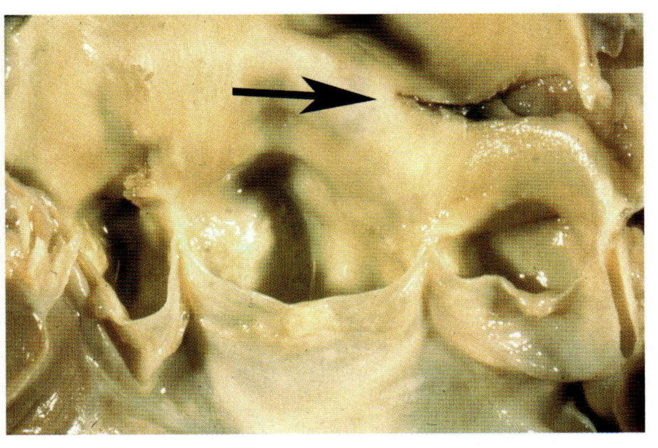

Fig. 9.8 Opened ascending aorta and aortic valve. The intimal tear (*arrow*) of the acute aortic dissection is located shortly after the valve. The ascending aorta is the most common site of the intimal tear in type A dissection

elastic fragmentation, accumulation of glycosaminoglycans, medionecrosis and medial fibrosis. It is the ground substance accumulation and the elastic fragmentation that are thought to lead to a propensity to aortic weakness and dissection. Some degree of medial degeneration is a normal age-related phenomenon that occurs unevenly throughout the aorta [13]. Systemic arterial hypertension accelerates these degenerative changes. The medial degenerative changes are also very marked in connective tissue disorders such as Marfan's, Ehlars Danlos and osteogenesis imperfecta. Mutations of collagen and fibrillin are implicated through their effects on transforming growth factor beta (TGF beta) activation [14].

In our experience, TEE is the preferred imaging modality as it has a good diagnostic accuracy and can be promptly performed at the bedside. Due to the intimate relationship between the thoracic aorta and the esophagus, the thoracic aorta can generally be very well imaged using the transesophageal approach. From a practical point of view, patients with suspected aortic dissection should have received optimal medical treatment before the TEE study. These treatments should include agents to blunt the hemodynamic responses. Adequate sedation is essential for the same reason.

The echocardiographic findings of aortic dissections are intimal flap, intimal tear, dilated aorta, increased aortic wall thickness and presence of aortic regurgitation [1, 15] (Figs. 9.9, 9.10). In patients with adequate images, these findings may be detected by transthoracic echocardiography. Beyond making a diagnosis, it is important to determine the locations of

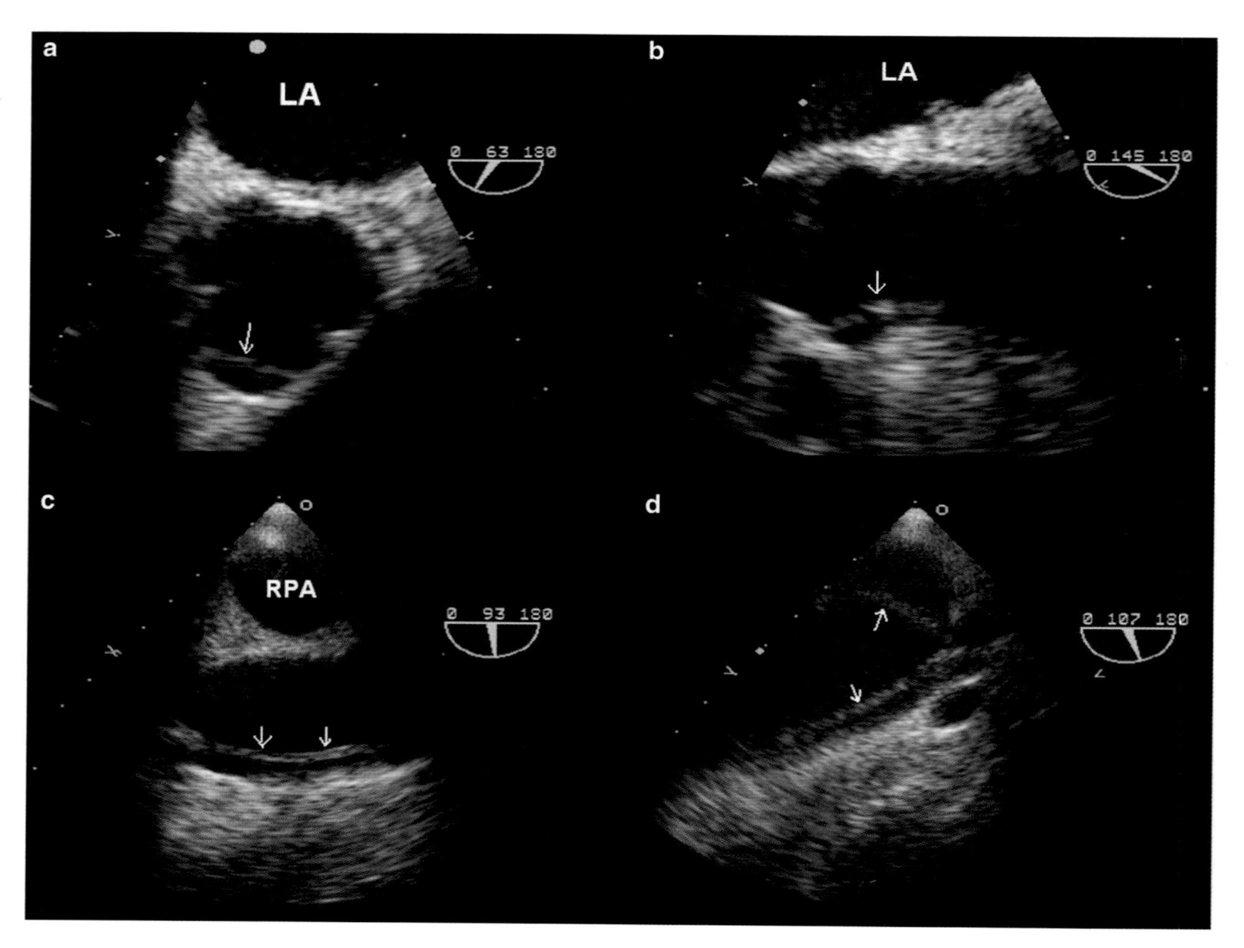

Fig. 9.9 The transesophageal views of a patient with type A aortic dissection are shown. The dissection flap (*arrow*) is imaged in multiple views. It starts in the right aortic sinus (**a**) and extends to involve the ascending aorta to the aortic arch (**b, c, d**). The intimal flap involves one of the arch vessels (**d**). *LA* left atrium, *RPA* right pulmonary artery

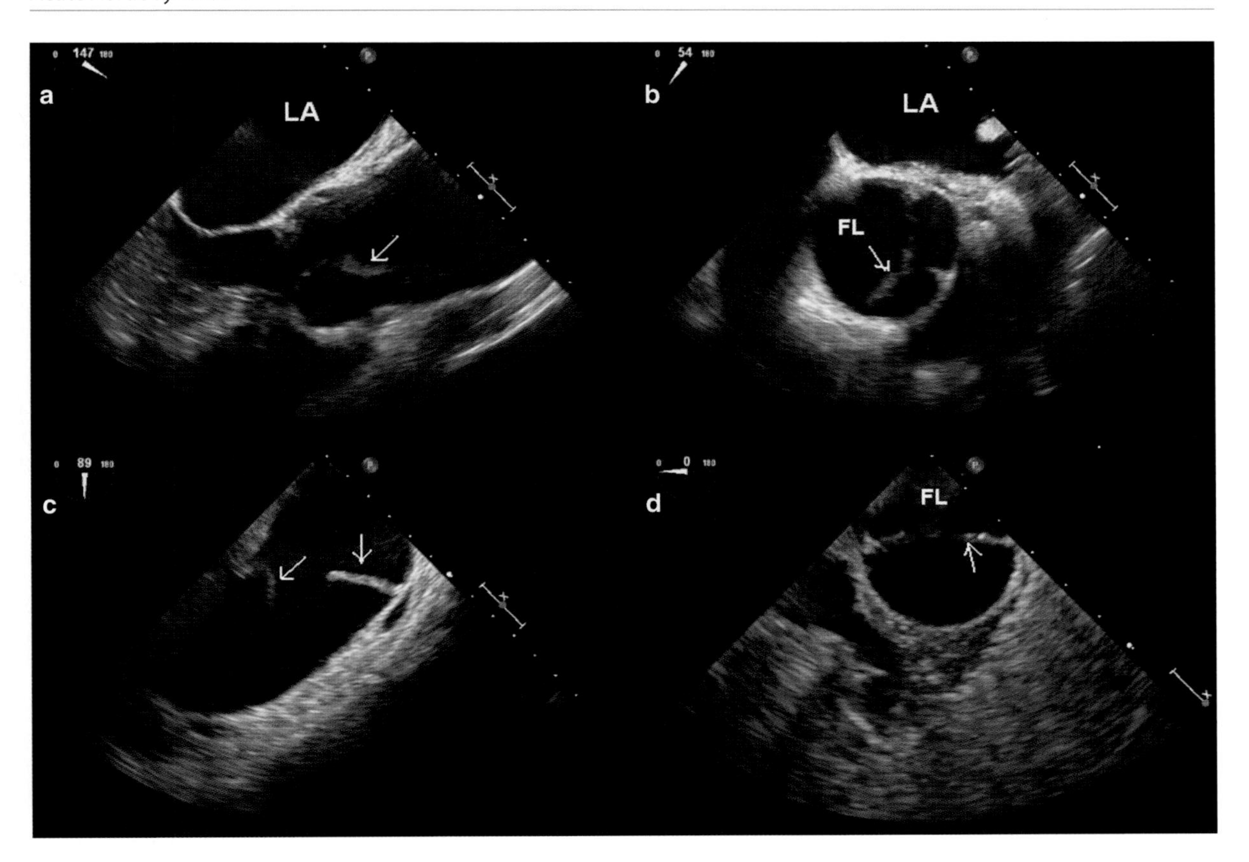

Fig. 9.10 In this patient with aortic dissection, the transesophageal echocardiographic views show that the dissection involves the entire ascending aorta (**a, b**). The aortic arch (**c**) and the descending thoracic aorta (**d**). The intimal flap (*arrow*) is imaged in all the different segments of the aorta. A large intimal tear is detected in the aortic arch (**c**)

the tears, the extent of the dissection flap, the status of the arch vessels, involvement of the coronary ostia, presence and severity of aortic regurgitation, and left ventricular function. Other serious complications of aortic dissection should also be assessed. These include aortic rupture with tamponade, severe disruption of aortic valvular function resulting in severe acute aortic regurgitation, and acute disruption of flow to vital organs such as the brain and the kidneys.

Elucidation of the mechanism of aortic regurgitation may allow the performance of valve sparing procedure with re-suspension of the aortic valve in selected patients (Figs. 9.11, 9.12) [16]. The dissection flap tends to involve the aortic lumen along its greater curvature such that the false lumen is more likely to be located anterior and rightward in the aortic root and posterior and leftward in the descending thoracic aorta. Other echo findings that are useful to differentiate the true lumen from the false lumen are summarized in the Table 9.5 (Fig. 9.13).

False-positive cases for aortic dissection have been encountered with computed tomography [17]. A linear density typical of an intimal flap may occasionally be seen in the ascending aorta just above the aortic valve in patients without dissection. This "intimal flap" is focal with the rest of the aorta appearing normal. This artifact is likely related to cardiac motion, and generally not present when the ECG-gated scan is performed (Figs. 9.14, 9.15). This is an important artifact to recognize, since computed tomography is frequently used in the assessment of patients with suspected dissection.

Intramural Hematoma

The presentation of aortic intramural hematoma simulates that of acute aortic dissection [18]. Indeed, in many instances of intramural hematoma, progression to aortic dissection takes place (Fig. 9.16) [19, 20].

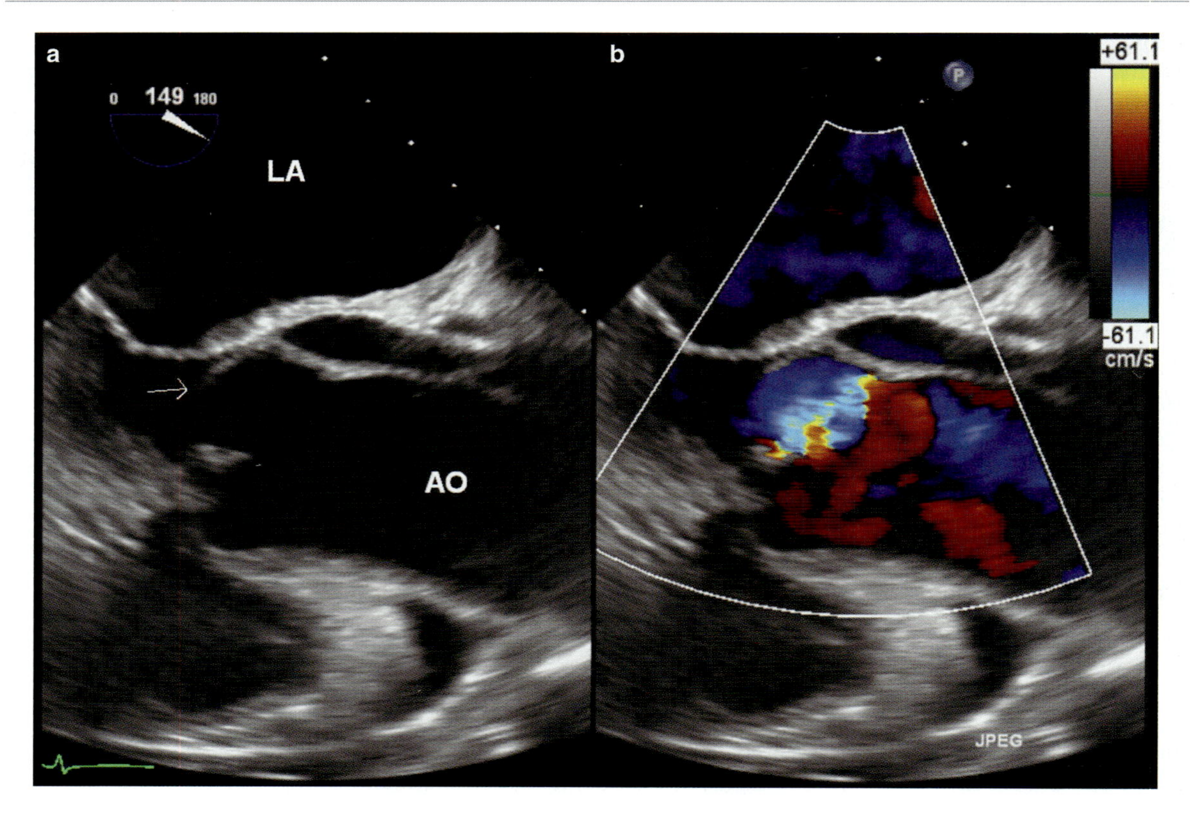

Fig. 9.11 In this patient with type A aortic dissection (**a, b**), the dissection flap extends down to the aortic annulus undermining the noncoronary cusp which demonstrates a marked degree of prolapse resulting in aortic regurgitation. *Ao* aorta, *LA* left atrium

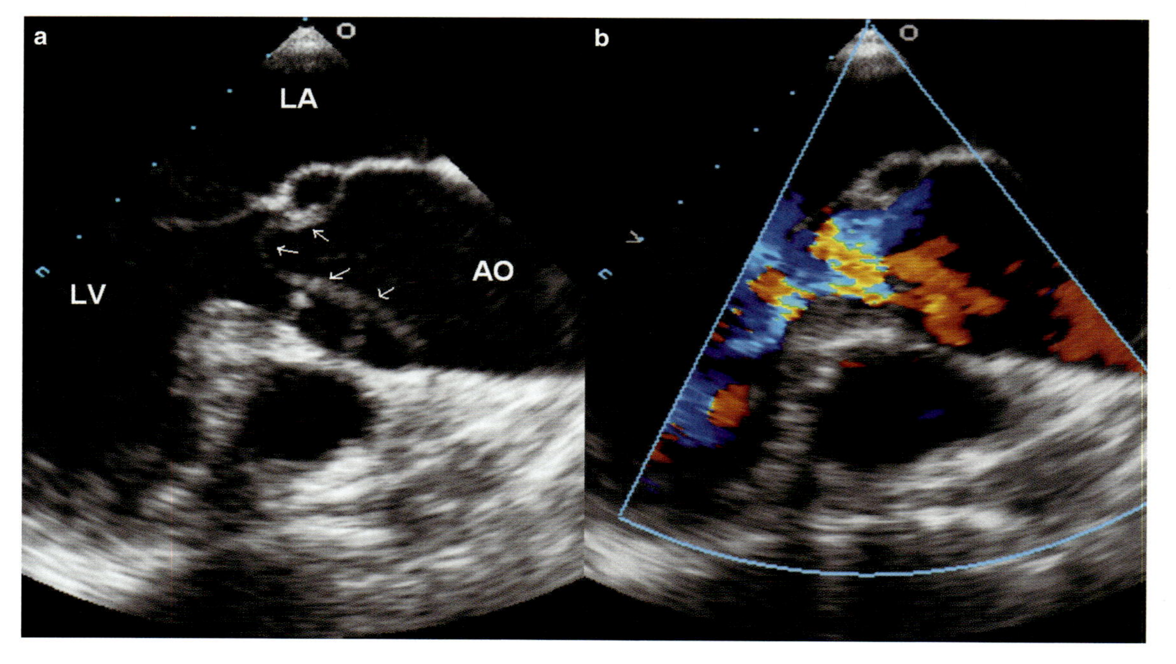

Fig. 9.12 In this patient with type A aortic dissection (**a, b**), the dissection flap is circumferential and protrudes into the aortic orifice during diastole resulting in aortic regurgitation. *Ao* aorta, *LA* left atrium, *LV* left ventricle

Table 9.5 Features differentiating a true lumen from a false lumen in aortic dissection

Location	• Rightward and anterior in the aortic root • Leftward and posterior in the descending aorta
Intimal flap	• Concave to the true lumen during systole
Intimal tear	• Flow into false lumen in systole and into true lumen in diastole
Spontaneous contrast	• More pronounced in the false lumen

This condition can account for up to 15% of patients presenting with acute aortic syndrome. The diagnosis of this condition is more difficult compared to typical aortic dissection. The typical echocardiographic findings are listed in the Table 9.6. In the early stage of this disease, the intramural hematoma may be limited and thus the crescent thickening of the aortic wall may be minimal (Fig. 9.17). Management of these patients is similar to patients with classic aortic dissection. If the aortic hematoma involves the ascending aorta, surgery should be considered, since up to half of these patients will progress to develop classic dissection. About 15–20% of the patients may proceed to develop rupture and up to 30% of patients may demonstrate resolution (Figs. 9.18, 9.19). Follow-up of these patients provides important prognostic information to guide the management. Gradual resolution of the aortic wall thickness supports the continuation of medical treatment [20]. On the other hand, extension of the intramural hematoma or cavitation forming a false lumen is a good indication that surgery may be necessary.

Aortic Rupture and Aortic Tear

Aortic rupture can be a complication resulting from aortic dissection or intramural hematoma. It may be a primary event on rare occasions. When the descending aorta is involved, aortic rupture is usually associated with penetrating atherosclerotic ulcer [21]. When the ascending aorta is involved, the best sign appears to be the detection of hematoma within the pericardium in the setting of a dilated ascending aorta, as the site of

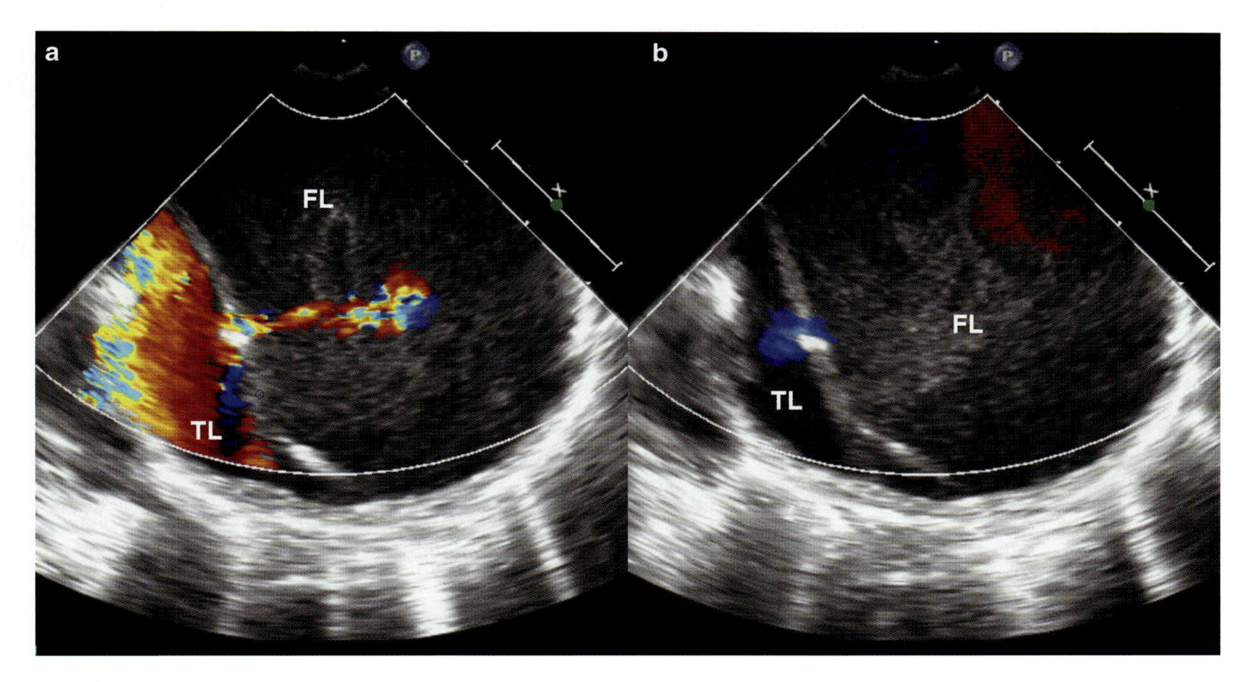

Fig. 9.13 The transesophageal images of the descending aorta show the presence of an intimal flap, a small true lumen, and a large false lumen. Systolic flow from the true lumen into the false lumen is shown in (**a**), and diastolic low velocity flow from the false lumen into the true lumen is shown in (**b**). *FL* false lumen, *TL* true lumen

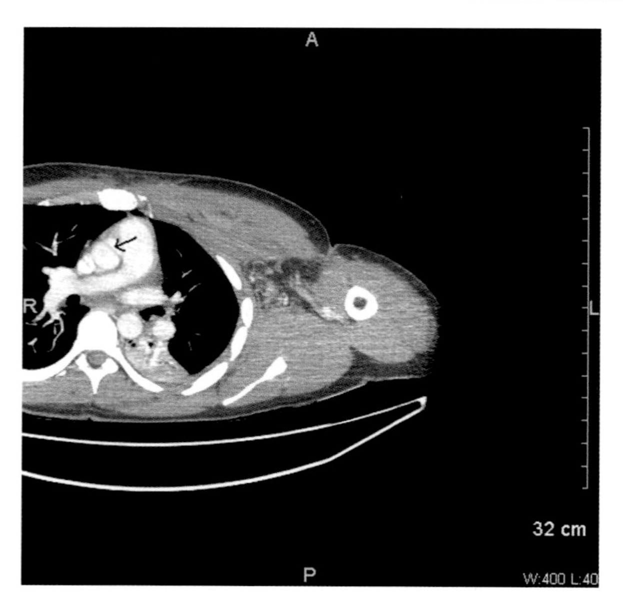

Fig. 9.14 This is a CT scan in a 22-year-old man presenting with chest pain. A linear density within the ascending aorta (*arrow*) is present. Based on the finding, the patient was taken into the Operating Room for aortic surgery. Intraoperative transesophageal echocardiogram showed no evidence of aortic dissection

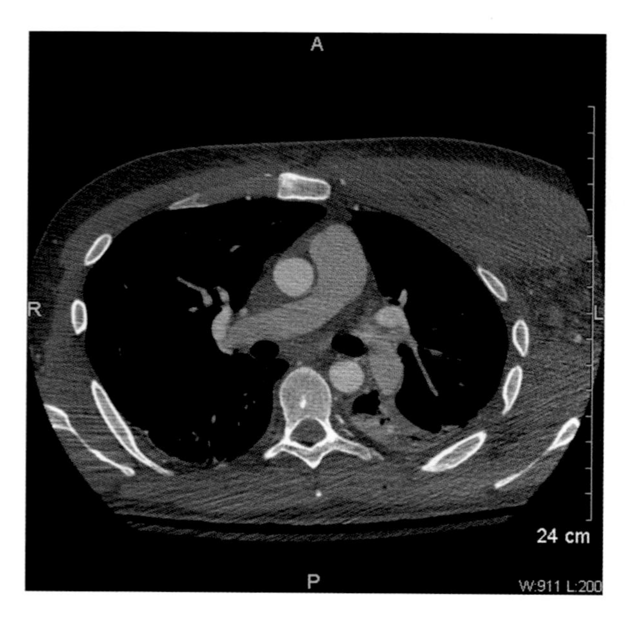

Fig. 9.15 This is the repeat ECG gated CT scan on the same patient as shown in Fig. 9.14. The aorta is normal with no evidence of intimal flap

rupture is frequently difficult to identify (Figs. 9.20, 9.21). Another related condition is aortic tear with localized hematoma but no obvious false lumen [22]. The aortic tear is usually located in the aortic root. The intimal tear can be difficult to identify since there is no associated false lumen. This condition can be difficult to diagnose even with the use of multiple different imaging modalities including angiography, computed tomography, and magnetic resonance imaging (Figs. 9.22, 9.23, 9.24). Careful attention to assess the integrity of the intima is essential if this condition is suspected.

Iatrogenic Aortic Dissection or Intramural Hematoma

Iatrogenic aortic dissection or intramural hematoma can result from invasive cardiac procedures including angiography and coronary intervention. Sakamoto et al. identified six cases after reviewing about 15,500 angiographic procedures [23]. The dissection can be focal or extensive. For patients with iatrogenic aortic injury related to coronary interventions, the dissection or intramural hematoma is generally localized to and near the coronary ostia (Fig. 9.25). There is a high likelihood of spontaneous resolution as the underlying aortic tissue is usually relatively normal (Fig. 9.26). These complications can also occur at the site of aortic cannulation, bypass graft ostia, or cross clamp site after cardiac surgery. TEE is the best modality to follow the progression or resolution of this condition, although computed tomography is also frequently used in these patients [23].

Penetrating Aortic Ulcer

Penetrating aortic ulcer generally involves the descending aorta [18, 21]. It is frequently associated with moderate or severe atherosclerotic plaques. Patients with this condition have a high prevalence of atherosclerotic risk factors including systemic arterial hypertension. This is an unusual condition accounting for less than 5% of patients presenting with acute aortic syndrome. In the proximal thoracic aorta the atheromatous plaque may develop a localized ulcer that is deeply penetrating through the aortic wall, eventually resulting in a false aneurysm (Figs. 9.27, 9.28). The penetrating

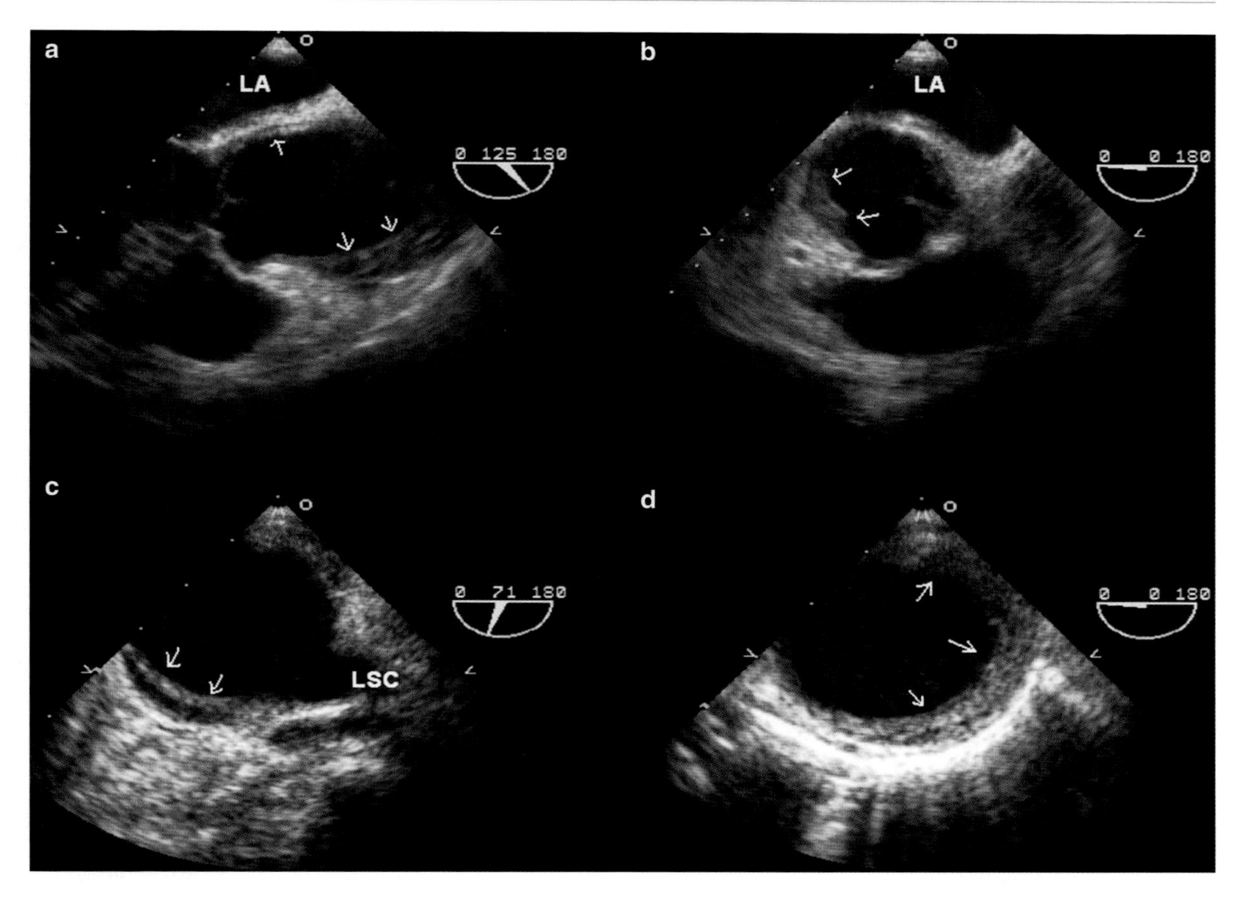

Fig. 9.16 This is a patient with extensive aortic intramural hematoma involving the ascending aorta (**a, b**). The aortic arch (**c**) and the descending thoracic aorta (**d**). The intramural hematoma (*arrows*) is crescentric in shape and somewhat echolucent. No false lumen is present. *LA* left atrium, *LSC* left subclavian artery

Table 9.6 Echocardiographic features of aortic intramural hematoma

• Circular or crescent thickening of aortic wall (>5 mm in thickness)
• May have echolucent areas within the thickening
• No intimal tear seen
• No communication with the aortic lumen
• Intimal calcification is displaced towards the lumen

aortic ulcer may present as an acute aortic syndrome and is associated with complications such as aortic rupture or dissection. By gross morphology the "ulcer" is a deep localized outpouching with an atheroma (Fig. 9.29). The penetrating ulcer may be flask-like in shape similar to other false aneurysms. Overhanging edges of the adjacent aorta may form a lip of the flask covering the underlying large protrusion which undermines the aorta.

Traumatic Aortic Injury

Traumatic aortic injury can present with a wide range of aortic manifestations ranging from localized intramural hematoma or dissection to transection [24]. The findings of intramural hematoma or dissection due to trauma are similar to the findings of nontraumatic cases, except that these findings are more focal and tend to be localized to the proximal descending aorta near the origin of the left subclavian artery (Fig. 9.30). In the case of transection, the aorta demonstrates an indistinct aortic wall at the region of the proximal

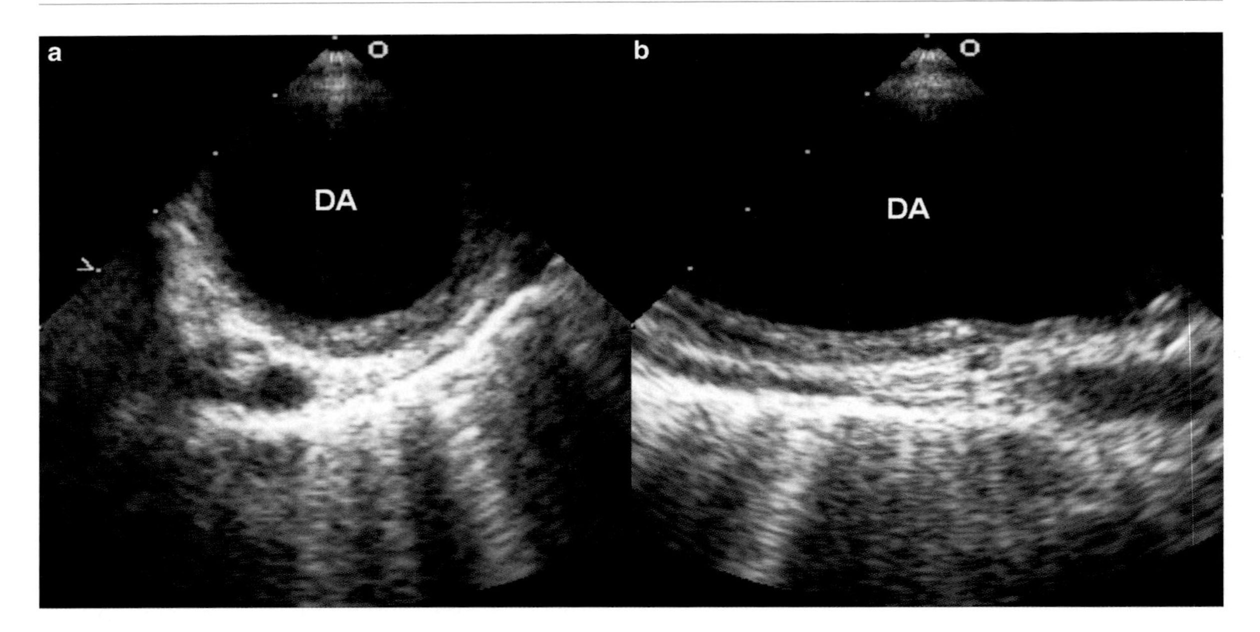

Fig. 9.17 The transesophageal transverse (**a**) and longitudinal (**b**) views in a patient with intramural hematoma show typical features involving the descending thoracic aorta. *DA* descending aorta

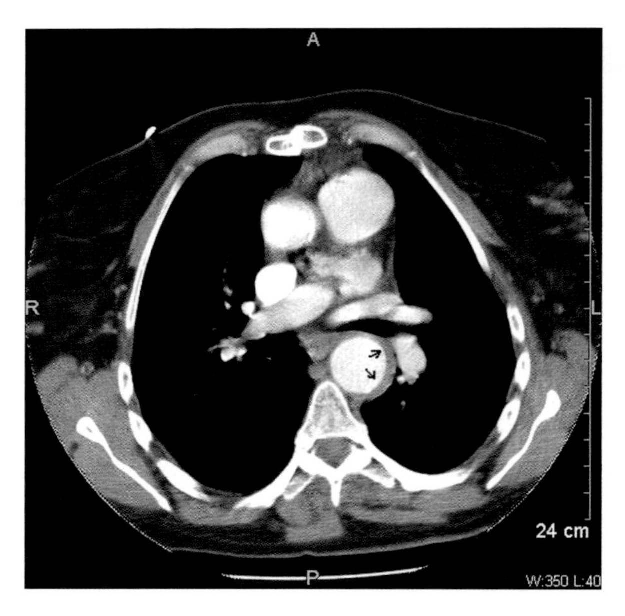

Fig. 9.18 The computed tomogram of a 46-year-old woman with Marfan syndrome and severe lower back pain shows crescentric thickness of the descending thoracic aorta (*arrows*) consistent with intramural hematoma

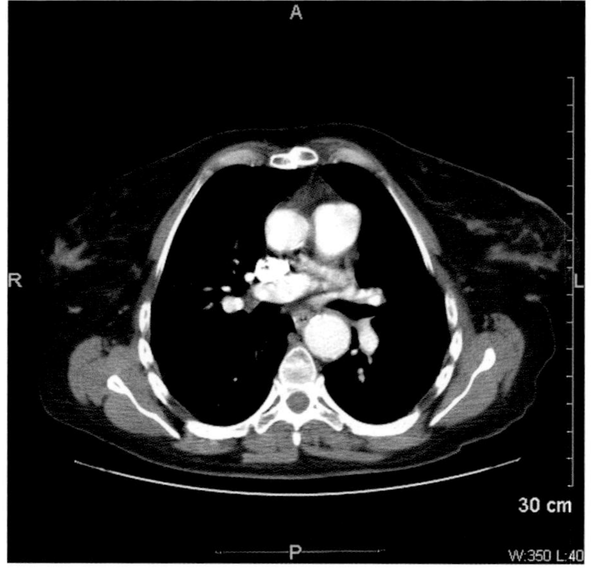

Fig. 9.19 A repeat computed tomogram 5 months later of the same patient in Fig. 9.18 shows complete resolution of the intramural hematoma

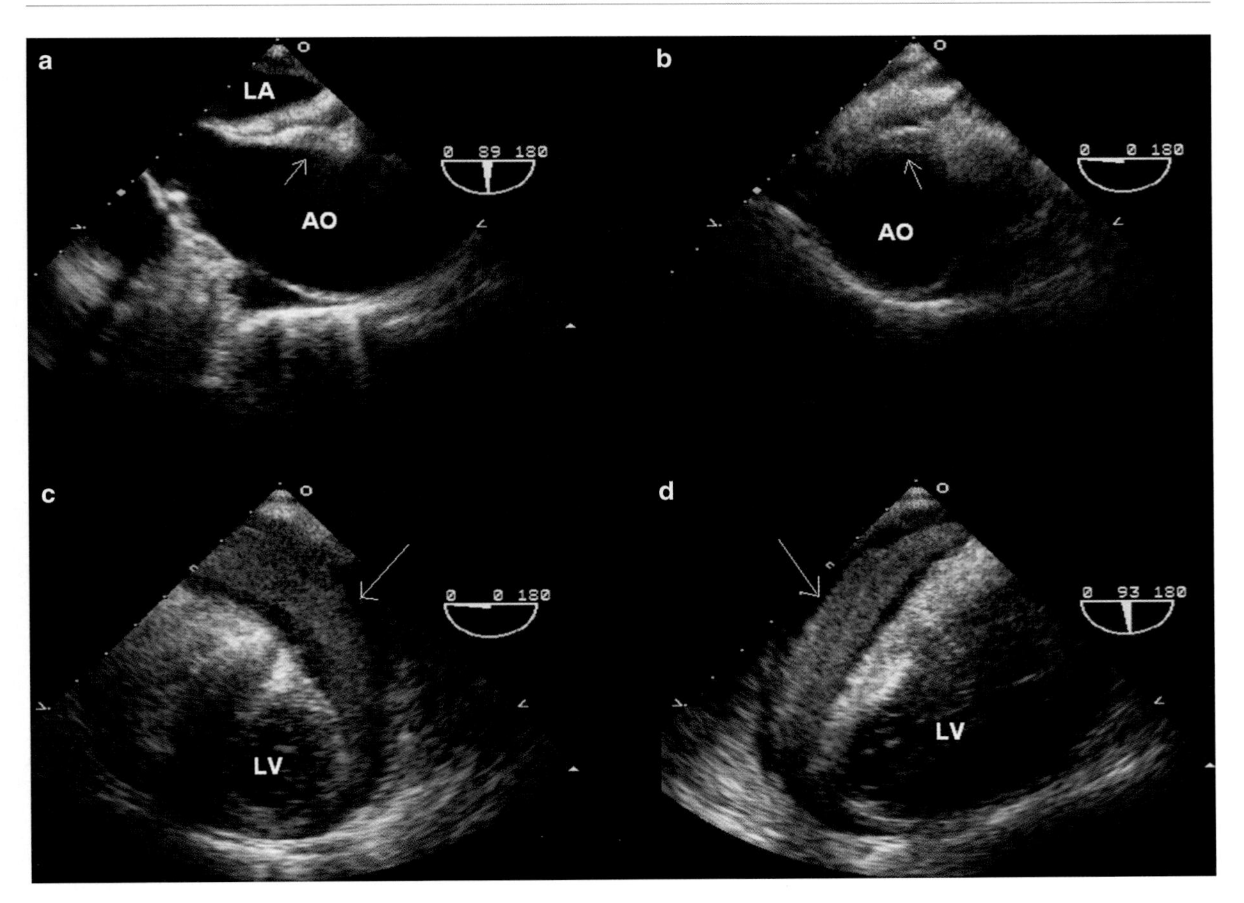

Fig. 9.20 Urgent transesophageal echocardiogram of a 79-year-old woman with shock and severe chest pain shows no false lumen or intimal flap. In the aortic long-axis (**a**) and short-axis (**b**) views a focal area of thickness involving the posterior aortic wall (*arrow*) is present. The transgastric short-axis (**c**) and long-axis (**d**) views show an echo dense pericardial effusion (*arrow*) consistent with hematoma. The left ventricle is small in size with normal systolic function. Primary aortic rupture with hemopericardium was confirmed at surgery. *Ao* aorta, *LA* left atrium, *LV* left ventricle

descending aorta and an increase in wall thickness associated with extrinsic hematoma. Like many of the other conditions in the acute aortic syndrome, a high index of suspicion is required to detect aortic transection which requires urgent surgical intervention.

In patients with suspected acute aortic syndrome, a negative imaging test, be it TEE or computed tomogram, may not necessarily rule out the diagnosis, as a number of the conditions such as aortic tear without false lumen or intramural hematoma may be difficult to detect with any one imaging modality. If the clinical suspicion is high, admission of the patient with follow-up imaging tests are indicated since the consequences of a missed diagnosis can be serious. After excluding acute aortic syndrome, acute coronary syndrome should be considered as, in our experience, it is the actual diagnosis in many of these patients [15]. It should be realized that the two may coexist because the aortic pathology may compromise the coronary artery ostia or result in severe acute aortic valve insufficiency leading to coronary insufficiency.

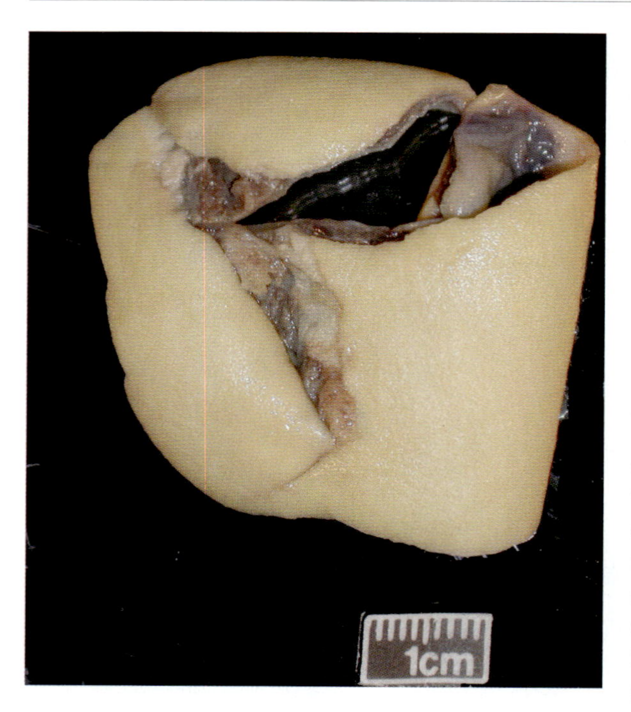

Fig. 9.21 The excised ascending aorta from patient in Fig. 9.20. The aorta has no intimal flaps but has extensive disruption of the intima with underlying blood. Interestingly the aorta only had mild medial degenerative changes. However, there was a congenitally bicuspid aortic valve with degenerative changes, also replaced at the same surgery

Chronic Aortic Diseases

Although diseases in this category such as aortitis may have an acute clinical onset, they are not considered to be an acute aortic syndrome, which includes only conditions that have a high immediate mortality and require prompt surgical intervention in most cases in addition to the acute presentation. TEE is also useful in patients with chronic aortic diseases due to its ability to provide a comprehensive assessment of the thoracic aorta.

Aortic Dissection Post-Repair

Patients who have had surgery for aortic dissection are an important patient group for close follow-up [25–27]. These patients remain at an increased risk for death and recurrent aortic complications such as extension of dissection, further aneurysmal expansion, pseudoaneurysm formation, aortic rupture, and progression of aortic valve insufficiency. A combined transthoracic and transesophageal approach should be used if the aortic involvement extends to involve the abdominal aorta. Many of these patients would also benefit from other imaging modalities, particularly computed tomography and magnetic resonance imaging.

Replacing the ascending aorta in a patient with extensive dissection of the entire thoracic aorta, including the aortic arch and descending thoracic aorta, should be considered a palliative procedure, because most of these patients will have persistent dissection beyond the distal anastomosis of the aortic tube graft and are at risk for complications associated with dissection (Figs. 9.31, 9.32). The double lumen aorta is prone to ongoing expansion, and invasive intentions, such as surgery or intravascular stenting, will need to be considered, as the risk of aortic rupture increases proportionally to the size of the aorta [28]. The intimal flap and intimal tear(s) can be important to patient management. Obstruction of flow in the true lumen may occur when there is a large proximal tear but no distal tears. Relief of the obstruction can be achieved by performing fenestration of the intimal flap. Progressive increase in thrombus formation in the false lumen may suggest future complete thrombosis of the false lumen, which is a good prognostic sign [28]. Table 9.7 summarizes the important TEE findings in these patients.

Chronic Aortic Aneurysm

An aneurysm is a localized abnormal dilatation of a vessel. This contrasts with vascular ectasia, which is a lengthier or more diffuse dilatation of a vessel. There are congenital cerebral berry aneurysms, but most other vascular aneurysms are acquired. Genetic predisposition is increasingly recognized as a common cause of aortic aneurysms and the abdominal aortic aneurysm is the most common site affected (Figs. 9.33, 9.34) [29]. Other causes of aneurysm are toxic/drug related, infectious, metabolic, immune/inflammatory, neoplastic, traumatic, and mechanical related.

Atherosclerosis is a common cause of ascending aortic aneurysm. The ascending aorta may become aneurysmal leading to aortic regurgitation as the valve cusps do not coapt any longer (Fig. 9.35). In the patients with aortic regurgitation in the setting of a

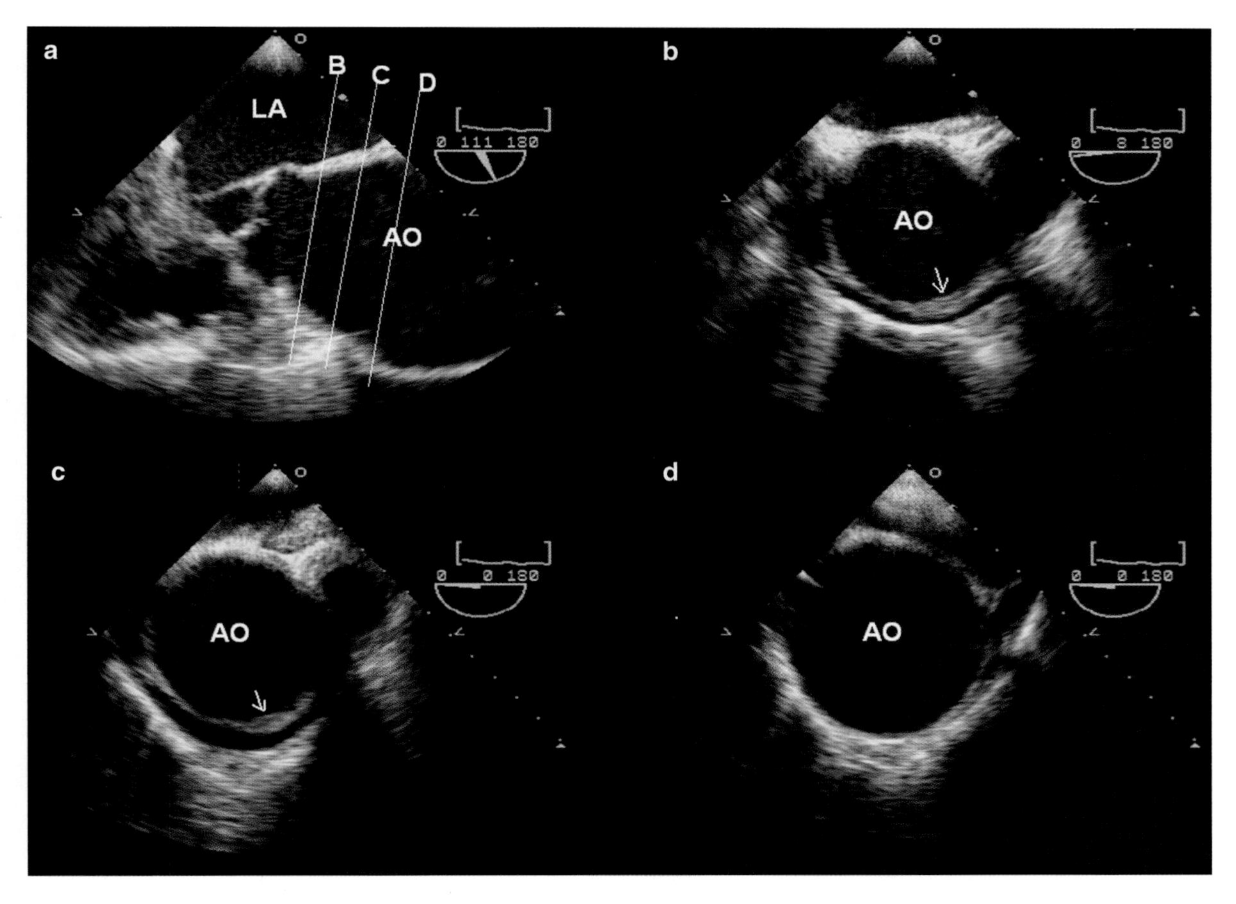

Fig. 9.22 Transesophageal echocardiogram in a 78-year-old woman with severe chest pain shows that the ascending aorta is aneurysmally dilated (**a**). Multiple short-axis views (**b, c, d**) of the ascending aorta show a focal thickening (*arrows*) of the anterior aortic wall just beyond the sinotubular junction (**b, c**). A small pericardial effusion is present. *Ao* aorta, *LA* left atrium

dilated aorta, careful assessment of the aortic valve is required because a valve sparing procedure may be feasible in many of these patients. Other complications of aneurysms include stasis, thrombosis, vascular obstruction, embolism, mass effect, and rupture. Aneurysms may also be true or false, and saccular or fusiform in shape.

Although Marfan patients frequently have ascending aortic aneurysms, most ascending aortic aneurysms are due to other causes including atherosclerosis, infectious, immune related or degenerative processes (Fig. 9.36). Atheroma may be marked in the aorta and if calcified may give rise to a "porcelain" aorta, a heavily calcified aorta on imaging. The ascending aorta is a source of embolic material–atheroma constituents or thrombus, and is often evaluated in a search for a source after a transient ischemic attack or a cerebral event.

Aortic Pseudoaneurysm

Aortic pseudoaneurysm may be an incidental finding since it may be a long-term complication of traumatic aortic injury such as closed chest trauma in a motor vehicle accident, if it is located at or near the proximal descending thoracic aorta (Fig. 9.37), or a complication of previous aortic surgery such as surgical correction for coarctation (Figs. 9.38, 9.39) [30, 31]. The pseudoaneurysm develops as a result of contained leakage at the site of the anastomosis of the surgical

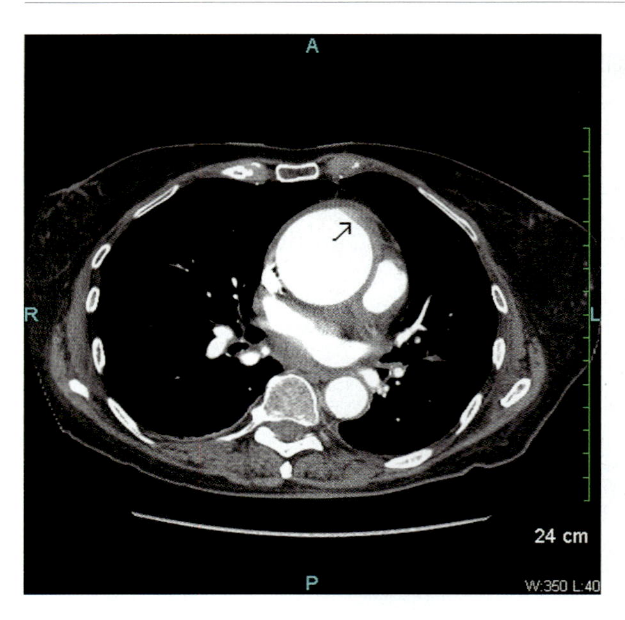

Fig. 9.23 Computed tomogram of the same patient as in Fig. 9.22 shows mild thickening of the anterior aortic wall (*arrow*). There is no intimal flap or false lumen

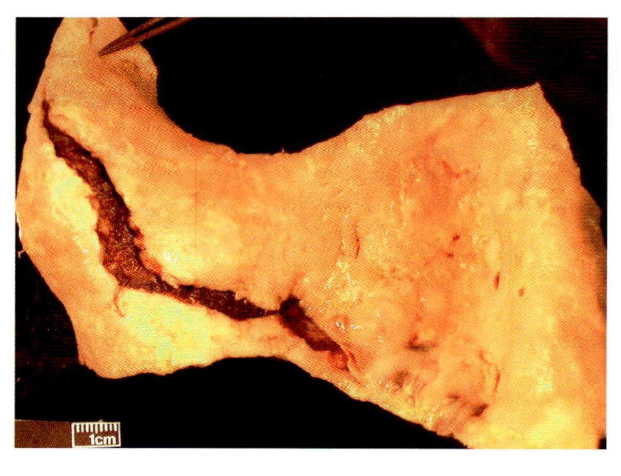

Fig. 9.24 Excised ascending aorta from same patient as Figs. 9.22 and 9.23. The aorta has a large horizontal tear with intimal disruption, but no intimal flap. The media had moderate to severe medial degenerative changes but no aortitis

patch or graft. Pseudoaneurysms may progressively enlarge (Fig. 9.40). Although the natural history of pseudoaneurysm is not well defined, invasive intervention is generally indicated to minimize the risk of acute rupture. The echo findings of the aortic pseudoaneurysm are summarized in the Table 9.8.

Aortitis

Ascending aortic aneurysms may also be infectious or immune related, a condition termed aortitis [32]. The typical echo finding is diffuse thickening of the aortic wall. With treatment there can be rapid resolution of the wall thickness. Aneurysm formation and localized narrowing may be the long-term sequelae. Aortitis causes medial destruction with subsequent aortic dilatation [33, 34]. Syphilis remains a common infectious cause of ascending aortic aneurysm worldwide. Aortic aneurysm is a manifestation of tertiary syphilitic disease. The intimal surfaces grossly show fibrous white thickening, a change termed "tree barking." The media is usually of normal thickness or it may be thin if there is significant aneurysm dilatation. By microscopy the infection causes a giant cell aortitis with medial destruction. The media tends to fibrose, so aortic dissection is not a complication. If large, the syphilitic aneurysm may erode into adjacent mediastinal structures or displace them. This can be manifest as hoarseness (recurrent laryngeal nerve displacement), dysphagia or dyspnea. Rupture leading to hemopericardium or hemothorax may be fatal.

Bacterial infections including tuberculosis and salmonella can cause aortitis (Fig. 9.41). Tuberculosis, still a common infection worldwide, may cause aortic aneurysms. The thoracic aorta is most often affected with thoracic aneurysms due to direct infection and destruction of the media. The aorta may also develop so-called "traction" aneurysms when the adjacent infected lymph nodes pull on the aortic adventitia and cause local dilation.

Immune-related aortitis has many causes [34]. Primary giant cell aortitis is a disease of unknown cause that may cause aneurysms and dissection. It occurs in individuals over the age of 50 and probably is autoimmune related. Some cases are associated with more generalized vasculitis, including temporal arteritis with polymyalgia rheumatica. Giant cell aortitis causes medial destruction and aortic weakness (Fig. 9.42). It causes tissue necrosis and little or no fibrosis, hence the propensity for aortic dilation and dissection. Patients with temporal arteritis need to be assessed for aortitis and vice versa [35].

Other autoimmune disease may be associated with aortitis (Fig. 9.43). For example, ankylosing spondylitis may cause giant cell aortitis and aneurysms and the aortic valve cusps may have scar retraction further

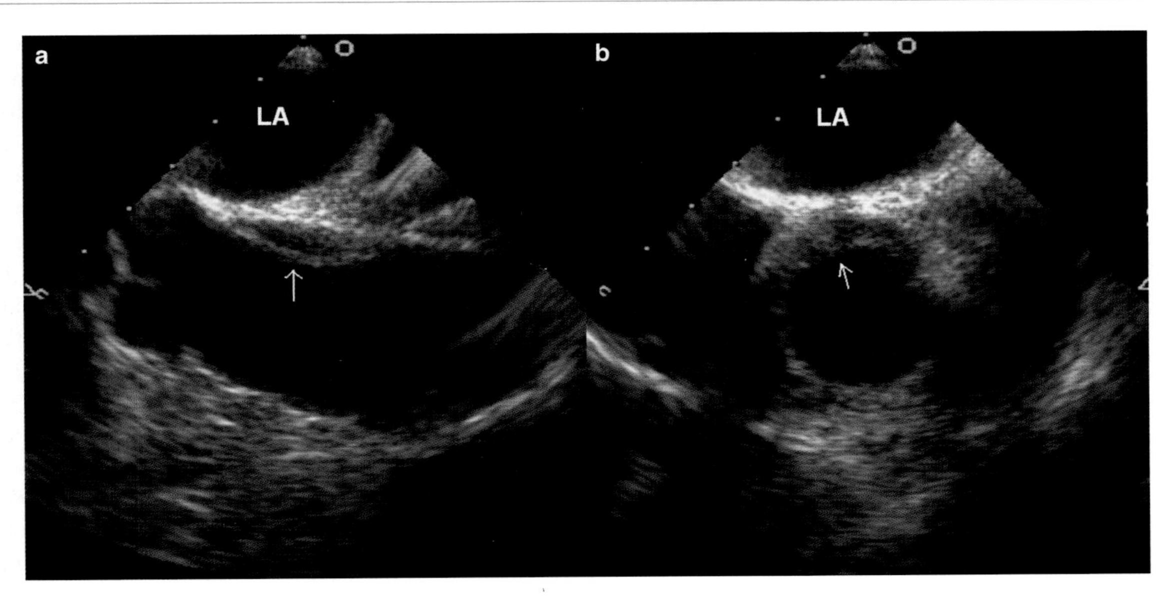

Fig. 9.25 This is a patient who develops focal aortic dissection involving the ascending aorta during cardiac catheterization. The focal dissection (*arrow*) is shown in the aortic long-axis (**a**) and short-axis (**b**) views. *LA* left atrium

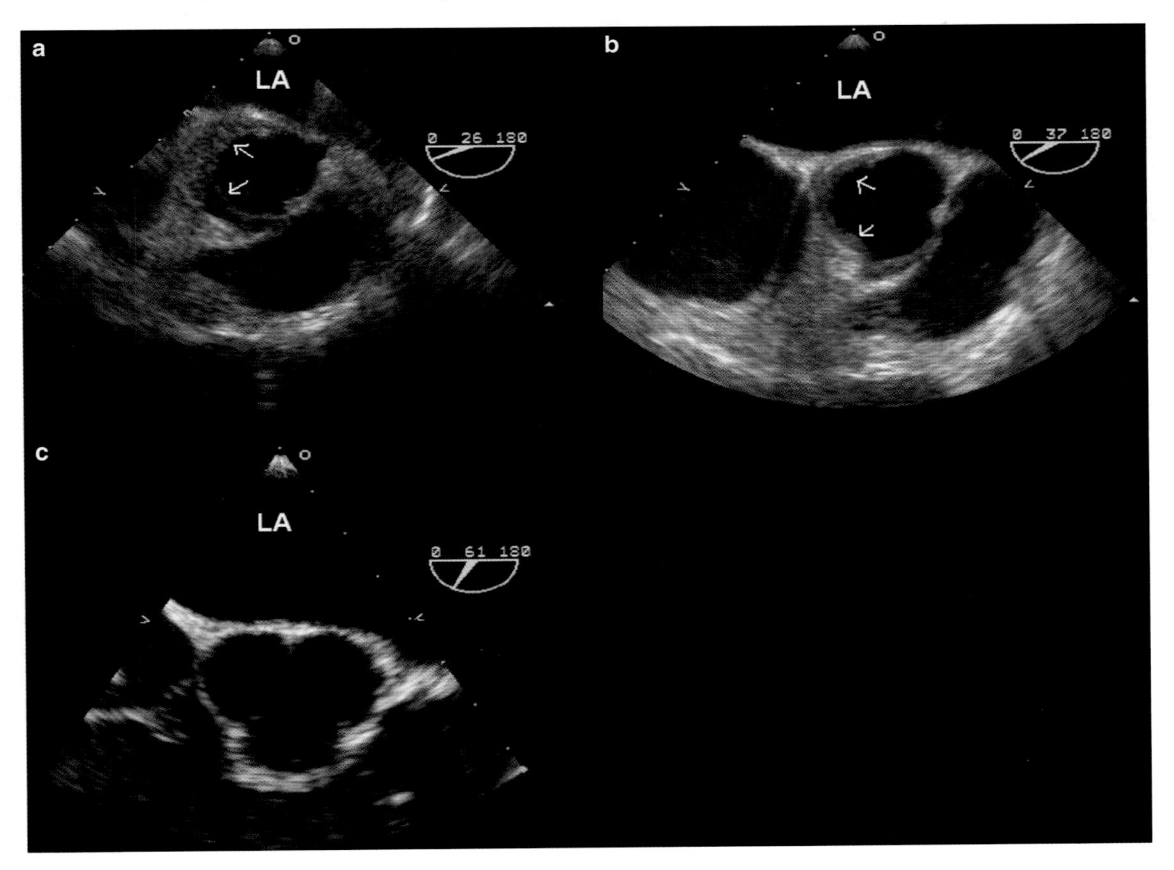

Fig. 9.26 The transesophageal short-axis view of the aortic root in a patient with aortic dissection caused by coronary intervention shows the evolutional changes. The image in (**a**) is obtained on the day of the procedure, (**b**) at 1 week after the procedure and (**c**) at 3 weeks after the procedure. There is progressive resolution of the intramural hematoma such that by 3 weeks, there is complete resolution

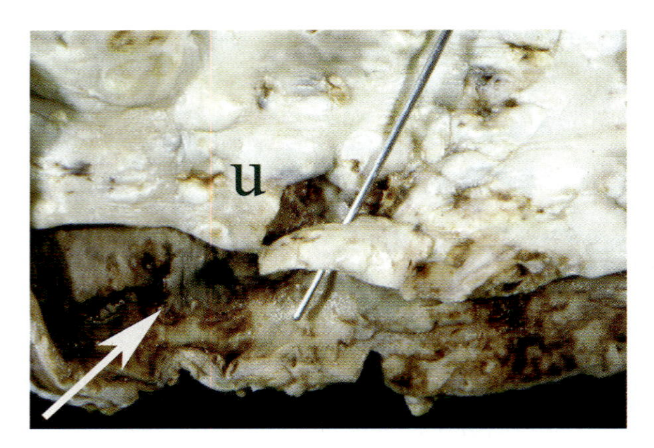

Fig. 9.27 Penetrating aortic ulcer (*U*) with probe within. This ulcer in the thoracic aorta was associated with a large chronic aortic dissection (*arrow*). Penetrating ulcers may rupture, penetrate, or dissect and are prone to complications

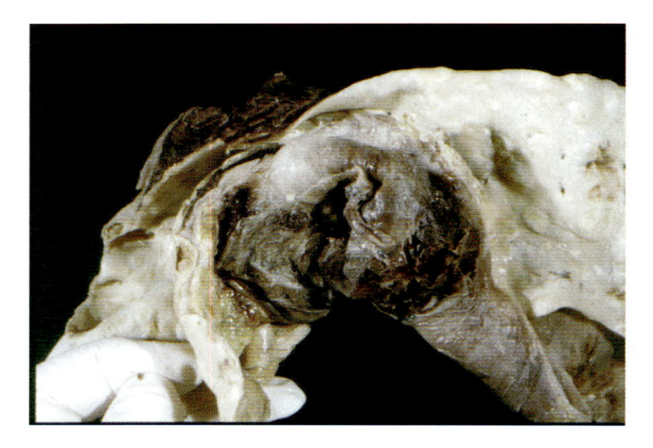

Fig. 9.28 Penetrating aortic ulcer with associated chronic dissection; the same patient as Fig. 9.27. This is the outside of the dissection which penetrated into the lung. The patient presented with fatal hemoptysis

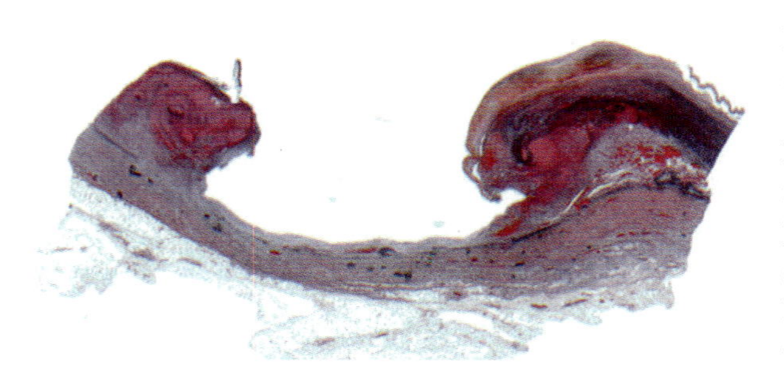

Fig. 9.29 Penetrating aortic ulcer microscopic appearance. The ulcer penetrates outward like a flask and thins the outer part of the wall making it prone to rupture

aggravating the aortic insufficiency. Systemic lupus erythematosus may be associated with giant cell aortitis. Rheumatoid arthritis may have arteritis and rheumatoid nodules may form.

Takayasu disease may involve the aorta or pulmonary trunk [36]. The ascending aorta is commonly involved (Fig. 9.44). The disease occurs in individuals under the age of 50 and may form aneurysms as well as obliterate the aortic branches (Fig. 9.45). The aortic wall has giant cell aortitis by pathology [37]. There is usually intimal thickening, medial destruction, and a prominent thickened and inflamed adventitia. The adventitia thickening is an important characteristic diagnostic feature of this disease. The cause of Takayasu disease is not known but it is associated with certain histocompatibility antigens [38]. Takayasu-related intimal fibrosis may occlude the ostial branches of the aorta. The arm, coronary, and neck arterial vessels gradually obliterate. Pulseless disease is the manifestation in the arms and coronary artery ostial obstruction may occur.

Aortic Plaques

Atherosclerotic plaques are commonly seen in elderly individuals and particularly in those with atherosclerotic risk factors [39–41]. Atherosclerotic plaque formation is not uniform in the aorta. The plaques tend to develop primarily in the abdominal aorta. The ascending aorta and arch are also commonly involved, although not as much as the abdominal segment. The predilection of plaque location is not well understood but it may be variable due to differing aortic diameter, smooth muscle medial embryological cell of origin, shear stress, and complexity of flow related to branches.

Plaques develop first as fatty intimal streaks. After puberty they complicate with progressive fibrosis forming fibrous and fibrofatty plaques that are raised intimal structures. Not all fatty streaks become plaques. Fibrofatty plaques have fibrous plaque caps and underlying soft cores of lipid and cellular debris. If these plaques lose their endothelium covering and become complicated, they may thrombose and components may embolize. In reality, even dysfunction of the endothelium is all that is necessary for thrombus to form. If the cap ruptures, with or without underlying plaque hemorrhage, the exposed plaque may cause marked thrombosis and embolism [42, 43]. Detecting significant atheroma is

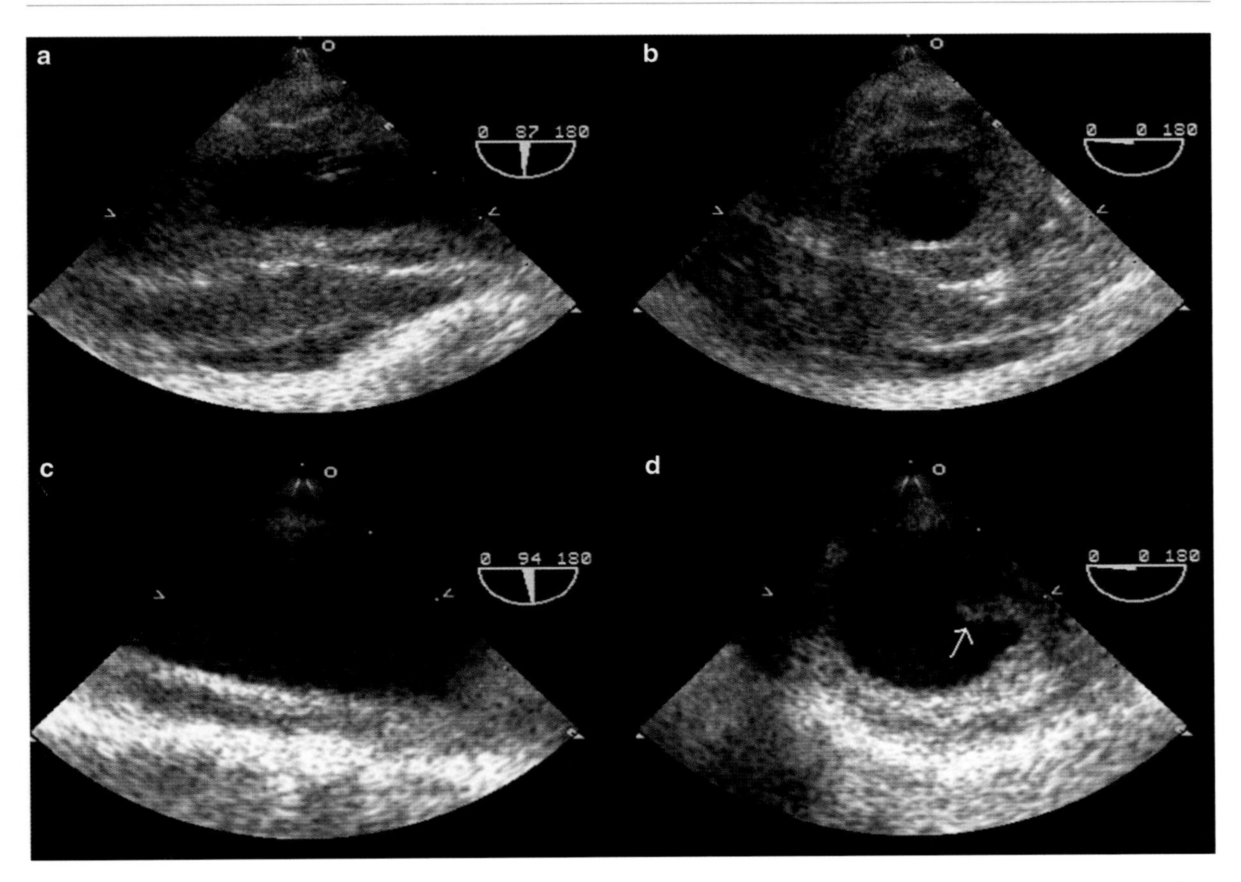

Fig. 9.30 This 22-year-old man was involved in a car accident. Transesophageal views of the proximal descending aorta show extensive and severe thickening of the aortic wall (**a, b**) consistent with aortic transection. Slightly distal to this region (**c, d**), the aortic wall is still thickened and a mobile intraluminal intimal flap (*arrow*) is present. These findings are consistent with aortic transection

important prior to intervention, especially if one is contemplating ascending aortic manipulation, cannulation or surgery. Visualization of ascending aortic plaque may lead to choice of off pump surgery if the plaque is significant, or at least allow the surgeon to more accurately avoid the plaque when manipulating the aorta.

When a pathologist grades the severity of atheroma they tend to estimate and grade the severity by evaluating the surface area. Alternately, one can grade atheroma by the Stary classification, which reflects the stage of atheroma development and the actual degree of complication of the plaques [43]. An aorta thus may have severe atheroma if the surface area is extensively involved or if the plaques are complicated, or both. The thickness of the plaque is probably a better indicator of risk than a simple surface area estimation that fails to take complexity of the plaque into consideration.

The severity of the aortic plaque can be semi-quantitated by echocardiography according to its thickness protruding into the lumen (Table 9.9) [40]. The thickness of the plaques carries prognostic significance. For plaques in the aortic arch, the odds ratio for stroke has been reported to be 13.8 for severe plaques and 3.9 for moderate plaques (Figs. 9.46, 9.47, 9.48). Complex morphology, such as mobile components, are associated with increased rates of thromboembolic events, which may be reduced with statin drugs or anticoagulation, although the management of this condition has not been well defined [41].

A large mobile mass can be the dramatic presentation in a small subset of patients who have embolic events [44–46]. Surgical removal is frequently performed, and will confirm it to be an organized thrombus arising from normal aortic wall or a small plaque (Figs. 9.49, 9.50).

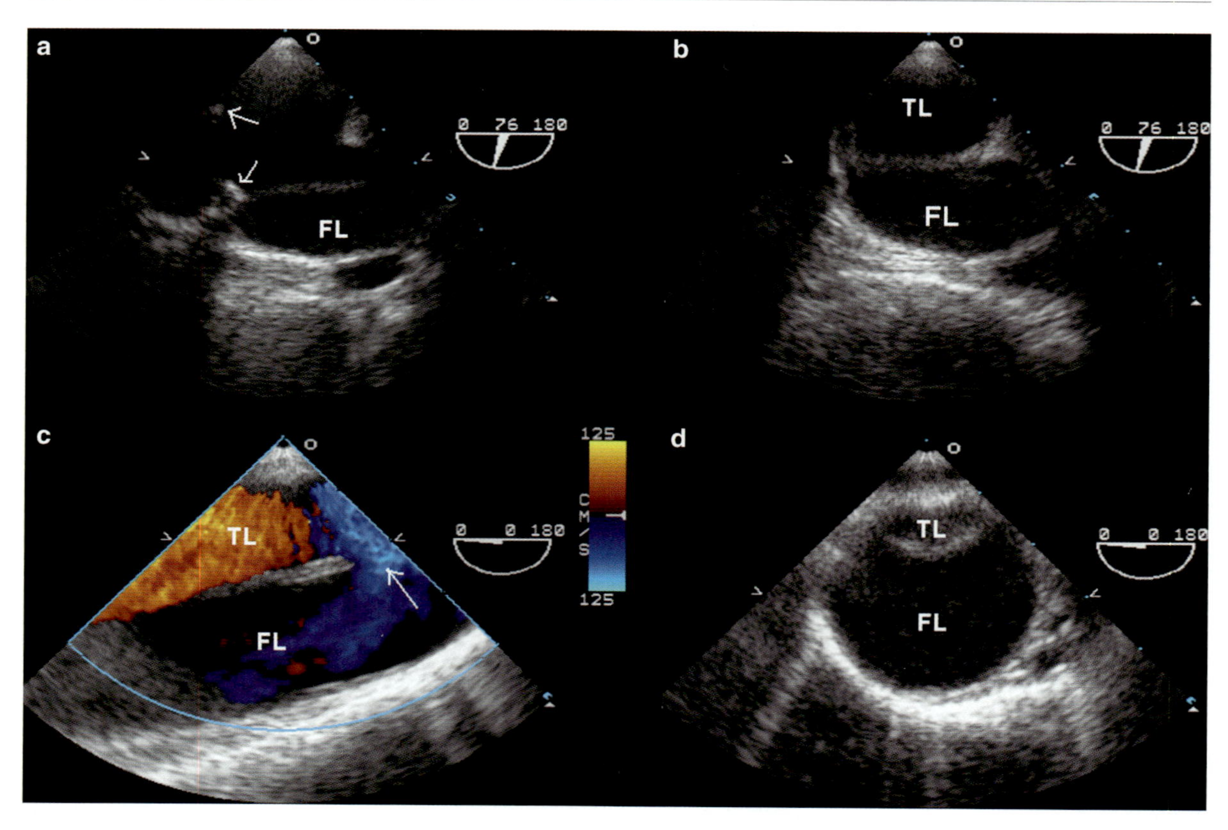

Fig. 9.31 This is a patient who had surgery for type A aortic dissection. A Bentall procedure was done with the ascending aorta replaced by a Dacron tube graft. These are the transesophageal views of the distal ascending aorta (**a, b**) and proximal descending aorta (**c**) and distal descending thoracic aorta (**d**). In the distal ascending aorta (**a**), the distal end of the tube graft (*arrows*) is detected. There is residual dissection beyond the anastomosis with the false lumen persisting in the aortic arch and descending thoracic aorta. A large intimal tear communicating the true lumen and false lumen is seen in the proximal descending thoracic aorta (*arrow*). In the distal descending aorta (**d**) the false lumen is much larger than the true lumen. *FL* false lumen, *TL* true lumen

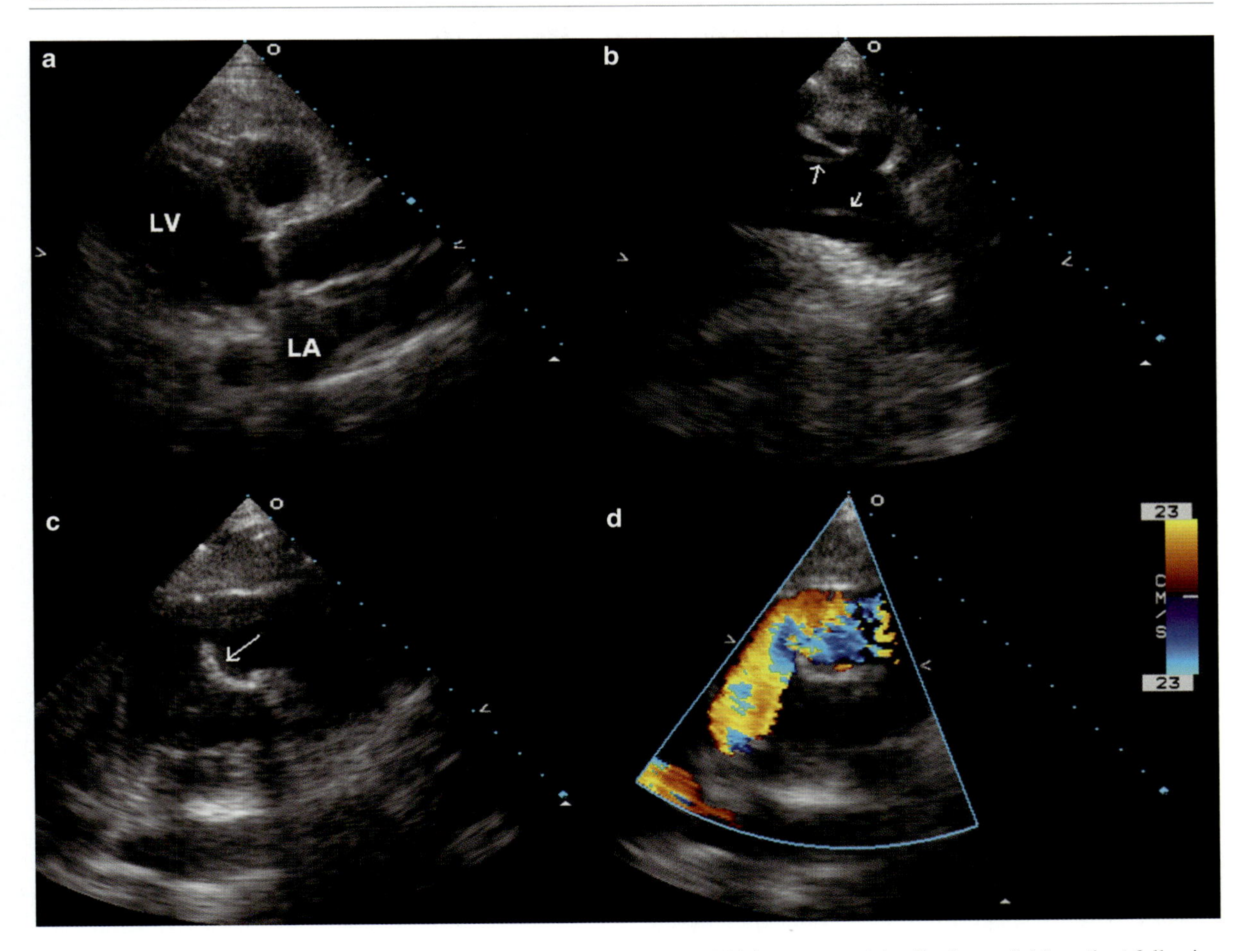

Fig. 9.32 The transthoracic parasternal long-axis (**a**) suprasternal (**b**) and high parasternal (**c, d**) views of this patient following Bentall procedure for type A aortic dissection show that there is residual dissection beyond the distal anastomosis with intimal flap (*arrows*) present in the aortic arch (**b**). The parasternal views with the transducer at the second intercostal space to the left of the sternum (**c**) shows that there is a kink at the distal end of the anastomosis of the prosthetic tube graft. The corresponding color-flow image showed acceleration of flow at the kink. *LA* left atrium, *LV* left ventricle

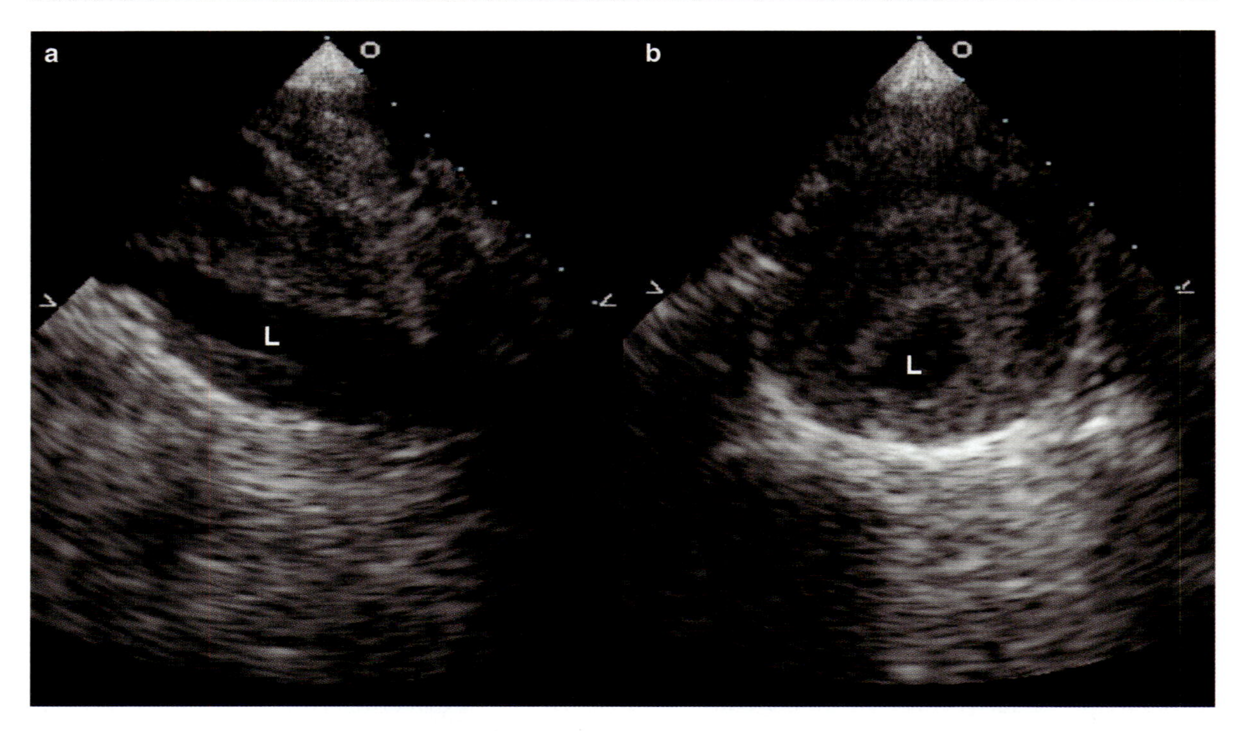

Fig. 9.33 The echo images of the abdominal aorta in long-axis (**a**) and in short-axis (**b**) demonstrates an abdominal aortic aneurysm about 6 cm in diameter. A large amount of laminated thrombus is present. *L* lumen

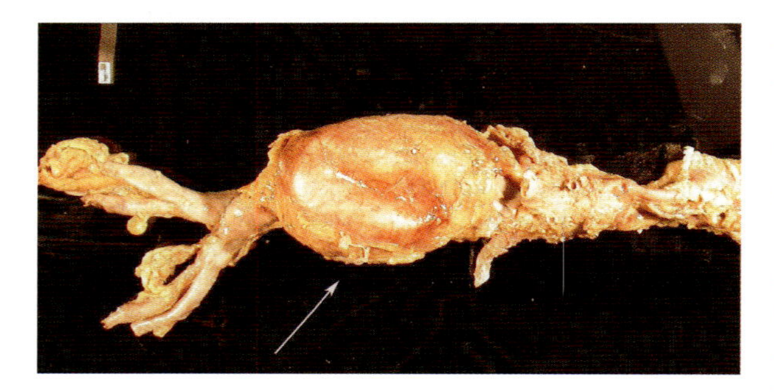

Fig. 9.34 Atherosclerotic abdominal aortic aneurysm (*arrow*); external posterior view

The rest of the aorta usually contains little or no additional plaques. The exact mechanism for the development of such a large thrombus and the long-term outcome of these patients are unclear.

Aortic Neoplasm

Primary aortic neoplasms are rare and are usually not associated with aneurysm. These tumors are usually intimal sarcomas or myxoid sarcomas [47]. They cause luminal narrowing and systemic emboli of the tumor fragments or associated thrombus.

Neoplasm-related aortic aneurysms may be caused by adjacent primary or secondary neoplasms in the mediastinum. These are usually primary lung or esophageal carcinomas or related to metastatic disease in para-aortic lymph nodes. The aorta itself is remarkably resistant to invasion and rupture, although this can rarely occur. Instead the aneurysms associated with neoplasms are usually traction aneurysms. The tumor invades the adventitia and causes a pulling or external traction (hence the name) on the aorta with an outpouching in this region.

Summary

TEE is a very useful tool in the assessment of aortic diseases, particularly in patients with acute aortic syndrome in whom a prompt and accurate diagnosis is crucial to the management. However, pitfalls of TEE need to be remembered (Table 9.10) [48], and there should be a very low threshold to perform ancillary investigations to confirm the diagnosis.

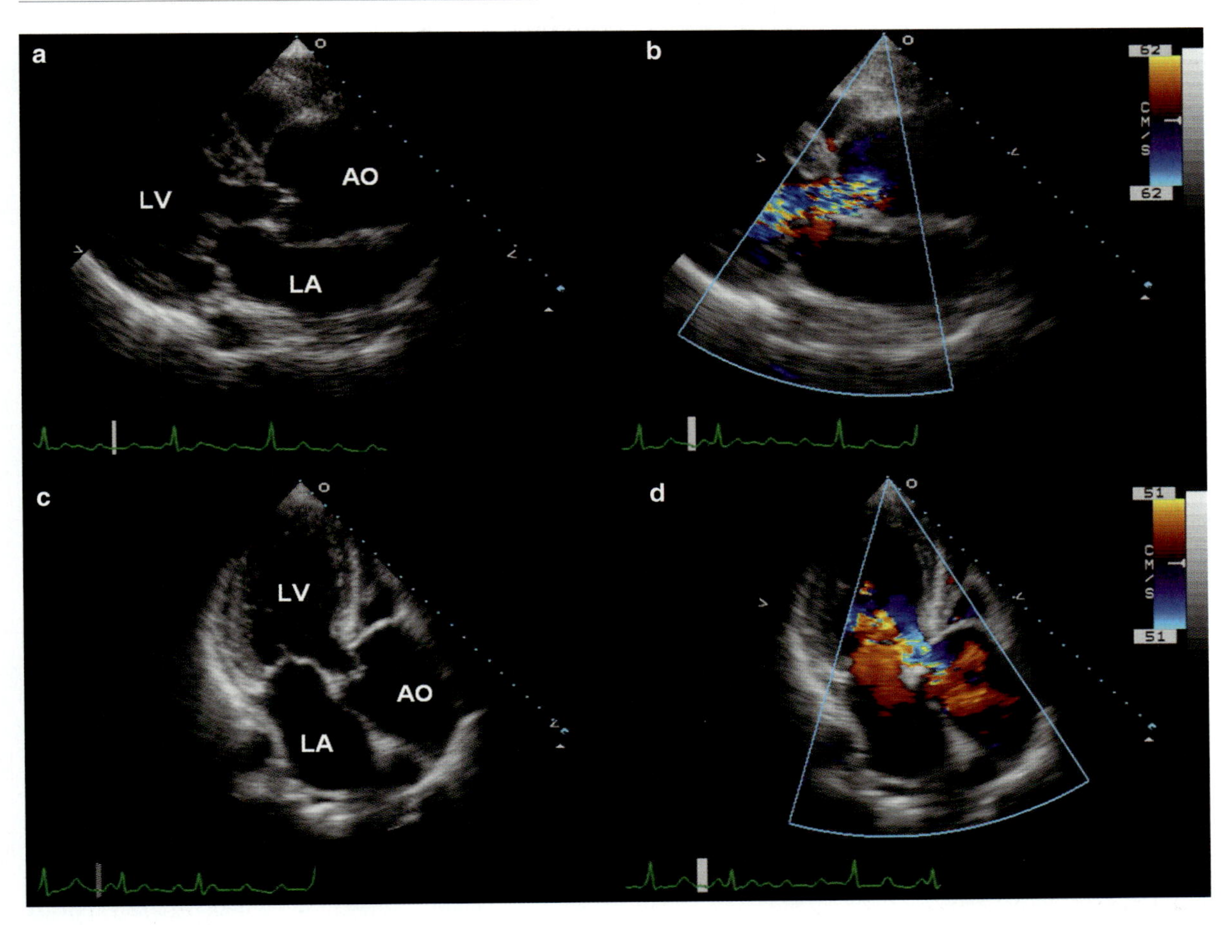

Fig. 9.35 The parasternal long-axis (**a, b**) and apical long-axis (**c, d**) views of this patient with dilated aorta shows that the aortic valve does not coapt properly resulting in aortic regurgitation. *Ao* aorta, *LA* left atrium, *LV* left ventricle

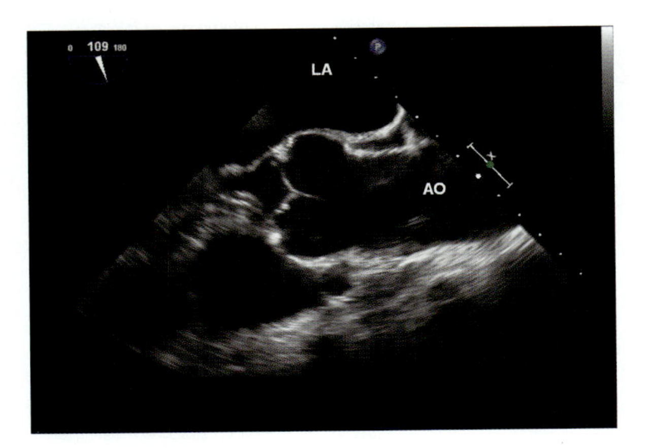

Fig. 9.36 The transesophageal aortic long-axis view shows the typical dilatation of the aortic root at a sinus level in a patient with Marfan syndrome. The rest of the ascending aorta is also mildly dilated. *Ao* aorta; *LA* left atrium

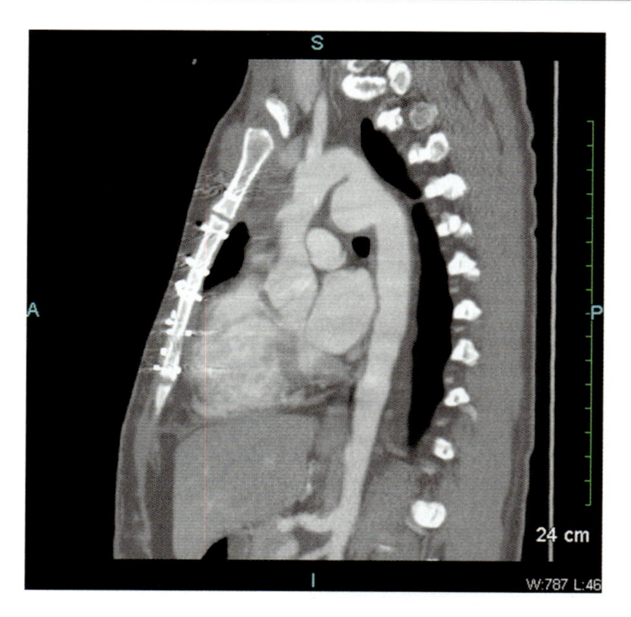

Fig. 9.37 This computed tomogram in a patient with a history of motor vehicle accident shows that there is localized aneurysmal dilatation involving the undersurface of the proximal descending thoracic aorta consistent with aortic pseudoaneurysm

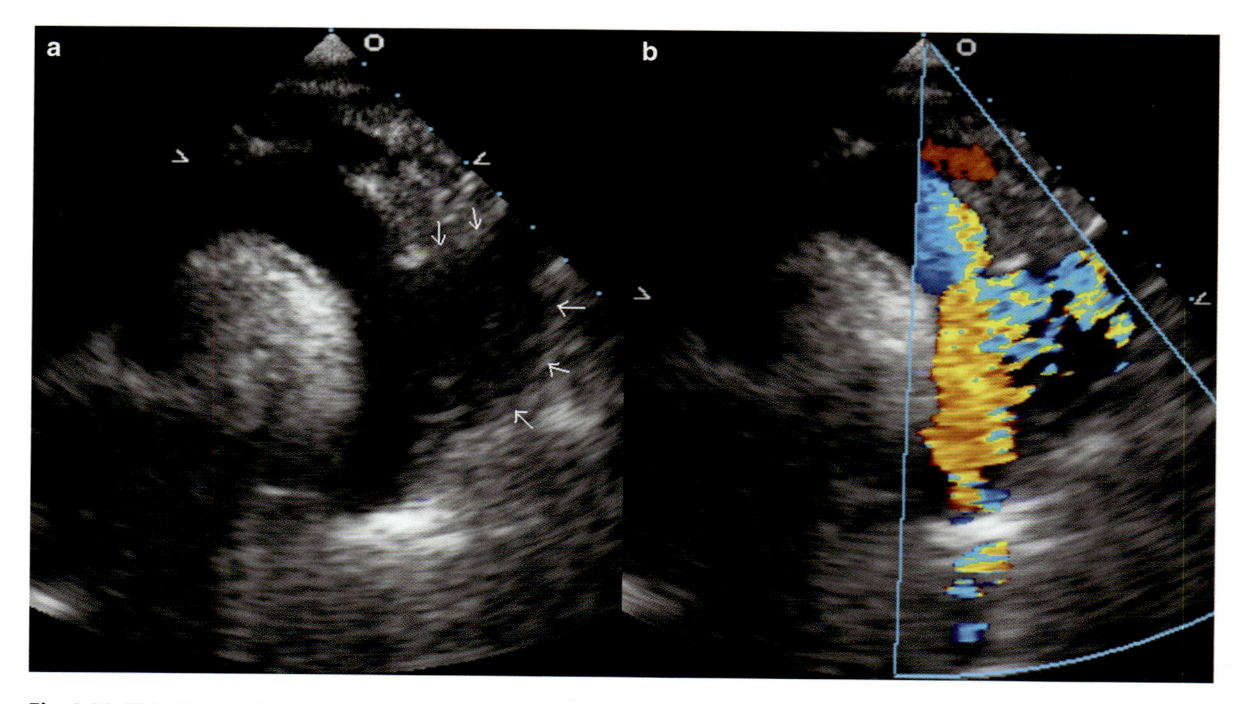

Fig. 9.38 This 19-year-old man has had surgery for coarctation. The suprasternal view (**a**) shows localized bulging (*arrows*) at the proximal descending thoracic aorta. Color flow imaging (**b**) confirms communication between this outpouching and the aorta

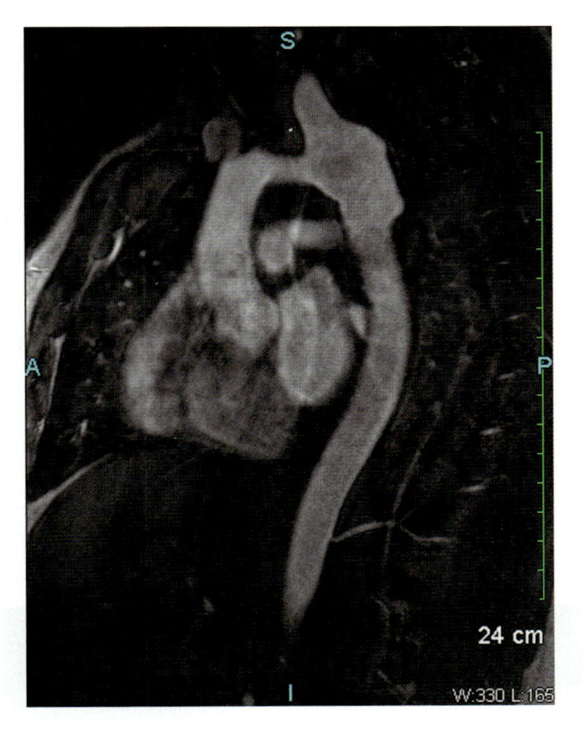

Fig. 9.39 This is the magnetic resonance image of the same patient shown in Fig. 9.38, confirming that its local aneurysmal dilatation involving the proximal descending thoracic aorta is consistent with pseudoaneurysm formation. This finding was confirmed at a subsequent operation

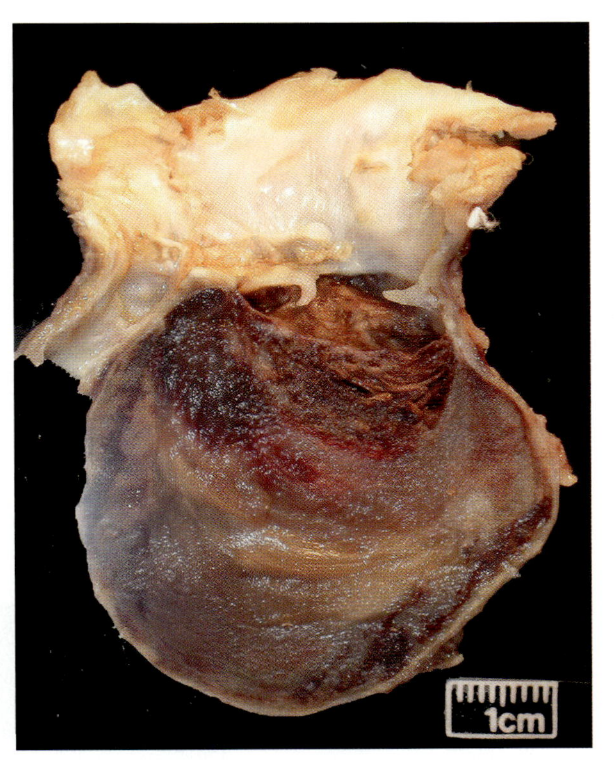

Fig. 9.40 Pseudoaneurysm of the arch of the aorta. The sac-like aneurysm has a thin wall and contains thrombus and clot. It originated in a small dissection of the aorta

Table 9.7 Important echocardiographic findings in patients who had undergone surgery for aortic dissection

• Dimensions of different aortic segments
• Presences and extent of intimal flap
• Number and locations of intimal tears
• Pseudo-dissection or coarctation due to enlargement or kinking of the native aorta
• Status of the arch vessels
• Presence and extent of thrombus in false lumen
• Integrity of the proximal and distal anastomosis of the aortic tube graft
• Status of the coronary ostia
• Native or prosthetic aortic valve function
• Left ventricular function

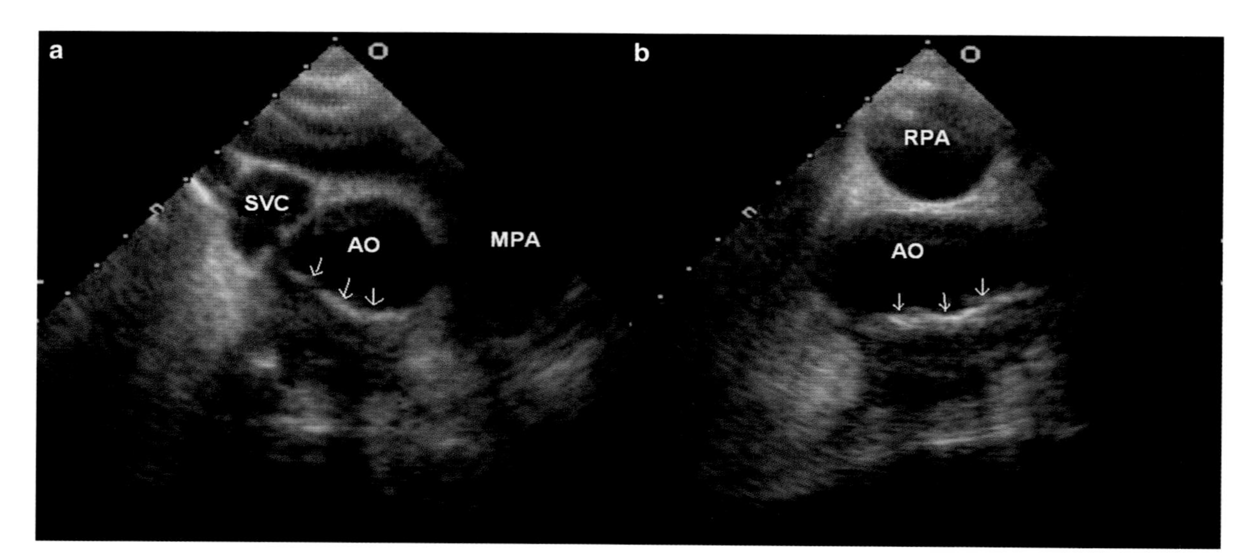

Fig. 9.41 This is a patient with Salmonella aortitis. The transesophageal transverse (**a**) and longitudinal (**b**) views show that there is diffuse thickening of the anterior surface of the ascending aorta (*arrows*). *Ao* aorta, *MPA* main pulmonary artery, *RPA* right pulmonary artery, *SVC* superior vena cava

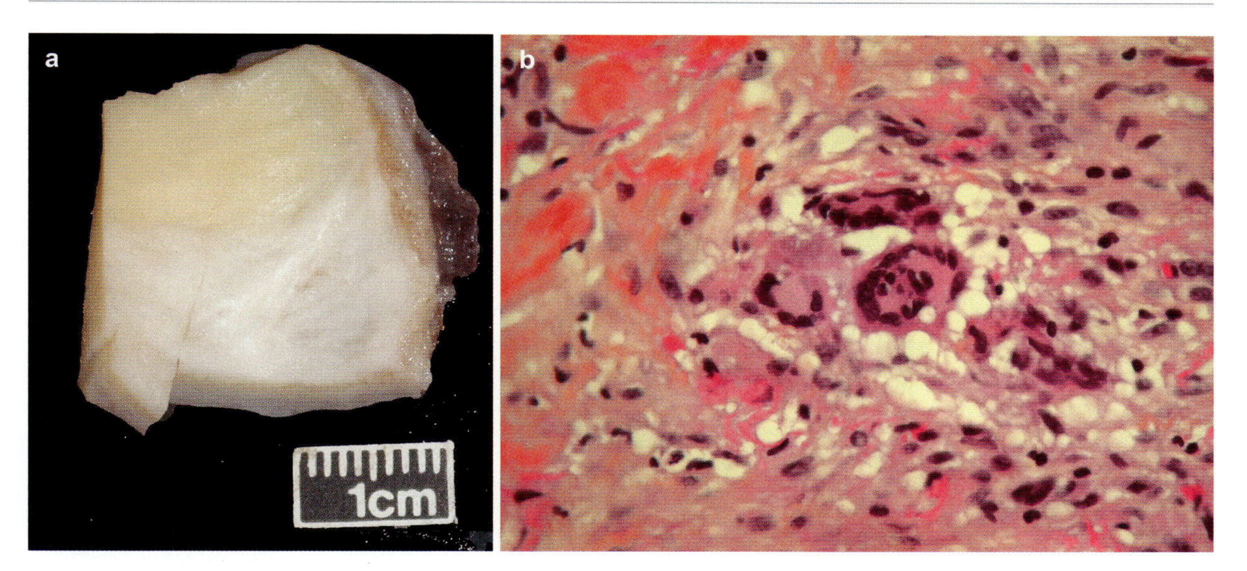

Fig. 9.42 (**a**) This is a segment of excised ascending aorta from an elderly patient with an ascending aortic aneurysm. The wall is thickened and the intima is white and discolored. (**b**) Microscopic examination revealed giant cell aortitis with medial destruction and the presence of numerous giant cells. Serology for syphilis was negative, as was serology for autoimmune diseases

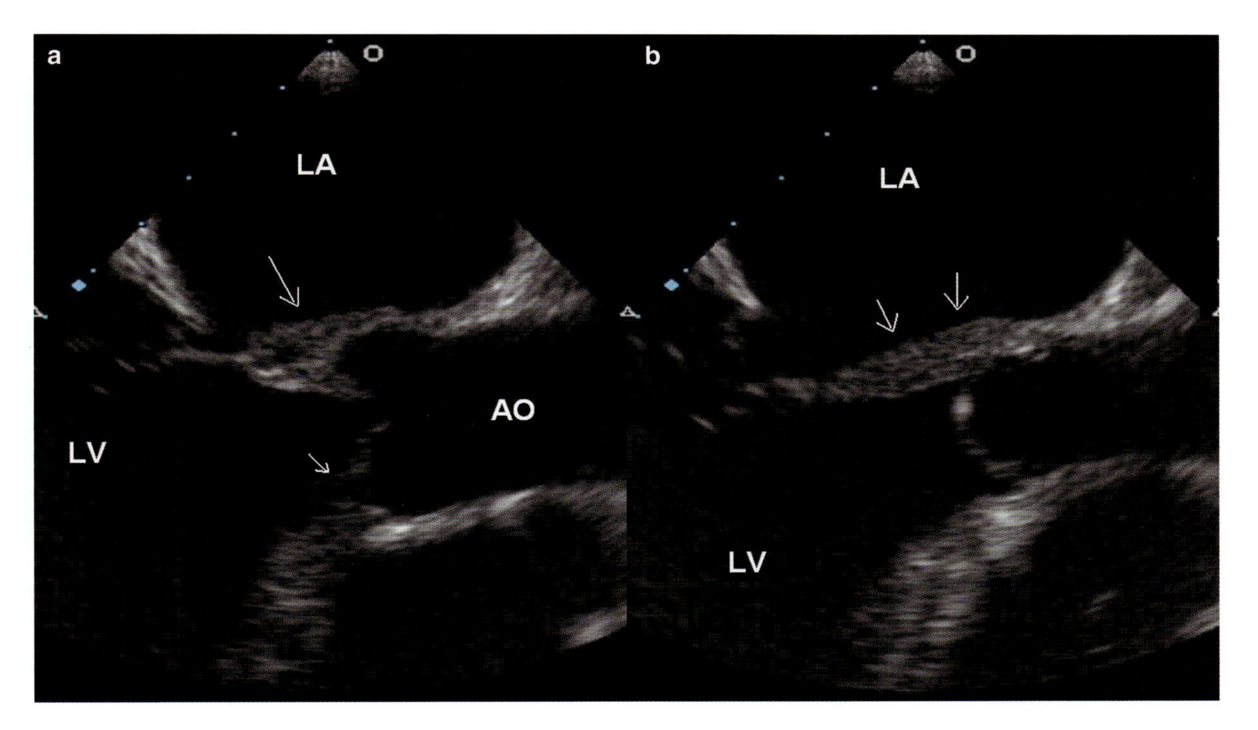

Fig. 9.43 This is a 54-year-old woman with aortitis. The transesophageal views of the long-axis of the aortic root (**a, b**) show diffuse thickening of the posterior aortic root extending onto the base of the anterior mitral leaflet (*arrows*). The base of the anterior aortic cusp is also involved (*short arrow*) as shown in (**a**). No specific cause for the aortitis has been established

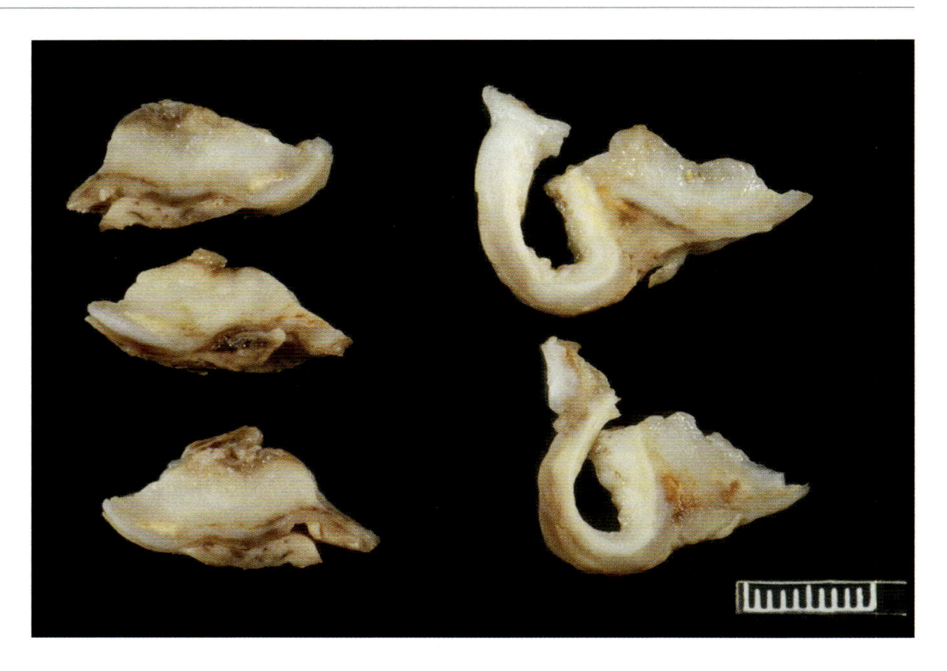

Fig. 9.44 Pieces of excised aorta from a young woman with Takayasu aortitis. The aorta wall was thickened and inflamed

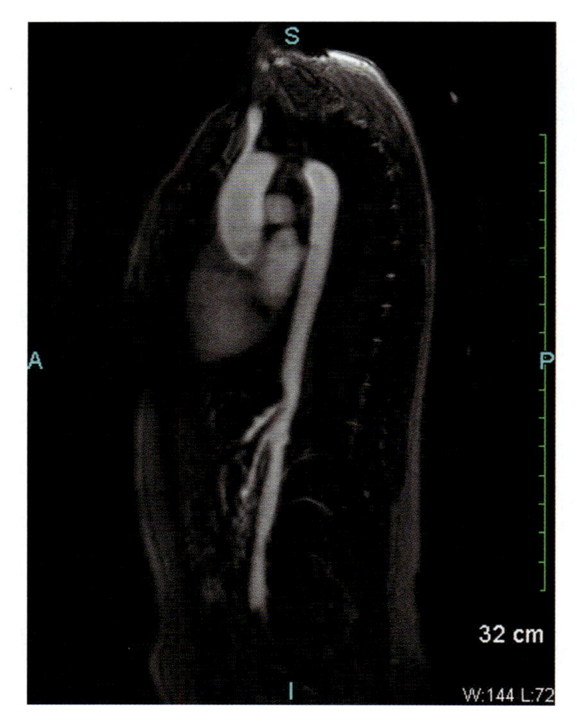

Fig. 9.45 This MRI scan is performed in a 34-year-old woman with Takayasu aortitis. Focal wall thickening and lumen narrowing of the proximal abdominal aorta are shown. The origin of the celiac artery is also narrowed

Table 9.8 Echocardiographic features of an aortic pseudoaneurysm

• Saccular, rather than fusiform
• Narrow mouth
• Usually lined with thrombus
• At previous site of surgery or trauma

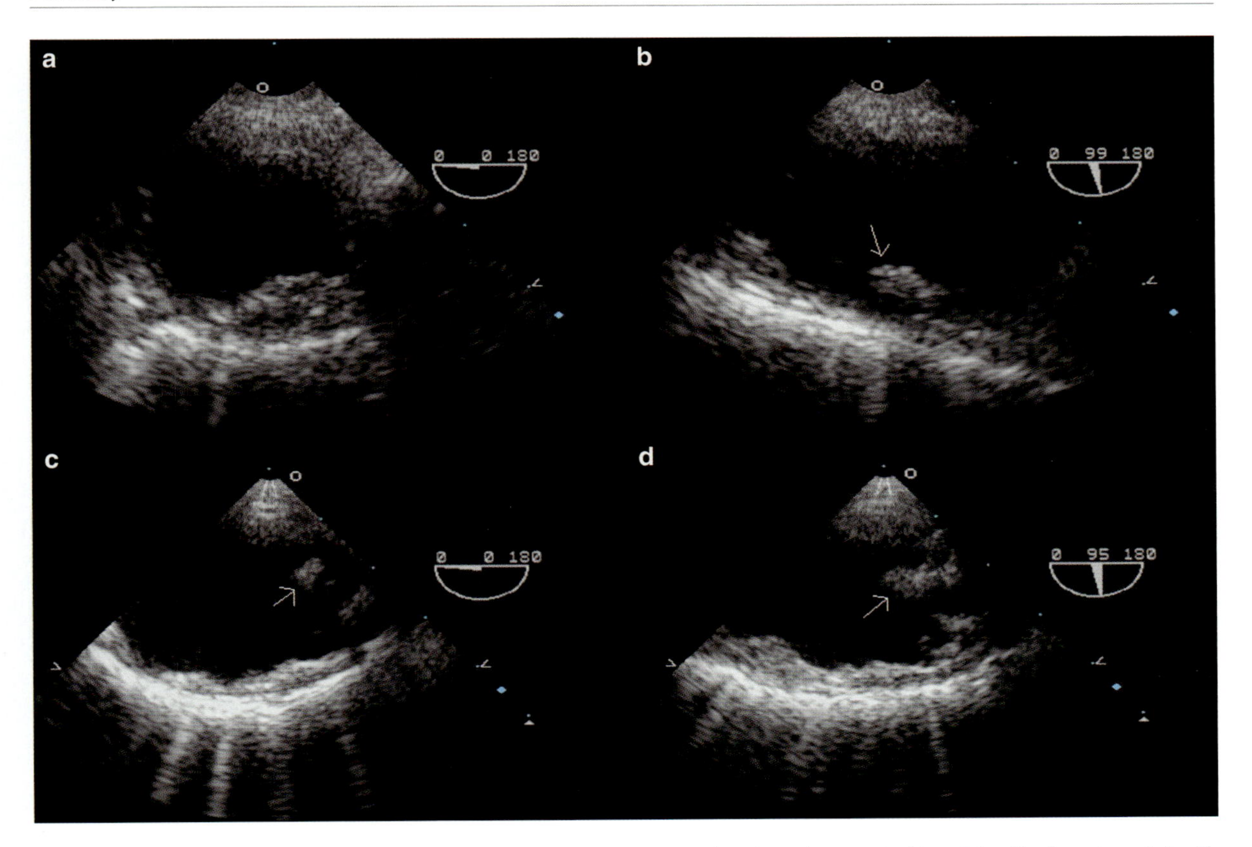

Fig. 9.46 This is a patient with severe aortic plaque involving the descending thoracic aorta (**a, b**) and the distal aortic arch (**c, d**). Some of the plaque is mobile (*arrow*)

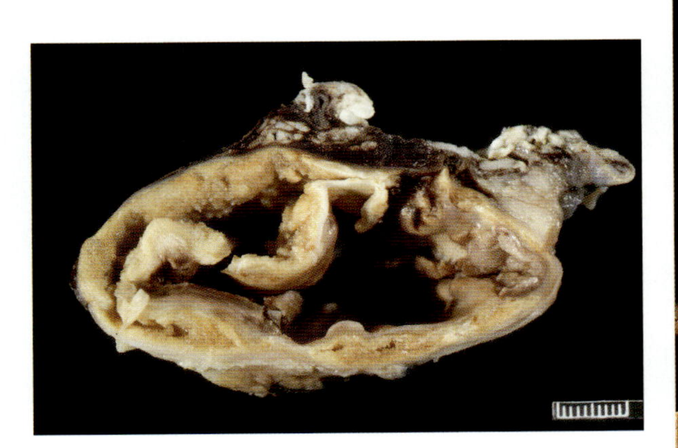

Fig. 9.47 Cross section of the thoracic aorta. Complicated thick atherosclerotic plaques are noted circumferentially. Thrombus is present on the aortic intimal surface (*arrow*)

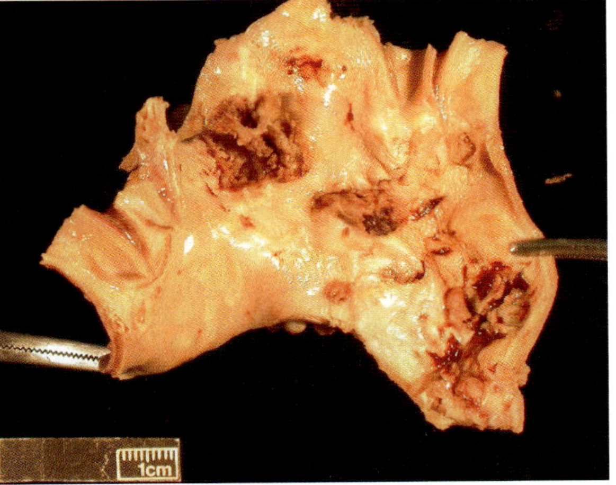

Fig. 9.48 The arch of the aorta is opened showing numerous ulcerated complicated atherosclerotic plaques

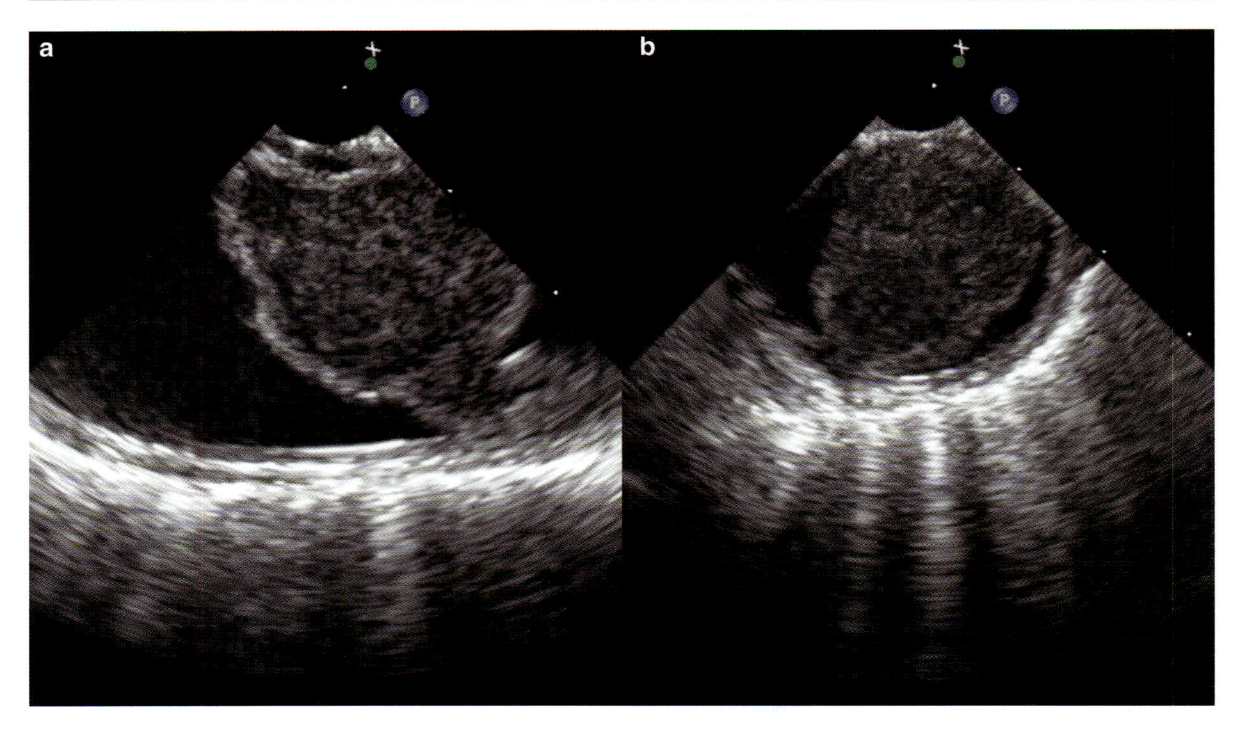

Fig. 9.49 The transesophageal views of the proximal descending aorta in long-axis (**a**) and short-axis (**b**) show that there is a large mass with a small stalk attaching to the posterior aortic wall

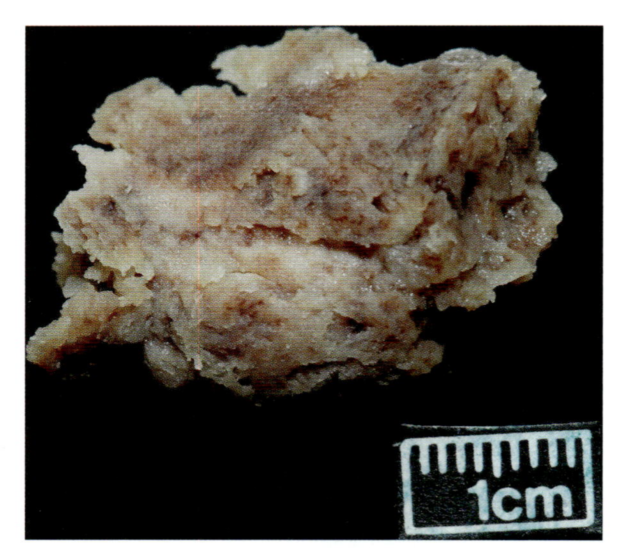

Fig. 9.50 This is a thoracic aortic mass removed surgically from the patient in Fig. 9.49. The patient was suspected to have an aortic neoplasm. At surgery there was an aortic plaque with a large adherent thrombus, as shown in the specimen

Table 9.9 Grading of severity of aortic plaques

Grade	Plaque thickness
Mild	<1.0
Moderate	1.0–3.9 mm
Severe*	≥4 mm

*Plaques with a mobile component would be graded severe even if the plaque thickness is < 4 mm

Table 9.10 Pitfalls in the echocardiographic diagnosis of aortic diseases

False positive studies
Dissection flap mimics
– Reverberation artifact
– Kinks in dilated and tortuous aorta
Intramural hematoma mimics
– Peri-aortic fat
– Atherosclerotic plaque
– Intraluminal thrombus in dilated aortas
False lumen mimics
– Transverse sinus
– Innominate vein
False negative studies
Poor image quality
Blind spots in ascending aorta and arch
Unusual variants
• Intramural hematoma
• Primary rupture
• Dissection with no hematoma

References

1. Erbel R, Engberding R, Daniel W, Roelandt J, Visser C, Rennollet H. Echocardiography in diagnosis of aortic dissection. *Lancet*. 1989 Mar 4;1(8636):457-461.
2. Nienaber CA, Spielmann RP, von Kodolitsch Y, et al. Diagnosis of thoracic aortic dissection. Magnetic resonance imaging versus transesophageal echocardiography. *Circulation*. 1992 Feb;85(2):434-447.
3. Nienaber CA, von Kodolitsch Y, Nicolas V, et al. The diagnosis of thoracic aortic dissection by noninvasive imaging procedures. *N Engl J Med*. 1993 Jan 7;328(1):1-9.
4. Shiga T, Wajima Z, Apfel CC, Inoue T, Ohe Y. Diagnostic accuracy of transesophageal echocardiography, helical computed tomography, and magnetic resonance imaging for suspected thoracic aortic dissection: systematic review and meta-analysis. *Arch Intern Med*. 2006 Jul 10;166(13):1350-1356.
5. Cigarroa JE, Isselbacher EM, DeSanctis RW, Eagle KA. Diagnostic imaging in the evaluation of suspected aortic dissection. Old standards and new directions. *N Engl J Med*. 1993 Jan 7;328(1):35-43.
6. DeSanctis RW, Doroghazi RM, Austen WG, Buckley MJ. Aortic dissection. *N Engl J Med*. 1987 Oct 22;317(17):1060-1067.
7. Larson EW, Edwards WD. Risk factors for aortic dissection: a necropsy study of 161 cases. *Am J Cardiol*. 1984;53:849-855.
8. de Sa M, Moshkovitz Y, Butany J, David TE. Histologic abnormalities of the ascending aorta and pulmonary trunk in patients with bicuspid aortic valve disease: clinical relevance to the ross procedure. *J Thorac Cardiovas Sur*. 1999 Oct; 118(4):588-594.
9. Nienaber CA, Eagle KA. Aortic dissection: new frontiers in diagnosis and management - Part I: from etiology to diagnostic strategies. *Circulation*. 2003;108(5):628-635.
10. Nienaber CA, Eagle KA. Aortic dissection: new frontiers in diagnosis and management - Part II: therapeutic management and follow-up. *Circulation*. 2003;108(6):772-778.
11. Miller DC. Acute dissection of the descending thoracic aorta. *Chest Surg Clin North Am*. 1992;2:347-378.
12. Parai JL, Masters RG, Walley VM, Stinson WA, Veinot JP. Aortic medial changes associated with bicuspid aortic valve: myth or reality? *Can J Cardiol*. 1999 Nov;15(11): 1233-1238.
13. Schlatmann TJ, Becker AE. Histologic changes in the normal aging aorta: implications for dissecting aortic aneurysm. *Am J Cardiol*. 1977;39:13-20.
14. Attias D, Stheneur C, Roy C, et al. Comparison of clinical presentations and outcomes between patients With TGFBR2 and FBN1 mutations in Marfan syndrome and related disorders. *Circulation*. 2009 Dec 22;120(25):2541-2549.
15. Chan KL. Usefulness of transesophageal echocardiography in the diagnosis of conditions mimicking aortic dissection. *Am Heart J*. 1991 Aug;122(2):495-504.
16. Movsowitz HD, Levine RA, Hilgenberg AD, Isselbacher EM. Transesophageal echocardiographic description of the mechanisms of aortic regurgitation in acute type A aortic dissection: implications for aortic valve repair. *J Am Coll Cardiol*. 2000 Sep;36(3):884-890.
17. Abe K, Mohri M, Ideno N, et al. Images in cardiovascular medicine. Chest pain and intimal flap detected by chest computed tomography scans. *Circulation*. 2006 Jul 25; 114(4):e64.
18. Sundt TM. Intramural hematoma and penetrating atherosclerotic ulcer of the aorta. *Annal Thorac Sur*. 2007 Feb; 83(2):S835-841.
19. Evangelista A, Mukherjee D, Mehta RH, et al. Acute intramural hematoma of the aorta: a mystery in evolution. *Circulation*. 2005 Mar 1;111(8):1063-1070.
20. Song JK, Yim JH, Ahn JM, et al. Outcomes of patients with acute type A aortic intramural hematoma. *Circulation*. 2009 Nov 24;120(21):2046-2052.
21. Stanson AW, Kazmier FJ, Hollier LH, et al. Penetrating atherosclerotic ulcers of the thoracic aorta: natural history and clinicopathologic correlations. *Ann Vasc Surg*. 1986;1: 15-23.
22. Svensson LG, Labib SB, Eisenhauer AC, Butterly JR. Intimal tear without hematoma: an important variant of aortic dissection that can elude current imaging techniques. *Circulation*. 1999 Mar 16;99(10):1331-1336.
23. Sakamoto I, Hayashi K, Matsunaga N, et al. Aortic dissection caused by angiographic procedures. *Radiology*. 1994 May;191(2):467-471.
24. Smith MD, Cassidy JM, Souther S, et al. Transesophageal echocardiography in the diagnosis of traumatic rupture of the aorta. *New Engl J Med*. 1995;332:356-362.
25. Mohr-Kahaly S, Erbel R, Rennollet H, et al. Ambulatory follow-up of aortic dissection by transesophageal two-dimensional and color-coded Doppler echocardiography. *Circulation*. 1989 Jul;80(1):24-33.
26. Erbel R, Oelert H, Meyer J, et al. Effect of medical and surgical therapy on aortic dissection evaluated by transesophageal echocardiography. Implications for prognosis and therapy. The European Cooperative Study Group on Echocardiography. *Circulation*. 1993 May;87(5): 1604-1615.

27. San Roman JA, Vilacosta I, Castilla JA. Role of transesophageal echocardiography in the assessment of composite aortic grafts for therapy in acute aortic dissection. *Am J Cardiol.* 1994;73:519-521.
28. Sueyoshi E, Sakamoto I, Hayashi K, Yamaguchi T, Imada T. Growth rate of aortic diameter in patients with type B aortic dissection during the chronic phase. *Circulation.* 2004 Sep 14;110(11 Suppl 1):II256-II261.
29. Kuivaniemi H, Shibamura H, Arthur C, et al. Familial abdominal aortic aneurysms: collection of 233 multiplex families. *J Vascul Sur.* 2003;37(2):340-345.
30. Knyshov GV, Sitar LL, Glagola MD, Atamanyuk MY. Aortic aneurysms at the site of the repair of coarctation of the aorta: a review of 48 patients. *Ann Thorac Surg.* 1996;61(3): 935-939.
31. Atik FA, Navia JL, Svensson LG, et al. Surgical treatment of pseudoaneurysm of the thoracic aorta. *J Thorac Cardiovas Surg.* 2006 Aug;132(2):379-385.
32. Evans JM, Bowles CA, Bjornsson J, Mullany CJ, Hunder GG. Thoracic aortic aneurysm and rupture in giant cell arteritis. A descriptive study of 41 cases. *Arthritis Rheum.* 1994 Oct;37(10):1539-1547.
33. Parums DV. The spectrum of chronic periaortitis. *Histopathology.* 1990;16:423-431.
34. Virmani R, Burke AP. Pathologic features of aortitis. *Cardiovas Pathol.* 1994;3(3):205-216.
35. Lie JT. Aortic and extracranial large vessel giant cell arteritis: a review of 72 cases with histopathologic documentation. *Seminars Arthritis Rheumat.* 1995;24(6):422-431.
36. Lie JT. Pathology of isolated nonclassical and catastrophic manifestations of Takayasu arteritis. *Int J Cardiol.* 1998 Oct 1;66(Suppl 1):S11-S21.
37. Lie JT. Occidental (temporal) and oriental (takayasu) giant cell arteritis. *Cardiovas Pathol.* 1994;3(3):227-240.
38. Numano F, Kishi Y, Tanaka A, Ohkawara M, Kakuta T, Kobayashi Y. Inflammation and atherosclerosis. Atherosclerotic lesions in Takayasu arteritis. *Annals NY Acad Sci.* 2000 May; 902:65-76.
39. Amarenco P, Cohen A, Baudrimont M, Bousser MG. Transesophageal echocardiographic detection of aortic arch disease in patients with cerebral infarction. *Stroke.* 1992 Jul;23(7):1005-1009.
40. Cohen A, Tzourio C, Bertrand B, Chauvel C, Bousser MG, Amarenco P. Aortic plaque morphology and vascular events: a follow-up study in patients with ischemic stroke. FAPS Investigators. French Study of Aortic Plaques in Stroke. *Circulation.* 1997 Dec 2;96(11):3838-3841.
41. Tunick PA, Nayar AC, Goodkin GM, et al. Effect of treatment on the incidence of stroke and other emboli in 519 patients with severe thoracic aortic plaque. *Am J Cardiol.* 2002 Dec 15;90(12):1320-1325.
42. Stary HC, Chandler AB, Glagov S, et al. A definition of initial, fatty streak, and intermediate lesions of atherosclerosis. A report from the Committee on Vascular Lesions of the Council on Arteriosclerosis, American Heart Association. *Circulation.* 1994;89:2462-2478.
43. Stary HC, Chandler AB, Dinsmore RE, et al. A definition of advanced types of atherosclerotic lesions and a histological classification of atherosclerosis. A report from the Committee on Vascular Lesions of the Council on Arteriosclerosis, American Heart Association. *Circulation.* 1995;92(5):1355-1374.
44. Choukroun EM, Labrousse LM, Madonna FP, Deville C. Mobile thrombus of the thoracic aorta: diagnosis and treatment in 9 cases. *Ann Vasc Surg.* 2002 Nov;16(6):714-722.
45. Blackshear JL, Jahangir A, Oldenburg WA, Safford RE. Digital embolization from plaque-related thrombus in the thoracic aorta: identification with transesophageal echocardiography and resolution with warfarin therapy. *Mayo Clin Proc.* 1993 Mar;68(3):268-272.
46. Wolfsohn AL, So DY, Chan K, et al. Thrombus of the ascending aorta: a rare cause of myocardial infarction. *Cardiovas Pathol.* 2005 Jul;14(4):214-218.
47. Burke AP, Virmani R. Sarcomas of the great vessels. *Cancer.* 1993;71:1761-1773.
48. Bansal RC, Chandrasekaran K, Ayala K, Smith DC. Frequency and explanation of false negative diagnosis of aortic dissection by aortography and transesophageal echocardiography. *J Am Coll Cardiol.* 1995 May;25(6): 1393-1401.

Pericardial Diseases

10

The pericardium surrounds the heart as the heart becomes enveloped in the developing pericardial sac during embryogenesis. There are two layers – the visceral pericardium, which is part of the epicardium and the parietal pericardium, which is a strong fibrous sac (Fig. 10.1) [1, 2]. Both are lined by mesothelial cells which have a secretory function and ensure that the pericardial space always has a small amount of fluid to allow for unimpeded cardiac motion throughout the cardiac cycle. The parietal pericardium fixes the heart in the chest and is attached to the diaphragm and the underlying sternum and separates the pericardial space from the pleural spaces. Between the two layers is a small volume (15–50 mL) of serous fluid. The function of the pericardium in health is uncertain, since its absence does not have significant adverse effects. On the other hand, diseases involving the pericardium can lead to serious hemodynamic consequences including shock.

The pericardium envelops the entire heart, the first few centimeters of the great vessels, and the caval and pulmonary veins [1, 3, 4]. It is important to remember that the proximal ascending aorta is within the pericardial space as rupture of the aorta in this location can cause hemopericardium and cardiac tamponade. Reflections of the pericardium create two normal sinuses. The transverse sinus is a pericardial space located behind the aorta and pulmonary trunk (Fig. 10.2). Surgeons may use this space to run bypass grafts through. The oblique sinus is at the posterior or base of the heart and is located between the reflections of the pericardium from the four pulmonary veins (Fig. 10.3). This space may be important in cases of occult tamponade where bleeding in this space may cause local left atrial compression and tamponade without an easily seen pericardial effusion.

Histologically, the parietal pericardium is composed of fibrous collagen. It is a strong structure not

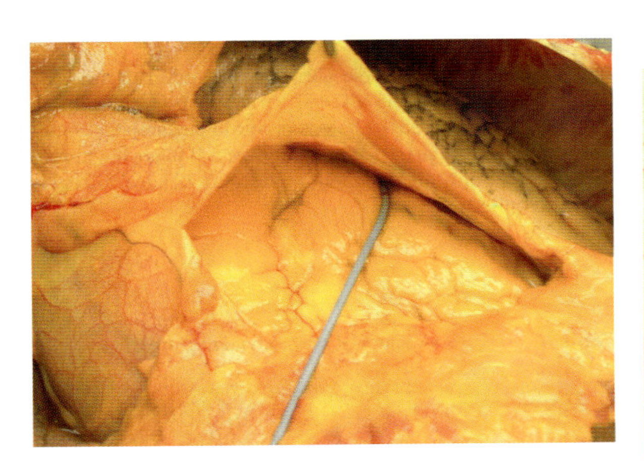

Fig. 10.1 The pericardial sac is opened at autopsy. The parietal pericardium (*top*) is held by forceps and a catheter has been placed in the space between the fibrous parietal pericardium and the visceral pericardium on the heart. A small amount of clear serous fluid is invariably present

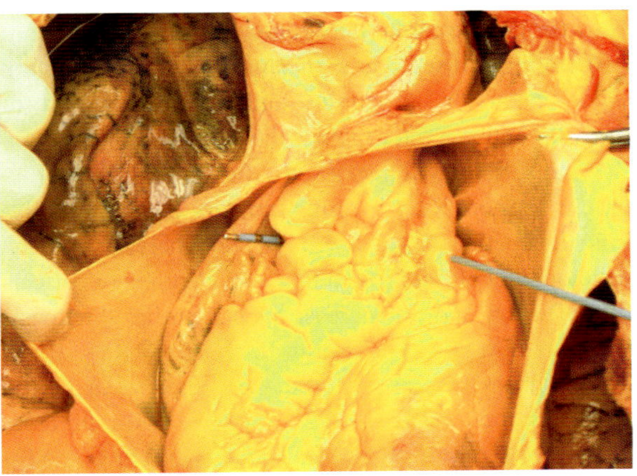

Fig. 10.2 The transverse sinus of the pericardium has a catheter placed in it. This is a normal space behind the aorta and the pulmonary trunk

K.-L. Chan and J.P. Veinot, *Anatomic Basis of Echocardiographic Diagnosis*,
DOI: 10.1007/978-1-84996-387-9_10, © Springer-Verlag London Limited 2011

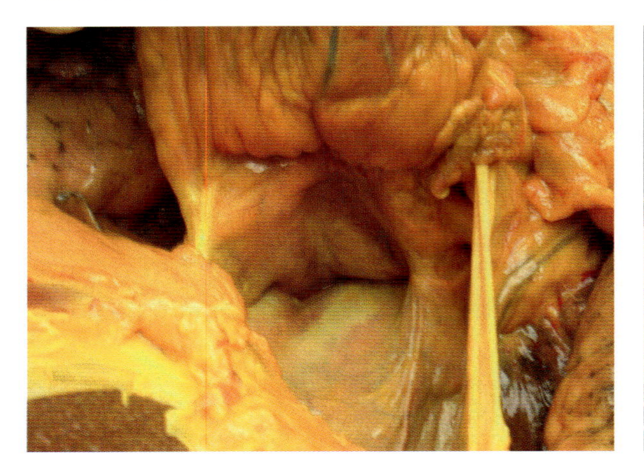

Fig. 10.3 The oblique sinus of the pericardium is seen when the heart is lifted up. This normal space lies between the normal left and right pulmonary veins as they enter the left atrium

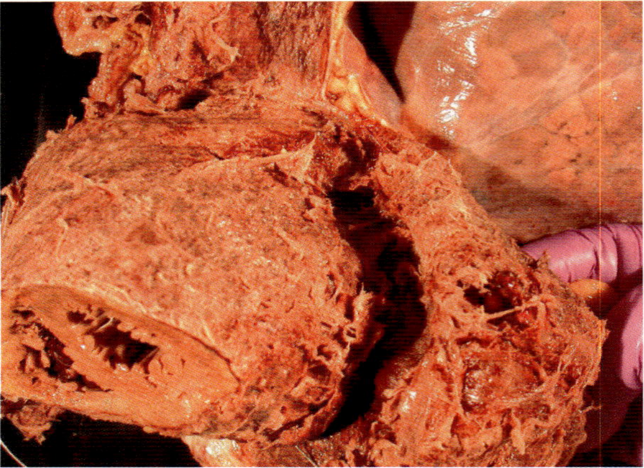

Fig. 10.4 Fibrinous pericarditis. The entire heart parietal and visceral pericardium is covered by shaggy red fibrinous material. This case also had hemopericardium contributing to the patient's death

easily distensible and resistant to acute stretching [2]. When fluid accumulates slowly in the pericardial space, the pericardium may gradually stretch and the volume of the fluid in the pericardial space can easily reach a liter without significant hemodynamic effects. Conversely, rapid accumulation of fluid is not tolerated. In cases of rapid accumulation, such as with infection or bleeding into the pericardial space (hemopericardium), as little as 100 mL of fluid accumulation is enough to cause compression of the thin right-sided heart chambers leading to hemodynamic derangement and cardiac tamponade. The classic clinical presentation is the Beck's triad – hypotension, muffled heart sounds, and an elevated jugular venous pressure. Common causes of acute hemopericardium include aortic or heart trauma (iatrogenic, penetrating and nonpenetrating closed chest trauma), aortic dissection (spontaneous or iatrogenic), and free wall rupture of the left ventricle after myocardial infarction [3].

The pathological response of the pericardium to disease is limited. Reactive inflammatory changes involving the pericardium result in an increase in the development of fluid (often fibrinous) leading to pericardial effusion and an increase in pericardial thickness, which is normally 1–2 mm in thick (Figs. 10.4, 10.5). These changes are nonspecific and can occur in a wide range of conditions including connective tissue diseases, viral infection, and myocardial infarction. The hemodynamic consequences of the pericardial changes depend on the interaction of various factors (Table 10.1). If the pericardium is intrinsically abnormal and noncompliant,

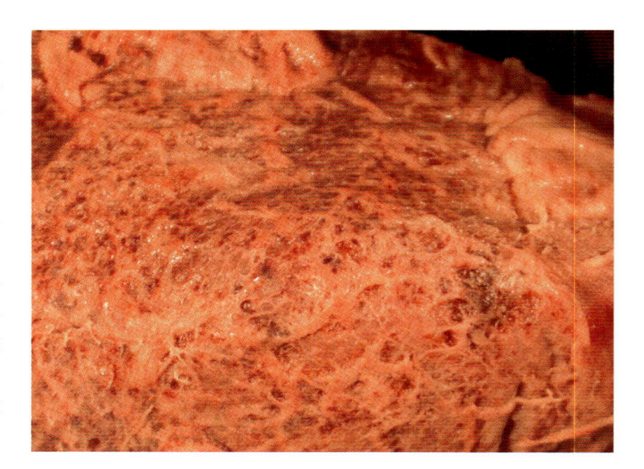

Fig. 10.5 Closer view of the fibrinous pericarditis of the same patient as Fig. 10.4. The visceral pericardium is ragged, red, irregular, and thickened. Pathology is able to diagnose the condition and assess the presence of malignancy. It is unable to provide the cause of benign fibrinous pericarditis. Clinical history is always required

Table 10.1 Determinants of hemodynamic significance of pericardial effusion

• Amount of effusion
• Property of the pericardium
• Rate of fluid accumulation
• Type of effusion (free fluid versus thrombus)
• Intravascular volume status

a small amount of pericardial effusion or even no effusion can cause limitation to ventricular filling and low cardiac output. If the pericardium is relatively unaffected, and the pericardial effusion builds up gradually; a large pericardial effusion can develop without much hemodynamic consequences. The type of pericardial effusion should be considered. Blood in the pericardium, such as following cardiac surgery, can become hematoma to cause local compression. Finally, the status of intracardiac pressures may mitigate or exacerbate the hemodynamic impact of pericardial effusion.

Pericarditis and Pericardial Effusion

Pericarditis is a common clinical problem. The most common causes include idiopathic causes, infection (viral, bacterial, Rickettsia, fungal, worms, and protozoa), autoimmune disease, primary and metastatic tumors, drugs and toxins, trauma (penetrating and blunt; iatrogenic and non-iatrogenic), radiation, and acute myocardial infarction/Dressler's phenomena [1, 3]. Pericarditis may be fibrinous, suppurative, and granulomatous (Figs. 10.4, 10.5). Granulomatous pericarditis may be caseating when the exudates in the pericardial space resemble soft cheese (Fig. 10.6).

Pericarditis may cause pericardial thickening and effusion accumulating fluid in the pericardial space. Usually this occurs slowly and an effusion may be clinically silent. If the effusion becomes hemorrhagic, there may be cardiac tamponade. As an effusion organizes, the pericardium may become thickened and fibrotic or the process may resolve without sequelae depending upon the initiating etiology of the effusion. Fibrinous pericarditis causes a friction rub which may be clinically detected by auscultation.

In some etiologies, the pericardial effusion may become "effusive-constrictive." In this clinical scenario, there are no tamponade signs and the clinical symptoms are not completely relieved by the removal of the pericardial fluid [3]. It is thought that the pericardium itself is causing constriction and compression of the heart chambers. It may be a confusing situation as the pericardium may not be thickened and the cause of the persistent cardiac dysfunction a mystery. Treatment may require pericardiectomy.

In assessing pericardial effusion, the size, extent, and hemodynamic consequences should be determined.

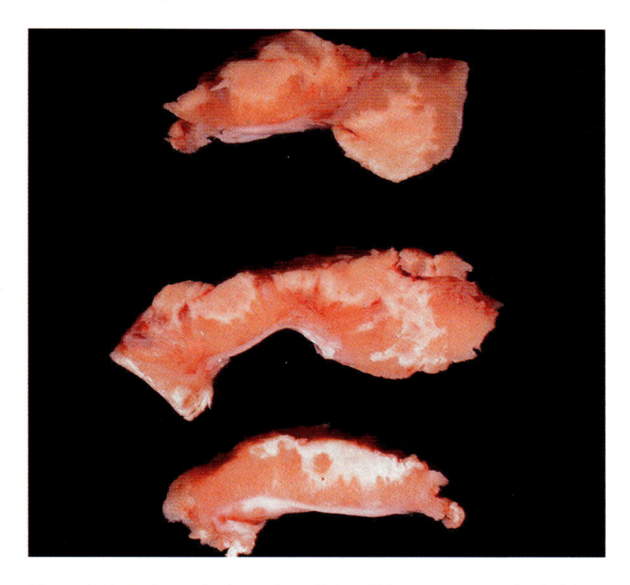

Fig. 10.6 Tuberculosis pericarditis. This young man had thickening of his right atrial wall and pericardium. He had bone lytic lesions. Caseous pericarditis and necrosis were confirmed by pathology, and culture eventually grew Mycobacterium. This is the surgically excised pericardium and atrial specimen

One common approach to semi-quantitate the amount of pericardial effusion is to assess the posterior pericardial separation in diastole at the mid ventricular level from the parasternal window. The pericardial effusion is small (<100 mL) if the separation is less than 1 cm. If the pericardial separation is greater than 2 cm, the pericardial effusion is large and generally more than 500 mL. The pericardial effusion is moderate when the pericardial separation is between 1 and 2 cm and the pericardial volume is between 100 and 500 mL. When the pericardial separation is mainly seen during systole, the amount of pericardial effusion is likely physiological, that is less than 50 mL. Trivial pericardial effusion is present if there is persistent pericardial separation in both diastole and systole and the separation is less than 0.5 cm in diastole.

Pericardial effusion was one of the first conditions to be identified by echocardiography and the diagnosis is easy to make in most circumstances [5]. If only an anterior pericardial separation is present, other diagnoses should be considered (Table 10.2). In such cases the diagnosis of pericardial effusion should be made with caution, as a pericardial effusion is generally more prominent posteriorly unless it is loculated (Fig. 10.7). If the "loculated pericardial effusion" is located only anteriorly and leftward, the possibility of

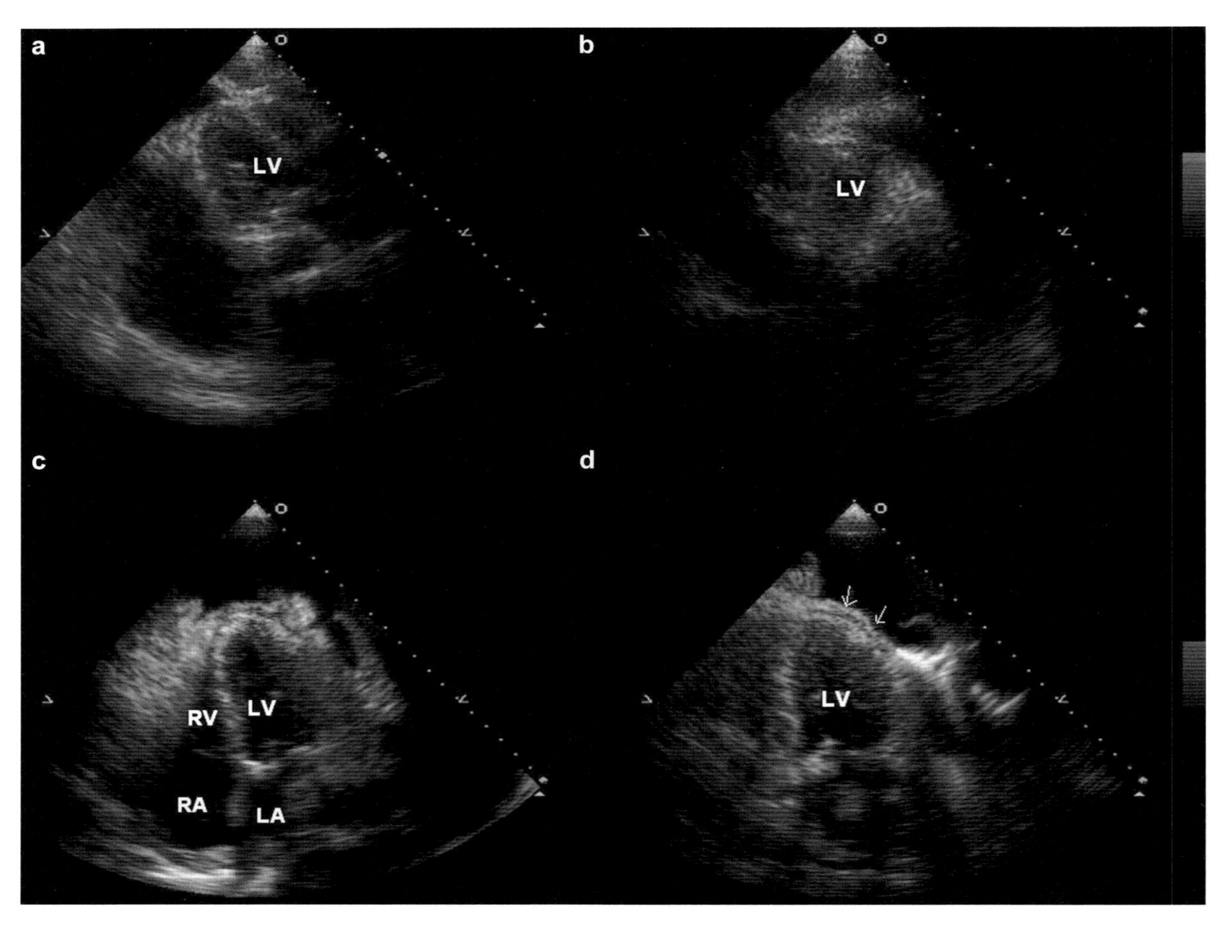

Fig. 10.10 A large left pleural effusion is demonstrated in multiple views including parasternal long-axis (**a**), short-axis (**b**), apical four-chamber (**c**), and apical two-chamber (**d**) views. This large pleural effusion may be confused with pericardial effusion. In the parasternal long-axis view (**a**), the effusion tracks behind the aorta consistent with pleural effusion. The pericardium (*arrows*) is well seen, particularly in the apical two-chamber view (**d**), confirming that there is no pericardial effusion. *LA* left atrium, *LV* left ventricle, *RA* right atrium, *RV* right ventricle

such that the pericardium is delineated between the two fluid spaces (Fig. 10.14). Although transesophageal echocardiography has been used to assess pericardial thickness, our experience suggests that it too has limitations [6]. Computed tomography (CT) is preferred over echocardiography in assessing pericardial thickness and the presence and extent of pericardial calcification (Figs. 10.15, 10.16). However, normal pericardial thickness by CT does not exclude the diagnosis of constrictive pericarditis [7]. Echocardiography has a limited role in the diagnosis of pericarditis. Although the presence of pericardial effusion is confirmatory in a patient suspected of pericarditis, the absence of pericardial effusion does not exclude the diagnosis.

Pericardial Tamponade

Tamponade refers to the condition in which the accumulation of pericardial effusion leads to limited ventricular filling resulting in diminished cardiac output [8]. The amount of pericardial effusion required to produce hemodynamic compromise is dependent on a number of factors described above. The mere presence of a large pericardial effusion does not necessarily indicate the presence of tamponade. In cardiac tamponade, there is an increase in intrapericardial pressure, thus restricting filling of the cardiac chambers during diastole. The elevated pericardial pressure can exceed the intracavitary pressures of the cardiac chambers at certain times

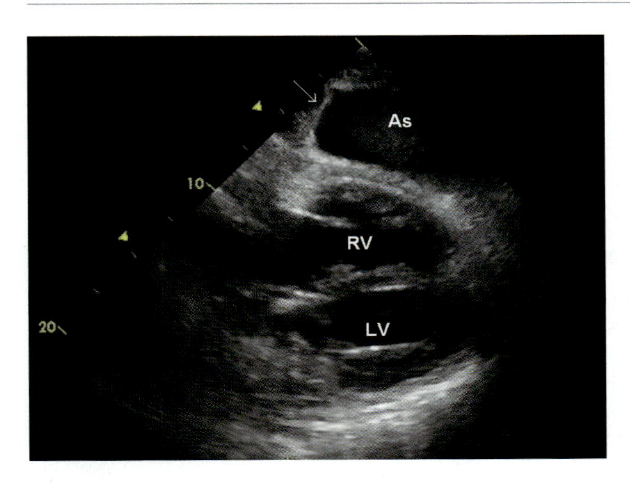

Fig. 10.11 The subcostal view shows that there is an echo lucent space anterior to the heart. There is echo linear density consistent with the falciform ligament (*arrow*). This echo lucent space is caused by ascites

of the cardiac cycle, as intracardiac pressures fluctuate during the cardiac cycle. When this happens, the positive transmural pressure gradient leads to compression of the free wall of the cardiac chamber. Thus, the cardiac chamber with the lowest intracavitary pressures is more liable to demonstrate compression at an earlier stage of the disease.

The early sign of tamponade is right atrial inversion occurring during atrial relaxation, which corresponds to late ventricular diastole or early systole (Fig. 10.17) [9]. Persistence of right atrial inversion over at least one third of the cardiac cycle enhances the specificity of the finding [10]. Right atrial inversion is best appreciated from the apical four-chamber view.

Early and mid-diastolic right ventricular collapse is another finding of tamponade (Fig. 10.17) [11]. The parasternal long and short axis view and the right

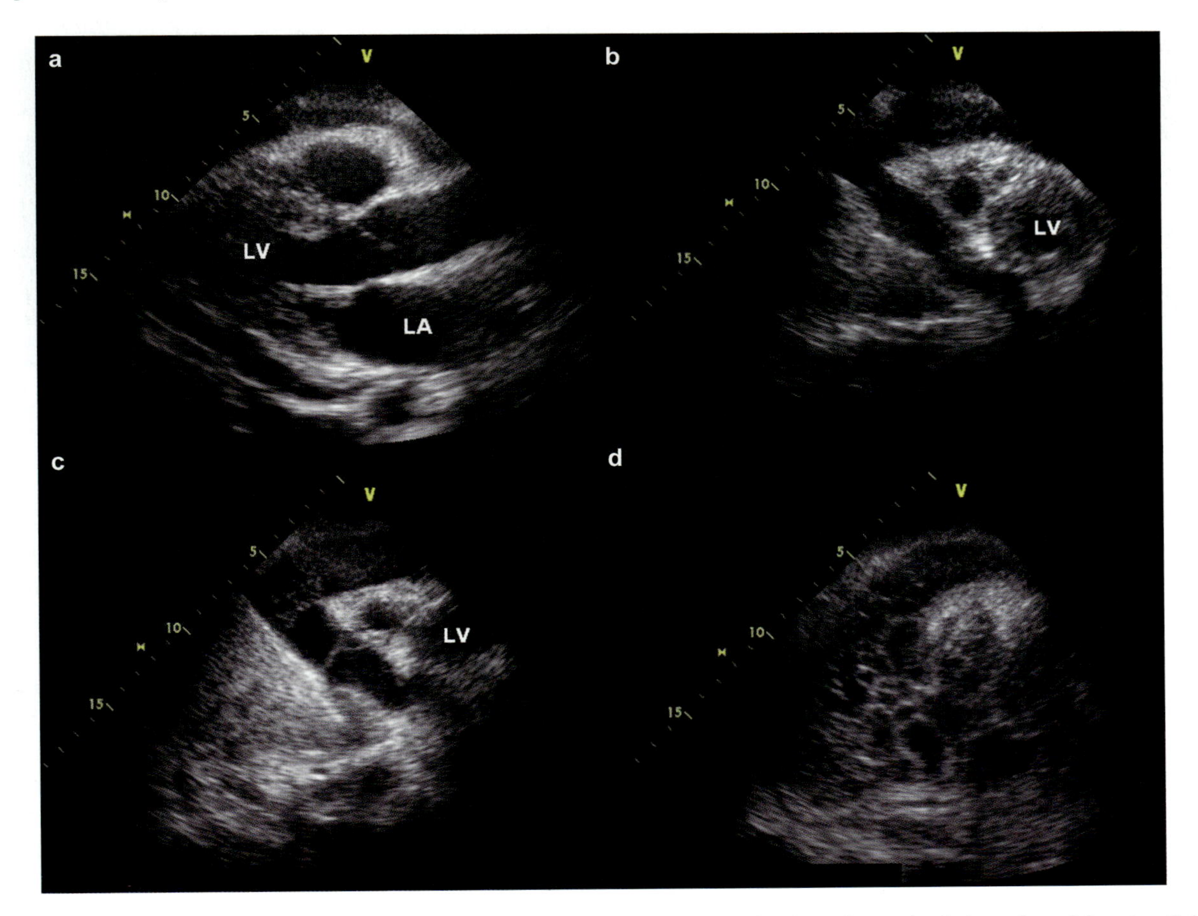

Fig. 10.12 This 31-year-old man has chronic idiopathic pericarditis for 18 months. A moderate sized circumferential pericardial effusion is seen in all views including the parasternal long-axis (**a**) and parasternal short-axis (**b–d**) views. Multiple linear densities are seen within the pericardial effusion particularly in (**c**) and (**d**). These likely represent fibrinous strands or bands. *LA* left atrium, *LV* left ventricle

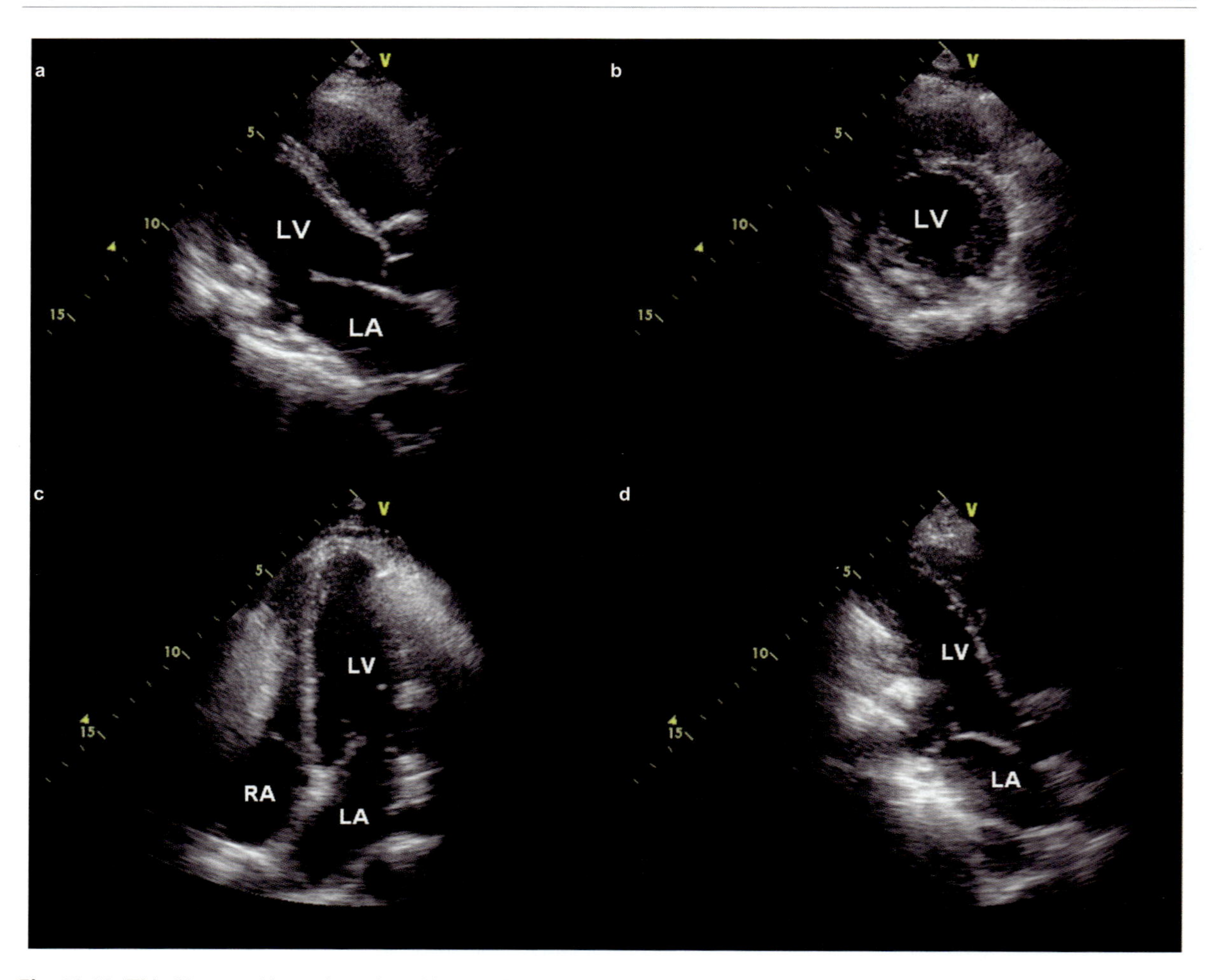

Fig. 10.13 This 51-year-old man has a long history of recurrent pericarditis. Prominent pericardial calcification is present posterior to the left ventricle (**a, b, d**) and over the right ventricular surface (**c**). *LA* left atrium, *LV* left ventricle

ventricular inflow view are used to assess this finding. Compared to right atrial inversion, right ventricular diastolic collapse is a more specific marker for tamponade. Loading conditions can affect the reliability of these findings. For instance, in the setting of tamponade and right ventricular hypertrophy, right ventricular collapse may not be present [12].

The total cardiac volume (right and left heart chambers) is limited by the pericardial effusion resulting in two important hemodynamic consequences. The increased intrapericardial pressure insulates the cardiac chambers from the fluctuations of intrathoracic pressure during respiration (Fig. 10.18) [8]. The limitation on the overall cardiac volume magnifies the effect of ventricular interdependence, which is reflected by the phasic changes in ventricular volume during the respiratory cycle. An increase in right ventricular volume during inspiration can only occur with leftward ventricular septal shift and a decrease in left ventricular volume, leading to a decrease in left ventricular stroke volume. This is the physiologic basis for pulsus paradoxus [13, 14].

During inspiration, the pressure within the extracardiac pulmonary veins decreases, but due to the elevated pericardial pressure the pressure within the intracardiac pulmonary veins is far less affected, thus reducing the driving pressure (Fig. 10.18). The pulmonary venous diastolic antegrade flow and mitral flow reflected by the mitral E velocity are both reduced. The decrease in left heart filling allows more right heart filling with shifting of the ventricular septum leftward, and the tricuspid flow reflected by the tricuspid E velocity is increased (Fig. 10.19). This prominent phasic variation of mitral and tricuspid inflow velocities is the basis for

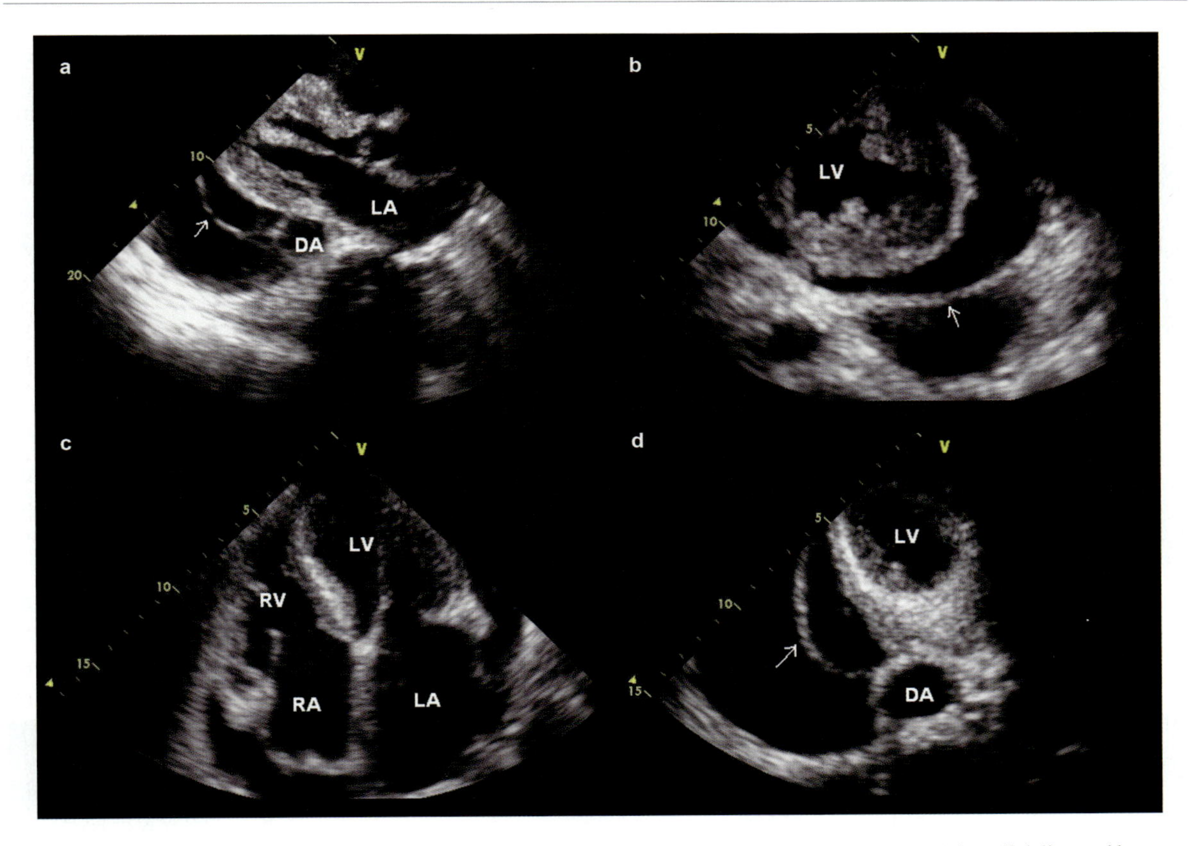

Fig. 10.14 In this patient with both pericardial effusion and left pleural effusion, the pericardium (*arrow*) is well delineated between the two fluid spaces in multiple parasternal and apical views (**a–d**). The pericardium is of normal appearance and thickness. *DA* descending aorta, *LA* left atrium, *LV* left ventricle, *RA* right atrium, *RV* right ventricle

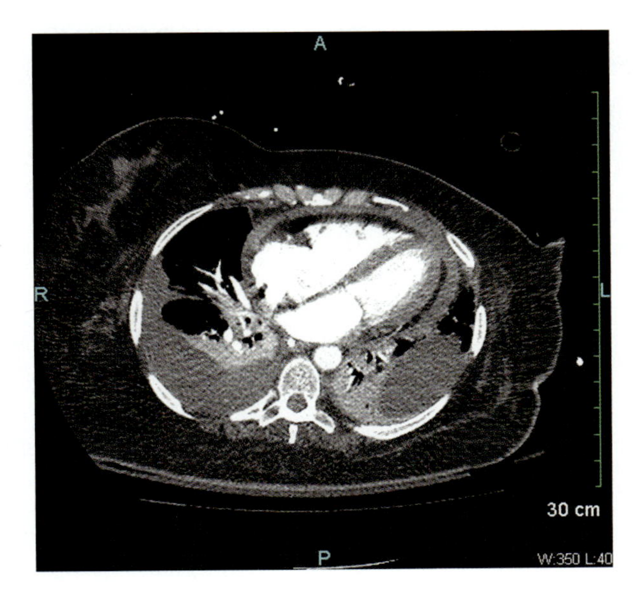

Fig. 10.15 On the computed tomogram, the pericardium shows severe diffuse thickening with no calcification. Bilateral pleural effusions are present

the diastolic septal bounce seen in this condition. Vena caval flow also demonstrates these respiratory phasic changes. This is demonstrated by pulsed wave Doppler with the sample volume in the hepatic vein. Expiration is usually accompanied by an increase in diastolic flow reversal. The inferior vena cava is dilated with no significant respiratory changes in size, as a result of elevated right atrial pressure [15].

Tamponade is a clinical diagnosis and it is not an "all or none" phenomenon, but instead it has a continuum of severity. Patients with mild symptoms may have some, but not all, of the echocardiographic features. Some of these features may not be apparent in the setting of hypovolemia. If hypovolemia is suspected, volume loading followed by repeat echo-Doppler assessment can be useful [16].

In patients with intrapericardial hematoma such as those following open heart surgery, the restriction to filling may be related to localized blood clot compressing one or two cardiac chambers, usually the right atrium

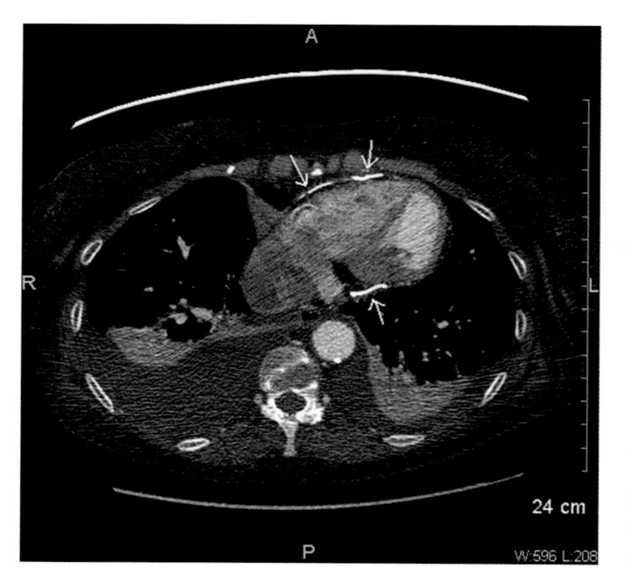

Fig. 10.16 The computed tomogram shows extensive calcification (*arrows*) involving both the anterior and posterior aspects of the pericardium. Bilateral pleural effusions are present

and/or the right ventricle. In this instance, the intrapericardial pressure is not evenly distributed, and the typical echo findings of tamponade may be absent. This diagnosis can be made by the evidence of limitation in ventricular filling and the demonstration of the compressive nature of the intrapericardial hematoma, which is well visualized by transesophageal echocardiography [17] (Fig. 10.20).

Constrictive Pericarditis

With resolution of acute pericarditis the pericardium may become thickened and calcified. The pericardial space is often obliterated with adherence of the pericardium to the visceral pericardium (Figs. 10.21, 10.22). This causes non-distensibility of the heart and may compress the thin right-sided chambers causing constriction. Clinically, this is manifest as chronic

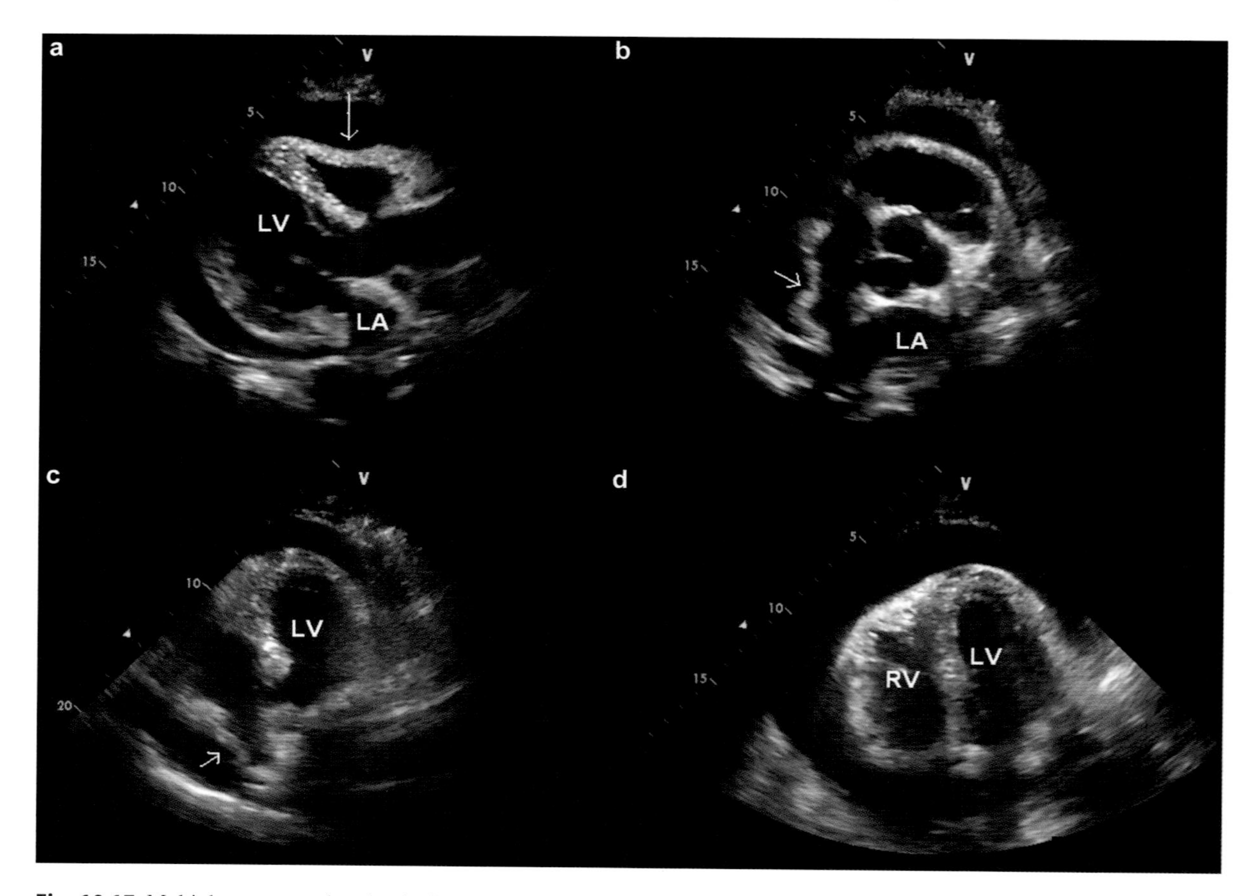

Fig. 10.17 Multiple parasternal and apical echocardiographic views (**a–d**) from a patient with cardiac tamponade showing the typical findings including right atrial inversion (*short arrow*) and right ventricular diastolic collapse (*long arrow*)

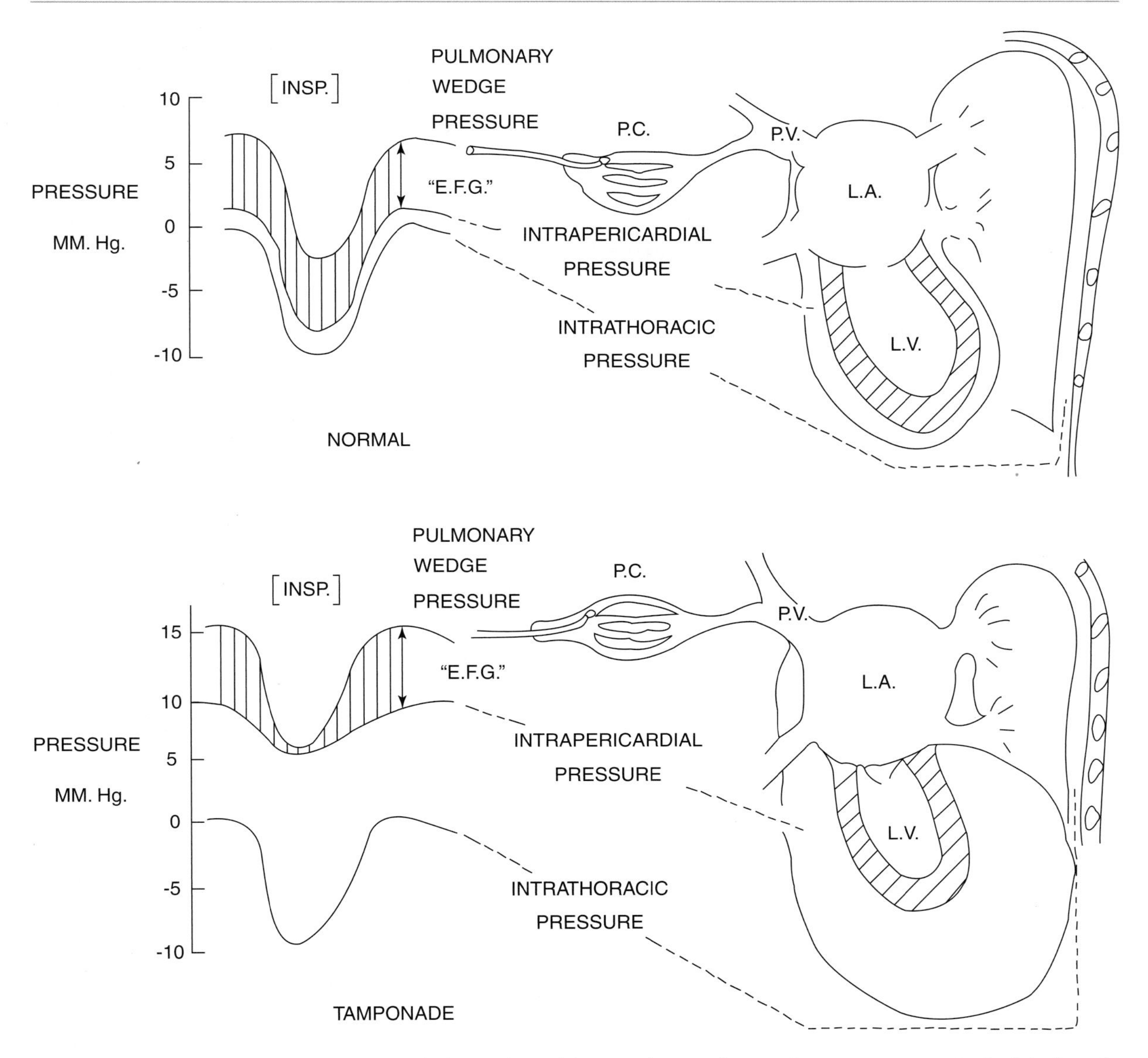

Fig. 10.18 In the normal setting (the *top* half of the schematic) concordant respiratory changes are present in the intrathoracic, intrapericardial, and pulmonary wedge pressures so that the effective filling gradient (*EFG*) of the left ventricle (*LV*) remains relatively stable during respiration, and little change in the mitral E velocity. In pericardial tamponade (the *bottom* half of the schematic), the intrapericardial pressure is elevated and the changes in intrathoracic pressure are poorly transmitted to the distended pericardial sac, thus reducing the effective filling gradient and a significantly diminished mitral E velocity on inspiration. (Reproduced by Sharp et al. [8]. With permission)

congestive heart failure, predominantly right sided, with signs and symptoms such as peripheral edema, ascites, and weight gain. Certain etiologies of pericarditis seem to be more prone to constrict than others. Tuberculosis was the most common cause and remains a common cause worldwide [18]. Purulent pericarditis and neoplastic pericarditis are also frequently associated with the development of constriction within 6 months after the diagnosis [19]. Iatrogenic causes such as poststernotomy or postradiation are now increasingly common causes of constrictive pericarditis in developed countries. On the other hand, about 20% of patients with idiopathic pericarditis may develop transient constriction, but they are unlikely to have long-term constriction [20, 21]. Constriction may be associated with an effusion, so called effusive–constrictive pericarditis, and,

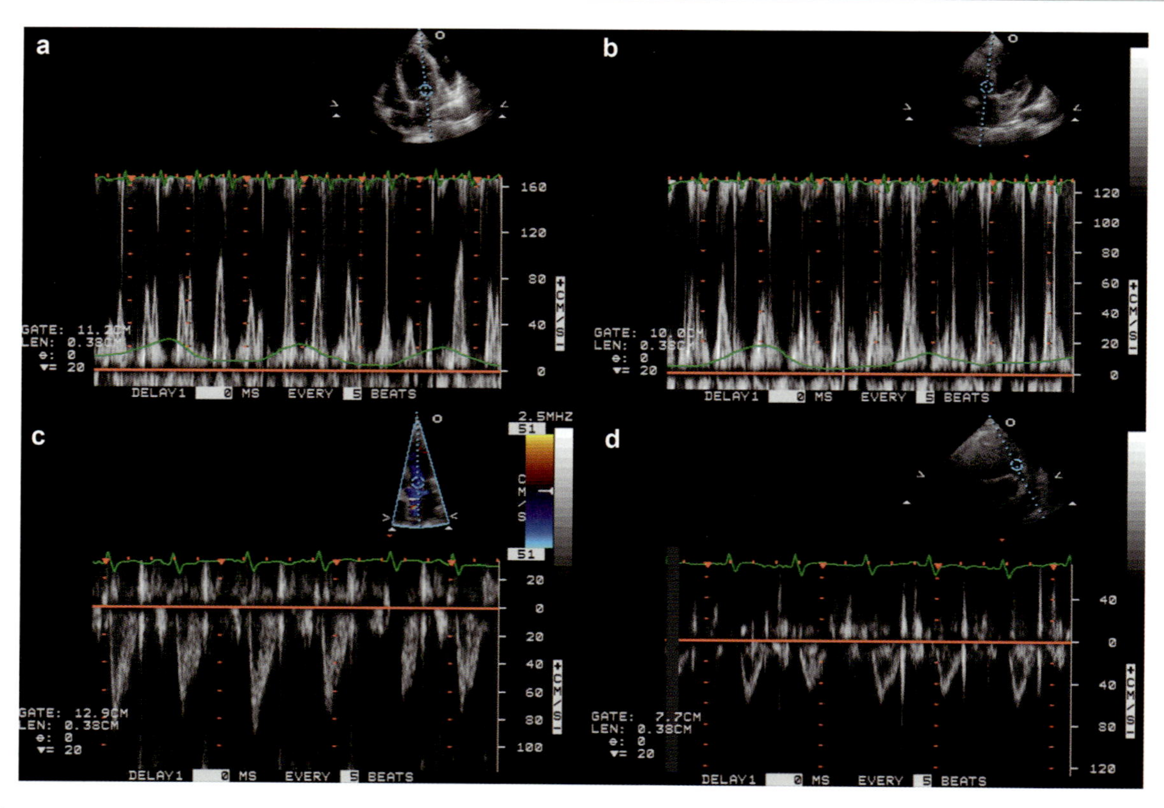

Fig. 10.19 In this 60-year-old woman with cardiac tamponade, severe degree of phasic variation in the mitral (**a**) and tricuspid (**b**) velocities is present. Respiratory phasic changes in the left ventricular (**c**) and right ventricular (**d**) stroke volumes are also present, consistent with the presence of pulsus paradoxus in this patient

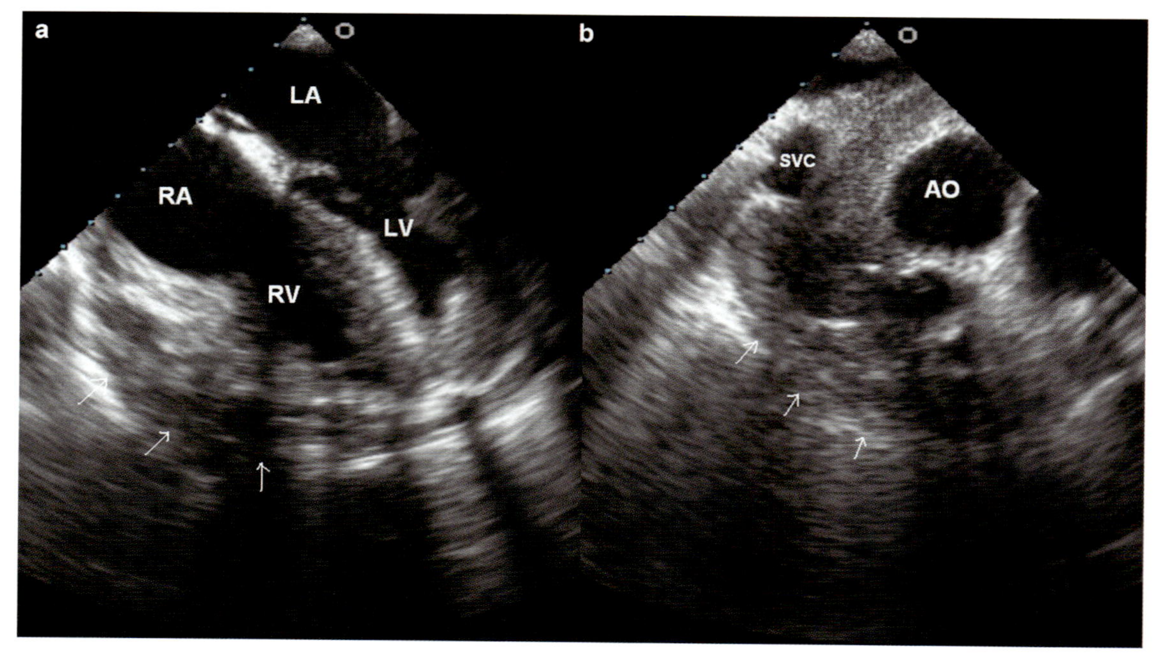

Fig. 10.20 The transesophageal echocardiogram is obtained in the recovery room in a patient with low cardiac output following cardiac surgery. Extensive mass consistent with hematoma (*arrows*) is present over the right atrial and right ventricular surface (**a**) and also surrounding the aorta and superior vena cava (**b**). *Ao* aorta, *LA* left atrium, *LV* left ventricle, *RA* right atrium, *RV* right ventricle, *SVC* superior vena cava

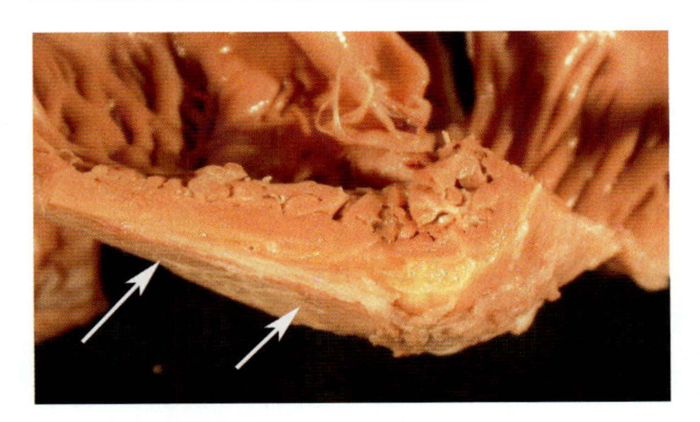

Fig. 10.21 Constrictive pericarditis in a patient after bypass grafting. The pericardial space is obliterated and the parietal pericardium (*arrows*) thickened and adherent to the heart

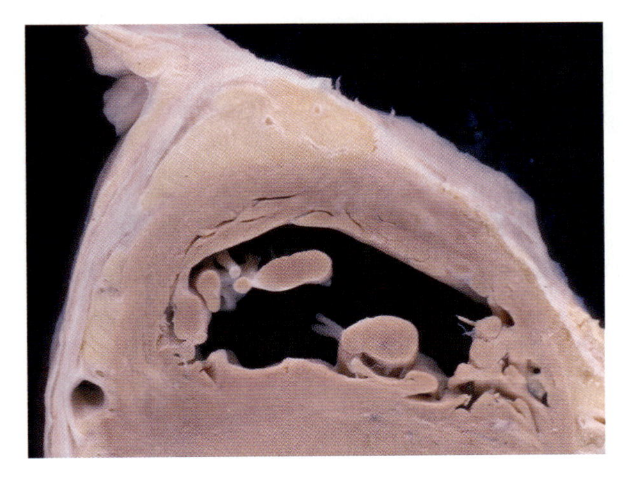

Fig. 10.22 Constrictive pericarditis after chest radiation. The pericardium is thick and adherent to the heart thus obliterating the normal pericardial space is some areas

in this setting, pericardiocentesis will have limited effect on the clinical outcome.

The limitation of cardiac volume is due to a noncompliant, thickened, or calcified pericardium encasing the heart. Although the underlying mechanism is different compared to tamponade, the hemodynamic effects are similar [22] (Fig. 10.23). The cardiac volume is small and fixed within the encasement of the noncompliant pericardium. Early diastolic filling is normal, but there is rapid termination of flow when the compliance of the pericardium is reached, leading to rapid equalization of pressures between atria and ventricles. The high intrapericardial pressure leads to a dissociation of the intrathoracic pressure with the intracardiac pressures. There is also enhancement of ventricular interdependence as a result of the fixed cardiac volumes, due to the restrictive effect of the noncompliant pericardium. An increase in right ventricular filling during inspiration is invariably associated with leftward displacement of the ventricular septum and a decrease in left ventricular filling.

The typical changes in constriction are (1)>25% decrease in mitral E velocity during inspiration, (2)>40% increase in tricuspid E velocity during inspiration, (3) a reduction in aortic velocity with inspiration, (4) decrease in isovolumic relaxation time with inspiration, and (5) an increase in tricuspid regurgitation velocity with inspiration [22, 23]. The pulmonary vein flow demonstrates similar phasic changes as the mitral velocities (Fig. 10.24). The pulmonary vein early diastolic velocity decreases on inspiration and increases on expiration. Mitral annular velocities remain relatively normal in this condition [24] (Fig. 10.25). It is recognized that these findings may not be present in some patients with proven constriction.

In our view, the pathophysiology is similar between constriction and tamponade. The difference between the two entities is largely quantitative rather than qualitative. In tamponade the cardiac volumes are much more reduced than those in constriction, leading to a greater degree of hemodynamic derangement.

Patients with chronic obstructive lung disease can have prominent phasic variation of mitral and tricuspid inflow velocities, due to the increased change in intrathoracic pressure during respiration. Superior vena cava flow velocities have been shown to be useful to differentiate chronic obstructive lung disease from constriction. In the former, there is respiratory variation in superior vena cava flow with significant increase in systolic antegrade velocity during inspiration, whereas in the latter there is little or no change from expiration to inspiration [25].

Constrictive Pericarditis Versus Restrictive Cardiomyopathy

It has been difficult to differentiate patients with constrictive pericarditis from patients with restrictive cardiomyopathy, as the clinical findings are similar (Table 10.3). The differentiation is important, as pericardiectomy can alleviate the symptoms in patients with constriction [26, 27]. The mitral velocities are also similar in both conditions with high mitral E velocity and short deceleration time. However, in patients with restrictive cardiomyopathy, there is normal association of intracardiac pressures with the intrathoracic pressure,

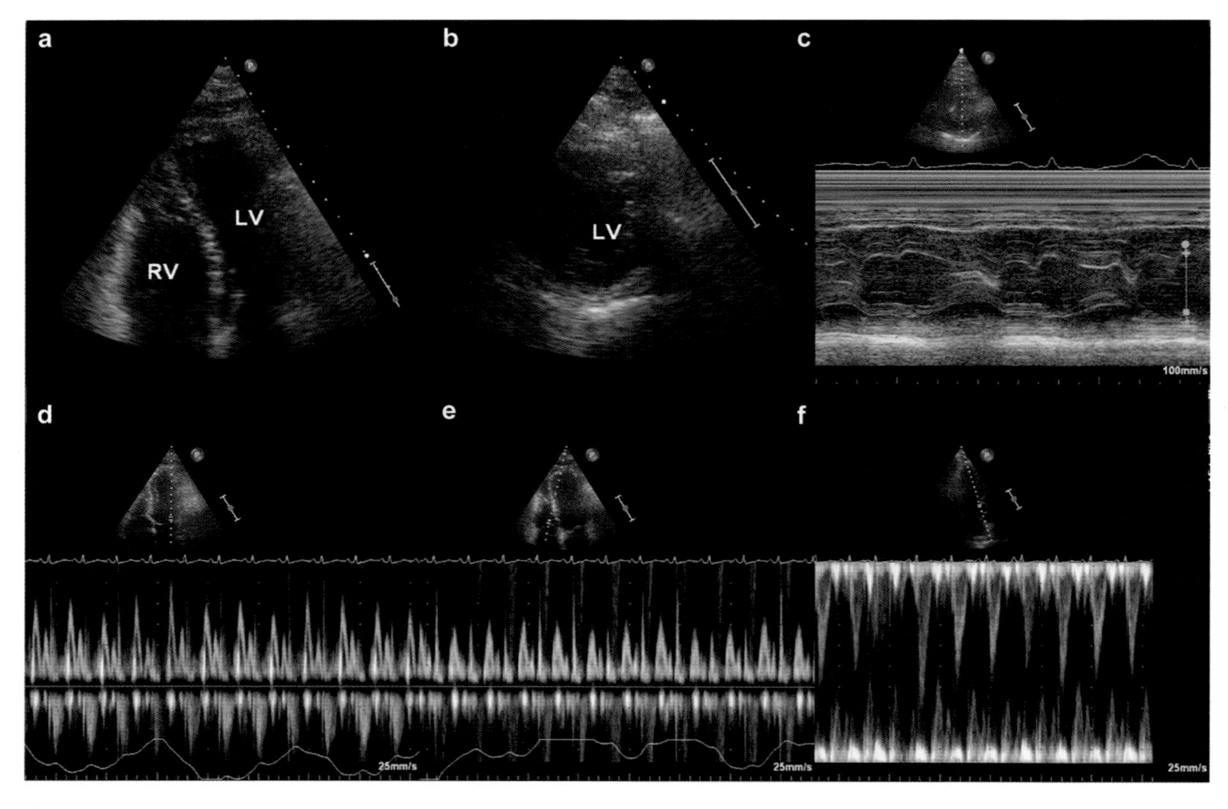

Fig. 10.23 In this 49-year-old man with constrictive pericarditis, the apical four-chamber (**a**) and parasternal short-axis (**b**) views show the abnormal septal bounce, which is better illustrated by the M-mode recording (**c**). The marked respiratory phasic changes of the mitral (**d**), tricuspid (**e**), and left ventricular outflow tract (**f**) velocities are present. *LV* left ventricle, *RV* right ventricle

such that the marked phasic changes in the mitral and tricuspid velocities are not seen. Furthermore, the annular early diastolic velocity is preserved in constriction, whereas it is generally markedly reduced in patients with restrictive cardiomyopathy due to the presence of intrinsic myocardial disease.

Endomyocardial biopsy may be important to distinguish pericardial constriction from restrictive myocardial disease, such as restrictive cardiomyopathy or amyloid [27]. In constrictive pericarditis the heart biopsy shows normal myocardium or atrophic fibers. In the restrictive disease there is myocardial pathology present and a pericardiectomy is inappropriate. For constrictive pericarditis the treatment is pericardiectomy. A total removal is often not possible due to the degree of fibrous adhesions. At surgery the pericardium is removed and the heart usually recovers function. Unfortunately some cases are detected too late and the myocardium has atrophied so that the ventricle does not recover. Ventricular failure and bleeding are important postoperative complications following pericardiectomy.

Pericardial Tumors

Tumors involving the pericardium may be primary or more commonly metastatic in nature [28]. Primary tumors are usually mesothelioma or angiosarcoma [29, 30]. Angiosarcoma is the most common primary malignant tumor involving the heart [31]. Typically, the tumor involves the pericardium and the right atrium. It is often associated with a bloody effusion and there may be tamponade. Grossly, there are large hemorrhagic masses or nodules associated with a bloody effusion. Microscopic examination shows that there are abnormal vascular channels either spindle-shaped cells, epitheloid, or poorly differentiated cells.

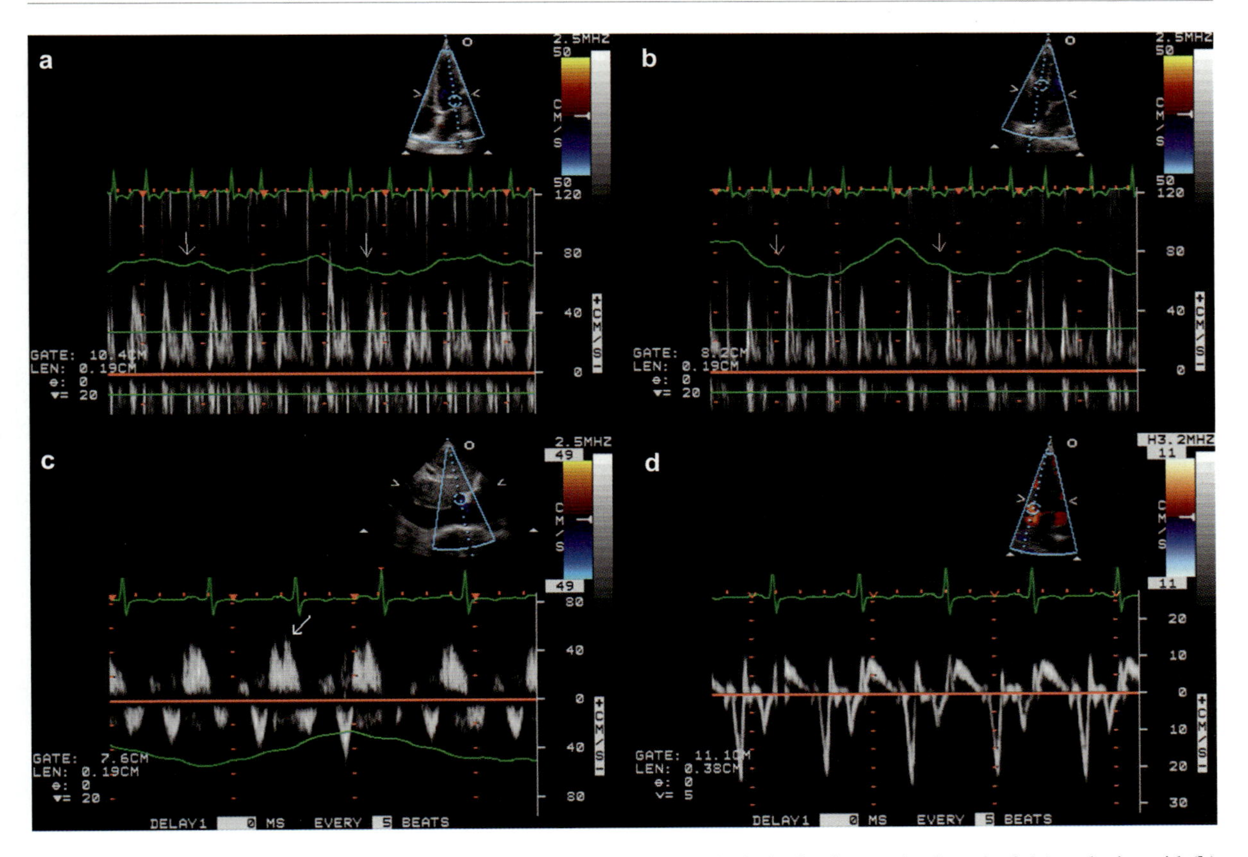

Fig. 10.24 In this 51-year-old man with constrictive pericarditis the marked phasic changes in the mitral (**a**) and tricuspid (**b**) velocities are present. There is a decrease in mitral velocities with a reciprocal increase in tricuspid velocities on inspiration (*arrows*). Hepatic vein flow shows an increase in diastolic flow reversal (*arrow*) on expiration. There is typical preservation of annular velocities (**d**), which are generally severely reduced in patients with restrictive cardiomyopathy

Patients with all types of angiosarcoma have poor prognosis. The tumor is often advanced at diagnosis and only palliation is possible. Eventually, the tumor will metastasize to visceral organs.

Mesothelioma of the pericardium is a rare tumor [32]. The pericardium becomes thickened on the visceral and parietal surfaces and the pericardial space may obliterate. Constrictive pericarditis is the usual outcome. Removing the pericardium or creating a pericardial window may relieve the associated effusion but the effect is transient and only palliative. All histological types of mesothelioma may occur – epitheloid, sarcomatoid, or biphasic. All mesotheliomas carry poor prognosis. In addition to primary mesothelioma, the pericardium may also be involved by spread of adjacent pleural mesothelioma.

Secondary or metastatic tumors may also involve the heart through local extension or invasion. Tumors may enter the heart locally via the endocardial route in the vena cava (renal cell carcinoma, gynecological tumor). There may be direct invasion from the adjacent primary tumor or lymph node deposits – common in lung and esophageal carcinoma and lymphomas (Fig. 10.26). The deposits may also result from spread via the blood or the lymphatics (carcinomas and melanomas).

Metastatic deposits may affect any layer of the heart but the pericardium is the most common layer to be involved [28]. Pericardial metastases may involve the visceral or the parietal pericardium. The pericardium may thicken, but sometimes despite being laden with tumor cells, the thickness may be normal. Pericardial effusion is very common, and constriction may occur. At pericardiectomy or pericardiocentesis a bloody effusion may suggest this possibility and cytological examination of the fluid or histological examination of tissues should be performed in order to make the

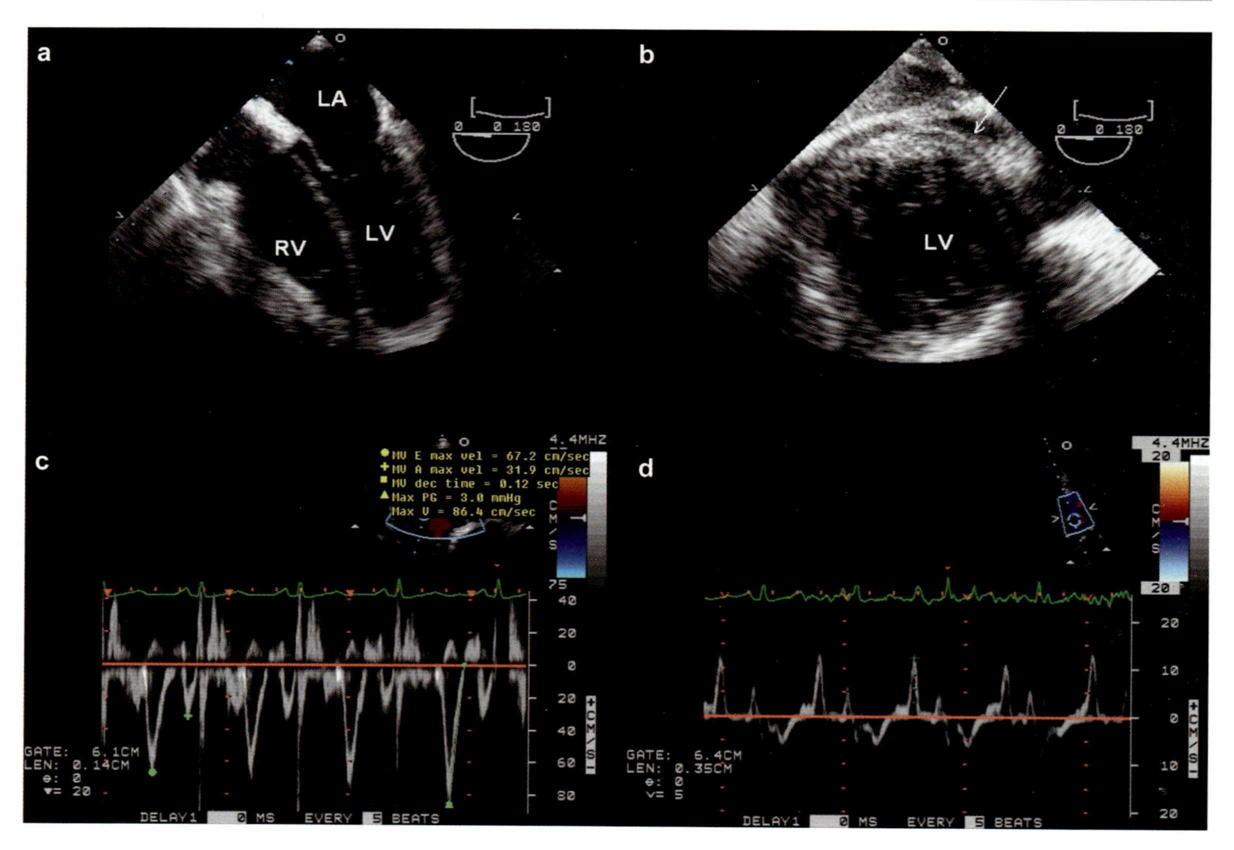

Fig. 10.25 This is the same patient shown in Fig. 10.24. Transesophageal four-chamber (**a**) and transgastric short-axis (**b**) views show that the pericardium is diffusely thickened (*arrow*). In addition to respiratory phasic variations, the mitral flow shows EA ratio>2 and a short deceleration time. The pulmonary vein velocities show similar respiratory phasic changes (**d**)

Table 10.3 Differentiating features of constrictive pericarditis versus restrictive cardiomyopathy

	Constrictive pericarditis	Restrictive cardiomyopathy
Pericardium	Normal or thickened	Normal
Left ventricular function	Normal	Normal or mildly reduced
Atrial size	Normal	Dilated atria
Tricuspid and mitral regurgitation	Absent or only mild	>Mild TR and MR are common
Mitral inflow velocities E>>A	Present	Present
Short mitral deceleration time	Present	Present
Abnormal respiratory phasic ventricular septal motion	Present	Absent
Increased respiratory phasic variation of mitral and tricuspid inflow velocities	Present	Absent
Mitral annular velocities	Normal or increased	Low

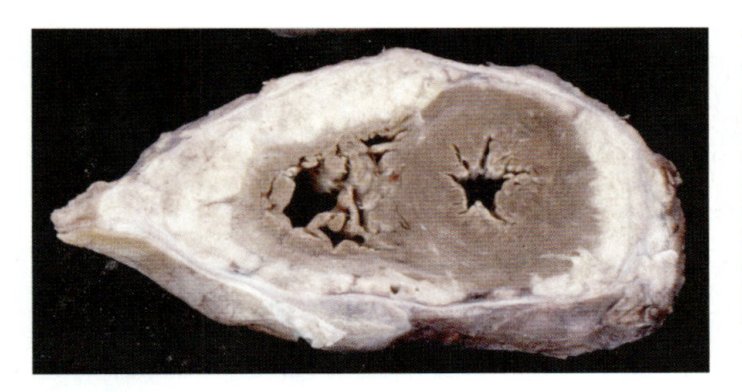

Fig. 10.26 Metastatic squamous cell carcinoma of the lung. The pericardium is white, thick, and adherent to the heart filling the pericardial space

diagnosis. Drainage of the fluid is palliative and a pericardial window to prevent tamponade may also be done for palliation.

Absence of the Pericardium

Congenital absence of the pericardium is an unusual condition with an estimated incidence of 5–10 per 100,000. It is more common to have complete absence of the left-sided pericardium [33]. Absence of the right-sided pericardium is rare. It is more common in men with a male to female ratio of 3:1. In about one third of the cases, there are associated cardiac anomalies. In complete absence of the pericardium, many of these patients are asymptomatic and the absence is detected as an incidental finding, although symptoms such as chest pain, dyspnea, or dizziness have been reported. In the setting of partial absence of the pericardium, constriction of cardiac structures such as the left atrium by the remaining pericardium is a rare complication. Chest X-ray shows levoposition of the heart, a narrow mediastinum and elongation of the left ventricular border. The echo findings of complete absence of the pericardium are listed in Table 10.4 [34, 35]. This condition needs to be considered, when the heart has an extremely transverse lie with the apical window near the axilla, particularly with the patient lying supine. The apical four-chamber view has a peculiar shape likened to a teardrop with the atria more streamlined and the ventricles more bulbous (Fig. 10.27). Due to the clockwise rotation of heart, it can simulate

Table 10.4 Echocardiographic features of complete absence of the pericardium

• Unusually lateral apical window
• Cardiac hypermobility
• Abnormal swinging motion
• Abnormal ventricular septal motion
• Teardrop shape

right ventricular volume overload. This condition can be readily confirmed by CT(Fig. 10.28). The prognosis in these patients is generally excellent and surgical intervention is rarely necessary except for patients with partial defects and cardiac symptoms.

Pericardial Cysts

The incidence of pericardial cysts is about 1 in 100,000. This is generally an incidental finding and not associated with symptoms. It is most commonly detected in the fourth decade and seen equally in both sexes. It is frequently located at the right or left costophrenic angle. It is a round or oval structure with smooth edges with an echo lucent center (Figs. 10.29, 10.30, 10.31). Surgical excision is rarely indicated because it generally does not cause significant compression to the surrounding structures. However, life-threatening complications such as tamponade have been reported [36, 37].

Echo-Guided Pericardiocentesis

Echo has an essential role in the performance of pericardiocentesis, as its use has reduced the complications associated with the procedure [38]. The principle of echo-guided pericardiocentesis is the localization of the largest pericardial separation with the least amount of interface between the chest wall and the pericardial separation. In addition to locating the optimal position on the chest wall for the pericardiocentesis, the exact angulation of the transducer should be noted. It is advisable to select a location at least 3 cm from the sternum so as to avoid inadvertent damage to the

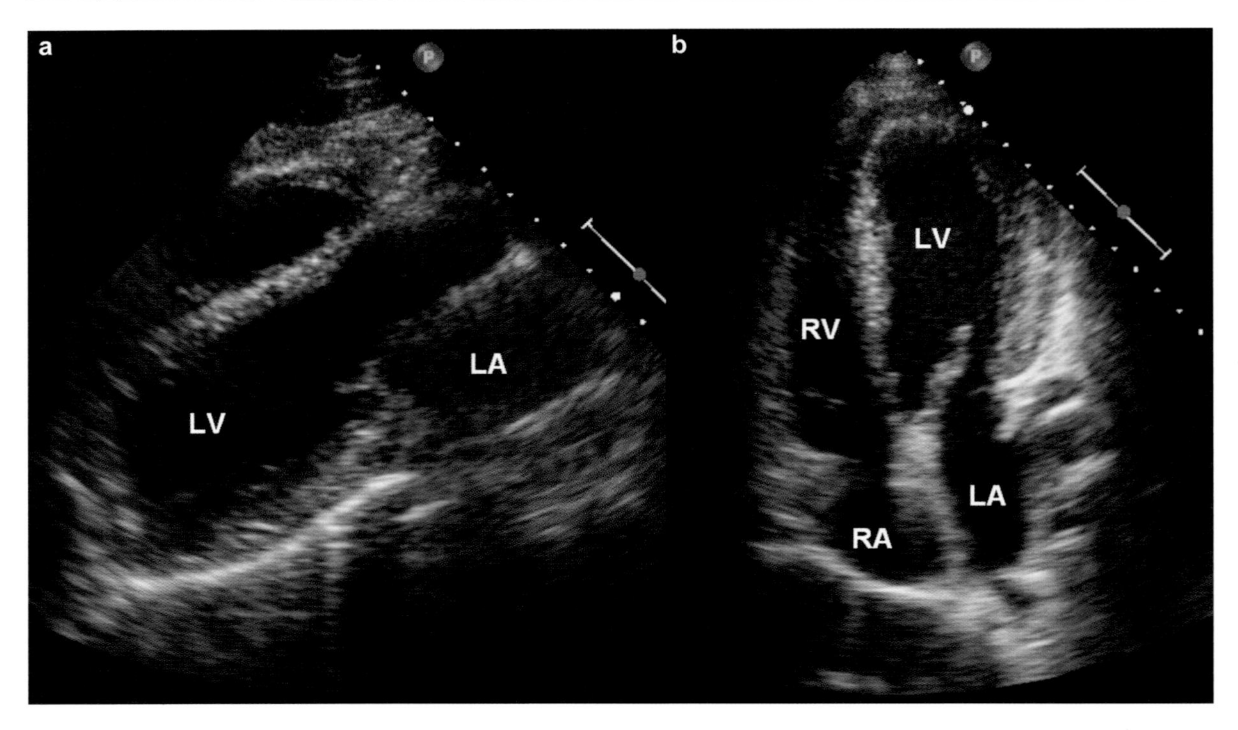

Fig. 10.27 The parasternal long-axis (**a**) and apical four-chamber (**b**) views in a 43-year-old man show typical findings of complete absence of the pericardium. The cardiac chambers have an unusual orientation. The apical four-chamber is obtained with the transducer at the left axilla with the patient lying supine as the apex of the heart is deviated extremely leftward and posterior. The four-chamber view has a typical teardrop shape. *LA* left atrium, *LV* left ventricle, *RA* right ventricle, *RV* right ventricle

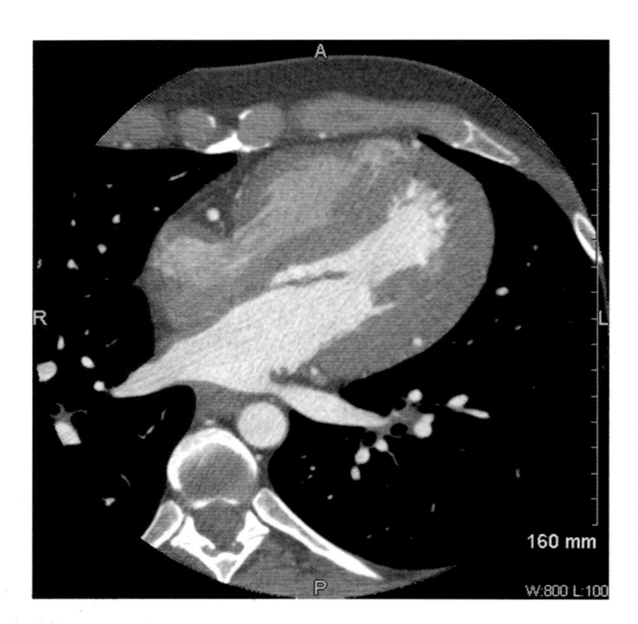

Fig. 10.28 The computed tomogram of the same patient shown in Fig. 10.27 confirms complete absence of the pericardium

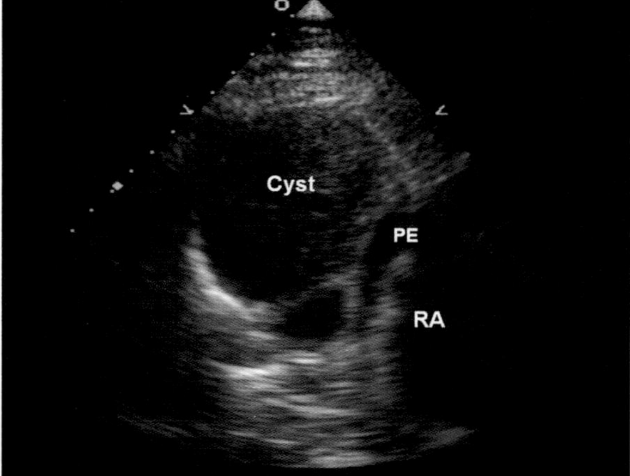

Fig. 10.29 This is a subcostal view showing a large echolucent mass at the right costophrenic angle consistent with a pericardial cyst. A small pericardial effusion is present. *PE* pericardial effusion, *RA* right atrium

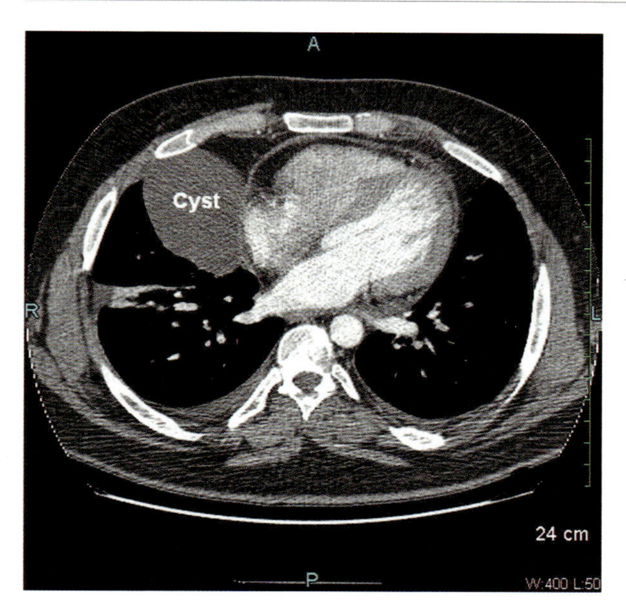

Fig. 10.30 A computed tomogram of the same patient as in Fig. 10.29 shows the large pericardial cyst to the right of the heart

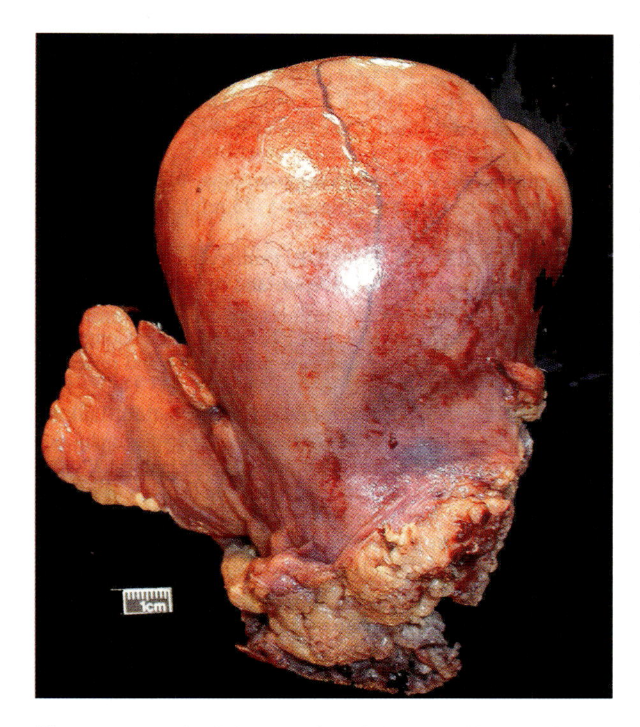

Fig. 10.31 Excised large pericardial cyst. This was full of fibrinous exudates and fluid. It was associated with adjacent fibrinous pericarditis in the pericardium surrounding the heart

internal thoracic artery. Selecting the chest wall location is the most critical step in the whole process.

Similar to the published data, our own experience shows that a para-apical location and not the subcostal location is the most common location for this procedure. When inserting the pericardiocentesis needle the operator should use the angulation similar to that of the echo transducer used to determine the optimal chest wall location. Monitoring the path of the needle is generally not necessary and in fact can be difficult as the ultrasound beam is usually oblique to the path of the needle. In order to ensure that the needle is in the pericardial space, injection of echo contrast into the pericardial space can be used to confirm its proper location. Echo-guided pericardiocentesis is the standard practice in our institution. Blindly using the subcostal approach can only be justified in emergency situations where echocardiography is not readily available.

Summary

Echocardiography is the primary tool in the detection of pericardial effusion. In pericardial tamponade and constrictive pericarditis, comprehensive Doppler assessment, particularly of the mitral and tricuspid velocities, has provided insight into the pathophysiology, and in constrictive pericarditis, it has a pivotal role in the diagnosis. Despite the advent of imaging modalities such as CT and magnetic resonance imaging, echocardiography is and will remain to be the imaging modality of choice in the assessment of patients with suspected pericardial disease.

References

1. Little WC, Freeman GL. Pericardial disease. *Circulation*. 2006 Mar 28;113(12):1622-1632.
2. Spodick DH. Macrophysiology, microphysiology, and anatomy of the pericardium: a synopsis. *Am Heart J*. 1992 Oct;124(4):1046-1051.
3. Ivens EL, Munt BI, Moss RR. Pericardial disease: the general cardiologist needs to know. *Heart*. 2007;93(8):993-1000.
4. Vaughan CM, D'Cruz IA. Applied anatomy of the pericardium:echocardiographic interpretation. *Primary Cardiol*. 1993;19(3):56-67.

Table 11.1 Early and late complications of prosthetic heart valves

Early complications (<1 month following implantation)		
All prostheses	Mechanical prostheses	Bioprosthesis
Paravalvular leak	Prosthesis malfunction due to suture overhang	Iatrogenic damage of prosthetic leaflet
Hemolysis	Suturing of valve orifice	
Infective endocarditis		
Valvular thrombosis		
Prosthesis malfunction		
left ventricular outflow tract (LVOT) obstruction		
Coronary ostial obstruction (AVR)		
Aortic dissection		
Thromboembolism		
Arrhythmia		
Heart block		
Chronic complications		
Thromboembolism Valvular thrombosis	Strut fracture	Leaflet degeneration
Pannus formation	Poppet variance	Leaflet tears
Perivalvular leak	Cloth wear and dehiscence	Leaflet perforation
Hemolysis		Stent creep
Patient–prosthesis mismatch		
Infective endocarditis		
LVOT obstruction		
LV free wall rupture (MVR)		
Heart block		
Arrhythmia		
Infective endocarditis		

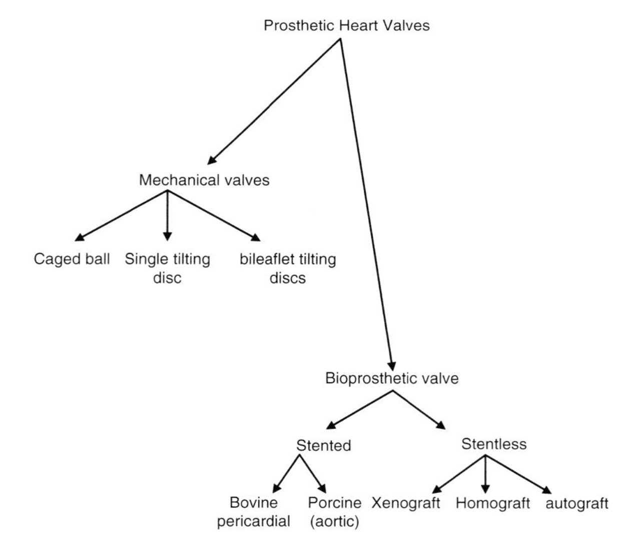

Fig. 11.1 Types of prosthetic heart valves

xenograft stentless valves usually are preparations of the porcine aortic root with the aortic valve in situ. They are developed to provide larger aortic orifices with lower transvalvular gradients. The Medtronic Freestyle and St. Jude Medical Toronto are two examples. They are technically demanding to implant. They can be fashioned to permit subcoronary implantation or to be implanted as a mini-root with reimplantation of the coronaries.

The same technical complexities apply to the homografts which are cryopreserved human aortas or pulmonary arteries. They are more limited in size and availability. An autograft is used mainly in young patients. This involves using the patient's own pulmonary valve to replace the dysfunctional aortic valve and implant a homograft in the pulmonary position. This procedure, commonly known as the Ross operation, is complex and technically demanding [7]. There is the potential of creating dysfunction of two valves (the aortic and pulmonary valves) to treat the dysfunction of one valve (the aortic valve), even if it is performed properly (Fig. 11.4).

It is useful to know the exact type, size and model of the prosthesis in order to properly interpret the hemodynamic findings obtained by Doppler echocardiography. For the tilting disc prosthesis (single disc or double disc), a small degree of regurgitation is a normal finding. With the Medtronic Hall valve, a single tilting disc with a central pivot, a small central valvular regurgitation is invariably present (Fig. 11.2). This normal regurgitant jet may not be appreciated by transthoracic echocardiography due to suboptimal images and reverberation artifact from the prosthetic valve, particularly those in the mitral or

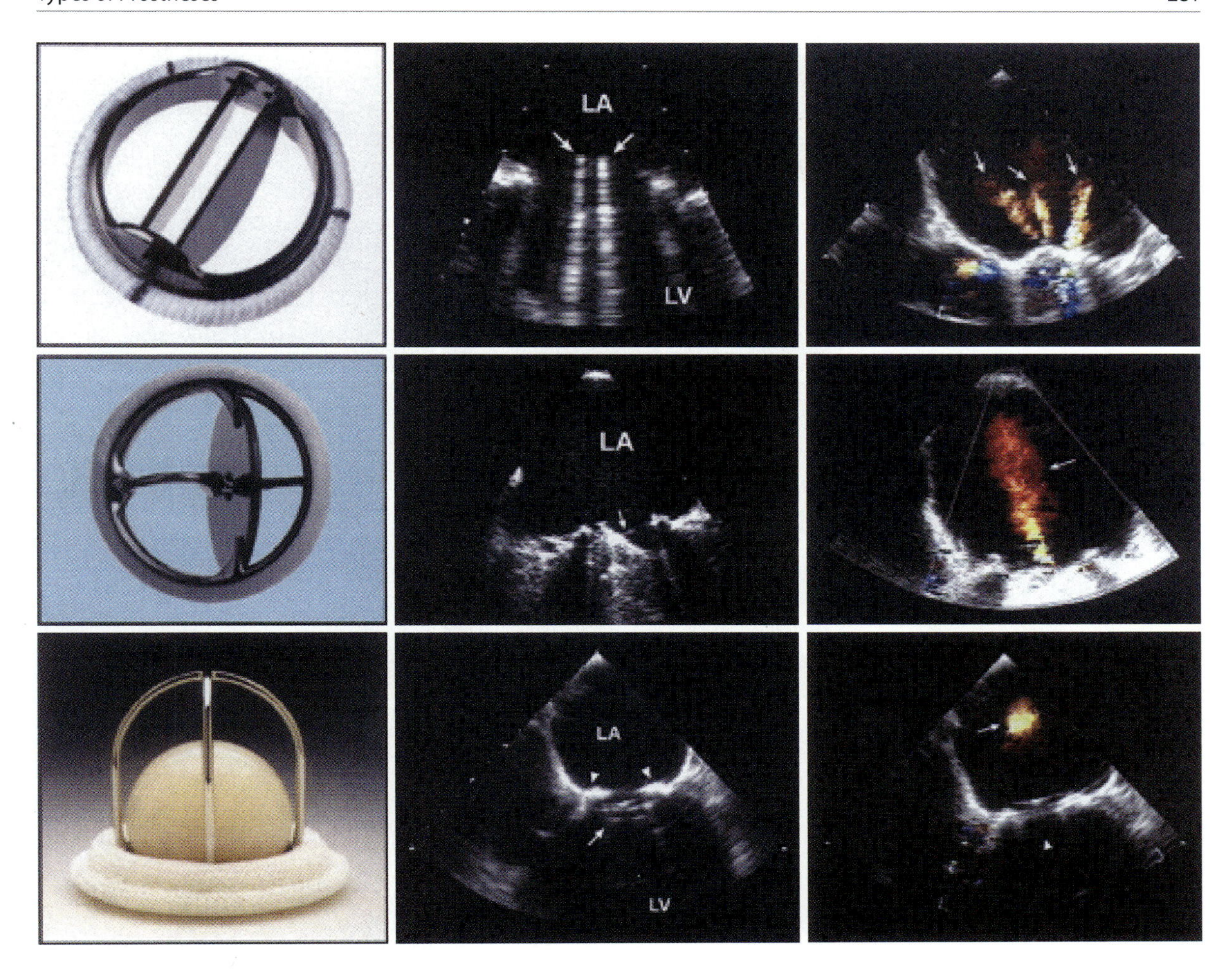

Fig. 11.2 The common types of mechanical heart valves with their corresponding transesophageal echocardiographic views during valve opening and typical color-flow images during closure. The St. Jude valve is shown on the top row, the Medtronic-Hall valve in the second row and the Starr-Edwards valve in the bottom row. *LA* left atrium, *LV* left ventricle (Reproduced from Zoghbi et al. [2]. With permission)

tricuspid position. In patients with bileaflet prosthetic valves, small valvular regurgitant jets emanating from the hinges are also a normal finding and thus eccentric regurgitant jets should not be used as an indication of perivalvular regurgitation in the setting of bileaflet mechanical valves. It is also not uncommon to have additional small regurgitant jets emanating from the central coaptation between the two leaflets [2].

In contrast, biological prosthetic valves generally do not have significant valvular regurgitation. Tiny jets of perivalvular regurgitation shortly following surgery can be detected and usually disappear on follow up. Anything other than trivial valvular regurgitation in a biologic valve should raise the possibility of pathologic changes such as degeneration of the prosthetic leaflets.

The absence of stents indicates that the biological valve is a type of stentless valve. In this situation, the ascending aorta should be examined to assess the distal anastomosis in case the mini-root technique is used, and since both coronary arteries may have been reimplanted onto the xenograft or homograft, the ostia of the coronary arteries should be carefully examined to detect complications such as dehiscence. It is not uncommon for the coronary ostia to appear dilated, due to the use of part of the aortic wall as a button in the reimplantation. Imaging the distal anastomosis in a patient with an aortic homograft will generally show that there is a size discrepancy between the homograft and the usually larger native distal ascending aorta.

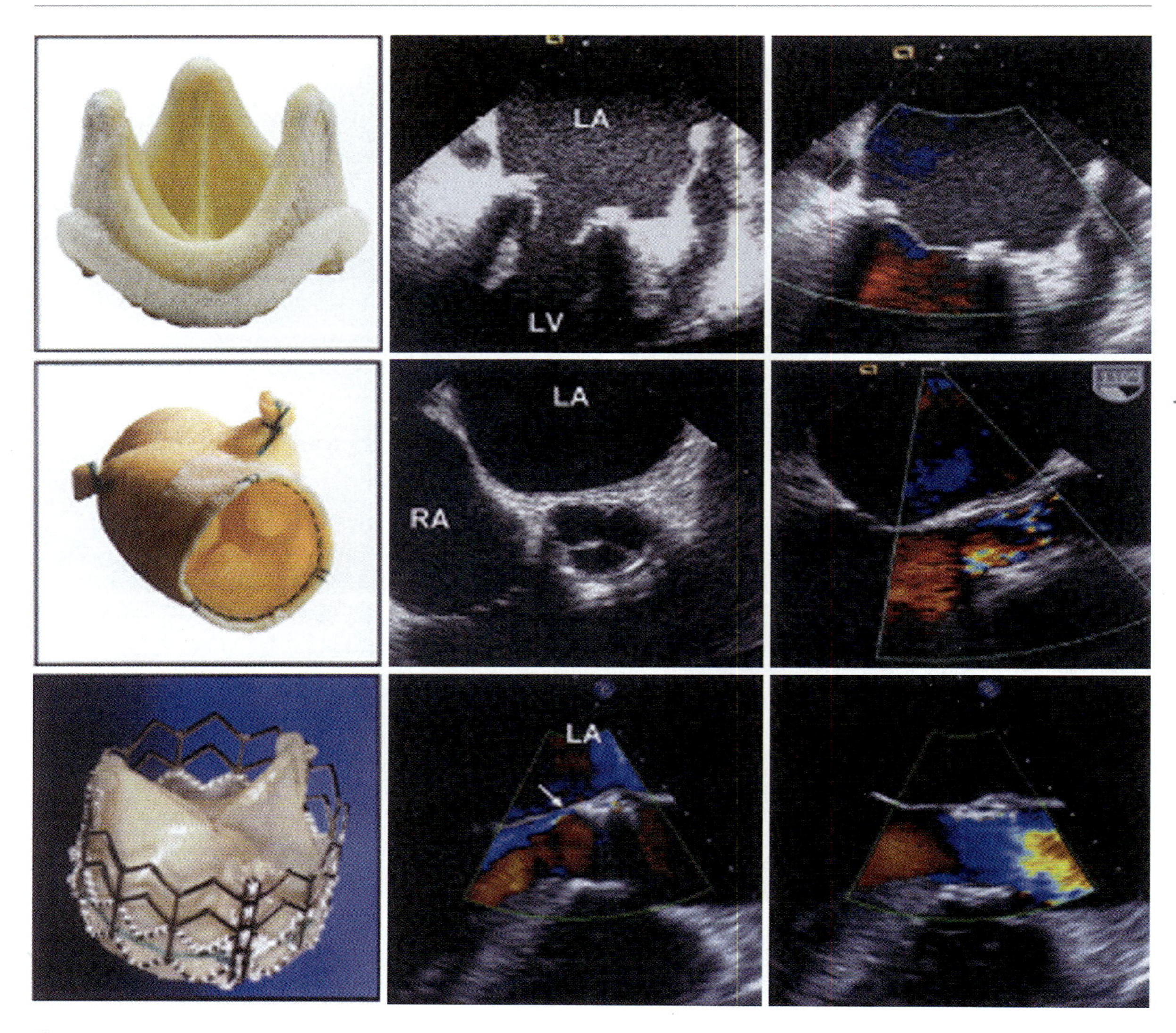

Fig. 11.3 The common bioprosthetic valves and their transesophageal echocardiographic views and color-flow findings are shown. The top row is a stented bioprosthetic valve, the middle row the stentless bioprosthetic valve, and the bottom row the Edwards Sapien valve which can be implanted percutaneously. *LA* left atrium, *LV* left ventricle, *RA* right atrium (Reproduced from Zoghbi et al. [2]. With permission)

As with native valves, there is an intimate relationship between valve morphology and function with prosthetic valves, but the challenge is that the valve morphology, particularly the mechanical prostheses, can be difficult to assess. The valve ring, stents, and fibrosis of adjacent cardiac structures due to valve surgery all contribute to the challenge for imaging the different components of the prosthetic valves. There should be a low threshold to perform transesophageal echocardiography (TEE) in this setting as TEE provides high quality images which are essential in the assessment of prosthetic valves. A comprehensive echo Doppler examination using pulsed wave, continuous wave and color flow imaging is the ideal non-invasive means to assess prosthetic valvular function. The examination should include measures of valvular stenosis, valvular regurgitation, right ventricular systolic pressure and the assessment of unusual intracardiac flow, such as a fistula communication between the aortic root and the right ventricular outflow tract. Since the prosthetic valves are intrinsically stenotic to some degree, the mere presence of high transvalvular

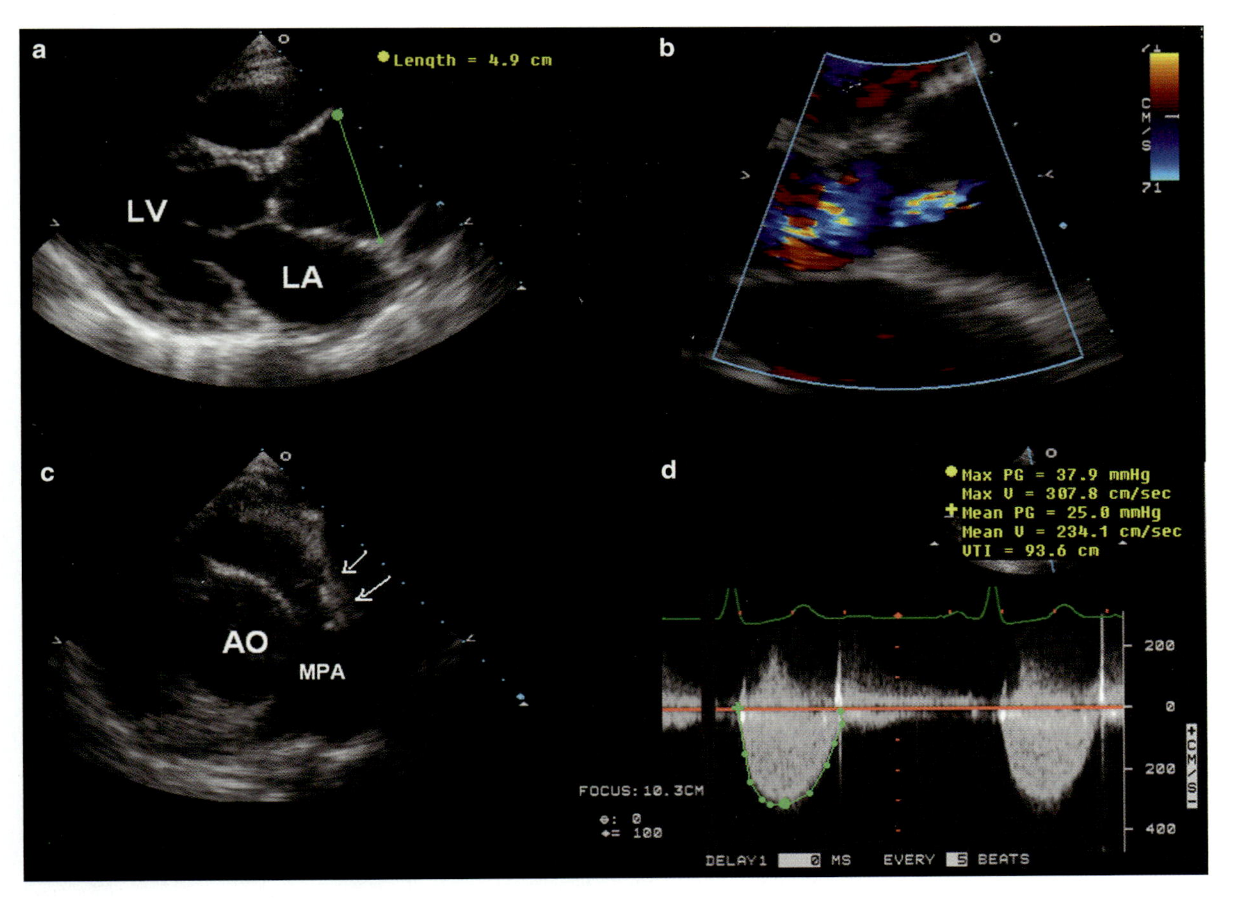

Fig. 11.4 This 32-year-old woman had the Ross procedure for congenital aortic stenosis at age 14. The parasternal long axis view (**a**) shows nodular thickening of the aortic valve and dilated ascending aorta of 4.9 cm in diameter. Color flow imaging (**b**) shows moderate aortic regurgitation. The pulmonary allograft (*arrows*) is diffusely narrowed (**c**). Continuous wave Doppler (**d**) confirms stenosis of the pulmonary allograft. *Ao* aorta, *LA* left atrium, *LV* left ventricle, *MPA* main pulmonary artery

gradient does not necessarily indicate dysfunction of the prosthetic valve. Comparison should be made with the expected gradients for the specific type and size of the prosthesis [2, 8, 9]. Other alternative explanations include the presence of subvalvular obstruction, perivalvular regurgitation and a high flow state.

Morphologic Assessment of Prosthetic Valves

The poppet(s) of a mechanical valve should have full unrestricted excursion during opening and proper coaptation with the valve ring during closure. The poppets of bileaflet valves can have a 90° opening angle such that the two semicircular poppets are parallel to each other during maximum opening (Fig. 11.5). The hinges of the bileaflet mechanical valve protrude above the valve ring and should not be confused with abnormal masses such as thrombus or vegetation. The Medtronic Hall valve has a single disc pivoted on a central strut with a maximum opening angle of about 70° (Fig. 11.6). The central strut can be quite prominently imaged above the sewing ring. The cage in a Starr Edwards valve has a high profile and protrudes prominently into the receiving chamber. The motion of the ball may be difficult to image as it is obscured by the cage (Fig. 11.7). Knowledge of the characteristics of the prosthetic valve is crucial to avoid improper interpretation of the echo findings.

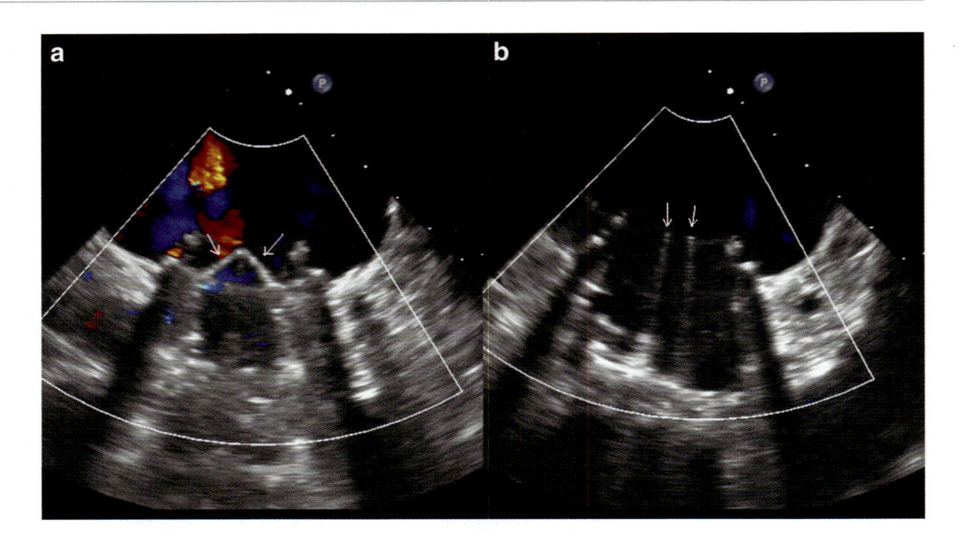

Fig. 11.5 Transesophageal views of a bileaflet mechanical valve in the mitral position showing normal leaflet closure (*arrows*) during systole (**a**) and a normal 90° opening of both leaflets (*arrows*) opening during diastole (**b**)

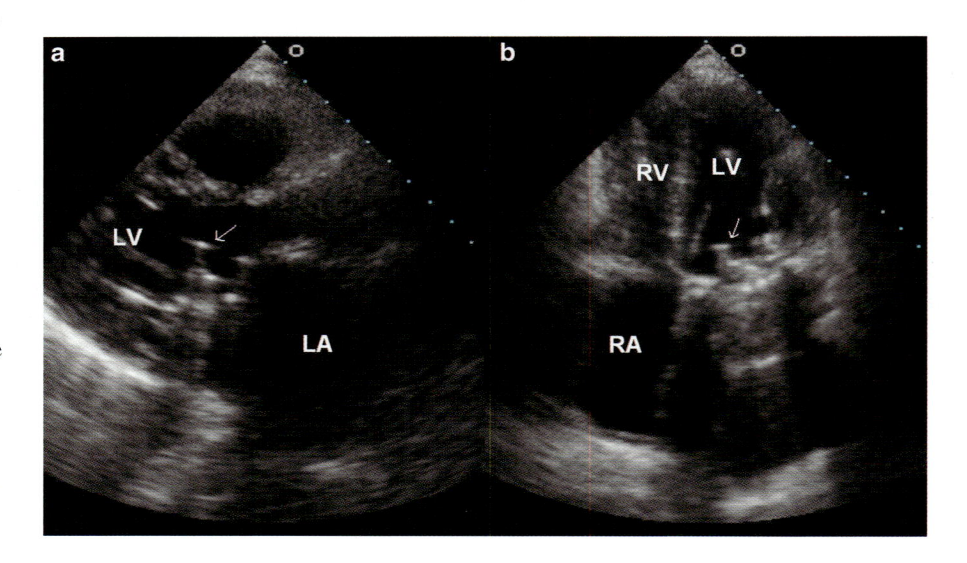

Fig. 11.6 Parasternal long-axis (**a**) and apical four-chamber (**b**) views of a normally functioning single leaflet mitral mechanical valve (Medtronic Hall) shows normal opening of the disc (*arrow*) to about 70°. Reverberation artifact is present in the left atrium in the four-chamber view. *LA* left atrium, *LV* left ventricle, *RA* right atrium, *RV* right ventricle

The poppet motion of either the single or double leaflet mechanical prosthetic valves can usually be imaged by transthoracic echocardiography. The best echocardiographic views to assess this motion are the parasternal long-axis and the apical views (Figs. 11.6, 11.8). The apical views can be adjusted so as to demonstrate the full motion of the poppet(s). In patients with a ball valve prosthesis, the excursion of the poppet can be difficult to appreciate because of the strong reflectivity of the cage and the poppet (Fig. 11.9). Sutures on the valve ring can be well imaged by TEE, particularly 3D TEE with mitral prostheses. Short mobile suture ends are not uncommon.

When the poppet is well seen and there is reduced poppet excursion, causes for the reduced poppet motion need to be carefully assessed. The two common causes are valvular thrombosis and pannus formation [10–12]. Transesophageal echocardiography has been used to differentiate these two conditions. Pannus is visualized as echo-dense tissue at the annulus encroaching into the inner opening of the sewing ring, as opposed to thrombus which is an echolucent sessile mass at the sewing ring extending to the adjacent atrial wall (Figs. 11.10, 11.11) [12]. It may be difficult to reliably differentiate these two conditions. Vegetations should always be considered when valvular masses are detected, although they are more likely to be pedunculated with excessive motion [13, 14]. The clinical context can be very useful. In a patient with sub-therapeutic anticoagulation and no clinical evidence of endocarditis, an echolucent

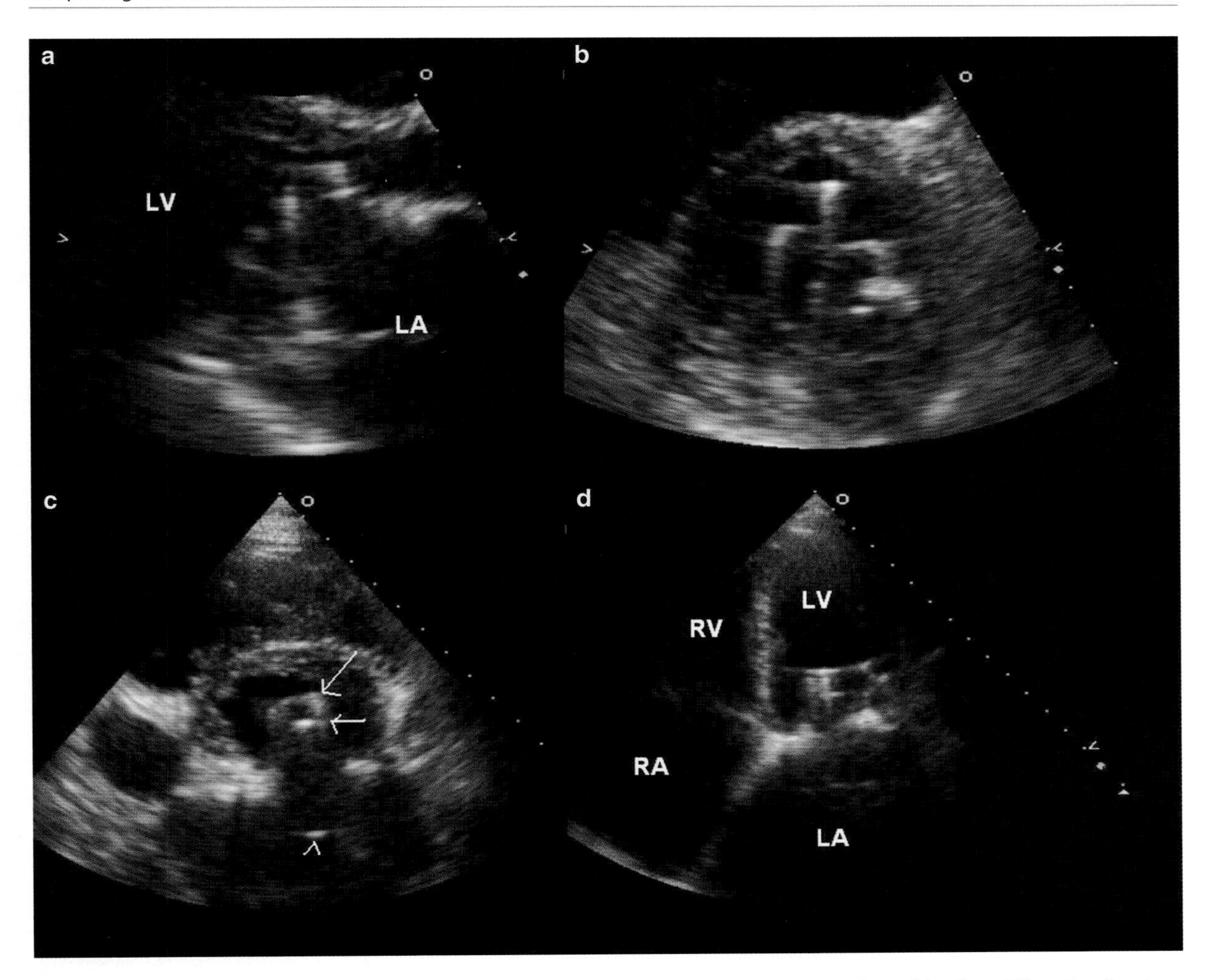

Fig. 11.7 Parasternal long-axis (**a**), short-axis (**b, c**) and apical four-chamber (**d**) views of a patient with a Starr-Edwards valve show that the high profile cage protrudes prominently into the left ventricle. The cage (*arrow*) is clearly seen but the ball cannot be clearly visualized. There is prominent reverberation artifact (*arrowhead*) in the left atrium. *LA* left atrium, *LV* left ventricle, *RA* right atrium, *RV* right ventricle

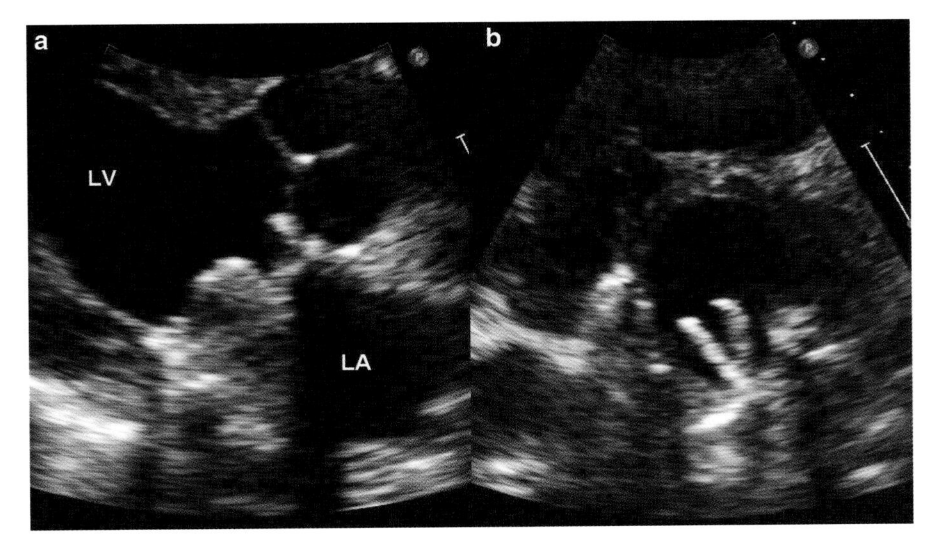

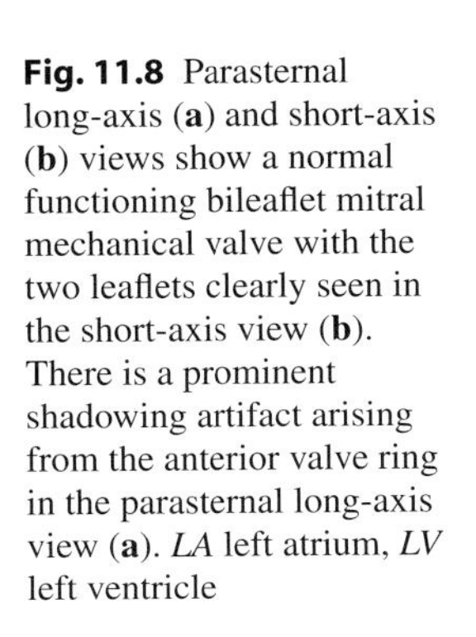

Fig. 11.8 Parasternal long-axis (**a**) and short-axis (**b**) views show a normal functioning bileaflet mitral mechanical valve with the two leaflets clearly seen in the short-axis view (**b**). There is a prominent shadowing artifact arising from the anterior valve ring in the parasternal long-axis view (**a**). *LA* left atrium, *LV* left ventricle

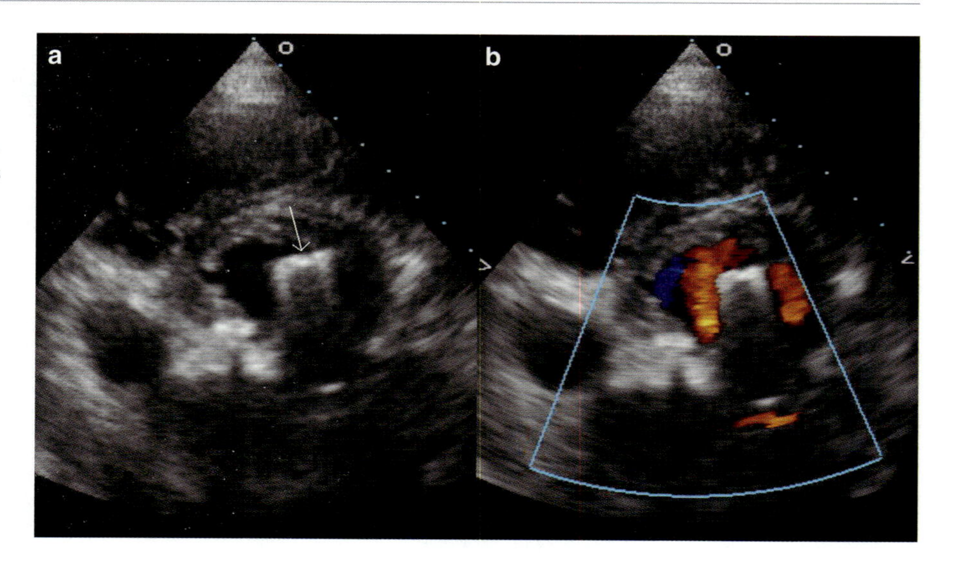

Fig. 11.9 Parasternal short axis view (**a**) shows the protruding cage of a mitral Starr-Edwards valve and the ball cannot be well seen. The color-flow imaging (**b**) shows normal flow coming into the left ventricle around the ball poppet

Fig. 11.10 (**a**) Transesophageal view of a bileaflet mitral mechanical valve showing immobility of the lateral leaflet and reduced mobility of the medial leaflet (*arrow*). Color-flow imaging (**b**) shows flow passing through only the medial orifice. At surgery extensive pannus formation impeding the motion of both leaflets is present. *LA*, left atrium

sessile mass on the sewing ring of a mechanical prosthetic valve is likely a thrombus. On the other hand, an echo dense mass at a similar location is likely pannus in a patient with adequate anticoagulation.

As discussed above, the current generation of single leaflet and bileaflet mechanical prosthetic valves are constructed in such a way that there are small jets of valvular regurgitation to reduce stasis and to wash out potential thrombus at the pivoting points (Fig. 11.2). These built in regurgitant jets are not well visualized by transthoracic echocardiography, which frequently confuses these jets with small paravalvular regurgitation jets. These jets can be well appreciated by TEE and can be differentiated from pathologic perivalvular jets by their typical location at the pivoting points, such as the two hinges in bileaflet valves, the small size of the jets and the origins of the jets located inside rather than outside of the sewing ring. Because of the good quality images, TEE should be readily used if there is any indication of prosthetic valvular dysfunction.

In stented bioprosthetic valves, the three stents can be quite prominent and obscure the leaflets (Figs. 11.12, 11.13). They must be differentiated from abnormal masses such as calcification. Mitral prostheses are

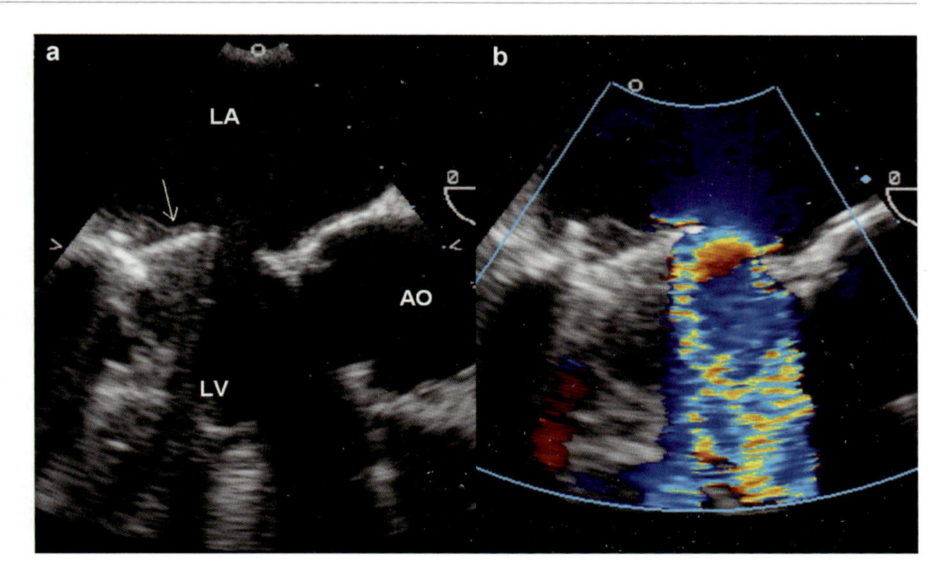

Fig. 11.11 (**a**) Transesophageal view of a bileaflet mitral mechanical valve shows that one of the leaflets (*arrow*) is immobile and there is echo density on the atrial surface of this immobile leaflet extending onto the atrial wall consistent with thrombus. The other leaflet demonstrates normal motion. Color-flow imaging (**b**) shows flow through the open half of the mitral orifice

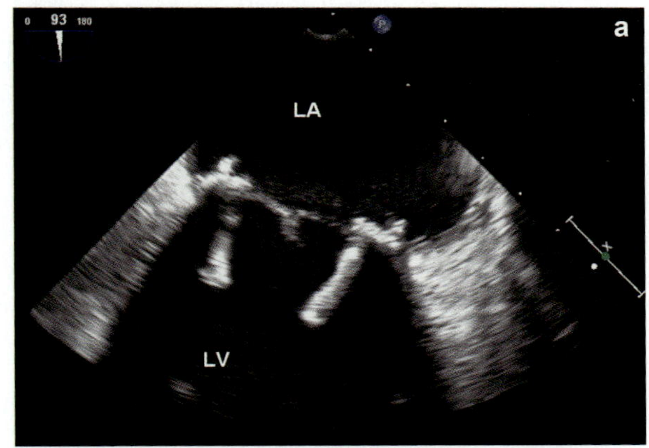

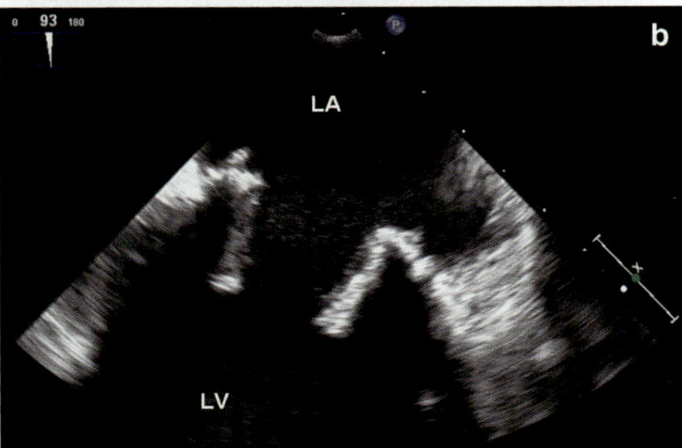

Fig. 11.12 (**a**) Transesophageal echo view of a normal functioning stented mitral bioprosthesis in systole shows that the leaflets coapt normally and the leaflets are thin with no localized nodule or brightness. (**b**) Tranesophageal view of the stented mitral bioprothesis in diastole shows that the leaflets are thin with full excursion and no doming. *LA* left atrium, *LV* left ventricle

positioned such that they are generally tilted anteriorly with the flow directed towards the septum. Although left ventricular outflow tract (LVOT) obstruction is possible with older high profile prostheses, this complication is very rare with the current prosthetic valves. The current stentless valves are exclusively for aortic valve replacement, and after implantation the only abnormal finding may be mild thickness at the aortic root. The leaflets are usually well seen without interference of the valve ring and stents (Fig. 11.14).

Biological prosthetic valves in general are easier to image, as compared to mechanical valves. The leaflets of the bioprosthetic valves are best imaged using the parasternal views. The imaging plane may need to be carefully adjusted so that it cuts between the valve stents in order to optimally visualize the leaflets. Normal bioprosthetic leaflets are thin and mobile with full excursion and proper coaptation. No regurgitation is present (Fig. 11.15). Doming of the leaflets indicates restricted motion and less than full excursion; and this is usually accompanied by degenerative changes with fibrin and lipid insudation leading to fibrosis, thickening and calcification of the leaflets [15, 16]. These changes can best be assessed by TEE (Fig. 11.16) [17]. When the degenerative changes become severe, the leaflet motion is further reduced resulting in valvular stenosis which can be assessed with an approach similar to that for native valve stenosis.

The coaptation of bioprosthetic leaflets should be carefully examined. The presence of leaflet prolapse is

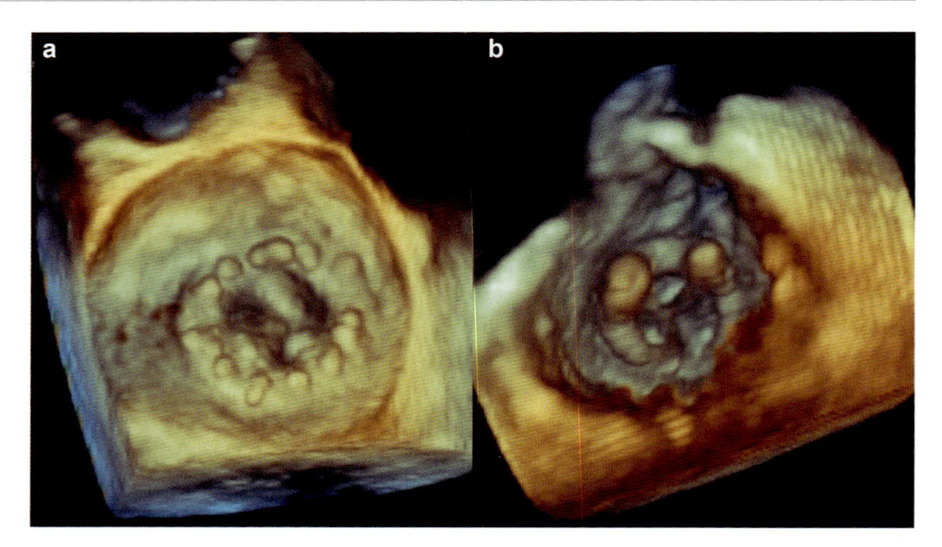

Fig. 11.13 Transesophageal 3D views of a normal stented mitral bioprosthetic valve from the left atrial (**a**) and left ventricular (**b**) perspectives. From the left atrial perspective, the sutures at the valve ring can be clearly seen. From the ventricular perspective, two of the stents are clearly seen while the remaining one is obscured. Proper coaptation of the three leaflets is present

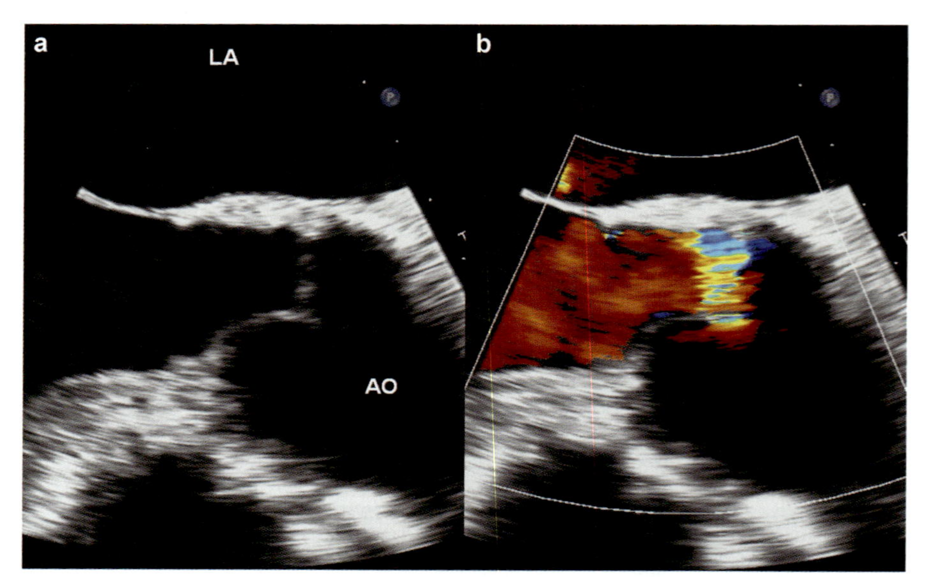

Fig. 11.14 (**a**) Tranesophageal longitudinal plane of a stentless aortic bioprosthesis shows a mild thickening of the aortic root but no evidence of stents. Color-flow imaging (**b**) show moderate aortic regurgitation which is posteriorly directed. *Ao* aorta, *LA* left atrium

an indication of the presence of a tear or tears in the leaflet (Figs. 11.17–11.19). Flail of the leaflet is diagnosed when the tip of the leaflet is everted pointing into the downstream chamber during leaflet coaptation, indicating that the leaflet tear(s) is large (Figs. 11.20, 11.21). Perforation of the leaflet can occur because of tissue degeneration at the base of the leaflet which is subjected to high mechanical stress. These morphologic features are important to detect because they are signs that the degeneration of the bioprosthetic valve is quite advanced and that significant valvular regurgitation is invariably present. Calcification can be particularly severe with homografts and when present can make assessment of leaflet excursion difficult (Figs. 11.22–11.24). We have observed that once moderate aortic regurgitation occurs in a patient with a calcified homograft, there is a high likelihood that further sudden increase in valvular regurgitation as a result of extension of the leaflet tear(s) may occur within the next 6–12 months. These patients need to be closely followed. During color flow examination, the regurgitant jet may be obscured by the prosthetic valve. Careful search for the presence of flow convergence on the upstream side of the valve helps to minimize the risks of missing significant regurgitation [18].

Normal prosthetic valves are well seated and move in unison with the surrounding cardiac structure. Excessive motion such as rocking of the sewing ring

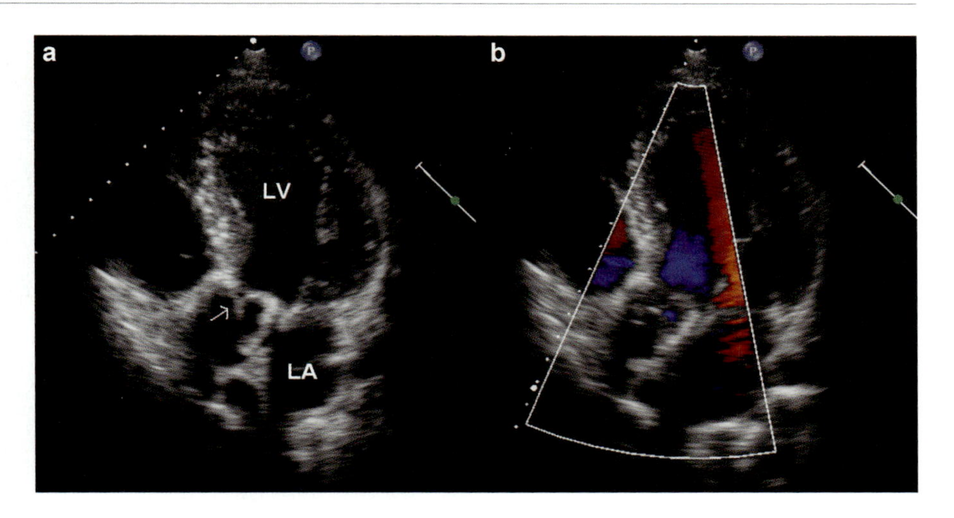

Fig. 11.15 Apical long-axis view (**a**) shows proper coaptation of the leaflets (*arrow*) of a stented aortic bioprosthetic valve. Color-flow imaging (**b**) shows no aortic regurgitation. *LA* left atrium, *LV* left ventricle

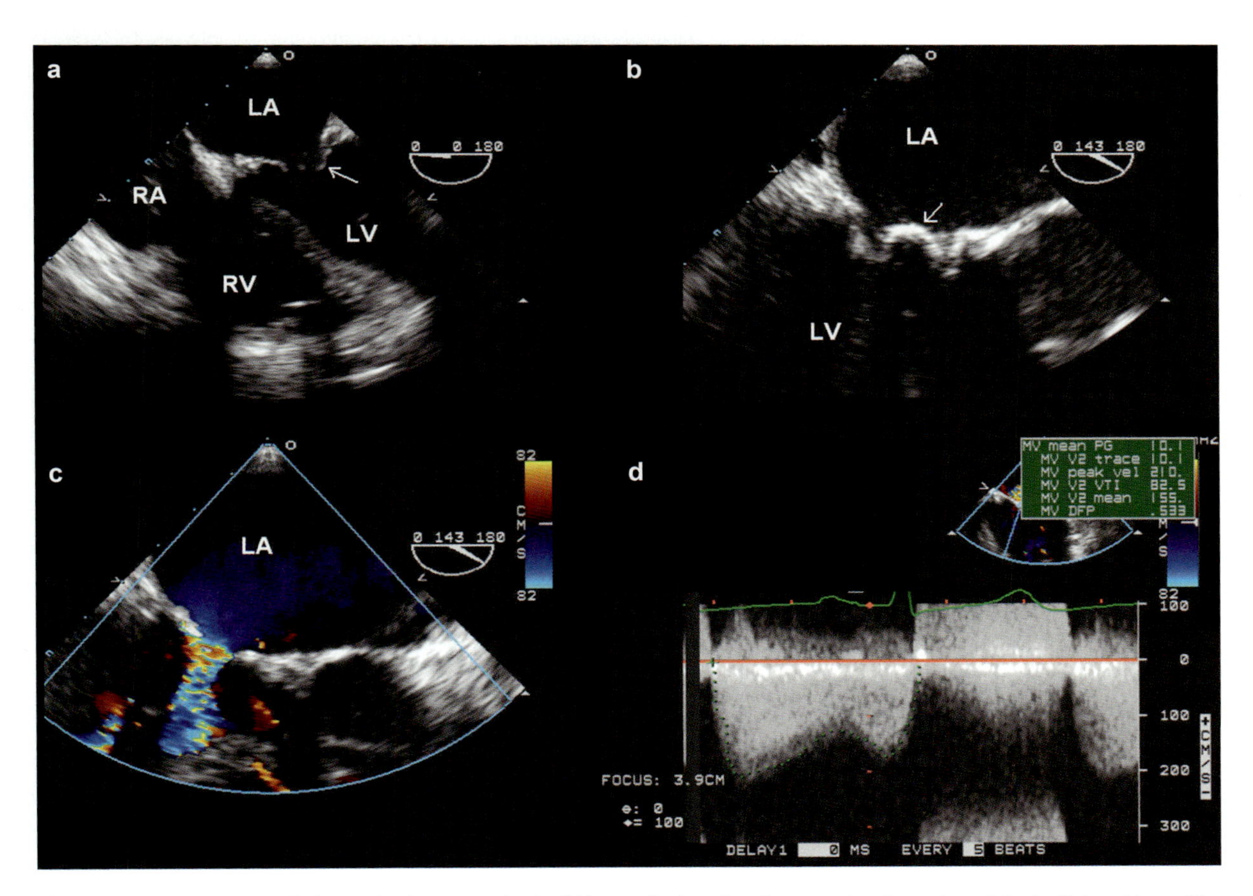

Fig. 11.16 Transesophageal views of a degenerated mitral bioprosthetic valve show restricted opening of the leaflets evidenced by doming (*arrow*) in (**a**). There is dense calcification on the leaflets (*arrow*) in (**b**). Color-flow imaging (**c**) shows a stenotic flow jet which is confirmed by continuous wave Doppler (**d**) showing a mean transprosthetic gradient of 10 mmHg. *LA* left atrium, *LV* left ventricle, *RA* right atrium, *RV* right ventricle

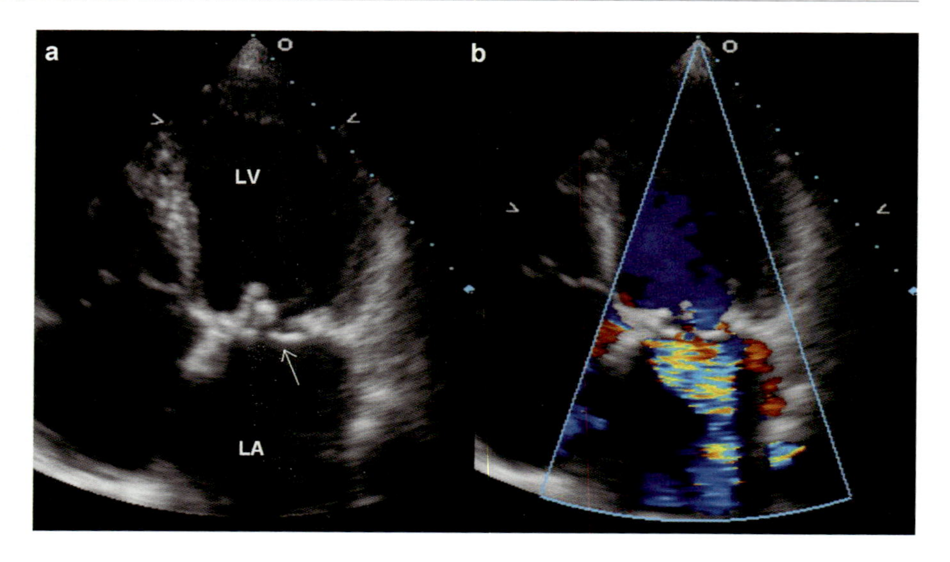

Fig. 11.17 Apical four-chamber view (**a**) in a patient with a stented mitral bioprosthesis shows prolapse of one of the leaflets (*arrow*). Color-flow imaging (**b**) confirms the presence of severe mitral regurgitation. *LA* left atrium, *LV* left ventricle

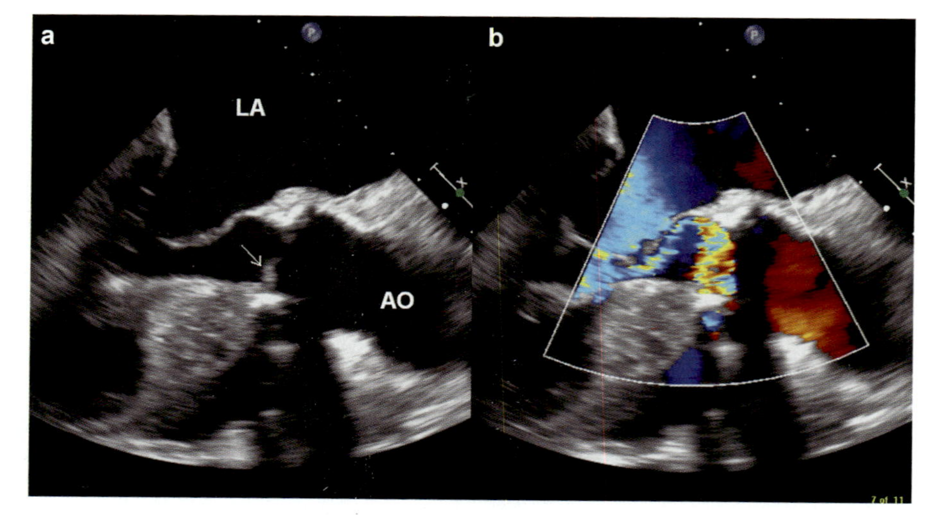

Fig. 11.18 Transesophageal view (**a**) of a stented aortic bioprosthetic valve shows prolapse of the anterior bioprosthetic leaflet (*arrow*). Color flow imaging (**b**) confirms significant aortic regurgitation which is directed posteriorly. *Ao* aorta, *LA* left atrium

indicates the presence of dehiscence. In these patients, perivalvular regurgitation is likely present and TEE should be performed if the transthoracic study fails to identify perivalvular regurgitation (Fig. 11.25).

Hemodynamic Assessment of Prosthetic Valves

A comprehensive assessment of the prosthetic heart valve comprises of a detailed examination of the different components of the valve, the motion of the moving poppet or the biological leaflets, and hemodynamic assessment including transvalvular gradients, calculated valve areas and the presence or absence of regurgitation. The blood pressure and heart rate of the patient need to be recorded and the left ventricular function carefully assessed in order to provide a proper understanding of the transvalvular hemodynamics, which are affected by preload and afterload [3]. An increase in stroke volume can accentuate the transvalvular gradients and similarly a decrease in stroke volume related to left ventricular dysfunction leads to reduced transvalvular gradients. Thus, assessment of stroke volume should be an integral part of an echo examination of patients with prosthetic valves.

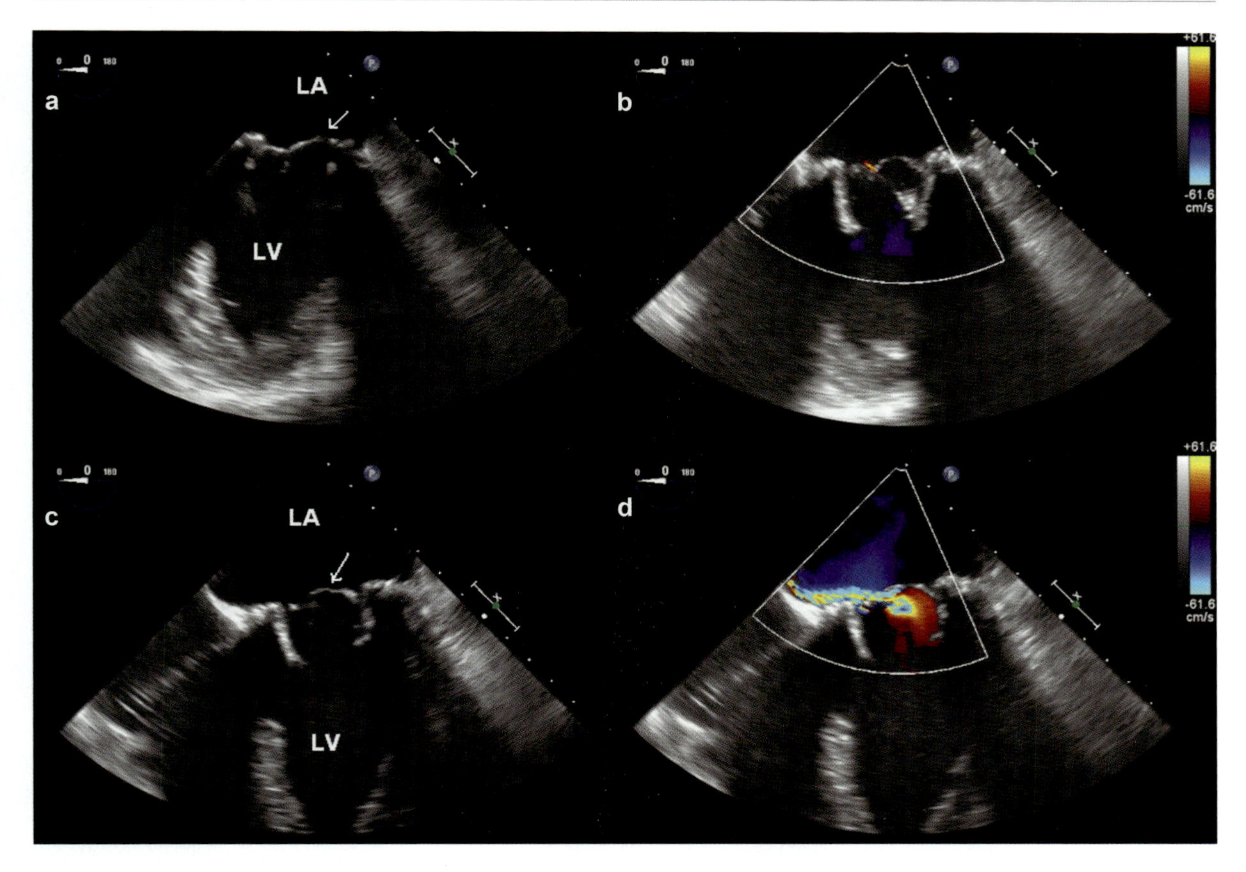

Fig. 11.19 Transesophageal view (**a**) of a bioprosthetic mitral valve shows prolapse of one of the bioprosthetic leaflets (*arrow*). Color-flow imaging (**b**) shows only trivial mitral regurgitation. Repeat study 2 years later (**c**) shows that the bioprosthetic leaflet is now flail (*arrow*). Color-flow image (**d**) shows eccentric mitral regurgitation of at least moderate severity. *LA* left atrium, *LV* left ventricle

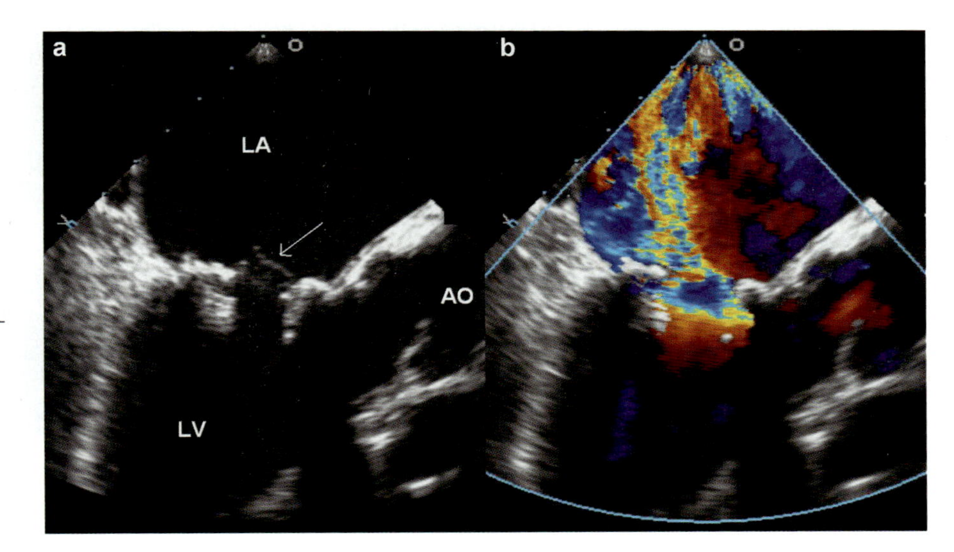

Fig. 11.20 (**a**) Transesophageal view of a mitral bioprosthetic valve shows flail of one of the bioprosthetic leaflets (*arrow*). Color-flow imaging (**b**) shows severe mitral regurgitation. *Ao* aorta, *LA* left atrium, *LV* left ventricle

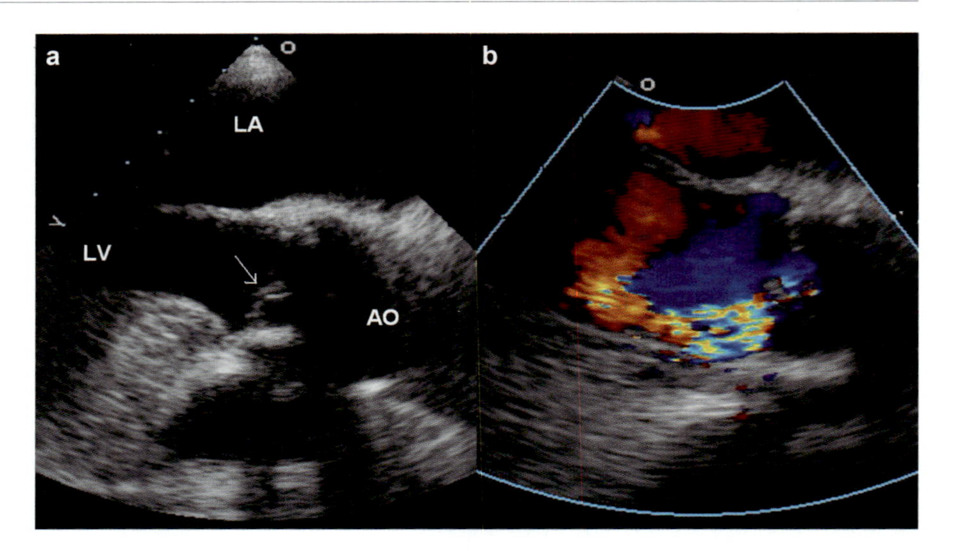

Fig. 11.21 (**a**) Transesophageal view of a stented aortic bioprosthetic valve shows flail of the posterior leaflet (*arrow*). Color-flow imaging (**b**) shows anterior directed aortic regurgitation. *Ao* aorta, *LA* left atrium, *LV* left ventricle

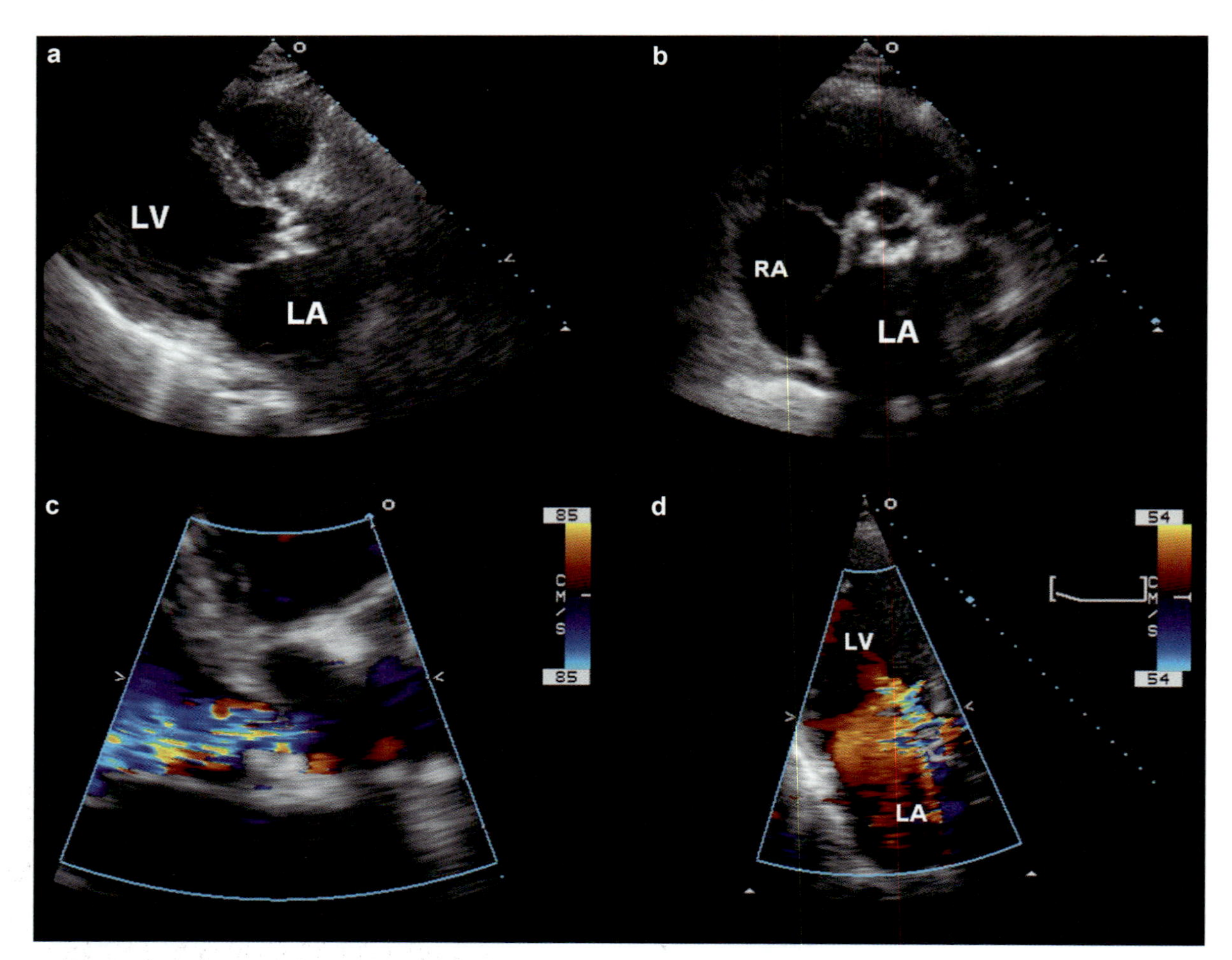

Fig. 11.22 Parasternal long-axis (**a**) and short-axis (**b**) views of a patient with an aortic homograft showed dense calcification involving the leaflets of the homograft as well as the base of the aortic root. Color-flow imaging in the parasternal long-axis (**c**) and apical long-axis (**b**) views confirmed severe aortic regurgitation. This patient went on to develop heart failure within 1 month following this study and required urgent repeat aortic valve replacement

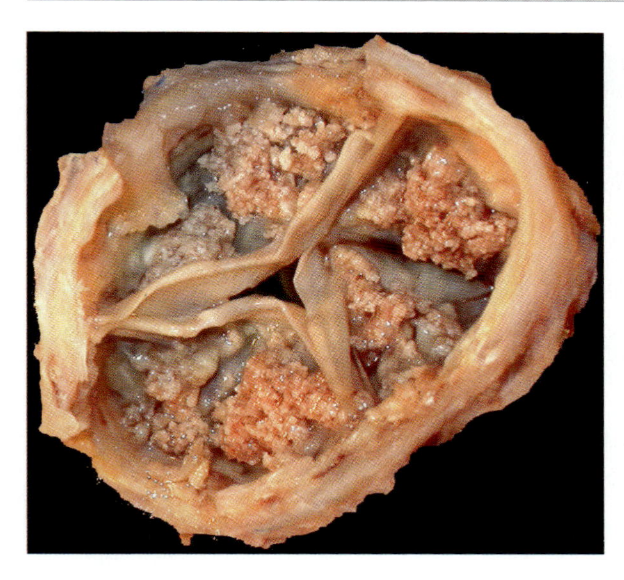

Fig. 11.23 Excised aortic homograft demonstrating severe calcification of the cusps

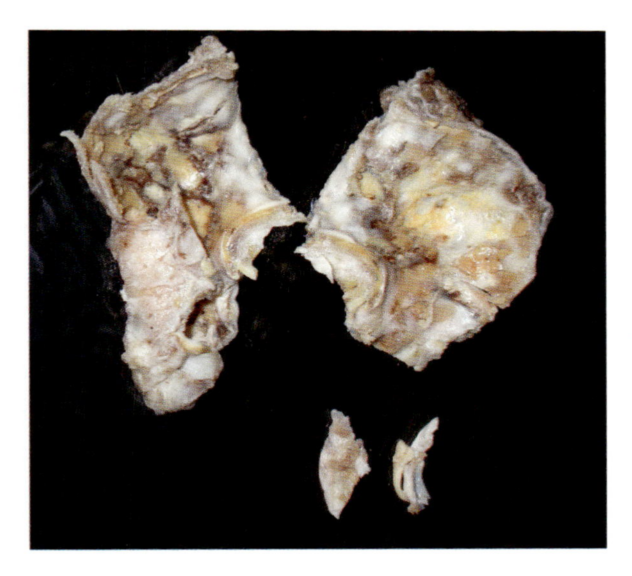

Fig. 11.24 Excised aortic homograft. The graft and cusps are removed in pieces due to the severe calcification and fibrosis. Calcified yellow plaques can be noted with white intimal tissues. Two distorted cusps are noted in the lower image

Prosthetic–Patient Mismatch

Despite improvement in the design of the valves, most prosthetic valves are intrinsically stenotic, particularly with prosthetic valves in the smaller size range. It is worth noting that the size of the prosthesis provided by the manufacturer refers to the outer diameter of the valve ring, and the inner diameter can be smaller by several millimeters. This difference may vary from one valve type to another [19, 20]. Proper interpretation of the hemodynamic performance of the prosthetic valves must take into consideration the type, the model and the size of the prosthesis. The normal ranges of transvalvular gradients and valve areas of the common prosthetic valves have been published [8, 9] (Appendices 11.1, 11.2). These values should be consulted and compared with those obtained in the patient. With the small sized valves, significant valvular obstruction as measured by transvalvular gradients and valve area can be present, despite the fact that the prosthetic valve is functioning normally. This is due to the smaller effective orifice area (EOA) of the prosthetic valve as compared to the normal native valve. This phenomenon has been termed "prosthesis–patient mismatch" and some degree of this is extremely common [21]. It has been shown that the hemodynamic consequence, as measured by the transvalvular gradient, sharply increases when the EOA indexed for body surface area is ≤ 0.85 cm^2/m^2 for the aortic prosthetic valves and ≤ 1.2 cm^2/m^2 for the mitral prosthetic valves (Fig. 11.26) [22, 23]. As expected, prosthesis–patient mismatch is more prevalent with smaller size valves implanted in large patients. The use of smaller size valves are generally necessitated by the presence of a small patient valve annulus. In this situation, the prosthetic valve is functioning normally but is just too small for the hemodynamic need of the patient. Prosthesis–patient mismatch has been shown to be associated with short-term and long-term adverse cardiovascular events [24–26]. With careful planning to choose the correct size and type of prosthesis and modification of the surgical technique, prosthesis–patient mismatch can be avoided.

High Transprosthetic Gradient and Prosthetic Dysfunction

A frequently encountered situation in patients with prosthetic valves is the detection of a high trans-prosthetic gradient, usually a peak velocity > 3 m/s and mean gradient > 20 mmHg for the aortic prostheses, and peak velocity > 1.9 m/s and mean gradient ≥ 5 mmHg for the mitral prostheses [2]. Prosthetic

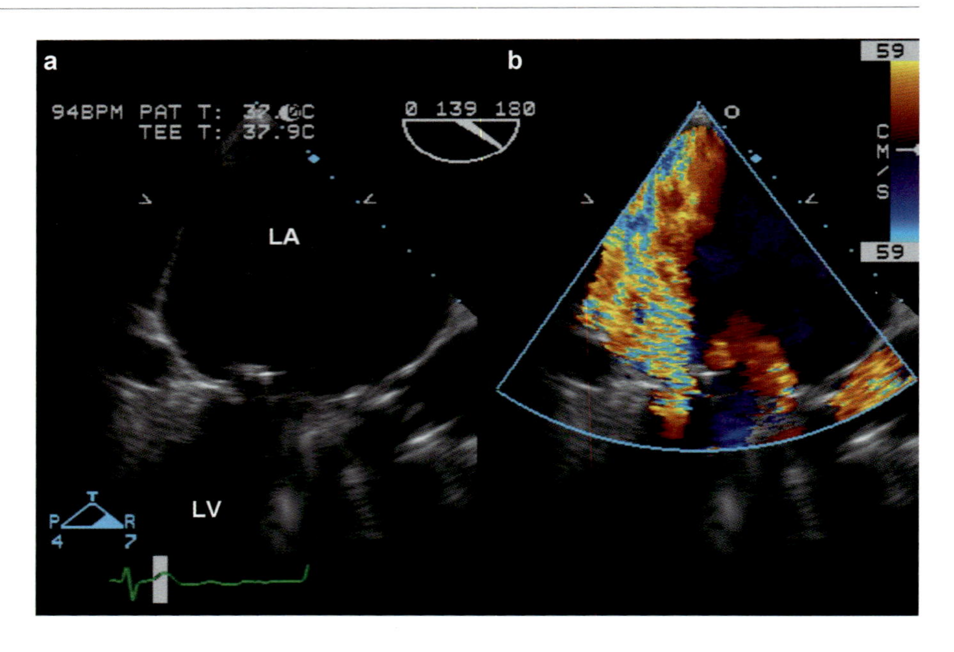

Fig. 11.25 Transesophageal view (**a**) of a mechanical bileaflet mitral valve shows excessive motion of the posterior sewing ring. Color-flow imaging (**b**) confirms severe paravalvular regurgitation. *LA* left atrium, *LV* left ventricle

valvular obstruction becomes a consideration. The algorithm in Fig. 27 is a practical approach to assess these patients [3]. As discussed above, information about the type, model and size of the prosthesis is crucial, and obtaining this information is the first step. This should be followed by calculating the EOA using the continuity equation. The stroke volume of the left ventricular outflow tract (LVOT) is usually the reference standard. Thus, EOA for aortic prosthesis (EOA_{AVR}) and mitral prosthesis (EOA_{MVR}) are:

$$EOA_{AVR} = \frac{\pi r^2_{LVOT} \times VTI_{LVOT}}{VTI_{AVR}},$$

and

$$EOA_{MVR} = \frac{\pi r^2_{LVOT} \times VTI_{LVOT}}{VTI_{MVR}},$$

where r_{LVOT} is the radius of the LVOT, VTI_{LVOT} the velocity time integral at LVOT, VTI_{AVR} the velocity time integral of the velocity at the aortic prosthetic

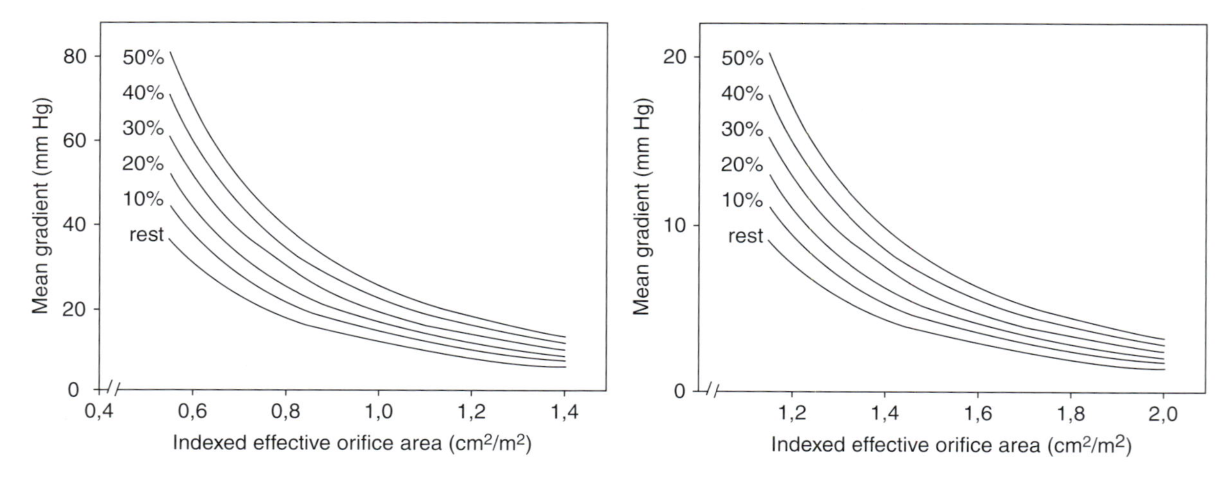

Fig. 11.26 The effect of 10–50% increase in stroke volume on the relationship between indexed effective orifice area and the trans-prosthetic gradient for the aortic bioprosthetic valves (**a**) and mitral bioprosthetic valves (**b**) studied in a physiologic pulse duplicator system (Reproduced from Dumesnil et al. [22]. With permission)

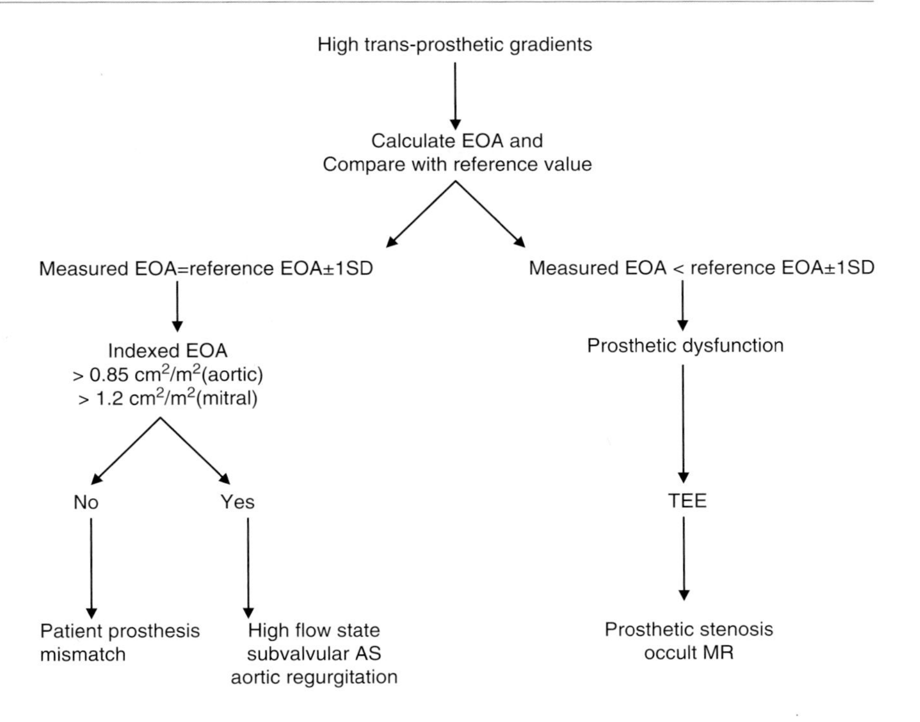

Fig. 11.27 A practical approach to assess high trans-prosthetic gradients. *AS* aortic stenosis, *EOA* effective orifice area, *MR* mitral regurgitation, *TEE* transesophageal echocardiography (Modified after Pibarot and Dumesnil [27])

valve and VTI_{MVR} the velocity time integral at the mitral prosthetic valve. The equation for EOA_{MVR} is not applicable, if there is significant concomitant aortic regurgitation or mitral regurgitation.

The gradients and EOA can then be compared with the published values for that particular prosthetic value of that particular size (Appendices 11.1, 11.2). If the measured EOA is smaller than the reference EOA, prosthetic valvular dysfunction is highly likely and our preference is to proceed with TEE to determine the etiology and to plan treatment. The TEE findings may help to differentiate thrombus from pannus, identify the poppet or leaflet motion, and assess the location and severity of valvular and paravalvular regurgitation. If the measured EOA is similar to the reference EOA, the EOA should then be indexed for the body surface area. An indexed EOA < 0.85 cm^2/m^2 for aortic prostheses or <1.2 cm^2/m^2 for mitral prostheses indicates that prosthesis–patient mismatch is the reason for the high trans-prosthesis gradients (Figs. 11.28, 11.29) [22, 23]. On the other hand, if the indexed EOA is clearly above these threshold values, one should consider causes for high flow in the LVOT such as subvalvular aortic stenosis, aortic regurgitation or a high flow state [2, 3].

The following caveats apply:

1. Consider left ventricular systolic function.

   The transprosthetic gradients should be interpreted in the context of LV systolic function. If there is severe LV dysfunction, prosthetic dysfunction may be present even with "normal" transprosthetic gradients. When there is LV systolic dysfunction, EOA should be routinely calculated in addition to the gradients and compared with the reference value.

2. Routine calculation of stroke volume.

   The LV stroke volume can be obtained readily by multiplying the velocity time integral of systolic flow in the LVOT with the area of the LVOT. Care should be taken to avoid placing the Doppler sample volume too close to the aortic prosthetic valve. Optimal LVOT pulsed wave Doppler signal should be laminar with a narrow spectrum and is usually obtained 1 cm from the aortic annulus. An accurate stroke volume measurement can be used to calculate the LV ejection fraction [27]. It is also the key component in calculating the prosthetic EOA.

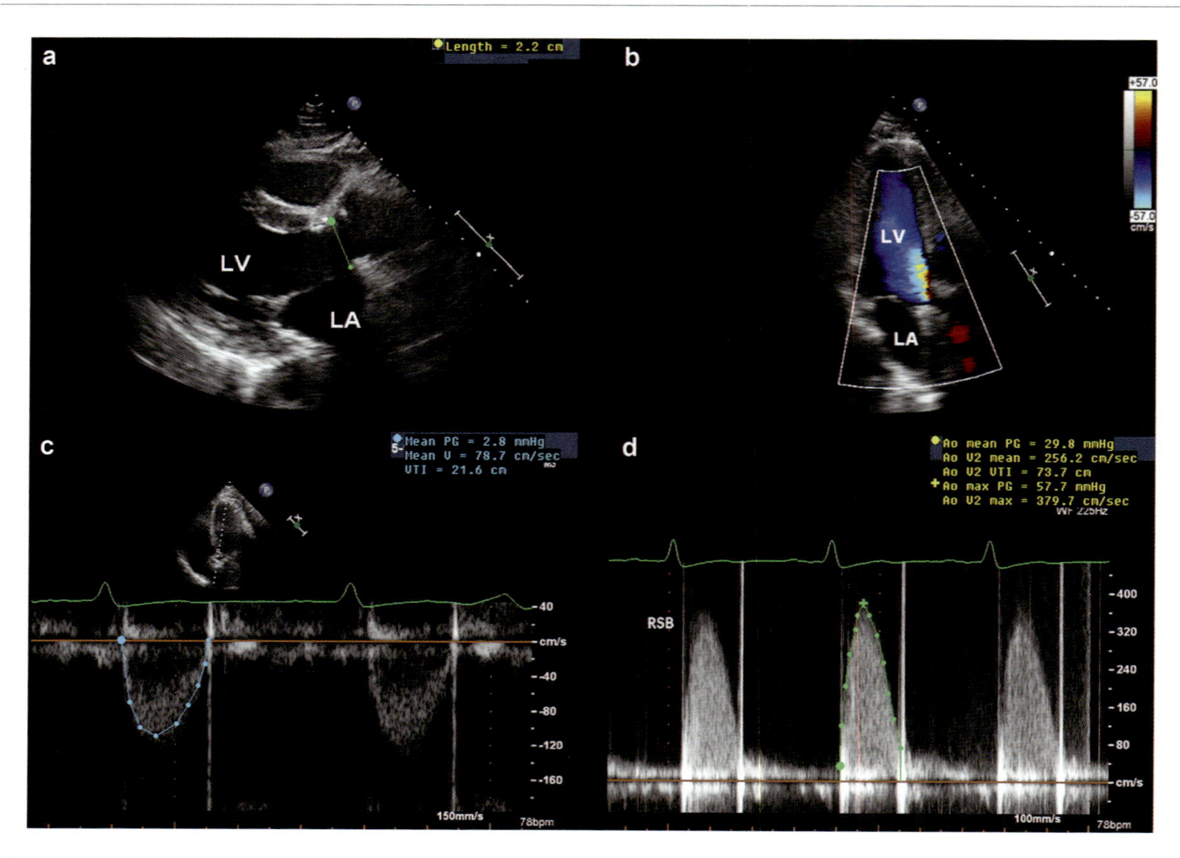

Fig. 11.28 (**a, b**) This 26-year-old man had enlargement of the aortic annulus and implantation of a mechanical bileaflet aortic valve (25 mm St. Jude valve) at age 12. (**c, d**) The transprosthetic peak and mean gradients are 58 and 30 mmHg. The Doppler velocity index is 0.29. The calculated effective orifice area is 1.11 cm^2 which is smaller than the reference value of 1.93 ± 0.45 cm^2, indicating that prosthetic dysfunction is present

3. Optimization of transprosthetic velocity.

   Similar to native aortic stenosis, the maximum velocity at the aortic prosthetic valve needs to be assessed from multiple acoustic windows to ensure that the highest velocity is obtained. The envelope of the Doppler signal should be optimized to avoid overestimation due to extraporation of a poorly defined spectral envelope.

4. Prosthetic size and model not available.

   When the size and model of the prosthetic valve are unavailable, there would be no appropriate reference values of pressure gradients or EOA for comparison. The dimensionless Doppler velocity index (DVI) can be useful in this setting [28]. DVI is a ratio of the peak velocity in the LVOT divided by the peak flow velocity through the aortic prosthesis. This ratio adjusts for high flow state such as aortic regurgitation which increases the flow velocities in the LVOT as well the aortic prosthesis. A DVI > 0.35 would indicate that the high transprosthetic gradient is related to high flow and not to prosthetic valve dysfunction. For the mitral prosthetic valve, a DVI > 0.45 cut-off has been suggested [3]. The routine calculation of stroke volume would likely have detected the possibility of the high flow state. A low DVI (<0.25) has been shown to be highly suggestive of aortic prosthetic stenosis, but it does not differentiate prosthesis–patient mismatch from other causes of prosthetic dysfunction (Figs. 11.28, 11.29) [29, 30].

5. Prosthetic leaflet or poppet mobility.

   When prosthetic dysfunction is suspected, the etiology should be investigated. In our experience, TEE is the preferred imaging modality, as it can identify abnormal leaflet or poppet motion, as well as the pres-

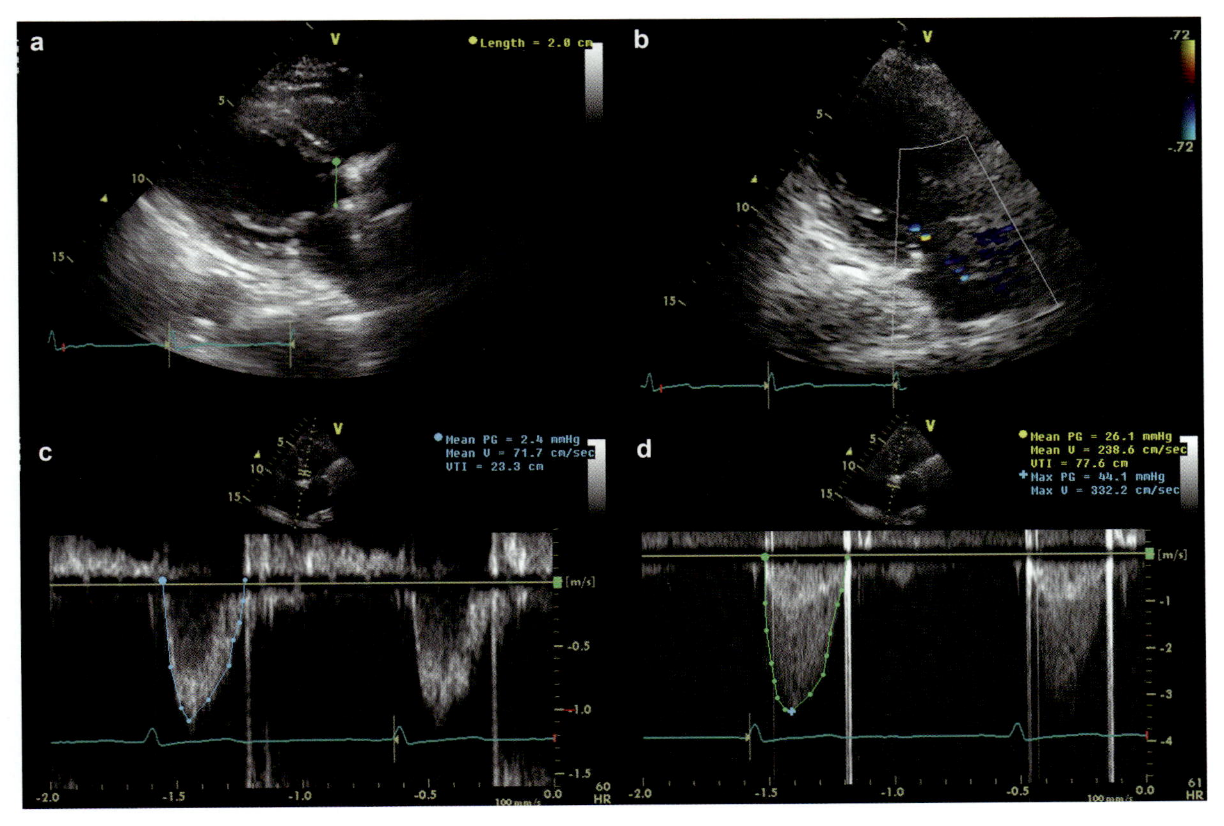

Fig. 11.29 This 62-year-old woman had aortic valve replacement with 19 mm St. Jude valve at age 44 for aortic stenosis. (**a, b, c, d**) The transprosthetic peak and mean gradients are 44 and 26 mmHg. The Doppler velocity index is 0.30. The calculated effective orifice area is 0.94 cm^2 which is similar to the reference value of 1.01 ± 0.24 cm^2, showing that it is functioning normally. The indexed valve area is 0.55 cm^2/m^2 indicating severe prosthesis–patient mismatch

ence and severity of valvular or paravalvular regurgitation. Our experience suggests that real-time 3D TEE is a powerful tool in assessing prosthetic valves (Figs. 11.30, 11.31). In mechanical prosthetic valves, cinefluoroscopy can be useful in assessing poppet motion, but not the etiology of the abnormal motion such as thrombus or pannus [3]. Occult prosthetic regurgitation also will not be detected by this means.

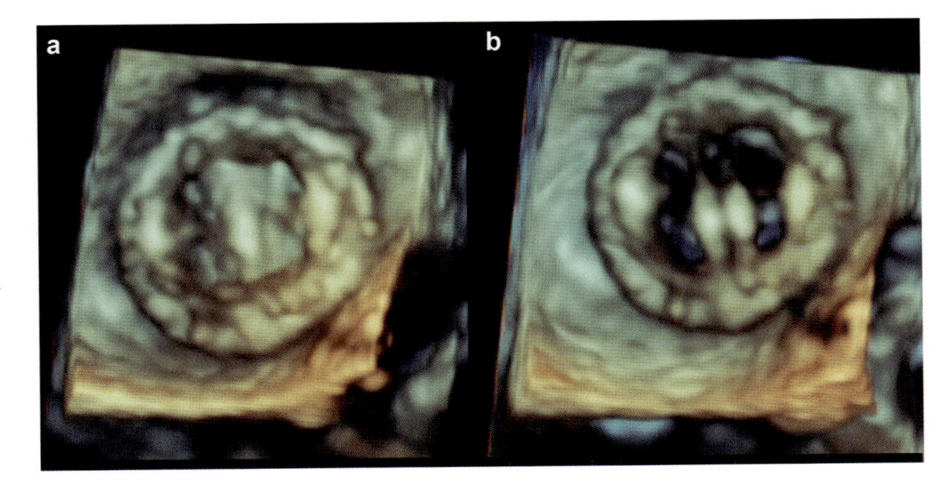

Fig. 11.30 Transesophageal 3D views of a bileaflet mitral mechanical prosthetic valve from the left atrial perspective in systole (**a**) and diastole (**b**) show normal leaflet closure and opening. Sutures at the valve ring can also be identified

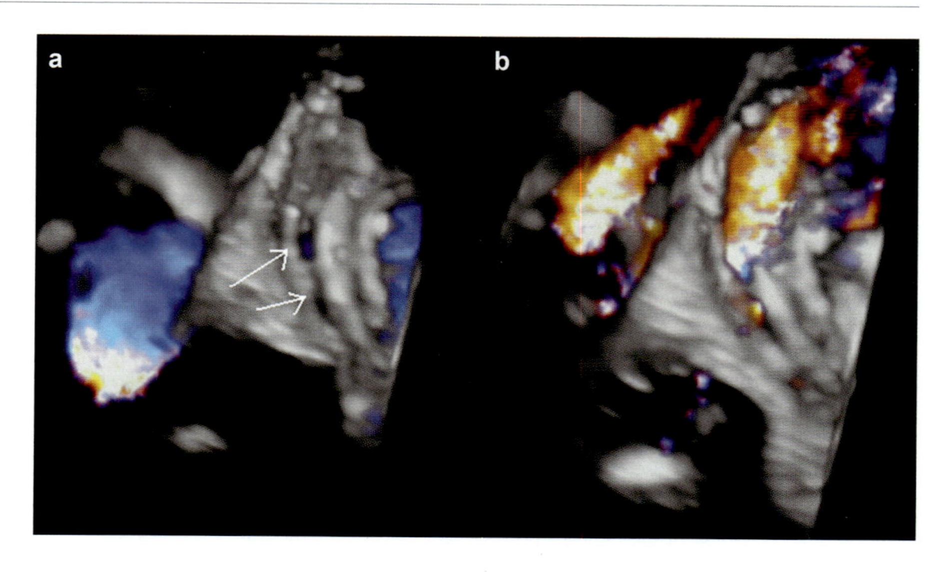

Fig. 11.31 Transesophageal 3D view of a bileaflet mitral mechanical valve shows two areas of dehiscence at the valve ring (*arrow*) in (**a**). Paravalvular regurgitation emanating from the areas of dehiscence is shown in (**b**)

6. Pressure recovery.

   Pressure recovery has been proposed to account for the discrepancy between the Doppler pressure gradients and catheter measured pressure gradients in bileaflet mechanical valves [31–33]. The magnitude of the difference is generally small, but may be substantial in the setting of a small size prosthesis and small aortic root (<3 cm in diameter). Calculations to correct the effect of pressure recovery have been published [33, 34].

7. Localized high gradient in bileaflet prosthesis.

   The bileaflet mechanical valve has three orifices with two larger side orifices and a smaller central orifice such that the velocity across the central orifice is slightly higher. Selective sampling of the velocity at the central orifice may yield a high transvalvular gradient which may be confused for an obstructed mechanical valve [3]. In our experience this phenomenon is quite rare. When this phenomenon is suspected, TEE should be performed to ensure that the leaflet motion is indeed normal.

8. Pressure half-time.

   In the follow-up of mitral prosthetic valves, an increase in the pressure half-time suggests the development of prosthetic obstruction and a decrease may indicate the development of mitral regurgitation. A substantial change in the pressure half-time should prompt a more detailed search for other findings of prosthetic dysfunction. However, it is invalid to use the pressure half-time to calculate the EOA based on the empirical formula developed for native mitral stenosis [22].

9. Comparison with prior studies.

   A baseline study of the prosthetic valve is very useful for comparison to detect subtle findings of prosthetic dysfunction, and should be performed within 6 months following surgery. An abrupt increase in the motion of the sewing ring may be a hint to the development of dehiscence, and reduction in the opening angle of the poppet an indication of valvular thrombosis [35]. Transprosthetic gradients can vary from study to study and should be interpreted in conjunction with other measures such as EOA, stroke volume and DVI.

10. Measurement errors.

    An echo Doppler study of the prosthetic valve provides multiple morphologic and functional measures which should show concordance in the diagnosis of prosthetic dysfunction. When discrepancies occur, it is important to re-examine the underlying measurements. For instance, a small prosthetic EOA may be due to an incorrect LVOT diameter measurement, as LVOT diameter is frequently underestimated. Overestimation of EOA can be caused by a spurious high flow velocity in the LVOT as a result of the Doppler sample volume being too close to the aortic prosthesis.

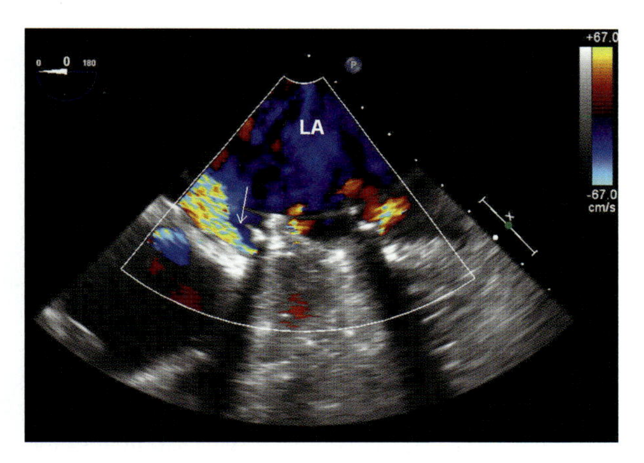

Fig. 11.32 Transesophageal view of a mechanical mitral bileaflet valve in systole shows the presence of paravalvular regurgitation at the medial valve ring (*arrow*)

11. Follow-up studies.

Doppler echocardiography is useful in the evaluation of patients with prosthetic valves and should be an integral part of the follow up of these patients. In addition to providing detailed information on prosthetic valvular function, it can also provide a comprehensive assessment of ventricular function. Optimal baseline studies are essential prior to discharge after valve replacement or at the first follow-up visit. Repeat studies should be performed at regular intervals [1]. For the biologic prosthesis, annual examination is reasonable, whereas for the mechanical prosthesis, examination once every 2 years is sufficient provided that the baseline study shows no abnormalities. On the other hand if the baseline study demonstrates abnormality, more frequent echocardiographic examinations should be performed.

Prosthetic Valvular Regurgitation

The approach to assess prosthetic valvular regurgitation is similar to that in native valvular regurgitation, although it is technically more demanding due to the artifacts from the highly echo-reflective components of the prosthetic valve. The reverberation artifact can mask part or whole of a regurgitant jet. This is a challenge when imaging for mitral regurgitation using transthoracic echocardiography but can be readily resolved by TEE (Fig. 11.32). Aortic prostheses do not obscure aortic regurgitation to the same extent. It is important to determine whether the regurgitation is valvular or paravalvular (Fig. 11.33). In bioprosthetic valves, eccentric jets arising from the sewing ring are an indication that the regurgitation is paravalvular, but this logic does not apply in assessing mechanical bileaflet valves as previously discussed. Quantitation of regurgitation is based on similar principles used in native valvular regurgitation which are discussed in Chaps. 3–5. It is important to look for flow convergence in the upstream chamber, and multiple flow convergences may be present when dealing with paravalvular regurgitation. Jet width and jet area are other parameters that are widely used to grade the severity of regurgitation.

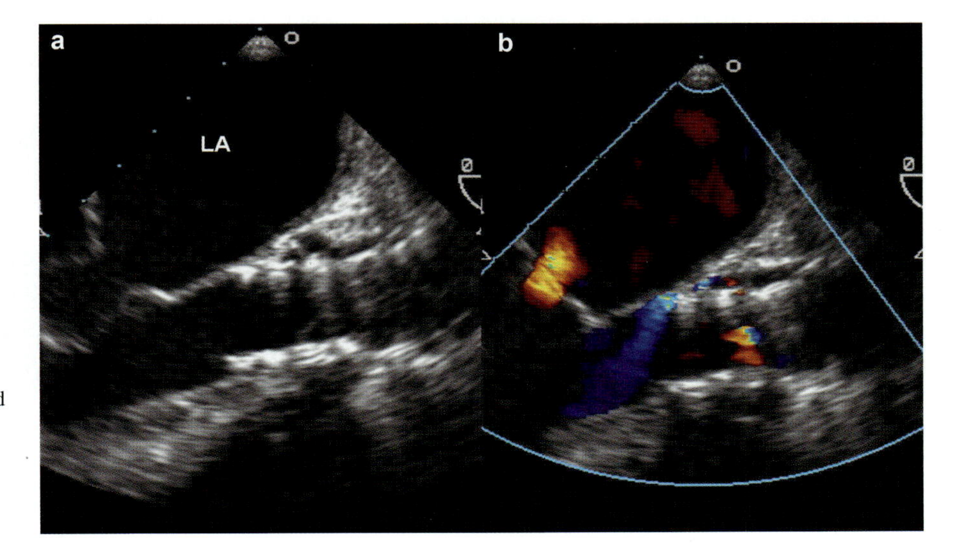

Fig. 11.33 Tranesophageal view (**a**) shows the presence of the CoreValve, which is a bioprosthetic valve imbedded in a nitinol frame, in the aortic position. Color-flow imaging (**b**) shows small perivalvular regurgitation posteriorly. *LA* left atrium

Stress Echocardiography

Stress echocardiography is increasingly used in the assessment of patients with valvular heart disease and can be very useful also in patients with suspected prosthetic dysfunction [36, 37]. Exercise is the preferred stress modality as it provides assessment of the physiologic responses to exercise. In patients who cannot exercise, pharmacologic stress, such as Dobutamine, can be used. Exercise echocardiography with a supine bicycle is best suited to assess patients with prosthetic heart valves due to its ability to assess intracardiac hemodynamics at different stages of exercise. There are two related indications for stress echocardiography: (a) to assess the functional significance of mild to moderate prosthetic dysfunction, and (b) to assess the cause of exertional symptoms. In patients with prosthetic stenosis particularly due to prosthesis–patient mismatch, it is a clinical challenge to decide if and when to replace the dysfunctional prosthesis because of the non-progressive nature of the condition, limited benefits of replacement with another prosthesis and increased risks associated with repeat surgery. On the other hand, regurgitation due to prosthetic valvular degeneration invariably progresses and will require repeat valve replacement. Thus exercise echocardiography is more commonly used to assess patients with prosthetic obstruction. During exercise, the transprosthetic gradients are measured at each stage of exercise, together with assessment of the right ventricular systolic pressure (Fig. 11.34). Other intracardiac hemodynamics to be assessed include presence and severity of subaortic obstruction, mitral regurgitation and tricuspid regurgitation (Fig. 11.35).

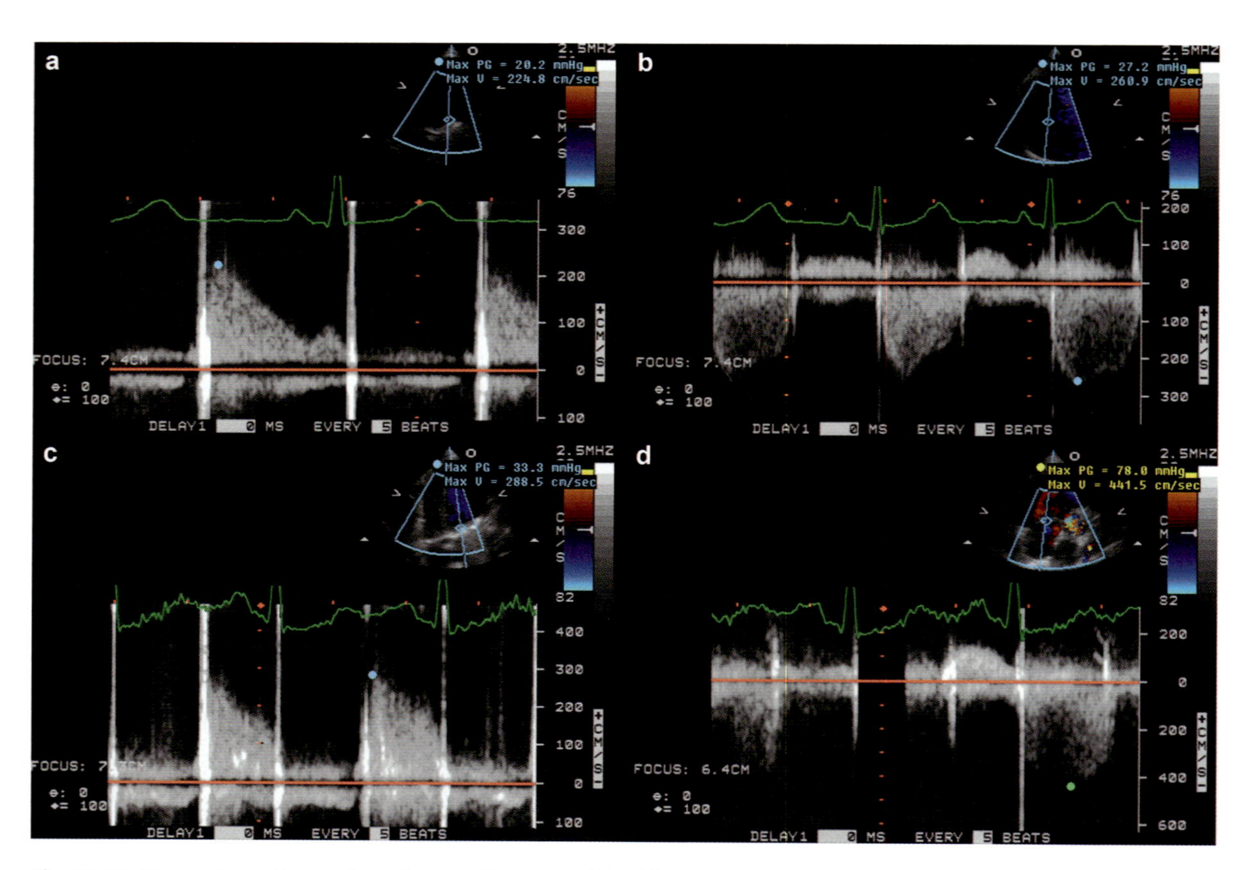

Fig. 11.34 Stress-echocardiogram in a 20-year-old woman with a 23 mm Medtronic Hall valve in the mitral position. The resting transprosthetic peak and mean gradients are 20 and 7 mmHg (**a**), and the right ventricular systolic pressure is 37 mmHg (**b**) assuming a right atrial pressure of 10 mmHg, at a heart rate of 83 beats/min. At peak exercise, the peak and mean transprosthetic gradients are 38 and 19 mmHg (**c**), and the right ventricular systolic pressure is 88 mmHg (**d**), at a heart rate of 118 beats/min associated with severe dyspnea. These findings confirm the clinical impression that the obstruction at the mitral prosthetic valve is significant and responsible for the patient's exercise intolerance

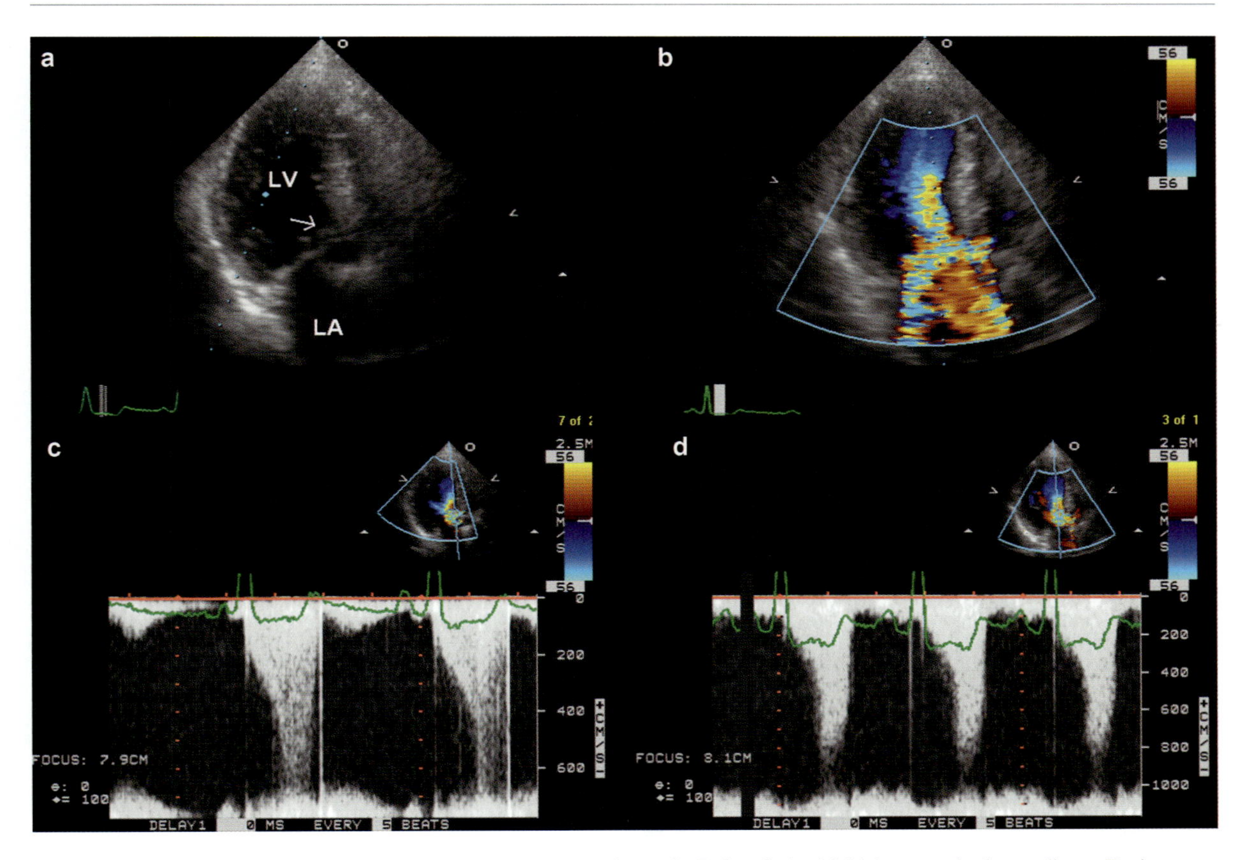

Fig. 11.35 This patient had a mechanical bileaflet aortic valve (19 mm St. Jude valve) with high transvalvular gradients. During exercise, systolic anterior motion of the mitral leaflets (*arrow*) was detected (**a**). Color-flow imaging (**b**) showed flow acceleration at the left ventricular outflow and severe mitral regurgitation which is posteriorly directed. Continuous wave Doppler examination (**c**, **d**) confirmed the presence of severe subaortic obstruction. The findings of the stress echocardiogram showed that the patient's exertional symptoms were due to the development of severe subaortic stenosis and severe mitral regurgitation. The patient went on to have aortic root enlargement, repeat aortic valve replacement with a larger size valve and myectomy of the basal septum. *LV* left ventricle

It has not been clearly defined as to what constitute a significant exercise-related increase for many of the intracardiac hemodynamic findings. It is reasonable to conclude that the prosthetic dysfunction is functionally significant when there are marked increases in transprosthetic gradients and/or right ventricular systolic pressure, particularly when they correlate with development of symptoms during the exercise.

Prosthesis-Related Complications

Prosthetic heart valves are associated with many complications both early following implantation and for the long term (Table 11.1) [38–42]. Some of the complications are associated with all types of valves (mechanical and bioprosthetic), some are valve design specific (such as the Bjork Shiley disc escape), and other complications are related to the surgical procedure and medical therapy such as anticoagulation. Valve prosthesis dysfunction and potential life-threatening sequelae continue to be the nemesis of all prosthetic valves. Currently available mechanical and bioprosthetic valves have a 11-year probability of valve-related complications of approximately 62–79% [43]. It should be recognized that many patients still have valve prostheses that are no longer being implanted. These prostheses may no longer be common but it is still important for echocardiographers and pathologists to recognize the complications specific for the valve type.

Early intra-operative or post-operative patient–prosthesis mismatch may become apparent if the valve size is not adequate. This can be recognized by

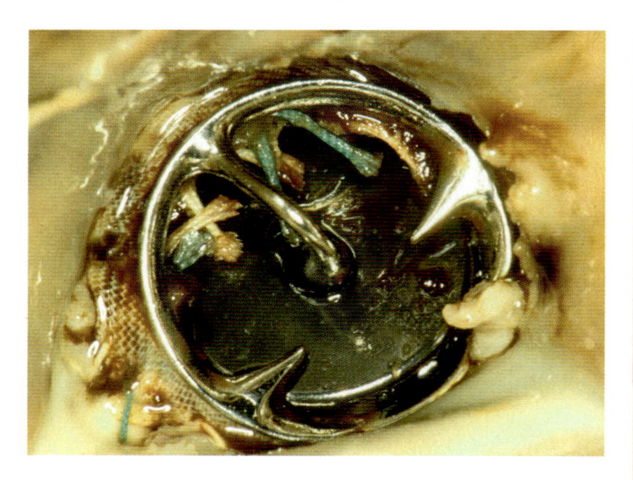

Fig. 11.36 Mechanical Medtronic Hall prosthesis with poor disc movement due to excessive suture material

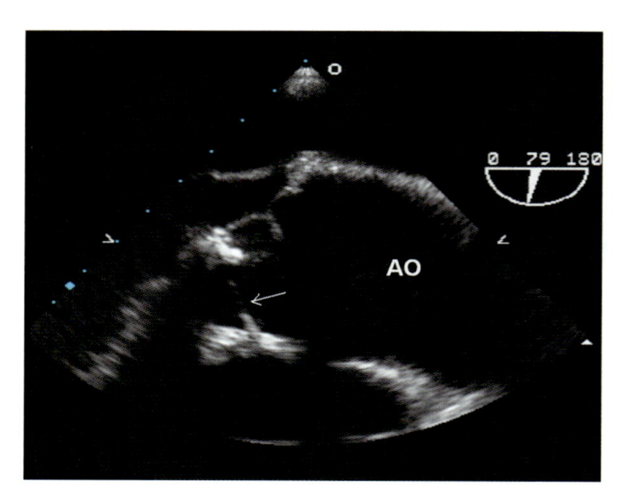

Fig. 11.37 Transesophageal view shows a stented aortic bioprosthetic valve which has an unusual orientation with the anterior sewing ring deviated into the left ventricular outflow tract (LVOT). A small intimal flap (*arrow*) is present at the anterior aortic root consistent with a localized dissection. *Ao* aorta

examining the reference EOA for the particular size and model of the prosthesis in relation to the body surface area of the patient [3, 23]. The valve ring number may actually be a different circumference for different valve types, that is a # 29 of one prosthesis may not be the same size as a # 29 of another valve type [19, 20]. The valve may be immediately obstructed if sutures are too long and overhang into the valve orifice and they interfere with disc movement (Fig. 11.36) or the sutures inadvertently suture the valve closed [44]. If the stents are poorly positioned a high profile mitral

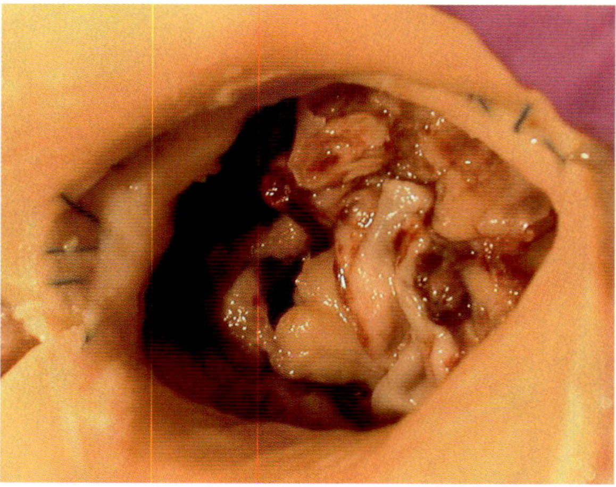

Fig. 11.38 Bioprosthesis with bacterial infective endocarditis involving the prosthesis leaflets

prosthesis may obstruct the left ventricle outflow tract. Previously observed ventricular free wall rupture from inadvertent ventricle free wall excision with the papillary muscles is no longer seen as the chordae are usually left intact to prevent negative ventricular remodeling. Atrioventricular groove disruption may still occur.

A poorly placed aortic prosthesis ring may obstruct the coronary ostia leading to ischemia or infarction of the heart. Aortic dissection may occur from many sites during or after valve surgery— from the local aortic valve site, the aortotomy incision, the cannulation site or the cross clamp region (Fig. 11.37). All may cause type A dissection.

All prostheses are at risk of infective endocarditis with an incidence of 3.4% within the first 6 months of implantation and thereafter about 0.68% per year [45]. Infections may involve the cusps of bioprostheses and the ring of both mechanical and bioprostheses (Fig. 11.38). Early infection is variably defined as infection less than a month or less than 6 months after surgery. These infections may be a result of the medical treatment (line or wound infections), sepsis from another infection (pneumonia or urinary tract infection) or residual infection if the prosthesis was implanted for treatment of infective endocarditis. Late infection has the same microbiological profile as community acquired endocarditis, with the addition of coagulase-negative staphylococci. The infections may destroy the bioprosthetic cusps, and thrombus may occur on both bioprostheses and mechanic prostheses. Thrombus may impede valve function or lead to

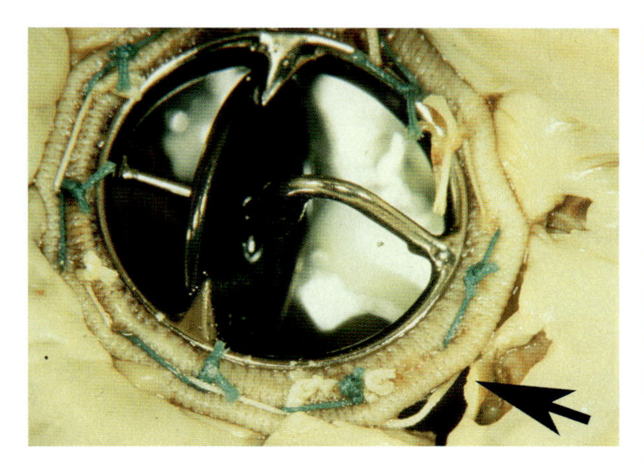

Fig. 11.39 Medtronic Hall mechanical prosthesis with a paravalvular leak that occurred after surgery. The defect is seen near the ring (*arrow*)

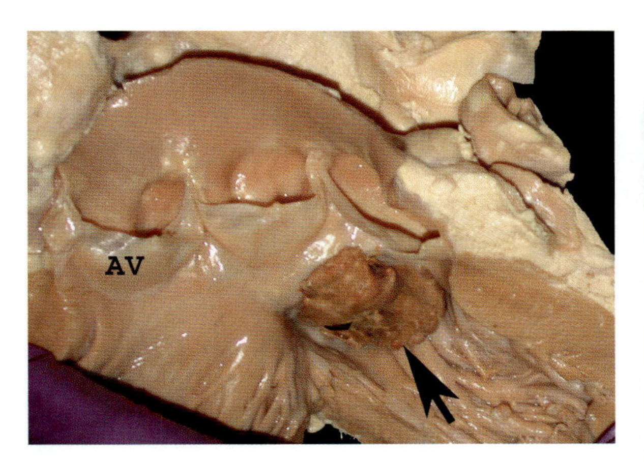

Fig. 11.40 The image shows a thrombosed mitral pericardial bioprosthesis (*arrow*). The heart is opened and the left ventricle outflow tract is seen with the aortic valve (*AV*). Abundant thrombus covered the prosthesis leaflets

emboli. Ring infection may lead to paravalvular leaks, fistulas or ring abscesses. These complications are elaborated upon in Chap. 12.

All prostheses may dehisce and/or have a paravalvular leak related to technical difficulties, tissue retraction during healing, or infective endocarditis (Fig. 11.39). Paravalvular leak may lead to valve regurgitation and heart failure, thrombosis and embolism or hemolysis.

Patients with prostheses, especially mechanical, have a significant risk of thrombosis, estimated at 0.1–5.7% per patient year [46]. Inadequate anti-coagulation plays a major role. Mechanical valve thrombosis remains the most common cause of mechanical valve obstruction (Figs. 11.40–11.42). The thrombus may interfere with the prosthesis function or be on the ring and present clinically as embolic events. Small thrombi may be clinically and functionally silent initially, but with growth they may obstruct the orifice, prevent prosthesis opening or closing, or embolize.

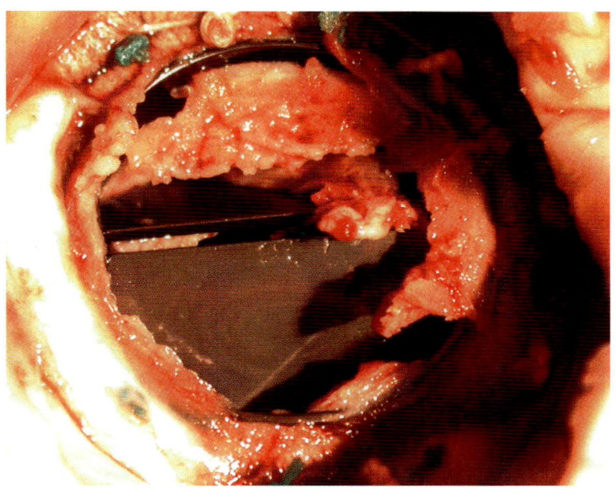

Fig. 11.41 Bi-leaflet mechanical prostheses, in aortic position, with thrombosis. The thrombus produced prosthesis stenosis and immobilized the leaflets. Thrombus is seen around the leaflets and in the hinge area

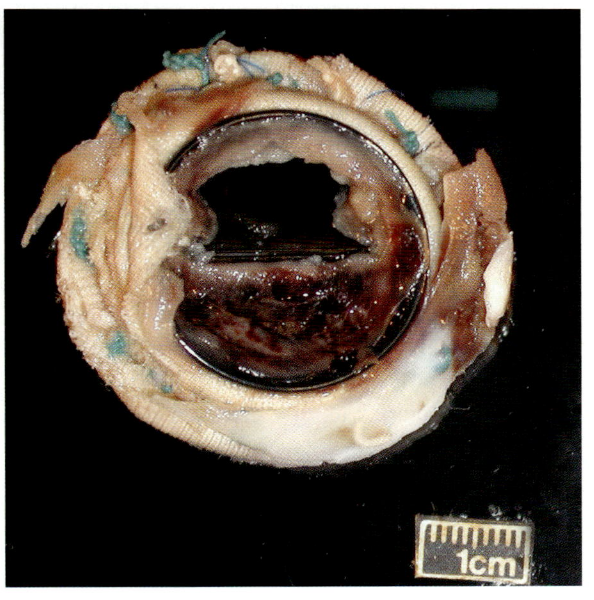

Fig. 11.42 Bi-leaflet mechanical prosthesis in aortic position that was excised for prosthesis stenosis. There is thrombus on the discs immobilizing it

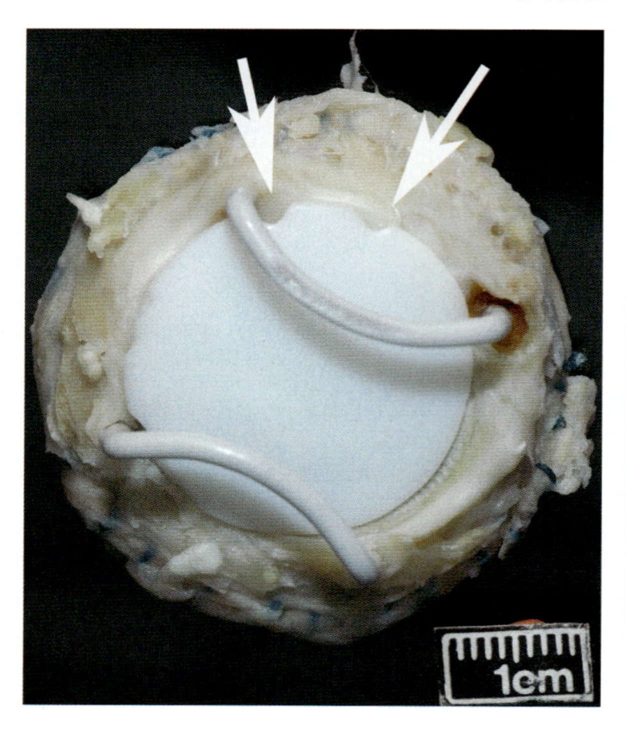

Fig. 11.43 Excised mechanical prosthesis with a plastic disc and struts. Repetitive movement has eroded pieces of the plastic disc where it hits the struts *(arrow)*

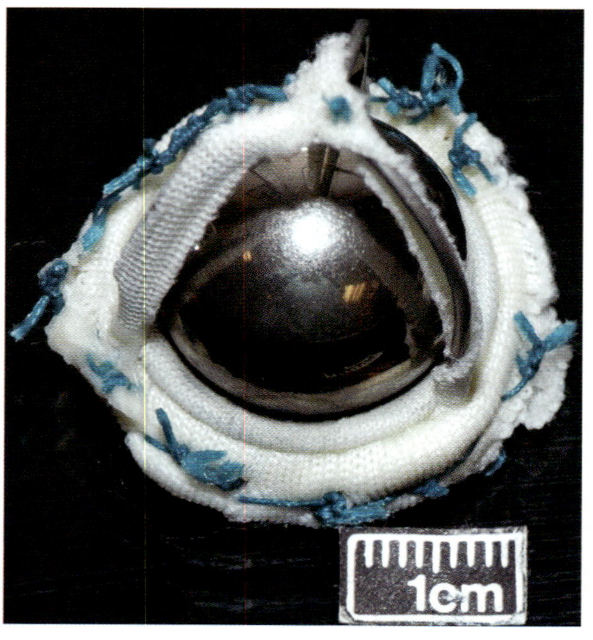

Fig. 11.44 Excised Starr Edwards mechanical ball and cage valve. The cloth has worn off the cage and appears loose and frayed

Mechanical prostheses may have defects in the valve structural components [39]. Plastic or silastic balls, seen in valves such as Starr Edwards valves, may absorb lipid leading to fragility. The ball may crack leading to emboli or the ball may escape. Plastic discs may wear on valve struts leading to emboli (Fig. 11.43). Metal struts may fracture with disc escape and embolization of the strut and the disc (such as occurred with Bjork Shiley valves). Cloth may wear off the struts or the valve ring and the cloth can embolize (Fig. 11.44). On the inner valve ring erosion of the cloth exposes sharp areas that can lead to hemolysis (Fig. 11.45). Rings may be coated with material such as silver in an attempt to decrease post-operative infections. This unfortunately is associated with a high incidence of paravalvular leak. Pannus may form on the valve ring leading to inflow obstruction of the orifice (Figs. 11.46–11.48). Some valve struts may gradually bend inwards leading to partial obstruction (stent or strut "creep") [47].

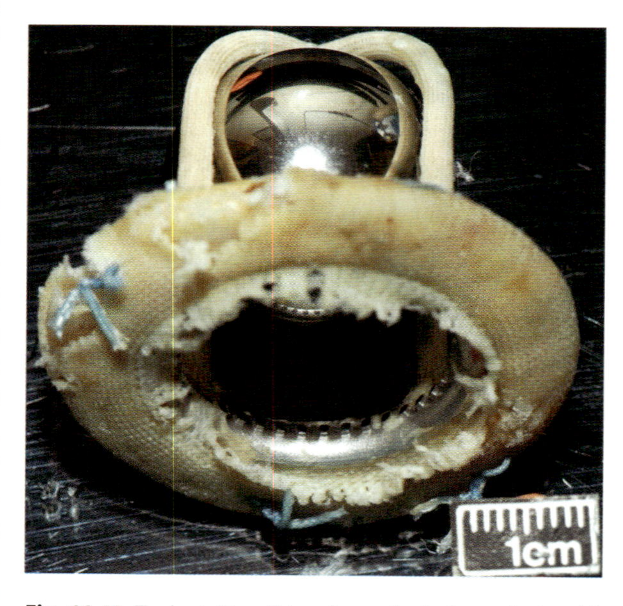

Fig. 11.45 Excised Starr Edwards mechanical prosthesis with cloth wear where the ball hits the ring. The cloth is frayed and irregular "teeth" are exposed. Such patients often have hemolysis

Bioprosthetic valves are at a lesser risk of thrombosis; hence the patient does not require long-term anticoagulation. However, structural failure limits the lifespan of bioprosthetic valves with a 10–20% failure rate for homografts and 30% for xenografts within 10–15 years [46]. The degeneration is a time dependent process. Tissue degeneration may be seen in all patient age groups, but is especially marked in

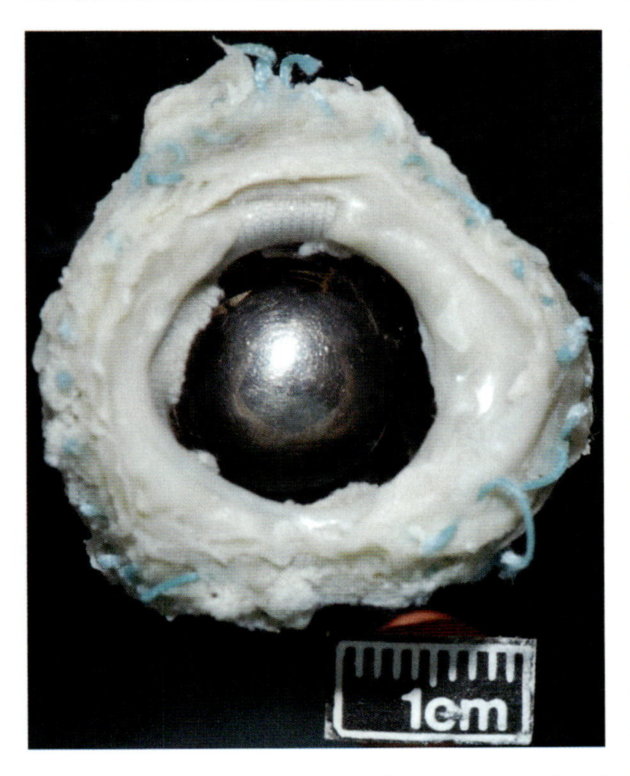

Fig. 11.46 Pannus white fibrotic material narrows the orifice of this Starr Edwards mechanical prosthesis

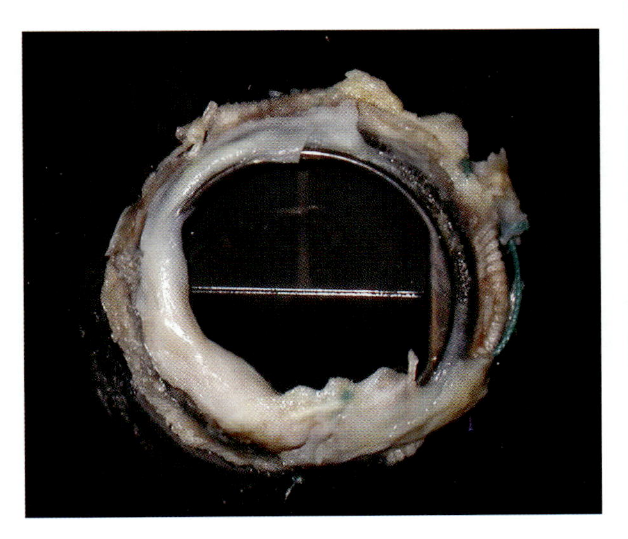

Fig. 11.47 Mechanical bileaflet prosthesis with poor disc movement due to white fibrosis pannus material

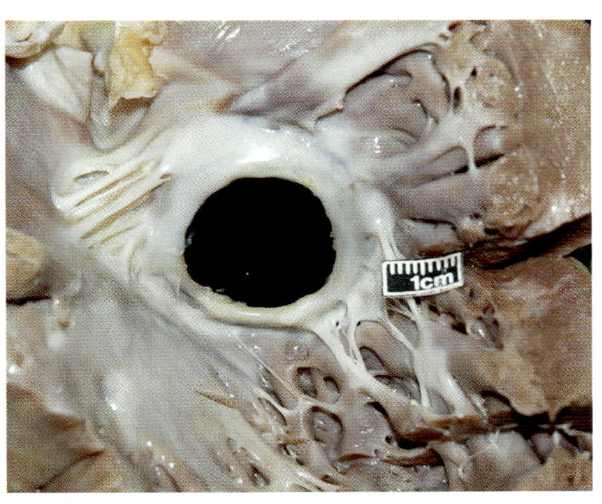

Fig. 11.48 Underside (ventricular) of a bi-leaflet mechanic prosthesis. There is severe pannus formation beneath the valve narrowing it. Abnormally inserted chordae remain from the patient's original atrioventricular septal valve defect

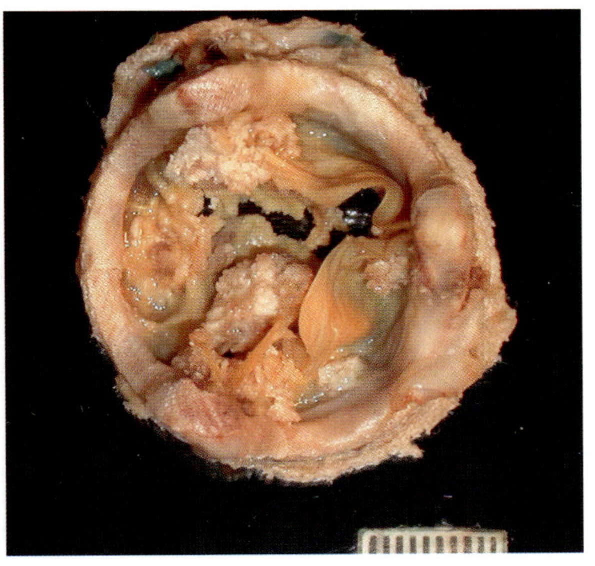

Fig. 11.49 Degenerated porcine bioprosthesis with cusp fibrosis and calcification

prostheses implanted in the young. Cusp degeneration, fibrosis, calcification and tearing are responsible for dysfunction, which may be stenosis, regurgitation or both (Figs. 11.49, 11.50) [43, 46]. Ionescu Shiley prostheses were prone to cusp tears at the anchoring stitch near the cusp stent commissures [48–50]. The tears can extend resulting in cusp prolapse or flail (Fig. 11.51). Pannus obstruction of the prosthetic orifice may occur and pannus may also immobilize or stiffen the cusps leading to prosthetic obstruction (Fig. 11.52). It is debatable whether the cusps illicit an immune response. They are fixed in gluteraldehyde,

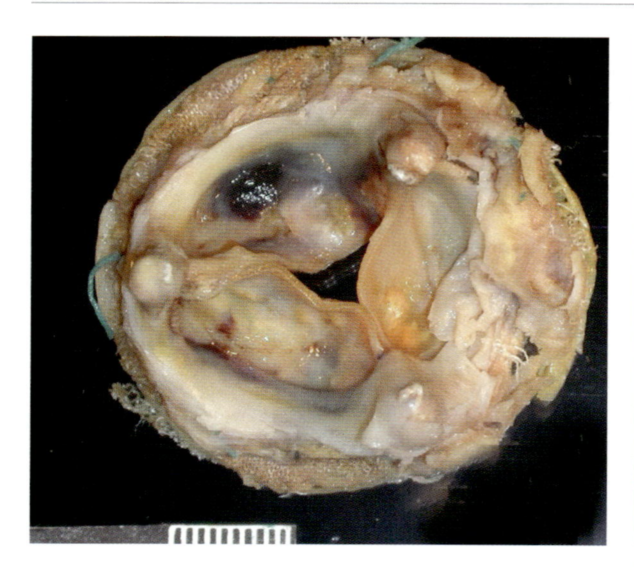

Fig. 11.50 Degenerated pericardial bioprosthesis with cusp fibrosis, calcification and fibrin accumulation. White pannus material is noted over the stents

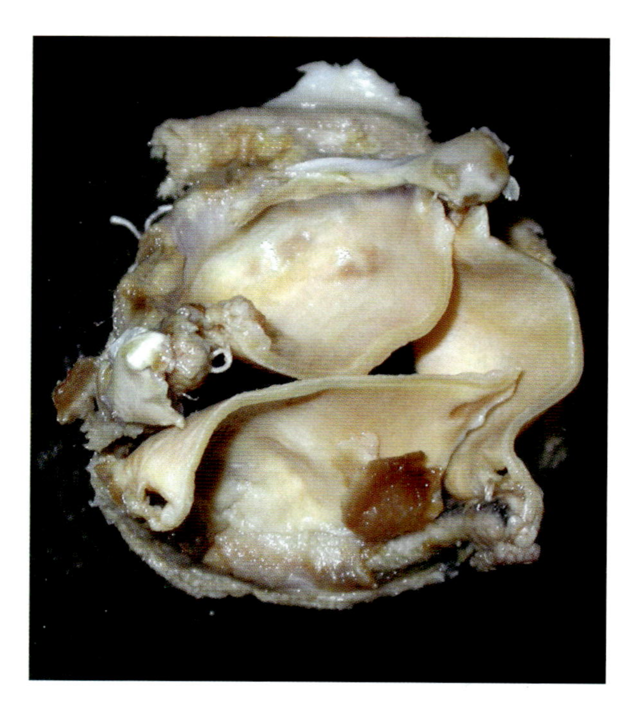

Fig. 11.51 Ionescu Shiley prosthesis with cusp fibrosis and calcification. Tears off the stents with leaflet prolapse and valve regurgitation are characteristic of the degenerative pattern of this bioprosthesis. Many of the tears started at an anchoring stitch near the stent

and some are treated with anti-calcification agents. They are washed prior to insertion but some local ring tissue toxicity from residual fixative is possible. Some prosthetic cusps may be under fixed so there is a

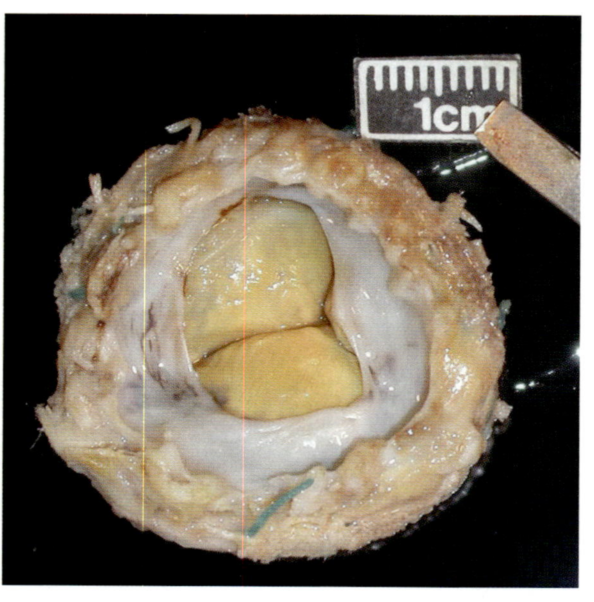

Fig. 11.52 Pannus inflow stenosis of a bioprosthesis by white pannus material. The prosthesis orifice is diminished and the leaflets are immobilized

possibility of residual immunogenicity. In the early postoperative period, the cusps have mild neutrophil infiltration and fibrin attachment, but generally the inflammatory cells disappear followed by the development of degenerative changes with lipid and fibrin insudation and calcification.

Summary

Patients with valvular heart diseases have benefited immensely from the development of prosthetic heart valves. Following implantation of a prosthetic heart valve, the patient needs to be regularly followed, as prosthetic valves are associated with acute and chronic complications. A complete echo Doppler study should be an integral part of the follow-up by providing detailed morphologic and functional assessments. There should be a low threshold to perform TEE in these patients as it provides high quality images and is more able to overcome the artifacts associated with prosthetic valves in the transthoracic study. A high transprosthetic gradient is a common finding in prosthetic valves, and a logical approach is useful to determine the etiology and to plan further investigation and management.

Appendix 11.1 Normal Doppler echocardiographic values for aortic valve prostheses

Valve	Size	N	Peak gradient (mmHg)	Mean gradient (mmHg)	Peak velocity (m/s)	Effective orifice area (cm²)
ATS Open Pivot AP	16	6	47.7 ± 12	27 ± 7.3	3.44 ± 0.47	0.61 ± 0.09
ATS open pivot	19	9	47 ± 12.6	26.2 ± 7.9	3.41 ± 0.43	0.96 ± 0.18
bileaflet	21	15	25.5 ± 6.1	14.4 ± 3.5	2.4 ± 0.39	1.58 ± 0.37
	23	8	19 ± 7	12 ± 4		1.8 ± 0.2
	25	12	17 ± 8	11 ± 4		2.2 ± 0.4
	27	10	14 ± 4	9 ± 2		2.5 ± 0.3
	29	5	11 ± 3	8 ± 2		3.1 ± 0.3
Biocor stentless	21	45	35.97 ± 4.06	18 ± 4		
bioprosthesis	23	115	29.15 ± 8.28	18.64 ± 7.14	3 ± 0.6	1.4 ± 0.5
	25	100	28.65 ± 6.6	17.72 ± 6.99	2.8 ± 0.5	1.6 ± 0.38
	27	55	25.87 ± 2.81	18 ± 2.8	2.7 ± 0.2	1.9 ± 0.46
	≥29	16	24 ± 2			
Biocor extended	19–21	12	17.5 ± 5.8	9.7 ± 3.5		1.3 ± 0.4
stentless bioprosthesis	23	18	14.8 ± 5.9	8.1 ± 3.1		1.6 ± 0.3
	25	20	14.2 ± 3.5	7.7 ± 1.9		1.8 ± 0.3
Bioflo pericardial	19	16	37.25 ± 8.65	24.15 ± 5.1		0.77 ± 0.11
stented bioprosthesis	21	9	28.7 ± 6.2	18.7 ± 5.5		1.1 ± 0.1
	23	4	20.7 ± 4	12.5 ± 3		1.3 ± 0.09
Björk Shiley monostrut	19	37	46.0	26.67 ± 7.87	3.3 ± 0.6	0.94 ± 0.19
tilting disc	21	161	32.41 ± 9.73	18.64 ± 6.09	2.9 ± 0.4	
	23	153	26.52 ± 9.67	14.5 ± 6.2	2.7 ± 0.5	
	25	89	22.33 ± 7	13.3 ± 4.96	2.5 ± 0.4	
	27	61	18.31 ± 8	10.41 ± 4.38	2.1 ± 0.4	
	29	9	12 ± 8	7.67 ± 4.36	1.9 ± 0.2	
Björk-Shiley spherical	17	1			4.1	
or not specified	19	2	27.0		3.8	1.1
tilting disc	21	18	38.94 ± 11.93	21.8 ± 3.4	2.92 ± 0.88	1.1 ± 0.25
	23	41	33.86 ± 11	17.34 ± 6.86	2.42 ± 0.4	1.22 ± 0.23
	25	39	20.39 ± 7.07	11.5 ± 4.55	2.06 ± 0.28	1.8 ± 0.32
	27	23	19.44 ± 7.99	10.67 ± 4.31	1.77 ± 0.12	2.6
	29	5	21.1 ± 7.1		1.87 ± 0.18	2.52 ± 0.69
	31	2			2.1 ± 0.14	
Carbomedics	17	7	33.4 ±13.2	20.1 ± 7.1		1.02 ± 0.2
bileaflet	19	63	33.3 ± 11.19	11.61 ± 5.08	3.09 ± 0.38	1.25 ± 0 36
	21	111	26.31 ± 10.25	12.68 ± 4.29	2.61 ± 0.51	1.42 ± 0.36
	23	120	24.61 ± 6.93	11.33 ± 3.8	2.42 ± 0.37	1.69 ± 0 29
	25	103	20.25 ± 8.69	9.34 ±4.65	2.25 ± 0.34	2.04 ± 0.37
	27	57	19.05 ± 7.0-1	8.41 ±2.83	2.18 ±0.36	2.55 ± 0.34
	29	6	12.53 ± 4.69	5.8 ± 3.2	1.93 ± 0.25	2.63 ± 0.38
Carbomedics reduced bileaflet	19	10	43.4 ± 1.8	24,4 ± 1,2		1.22 ± 0.08
Carbomedies	19	4	29.04 ± 10.1	19.5 ± 2.12	1.8	1 ± 0.18

(continued)

Appendix 11.1 (continued)

Valve	Size	N	Peak gradient (mmHg)	Mean gradient (mmHg)	Peak velocity (m/s)	Effective orifice area (cm²)
supraannular top hat	21	30	29.61 ±8 95	16.59 ± 5.79	2.62 ± 0.35	1.18 ± 0.33
bileaflet	23	30	24.38 ±7.53	13.29 ± 3.73	2.36 ± 0.55	1.37 ± 0.37
	25	1	22.011.0	2.4		
Carpentier-Edwards	19	56	43.48 ±12.72	25.6 ± 8.02		0.85 ± 0.17
stented bioprosthesis	21	73	27.73 ±7.6	17.25 ± 6.24	2.37 ± 0.54	1.48 ± 0.3
	23	100	28.93 ±7.49	15.92 ± 6.43	2.76 ± 0.4	1.69 ± 0.45
	25	85	23.95 ±7.05	12.76 ± 4.43	2.38 ± 0.47	1.94 ± 0.45
	27	50	22.14 ± S 24	12.33 ± 5.59	2.31 ± 0.39	2.25 ± 0.55
	29	24	22.09.92 ± 2.9	2.44 ± 0,43	2.84 ± 0.51	
	31	4			2-41 ±0.13	
Carpentier-Edwards	19	14	32.13 ± 3.35	24.19 ±8.6	2.83 ± 0.14	1.21 ± 0.31
pericardial	21	34	25.69 ± 9.9	20.3 ± 9.08	2.59 ± 0.42	1.47 ± 0.36
stented bioprosthesis	23	20	21.72 ± 8.57	13.01 ± 5.27	2.29 ± 0.45	1.75 ± 0.28
	25	5	16.46 ± 5.41	9.04 ± 2.27	2.02 ± 0.31	
	27	1	19,2 ± 0	5.6	1.6	
	29	1	17.6 ± 0	1 1.6	2.1	
Carpentier-Edwards	19	15	34.1 ± 2.7			1.1 ± 0.09
supraannular AV (CE-SAV)	21	8	25 ± 8	14 ± 5		1.06 ± 0.16
stented bioprosthesis						
CryoLife-O'Brien	19	47		12 ±4.8		1.25 ± 0.1
stentless	21	163		10.33 ± 2		1.57 ± 0.6
bioprosthesis	23	40		8.5		2.2
	25	40		7.9		2.3
	27	39		7.4		2.7
Duromedics (Tekna)	19	1			3.6	
bileaflet	21	3	19.08 ± 16	8.98 ± 5		1.3
	25	12	19.87 ± 7	7 ± 2	2.64 ± 0.27	
	25	18	21 ± 9	5 ± 2	2.34 ± 0.38	
	27	15	22.5 ± 12	6 ± 3	1.88 ± 0.6	
	29	1	13.0	3.4	2.1	
Edwards Prima stentless	19	7	30.9 ± 11.7	15.4 ± 7.4		1 ± 0.3
bioprosthesis	21	30	31.22 ± 17.35	16.36 ± 11.36		1.25 ± 0.29
	23	62	23.39 ± 10.17	11.52 ± 5.26	2.8 ± 0.4	1.49 ± 0.46
	25	97	19.74 ± 10.36	10.77 ± 9.32	2.7 ± 0.3	1.7 ± 0.55
	27	46	15.9 ± 7.3	7.1 ± 3.7		2 ± 0.6
	29	11	11.21 ± 8.6	5.03 ± 4.53		2.49 ± 0.52
Hancock I	21	1			3.5	
stented bioprosthesis	23	14	19.09 ±4.35	12.36 ± 3.82	2.94 ± 0.24	
	25	26	17.61 ± 3.13	11 ± 2.85	2.36 ± 0.37	
	27	20	18.11 ± 6.92	10 ± 3.46	2.4 ± 0.36	
	29	2			2.23 ± 0.04	

Appendix 11.1 (continued)

Valve	Size	N	Peak gradient (mmHg)	Mean gradient (mmHg)	Peak velocity (m/s)	Effective orifice area (cm²)
	31	1			2.0	
Hancock II	21	39	20 ±4	14.8 ±4.1		1.23 ± 0.27
stented bioprosthesis	23	119	24.72 ± 5.73	16.64 ± 6.91		1.39 ± 0.23
	25	114	20 ± 2	10.7 ± 3		1,47 ± 0.19
	27	133	14 ± 3			1.55 ± 0.18
	29	35	15 ± 3			1.6 ± 0.15
Ionescu-Shiley	17	11	42.0	21.1 ± 3.21		0.86 ± 0.1
stented bioprosthesis	19	63	23.17 ± 6.58	20.44 ± 8.47	2.63 ± 0.32	1.15 ± 0.18
	21	11	27.63 ± 8.34	15.1 ± 1.56	2.75 ± 0.25	
	23	5	18.09 ± 6.49	9.9 ± 2.85	2.1 ± 0.38	
	25	1	18,0			
	27	3	14.75 ± 2.17	8.97 ± 0.57	1.92 ± 0.14	
	29	1	16.0	7.3 ± 0	2.0	
Jyros bileaflet	22	4	17.3	10.8		1.5
bileaflet	24	7	18.6	11 4		1.5
	26	8	14.4	8.4		1.7
	28	3	10.0	5.7		1.9
	30	1	8.0	6.0		1.6
Lillehei-Kaster	14	1			2.7	
tilting disc	16	2			3.43 ± 0.39	
	18	2			2.85 ± 0.21	
	20	1			1.7	
Medtronic Freestyle	19	11		13.0		
	21	85		7.99 ± 2.6		1.6 ± 0.32
stentless bioprosthesis	23	141		7.24 ± 2.5		1.9 ± 0.5
	25	164		5.35 ± 1.5		2.03 ± 0.41
	27	105		4.27 ± 1.6		2.5 ± 0.47
Medtronic-Hall	20	24	34.37 ± 13.06	17.08 ± 5.28	2.9 ± 04	1.21 ± 0.45
tilting disc	21	30	26.86 ± 10.54	14.1 ± 5.93	2.42 ± 0.36	1.08 ± 0.17
	23	27	26.85 ± 8.85	13.5 ± 4.79	2.43 ± 0.59	1.36 ± 0.39
	25	17	17.13 ± 7.04	9.53 ± 4.26	2.29 ± 0.5	1.9 ± 0.47
	27	8	18.66 ± 9.71	8.66 ± 5.56	2.07 ± 0.53	1.9 ± 0.16
	29	1			1.6	
Medtronic intact	19	16	39.43 ± 15.4	23.71 ± 9.3	2.5	
stented bioprosthesis	21	55	33.9 ± 12.69	18.74 ± 8.03	2.73 ± 0.44	1.55 ± 0.39
	23	110	31.27 ± 9.62	18.88 ± 6.17	2.74 ± 0.37	1.64 ± 0.37
	25	41	27.34 ± 10.59	16.4 ± 6.05	2.6 ± 0.44	1.85 ± 0.25
	27	16	25.27 ± 7.58	15 ± 3.94	2.51 ± 0.38	2.2 ± 0.17
	29	5	31.0	15.6 ± 2.1	2.8	2.38 ± 0.54
Medtronic mosaic	21	51		12.43 ± 7.3		1.6 ± 0.7
porcine	23	121		12.47 ± 7.4		2.1 ± 0.8
stented bioprosthesis	25	71		10.08 ± 5.1		2.1 ± 1.6

(continued)

Appendix 11.2 Normal Doppler echocardiographic values for mitral prostheses [9]

Valve	Size	n	Peak gradient (mmHg)	Mean gradient (mmHg)	Peak velocity (m/s)	Pressure half-time (ms)	Effective orifice area (cm²)
Biocor	27	3	13 ± 1				
stentless bioprosthesis	29	3	14 ± 2.5				
	32	8	11.5 ± 0.5				
	33	9	12 ± 0.5				
Bioflo pericardial	25	3	10 ± 2	6.3 ± 1.5			2 ± 0.1
stented bioprosthesis	27	7	9.5 ± 2.6	5.4 ± 1.2			2 ± 0.3
	29	8	5 ± 2.8	3.6 ± 1			2.4 ± 0.2
	31	1	4.0	2.0			2.3
Björk-Shiley	23	1			1.7	115	
tilting disc	25	14	12 ± 4	6 ± 2	1.75 ± 0.38	99 ± 27	1.72 ± 0.6
	27	34	10 ± 4	5 ± 2	1.6 ± 0.49	89 ± 28	1.81 ± 0.54
	29	21	7.83 ± 2.93	2.83 ± 1.27	1.37 ± 0.25	79 ± 17	2.1 ± 0.43
	31	21	6 ± 3	2 ± 1.9	1.41 ± 0.26	70 ± 143	2.2 ± 0.3
Björk-Shiley monostrut	23	1		5.0	1.9		
tilting disc	25	102	13 ± 2.5	5.57 ± 2.3	1.8 ± 0.3		
	27	83	12 ± 2.5	4.53 ± 2.2	1.7 ± 0.4		
	29	26	13 ± 3	4.26 ± 1.6	1.6 ± 0.3		
	31	25	14 ± 4.5	4.9 ± 1.6	1.7 ± 0.3		
Carbomedics	23	2			1.9 ± 0.1	126 ± 7	
bileaflet	25	12	10.3 ± 2.3	3.6 ± 0.6	1.3 ± 0.1	93 ± 8	2.9 ± 0.8
	27	78	8.79 ± 3.46	3.46 ± 1.03	1.61 ± 0.3	89 ± 20	2.9 ± 0.75
	29	46	8.78 ± 2.9	3.39 ± 0.97	1.52 ± 0.3	88 ± 17	2.3 ± 0.4
	31	57	8.87 ± 2.34	3.32 ± 0.87	1.61 ± 0.29	92 ± 24	2.8 ± 1.14
	33	33	8.8 ± 2.2	4.8 ± 2.5	1.5 ± 0.2	93 ± 12	
Carpentier-Edwards	27	16		6 ± 2	1.7 ± 0.3	98 ± 28	
stented bioprosthesis	29	22		4.7 ± 2	1.76 ± 0.27	92 ± 14	
	31	22		4.4 ± 2	1.54 ± 0.15	92 ± 19	
	33	6		6 ± 3		93 ± 12	
Carpentier-Edwards	27	1		3.6	1.6	100	
pericardial	29	6		5.25 ± 2.36	1.67 ± 0.3	110 ± 15	
stented bioprosthesis	31	4		4.05 ± 0.83	1.53 ± 0.1	90 ± 11	
	33	1		1.0	0.8	80	
Duromedics	27	8	13 ± 6	5 ± 3	161 ± 40	75 ± 12	
bileaflet	29	14	10 ± 4	3 ± 1	140 ± 25	85 ± 22	
	31	21	10.5 ± 4.33	3.3 ± 1.36	1.38 ± 27	81 ± 12	
	33	1	11.2	2.5		85	
Hancock I or not specified	27	3	10 ± 4	5 ± 2			1.3 ± 0.8
stented bioprosthesis	29	13	7 ± 3	2.46 ± 0.79		115 ± 20	1.5 ± 0.2
	31	22	4 ± 0.86	4.86 ± 1.69		95 ± 17	1.6 ± 0.2
	33	8	3 ± 2	3.87 ± 2		90 ± 12	1.9 ± 0.2
Hancock II	27	16					2.21 ± 0.14
stented bioprosthesis	29	64					2.77 ± 0.11

Appendix 11.2 (continued)

Valve	Size	n	Peak gradient (mmHg)	Mean gradient (mmHg)	Peak velocity (m/s)	Pressure half-time (ms)	Effective orifice area (cm²)
	31	90					2.84 ± 0.1
	33	25					3.15 ± 0.22
Hancock pericardial	29	14		2.61 ± 1.39	1.42 ± 0.14	105 ± 36	
stented bioprosthesis	31	8		3.57 ± 1.02	1.51 ± 0.27	81 ± 23	
Ionescu-Shiley	25	3		4.87 ± 1.08	1.43 ± 0.15	93 ± 11	
stented bioprosthesis	25	3		4.87 ± 1.08	1.45 ± 0.15	93 ± 11	
	27	4		3.21 ± 0.82	1.31 ± 0.24	100 ± 28	
	29	6		3.22 ± 0.57	1.38 ± 0.2	85 ± 8	
	31	4		3.63 ± 0.9	1.45 ± 0.06	100 ± 36	
Ionescu-Shiley low profile	29	13		3.31 ± 0.96	1.36 ± 0.25	80 ± 30	
stented bioprosthesis	31	10		2.74 ± 0.37	1.33 ± 0.14	79 ± 15	
Labcor-Santiago	25	1	8.7	4.5		97	2.2
pericardial	27	16	5.6 ± 2.3	2.8 ± 1.5		85 ± 18	2.12 ± 0.48
stented bioprosthesis	29	20	6.2 ± 2.1	3 ± 1.3		80 ± 34	2.11 ± 0.73
Lillehei-Kaster	18	1			1.7	140	
tilting disc	20	1			1.7	67	
	22	4			1.56 ± 0.09	94 ± 22	
	25	5			1.38 ± 0.27	124 ± 46	
Medtronic-Hall	27	1			1.4	78	
tilting disc	29	5			1.57 ± 0.1	69 ± 15	
	31	7			1.45 ± 0.12	77 ± 17	
Medtronic Intact	29	3		3.5 ± 0.51	1.6 ± 0.22		
porcine	31	14		4.2 ± 1.44	1.6 ± 0.26		
stented bioprosthesis	33	13		4 ± 1.3	1.4 ± 0.24		
Mitroflow	25	1		6.9	2.0	90	
stented bioprosthesis	27	3		3.07 ± 0.91	1.5	90 ± 20	
	29	15		3.5 ± 1.65	1.43 ± 0.29	102 ± 21	
	31	5		3.85 ± 0.81	1.32 ± 0.26	91 ± 22	
Omnicarbon	23	1		8.0			
tilting disc	25	16		6.05 ± 1.81	1.77 ± 0.24	102 ± 16	
	27	29		4.89 ± 2.05	1.63 ± 0.36	105 ± 33	
	29	34		4.93 ± 2.16	1.56 ± 0.27	120 ± 40	
	31	58		4.18 ± 1.4	1.3 ± 0.23	134 ± 31	
	33	2		4 ± 2			
On-X	25	3	11.5 ± 3.2	5.3 ± 2.1			1.9 ± 1.1
bileaflet	27–29	16	10.3 ± 4.5	4.5 ± 1.6			2.2 ± 0.5
	31–33	14	9.8 ± 3.8	4.8 ± 2.4			2.5 ± 1.1
Soring Allcarbon	25	8	15 ± 3	5 ± 1	2 ± 0.2	105 ± 29	2.2 ± 0.6

(continued)

Appendix 11.2 (continued)

Valve	Size	n	Peak gradient (mmHg)	Mean gradient (mmHg)	Peak velocity (m/s)	Pressure half-time (ms)	Effective orifice area (cm²)
tilting disc	27	20	13 ± 2	4 ± 1	1.8 ± 0.1	89 ± 14	2.5 ± 0.5
	29	34	10 ± 2	4 ± 1	1.6 ± 0.2	85 ± 23	2.8 ± 0.7
	31	11	9 ± 1	4 ± 1	1.6 ± 0.1	88 ± 27	2.8 ± 0.9
Sorin Bicarbon	25	3	15 ± 0.25	4 ± 0.5	1.95 ± 0.02	70 ± 1	
bileaflet	27	25	11 ± 2.75	4 ± 0.5	1.65 ± 0.21	82 ± 20	
	29	30	12 ± 3	4 ± 1.25	1.73 ± 0.22	80 ± 14	
	31	9	10 ± 1.5	4 ± 1	1.66 ± 0.11	83 ± 14	
St Jude Medical	23	1		4.0	1.5	160	1.0
bileaflet	25	4		2.5 ± 1	1.34 ± 1.12	75 ± 4	1.35 ± 0.17
	27	16	11 ± 4	5 ± 1.82	1.61 ± 0.29	75 ± 10	1.67 ± 0.17
	29	40	10 ± 3	4.15 ± 1.8	1.57 ± 0.29	85 ± 10	1.75 ± 0.24
	31	41	12 ± 6	4.46 ± 2.22	1.59 ± 0.33	74 ± 13	2.03 ± 0.32
Starr-Edwards	26	1		10.0			1.4
ball-and-cage	28	27		7 ± 2.75			1.9 ± 0.57
	30	25	12.2 ± 4.6	6.99 ± 2.5	1.7 ± 0.3	125 ± 25	1.65 ± 0.4
	32	17	11.5 ± 4.2	5.08 ± 2.5	1.7 ± 0.3	110 ± 25	1.98 ± 0.4
	34	1		5.0			2.6
Stentless quadrileaflet	26	2		2.2 ± 1.7	1.6	103 ± 31	1.7
bovine pericardial	28	14			1.58 ± 0.25		1.7 ± 0.6
stentless bioprosthesis	30	6			1.42 ± 0.32		2.3 ± 0.4
Wessex	29	9		3.69 ± 0.61	1.66 ± 0.17	83 ± 19	
stented bioprosthesis	31	22		3.31 ± 0.83	1.41 ± 0.25	80 ± 21	

Source: Reproduced from Rosenhek et al. [9]. With permission

References

1. Bonow RO, Carabello BA, Chatterjee K, et al. ACC/AHA 2006 guidelines for the management of patients with valvular heart disease. *Circulation*. 2006;114(5):E84-E231.
2. Zoghbi WA, Chambers JB, Dumesnil JG, et al. Recommendations for evaluation of prosthetic valves with echocardiography and doppler ultrasound: a report From the American Society of Echocardiography's Guidelines and Standards Committee and the Task Force on Prosthetic Valves, developed in conjunction with the American College of Cardiology Cardiovascular Imaging Committee, Cardiac Imaging Committee of the American Heart Association, the European Association of Echocardiography, a registered branch of the European Society of Cardiology, the Japanese Society of Echocardiography and the Canadian Society of Echocardiography, endorsed by the American College of Cardiology Foundation, American Heart Association, European Association of Echocardiography, a registered branch of the European Society of Cardiology, the Japanese Society of Echocardiography, and Canadian Society of Echocardiography. *J Am Soc Echocardiogr*. 2009 Sept; 22(9):975-1014.
3. Pibarot P, Dumesnil JG. Prosthetic heart valves selection of the optimal prosthesis and long-term management. *Circulation*. 2009;119(7):1034-1048.
4. Zabalgoitia M. Echocardiographic assessment of prosthetic heart valves. *Curr Probl Cardiol*. 1992;17:265-325.
5. Grube E, Schuler G, Buellesfeld L, et al. Percutaneous aortic valve replacement for severe aortic stenosis in high-risk patients using the second- and current third-generation self-expanding CoreValve prosthesis – Device success and 30-day clinical outcome. *J Am Coll Cardiol*. 2007;50(1):69-76.
6. Webb JG, Chandavimol M, Thompson CR, et al. Percutaneous aortic valve implantation retrograde from the femoral artery. *Circulation*. 2006;113(6):842-850.
7. Sievers HH, Hanke T, Stierle U, et al. A critical reappraisal of the Ross operation – renaissance of the subcoronary implantation technique? *Circulation*. 2006;114:I504-I511.
8. Rajani R, Mukherjee D, Chambers JB. Doppler echocardiography in normally functioning replacement aortic valves: a review of 129 studies. *J Heart Valve Dis*. 2007 Sept;16(5): 519-535.
9. Rosenhek R, Binder T, Maurer G, Baumgartner H. Normal values for Doppler echocardiographic assessment of heart valve prostheses. *J Am Soc Echocardiogr*. 2003 Nov; 16(11):1116-1127.

10. Gueret P, Vignon P, Fournier P, et al. Transesophageal echocardiography for the diagnosis and management of nonobstructive thrombosis of mechanical mitral valve prosthesis. *Circulation*. 1995 Jan 1;91(1):103-110.
11. Dzavik V, Cohen G, Chan KL. Role of transesophageal echocardiography in the diagnosis and management of prosthetic valve thrombosis. *J Am Coll Cardiol*. 1991 Dec; 18(7):1829-1833.
12. Barbetseas J, Nagueh SF, Pitsavos C, Toutouzas PK, Quinones MA, Zoghbi WA. Differentiating thrombus from pannus formation in obstructed mechanical prosthetic valves: an evaluation of clinical, transthoracic and transesophageal echocardiographic parameters. *J Am Coll Cardiol*. 1998 Nov; 32(5):1410-1417.
13. Daniel WG, Mugge A, Grote J, et al. Comparison of transthoracic and transesophageal echocardiography for detection of abnormalities of prosthetic and bioprosthetic valves in the mitral and aortic positions. *Am J Cardiol*. 1993 Jan 15; 71(2):210-215.
14. Shively BK, Gurule FT, Roldan CA, Leggett JH, Schiller NB. Diagnostic value of transesophageal compared with transthoracic echocardiography in infective endocarditis. *J Am Coll Cardiol*. 1991 Aug;18(2):391-397.
15. Schoen FJ, Levy RJ. Calcification of tissue heart valve substitutes: progress toward understanding and prevention. *Ann Thorac Surg*. 2005 Mar;79(3):1072-1080.
16. Srivatsa SS, Harrity PJ, Maercklein PB, et al. Increased cellular expression of matrix proteins that regulate mineralization is associated with calcification of native human and porcine xenograft bioprosthetic heart valves. *J Clin Invest*. 1997 Mar 1;99(5):996-1009.
17. Bach DS. Transesophageal echocardiographic (TEE) evaluation of prosthetic valves. *Cardiol Clin*. 2000 Nov;18(4): 751-771.
18. Cohen GI, Davison MB, Klein AL, Salcedo EE, Stewart WJ. A comparison of flow convergence with other transthoracic echocardiographic indexes of prosthetic mitral regurgitation. *J Am Soc Echocardiogr*. 1992 Nov;5(6):620-627.
19. Christakis GT, Buth KJ, Goldman BS, et al. Inaccurate and misleading valve sizing: a proposed standard for valve size nomenclature. *Ann Thorac Surg*. 1998 Oct;66(4):1198-1203.
20. Chambers JB, Oo L, Narracott A, Lawford PM, Blauth CI. Nominal size in six bileaflet mechanical aortic valves: a comparison of orifice size and biologic equivalence. *J Thorac Cardiovasc Surg*. 2003 June;125(6):1388-1393.
21. Pibarot P, Dumesnil JG. Prosthesis-patient mismatch: definition, clinical impact, and prevention. *Heart*. 2006; 92(8):1022-1029.
22. Dumesnil JG, Yoganathan AP. Valve prosthesis hemodynamics and the problem of high transprosthetic pressure gradients. *Eur J Cardiothorac Surg*. 1992;6(Suppl 1):S34-S37.
23. Pibarot P, Dumesnil JG. Hemodynamic and clinical impact of prosthesis-patient mismatch in the aortic valve position and its prevention. *J Am Coll Cardiol*. 2000 Oct;36(4):1131-1141.
24. Magne J, Mathieu P, Dumesnil JG, et al. Impact of prosthesis-patient mismatch on survival after mitral valve replacement. *Circulation*. 2007;115(11):1417-1425.
25. Lam BK, Chan V, Hendry P, et al. The impact of patient-prosthesis mismatch on late outcomes after mitral valve replacement. *J Thorac Cardiovasc Surg*. 2007 June; 133(6):1464-1473.
26. Ruel M, Rubens FD, Masters RG, et al. Late incidence and predictors of persistent or recurrent heart failure in patients with aortic prosthetic valves. *J Thorac Cardiovasc Surg*. 2004 Jan;127(1):149-159.
27. Dumesnil JG, Dion D, Yvorchuk K, Davies RA, Chan K. A new, simple and accurate method for determining ejection fraction by Doppler echocardiography. *Can J Cardiol*. 1995 Dec;11(11):1007-1014.
28. Fernandes V, Olmos L, Nagueh SF, Quinones MA, Zoghbi WA. Peak early diastolic velocity rather than pressure half-time is the best index of mechanical prosthetic mitral valve function. *Am J Cardiol*. 2002 Mar 15; 89(6):704-710.
29. Saad RM, Barbetseas J, Olmos L, Rubio N, Zoghbi WA. Application of the continuity equation and valve resistance to the evaluation of St. Jude Medical prosthetic aortic valve dysfunction. *Am J Cardiol*. 1997 Nov 1;80(9):1239-1242.
30. Chafizadeh ER, Zoghbi WA. Doppler echocardiographic assessment of the St. Jude Medical prosthetic valve in the aortic position using the continuity equation. *Circulation*. 1991 Jan;83(1):213-223.
31. Baumgartner H, Khan S, DeRobertis M, Czer L, Maurer G. Discrepancies between Doppler and catheter gradients in aortic prosthetic valves in vitro. A manifestation of localized gradients and pressure recovery. *Circulation*. 1990 Oct; 82(4):1467-1475.
32. Baumgartner H, Khan S, DeRobertis M, Czer L, Maurer G. Effect of prosthetic aortic valve design on the Doppler-catheter gradient correlation: an in vitro study of normal St. Jude, Medtronic-Hall, Starr-Edwards and Hancock valves. *J Am Coll Cardiol*. 1992 Feb;19(2):324-332.
33. Baumgartner H, Stefenelli T, Niederberger J, Schima H, Maurer G. "Overestimation" of catheter gradients by Doppler ultrasound in patients with aortic stenosis: a predictable manifestation of pressure recovery. *J Am Coll Cardiol*. 1999 May;33(6):1655-1661.
34. Garcia D, Pibarot P, Dumesnil JG, Sakr F, Durand LG. Assessment of aortic valve stenosis severity: a new index based on the energy loss concept. *Circulation*. 2000 Feb 22;101(7):765-771.
35. Muratori M, Montorsi P, Teruzzi G, et al. Feasibility and diagnostic accuracy of quantitative assessment of mechanical prostheses leaflet motion by transthoracic and transesophageal echocardiography in suspected prosthetic valve dysfunction. *Am J Cardiol*. 2006 Jan 1;97(1): 94-100.
36. Pibarot P, Dumesnil JG, Jobin J, Cartier P, Honos G, Durand LG. Hemodynamic and physical performance during maximal exercise in patients with an aortic bioprosthetic valve: comparison of stentless versus stented bioprostheses. *J Am Coll Cardiol*. 1999 Nov 1;34(5):1609-1617.
37. Picano E, Pibarot P, Lancellotti P, Monin JL, Bonow RO. The emerging role of exercise testing and stress echocardiography in valvular heart disease. *J Am Coll Cardiol*. 2009 Dec 8;54(24):2251-2260.
38. Ferrans VJ, Tomita Y, Hilbert SL, Jones M, Roberts WC. Pathology of bioprosthetic cardiac valves. *Hum Pathol*. 1987;18:586-595.
39. Silver MD, Butany J. Mechanical heart valves: methods of examination, complications, and modes of failure. *Hum Pathol*. 1987;18:577-585.

40. Silver MD. Late complications of prosthetic heart valves. *Arch Pathol Lab Med.* 1978;102:281-284.
41. Silver MD. Pathology of prosthetic cardiac valves. *Am J Cardiovasc Pathol.* 1988;1:335-338.
42. Walley VM, Masters RG. Complications of cardiac valve surgery and their autopsy investigation. *Cardiovasc Pathol.* 1995;4(4):269-286.
43. Hammermeister KE, Sethi GK, Henderson WG, Oprian C, Kim T, Rahimtoola S. A comparison of outcomes in men 11 years after heart-valve replacement with a mechanical valve or bioprosthesis. Veterans Affairs Cooperative Study on Valvular Heart Disease. *N Engl J Med.* 1993 May 6;328(18): 1289-1296.
44. Starek PJK. Immobilization of disc heart valves by unraveled sutures. *Ann Thorac Surg.* 1981;31:66-69.
45. Puvimanasinghe JP, Steyerberg EW, Takkenberg JJ, et al. Prognosis after aortic valve replacement with a bioprosthesis: predictions based on meta-analysis and microsimulation. *Circulation.* 2001 Mar 20;103(11):1535-1541.
46. Vongpatanasin W, Hillis LD, Lange RA. Prosthetic heart valves. *N Engl J Med.* 1996 Aug 8;335(6):407-416.
47. Akiyama K, Sawatani O, Imamura E, Endo M, Hashimoto A, Koyanagi H. Stent creep of porcine bioprosthesis in the mitral position. *Ann Thorac Surg.* 1988;46:73-78.
48. Walley VM, Bedard P, Brais M, Keon WJ. Valve failure caused by cusp tears in low-profile Ionescu-Shiley bovine pericardial bioprosthetic valves. *J Thorac Cardiovasc Surg.* 1987;93:583-586.
49. Walley VM, Keon CA, Khalili M, Moher D, Campagna M, Keon WJ. Ionescu-Shiley valve failure I: experience with 125 standard-profile explants. *Ann Thorac Surg.* 1992;54:111-116.
50. Walley VM, Keon CA, Khalili M, Moher D, Campagna M, Keon WJ. Ionescu-Shiley valve failure II: experience with 25 low-profile explants. *Ann Thorac Surg.* 1992;54:117-122.

12 Infective Endocarditis and Related Conditions

Endocarditis, as a pathological entity, has been traditionally classified into infective endocarditis (IE), verrucous endocarditis, and nonbacterial thrombotic endocarditis (NBTE). Infective endocarditis can be subdivided into culture negative or culture positive endocarditis. NBTE has been associated with connective tissue diseases, chronic inflammatory processes, burns, and malignancy [1, 2]. Rheumatic verrucous endocarditis is observed in acute rheumatic fever, but seldom clinically recognized or diagnosed by imaging.

Infective endocarditis (IE) is an active intracardiac infection involving one or more heart valve surfaces. Other cardiac structures may become primarily or secondarily involved including myocardium, chordae, endocardium, and pericardium. The causal organism is usually bacterial, fungal, or Rickettsial. The clinical distinction between acute and subacute types has little current value, and it is preferable to think in terms of active and healed endocarditis. Practically, the anatomical location of the infection and the identity of the infective agent are probably the most important factors that determine the prognosis.

Predisposing Factors

Infective endocarditis may be increasing due to the increased aging population, nosocomial infections, use of cardiovascular prostheses, immunosuppression, and intravenous drug use (IVDU). The pathobiology depends upon both individual immune responses and virulence factors of the organism. Rheumatic valve disease was traditionally the most common valve lesion underlying IE. Today, three broad groups of individuals are affected: (a) younger individuals with rheumatic valve disease, congenital heart lesions and IVDU; (b) older individuals with degenerative cardiac lesions including mitral valve prolapse, age-related aortic stenosis, and mitral annular calcification (MAC); and (c) patients with prosthetic heart valves.

Endocarditis may arise on normal valves, or more commonly in patients with abnormal cardiac anatomy. The most common preexisting valvular lesions are left-sided including aortic stenosis (particularly congenitally bicuspid aortic valve), aortic insufficiency, and mitral insufficiency. Many hearts have congenital heart disease including ventricular septal defect, patent ductus arteriosus, coarctation, transposition of the great arteries, tricuspid and pulmonary atresia or stenosis, and tetralogy of Fallot. Hypertrophic cardiomyopathy and prosthetic grafts or valves may also predispose to IE.

For bacterial IE to occur there must be valvular thrombus, circulating bacteria, and bacterial growth on the valve. Hearts may develop valvular thrombus due to abnormal blood flow and valve or intracardiac anatomy. Invasive procedures may cause valvular thrombi (pacemakers, indwelling heart catheters, grafts, and other prostheses). Thrombus may develop due to jet lesions or on contact surfaces or other areas of mechanical trauma. Intravenous drug use (IVDU) may result in a repetitive bacterial challenge to the body. Bacteria may originate from a variety of sources including teeth, tonsils, bowel, genitourinary tract, bone, biliary tract, uterus, lung, and skin. In IVDU, skin and gastrointestinal organisms predominate.

The clinical diagnosis of IE may be challenging with combinations of fever, a new heart murmur, emboli (Osler nodes, Janeway lesions, Roth spots),

K.-L. Chan and J.P. Veinot, *Anatomic Basis of Echocardiographic Diagnosis*,
DOI: 10.1007/978-1-84996-387-9_12, © Springer-Verlag London Limited 2011

petechiae and subungual hemorrhages. Renal failure may be present due to infarct, abscess, pyelonephritis, and focal necrotizing, or diffuse proliferative glomerulonephritis. Congestive heart failure due to major coronary emboli with infarct, microemboli, myocarditis, or (most commonly) valvular destruction may also be prominent.

Diagnostic Approach

Detection of vegetations at surgery or necropsy has long been considered the definitive evidence of the disease. A noninvasive and reliable means to detect vegetation is essential to the early diagnosis of IE. Echocardiography has been used in the diagnosis of endocarditis for at least 3 decades and incorporated in the widely used Duke criteria for the diagnosis of IE (Table 12.1) [3]. The typical echo features of a vegetation is an echogenic mass distinct from the underlying cardiac structure, adherent to valves, endothelial surfaces or intracardiac prosthetic devices, and frequently associated with oscillatory motions (Fig. 12.1) [4]. It should be visible throughout the cardiac cycle and in multiple views. An abscess is a localized abnormal echo lucent area within the perivalvular tissue that does not communicate with the circulation, and it may have a nonhomogeneous echo appearance (Fig. 12.2) [4, 5]. Among the many technological advancements, the development of transesophageal echocardiography (TEE) has been the most important in this regard, as it can detect smaller vegetations as compared to transthoracic echocardiography (TTE). TEE has an axial resolution of 1 mm and can reliably detect vegetations 2–5 mm in size, whereas TTE detects only 25% of vegetation <5 mm and about 50% of vegetations between 5 and 10 mm [6, 7]. For the detection of vegetations, TEE has a sensitivity of 87–100% and a specificity of 91–100%. The sensitivity and specificity of TTE are 30–63% and 83–100%, respectively (Fig. 12.3) [6–11]. TEE also demonstrates superiority in the detection of perivalvular complications with a sensitivity of 78–100% and specificity of 92% in the diagnosis of perivalvular abscess, whereas TTE has a sensitivity of 28–86% and specificity of 85–90% for the same indication [12–19].

In patients suspected to have IE, many centers use TEE exclusively, as a missed diagnosis or even a delayed diagnosis can adversely affect patient outcome. Our approach as to when to use TEE instead of TTE is summarized in Fig. 12.4. The relative value of TEE versus TTE in the diagnosis of IE depends very much on the likelihood of the disease in a particular patient. We consider patients with positive blood culture fulfilling the Duke Major criterion to be at an intermediate to high likelihood for IE and those patients with only Duke minor criteria (one or several) to be at a low risk for IE. In patients with a low likelihood of the disease, TTE is generally adequate, while in patients with intermediate or high probability of the disease, a negative TEE may not be sufficient to exclude the disease, due to the lower sensitivity of the transthoracic approach. In the patients with a low clinical suspicion for endocarditis, if TTE shows no evidence of IE, alternate diagnosis should be considered and pursued. On the other hand a positive TTE in these patients should be interpreted with caution and put into the proper clinical context, as there are many echocardiographic conditions that mimic vegetations (Table 12.2). If a mimic of vegetation is suspected, TEE can be considered to

Table 12.1 The modified Duke criteria for the diagnosis of infective endocarditis[a]

Major criteria
Positive blood culture
• Two separate blood cultures positive for typical organisms without a primary source
• Persistently positive blood cultures
• Single culture or positive serology of Coxiella burnetti
Endocardial involvement
• New valvular regurgitation
• Typical echocardiographic evidence of vegetation, abscess or new prosthetic dehiscence
Minor criteria
Predisposing heart condition or intravenous drug use
Fever (>38°C)
Vascular phenomena
Immunologic phenomena
Microbiologic evidence (positive blood culture or serology) not meeting major criterion

[a]Definite endocarditis requires two major criteria or one major and three minor criteria or five minor criteria
Source: Adapted from Li et al. [3]

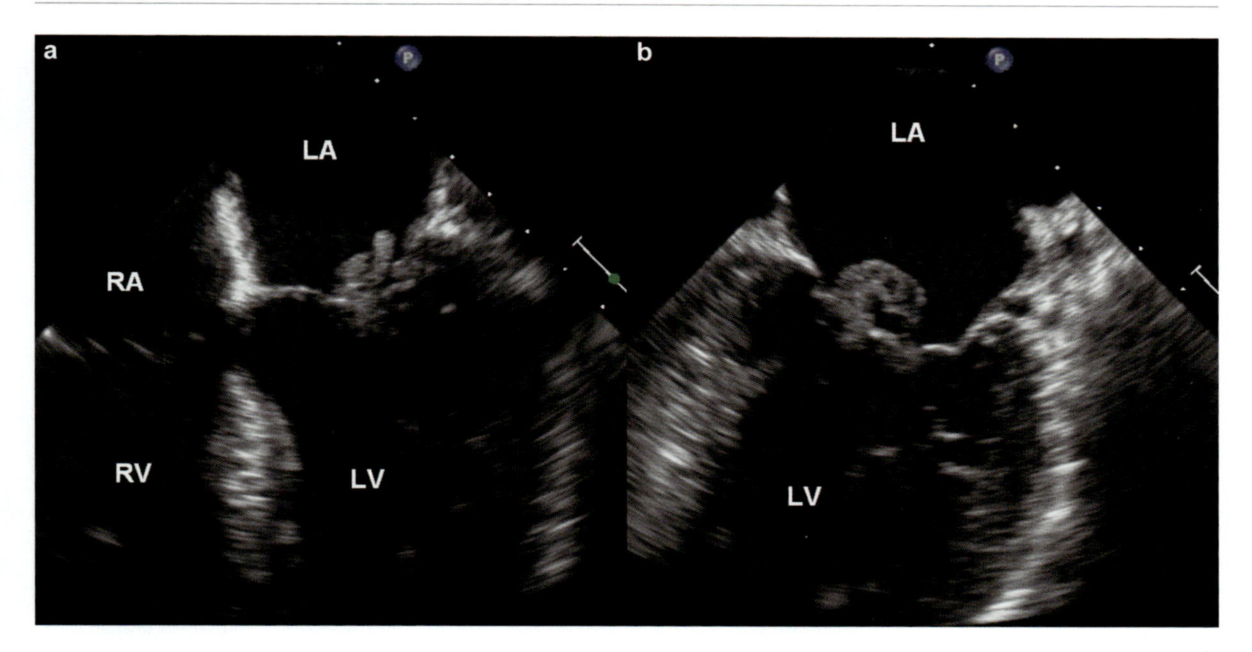

Fig. 12.1 Transesophageal transverse (**a**) and longitudinal (**b**) views demonstrate a multi-lobulated mass, typical of vegetation, on the mitral valve. *LA* left atrium, *LV* left ventricle, *RA* right atrium, *RV* right ventricle

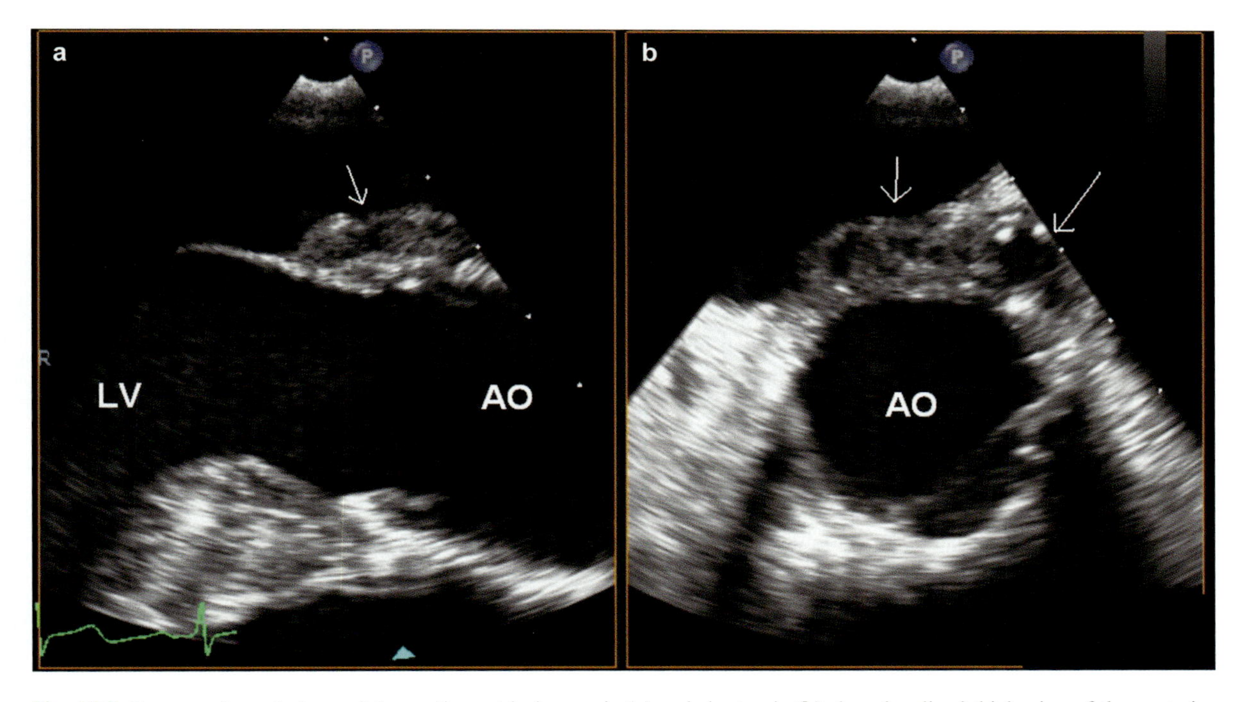

Fig. 12.2 Transesophageal views of the aortic root in long-axis (**a**) and short-axis (**b**) show localized thickening of the posterior aortic root up to 1 cm in thickness with a nonhomogenous appearance and localized area of echo-lucency (*arrows*) typical of a perivalvular abscess. *Ao* aorta, *LV* left ventricle

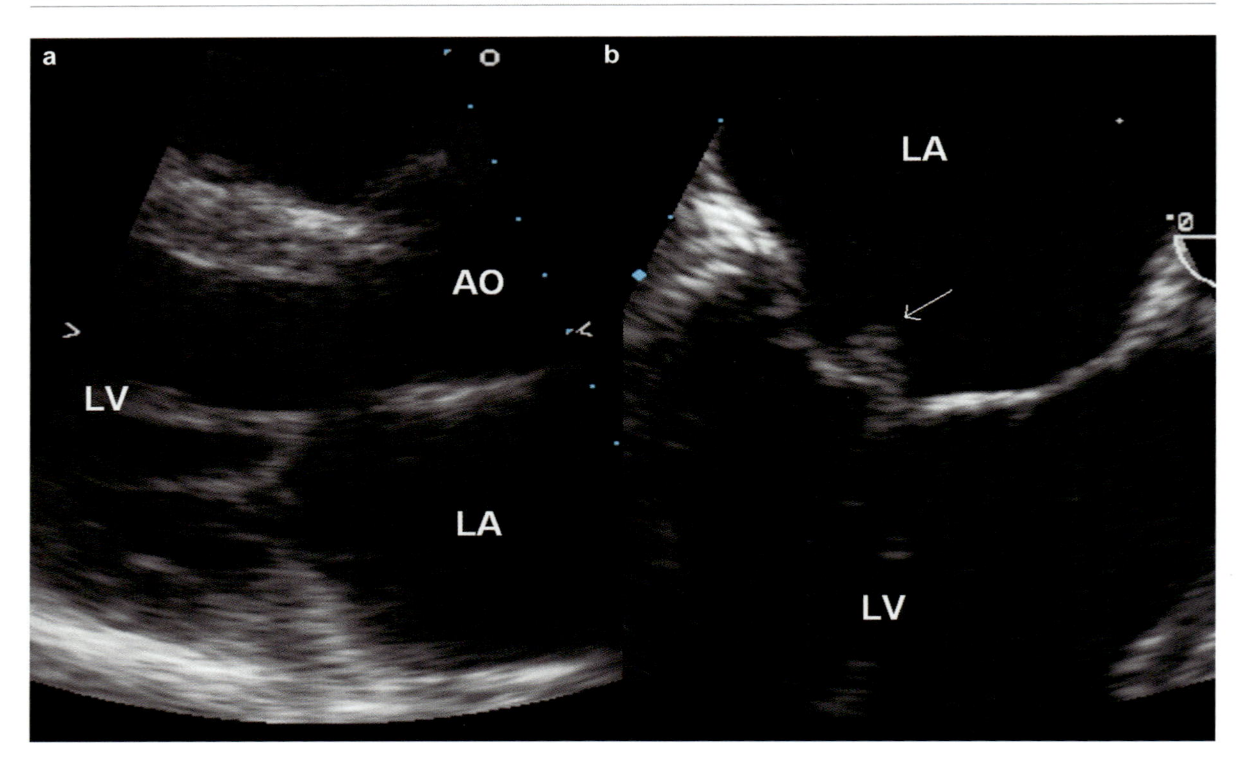

Fig. 12.3 In this patient with mitral valve infective endocarditis, the mitral vegetation is not detected by transthoracic echocardiogram illustrated by the parasternal long-axis view (**a**). The transesophageal view (**b**) shows the vegetation (*arrow*) on the atrial surface of the posterior mitral leaflet. This is not unusual since transesophageal echocardiography has a higher sensitivity in detecting vegetations as compared to transthoracic echocardiography. *Ao* aorta, *LA* left atrium, *LV* left ventricle

provide additional anatomic details useful in the differential diagnosis.

When the clinical suspicion of IE is intermediate or high, proceeding directly to TEE may be cost-effective due to the higher sensitivity of TEE in the detection of vegetation of abscess [20], provided TEE can be performed readily without delay and the echocardiographer is experienced and able to perform a goal-oriented TEE with a very low complication rate. TTE should be performed if there is any contraindication to or any significant delay in performing TEE. In uncooperative or confused patients, it is appropriate to perform TTE, but it is important to remember that a negative TTE does not necessarily rule out the diagnosis. For instance in a series of patients with Staphylococcal bacteremia, TEE detected vegetation in 19% of patients with negative TTE [21]. There should be a low threshold to perform TEE if the clinical suspicion persists despite a negative TTE.

In patients with high risk features such as those with prosthetic heart valves and those with Staphylococcal bacteremia, even a negative TEE may not exclude the diagnosis as patients may be at an early stage of IE before the vegetation becomes large enough to be detectable. A repeat study in 7–10 days should be considered to look for evolving evidence of endocarditis, which is a dynamic process [22]. Despite the high image quality provided by TEE, false-positive and false-negative studies can occur (Table 12.2). False negative studies are more likely if the quality of TEE is suboptimal or preexisting valvular abnormalities are present.

Complications

The complications of IE can be grouped into local, paravalvular, and systemic categories. Systemic

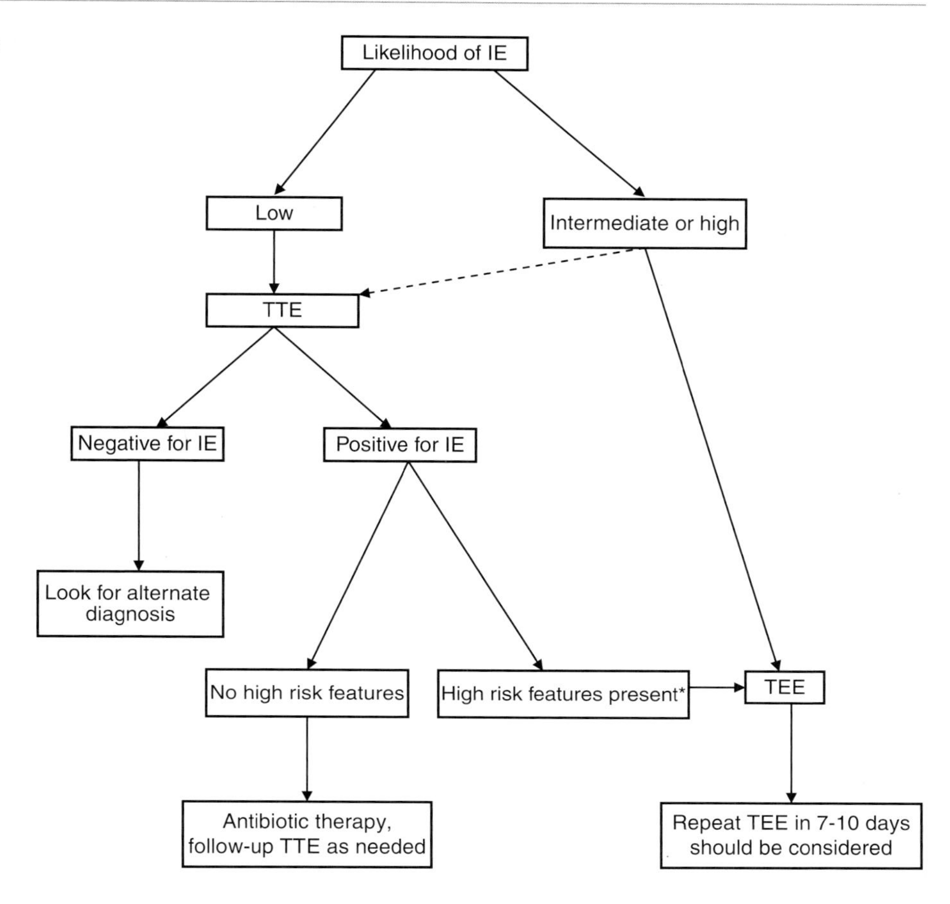

Fig. 12.4 Echocardiographic evaluation of patients with suspected infective endocarditis. *High risk features include prosthetic heart valves, virulent organisms such as Staphylococcus aureus, and probable perivalvular involvement

complications are common and should be looked for in all patients with IE (Table 12.3).

Local

Infective endocarditis may give rise to a variable array of valvular findings including infected thrombi (vegetations) and sequelae of valvular destruction. Hearts may be examined at pathology when there has been clinical suspicion of endocarditis, or an unexpected valvular lesion may be encountered. Regardless of the situation, before immersion in fixative, an attempt should be made to visualize the valves. If a suspicious lesion is encountered, sterile instruments should be used for the remainder of the examination and portions of the thrombus should be submitted for culture. Swabs are not recommended. Excised valves may be picked up fresh from the operating suite and portions of thrombus or mass are selected by pathology personnel for culture. Cultures should never be interpreted in isolation. Microscopy of the valve or thrombus to confirm the presence of infective microorganisms is essential. Clinical history and premortem or preoperative blood cultures should also be consulted.

Infected vegetations of variable size are detected along the lines of valve closure or at the low pressure end of jet lesions. Common sites include the atrial side of the mitral valve or the left atrial endocardium in cases of mitral insufficiency, the ventricular side of the aortic valve, the ventricular septum or the anterior mitral leaflet in aortic insufficiency, and on the right ventricular endocardium in the setting of membranous

Table 12.2 Conditions that can mimic a vegetation on echocardiography

Preexisting valvular abnormalities • Flail leaflet • Calcified nodules • Fibrin strands
Sequelae of prior valve surgery • Sutures • Annuloplasty ring • Peri-annular hematoma
Components of prosthetic valves • Sewing ring and stents • Prosthetic poppet
Normal structures • Lambl's excrescence • Ruptured fenestration
Thrombi
Tumor – myxoma and papillary fibroelastoma
Extrinsic mediastinal masses
Artifacts

Table 12.3 Systemic complications of infective endocarditis

• Sepsis • Immune complex related • Leucocytoclastic vasculitis • Glomerulonephritis • Osler node (painful nodules on pads of fingers and toes) • Roth spots (oval retinal lesions with pale centers and surrounding hemorrhages) • Arthritis • Right sided emboli – pulmonary emboli, abscess, empyema • Paradoxical embolus through patent foramen ovale • Left-sided emboli – systemic organ infarct (including cerebral and myocardial infarcts), organ ischemia, atrophy, infected/mycotic aneurysm, infective vasculitis

ventricular septal defect. Left-sided lesions are more common than right sided, except for cases related to interventional devices, catheters, or IVDU. Both right- and left-sided valve lesions may be found in IVDU [23, 24]. Vegetations are usually gray, pink, or brown and are often friable. They may be single or multiple and affect more than one valve. Infection may also involve the intima of a blood vessel distal to a coarctation or involve the pulmonary artery side of an infected patent ductus arteriosus.

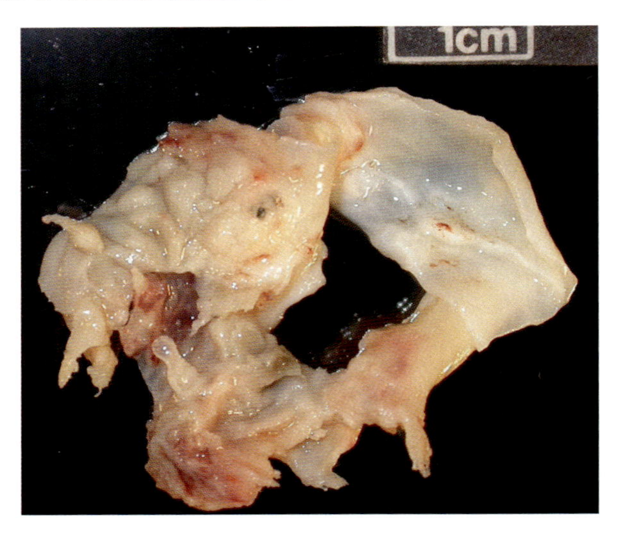

Fig. 12.5 Excised aortic valve with bacterial infective endocarditis. The valve originally had three cusps but only one is still identifiable. The others are destroyed by tan color infected thrombus vegetation. Valve destruction is a characteristic feature of infective endocarditis

Vegetations may be located anywhere on the valve cusp or leaflet or endocardial surface (Fig. 12.5). In fact this is an important distinguishing feature to note, as valve thrombi associated with nonbacterial thrombotic endocarditis (NBTE) and those verrucous thrombi related to rheumatic fever do not have this variability in location, and are usually only along the lines of valve closure. Libman Sacks – lupus anticoagulant lesions may be on both sides of the valve, but are still centered on the line of closure. Thrombi from NBTE, rheumatic fever, Libman Sacks are not associated with valve destruction.

Infected valves usually have destructive ulcers, defects, perforations, aneurysms, erosions, and chordal ruptures (Figs. 12.6–12.9, Table 12.4). The amount of thrombus and valve destruction may mask the underlying predisposing valve disease. With spread of the infection onto the chordae or papillary muscles, these structures may rupture. If an aneurysm sac tip ruptures, the valve may become severely regurgitant due to defects (Figs. 12.10, 12.11). Thrombi may obstruct the valvular orifice creating stenosis, although this is rare compared to insufficiency. Vegetations may cause valve dysfunction due to interference with efficient valve coaptation and closure. This is especially true of culture negative endocarditis with large vegetations including HACEK organisms (Hemophilus, Actinobacillus,

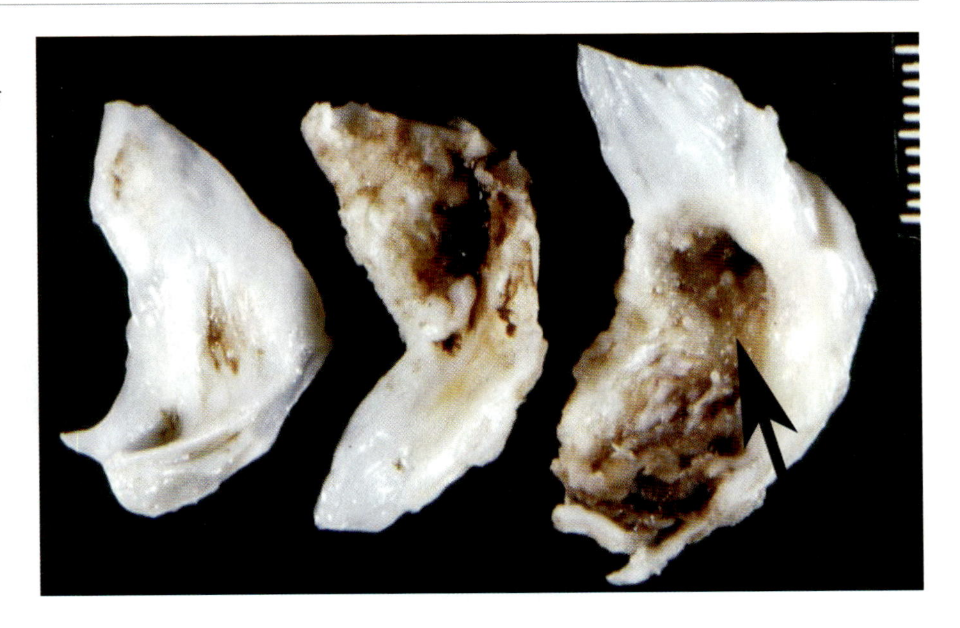

Fig. 12.6 Excised aortic valve with adherent dark infected thrombus. On one of the cusps, an aneurysm or outpouching is forming (*arrow*)

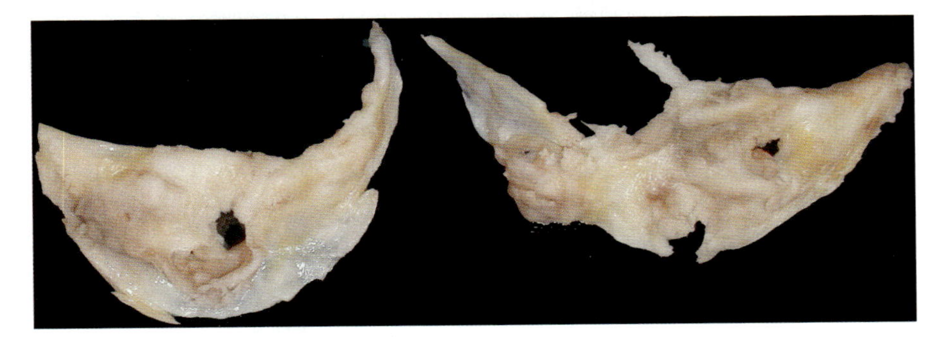

Fig. 12.7 Excised congenitally bicuspid aortic valve. There is abundant shaggy infected thrombus with valve holes from the infection

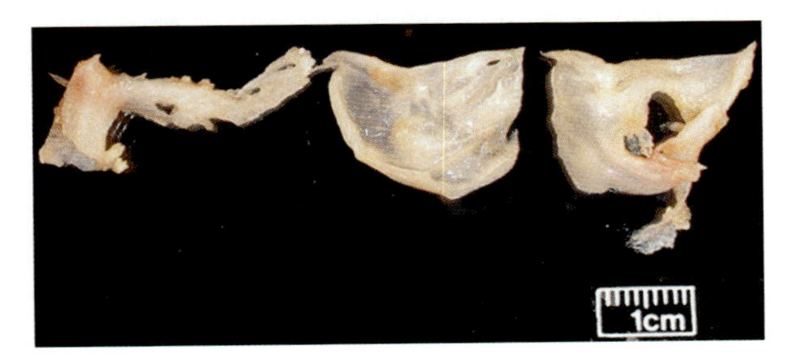

Fig. 12.8 Excised aortic valve with cusp destruction from infection

Cardiobacterium, Eikenella, and Kingella) and fungal endocarditis.

Extension of the infection to adjoining local structures is common (aortic valve to anterior mitral leaflet, posterior leaflet mitral valve to left atrial endocardium, and aortic valve to ascending aorta), including "kissing" lesions where adjacent valves touch. Fistulas from the aortic valve to the right and left atria and the right ventricle may occur. Extension into the myocardium and the conduction system may occur when the infection involves the valve ring or annulus. Jet lesions, as a result of valvular insufficiency, may cause endocardial lesions to form.

By microscopy, the appearance of the vegetation which is essentially an "infected thrombus" depends upon both the virulence and destructiveness of the organism, and upon the time at which the vegetation is examined. Early in the disease course, or with very virulent organisms, there is fibrin, acute inflammation, and clumps of organisms. With therapy the organisms may calcify, and the thrombi organize from the base. One may be left with an organizing thrombus, acute and chronic inflammation with neovascularization, and

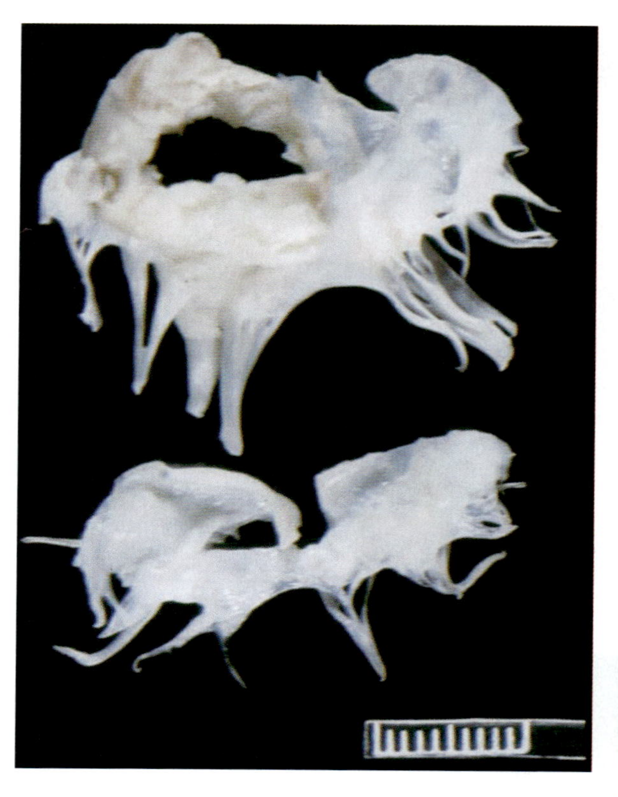

Fig. 12.9 Excised mitral valve with adherent thrombus. The infection has produced leaflet holes

Table 12.4 Pathology of valvular sequelae of infective endocarditis

Acute
- Vegetations – infected thrombi
- Valve ulcers or erosions
- Aneurysms
- Chord rupture
- Annular and ring abscess
- Endocardial jet lesions
- Flail leaflet or cusp

Chronic
- Perforations
- Calcified nodules
- Valve tissue defects
- Valve fibrosis

fibroblastic proliferation but no easily recognizable organisms. Giant cells may be seen and if prominent one should consider Coxiella, mycobacteria, or fungi. Foamy macrophages may suggest Whipple disease. Electron microscopy, immunofluorescence, polymerase chain reaction, or molecular techniques are contributory in the diagnosis [25–28].

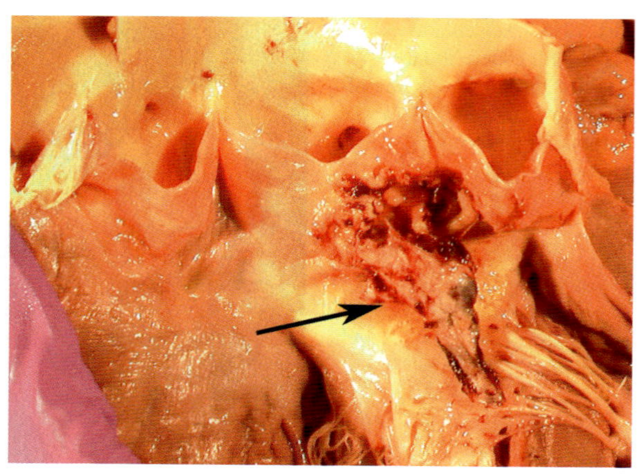

Fig. 12.10 Heart from autopsy of a patient who died of sepsis and heart failure. The aortic valve has a large diverticulum which has ruptured. At autopsy the defect had a long windsock of thrombus attached to it (*arrow*)

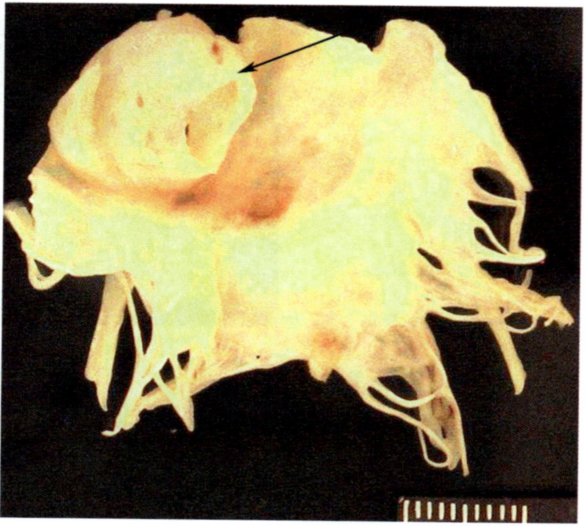

Fig. 12.11 Excised mitral valve. The infection produced an aneurysm which has ruptured and left a defect (*arrow*)

Special stains are useful to detect microorganisms. Treatment with antimicrobials alters the utility of these stains. Gram stain is useful to detect bacteria, but with therapy after a few weeks the organisms may not stain. Silver stains should always be performed, not only to detect fungi, but also to detect bacteria that have lost their Gram positive staining, yet still stain their cell walls with silver stain. Giemsa stain may be done to detect Rickettsia. Periodic acid-schiff (PAS) stain is useful to diagnose Whipple disease.

Correlation with culture results from preoperative or premortem blood cultures and from cultures at surgery is essential. Communication with the clinicians may save much frustration if the stains are negative and the organism is already known from cultures at another health care institution. In cases that are culture negative, the common culprit organisms include Eikenella, Brucella, Neisseria, fungi, Chlamydia, acid-fast bacilli or right-sided endocarditis where the lungs filter out the organisms. HACEK (Hemophilus, Actinobacillus, Cardiobacterium, Eikenella, Kingella) organisms may be particularly difficult to grow. Clinical history may also give clues to possible infective etiology as certain infections are associated with occupations, travel, exposures, or lifestyles. Serology may be informative for infections such as Bartonella, Brucella, or Q fever (Coxiella).

Commonly there are destructive sequelae with healed valve infection (Table 12.4). The infected vegetations organize forming calcific valve nodules. The valve may have defects at the edges or central defects with irregular perforations (Figs. 12.12, 12.13). Around the holes or perforation there may be nodules of organisms that eventually form fibrocalcific nodules. Staining for microbes is still useful even for what appear to be only calcific nodules.

The destruction of the valve tissue may lead to defects at the margins with resulting poor valve closure. Distinguishing a post-IE perforation from a congenital accessory orifice may be difficult. Atrioventricular valve congenital orifices should have surrounding chordae, while a post-IE perforation would not. Semilunar valve cusp fenestrations, an age-related finding, are also confused with perforations. Fenestrations are located laterally on the semilunar valve cusps near the commissures and are always above the line of valve closure. Chordae may be ruptured resulting in flail leaflets and valve regurgitation. The ruptured chords may knot and calcify along with the organizing infected thrombi. The valve leaflet itself may thicken and the chords may fuse. All these are significant contributors to chronic valve regurgitation.

Ventricular papillary muscles may rupture for multiple reasons with IE. The infection may extend from an adjacent chord and cause myocardial necrosis and rupture. A coronary arterial embolus may cause a myocardial infarct with papillary muscle rupture, similar to any acute myocardial infarct. Finally an embolus may lead to a papillary muscle myocardial abscess with local tissue destruction and muscle rupture.

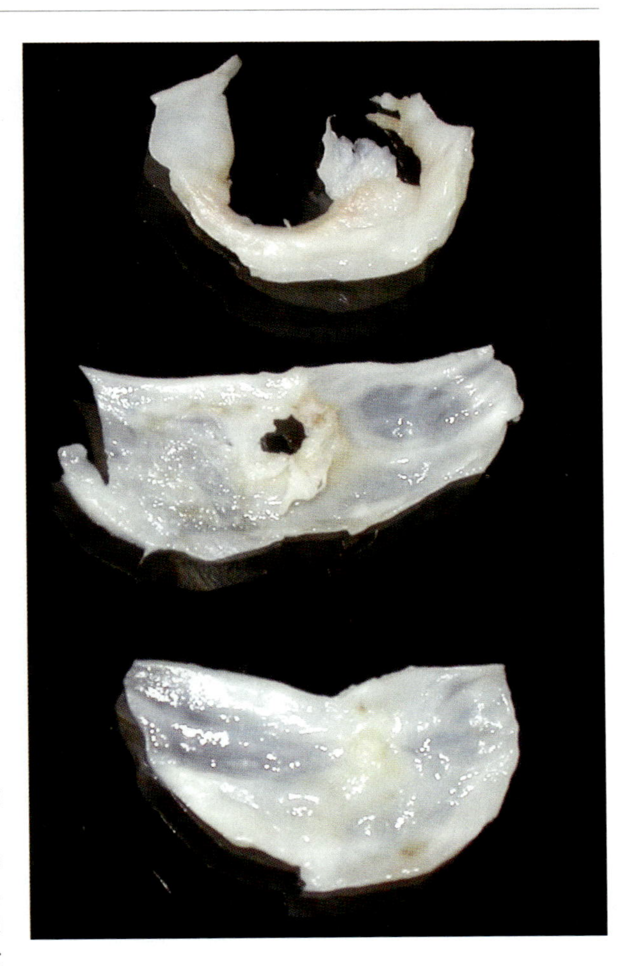

Fig. 12.12 Excised aortic valve. Prior infection is organizing leaving defects (*top* cusp) and a cusp hole (*middle* cusp) that cause valve regurgitation

Echocardiographic Correlates

An active vegetation is an echo lucent mass with an irregular shape. It is usually located at the upstream side and near the tips of the valvular leaflets. It can be sessile or pedunculated. When it is pedunculated, it demonstrates high frequency motion independent of the underlying cardiac structure (Figs. 12.1, 12.14, 12.15). Satellite vegetations should be looked for along the path of the entire "infected" flow jet, such as aortic regurgitation flow jet in the setting of aortic valve endocarditis. In these patients, satellite lesions can be present on the ventricular surface of the anterior mitral leaflet, the supporting valvular structure and even the left ventricular myocardium if the aortic regurgitant jet

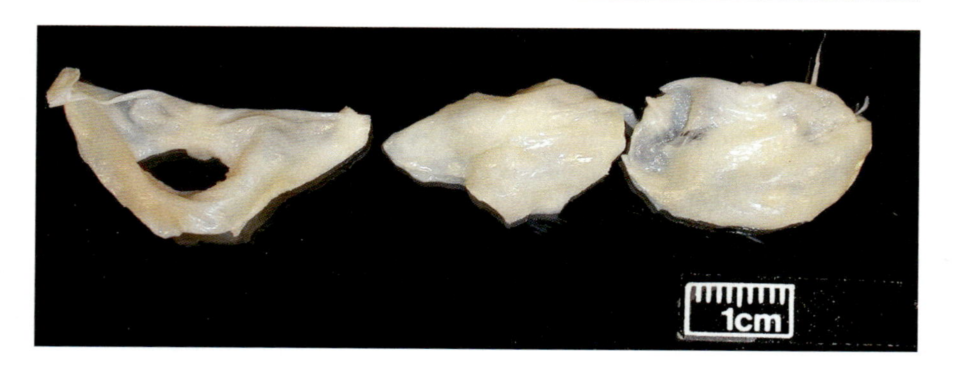

Fig. 12.13 Excised aortic valve. The infection has resulted in a large cusp hole

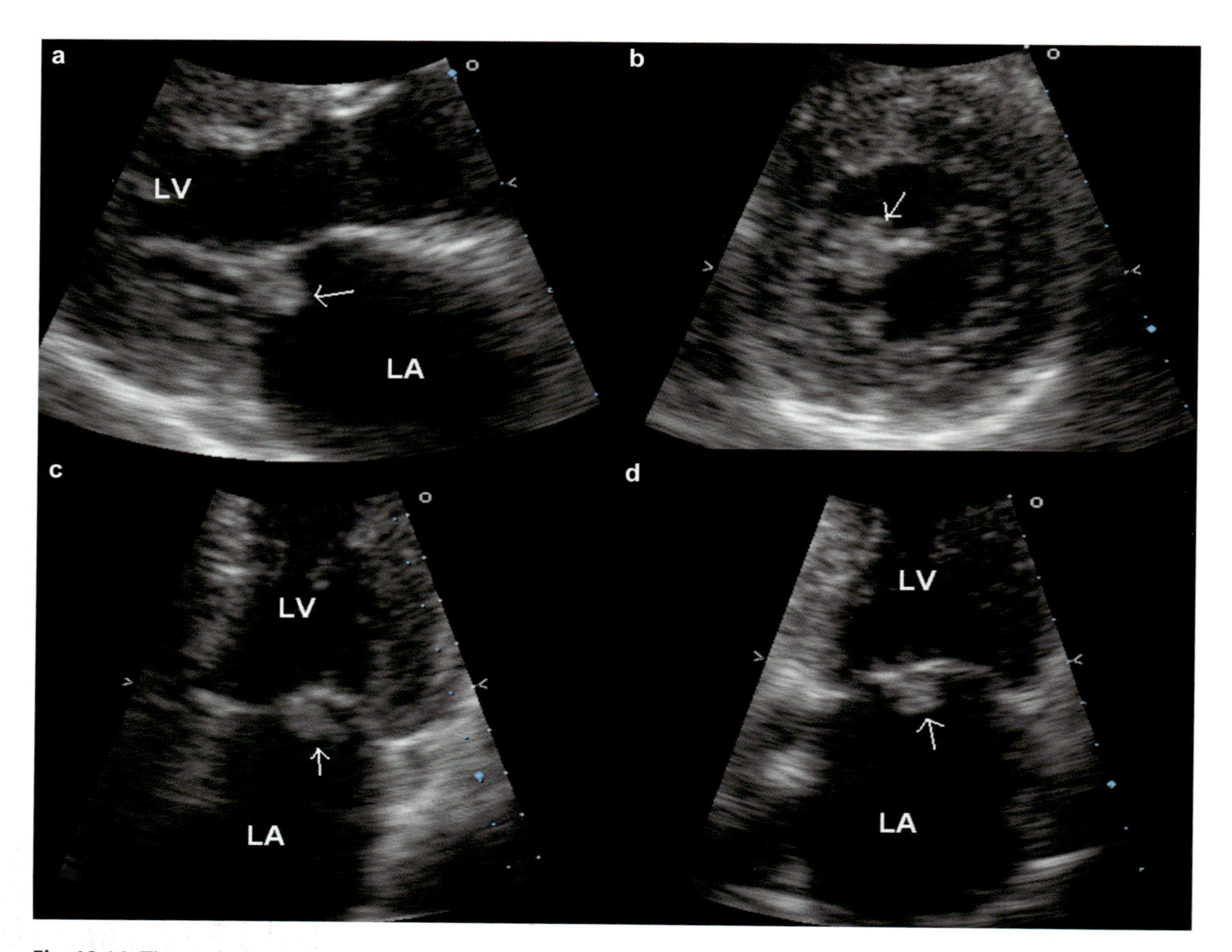

Fig. 12.14 The vegetation (*arrow*) on the medial scallop of the anterior mitral leaflet can be detected in the parasternal long-axis (**a**), short-axis (**b**), apical four-chamber (**c**) and apical two-chamber (**d**) views. *LA* left atrium, *LV* left ventricle

is directed posteriorly. On the other hand if the aortic regurgitant jet is directed anteriorly, satellite vegetation can occur on the myocardium of the anterior ventricular septum. In the setting of mitral valve endocarditis with mitral regurgitation, a satellite lesion can form on the left atrial wall along the path of the mitral regurgitant jet.

Vegetations undergo evolution with drug treatment. As a general rule, vegetations regress in size and become more echodense [29] (Figs. 12.16, 12.17).

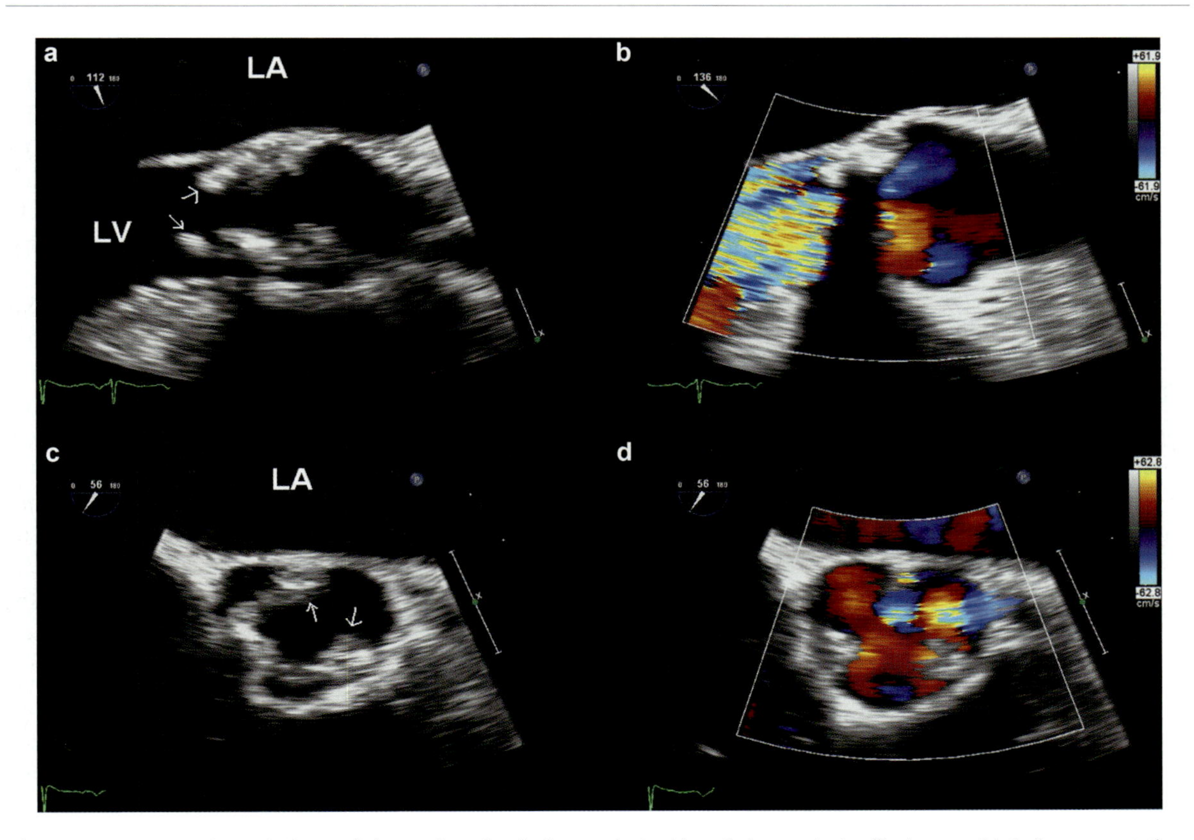

Fig. 12.15 Transesophageal views of the aortic valve in long-axis (**a**, **b**) and short-axis (**c**, **d**) show multiple large vegetations (*arrows*) on the aortic valve. The vegetations prolapse into the left ventricular outflow tract during diastole, associated with severe aortic regurgitation on color-flow imaging. *LA* left atrium, *LV* left ventricle

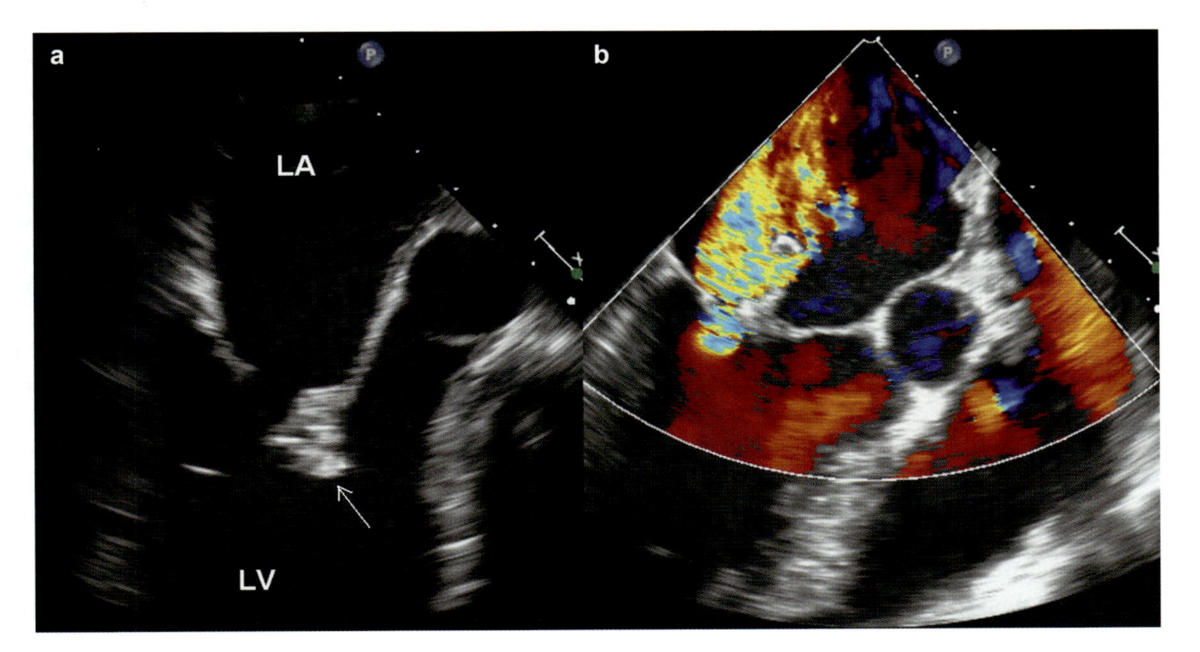

Fig. 12.16 Transesophageal views (**a**, **b**) of the mitral valve showing a large mass (*arrow*) on the anterior mitral leaflet, associated with severe mitral regurgitation. The mass appears to be echodense consistent with a healed vegetation. *LA* left atrium, *LV* left ventricle

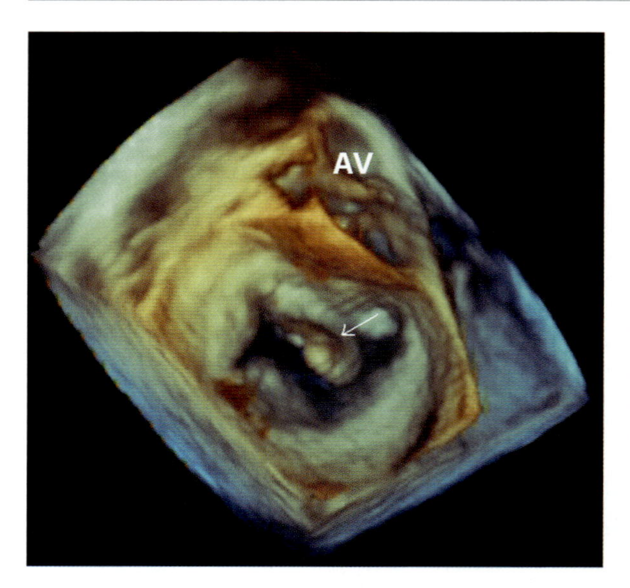

Fig. 12.17 Transesophageal 3D view of the mitral valve from the left atrial perspective in the same patient as in Fig. 12.16 shows the large healed vegetation (*arrow*) on the anterior mitral leaflet. *AV* aortic valve

Valvular dysfunction is the norm following endocarditis, and indeed less than 10% of affected valves will retain normal function despite successful medical treatment for IE [30]. If there is no significant valvular dysfunction, the mere persistence of vegetation does not appear to predict a poor prognosis.

There are multiple mechanisms for the development of valvular regurgitation in IE. In the acute stage, the proper coaptation of the leaflets may be interfered with by the presence of vegetation or by erosion of the leaflet as a result of the vegetative process. In the chronic setting, fibrosis and retraction of the leaflets are the most likely cause of valvular insufficiency. Vegetations may also erode the subvalvular chords leading to a flail leaflet.

The vegetative process can also lead to perforation if the vegetation is located away from the site of leaflet coaptation. Thus, perforation should be suspected if the regurgitant jet is located away from the site of leaflet coaptation (Fig. 12.18). The development of leaflet aneurysm or acquired diverticulum may be a prelude to perforation (Figs. 12.6, 12.10, 12.11). Indeed, IE is usually the cause of an acquired leaflet diverticulum or aneurysm, as a result of localized inflammation and destruction of the structural components of the valvular leaflet (Fig. 12.19). Not surprisingly concomitant perforation of the aneurysm is common [31]. Valve aneurysms without perforation can be a source of embolism. Elucidation of the mechanism of valvular insufficiency is useful to management since mitral valve repair may be very feasible in situations such as perforation in patients whose infection has been successfully treated by antibiotic therapy.

Several morphologic features of the vegetation have been examined in predicting the risks of embolic events. Many studies have shown that the size of the vegetation is the most consistent feature that relates to the risk of embolic events [32] (Fig. 12.20). However, vegetation size may be of limited clinical utility, since there is a considerable overlap in vegetation size between patients with and without embolic events [33]. Thus, clinical decision as to whether to proceed with surgical intervention to prevent embolism should not be based on echocardiographic findings alone.

Paravalvular Complications

Paravalvular lesions include leaks, fistulas, and abscesses (Table 12.5). Paravalvular leaks due to tissue destruction and paravalvular abscess may be seen with native valve IE (aortic more than mitral), but are especially common adjacent to infected valve prostheses [34] (Figs. 12.21–12.23). These leaks may cause clinically significant congestive heart failure and hemolysis. Extension of the valve infection into surrounding structures predicts a high mortality, a high risk of significant heart failure and the need for cardiac surgery [25]. Paravalvular lesions may be acute or become chronic. They are not static complications and may be progressive.

Extension of an active valve infection to adjacent intracardiac structures is common including infected lesions where adjacent valves touch or are contiguous, such as the aortic valve to the back of anterior mitral leaflet, the posterior leaflet mitral valve to the left atrial endocardium, and the aortic valve to the ascending aorta [35]. Jet lesions as a result of valvular insufficiency may cause infected endocardial lesions to form [23, 35].

Infections may extend from the mitral and aortic valves to the valve annuli [36]. This complication is considerably more common in the aortic position as

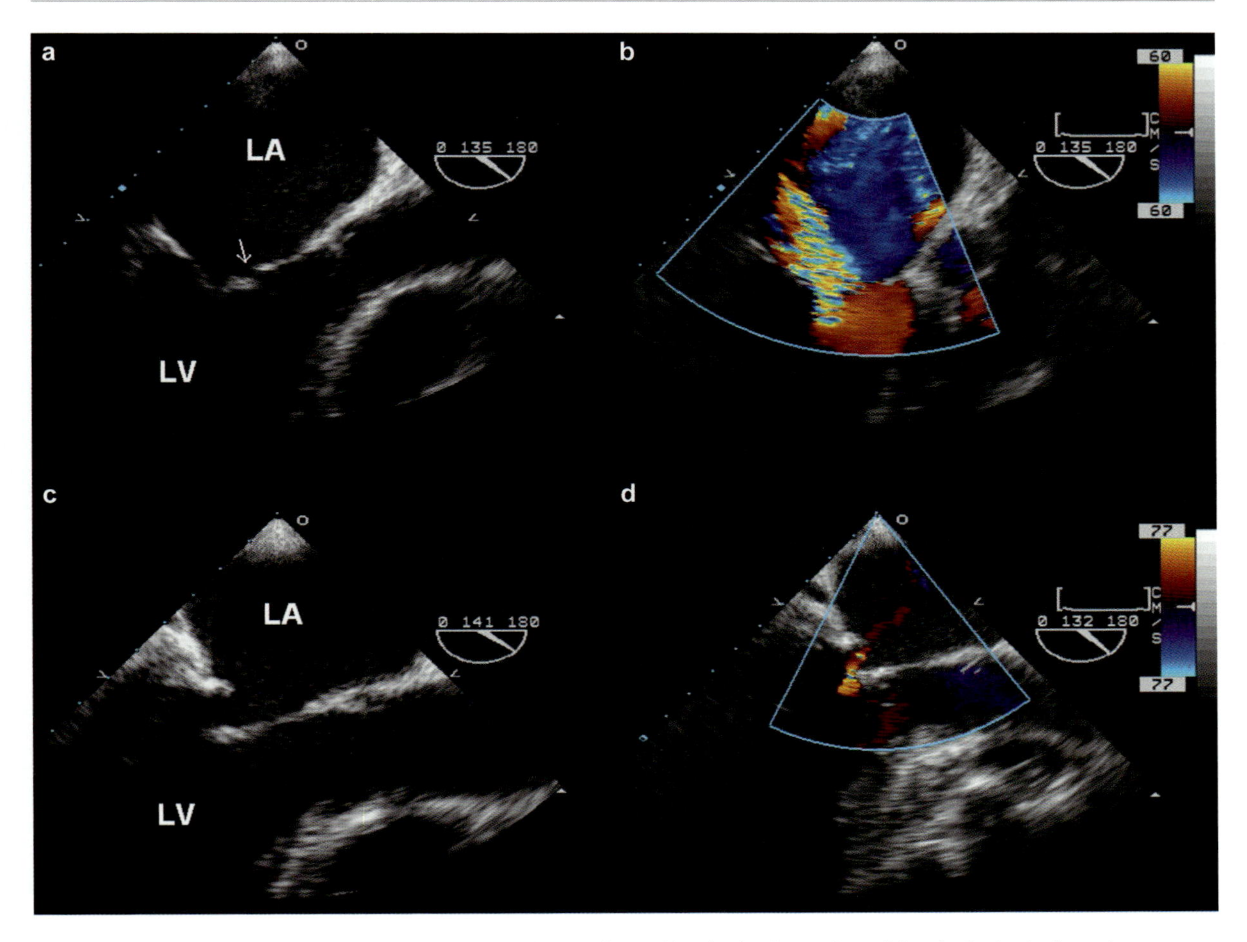

Fig. 12.18 Transesophageal views of the mitral valve in a patient with mitral valve endocarditis who had mitral repair surgery to correct mitral regurgitation. In the preoperative images (**a**, **b**) no vegetation was detected but there was a perforation (*arrow*) at the anterior mitral leaflet. Color-flow image (**b**) shows that there was mitral regurgitation from the coaptation site and from the perforation. Images post-surgery (**c**, **d**) show that the perforation has been successfully patched with only trivial residual mitral regurgitation (**d**). *LA* left atrium, *LV* left ventricle

compared to the mitral. This may manifest as an aortic root abscess, or the mitral annulus or mitral annular calcification (MAC) may become infected.

MAC may ulcerate giving rise to thrombus deposition with potential for embolization and infection. If infected, there is usually leaflet perforation and myocardial abscess [37]. If the infection spreads into the lateral atrioventricular groove the circumflex coronary artery may become distorted from local effects of the infection, and may become inflamed with an arteritis leading to thrombosis. Annular abscesses may also erode to the free pericardial surface producing fibrinous or suppurative pericarditis and hemopericardium.

Aortic root abscesses may be a source of embolic material and may compress structures around the aortic root. If the proximal coronary arteries are distorted, myocardial ischemic sequelae may result. The formation of a root or annular abscess is not an end event. Rather these structures are progressive with potential formation of perforations or fistulas.

Due to the central position of the aortic valve, infection of this valve may form fistulas with practically any cardiac chamber (Figs. 12.21–12.23, Table 12.6) [38]. Infection in the left aortic cusp or sinus may spread through the aortic wall and cause pericarditis or tamponade, or a fistula may extend into the left atrium. Infection of the posterior (noncoronary) aortic cusp or sinus may cause a fistula to either the left or right atrium. Infection of the right aortic cusp or sinus may cause a fistula to the right atrium, and the right

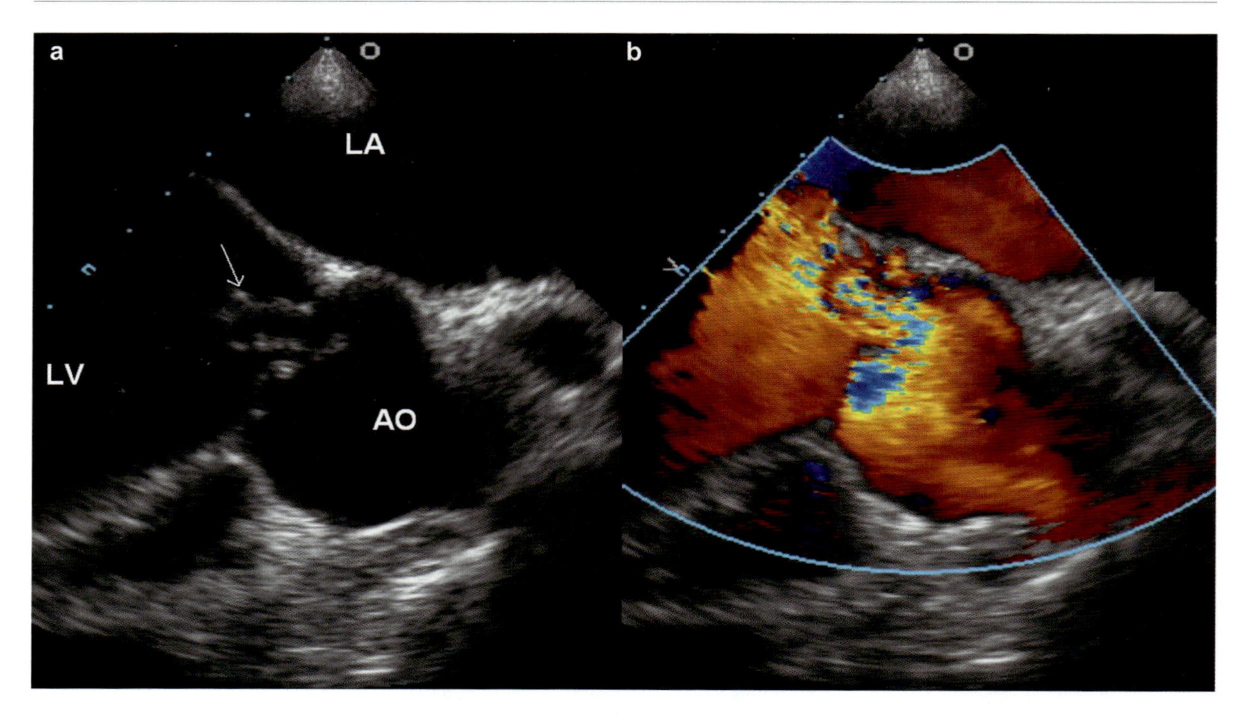

Fig. 12.19 In this patient with Staphylococcal endocarditis, the transesophageal view (**a**) shows a large tubular diverticulum (*arrow*) arising from the posterior aortic cusp. The tip of the diverticulum is perforated. Color-flow image (**b**) shows aortic regurgitation traversing the diverticulum into the left ventricle during diastole. Acquired valvular diverticulum is invariably due to endocarditis and is usually associated with perforation. *Ao* aorta, *LA* left atrium, *LV* left ventricle

Study	Vegetation Size ⩾10 mm n/N	Vegetation Size <10 mm n/N	Weight (%)	OR (fixed) 95% CI
Buda 1986	6/11	10/31	3.97	2.52 [0.62, 10.28]
De Castro 1997	16/31	9/26	7.90	2.01 [0.69, 5.89]
Deprele 2004	20/35	10/45	6.26	4.67 [1.77, 12.32]
Di Salvo 2001	40/67	26/111	13.16	4.84 [2.51, 9.34]
Erbel 1988	3/14	11/82	4.21	1.76 [0.42, 7.33]
Hwang 1993	7/31	2/10	3.91	1.17 [0.20, 6.80]
Jaffe 1990	8/32	2/18	3.20	2.67 [0.50, 14.22]
Lutas 1986	9/26	8/50	5.97	2.78 [0.92, 8.40]
Mangoni 2003	28/51	15/43	12.25	2.27 [0.99, 5.24]
Mugge 1989	22/47	11/58	8.74	3.76 [1.57, 8.99]
Sanfilippo 1991	28/58	26/90	17.59	2.30 [1.15, 4.57]
Stafford 1985	21/41	2/21	2.15	9.98 [2.05, 48.45]
Stewart 1980	14/47	4/40	5.06	3.82 [1.14, 12.77]
Wann 1979	4/7	3/14	1.43	4.89 [0.68, 34.96]
Wong 1983	3/16	3/15	4.20	0.92 [0.16, 5.49]
Total (95% CI)	514	654	100.00	3.09 [2.35, 4.05]

Total events: 229 (large >/=10 mm), 142 (small < 10 mm)
Test for heterogeneity: Chi² = 10.65, df = 14 (P = 0.71), I² = 0%
Test for overall effect: Z = 8.16 (P < 0.00001)

OR 95% CI: 0.1 0.2 0.5 1 2 5 10
<10 mm less risk ⩾10 mm more risk

Fig. 12.20 Pooled analysis of the association of vegetation size and the risk of systemic embolism. *CI* confidence interval, *OR* odds ratio (Reproduced from Salehian and Chan (32). With permission)

Table 12.5 Pathology of paravalvular sequelae of infective endocarditis

- Paravalvular leaks
- Prosthesis dehiscence
- Annular and root abscess
- Fistula or sinus formation
- Pseudoaneurysm
- Conduction system destruction
- Myocardial abscess
- Pericarditis
- Hemopericardium
- Coronary artery compression
- Coronary artery erosion, thrombosis, or rupture
- Spread to the chords or papillary muscle with rupture – important to remember the fibrous continuity of the aortic and mitral valves

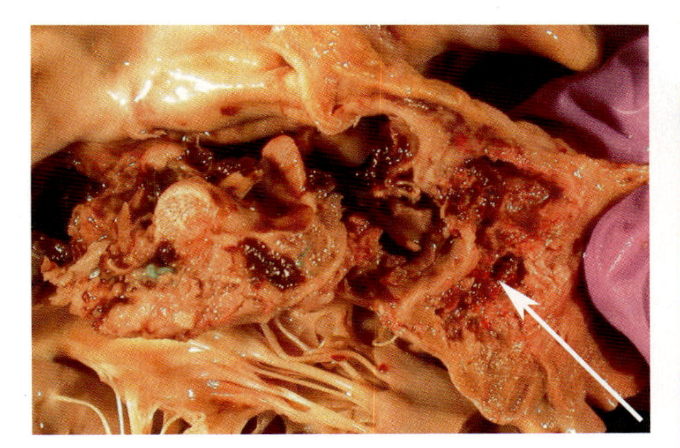

Fig. 12.21 Aortic root abscess around an infected valve prosthesis. When the aorta was opened the valves detached from the underlying tissues. The adjacent abscess contains inflamed thrombus (*arrow*)

ventricle/right ventricular outflow tract. An aorto-right ventricular fistula is possible due to the presence of the atrioventricular component of the interventricular septum. Extension into the underlying myocardium and the conduction system may be found when the infection involves the valve ring or annulus.

IE may involve the coronary arteries due to distortion from an aortic root abscess or they may become directly infected by local extension through the coronary ostia or by formation of mycotic/infected aneurysms. Mycotic aneurysms may occur in normal arteries but also there may be infection of an underlying atherosclerotic plaque. Mycotic aneurysms may

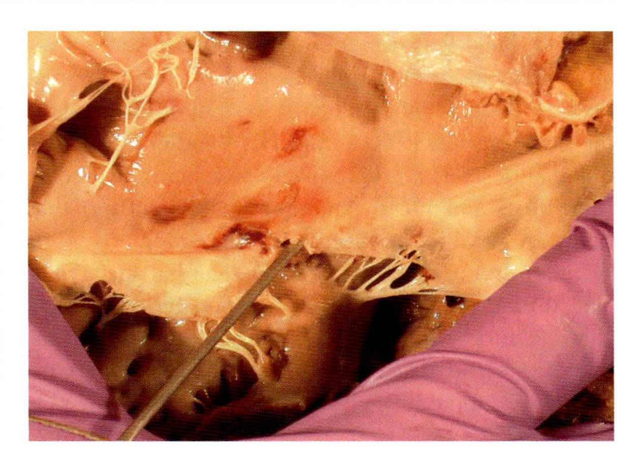

Fig. 12.22 Same patient as Fig. 12.21. Aortic root abscess has produced a fistula between the aortic root and the right atrium. The probe is passed just above the septal anterior commissure of the tricuspid valve

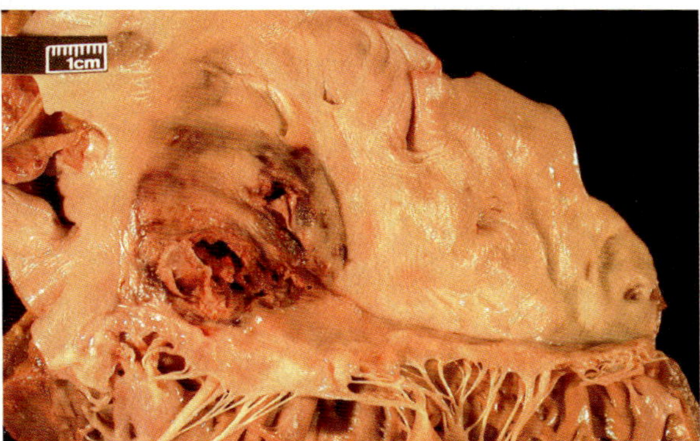

Fig. 12.23 Same patient as Fig. 12.21. The aortic root abscess has produced a fistula between the root and the left atrium. The opened left atrium with an irregular defect is seen

Table 12.6 Aortic root fistulae

- Right cusp infections may connect with the right atrium and ventricle and also with the epicardium causing tamponade
- Left cusp infections may connect to the left atrium and to the epicardium with tamponade
- Noncoronary (posterior) cusp infection may connect to both the right and left atria

thrombose and infected thrombi may seed the myocardium leading to myocardial abscesses.

Myocardial abscesses may be embolic or form as a result of local extension of the valvular infective process into the adjacent myocardium. Aortic root abscesses and myocardial abscesses may impinge upon or destroy the conduction system in the areas of the atrioventricular node and His bundle. Clinically, this manifests as a progressively worsening degree of heart block and may be an important clinical sign that treatment is failing or disease is progressing.

Extension of infection to the pericardial space may lead to hemopericardium and tamponade or to pericarditis. Fibrinous pericarditis is a common finding with IE, but the pericardium may also become infected leading to suppurative pericarditis.

Echocardiographic Correlates

On echocardiography, a perivalvular abscess can be identified by the detection of a localized abnormal thickening of the perivalvular tissue [5] (Fig. 12.24). This condition is far more common with aortic valve endocarditis than with mitral valvular endocarditis. Abscess formation is a dynamic process so patients with suspected or known perivalvular abscess should be closely followed by echocardiography (Figs. 12.24, 12.25). These patients have a worse prognosis compared to patients without abscess formation. Although

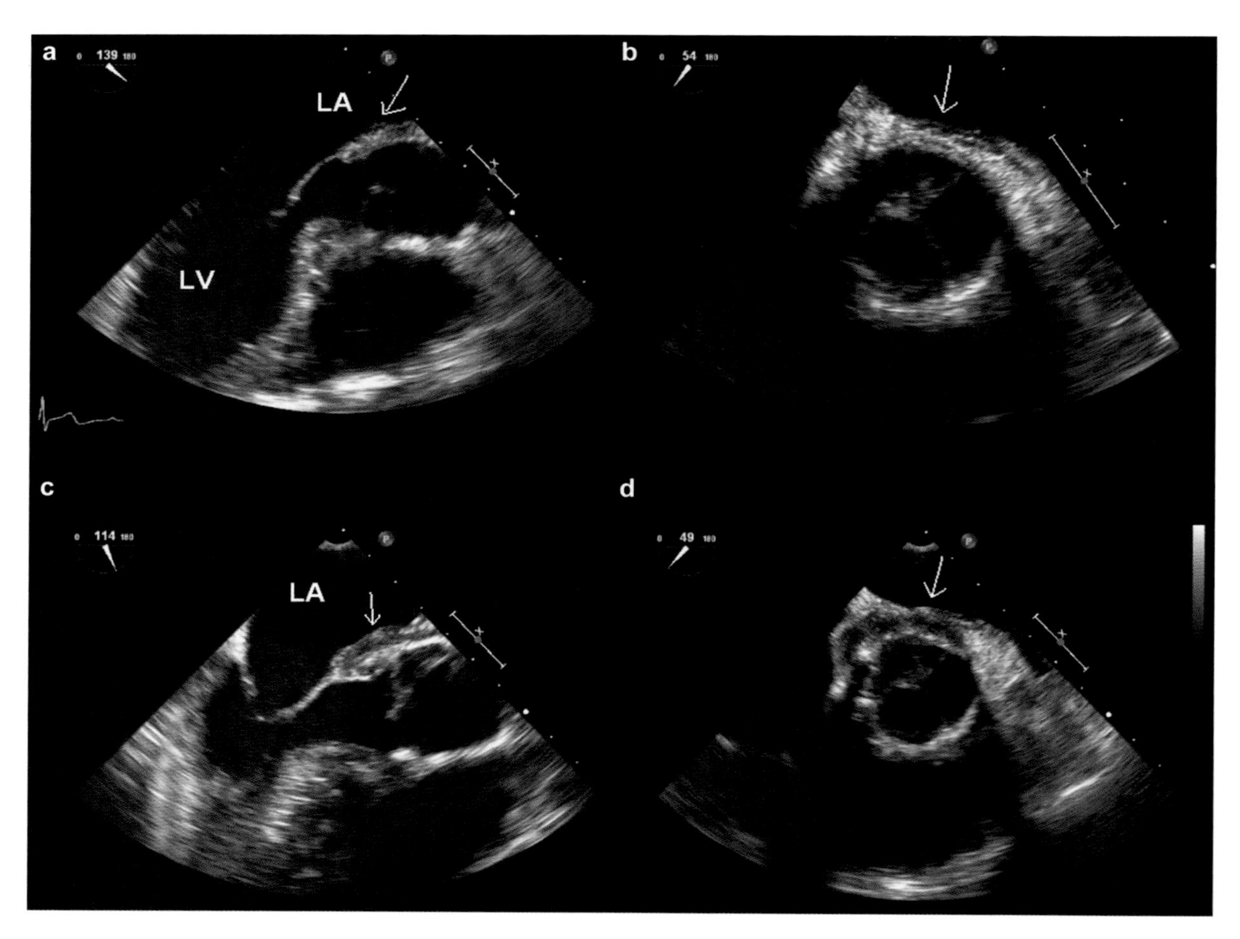

Fig. 12.24 Transesophageal echocardiograms in a patient with Staphylococcal endocarditis. The first study (**a**, **b**) show mild thickening (*arrow*) of the posterior aortic root. The second study (**c**, **d**) 1 week later shows an increase in the thickness of the posterior aortic root (*arrows*). There are areas of echo-lucency within the thickening best seen in the short-axis view (**d**). These evolutional changes confirm that there was a posterior aortic root abscess. *LA* left atrium, *LV* left ventricle

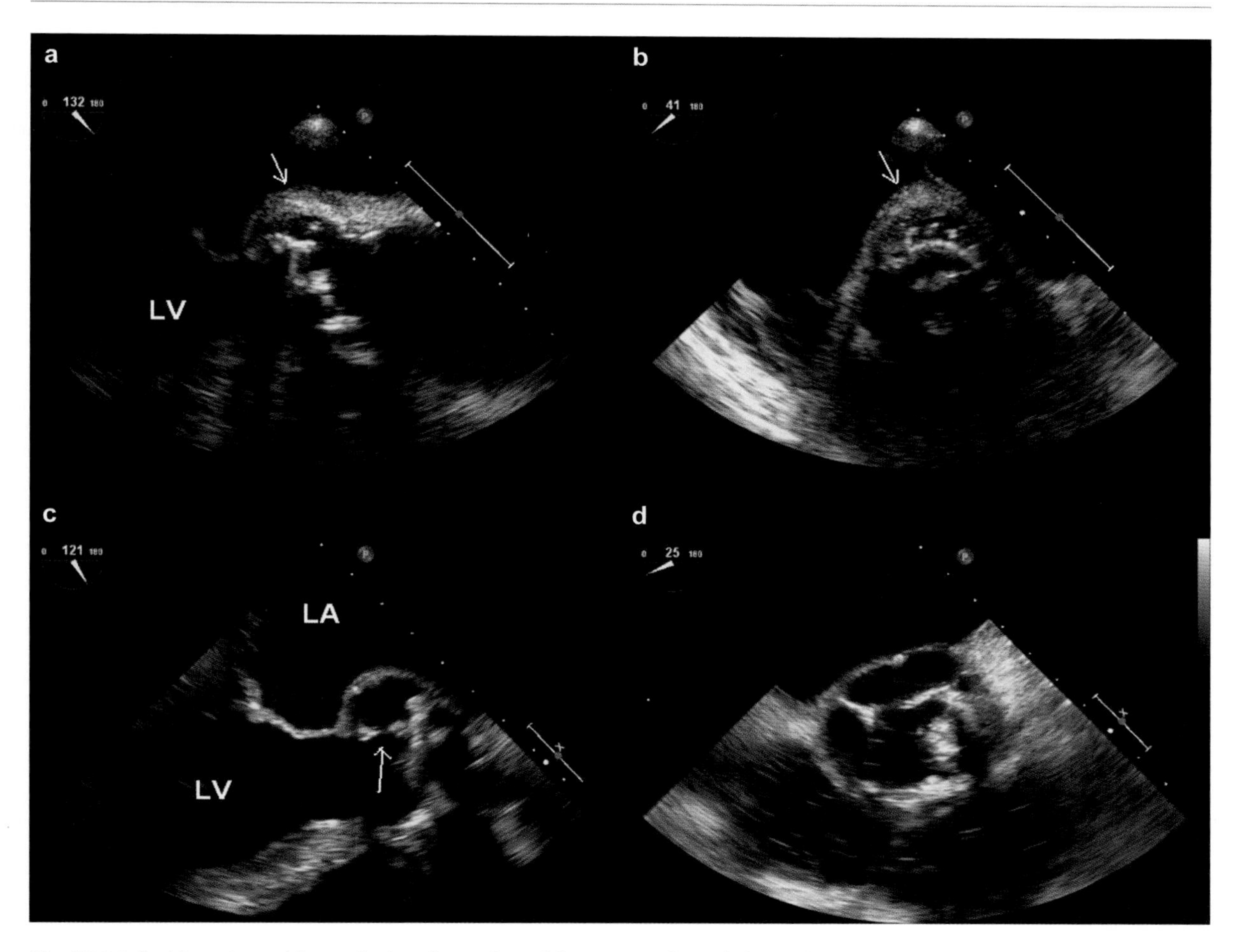

Fig. 12.25 In this patient with prosthetic valve endocarditis, transesophageal views of the aorta in long-axis (**a**) and short-axis (**b**) show increased thickness of the posterior aortic root consistent with abscess. The patient was treated medically due to his comorbidities. Repeat transesophageal echocardiogram (**c**, **d**) was performed 2 months later, showing that the abscess had drained and there was a pseudoaneurysm at the posterior aortic root with a communication (*arrow*) with the left ventricular outflow tract. These changes illustrate the progression of paravalvular abscess and the perivalvular complications in this setting

surgical intervention is frequently performed in these patients, some patients may respond to medical treatment alone [5].

Echocardiography has provided new insight regarding the evolution of perivalvular abscess. This information is mainly derived from echocardiographic follow-up studies in patients with perivalvular abscess who were considered to be too high-risk for surgical intervention and received medical treatment only [5]. A part of the abnormal thickening, usually the central portion, becomes more echo lucent followed by cavitation and communication with an adjacent cardiac chamber. In periaortic abscess, the communication is usually with the aortic root or the left ventricular outflow tract. The area of lucency increases in size and the abscess wall becomes more defined and echodense (Fig. 12.25). The end result is a localized bulge at the aortic root which expands in diastole, if it communicates with the aortic root, and expands in systole if it communicates with the left ventricular outflow tract (Fig. 12.26). The evolution of the perivalvular abscess can result in the communication between two adjacent cardiac chambers leading to the formation of a fistula (Figs. 12.27, 12.28). The location of the periaortic abscess predicts the path of the fistula, as

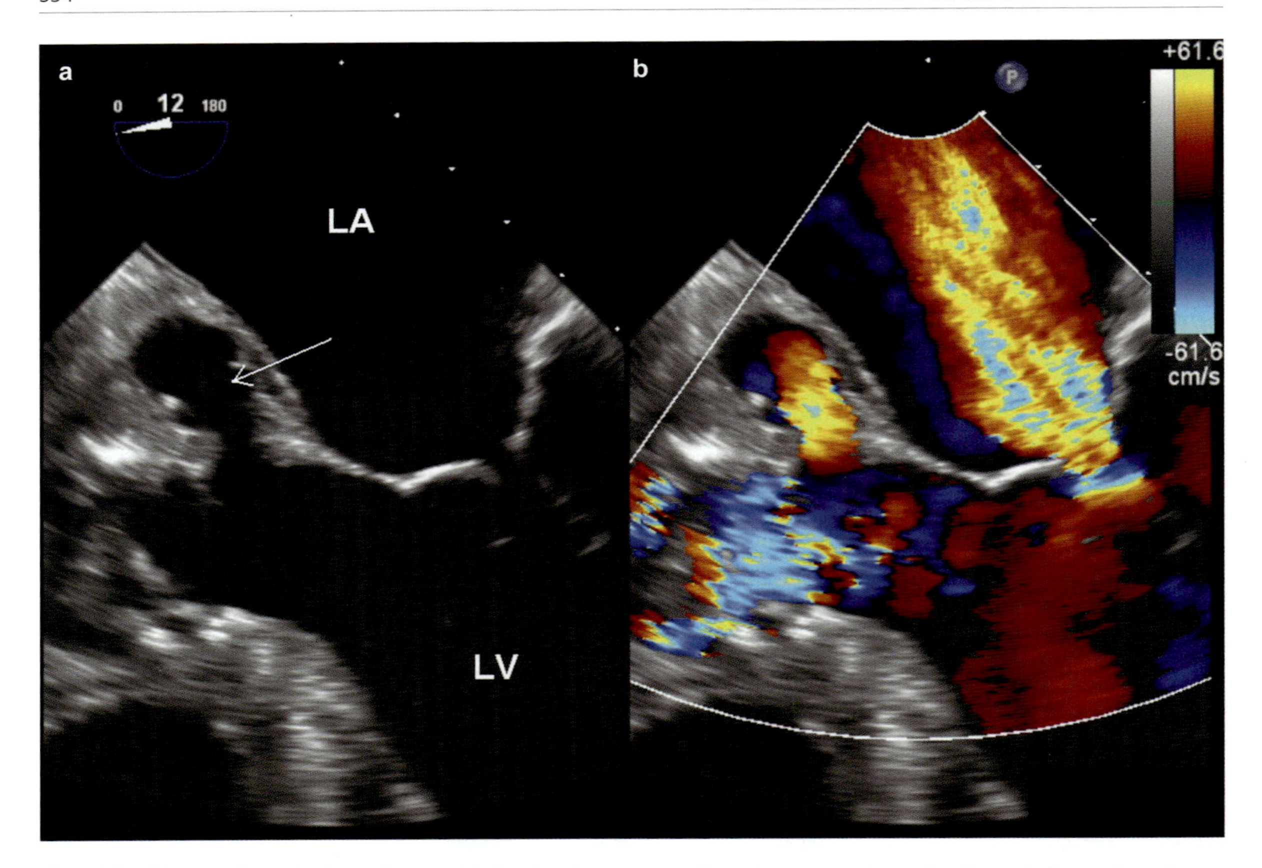

Fig. 12.26 Transesophageal echocardiogram (**a**) showing the presence of pseudoaneurysm (*arrow*) at the posterior aortic root communicating with left ventricular outflow tract. The color-flow image (**b**) shows low velocity flow from the left ventricular outflow tract into the pseudoaneurysm. Severe mitral regurgitation is also present. *LA* left atrium, *LV* left ventricle

discussed above. Concomitant valvular destruction is very common in these patients and thus careful assessment of the color-flow images often utilizing frame-to-frame analysis is important to distinguish flow jets due to valvular regurgitation from other abnormal flow jets due to perivalvular regurgitation and fistula formation (Figs. 12.28, 12.29).

Right-Sided Endocarditis

Right-sided endocarditis usually occurs in patients with IVDU or in patients with indwelling catheters or pacemaker leads. However, IVDU patients frequently have left-sided IE which is important to recognize due to its worse prognosis as compared to right-sided IE (Fig. 12.30). The in-hospital mortality of right-sided IE is <5% compared to 10–20% in left-sided IE [33, 39]. Levine et al. reported left-sided involvement in 57% of IVDU patients [40], although the tricuspid valve was also involved in many of these patients. Overall the tricuspid valve is the most common valve to be affected in IVDU patients who are generally younger and have a lower incidence of underlying heart disease as compared to patients with left-sided IE. The incidence of IE in IVDU patients is about 1–5% per year and they account for about 5–20% of the IE cases in most centers [39]. *Staphylococcus aureus* is the most common etiologic agent, accounting for about two thirds of the cases. Fungal endocarditis is also common.

There is concern regarding valve replacement in IVDU patients due to the risk of future IE. The event-free survival following valve replacement in these

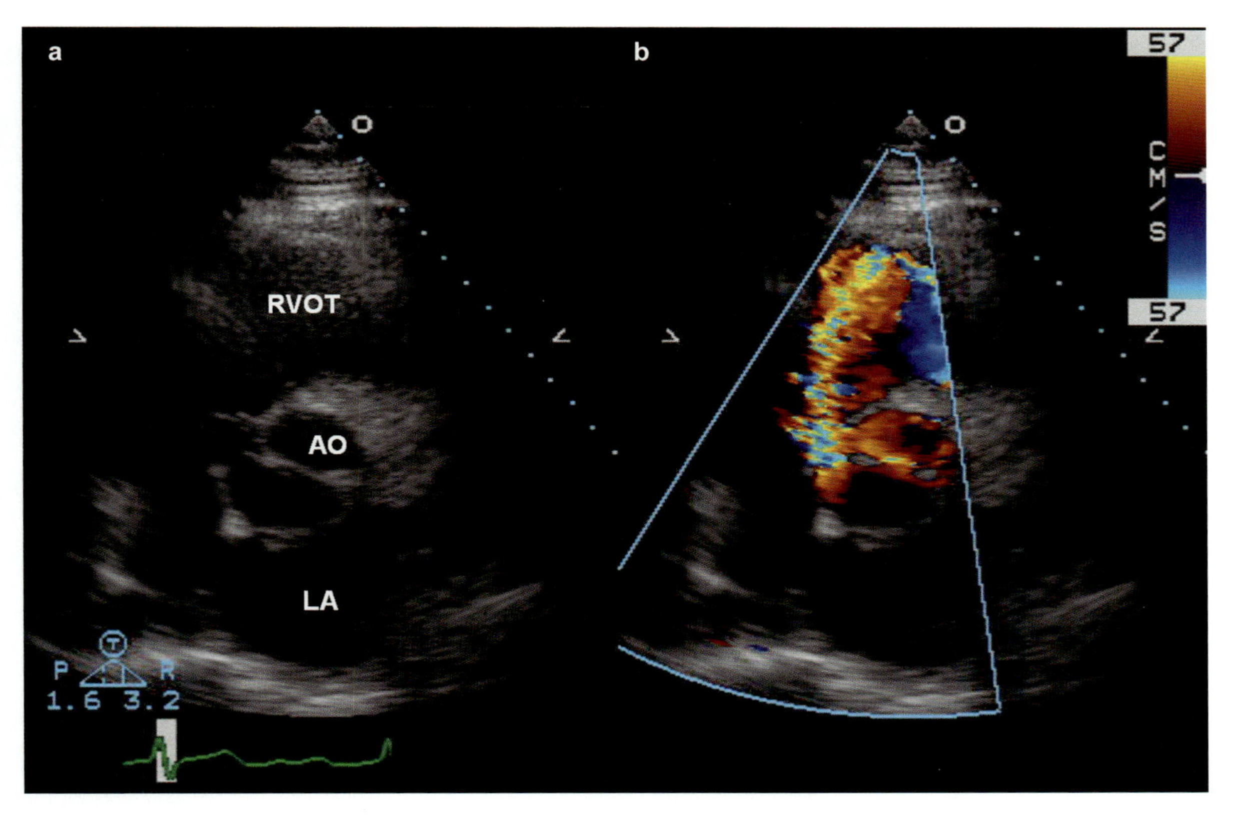

Fig. 12.27 The parasternal short-axis (**a**) shows the presence of a fistula at the posterior aortic root in a patient with endocarditis. Color-flow image (**b**) shows flow into the right ventricle during systole confirming that the fistula is communicating between the left ventricular outflow tract and the right ventricle. *Ao* aorta, *LA* left atrium, *RVOT* right ventricular outflow tract

patients has been reported to be 0.65 at 36 months and 0.52 at 60 months [41]. These are discouraging numbers but need to be balanced with the likely 100% mortality without surgery. The main indications for valve replacement in IVDU patients are similar to patients with left-sided IE. They are refractory heart failure (in this case right-sided failure), persistent sepsis despite antibiotic therapy and recurrent embolization [41]. Patients with tricuspid valve vegetation >2 cm and with a dilated right heart may also benefit from valve surgery [42].

Right-sided IE can be readily diagnosed by TTE, since tricuspid valve vegetations tend to be large (>1 cm) and are readily detected [43] (Fig. 12.31). Pulmonary valve cusp vegetations can also be readily detected by TTE, although the number of reported cases in small [44] (Fig. 12.32). In general, TEE is not required for the detection of vegetation to make the diagnosis, but TEE can provide important information when intracardiac complications are suspected [43].

Prosthetic Valve Endocarditis

Valve prostheses may become infected early after surgery or infected after hospital discharge [45–48]. Prosthetic IE can be divided into early (less than 1 year) and late (greater than 1 year) time periods with differing causes and organisms. Early endocarditis is usually due to infection at the time of surgery, re-occurrence of residual infection, if the indication for valve replacement was endocarditis to start with, or new infection due to the invasive treatment including catheters and indwelling lines. Early organisms are often fungi or skin flora, most commonly Staphylococci. Late prosthetic endocarditis is usually similar in pathoetiology and microbiology to community-acquired native valve endocarditis, with Streptococci being common. Coagulase-negative Staphylococci can be the etiologic agent for both early and late prosthetic IE due to their high affinity to prosthetic material.

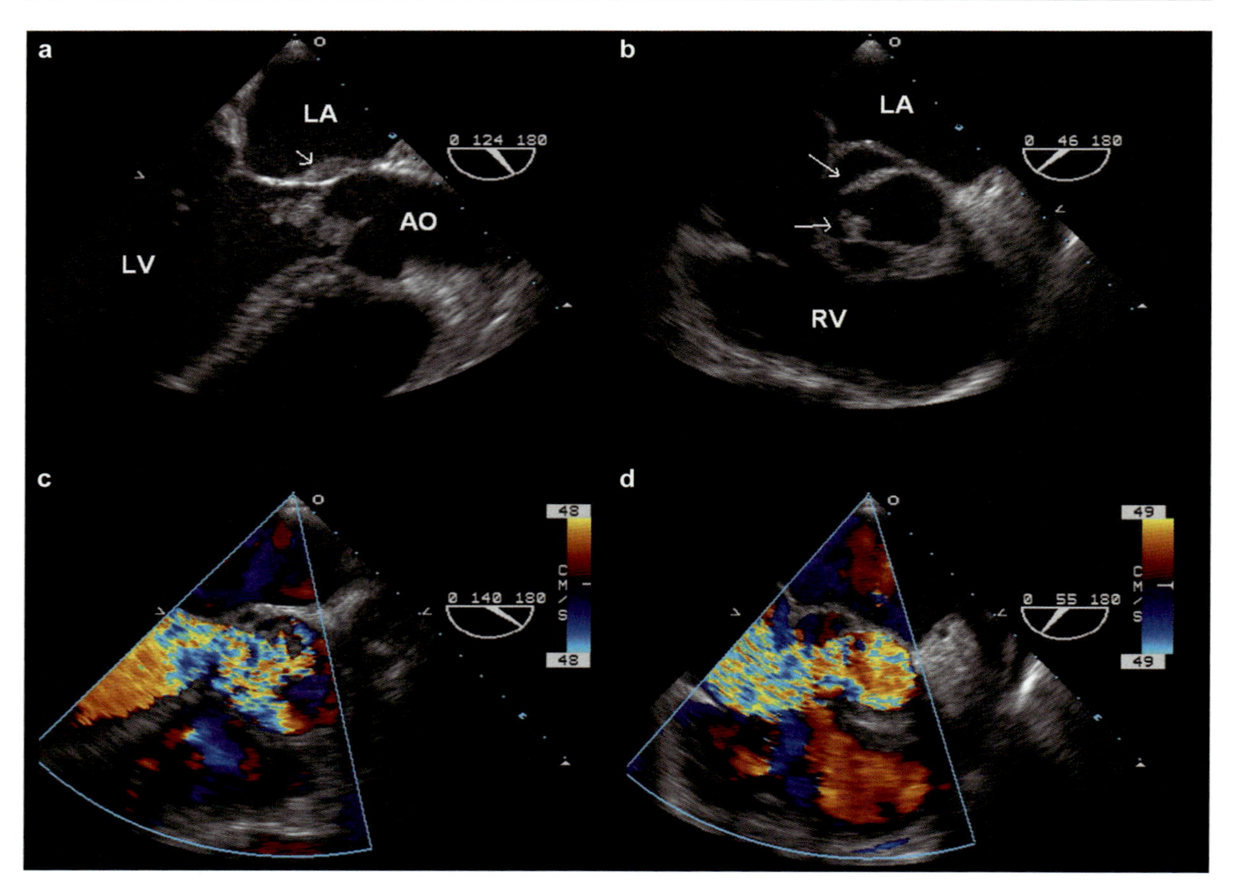

Fig. 12.28 Transesophageal echocardiogram of the aorta in long-axis (**a**, **c**) and short-axis (**b**, **d**) show large vegetations involving the aortic valve. There is also a pseudoaneurysm (*arrows*) involving the posterior and medial aspect of the aortic root. Color-flow images (**c**, **d**) show the presence of severe aortic regurgitation and fistula communication between the aorta and the right atrium. *Ao* aorta, *LA* left atrium, *LV* left ventricle, *RV* right ventricle

Invariably prosthetic endocarditis leads to infection of the prosthetic ring, which may lead to valve dehiscence or a paravalvular leak. Annular abscess is not uncommon, with complications similar to native root abscess (Figs. 12.21–12.23). With bioprostheses, the actual cusp tissue may be destroyed leading to cusp thrombi, destruction, erosions, and perforations similar to native valves. Mechanical prostheses may get variable sized thrombi, but the actual prosthesis usually remains intact and the infection is mainly in the sewing ring and surrounding tissues. The thrombi on a mechanical or a bioprosthesis may interfere with normal function and the prosthesis may become dysfunctional with disc or cusp immobility or the bioprosthetic cusp destruction causes regurgitation [23, 49].

The development of new perivalvular regurgitation is usually indicative of IE, underscoring the importance of a baseline echocardiographic study after valve replacement. Echocardiographic evaluation of a patient with suspected prosthetic valve IE can be challenging, because of the presence of preexisting perivalvular abnormalities related to the underlying valve disease and the effects of surgery, the confusing findings of the different components of the prosthetic valve and reverberation artifacts caused by the prosthetic material. TEE is superior to TTE in this clinical setting and should be performed even when a good quality TTE shows no evidence of infection (Figs. 12.33, 12.34). The sensitivity of TTE in the diagnosis of prosthetic valve IE is 25–36%, lower than that of TEE which is 77–100% (Fig. 12.34) [33, 50, 51]. Aortic prosthetic valves are more difficult to image optimally by TEE, accounting for the majority of the false-negative cases (Fig. 12.35) [51].

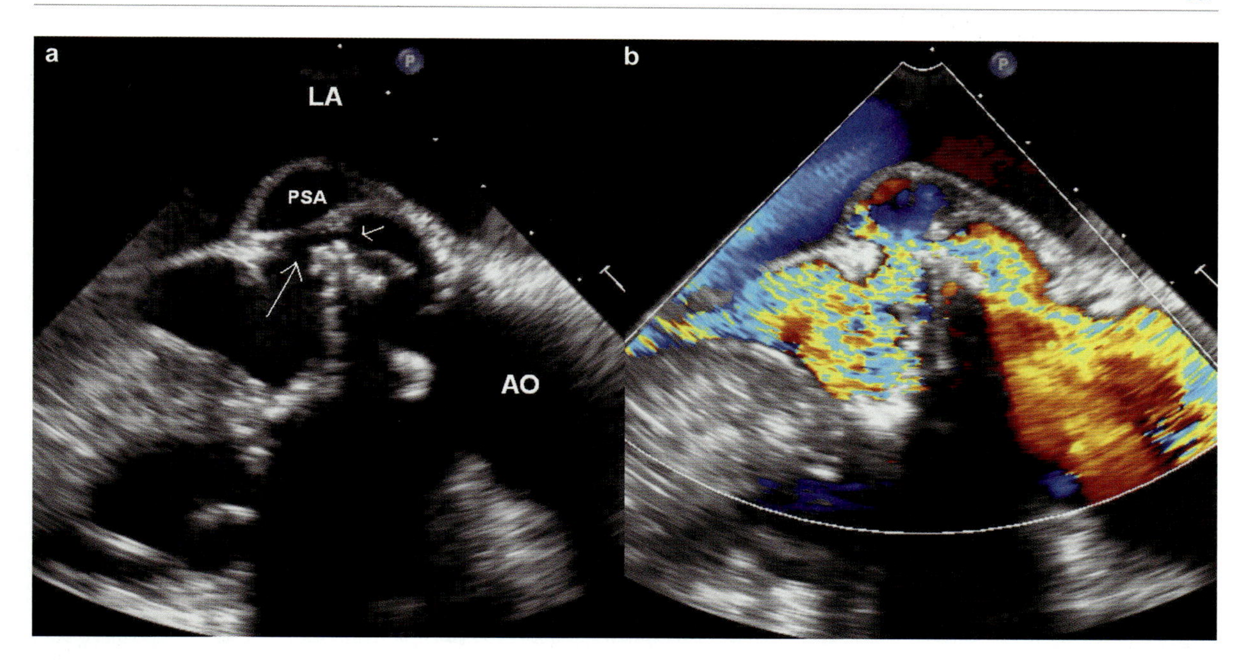

Fig. 12.29 In this patient with bioprosthetic aortic valve and aortic root abscess, the abscess has cavitated and developed into a pseudoaneurysm (**a**). There is dehiscence of the posterior sewing ring (*arrows*) with severe paravalvular aortic regurgitation (**b**). *Ao* aorta, *LA* left atrium, *PSA* pseudoaneurysm

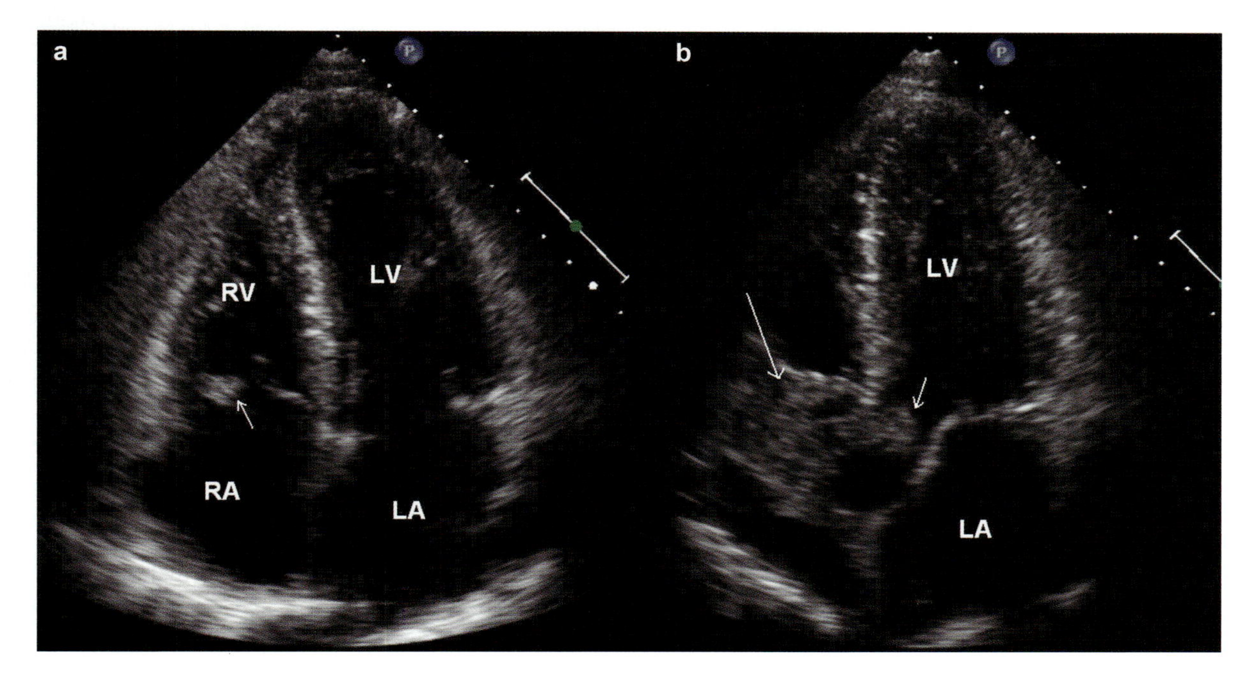

Fig. 12.30 Apical four-chamber (**a**) and five-chamber (**b**) views in a patient with intravenous drug use and Staphylococcal endocarditis show that in addition to vegetation (*arrow*) on the tricuspid valve in the four-chamber view (**a**), there is a large vegetation involving the aortic valve (short *arrow*) and a large aortic root abscess (long *arrow*) in the apical five-chamber view (**b**). *LA* left atrium, *LV* left ventricle, *RA* right atrium, *RV* right ventricle

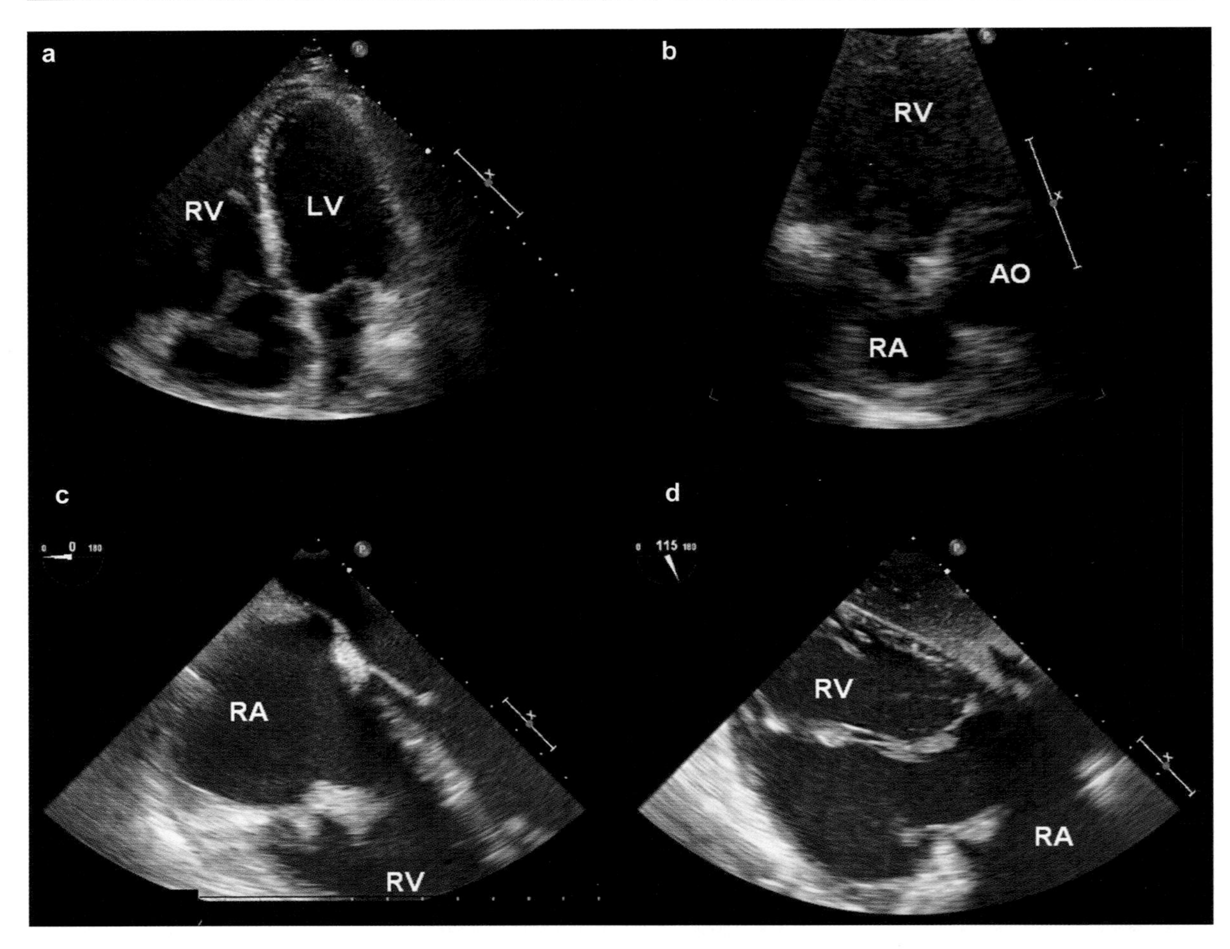

Fig. 12.31 Transthoracic apical four-chamber (**a**) and parasternal short-axis (**b**) views in a patient with intravenous drug use and endocarditis showing vegetations involving the tricuspid valve. Transesophageal views of the same patient (**c**, **d**) show similar findings. In patients with tricuspid valve endocarditis, the sensitivity of transthoracic study is similar to that of transesophageal studies because the vegetations generally are quite large and usually well seen. *LA* left atrium, *LV* left ventricle, *RA* right atrium, *RV* right ventricle

Both bacterial and fungal organisms are important causes of prosthetic IE [52]. Peripheral emboli are not uncommon [45]. Although a paravalvular leak may be technically related to poor tissues, suture unraveling, suture tissue cut through, and other technical matters, it is important to keep the possibility of IE in mind with all paravalvular leaks. Annular abscess and fistulas are much more common with prostheses, as compared to native valves. It is a disturbing and memorable experience to image a near totally dehisced valve prosthesis by echocardiography and for the surgeon to be able to remove the prosthesis from a patient without much need to cut tissue or sutures as all have been destroyed by the infection. Sutures, pledgets, and the aortotomy site may also become infected.

Chronically, paravalvular defects and paravalvular leaks may form and become clinically significant with regurgitation, heart failure, or hemolysis. Destruction of the adjacent tissues may lead to intracardiac fistulas, conduction system destruction and arrhythmias, and coronary artery inflammation and thrombosis [45]. The mortality of prosthetic IE remains high, with or without surgery. Fungal infection of prosthesis is a surgical indication due to near total mortality without surgery [46, 53, 54].

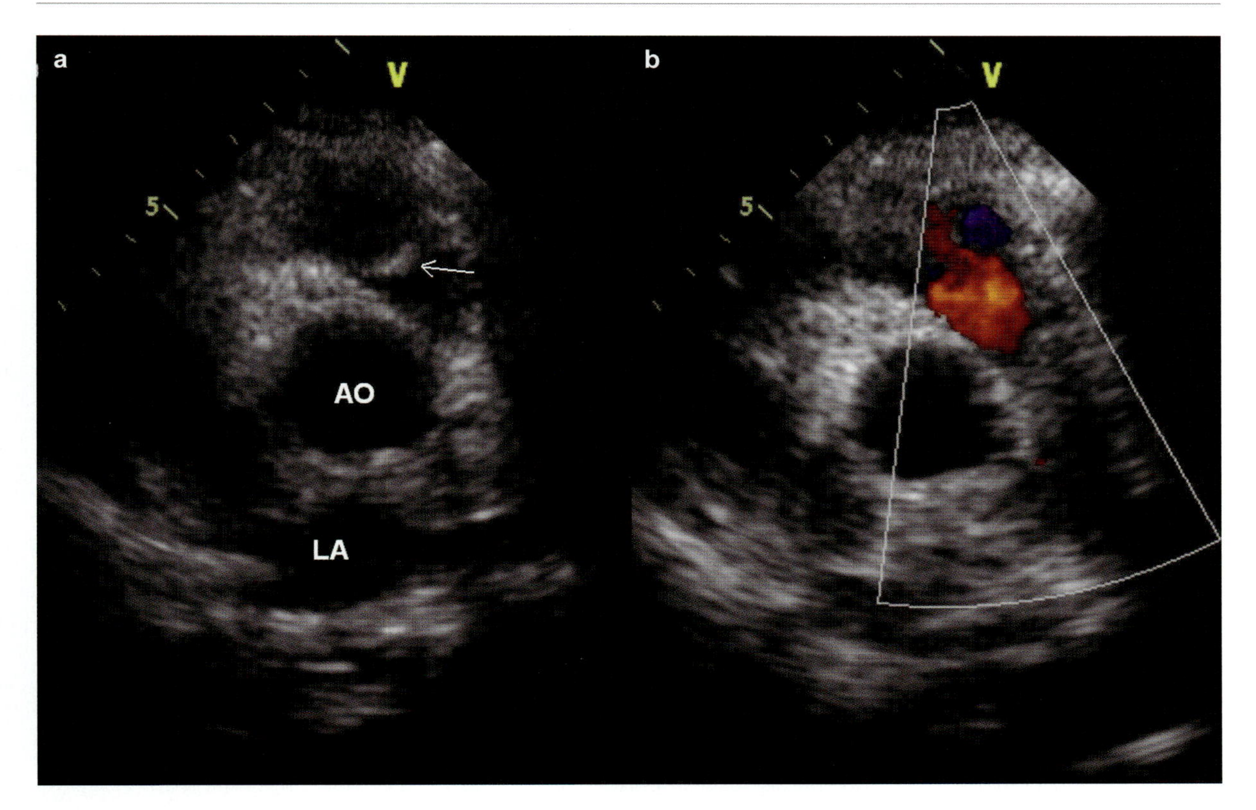

Fig. 12.32 Parasternal short-axis view (**a**) in a patient with vegetation (*arrow*) involving the pulmonic valve. Color-flow image (**b**) shows no significant pulmonic regurgitation. *Ao* aorta, *LA* left atrium

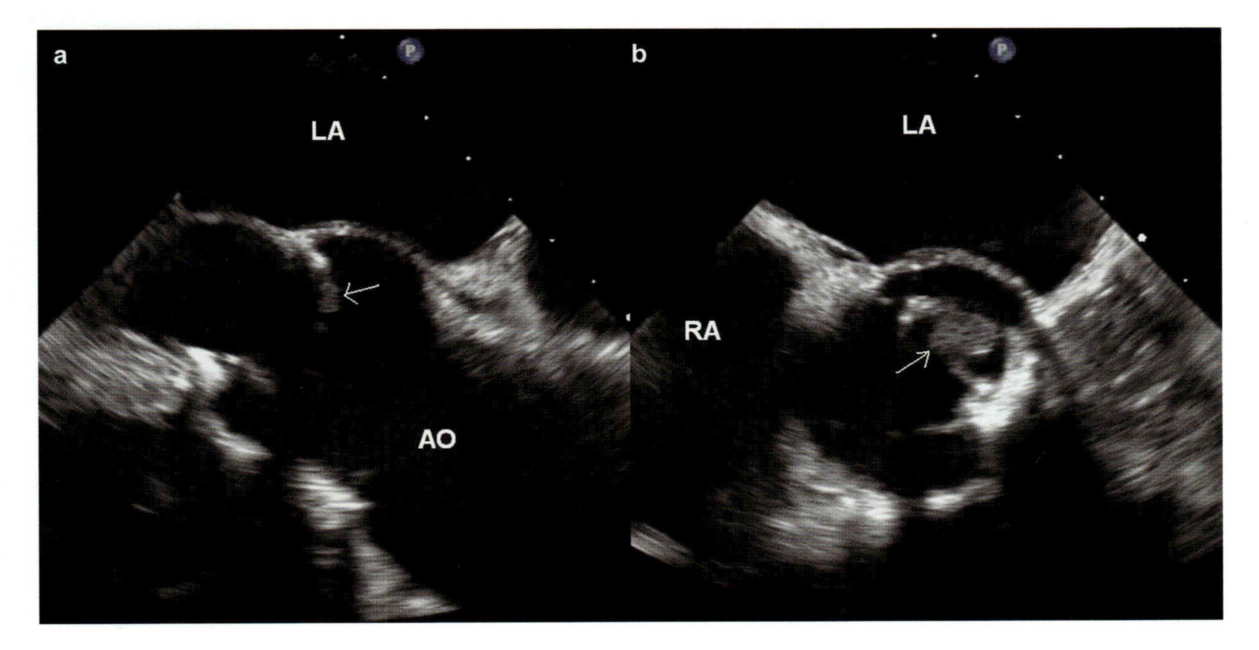

Fig. 12.33 Transesophageal views of the aortic bioprosthetic valve in long-axis (**a**) and short-axis (**b**) show the presence of a large vegetation (*arrow*) involving one of the prosthetic leaflets. This vegetation is not imaged on the transthoracic study

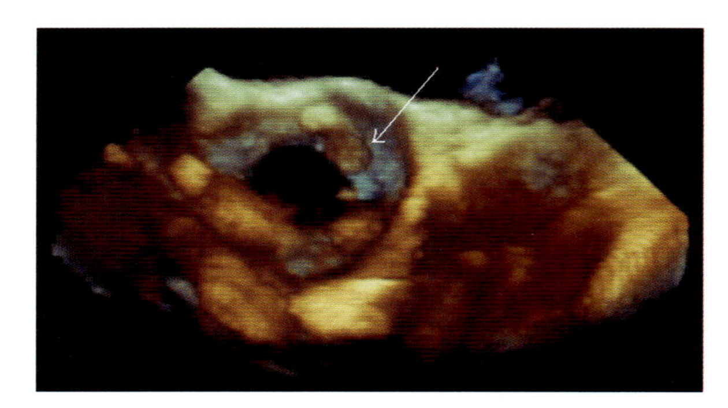

Fig. 12.34 Transesophageal 3D image of the bioprosthetic valve from the aortic perspective shows the large vegetation (*arrow*) attached to one of the posterior bioprosthetic leaflets. This is the same patient as in Fig. 12.33

Culture Negative Endocarditis

Patients with clinical and echocardiographic evidence of native or prosthetic valve endocarditis with persistently negative blood cultures should be investigated for possible fungal endocarditis and endocarditis secondary to other unusual or fastidious microorganisms, including HACEK group bacteria, Bartonella, Brucella, Chlamydia, Coxiella, Corynebacterium, Legionella, Listeria, Mycobacterium, Mycoplasma, Neisseria, Nocardia, and nutritionally variant Streptococci. Special media (hypertonic, B6 and cysteine-enriched), lysis centrifugation techniques, and resin treatment to remove antibiotics have been recommended. A minimum 3-week incubation of blood cultures has been recommended for all patients with culture negative endocarditis. Serology and molecular techniques are also useful [55]. Histopathologic examination of embolic material along with culture has been helpful in confirming fungal etiologies for both prosthetic and native valve endocarditis. This is one of the reasons that all extracted emboli should be examined microscopically by a pathologist. In this clinical setting, echocardiographic findings assume even greater importance in making the diagnosis.

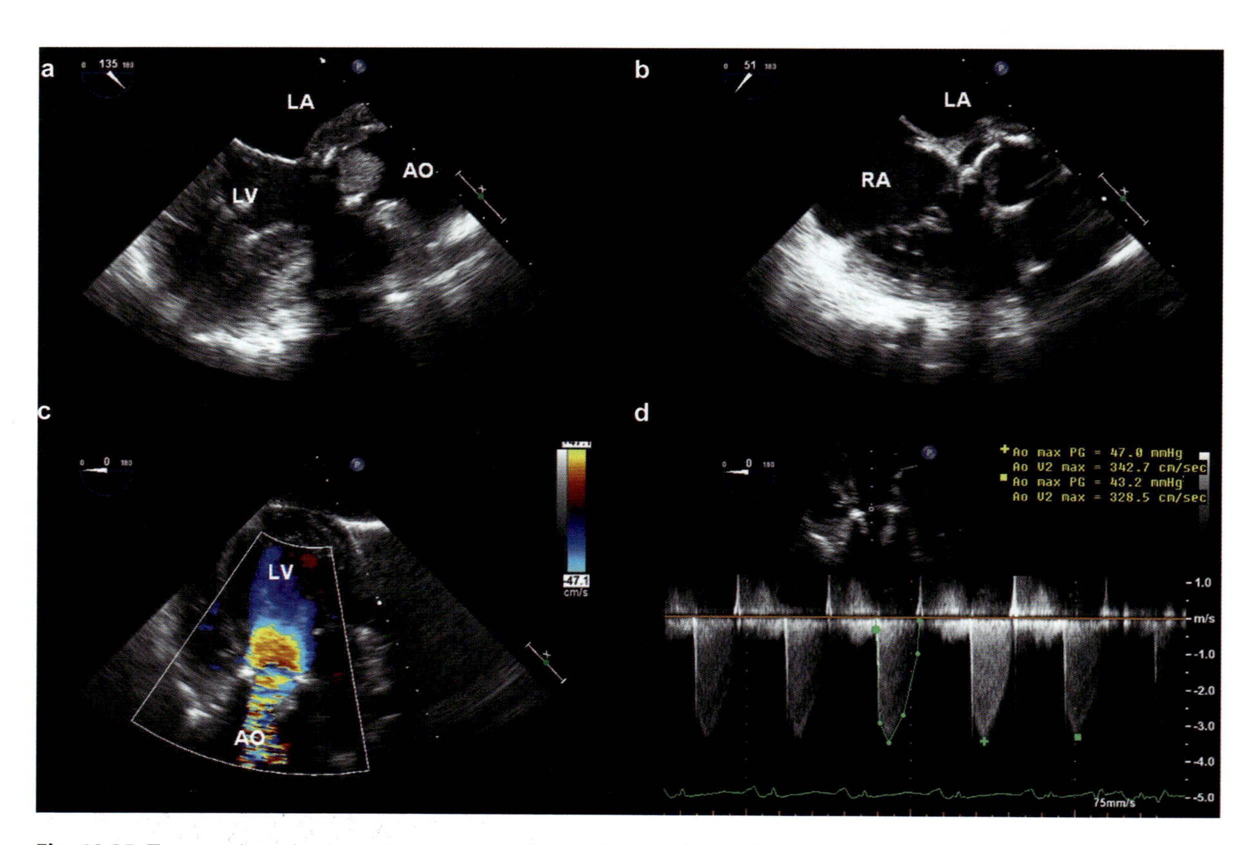

Fig. 12.35 Transesophageal echocardiogram in a patient with Staphylococcal prosthetic valve endocarditis shows a large mass involving the aortic valve (**a**, **b**). There is also increase in thickness of the posterior aortic root consistent with abscess. The large size of the vegetation leads to aortic stenosis with turbulent flow distal to the aortic valve (**c**) and a peak transvalvular gradient of 45 mmHg (**d**)

Fungal Endocarditis

Fungal endocarditis is usually encountered with IVDU, postsurgically or with immunosuppression [56]. Fungi represent 1–10% of the infectious pathogens causing infective endocarditis. About 5–15% of prosthetic IE and 12–20% of intravenous drug-related IE is fungal in etiology. *Candida albicans*, non-albicans *Candida* and *Aspergillus* species are the most common etiologic agents. Immunocompromised hosts may not develop classic valvular endocarditis, but instead may have non-valvular and mural sites of endocardial infection. Fungal vegetations are usually quite large and friable (Figs. 12.36, 12.37). Valve stenosis and embolic events are common. Both native and prosthetic valve fungal endocarditis are associated with severe complications, including disseminated infection, large and friable valvular vegetations with a propensity to embolize, and valve ring and myocardial abscesses.

Fungal endocarditis is difficult to diagnose as fungemia occurs in only 50% of cases. Fungi tend to form mycelial masses and have a tendency for vascular invasion, thus decreasing their identification in blood. Documented fungemia is rare for Aspergillus, Histoplasma, and Mucor, as these fungi are uncommonly grown in routine blood cultures.

Histopathologic examination of embolic material with culture has been helpful in confirming fungal etiology. Unfortunately, this diagnostic procedure is dependent on a complication of fungal endocarditis that all clinicians would like to avoid. In cases of Aspergillus endocarditis, histopathologic examination and fungal cultures of skin lesions have been effective. Choroiditis may be present. The diagnosis

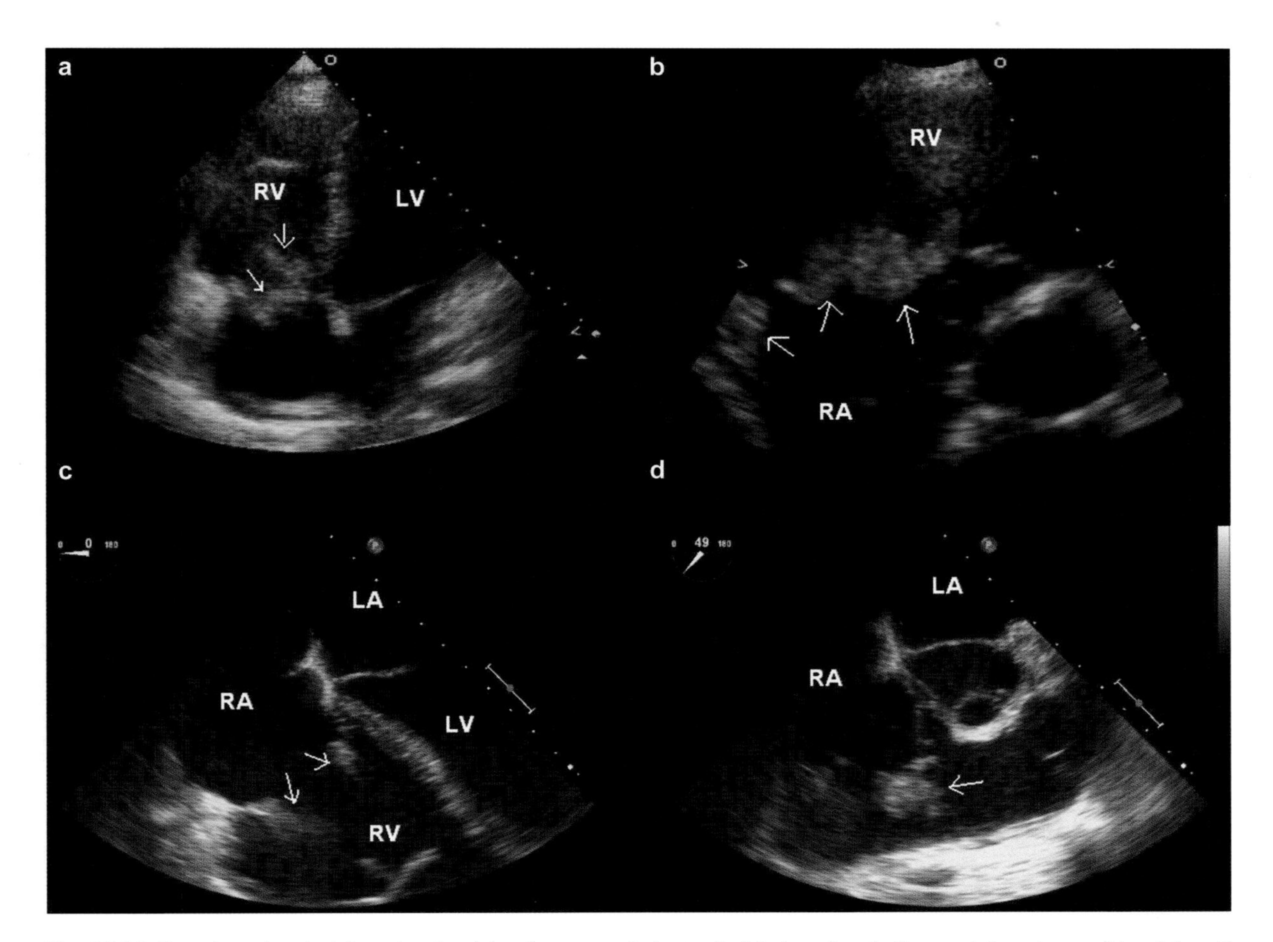

Fig. 12.36 Transthoracic apical four-chamber (**a**) and parasternal short-axis (**b**) views how bulky vegetations (*arrows*) involving all three tricuspid leaflets in a patient with intravenous drug use and Candida endocarditis. Transesophageal views of the same patient (**c**, **d**) show similar findings. *LA* left atrium, *LV* left ventricle, *RA* right atrium, *RV* right ventricle

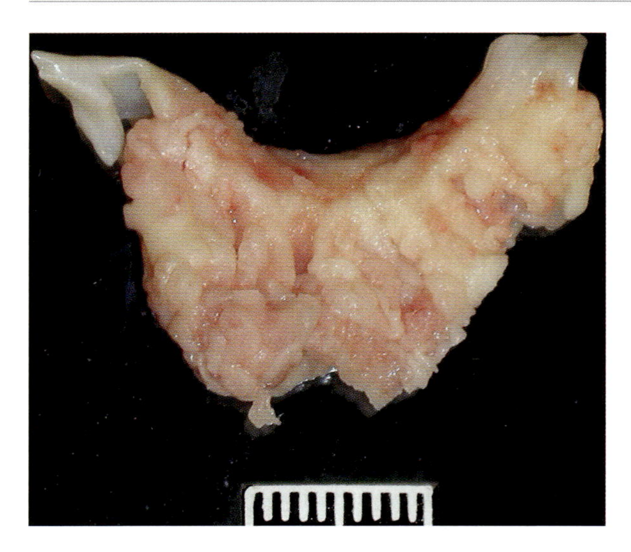

Fig. 12.37 Excised aortic valve cusp with fungal endocarditis. The infected thrombus is large, bulky, and obscures the underlying valve cusp

of Histoplasma endocarditis has been established through surgical biopsy and fungal cultures of bone marrow, liver, and oropharyngeal ulcers [49]. Serological tests are of limited value in the diagnosis of fungal endocarditis, but may be useful in confirming endocarditis due to Cryptococcus and Histoplasma. Candida serological tests are unreliable and false-positive tests for Candida precipitins occur commonly in post-cardiac surgery patients with no evidence of endocarditis [54].

Although rare cases of fungal endocarditis have been successfully treated with antimycotic therapy alone, most clinicians advocate aggressive debridement and antimycotic therapy, regardless of whether the involved cardiac valves are native or prosthetic. About 10% of patients thought to be free of fungal endocarditis will subsequently re-develop it. Some advocate that the optimum treatment of fungal native or prosthetic valve endocarditis includes life-long, suppressive, antimycotic therapy.

Nonbacterial Thrombotic Endocarditis

Nonbacterial thrombotic endocarditis (NBTE) is also known as thrombo-endocarditis and marantic endocarditis. This type of valve lesion describes deposition of fibrin and platelets on cardiac valves in the absence of microorganisms [57]. Association with malignancy and debilitation was noted early. Deppisch et al. reported a retrospective clinicopathological analysis of 4,096 autopsies at Mount Sinai hospital from 1965 to 1974 [58]. Of 102 patients diagnosed premortem with NBTE, only 65 had pathological confirmation. Of these 65 patients, the most common underlying associated condition was malignancy (51 patients) and of all the malignancies adenocarcinoma, by itself, or with a second malignancy, was the most common neoplasm. The other 14 patients had no malignancy, but had chronic debilitating diseases including systemic lupus erythematosus (SLE), and cirrhosis [58]. The other etiological mechanism of NBTE is the presence of a hypercoagulable state. The association of thrombosis (hypercoagulable state) and disseminated intravascular coagulation and malignancy was first noted by Trousseau [59, 60]. This association was also seen with other underlying systemic diseases including chronic inflammatory conditions, stress from burns, or dehydration [60]. The hypercoagulable state has been attributed to production of procoagulants, tumor mucin release or elevated clotting factors, fibrin degradation products, or thrombocytosis, or platelet activation through platelet activating factors released secondary to the localized valvular injury and fibrin depositions [2].

Before the wide availability of echocardiography, NBTE was most commonly discovered at postmortem examination [1]. Lopez reviewed the autopsy and echocardiographic records from Cedars-Sinai Medical Center between 1982 and 1984 [61]. Six patients had confirmed postmortem pathological diagnosis of NBTE and also an adequate premortem echocardiographic assessment by M-mode and 2D echocardiography within 45 days of death. Five of the six patients were diagnosed with valvular vegetations by 2D echocardiography. There was excellent correlation between the echocardiographic measurements and the autopsy findings.

The most common morphologic finding of NBTE is a vegetation-like lesion, a localized mobile echogenic mass attached to a normal appearing valve [1]. These lesions are located along the lines of valve closure and there is no associated underlying valve destruction (Fig. 12.38). The common sites are the atrial side of the atrioventricular valves and the ventricular side of the semilunar valves [1, 62]. Vegetation size can vary from small 2–3 to 10 mm.

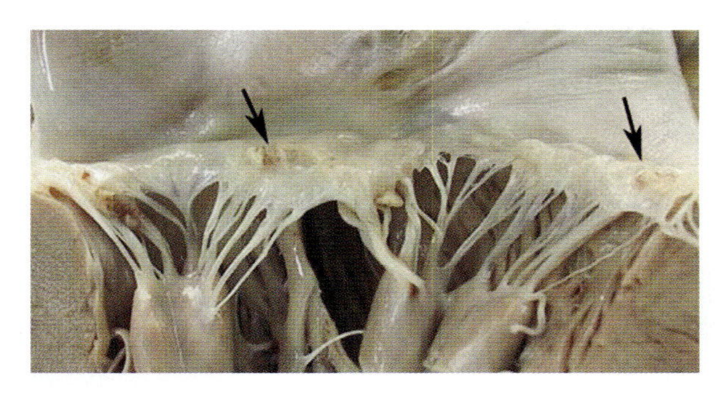

Fig. 12.38 Opened mitral valve with nonbacterial thrombotic endocarditis. This patient had malignancy. The tan small thrombi are located on the atrial side of the valve leaflets along the line of closure (*arrows*)

Left heart valves are almost exclusively affected with the aortic and mitral valves equally affected. The majority of the NBTE vegetations were associated with some degree of valvular insufficiency (54%), but two thirds had only mild insufficiency and only 2–3% needed surgery [1]. NBTE may still be clinically significant as the vegetation still has a propensity for embolic events including stroke, myocardial infarct, and systemic organ ischemia.

Rheumatic Fever Verrucous Endocarditis

Rheumatic fever is a pancarditis including endocarditis and valve involvement [63]. Chronic rheumatic valve disease is an important cause of aortic and mitral valve disease. The acute valve lesions of rheumatic fever are less recognized as they are clinically silent and usually undetectable by imaging.

Grossly, in the acute phase of rheumatic fever, the valves become thickened and less translucent. Tiny 1–2 mm thrombi (verrucae) are present at the lines of closure – on the atrial surface of the atrioventricular valves and the ventricular surfaces of the semilunar valves. Thrombi may also be present on the chords, left ventricular papillary muscles, or the left atrial endocardial surface. Chordal rupture may occur. The mitral valve is most often affected, followed by the mitral and aortic valves together, and lastly the aortic valve alone. Commonly, there is mitral insufficiency; however, this is usually due to ventricular dilatation (from heart failure and myocarditis related to the rheumatic fever). These valve changes are usually too small to be detected by imaging, but may be noted at surgery or pathology examination.

By microscopic examination, the earliest changes that occur at the valve rings are swelling, edema, and accumulation of acid mucopolysaccharides. There may be acute and chronic inflammation, including plasma cells, neovascularization with capillary proliferation, fibroblasts, and fibrinoid necrosis of collagen. Structures resembling Aschoff bodies may rarely be present [64].

Libman Sacks Endocarditis, Antiphospholipid, and Anticardiolipin Antibody Syndrome

Valve lesions, both focal and diffuse, are seen in systemic lupus erythematosus (SLE) with or without the presence of antiphospholipid antibodies. The antiphospholipid syndrome (APS) is defined by the presence of these antibodies and thrombocytopenia, repeated abortion, and arterial and/or venous thrombosis. About half the cases are primary and the other half secondary to SLE. These antibodies, which are heterogeneous in type and nature, may be present in disease states other than SLE (other autoimmune diseases, malignancy, or drug induced) or they may be part of a primary syndrome. The antibody may cause endothelial dysfunction allowing valvular thrombosis to occur or the mechanism may involve antibody deposition and an immune reaction [65, 66].

The valvular pathology described in SLE and the APS is variable [66]. Most of the older studies of these processes are postmortem based, while in modern studies, assessment with imaging modalities are common. These divergent studies give different results. There is also a bias in the older literature, as the presence of the valvular thrombi was considered to be one of the major specific autopsy criteria for SLE. Less overt valve lesions are seen in current patients and this may reflect a change in the medical management of SLE.

The classic valve lesions are termed Libman Sacks endocarditis. These small sterile thrombi may occur anywhere on the endocardial surface, but have a propensity for left-sided valves. The thrombi are sessile and usually about 3–4 mm, although lesions up to

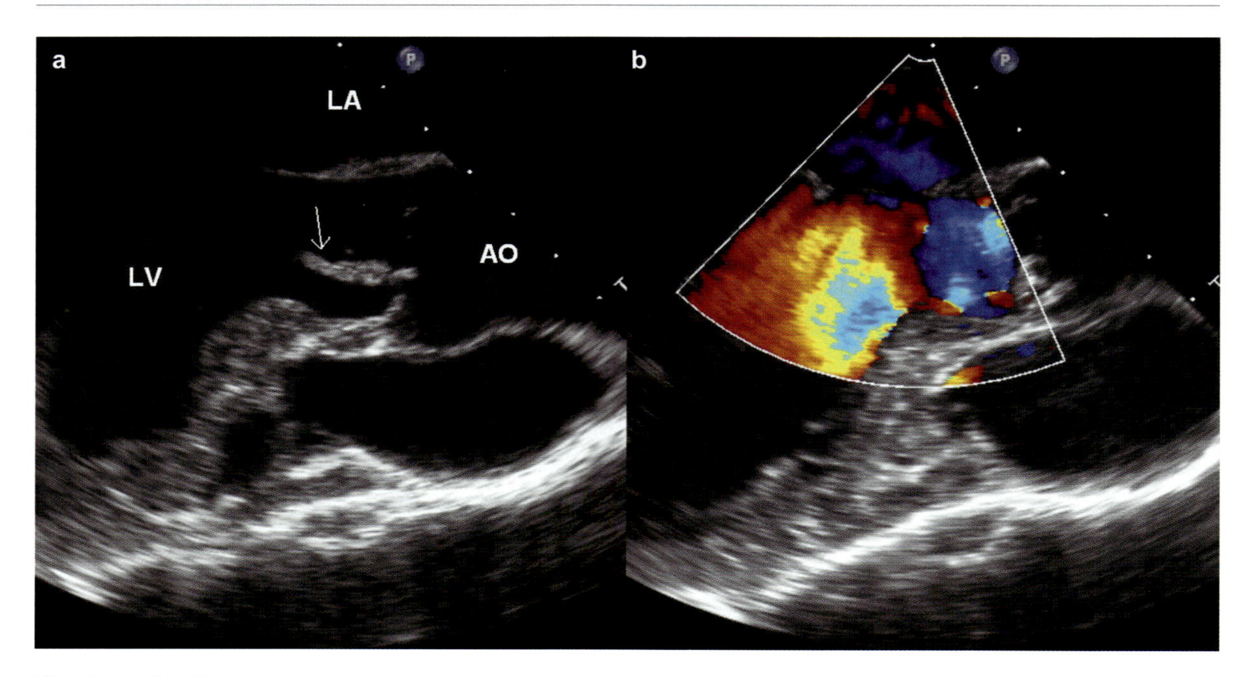

Fig. 12.39 This 64-year-old woman had systemic lupus erythematosus and markedly elevated antiphospholipid antibody level. She had no clinical evidence of endocarditis and blood cultures are negative. The transesophageal image (**a**) showed a large mobile mass on the aortic valve protruding into the left ventricular outflow tract during diastole. The color-flow image (**b**) showed no aortic regurgitation, strongly suggesting that this is not an infective vegetation. *Ao* aorta, *LA* left atrium, *LV* left ventricle

1.4 cm have been seen. They are present in about 10% of lupus patients, and the prevalence is associated with disease duration, disease activity, and antiphospholipid antibodies [67]. The valvular lesions can be quite large when there is associated antiphospholipid syndrome (Fig. 12.39). The most common location is along the line of valve closure and the opposite corresponding area on the other side of the leaflet or cusp. No valve destruction is present, an important fact to distinguish these thrombi from those of infective endocarditis (Fig. 12.40). Microscopy reveals bland thrombi with little chronic inflammation. In earlier reports, before the use of steroids, more inflammation, fibrinoid necrosis, and hematoxylin bodies were described. Special stains to rule out the presence of infective endocarditis are important.

Although clinically silent from a valvular dysfunction point of view, the thrombi may be responsible for embolic events including stroke, myocardial infarct, and systemic organ ischemia. Some of the clinical manifestations of SLE may not be vasculitic, but rather thromboembolic in nature.

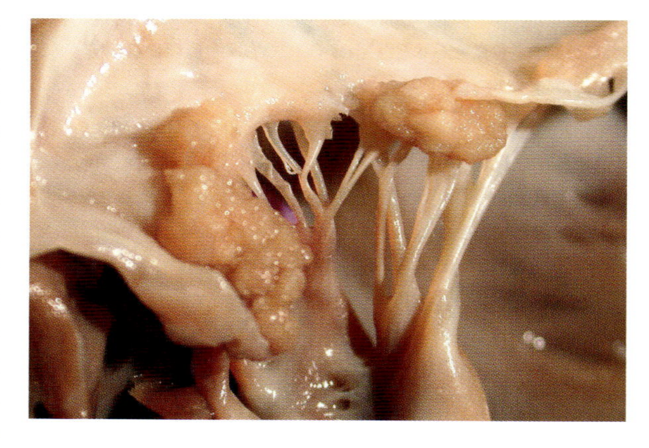

Fig. 12.40 Large Libman Sacks vegetations that were quite large and friable but did not destroy the underlying valve leaflet

Summary

Infective endocarditis has protean manifestations and may mimic many diseases. Prompt and accurate diagnosis is essential to the management of these patients.

The pivotal role of echo in the diagnosis of IE is recognized by the widely used Duke criteria for IE. It is the only noninvasive means to reliably detect valve vegetation, which is the hallmark of the disease. Transthoracic echo has a limited sensitivity in the detection of vegetation, and in up to 20% of patients TTE provides suboptimal images due to poor acoustic windows from chest deformity, obesity, pulmonary disease, or preexisting valvular abnormalities including the presence of prosthetic heart valves. In these situations, TEE is preferred since it can consistently provide high quality images and has been demonstrated to have a high sensitivity in the detection of vegetations and abscesses. TEE should be performed in high-risk patients even in the setting of a negative TTE to detect evidence of IE and in the setting of a positive TTE to assess local complications such as intracardiac pseudoaneurysm or fistula. Echocardiography has also provided valuable insight into the natural history of perivalvular abscess.

References

1. Reisner SA, Brenner B, Haim N, Edoute Y, Markiewicz W. Echocardiography in nonbacterial thrombotic endocarditis: from autopsy to clinical entity. *J Am Soc Echocardiogr.* 2000 Sept;13(9):876-881.
2. Lopez JA, Ross RS, Fishbein MC, Siegel RJ. Nonbacterial thrombotic endocarditis: a review. *Am Heart J.* 1987 Mar;113(3):773-784.
3. Li JS, Sexton DJ, Mick N, et al. Proposed modifications to the Duke criteria for the diagnosis of infective endocarditis. *Clin Infect Dis.* 2000 Apr;30(4):633-638.
4. Sachdev M, Peterson GE, Jollis JG. Imaging techniques for diagnosis of infective endocarditis. *Cardiol Clin.* 2003 May;21(2):185-195.
5. Chan KL. Early clinical course and long-term outcome of patients with infective endocarditis complicated by perivalvular abscess. *CMAJ.* 2002 July 9;167(1):19-24.
6. Erbel R, Rohmann S, Drexler M, et al. Improved diagnostic value of echocardiography in patients with infective endocarditis by transoesophageal approach. A prospective study. *Eur Heart J.* 1988 Jan;9(1):43-53.
7. Reynolds HR, Jagen MA, Tunick PA, Kronzon I. Sensitivity of transthoracic versus transesophageal echocardiography for the detection of native valve vegetations in the modern era. *J Am Soc Echocardiogr.* 2003 Jan;16(1):67-70.
8. Shively BK, Gurule FT, Roldan CA, Leggett JH, Schiller NB. Diagnostic value of transesophageal compared with transthoracic echocardiography in infective endocarditis. *J Am Coll Cardiol.* 1991 Aug;18(2):391-397.
9. Birmingham GD, Rahko PS, Ballantyne F III. Improved detection of infective endocarditis with transesophageal echocardiography. *Am Heart J.* 1992 Mar;123(3):774-781.
10. Shapiro SM, Young E, De GS, et al. Transesophageal echocardiography in diagnosis of infective endocarditis. *Chest.* 1994 Feb;105(2):377-382.
11. Lowry RW, Zoghbi WA, Baker WB, Wray RA, Quinones MA. Clinical impact of transesophageal echocardiography in the diagnosis and management of infective endocarditis. *Am J Cardiol.* 1994 June 1;73(15):1089-1091.
12. Ellis SG, Goldstein J, Popp RL. Detection of endocarditis-associated perivalvular abscesses by two-dimensional echocardiography. *J Am Coll Cardiol.* 1985 Mar;5(3): 647-653.
13. Daniel WG, Mugge A, Martin RP, et al. Improvement in the diagnosis of abscesses associated with endocarditis by transesophageal echocardiography. *N Engl J Med.* 1991 Mar 21;324(12):795-800.
14. Aguado JM, Gonzalez-Vilchez F, Martin-Duran R, Arjona R, Vazquez de Prada JA. Perivalvular abscesses associated with endocarditis. Clinical features and diagnostic accuracy of two-dimensional echocardiography. *Chest.* 1993 July; 104(1):88-93.
15. Tingleff J, Egeblad H, Gotzsche CO, et al. Perivalvular cavities in endocarditis: abscesses versus pseudoaneurysms? A transesophageal Doppler echocardiographic study in 118 patients with endocarditis. *Am Heart J.* 1995 July;130(1): 93-100.
16. Blumberg EA, Karalis DA, Chandrasekaran K, et al. Endocarditis-associated paravalvular abscesses. Do clinical parameters predict the presence of abscess? *Chest.* 1995 Apr;107(4):898-903.
17. San Roman JA, Vilacosta I, Sarria C, et al. Clinical course, microbiologic profile, and diagnosis of periannular complications in prosthetic valve endocarditis. *Am J Cardiol.* 1999 Apr 1;83(7):1075-1079.
18. Choussat R, Thomas D, Isnard R, et al. Perivalvular abscesses associated with endocarditis; clinical features and prognostic factors of overall survival in a series of 233 cases Perivalvular Abscesses French Multicentre Study. *Eur Heart J.* 1999 Feb;20(3):232-241.
19. Graupner C, Vilacosta I, SanRoman J, et al. Periannular extension of infective endocarditis. *J Am Coll Cardiol.* 2002 Apr 3;39(7):1204-1211.
20. Heidenreich PA, Masoudi FA, Maini B, et al. Echocardiography in patients with suspected endocarditis: a cost-effectiveness analysis. *Am J Med.* 1999 Sept;107(3):198-208.
21. Fowler VG Jr, Li J, Corey GR, et al. Role of echocardiography in evaluation of patients with Staphylococcus aureus bacteremia: experience in 103 patients. *J Am Coll Cardiol.* 1997 Oct;30(4):1072-1078.
22. Sochowski RA, Chan KL. Implication of negative results on a monoplane transesophageal echocardiographic study in patients with suspected infective endocarditis. *J Am Coll Cardiol.* 1993 Jan;21(1):216-221.
23. Atkinson JB, Virmani R. Infective endocarditis: changing trends and general approach for examination. *Hum Pathol.* 1987;18:603-608.
24. LeSaux N, Veinot JP, Masters RG, Stinson WA, Walley VM. The surgical pathology of infective endocarditis. *J Surg Path.* 1997;2:223-232.
25. Bayer AS, Bolger AF, Taubert KA, et al. Diagnosis and management of infective endocarditis and its complications. *Circulation.* 1998 Dec 22;98(25):2936-2948.

Left ventricular intramural tumors may be asymptomatic or present with a mass effect. With protrusion into the endocardial cavity, hemodynamic compromise may result [9]. Local extension of the tumor may cause conduction or coronary artery compromise with chest pain, myocardial infarction, arrhythmia, heart block, or sudden death.

Some tumors, such as myxoma, have associated constitutional symptoms including anorexia, weight loss, fatigue, and malaise which may mimic a variety of systemic disorders [2, 12, 14, 15]. Interestingly, there may be hematological abnormalities, including anemia, polycythemia, leukocytosis, thrombocytosis, and elevated sedimentation rate [9]. Tumor production of mediators, including interleukins, has been reported [15].

Echocardiographic Approach

Echocardiographic detection of a cardiac tumor is a rare occurrence and is frequently associated with considerable excitement given the dramatic echocardiographic features of many cardiac tumors. Cardiac tumors can be difficult to diagnose as they have different presentations including systemic symptoms and embolic events. In many instances, the diagnosis of cardiac tumor may be an incidental finding. For instance, about a third of patients with myxoma in our centre were asymptomatic and the diagnosis was an incidental finding during an echocardiographic examination for another indication [16].

The most common echocardiographic feature of a cardiac tumor is the presence of an abnormal intracardiac mass. Clearly, not all intracardiac masses are tumors, and not all cardiac tumors present as an intracardiac mass. When an intracardiac mass is detected by echocardiography, a systematic approach is essential to arrive at the correct diagnosis. Many other possible conditions should be excluded before one makes the diagnosis of cardiac tumor. A critical evaluation of the echocardiographic findings is particularly important, since it is the imaging modality that is most frequently used in the detection of cardiac tumor. In the series of 546 cardiac tumors by Blondeau et al., echocardiography was utilized in about 80% of the cases, whereas computed tomography was used in only 7% of the cases [17]. Although other imaging modalities such as magnetic resonance imaging (MRI) may assume a larger role, echocardiography will remain the gold standard in the diagnosis of most cardiac tumors because of its noninvasive nature and superior temporal resolution.

Our approach in the evaluation of intracardiac mass is to start with a broad perspective bearing in mind that tumor is but one of many potential causes of an intracardiac mass. The most common causes of an echocardiographic mass are listed in Table 13.1. Artifacts should always be one of the first conditions to consider in dealing with an intracardiac mass. Reverberation artifact arising from a mechanical mitral valve can give the impression of a mass within the left atrium and conversely, the reverberation artifact can mask the presence of a left atrial mass (Fig. 13.1). Other common artifacts include acoustic shadowing from a very bright echo reflector, beam width artifact, and side lobe artifacts. Artifacts are particularly common in patients with suboptimal images. Multiple image windows including the use of the transesophageal window may be needed to exclude these artifacts.

Extracardiac masses may appear to be intracardiac. Sequential images with slight transducer angulation should be used to demonstrate the extent of the mass and its relationship to the cardiac structures in order to avoid confusing an extrinsic mass with an intracardiac mass (Fig. 13.2). The right and left atria are more prone to the effect of extrinsic compression by an extracardiac mass, and thus, extracardiac masses should be carefully excluded when a left atrial or right atrial mass is detected by echocardiography. Extrinsic cardiac conditions that can simulate an intracardiac mass include pectus excavatum, the spine, hiatus hernia, hematoma, pericardial cyst, bronchogenic cyst, and noncardiac tumors such as lymphoma and posterior mediastinal neurogenic tumors (Figs. 13.3–13.5). It is

Table 13.1 Differential diagnosis of a cardiac mass

- Artifact
- Extracardiac mass
- Normal structure or variants
- Thrombus
- Vegetation
- Tumors
- Infections

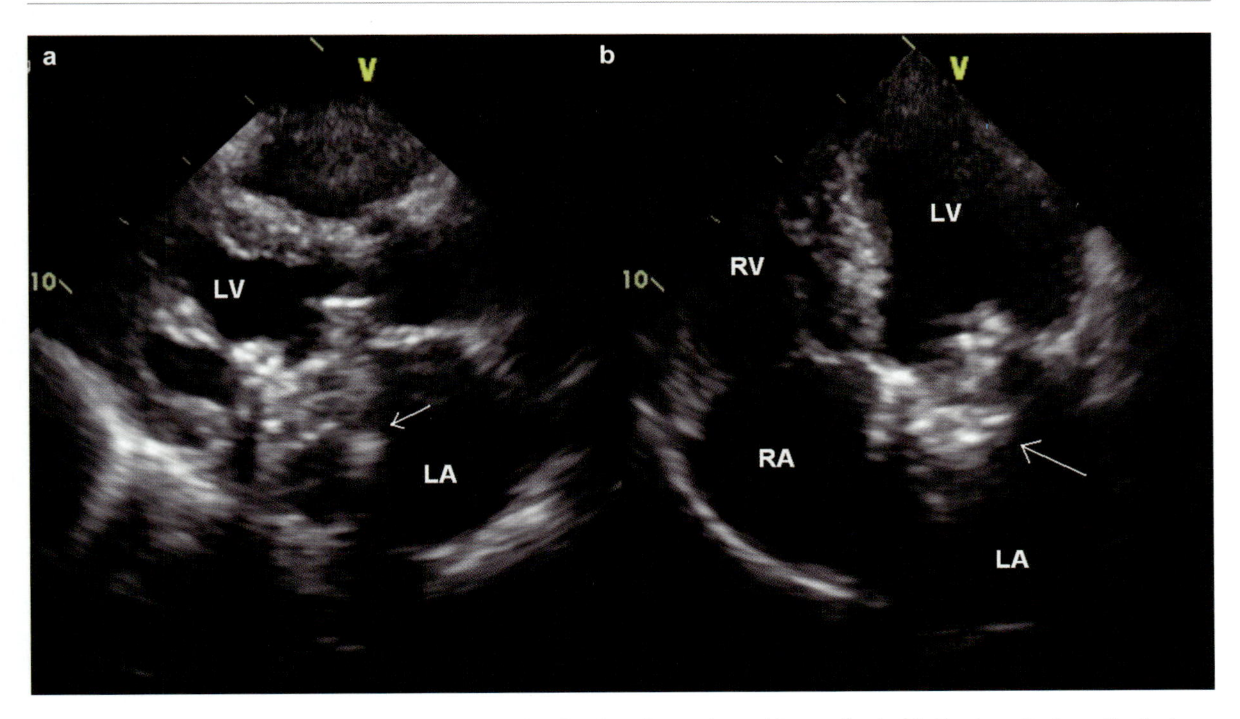

Fig. 13.1 The parasternal long-axis (**a**) and four-chamber (**b**) views in a patient with a mechanical ball valve mitral prosthesis showing reverberation artifacts (*arrow*) in the left atrium, which may be confused for left atrial masses. *LA* left atrium, *LV* left ventricle, *RA* right atrium, *RV* right ventricle

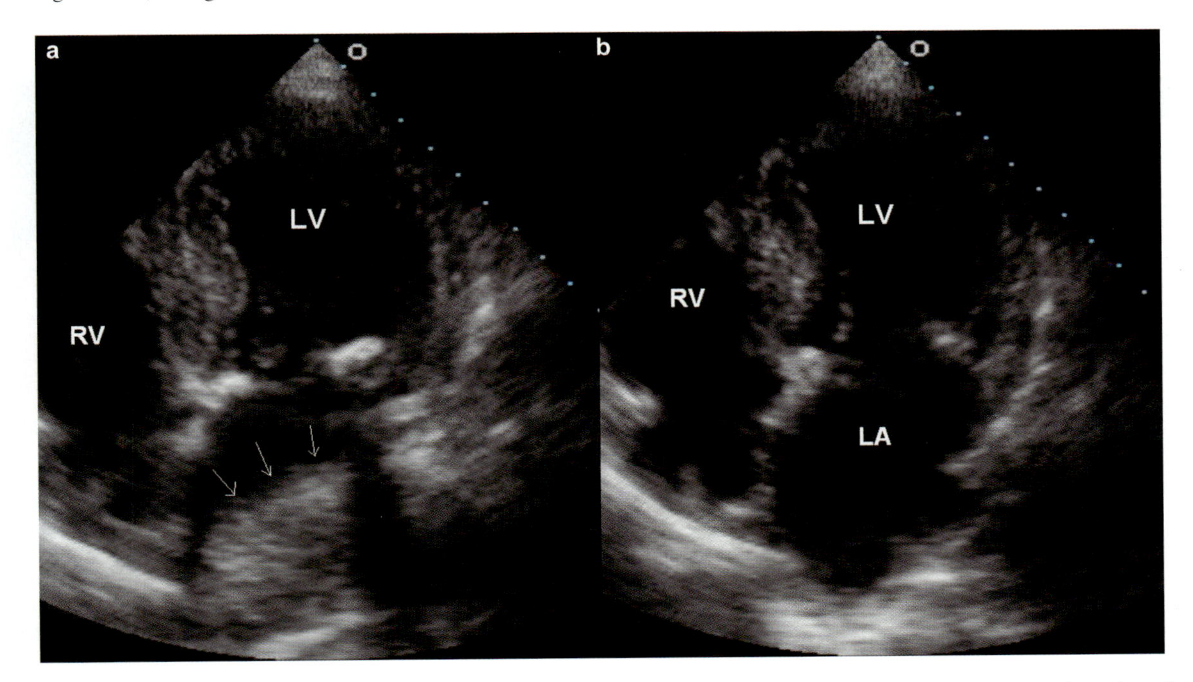

Fig. 13.2 This is a patient with a known hiatus hernia. The apical four-chamber views obtained on two separate occasions show that there is an apparent large mass (*arrows*) in the left atrium (**a**), which is not seen in (**b**). A sliding hiatus hernia may move into the thorax and indent the left atrium such that it is imaged on one occasion and not the other. If hiatus hernia is suspected, the diagnosis can be confirmed by the detection of enhanced echogenicity following ingestion of a carbonated drink. *LA* left atrium, *LV* left ventricle, *RV* right ventricle

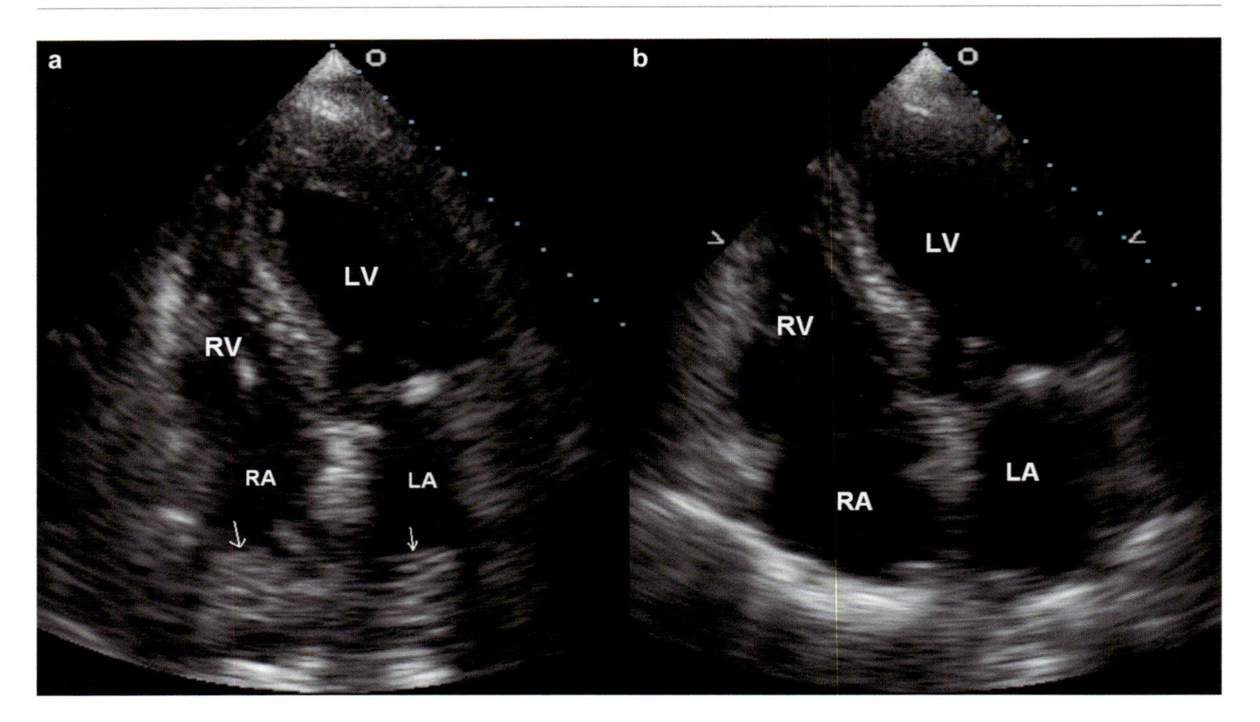

Fig. 13.3 This apical four-chamber view (**a**) was obtained in a patient with low cardiac output following cardiac surgery. Large masses appear to be within the right and left atria (*arrows*). These masses were correctly diagnosed to be extracardiac hematomas indenting the atria. After evacuation of the pericardial hematoma, the apparent atrial masses were no longer seen (**b**). *LA* left atrium, *LV* left ventricle, *RA* right atrium, *RV* right ventricle

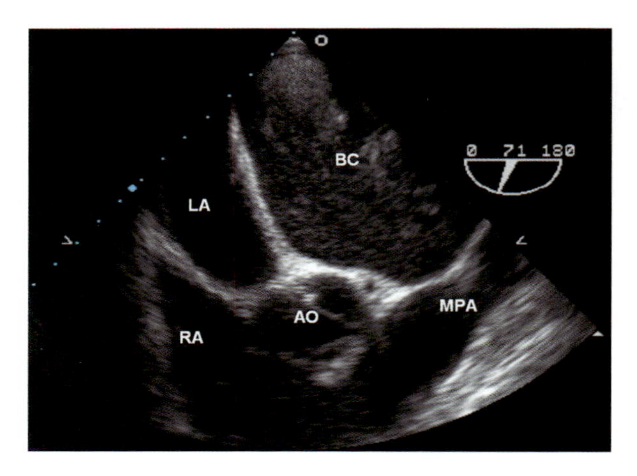

Fig. 13.4 This is a transesophageal view in a patient with a bronchogenic cyst in the posterior mediastinum indenting and displacing the adjacent cardiac structure. *Ao* aorta, *BC* bronchogenic cyst, *LA* left atrium, *MPA* main pulmonary artery, *RA* right atrium

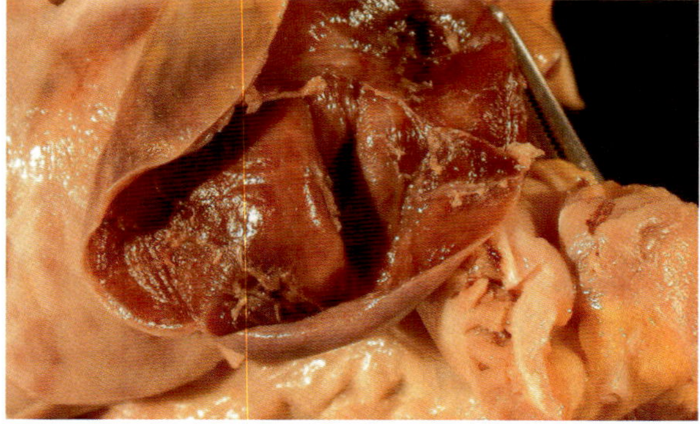

Fig. 13.5 This is a 5 cm pericardial cyst located on the anterior heart near the left atrial appendage. It was an incidental finding at autopsy. The cyst is opened demonstrating red brown fibrin on the inside. Pericardial cysts may be located all around the heart. Pathologists, surgeons, and cardiologists gain an appreciation of the many neoplastic and nonneoplastic mediastinal lesions that exist. Ectopic thyroid tissue has even been reported near the heart

worth emphasizing that a solid tumor in the far view can appear cystic. In our experience this is particularly the case with lymphoma.

Normal cardiac structures can be quite prominent and confused with an abnormal mass (Table 13.2). The partition between the left upper pulmonary vein and the left atrial appendage can be quite bulbus, but the correct diagnosis can be made by its typical location and appearance (Fig. 13.6). Similarly, the crista terminalis can be

Table 13.2 Normal cardiac structures mimicking an intracardiac mass

- Crista terminalis
- Eustachian valve
- Thebesian valve
- Chiari network
- Bulbous partition between left atrial appendage and left pulmonary vein
- Moderator band
- Accessory papillary muscle
- False tendon – pseudotendon
- Ventricular trabeculation
- Lipomatous hypertrophy of atrial septum
- Age-related valve nodules on closing margin
- Prominent interatrial septal mobility

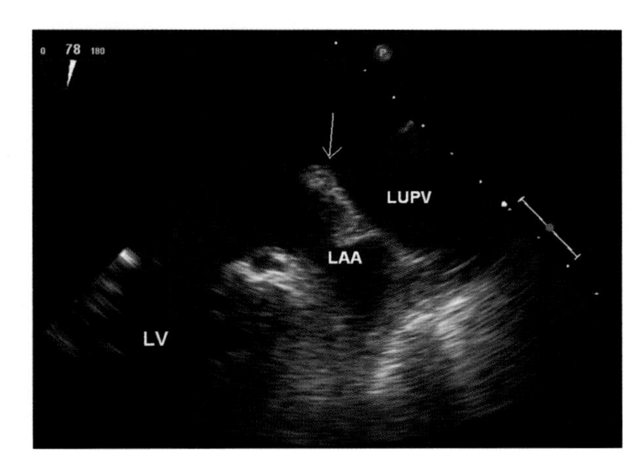

Fig. 13.6 This transesophageal echocardiogram shows an apparent intracardiac mass (*arrow*) which represents the bulbous partition between the left atrial appendage and the left upper pulmonary vein. This is a normal anatomical variant. *LAA* left atrial appendage, *LV* left ventricle, *LUPV* left upper pulmonary vein

prominent in some patients and should not be confused with an abnormal right atrial mass (Fig. 13.7). Additional images should be used to show the typical course of this muscle bundle running from the origin of the superior vena cava down the right side of the vena cava and curving toward the tricuspid orifice, thus dividing the trabeculated atrial appendage from the posterior smooth-wall right atrial cavity. A mobile and redundant atrial septum can mimic an atrial myxoma due to tangential section of the atrial septum (Fig. 13.8). In the elderly, mitral annular calcification can be quite large with central liquefaction and should not be confused for a cardiac tumor (Figs. 13.9, 13.10). Unusual infections caused by actinomycetes or mycobacteria may affect the myocardium and give rise to an intracardiac mass (Figs. 13.11, 13.12). Hydatid cyst is a rare condition which is usually intramyocardial involving the ventricular septum or the left ventricular free wall. This possibility needs to be considered when an intracardiac cystic mass is encountered in a patient from a sheep-raising country, where echinococcal infection may be endemic.

After excluding artifacts, extracardiac masses, and normal structures, the diagnosis of an abnormal intracardiac mass can be made, and the differential diagnoses then include thrombus, vegetation, or tumor. The differentiation of these three entities is largely based on the location and morphologic characteristics. Associated findings, such as evidence of stasis, and clinical correlation, such as the presence of fever, are very useful. Similarly, evolutional changes over time or with treatment may also be helpful. The typical features of thrombus and vegetation are listed in Table 13.3. Thrombus occurs in areas of stasis and is more common in the left atrial appendage or the left ventricular apex in the setting of anterior wall myocardial infarction. Thrombus tends more likely to be single and well defined. Mobile thrombus is less common. Old thrombi may appear echo dense.

Valve vegetations are located on or near the coaptation area on the upstream side of the cardiac valves. They can be single or multiple and are usually highly mobile. Old vegetations can be echogenic in appearance. The presence of leaflet destruction or paravalvular extension is a good indication that one is dealing with a destructive process such as vegetation rather than thrombus.

Differentiating a tumor from a vegetation or thrombus can be difficult, and it is crucial to interpret echo findings in light of the clinical setting. A cardiac tumor should be suspected when a cardiac mass is detected without clinical evidence of infection or predisposing conditions for intracardiac stasis. The location and morphologic features are very helpful. The useful features to differentiate a benign primary cardiac tumor from malignant or secondary cardiac tumors are listed in Table 13.4.

Benign primary cardiac tumors obey the anatomic confines. For instance, a left atrial myxoma does not invade the pulmonary veins, the underlying left atrial wall, or the left ventricle. Benign tumors are usually well circumscribed and do not involve the pericardium.

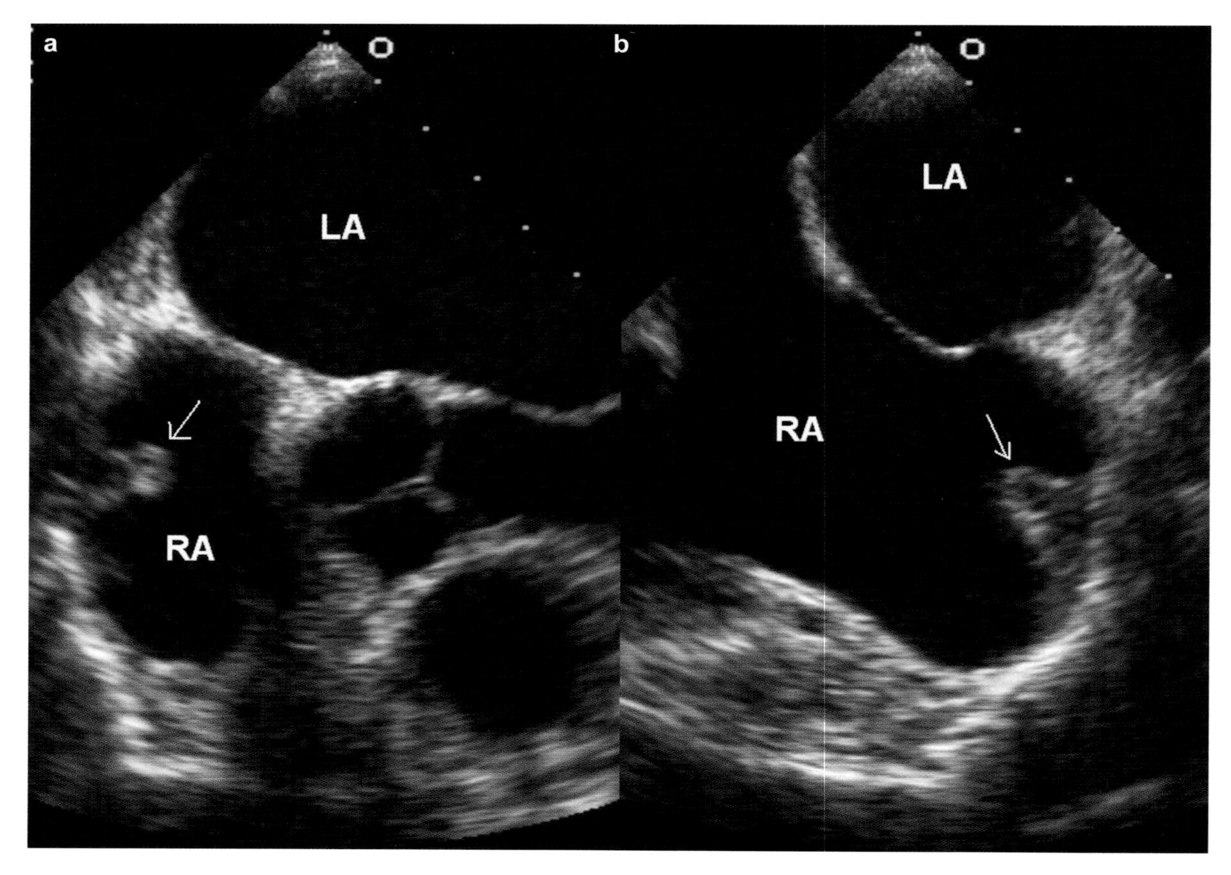

Fig. 13.7 The transesophageal echocardiogram in the transverse plane (**a**) shows a mass (*arrow*) in the right atrium. The longitudinal plane (**b**) shows that this mass (*arrow*) is located at the entrance of the superior vena cava. Additional images (not shown) show that this is the crista terminalis, which runs from the origin of the superior vena cava down to the tricuspid orifice

On the other hand, malignant or secondary tumors frequently invade beyond the anatomic borders of any one cardiac chamber. They are poorly demarcated and the pericardium is frequently involved. The most common metastatic tumors that involve the heart are lymphoma, breast carcinoma, lung carcinoma, and malignant melanoma. Angiosarcoma is the most common primary malignant cardiac tumor.

Primary Benign Cardiac Tumors

Primary benign cardiac tumors are rare but receive most attention because of their unique morphologic features. The location and morphology are important clues to identify the type of cardiac tumor (Table 13.5). The two most common benign cardiac tumors are myxoma and papillary fibroelastoma (PFE). Their features are compared in the Table 13.6.

Cardiac Myxoma

Cardiac myxoma is the most common benign cardiac tumor. Myxomas occur more often in women than men [18]. A recent analysis of multiple surgical-based series including 1,195 individuals having surgical excision of myxomas found 67% female patients and 33% male patients. In the same review, three series that included autopsy patients found 71% females and 29% males [18]. The Armed Forces Institute of Pathology (AFIP) reports more male patients, but this likely reflects a referral pattern [7, 18].

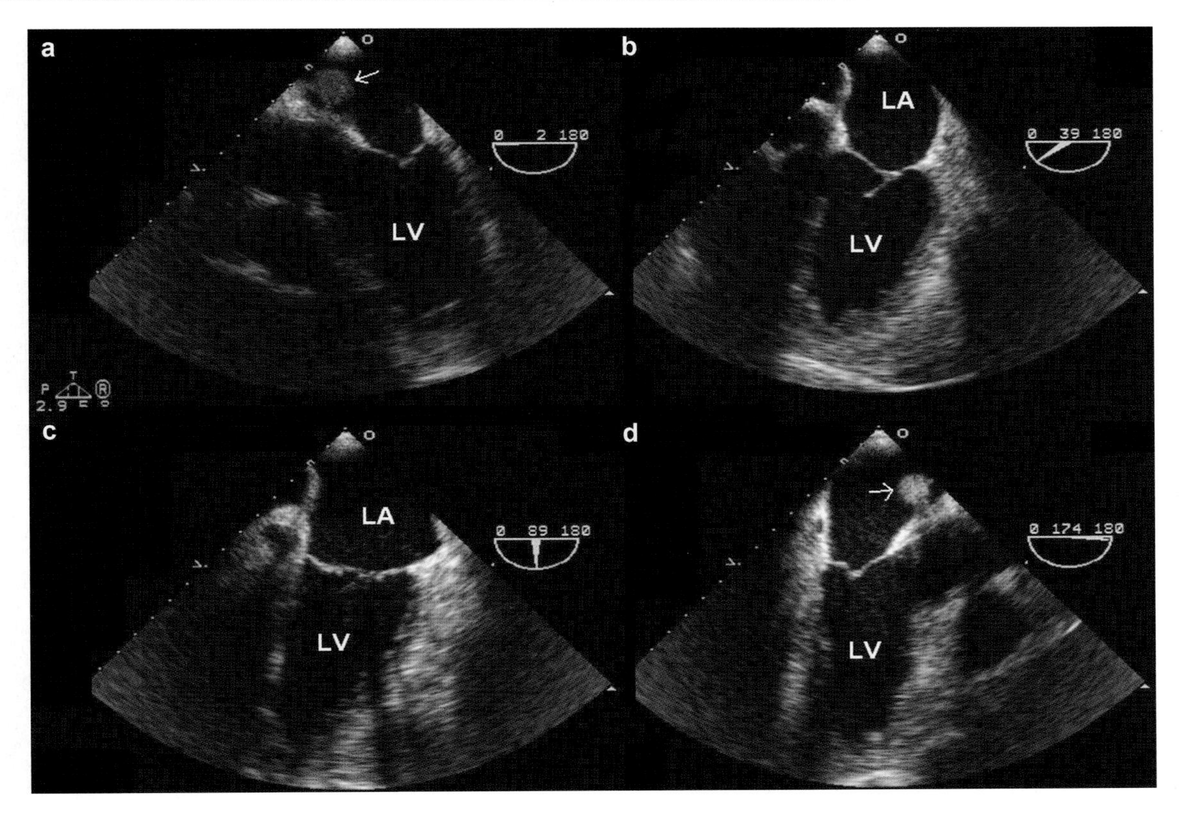

Fig. 13.8 This is a patient with a redundant and mobile atrial septum. The atrial septum is imaged tangentially such that it appears as a mass (*arrow*) attaching to the atrial septum (**a**, **d**). Additional views are important to show that this apparent mass is due to the mobile atrial septum (**b**, **c**). *LA* left atrium, *LV* left ventricle, *RA* right atrium

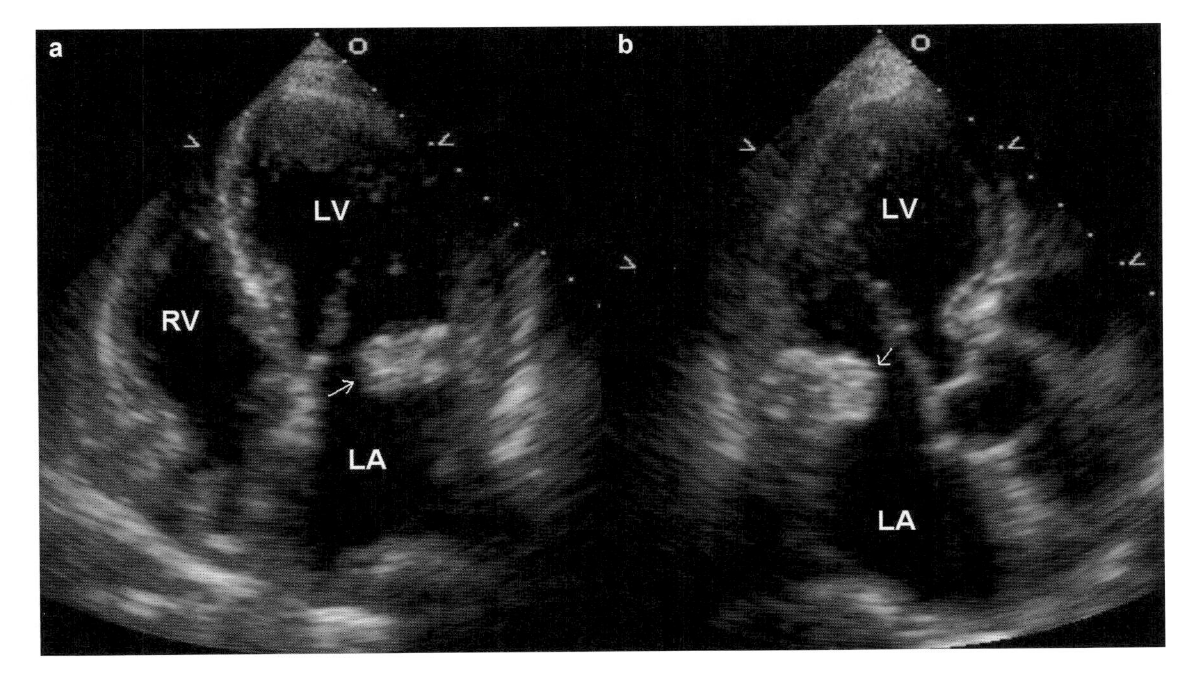

Fig. 13.9 The apical four-chamber (**a**) and long-axis (**b**) view in an 82-year-old woman show very prominent mitral annular calcification (*arrow*) with some degree of central liquefaction. The typical location is a key feature differentiating mitral annular calcification from other intracardiac masses. *LA* left atrium, *LV* left ventricle, *RV* right ventricle

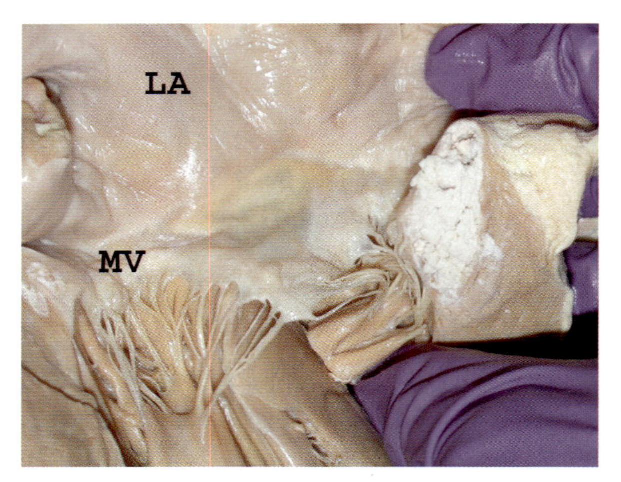

Fig. 13.10 Elderly woman with renal failure. The mitral annular calcification in the left atrioventricular groove is soft and caseous like. It produced a left atrial mass. When this is encountered there is confusion with an abscess as the white material is soft and may protrude out when the heart is opened or when the valve is removed. Microscopic examination provides clarification. Similar changes may occur surrounding the aortic root. *LA* left atrium, *MV* mitral valve

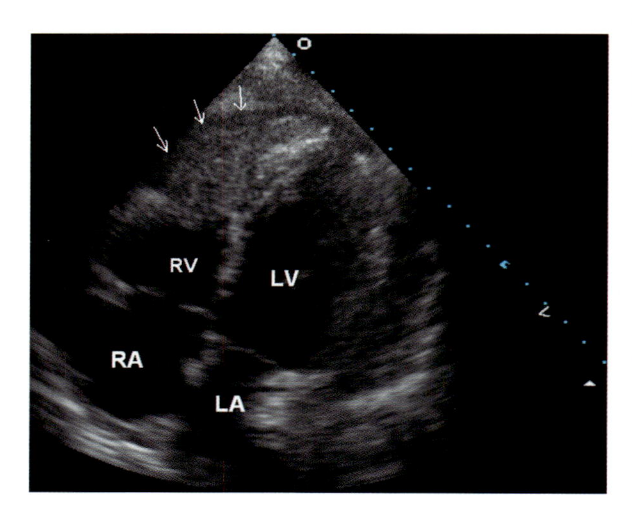

Fig. 13.11 This 51-year-old man developed fever and a pericardial effusion which was drained. The apical four-chamber view showed a large mass involving the right ventricular apex and right ventricular free wall (*arrows*). Endocardial biopsy confirmed abscess with Actinomycosis infection. *LA* left atrium, *LV* left ventricle, *RA* right atrium, *RV* right ventricle

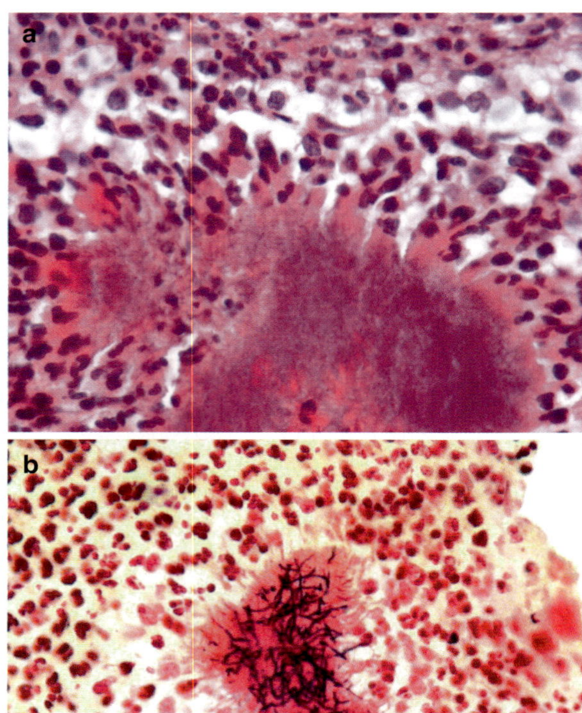

Fig. 13.12 Endomyocardial biopsy from patient in Fig. 13.11. (**a**) Shows purulent cellular material and a large purple filamentous structure typical of Actinomyces. If appreciated on gross exam, these are termed sulfur granules due to their yellow color. (**b**) Is the Gram stain demonstrating the Gram-positive filamentous organisms. This patient had been scheduled to receive chemotherapy for a sarcoma. After this diagnosis he received antibiotics and recovered

Patient age ranges from 2.5 to 97 years, 90% between the ages of 30 and 60 years [18]. Myxomas occur only rarely in children. The familial myxoma syndrome has been reported under the acronyms NAME (nevi, atrial myxoma, myxoid neural fibroma, ephelides), LAMB (lentigines, atrial myxoma, mucocutaneous myxomas, blue nevi), and the Carney syndrome (cardiac myxomas and extracardiac manifestations including skin pigmentation, testicular tumors, cutaneous myxomas, myxoid breast fibroadenomas, cortical adrenal hyperplasia, and pituitary hyperactivity) [19]. Familial myxomas are more than often multiple, recurrent, and right sided as compared to sporadic myxomas. The affected patients are younger than those with sporadic myxoma.

Myxomas usually present as embolic events with transient ischemic attacks or strokes. Peripheral emboli are possible. Tumors may obstruct the left atrial chamber

Table 13.3 Echo features of thrombus and vegetation

	Thrombus	Vegetation
Location	• Area of stasis, i.e., LV apex and LA appendage	• On or near coaptation area on the upstream side of the valves
Morphology	• Usually single • Mobile fronds less common • Echo-dense when chronic	• Frequently multiple • Mobile fronds are common • Echo-dense when chronic
Associated findings	• Cause for stasis, i.e., dilated LV • Underlying wall motion abnormalities	• Leaflet destruction and regurgitation • Perivalvular involvement

LA left atrium, *LV* left ventricle

Table 13.4 Echo features of benign and malignant cardiac tumors

Benign tumors • Obey anatomic boundaries • Well circumscribed • Pericardium not involved
Malignant or secondary tumors • Invade beyond anatomic boundaries • Poorly demarcated • Involvement of the pericardium

Table 13.5 Diagnostic features of cardiac tumors

Location • Atria versus ventricles • Intracavitary versus intramural
Morphology • Sessile versus pedunculated • Smooth surface versus mobile fronds • Echo-lucent versus echo-dense

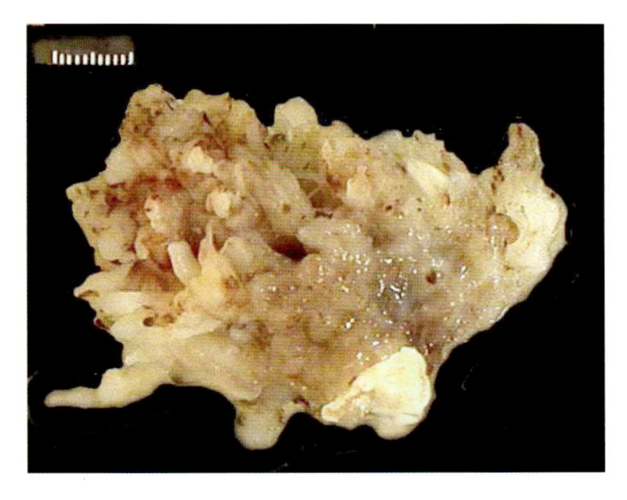

Fig. 13.13 This left atrial myxoma is soft, gelatinous, and multilobulated. It is easy to understand why such tumors may prolapse into the mitral valve, entrap thrombi, and embolize pieces of tumor and thrombus.

Table 13.6 Comparison of myxoma with papillary fibroelastoma

	Myxoma	Fibroelastoma
Location	• Attached to fossa ovalis	• On cardiac valves
Pedicle	• Sometimes present	• Present
Surface	• Smooth, can have mobile fronds	• Central core with multiple mobile fronds
Size	• Variable, often large	• Usually small, less than 1 cm in size

and mimic mitral stenosis with congestive heart failure. Myxomas may be clinically silent and some are detected at autopsy as an incidental finding or as a regressed atrial nodule.

Myxomas are endocardial-based lesions that do not infiltrate into the underlying tissue. They are commonly located on the left atrial side of the interatrial septum. They can be firm and lobulated, myxoid and gelatinous, or friable and irregular (Figs. 13.13–13.15). They do not occur often on the free wall of the atrium. They do not invade the underlying myocardium and do not invade into the adjacent pulmonary veins. The location and noninvasiveness are important benign features.

The cells of the myxoma possess an abundant eosinophilic cytoplasm and have indistinct cell borders. They arise in a myxoid background. Fibrosis, calcification, and hemorrhage are common, and extramedullary hematopoiesis may occur. Calretinin immunostain is a useful stain that is positive in most myxomas. This may be useful in tumors that have regression or are covered with thrombus. Vascular immunostains, such as CD31 and factor VIII, mark the blood vessels within the tumor.

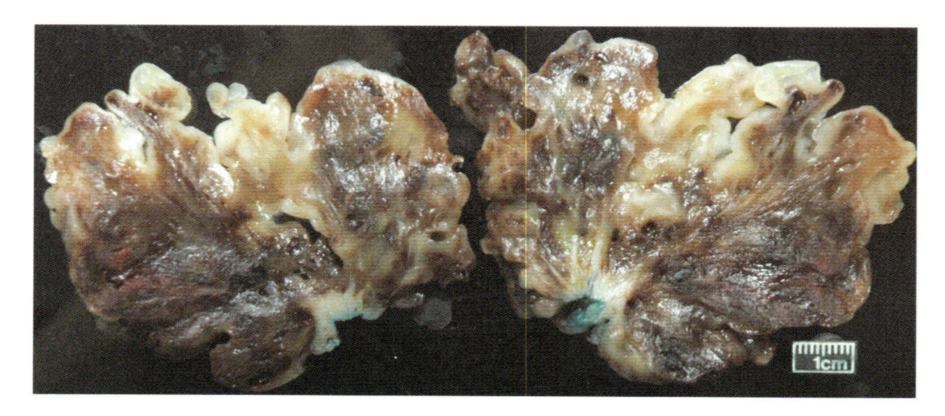

Fig. 13.14 This is a large left atrial myxoma that had mitral stenosis-like symptoms due to its size. It has been bisected to demonstrate the mottled red and dark appearance from a large amount of hemorrhage in the tumor. Such degenerative changes including hemorrhage, calcification, and bone formation are not uncommon

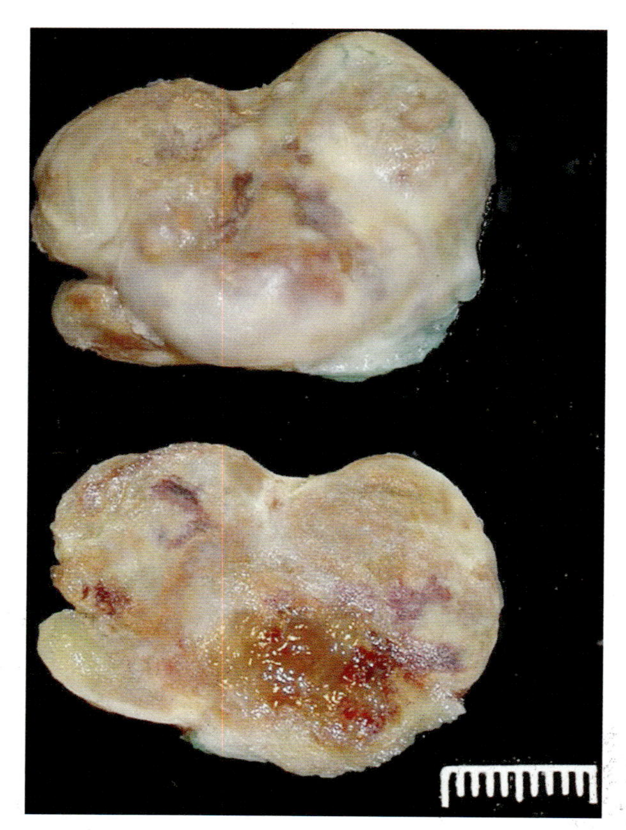

Fig. 13.15 This is a left atrial myxoma of another common gross morphology. This tumor has been bisected. The outer surface is seen on the *top* of the picture, and the cut surface on the lower. The myxoma is smooth, hard, and compact. Degenerative changes with fibrosis, calcification, and organized hemorrhage predominate. It may be difficult to find residual myxoma cells

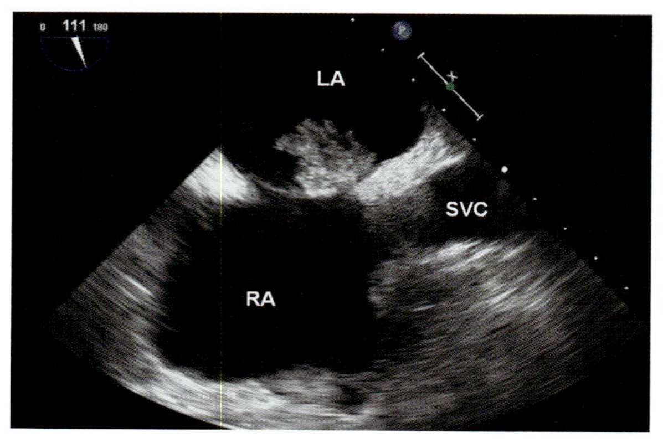

Fig. 13.16 A small myxoma is demonstrated in the transesophageal longitudinal plane showing the typical attachment to the foramen ovale. *LA* left atrium, *RA* right atrium, *SVC* superior vena cava

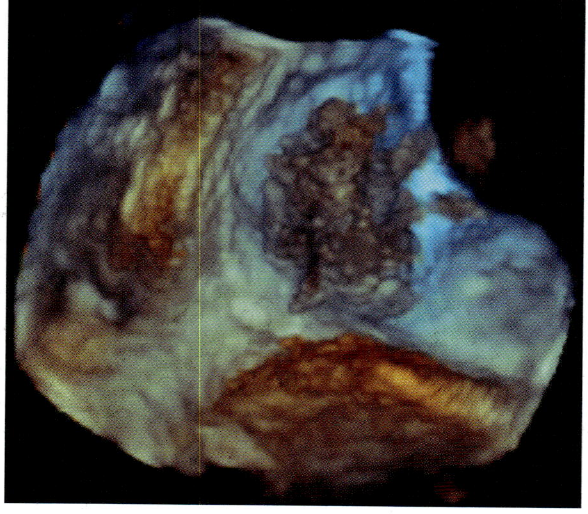

Fig. 13.17 Transesophageal 3D view of the myxoma in the same patient shown in Fig. 13.16, demonstrating the multiple fronds on the surface of the myxoma

Cardiac myxoma is typically located in the left atrium with attachment to or near the fossa ovalis (Figs. 13.16, 13.17). It generally has a smooth surface but can have mobile components (Figs. 13.18, 13.19).

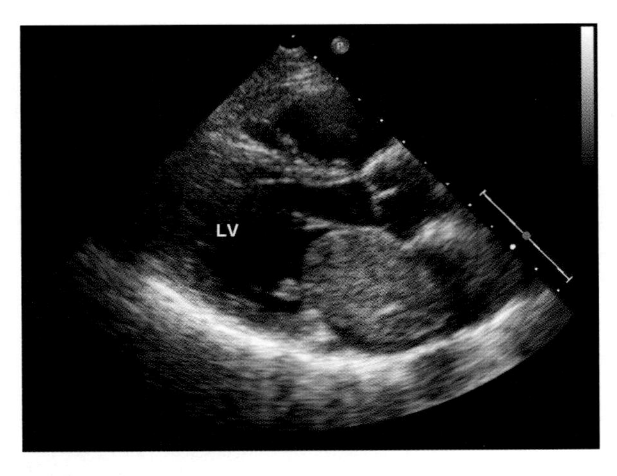

Fig. 13.18 The parasternal long-axis view shows a large left atrial myxoma with a smooth surface obstructing the mitral inflow leading to mitral stenosis and heart failure. *LV* left ventricle

It has a slightly echo-lucent appearance and there may be heterogeneous acoustic pockets within the myxoma. The size can vary, although it can be quite large when they are detected and can cause obstructive symptoms (Figs. 13.18, 13.19).

Right atrial myxoma may occur (Fig. 13.20). If the myxoma is right sided or multiple, the possibility of a familial myxoma syndrome should be entertained. Valve myxomas are rare [20]. There has been confusion in the past with some myxomas of the valves actually representing hamartomas or papillary fibroelastomas.

The treatment of a myxoma is by resection of the mass with a cuff of underlying atrial septal wall (Fig. 13.21). Patch repair of the residual septal defect is performed. With a good margin, the surgery should be curative. Myxomas that are soft may embolize and cause cerebral or systemic emboli and ischemia. Malignant myxomas reported in the literature may be embolic foci that have become attached to the vessels and grown locally.

Cardiac Rhabdomyoma

Cardiac rhabdomyoma is the most common primary pediatric tumor of the heart and is a hamartoma of developing cardiac myocytes [21–23]. These lesions

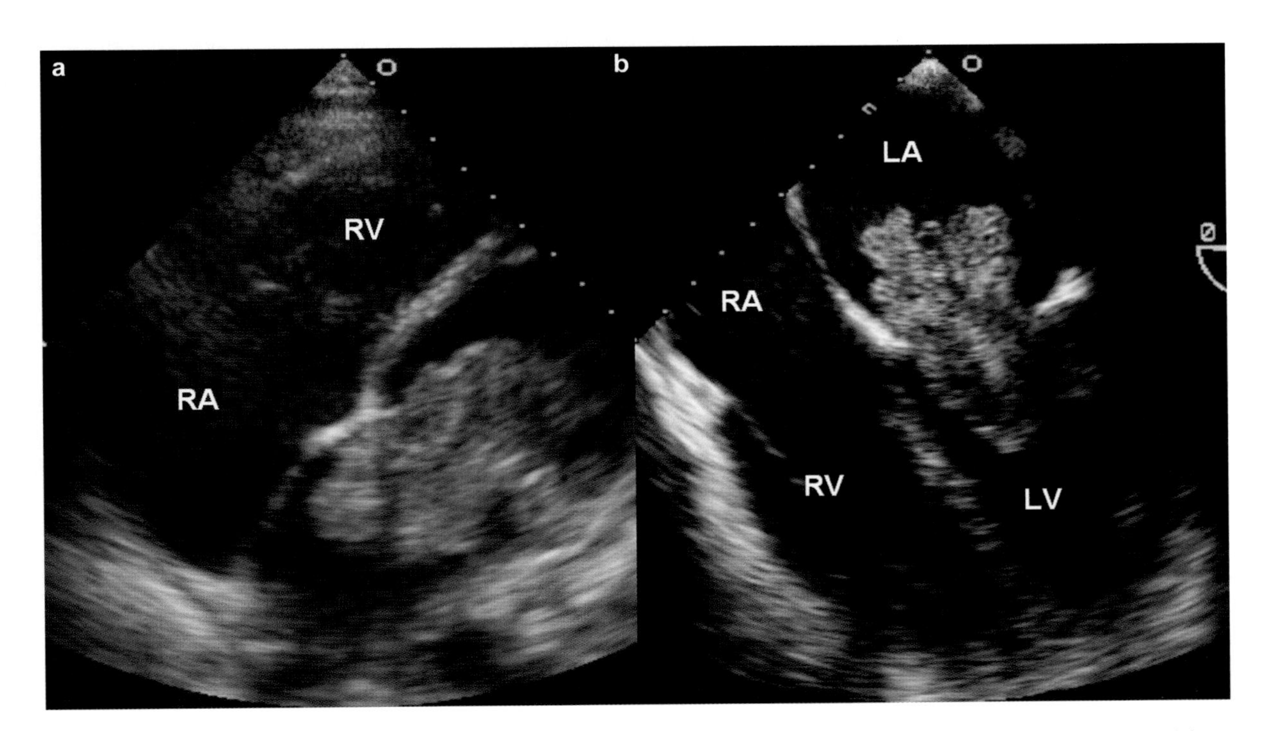

Fig. 13.19 A large left atrial myxoma is shown in the transthoracic modified four-chamber view (**a**) and the transesophageal four-chamber view (**b**). The myxoma obstructs the mitral inflow. It is polypoid in shape with multiple fronds on its surface. *LA* left atrium, *LV* left ventricle, *RA* right atrium, *RV* right ventricle

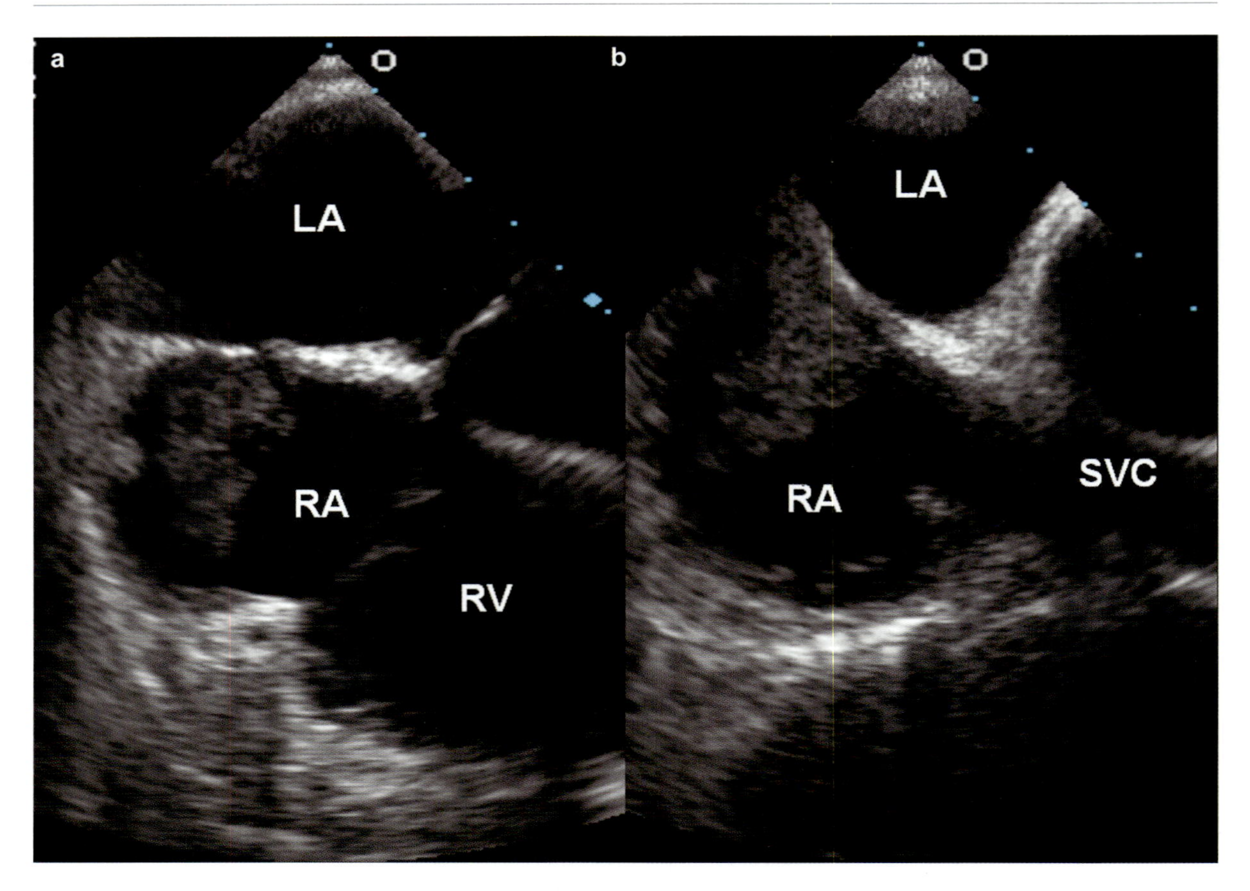

Fig. 13.20 This 55-year-old woman was investigated for pulmonary hypertension. The transesophageal transverse plane (**a**) and longitudinal plane (**b**) showed the presence of a right atrial myxoma with typical attachment near the foramen ovale. *LA* left atrium, *RA* right atrium, *RV* right ventricle, *SVC* superior vena cava

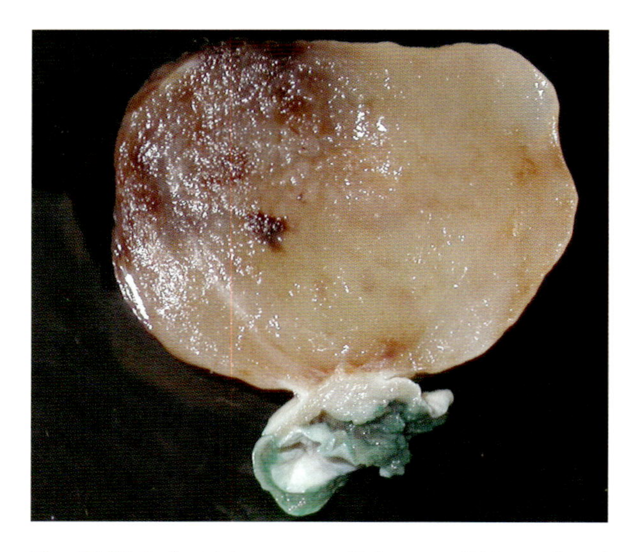

Fig. 13.21 Left atrial myxoma which was solid but soft and gelatinous. It showed a stalk and was excised with a cuff of atrial septum where it was attached

lack the capacity for metastasis or invasion. Although the behavior of the cardiac rhabdomyoma is benign, its positioning within critical areas in the heart can lead to lethal arrhythmias and chamber obstruction. The natural history of these lesions is to spontaneously regress. Rhabdomyomas are usually detected prenatally or during the first year of life. They account for over 60% of all primary cardiac tumors. Studies have demonstrated that the incidence of cardiac rhabdomyoma is 0.002–0.25% at autopsy, 0.02–0.08% in liveborn infants, and 0.12% in prenatal reviews [24]. There is an increasing clinical recognition of cardiac rhabdomyomas in utero due to use of ultrasound imaging as part of routine prenatal screening.

Cardiac rhabdomyomas frequently occur in association with tuberous sclerosis, an autosomal dominant inherited or sporadically occurring disorder characterized by widespread hamartomas that variably involve the brain, kidneys, heart, skin, and other organs. Half the individuals with tuberous sclerosis will develop a cardiac rhabdomyoma. Similarly, approximately, about half the children diagnosed with cardiac rhabdomyomas will demonstrate clinical or radiological evidence of tuberous sclerosis or have a positive family history. Genetic analysis has identified two disease genes: TSC-1 on chromosome 9q34 encodes for the protein hamartin and TSC-2 on 16p13 encodes for tuberin [23]. These proteins are both tumor suppressor genes that appear to assist in the regulation of growth and differentiation of developing cardiomyocytes.

Cardiac rhabdomyomas range from 1 mm to 10 cm in greatest dimension and can be single or multiple (Fig. 13.22). Cardiac rhabdomyomas most frequently arise in the ventricular myocardium, but may be located in the atria, epicardial surface, or cavo-atrial junction. Larger lesions can lead to obstruction of inflow or outflow tracts. Rhabdomyomas are round or lobulated and grossly well circumscribed. They possess a solid tan-white homogeneous consistency and are often watery and glistening on cut surface. Calcification and hemorrhage are infrequent. Intracavitary extension can occur in as many as half of the cases.

By microscopy, rhabdomyomas are well-circumscribed nodules that lack a capsule, but are distinct from the normal surrounding myocardium. The rhabdomyoma cells are round or polygonal in shape and are enlarged with clear cytoplasm. The clear cytoplasm is secondary to loss of glycogen that occurs during standard slide preparation techniques. Glycogen reacts strongly with periodic acid Schiff (PAS) stain. The nuclei of the rhabdomyoma cells are central or eccentrically located. In some cells, eosinophilic septae stretch from the cell membrane to a centrally placed nucleus, imparting a "spider-like" appearance to the cell. These "spider cells" are pathognomonic for cardiac rhabdomyomas. The septae of spider cells stain strongly for ubiquitin by immunostaining. The ubiquitin pathway facilitates myofilament degradation, intracytoplasmic glycogen vacuolization, and the production of spider cells. Spider cells then undergo apoptosis, myxoid degeneration, and regression of the rhabdomyoma. The myogenous origin of rhabdomyoma cells is demonstrated by the strong expression of striated muscle markers including actin, myoglobin, vimentin, and desmin. Ubiquitin, hamartin, and tuberin are also positive. Proliferation markers such as MIB-1 are negative.

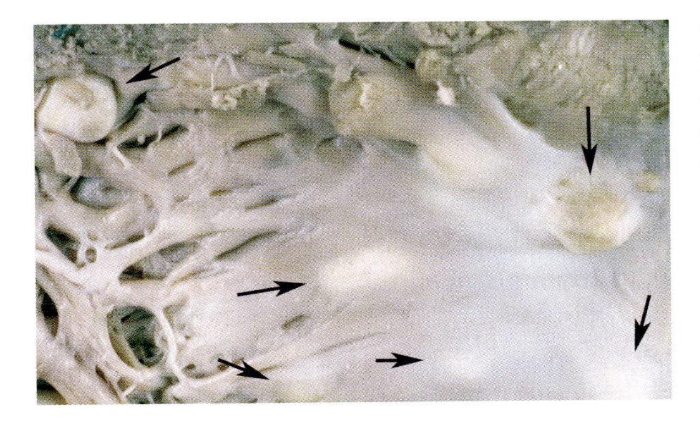

Fig. 13.22 Opened ventricle of a child with multiple rhabdomyomas. These are small white myocardial nodules seen under the endocardium and also protruding into the endocardial cavity (*arrows*)

The clinical features of cardiac rhabdomyomas are variable and are dependent upon the location, size, and number of lesions [21–23]. Symptoms arise due to chamber or valve obstruction, arrhythmias or failure from extensive myocardial involvement. Tumors obstructing the right-sided inflow or the outflow of the ventricles can lead to decreased cardiac output, atrial and caval hypertension, hydrops fetalis, and death. Arrhythmias, both ventricular and atrial, are not uncommon. Wolff–Parkinson–White syndrome has been observed in a higher proportion of patients with tuberous sclerosis, as compared to the general population. Death may occur due to obstruction of ventricular blood flow, arrhythmias, valve stenosis, or from loss of functional myocardium secondary to extensive tumor involvement.

Rhabdomyomas are frequently diagnosed by fetal echocardiography during the prenatal period. Multiple lesions are often associated with tuberous sclerosis. Cardiac rhabdomyomas appear as well-circumscribed homogenous hyperechoic masses that most frequently involve the ventricles, but can be found at any location in the heart (Fig. 13.23). They frequently regress spontaneously (Fig. 13.24). Small multiple lesions may manifest as a thickened myocardium on ultrasound and magnetic resonance imaging (MRI). MRI is utilized if the results of echocardiography are inconclusive or if aggressive surgical management is being planned. On MR imaging, rhabdomyomas have a signal intensity similar to that of myocardium on T1-weighted images. On T2-weighted images, the signal intensity is increased. MRI is also used to evaluate the presence of tuberous sclerosis involving the brain, kidneys, and liver.

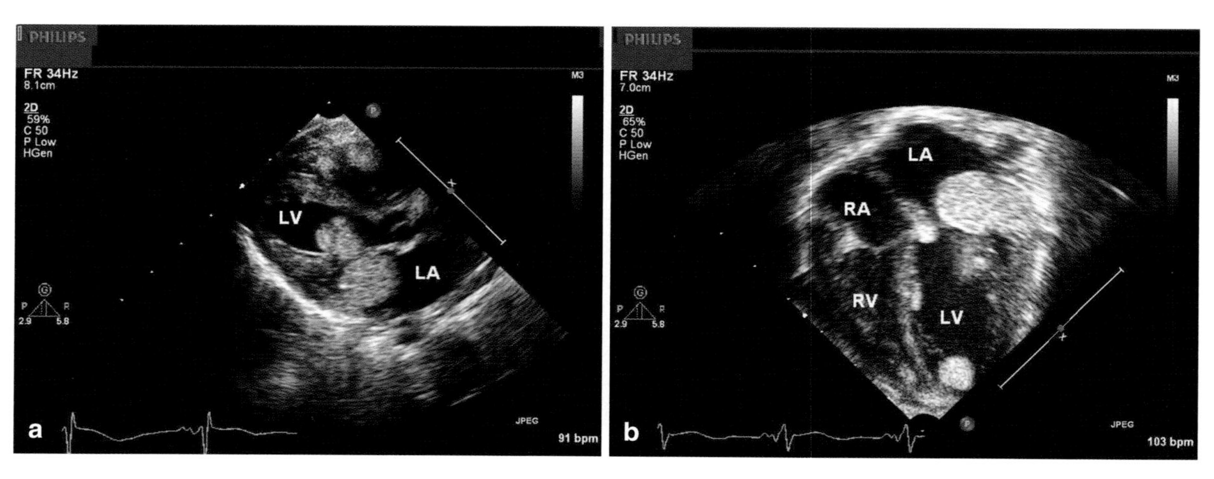

Fig. 13.23 (**a**) Parasternal long-axis view in a neonate showing multiple intracardaic masses consistent with rhabdomyomas. Tumors are present in the right ventricle, left atrium, and left ventricle. (**b**) Apical four-chamber views show an additional tumor in the left ventricular apex (Figures provided by Dr. J. Lougheed). *LA* left atrium, *LV* left ventricle

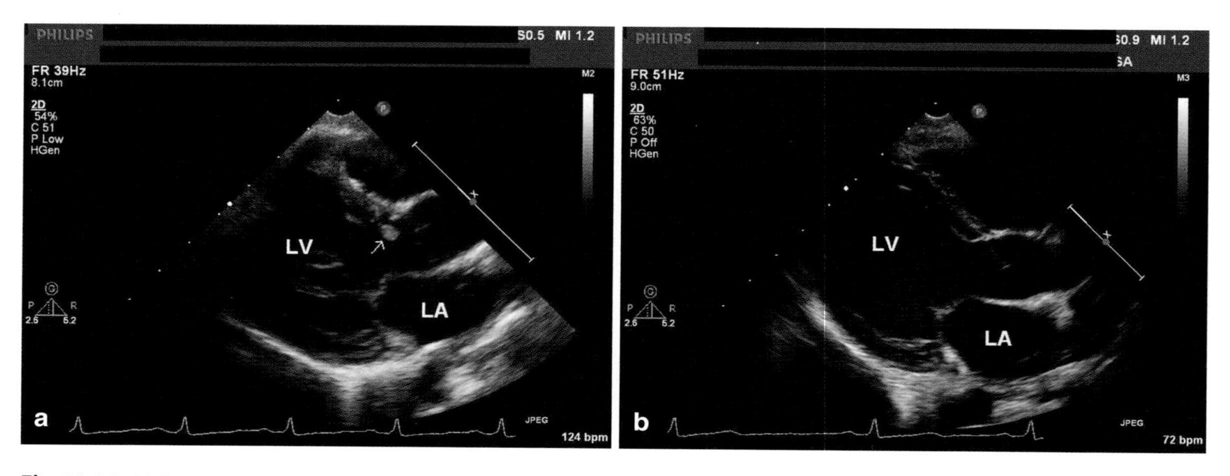

Fig. 13.24 (**a**) Parasternal long-axis view in a child shows a mass (*arrow*) in the left ventricular outflow tract. (**b**) A follow-up study shows that the mass has spontaneously regressed (Figures provided by Dr. J. Lougheed). *LA* left atrium, *LV* left ventricle

Papillary Fibroelastoma

Cardiac papillary fibroelastoma (PFE) is the second most common benign tumor of the heart, commonly occurring on heart valves [25]. PFE is the most common primary tumor of cardiac valves. PFE can occur in any age-group, with the majority occurring in adults and the highest prevalence in the eighth decade. They occur most frequently on valvular surfaces, particularly on aortic and mitral valves.

The majority are asymptomatic. Common presenting symptoms include stroke or transient ischemic attack, followed by angina, myocardial infarction, sudden death, heart failure, and embolism. Large tumor size, left-sided location, and particularly increased tumor mobility are echocardiographic features associated with embolism [26].

PFEs consist of multiple fibroelastic papillae originating from a stalk. They resemble a polyp or a sea anemone (Figs. 13.25–13.27). They are usually solitary but multiple lesions have been reported after radiation or open heart surgery. Histologically, these avascular papillary fronds consist of collagen, proteoglycans, and elastic fibers. The resemblance to Lambl's excrescences has led to the suggestion of a common pathoetiology, perhaps from trauma or organized thrombus. Other

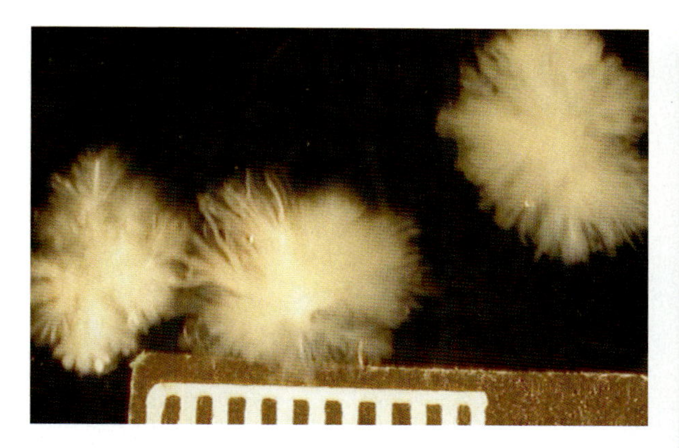

Fig. 13.25 These are multiple aortic valve papillary fibroelastomas. They are photographed in water allowing demonstration of their multiple thin sea anemone-like fronds

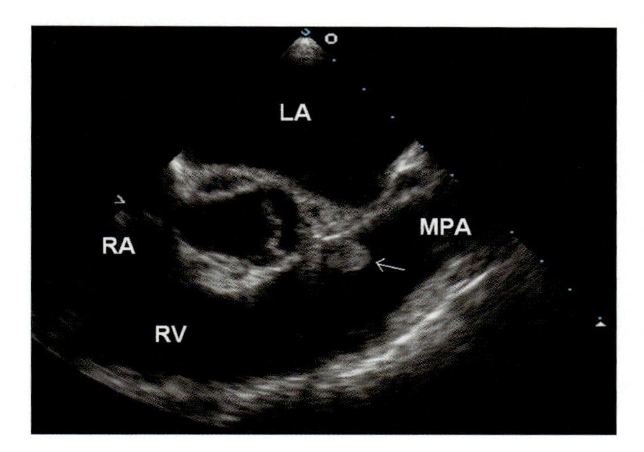

Fig. 13.26 There is a mobile mass (*arrow*) attached to the pulmonic valve in this 64-year-old woman. She had a history of malignant melanoma which had been resected. The pulmonic valvular mass was excised and was a papillary fibroelastoma. *LA* left atrium, *MPA* main pulmonary artery, *RA* right atrium, *RV* right ventricle

suggested etiologies include congenital origin, or complications of valve degeneration, cytomegalovirus, or cardiac surgery.

If a PFE is detected, it is usually surgically resected [27]. The treatment of an asymptomatic patient or an incidentally found lesion is less clear. Large, left-sided mobile tumors should be excised to prevent sudden death and emboli. Small, nonmobile tumors may be followed with serial echocardiography and removed if they increase in size, become mobile or symptomatic (Fig. 13.28).

PFEs are usually pedunculated and can be easily surgically removed with associated endocardial tissue.

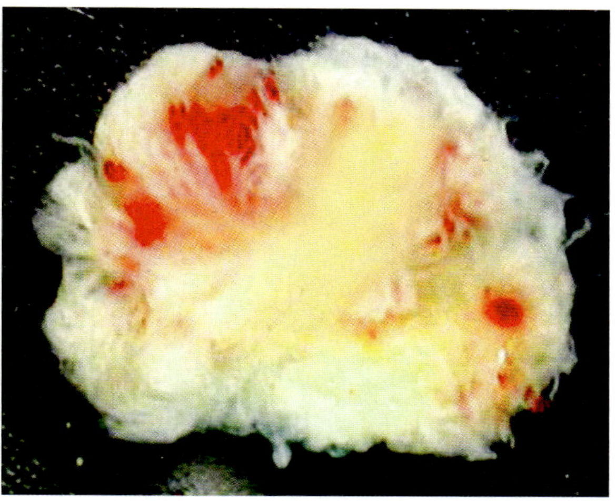

Fig. 13.27 This is the papillary fibroelastoma removed from the pulmonary valve of the patient in Fig. 13.26. This was a relatively large compact tumor, but when put in water, the multiple fronds were evident

Valve shaving can be done with little removal of the underlying valve. Care should be taken to avoid fragmentation to prevent embolization. Any resulting valve defects can be closed primarily or with autologous pericardium. Valve repair is preferred. Surgical resection is curative, safe, and well tolerated.

Patients who are not surgical candidates can be treated with systemic anticoagulation or antiplatelet agents to reduce thrombus formation, although there is no clear evidence to support this. Some think that the embolic events associated with a PFE are not due to the tumor itself, but rather due to thrombus that gets entrapped in the fronds of the PFE [28]. Antiplatelet agents may thus be indicated.

Other Benign Neoplasms

Lipomas are usually intramyocardial tumors which affect both sexes equally. They have a typical echodense appearance and have been associated with cardiac arrhythmia (Fig. 13.29).

Fibromas are more commonly seen in children. They are intramyocardial and generally affect the ventricular septum or the left ventricular free-wall. They tend to be solitary and can be large [29]. Cardiac fibromas may be a neoplasm, or some consider them to be a fibrous hamartoma. They may present with ventricular

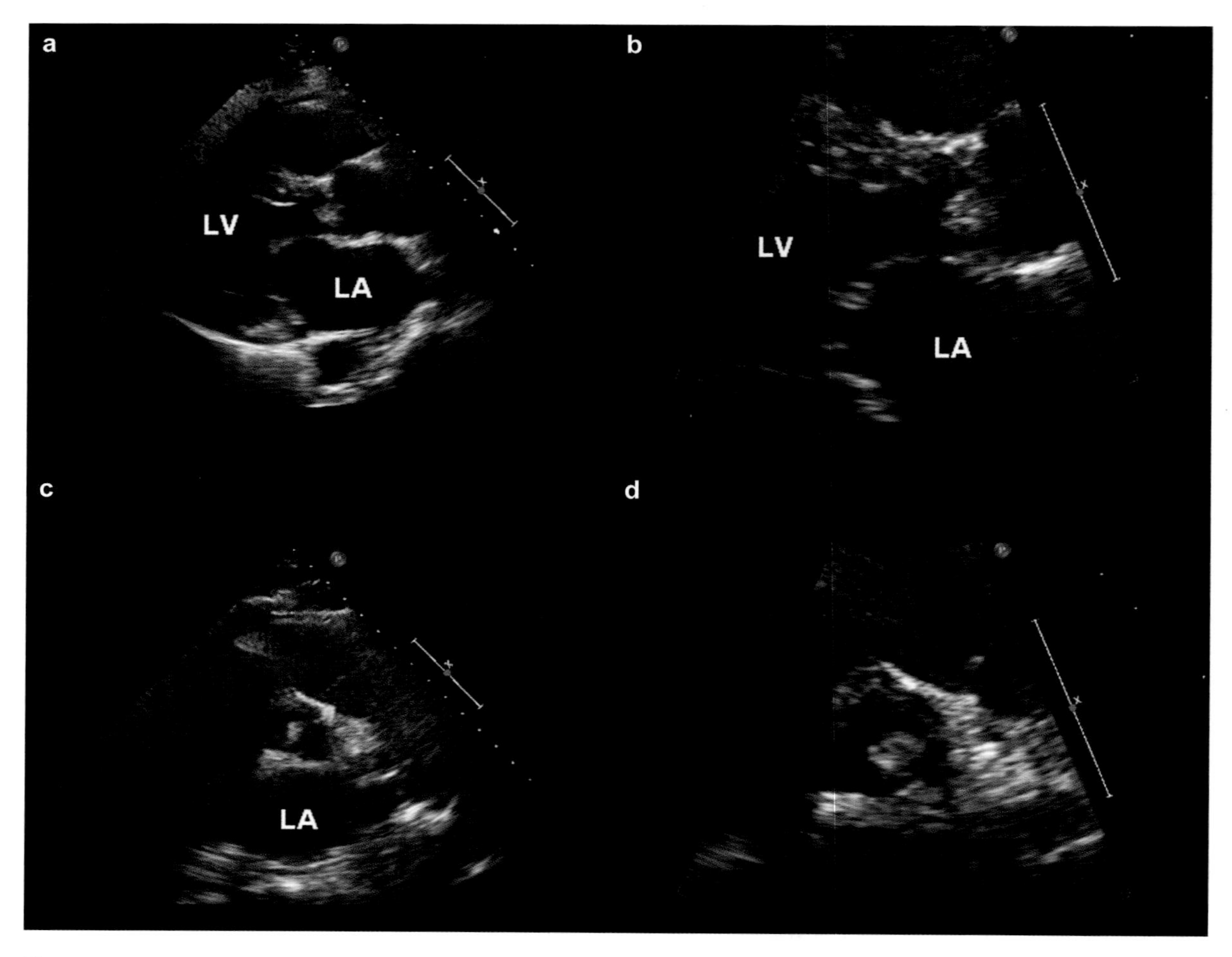

Fig. 13.28 The parasternal long-axis (**a**, **d**) and short-axis (**c**, **d**) views show that there is a small sessile mass on the left coronary cusp of the aortic valve consistent with a papillary fibroelastoma. This is an incidental finding in a 72-year-old woman who has not had surgical excision of this aortic valvular mass. *LA* left atrium, *LV* left ventricle

arrhythmias or become large enough to distort the ventricle causing flow obstruction or heart failure [30]. Cardiac fibromas often bulge into the chamber lumen. They are firm or rubbery and do not demonstrate hemorrhage or necrosis (Fig. 13.30). They are usually white or tan in color and seem well circumscribed and distinct from the surrounding myocardium. Calcifications are typically present, a useful finding on routine imaging. The microscopic features of fibromas show fibroblasts and dense mature collagen. Elastic fibers can be identified with the use of special stains. The fibroblast cells are not atypical and the mitotic rate is low, if any are found. There is no necrosis but calcification is frequently observed. At the edge, the tumor interdigitates with the adjacent normal myocardium and the neoplasm is not actually circumscribed.

Treatment of a fibroma is usually by surgical excision [30]. It may be tempting for the surgeon just to shell these hard masses out of the myocardium, but this would lead to incomplete resection and possible recurrence. As complete as possible excision is recommended but leaving tumor at the margin is common. The fibroma could recur but they are slow growing.

A cardiac hamartoma is composed of an overgrowth of mature cells and tissue. Vascular, mesenchymal, and hamartoma of mature cardiac myocytes are possible [31]. These are usually intramyocardial and do not become invasive. They can be associated with arrhythmia. The

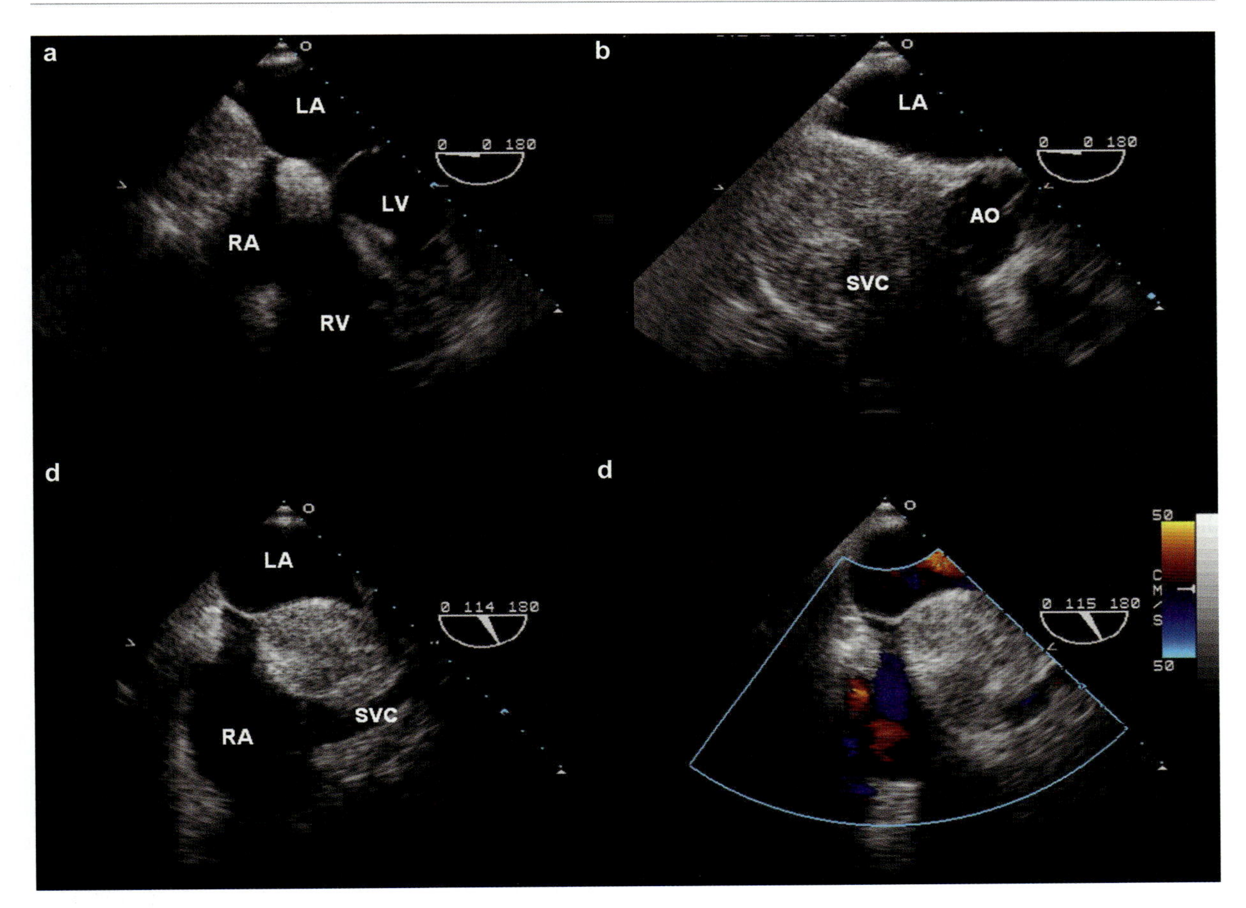

Fig. 13.29 The transesophageal views (**a, b, c**) show that the atrial septum is echo-dense and massively hypertrophied with sparing of the foramen ovale. These findings are consistent with lipomatous hypertrophy of the atrial septum. Despite the severe nature of lipomatous infiltration of the atrial septum and right atrial wall, there is no obstruction to intracardiac blood flow (**d**). *LA* left atrium, *LV* left ventricle, *RA* right atrium, *RV* right ventricle, *SVC* superior vena cava

echo features of hamartoma are similar to those of fibroma (Figs. 13.31, 13.32a, b).

Primary Malignant Cardiac Tumors

Sarcoma

Up to a quarter of the primary cardiac tumors can be malignant. Cardiac sarcomas represent a significant diagnostic challenge. They frequently involve the atria, and pericardial invasion is common. Pericarditis is a typical clinical presentation. Careful echocardiographic examination will show that the tumor is generally wide based and extends beyond anatomic boundaries. For instance, a left atrial sarcoma can usually involve adjacent pulmonary vein and invade the right atrium or pericardium. Sarcomas are the most common primary malignancy, accounting for 70–80% or more of malignancies in some series [2, 5, 7, 32]. Like lymphomas, the classification of sarcomas has changed with modern diagnostic immunohistochemical and molecular modalities, and thus reclassification of some cases in the literature is possible and not unexpected.

There are predominantly three groups of cardiac sarcomas that pose a diagnostic challenge: (a) spindle cell neoplasms, (b) pleomorphic or giant cell neoplasms, and (c) small cell or round cell neoplasms. Spindle cell carcinoma can usually be ruled out either by sampling or immunohistochemistry. Lymphomas, carcinomas, and mesothelioma may mimic giant cell or pleomorphic sarcoma. A panel of immunostains

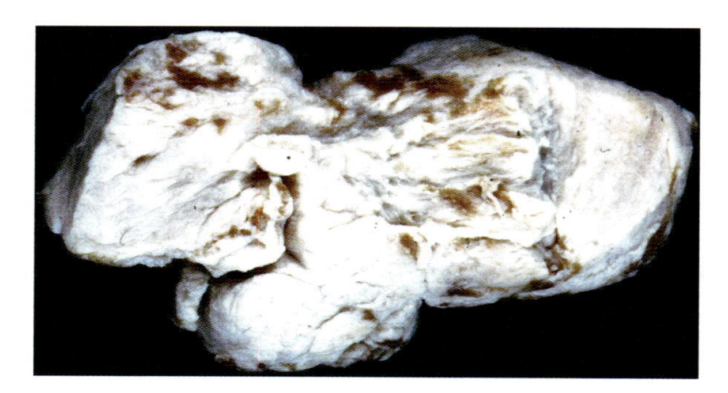

Fig. 13.30 This large cardiac fibroma tumor was removed from the left ventricle. It was white on cut surface. It had small calcifications which were noted on chest X-ray. Small pieces of red myocardium remain on the surface

that includes leukocyte common antigen (LCA), cytokeratins AE1/AE3, B72.3, epithelial membrane antigen (EMA), carcinoembryonic antigen (CEA), and vimentin are invaluable in the distinction. Round cell sarcomas can be confused with hematogenous malignancies, and small cell carcinoma. Many of these neoplasms may be distinguished by electron microscopy or molecular diagnosis for specific chromosomal or gene product detection. Some of these ancillary studies could be done retrospectively on paraffin-embedded tissue, while others require fresh tissue.

Angiosarcoma is the most common sarcoma encountered in the heart. It is typically on the right side of the heart with pericardial involvement [33] (Figs. 13.33, 13.34). The tumor forms bulky hemorrhagic masses often with bloody pericardial effusion (Fig. 13.35). The heart may seem to be encased with the hemorrhagic mass. By microscopy, the histological pattern may be as variable as soft tissue extracardiac angiosarcoma. Some are spindle cell neoplasms. Some have atypical endothelial cells with vascular spaces full of blood. Others may be high grade, or epitheloid. Factor VIII or CD31 immunostains are usually positive. Angiosarcomas are usually unresectable. They may be treated with a pericardial window or a limited pericardiectomy. Metastases may occur outside the heart. Often, death is from heart failure, constriction, and tamponade.

Left-sided sarcomas may clinically mimic atrial myxomas and thus be encountered by the surgical pathologist [34]. They are soft and polypoid but unlike myxoma, they are located away from the interatrial septum and may invade the atrial wall, the extracardiac soft tissues, or extend into the pulmonary veins (Fig. 13.36). These are often spindle cell sarcomas, resembling malignant fibrous histiocytoma, leiomyosarcoma, fibrosarcoma, myxoid fibrosarcoma, osteosarcoma, or

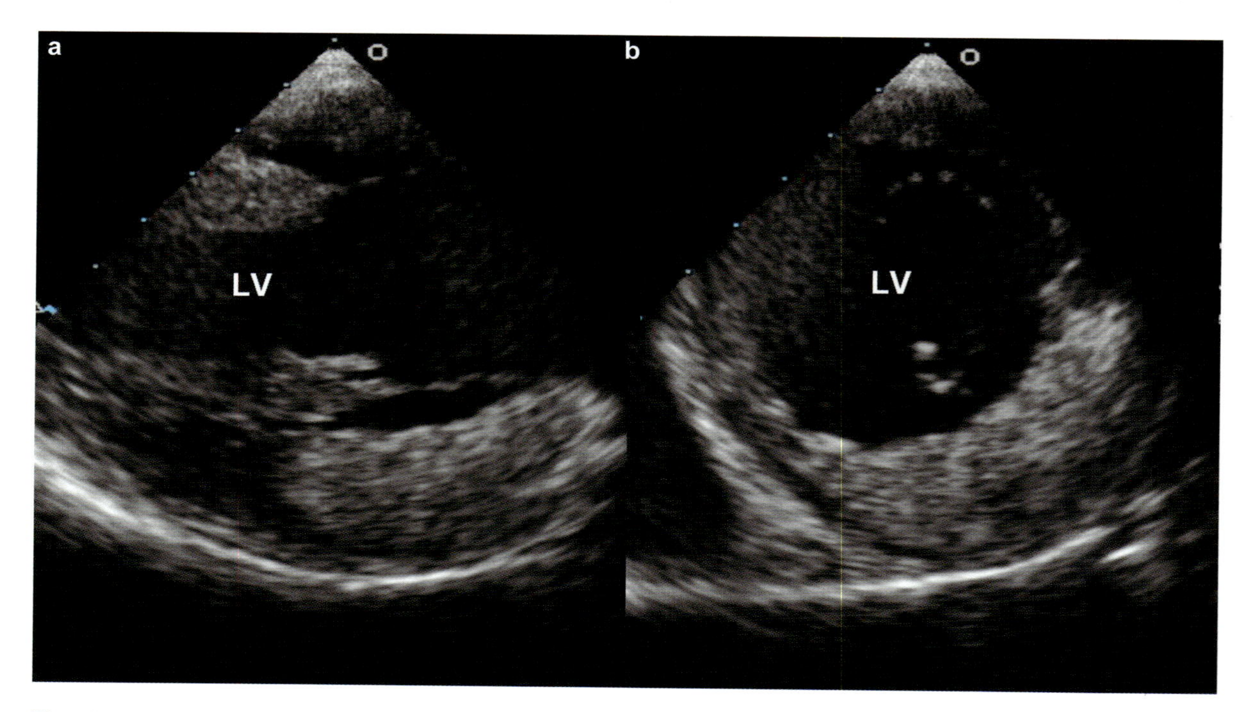

Fig. 13.31 This young woman presented with a cardiac arrest and ventricular arrhythmias. The transesophageal transgastric views of the left ventricle in long-axis (**a**) and short-axis (**b**) demonstrated a well-defined intramyocardial mass in the basal and mid anterior wall of the left ventricle. She had surgery and this was a hamartoma. *LV* left ventricle

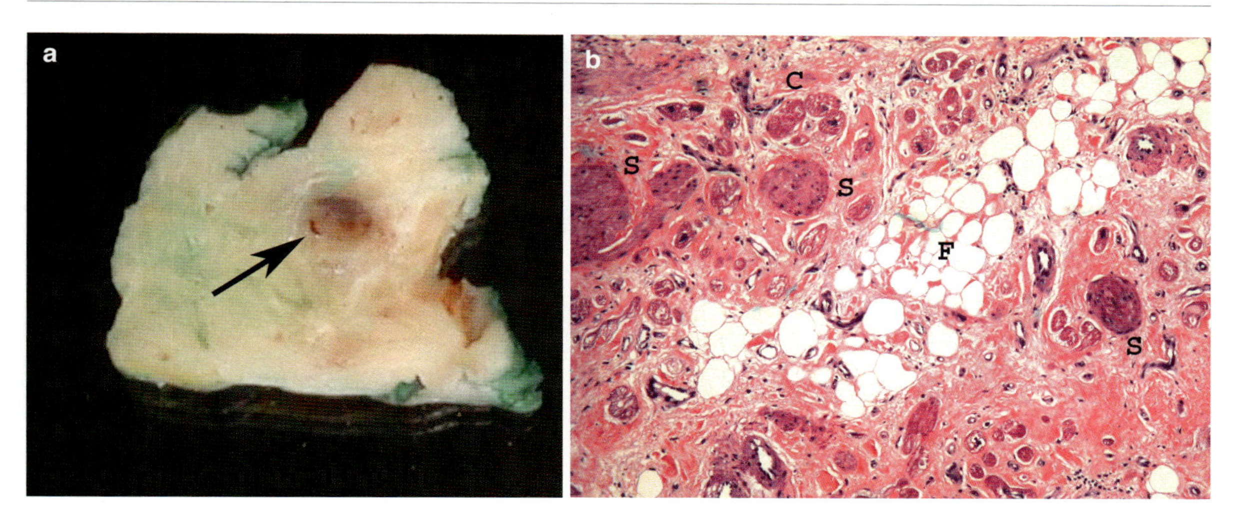

Fig. 13.32 (**a**) This is the left ventricle hamartoma removed from the patient in Fig. 13.31. It was soft, tan, and had red nodular areas (*arrow*). (**b**) By microscopy, this is a mesenchymal hamartoma composed of cardiac myocytes (*C*), smooth muscle (*S*), blood vessels, nerves, and fat (*F*). These are all mature elements and such a hamartoma is benign

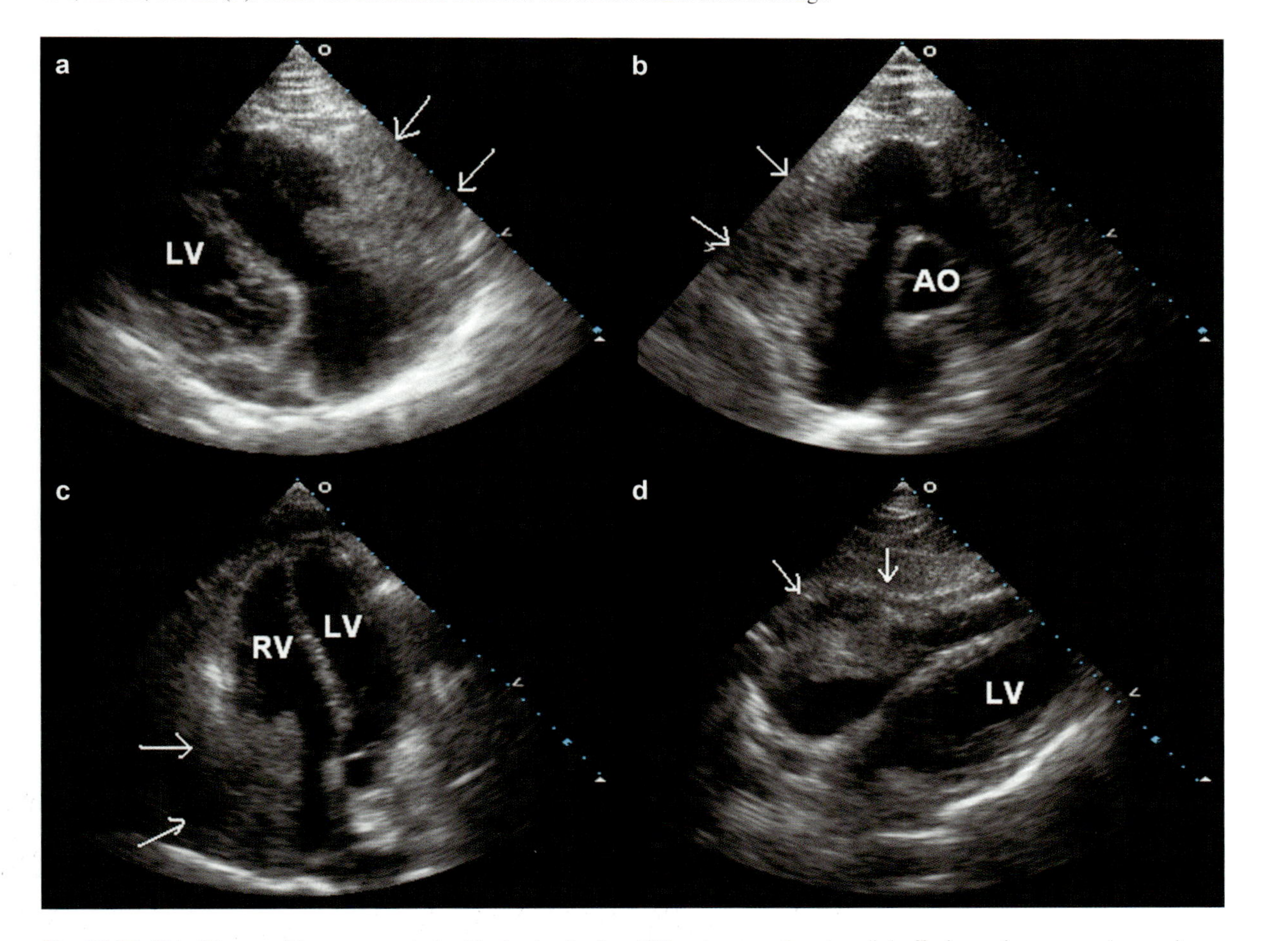

Fig. 13.33 This 30-year-old man presented with chest pain. In addition to a small pericardial effusion, a large mass (*arrows*) was present involving both the right atrial and right ventricular free-wall, with protrusion into the right atrium. The mass is imaged in the right ventricular inflow (**a**), parasternal short-axis (**b**), apical four-chamber (**c**), and subcostal (**d**) views. Involvement of the pericardium (*arrows*) by this large mass is clearly demonstrated in the subcostal view (**d**). Biopsy confirmed that this was an angiosarcoma. *Ao* aorta, *LV* left ventricle, *RV* right ventricle

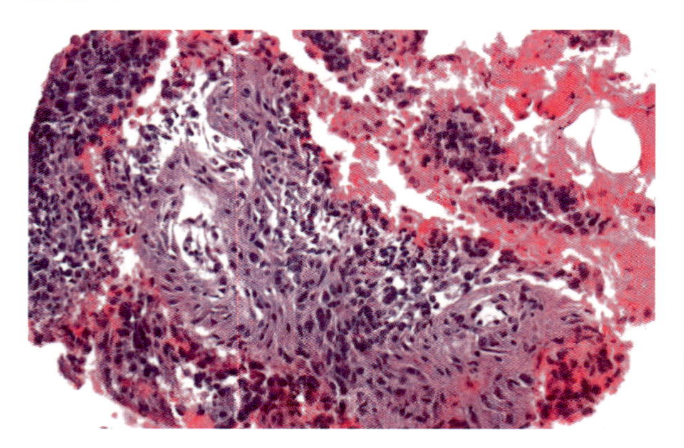

Fig. 13.34 This is the angiosarcoma tissue from the same patient in Fig. 13.33. The cytology examination of the pericardial fluid demonstrated clusters of malignant spindle cells with blood vessels and blood. Immunostaining was positive for endothelial cell markers such as CD 31, confirming the vascular nature of the sarcoma

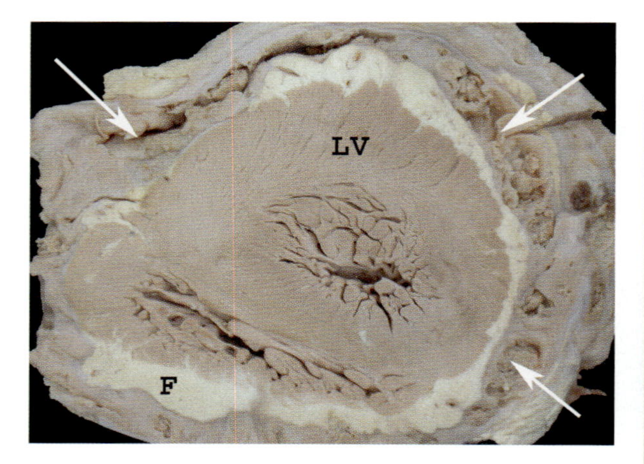

Fig. 13.35 Autopsy heart cut in short axis. This is a patient with angiosarcoma. The heart is surrounded by tan, soft, sarcoma tumor mass involving the pericardium (*arrows*). *F* epicardial fat, *LV* left ventricle

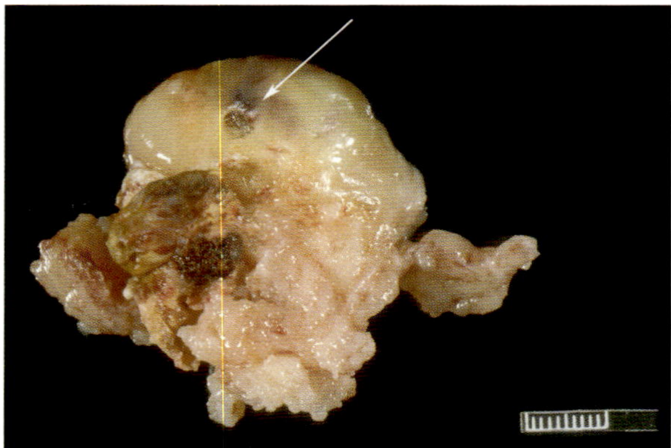

Fig. 13.36 This is a left atrial myxosarcoma surgically excised for relief of mitral stenosis-like symptoms. This sarcoma was on the posterior wall and infiltrated through the atrial wall and extended up and occluded an adjacent pulmonary vein. The surface defect (*arrow*) is from an endomyocardial biopsy done before the surgery. This transseptal biopsy confirmed the tissue diagnosis preoperatively. The patient's symptoms improved but metastatic disease followed

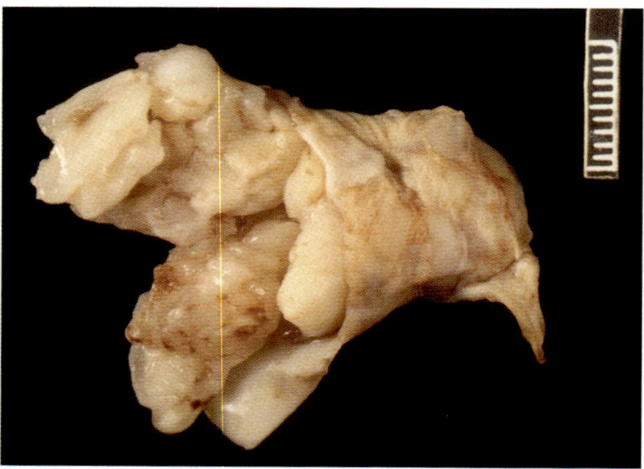

Fig. 13.37 This is a pulmonary artery myxosarcoma removed during pulmonary thromboendarterectomy procedure. The patient had dyspnea and was thought to have chronic thromboembolic pulmonary hypertension. The soft tumor fills the lumen. These sarcomas are of many tissue types and almost all patients do poorly

chondrosarcoma. Mitotic counts, cellularity, pleomorphism, and tumor necrosis are very important parameters in the grading and assessment of some of these tumors [35, 36]. Resection with atrial reconstruction may be attempted. Pulmonary resection may be necessary. Reoccurrence is common and these tumors also have a poor prognosis.

Tumors located in the right ventricle outflow tract are often in continuity with pulmonary trunk sarcoma (Fig. 13.37). Most of these are "intimal sarcomas" with no differentiation noted (myxosarcomas). Other types of sarcomas are also seen, including leiomyosarcomas, osteosarcomas, and chondrosarcomas. These right ventricle–pulmonary trunk sarcomas are usually soft, polypoid, and obstructive and are often associated with pulmonary embolic events. Growth along the great arteries or retrograde into the ventricle has been observed. Pulmonary metastases are common. They may clinically mimic pulmonary thromboembolism, saddle or chronic, and are associated with pulmonary hypertension [37, 38]. Sudden death from massive tumor embolization is possible. Resection may be attempted, often with lung segmentectomy or lobectomy, but the prognosis is still poor.

Metastatic Secondary Tumors

Metastatic disease of the heart is much more common than primary benign or malignant cardiac tumors [3]. Regardless of origin, the neoplasms may be clinically silent or present with signs and symptoms reflecting the location of the deposits. The common tumors that metastasize to the heart include breast carcinomas, gastric carcinoma, lung carcinoma, lymphomas, esophageal carcinomas, and melanomas [8]. Many of these are in close proximity and the metastasis may actually be local tumor invasion directly into the myocardium and the great arteries (Figs. 13.38, 13.39). Tumor may also extend into the heart via the caval veins or pulmonary veins. Renal cell carcinoma and hepatoma frequently invade the right atrium via the inferior vena cava (Fig. 13.40). Thus if a right atrial mass is present, careful scanning of the inferior vena cava should be performed. Finally, local lymph node metastatic deposits may enter the heart by direct invasion or via lymphatics.

Pericardial deposits are the most common metastatic location observed (Figs. 13.41, 13.42). These deposits cause pericarditis, hemorrhagic effusions, effusive constrictive pericarditis, or pericardial constriction. Hemopericardium with tamponade may occur. A pericardiectomy or a pericardial window may be required for treatment and diagnosis.

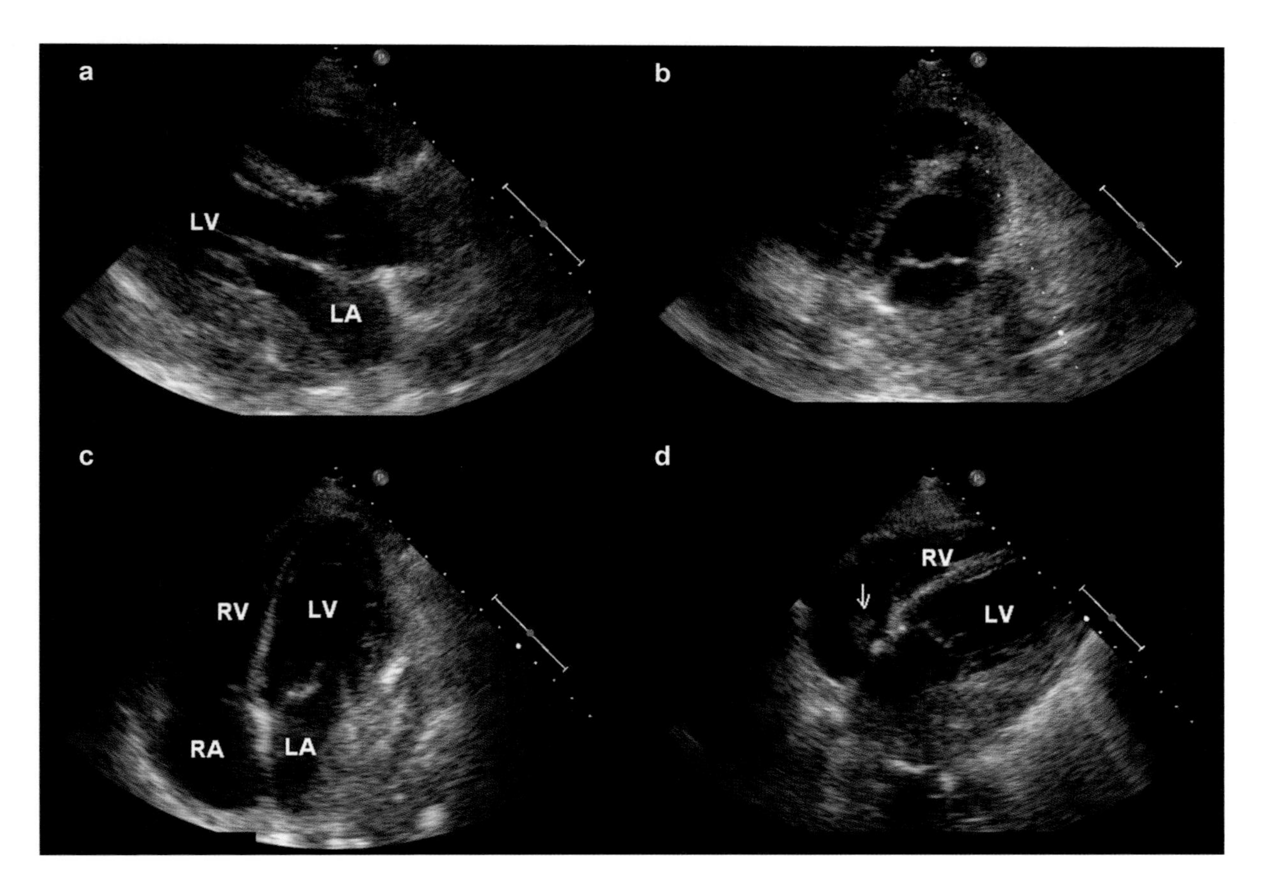

Fig. 13.38 In this patient with squamous cell lung carcinoma, metastatic invasion of the left atrium and left ventricle is demonstrated in the parasternal long-axis (**a**), short-axis (**b**), apical four-chamber (**c**), and subcostal four-chamber (**d**) views. Invasion into the right atrium (*arrow*) is detected in the subcostal view (**d**). *LA* left atrium, *LV* left ventricle, *RA* right atrium, *RV* right ventricle

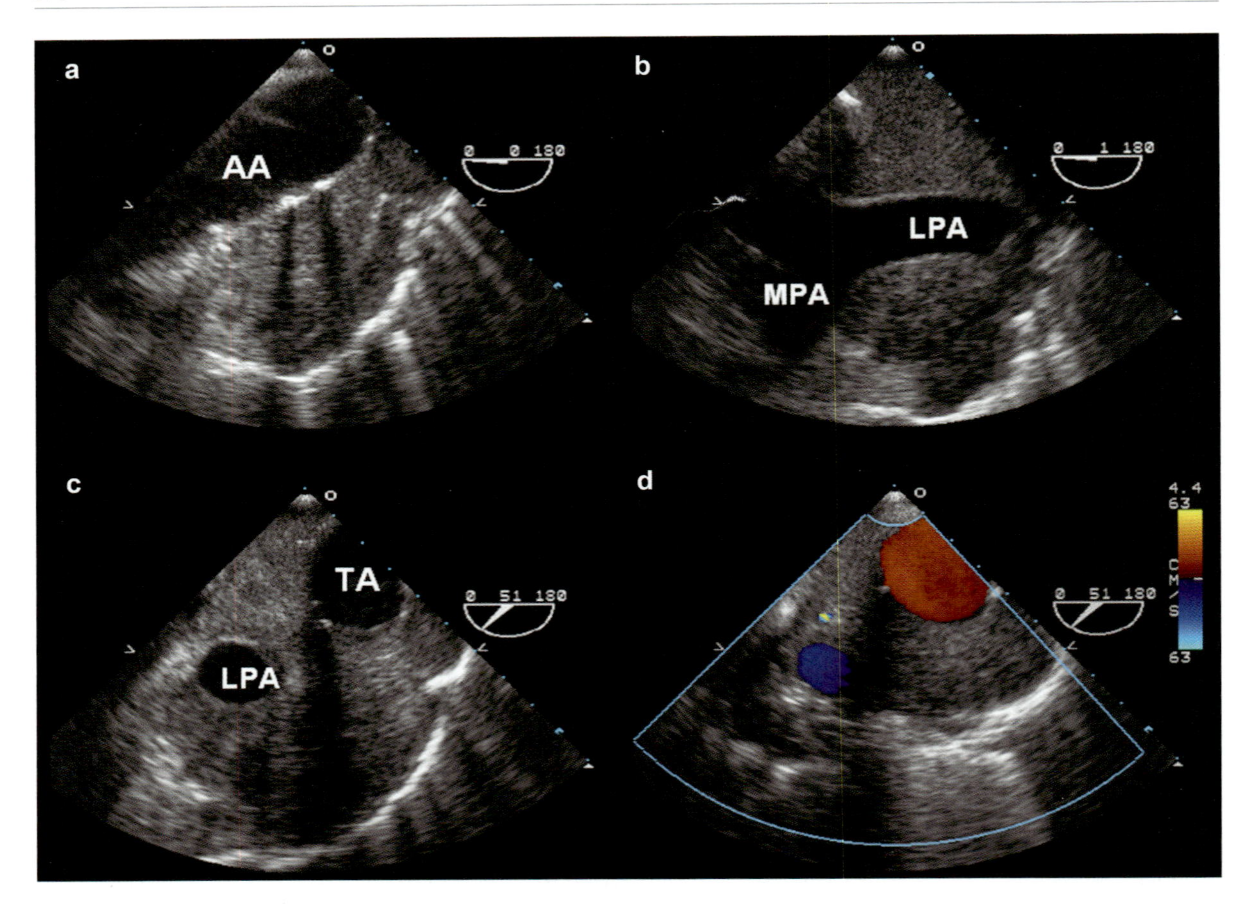

Fig. 13.39 In this patient with small cell carcinoma of the lung, extension of the tumor to involve the ascending aorta (**a**), the aortic arch (**c**), and the pulmonary arteries (**b**, **d**) is demonstrated by transesophageal echocardiography. No obstruction to aortic or pulmonary blood flow is detected. *AA* ascending aorta, *LPA* left pulmonary artery, *MPA* main pulmonary artery, *TA* transverse aorta

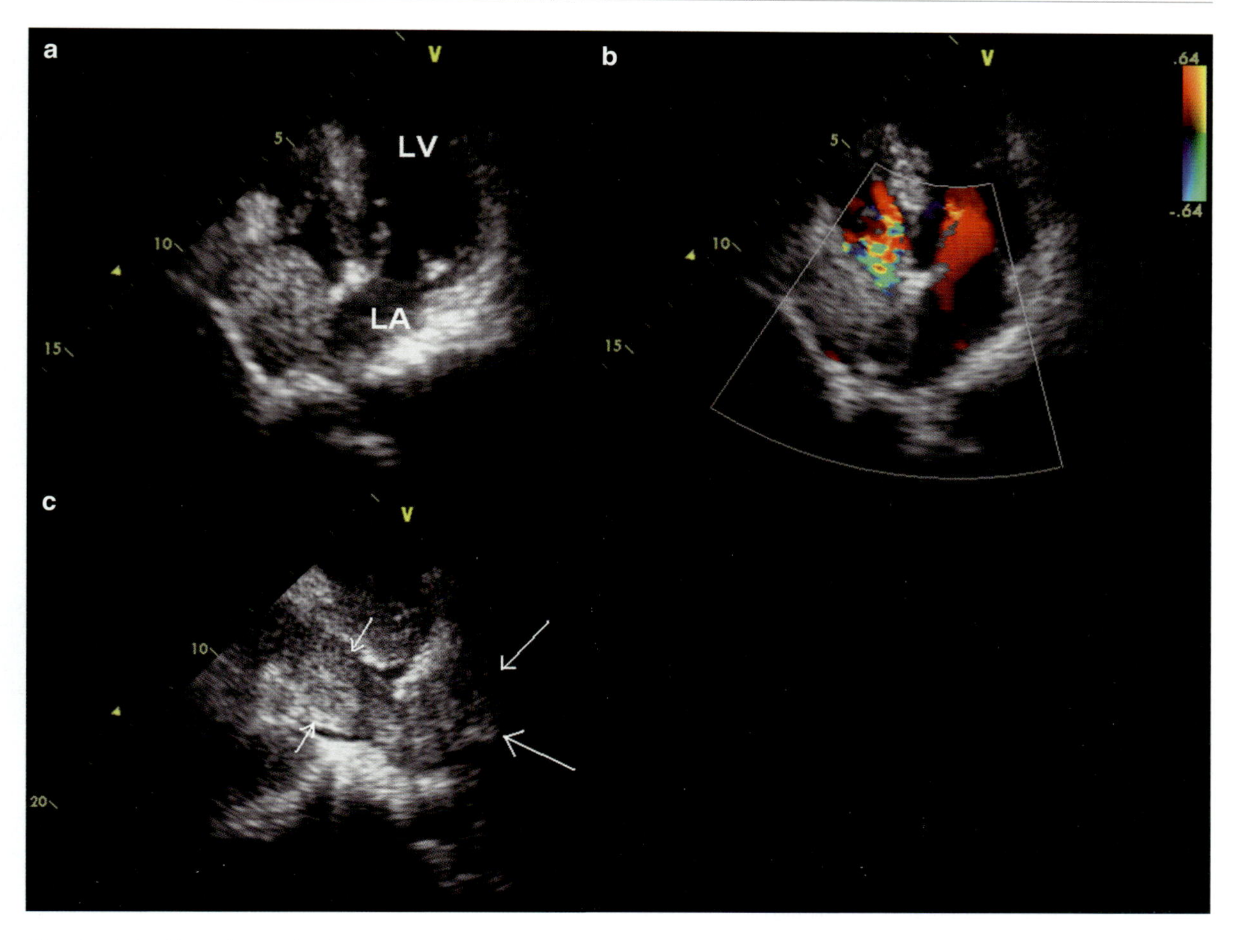

Fig. 13.40 In this patient with a hepatoma (hepatocellular carcinoma), there is a large mass in the right atrium in the four-chamber view (**a**). Color-flow imaging (**b**) shows that there is obstruction to venous flow into the right atrium. The subcostal view (**c**) shows that there is tumor infiltration of the inferior vena cava (*short arrows*) with protrusion into the right atrium (*long arrows*). *LA* left atrium, *LV* left ventricle

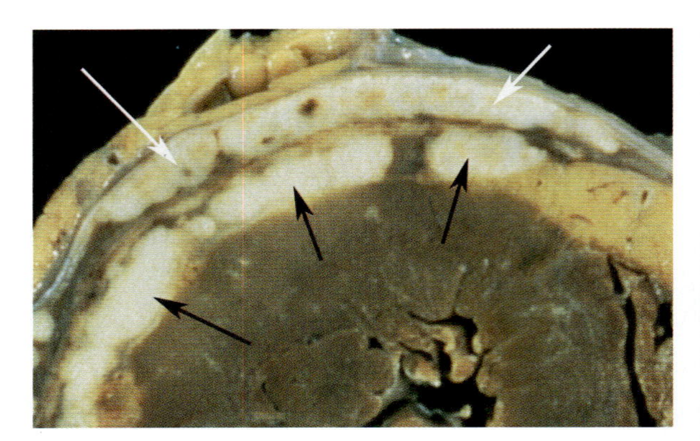

Fig. 13.41 Heart with metastatic carcinoma involving the pericardial surfaces (*arrows*). Such tumor deposits may cause effusion or constriction

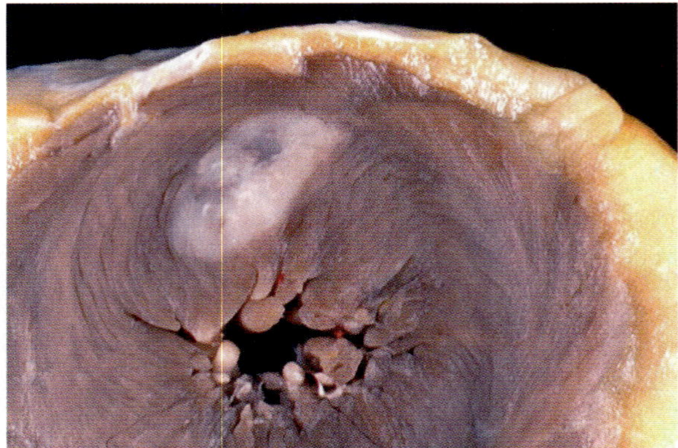

Fig. 13.43 Short axis cut showing the left ventricle with a well-circumscribed white deposit of lung carcinoma. Other metastatic deposits were present in the body

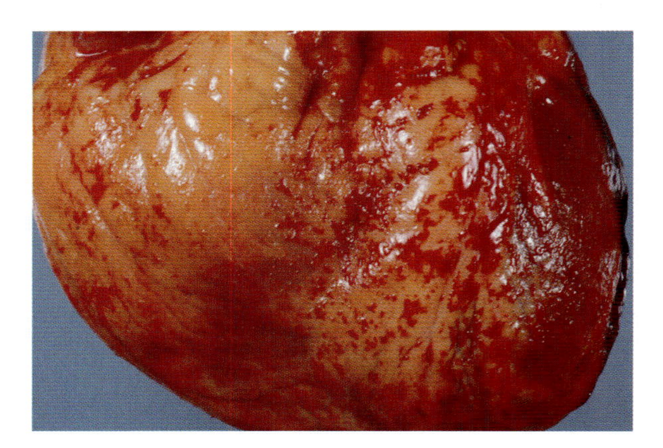

Fig. 13.42 External surface of the heart with metastatic carcinoma. There are multiple microscopic pericardial deposits that are seen only by microscopy. No masses are seen. The surface is bloody and there was a bloody pericardial effusion

Myocardial metastases are seen with melanomas and carcinomas (Fig. 13.43). They may be silent, cause arrhythmias, or form a mass lesion that interferes with ventricular function. Endocardial lesions may be polypoid. They may obstruct the chamber if they get large enough. Often, this type of metastatic deposit extends in from a vein.

Cardiac metastatic deposits are often accompanied by other extracardiac deposits. Resection is rarely attempted.

Summary

In the echocardiographic assessment of an intracardiac mass, a systematic approach is important to exclude artifacts, extracardiac mass, and normal structures. The location and morphologic features are helpful to differentiate thrombus from vegetation and from tumor. Associated findings and the clinical settings are very useful to the differential diagnosis. It is important to be aware of artifacts and learn how to avoid them. Always be mindful of extrinsic masses, which can be quite confusing. The location and typical morphologic features can be helpful, but need to be considered in the clinical context.

References

1. Wold LE, Lie JT. Cardiac myxomas: a clinicopathologic profile. *Am J Pathol*. 1980 Oct;101(1):219-240.
2. Chitwood WR Jr. Cardiac neoplasms: current diagnosis, pathology, and therapy. *J Card Surg*. 1988;3:119-154.
3. Lam KY, Dickens P, Chan ACL. Tumors of the heart: a 20-year experience with a review of 12, 485 consecutive autopsies. *Arch Pathol Lab Med*. 1993;117:1027-1031.
4. Reynen K. Frequency of primary tumors of the heart. *Am J Cardiol*. 1996;77:107.
5. Molina JE, Edwards JE, Ward HB. Primary cardiac tumors: experience at the University of Minnesota. *Thorac Cardiovasc Surg*. 1990;38:183-191.
6. Wiatrowska BA, Walley VM, Masters RG, Goldstein W, Keon WJ. Surgery for cardiac tumours: the University of Ottawa Heart Institute experience (1980–91). *Can J Cardiol*. 1993;9:65-72.
7. Burke A, Virmani R. Classification and incidence of cardiac tumors. Tumors of the heart and great vessels. Third series ed. Bethesda, MD: Armed Forces Institute of Pathology; 1996:1–12.
8. Abraham DP, Reddy V, Gattuso P. Neoplasms metastatic to the heart: review of 3314 consecutive autopsies. *Am J Cardiovasc Pathol*. 1990;3:195-198.

9. Majano-Lainez RA. Cardiac tumors: a current clinical and pathological perspective. *Crit Rev Oncog.* 1997;8(4): 293-303.
10. Shapiro LM. Cardiac tumours: diagnosis and management. *Heart.* 2001 Feb;85(2):218-222.
11. Veinot JP, Burns BF, Commons AS, Thomas J. Cardiac neoplasms at the Canadian Reference Centre for Cancer Pathology. *Can J Cardiol.* 1999 Mar;15(3):311-319.
12. Grebenc ML, Rosado de Christenson ML, Burke AP, Green CE, Galvin JR. Primary cardiac and pericardial neoplasms: radiologic-pathologic correlation. *Radiographics.* 2000 July; 20(4):1073-1103.
13. Perchinsky MJ, Lichtenstein SV, Tyers GF. Primary cardiac tumors: forty years' experience with 71 patients. *Cancer.* 1997;79(9):1809-1815.
14. Vaughan CJ, Veugelers M, Basson CT. Tumors and the heart: molecular genetic advances. *Curr Opin Cardiol.* 2001 May; 16(3):195-200.
15. Seguin JR, Beigbeder JY, Hvass U, et al. Interleukin 6 production by cardiac myxomas may explain constitutional symptoms. *J Thorac Cardiovasc Surg.* 1992 Mar;103(3): 599-600.
16. Scott N, Veinot JP, Chan KL. Symptoms in cardiac myxoma. *Chest.* 2003 Dec;124(6):2408.
17. Blondeau P. Primary cardiac tumors – French studies of 533 cases. *Thorac Cardiovasc Surg.* 1990 Aug;38(Suppl 2): 192-195.
18. Yoon DH, Roberts W. Sex distribution in cardiac myxomas. *Am J Cardiol.* 2002 Sept 1;90(5):563-565.
19. Carney JA. The Carney complex (myxomas, spotty pigmentation, endocrine overactivity, and schwannomas). *Dermatol Clin.* 1995 Jan;13(1):19-26.
20. Pessotto R, Santini F, Piccin C, Consolaro G, Faggian G, Mazzucco A. Cardiac myxoma of the tricuspid valve: description of a case and review of the literature. *J Heart Valve Dis.* 1994;3:344-346.
21. Burke AP, Virmani R. Cardiac rhabdomyoma: a clinicopathologic study. *Mod Pathol.* 1991 Jan;4(1):70-74.
22. Burke A, Virmani R. Pediatric heart tumors. *Cardiovasc Pathol.* 2008 Jul;17(4):193-198.
23. Jozwiak J, Sahin M, Jozwiak S, et al. *Cardiac rhabdomyoma in tuberous sclerosis: hyperactive Erk signaling Int J Cardiol.* 2009;132:145-147.
24. Isaacs H Jr. Fetal and neonatal cardiac tumors. *Pediatr Cardiol.* 2004 May;25(3):252-273.
25. Roberts WC. Papillary fibroelastomas of the heart [editorial]. *Am J Cardiol.* 1997 Oct 1;80(7):973-975.
26. Gowda RM, Khan IA, Nair CK, Mehta NJ, Vasavada BC, Sacchi TJ. Cardiac papillary fibroelastoma: a comprehensive analysis of 725 cases. *Am Heart J.* 2003 Sept;146(3): 404-410.
27. Boodhwani M, Veinot JP, Hendry PJ. Surgical approach to cardiac papillary fibroelastomas. *Can J Cardiol.* 2007 Mar 15;23(4):301-302.
28. Veinot JP. Fibroelastoma and embolic stroke. *Circulation.* 1999 May 25;99(20):2709-2712.
29. Veinot JP, O'Murchu B, Tazelaar HD, Orszulak TA, Seward JB. Cardiac fibroma mimicking apical hypertrophic cardiomyopathy: a case report and differential diagnosis. *J Am Soc Echocardiogr.* 1996;9(1):94-99.
30. Burke AP, Rosado-de-Christenson M, Templeton PA, Virmani R. Cardiac fibroma: clinicopathologic correlates and surgical treatment. *J Thorac Cardiovasc Surg.* 1994; 108:862-870.
31. Burke AP, Ribe JK, Bajaj AK, Edwards WD, Farb A, Virmani R. Hamartoma of mature cardiac myocytes. *Hum Pathol.* 1998 Sep;29(9):904-909.
32. Murphy MC, Sweeney MS, Putnam JBJ, et al. Surgical treatment of cardiac tumors: a 25-year experience. *Ann Thorac Surg.* 1990;49:612-618.
33. Butany J, Yu W. Cardiac angiosarcoma: two cases and a review of the literature. *Can J Cardiol.* 2000 Feb;16(2): 197-205.
34. Chan KL, Veinot J, Leach A, Bedard P, Smith S, Marquis JF. Diagnosis of left atrial sarcoma by transvenous endocardial biopsy. *Can J Cardiol.* 2001 Feb;17(2):206-208.
35. Burke AP, Cowan D, Virmani R. Primary sarcomas of the heart. *Cancer.* 1992;69:387-395.
36. Raaf HN, Raaf JH. Sarcomas related to the heart and vasculature. *Semin Surg Oncol.* 1994 Sep;10(5):374-382.
37. Dennie CJ, Veinot JP, McCormack DG, Rubens FD. Intimal Sarcoma of the pulmonary arteries seen as a mosaic pattern of lung attenuation on high-resolution CT. *AJR Am J Roentgenol.* 2002 May;178(5):1208-1210.
38. Burke AP, Virmani R. Sarcomas of the great vessels. A clinicopathologic study. *Cancer.* 1993 Mar 1;71(5):1761-1773.

Table 14.1 Segmental analysis in patients with suspected congenital heart disease

Location of atria (situs) Solitus – RA on right side Inversus – RA on left side Ambiguous – undifferentiated atria/two similar atria
Location and relationship of ventricles D-loop – morphologic RV anterior and to the right L-loop – morphologic RV posterior and to the left
Relationship and connections of the great arteries Concordant – aorta arising from LV and pulmonary artery from RV Discordant (transposition) – aorta arising from RV and pulmonary artery from LV Double outlet – both aorta and pulmonary artery arising from RV or LV

RA right atrium, *RV* right ventricle, *LV* left ventricle

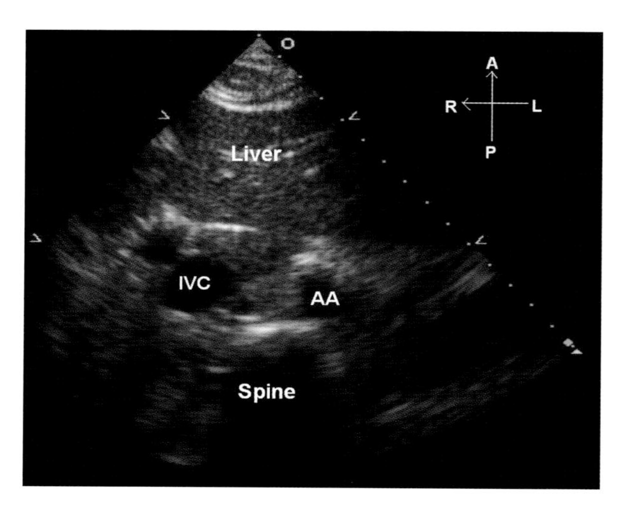

Fig. 14.1 The subcostal view is used to demonstrate cardiac situs. This short-axis view in situs solitus shows that the abdominal aorta is located leftward and slightly posterior to the inferior vena cava. *A* anterior, *AA* abdominal aorta, *IVC* inferior vena cava, *L* left, *P* posterior, *R* right

functions as the systemic ventricle, and assumes an ellipsoid shape, while the left ventricle is more crescentic in shape. Distinguishing anatomic structures such as the infundibular septum (right ventricle), the continuity of the aortic and mitral valves (left ventricle), and large ventricular trabeculae carnae (right ventricle) are more useful for true anatomic distinction (Figs. 14.3–14.6).

In relation to the pulmonary valve, the aortic valve is posterior, inferior, and to the right. The aortic root ascends to the right of the main pulmonary artery, courses superiorly, and then curves leftward and posteriorly to give rise to the left aortic arch. The main pulmonary artery has a more immediate posterior course to bifurcate into the right and left pulmonary arteries. The ductus arteriosus arises at the pulmonary bifurcation near the origin of the left pulmonary artery to connect to the undersurface of the distal aortic arch. The coronary arteries arise from the aortic sinuses in the aortic root. The aorta and pulmonary artery are identified not by their position, but by their connections to their respective branch vessels.

When performing an echocardiographic examination, detailed anatomic information should be obtained from all the available imaging windows, including transesophageal windows if necessary. Due to the tremendous variability in cardiac anatomy, it is important not to restrict the examination to only the conventional views and standard transducer orientations. Indeed, both the views and transducer orientation should be modified to provide the most diagnostic information, with the aim that the location, relationship, and connections of the cardiac chambers, veins, and great arteries are clearly demonstrated to provide the diagnosis.

Table 14.2 Morphologic features of the ventricles

	Left ventricle	Right ventricle
Atrioventricular valve	• Bileaflet (mitral valve) • Septal insertion closer to crux • Contiguous with semilunar valve	• Trileaflet (tricuspid valve) • Septal insertion more apically displaced • Discontiguous with semilunar valve; infundibular septum present
Trabecular pattern	• Fine trabeculations • Smooth septum	• Coarse trabeculations • Moderator band present
Papillary muscle	• Two papillary muscles on free wall	• Multiple, with papillary muscles(s) on septum

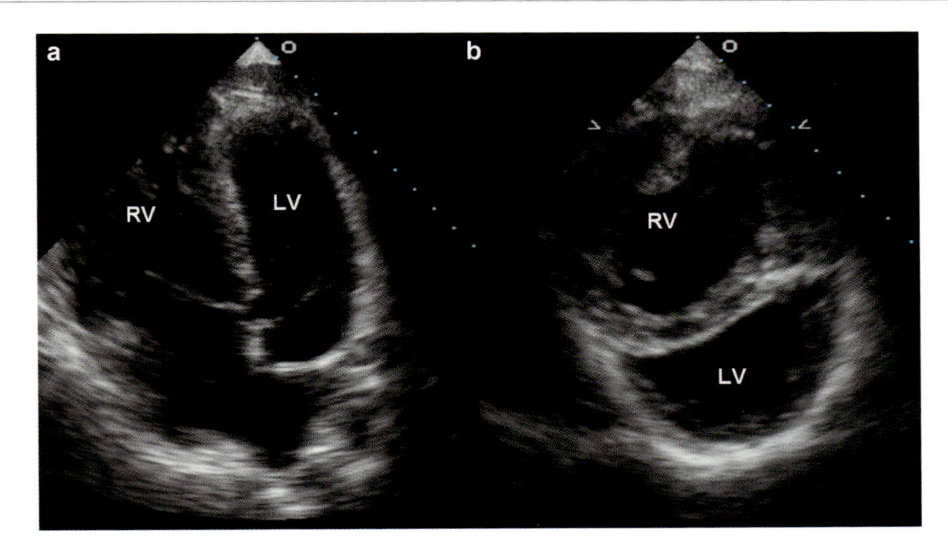

Fig. 14.2 This is a patient with complete transposition of the great arteries with a Mustard procedure. The morphologic right ventricle is the systemic ventricle which is hypertrophied and larger than the left ventricle shown in the apical two-chamber (**a**) and the parasternal short-axis (**b**) views. In the parasternal short-axis view (**b**), the ventricular septum is flattened and the morphologic left ventricle assumes a "D" shape. The shape of the ventricle is not a reliable identifying anatomical feature of the underlying ventricle

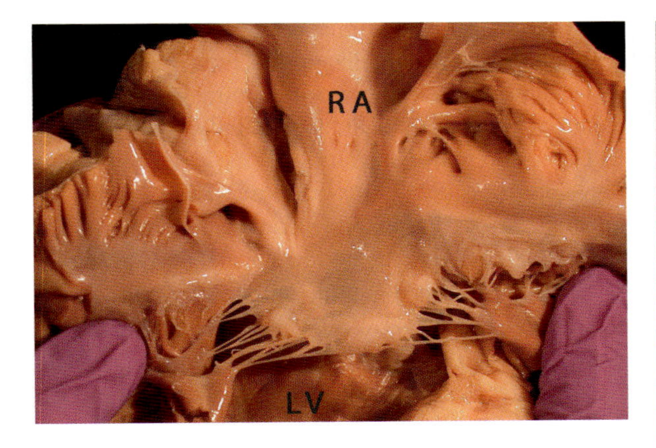

Fig. 14.3 Corrected transposition of great arteries. The right heart connects the right atrium to the morphological left ventricle with a morphological mitral valve in between. The morphological right atrium (*RA*) has pectinate muscles. The left ventricle (*LV*) has a morphological mitral valve with two leaflets

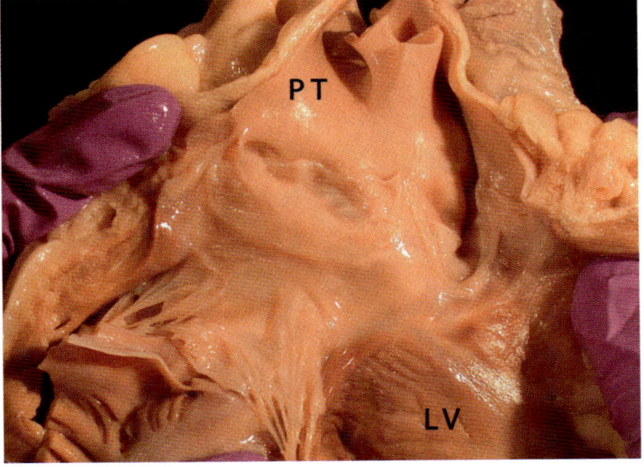

Fig. 14.4 Corrected transposition of great arteries. The right-sided outflow consists of a morphologic left ventricle (*LV*) and the pulmonary trunk (*PT*). Note that the pulmonic valve and the mitral valve have continuity – a feature of a morphological left ventricle

Unrepaired Lesions

Atrial Septal Defect

There are three main types of atrial septal defect, as defined by the location of the defect [5] (Fig. 14.7). The most common type is the secundum atrial septal defect which involves the primum septum and located where we expect the foramen ovale (Figs. 14.8, 14.9). This may be congenital or secondary to a dilated left atrium which stretches the septum (as in mitral stenosis-Lutembacher syndrome). Primum atrial septal defect involves the atrial septum near the internal crux of the heart and forms a part of an atrioventricular

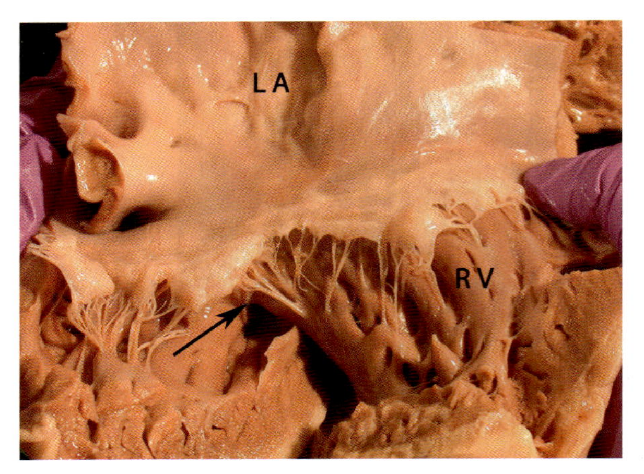

Fig. 14.5 Corrected transposition of great arteries. The left atrium (*LA*) connects to the morphological right ventricle (*RV*) with an intervening tricuspid valve. The morphological left atrium is smooth and has no pectinate muscles. The tricuspid valve has the expected septal chordal attachments (*arrow*). The right ventricle is hypertrophied as this is the systemic ventricle

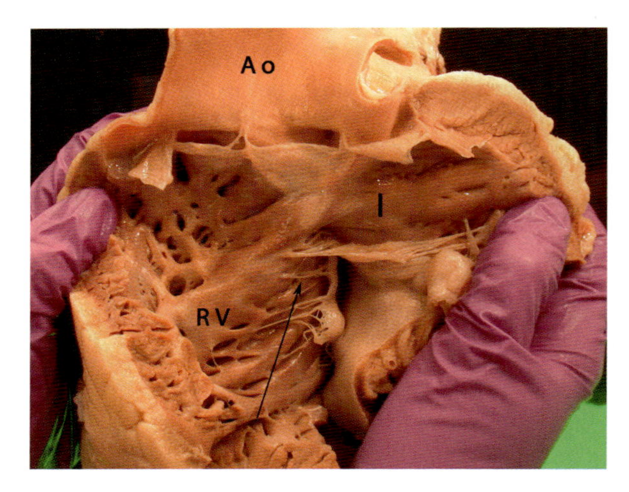

Fig. 14.6 Corrected transposition of great arteries. The left-sided outflow tract connects a morphological right ventricle (*RV*) to the aorta (*Ao*). As this is an anatomical right ventricle, there is discontinuity between the tricuspid valve and the semilunar aortic valve due to the presence of an infundibular septum (*I*). Septal chordal attachments are also seen (*arrow*)

septal (atrioventricular canal) defect (Fig. 14.10). The last type is the sinus venosus atrial septal defect which can be located superiorly near the entrance of the superior vena cava or inferiorly just above the entrance of the inferior vena cava (Fig. 14.11).

Transthoracic echocardiography has a sensitivity of about 90% in the detection of secundum atrial septal

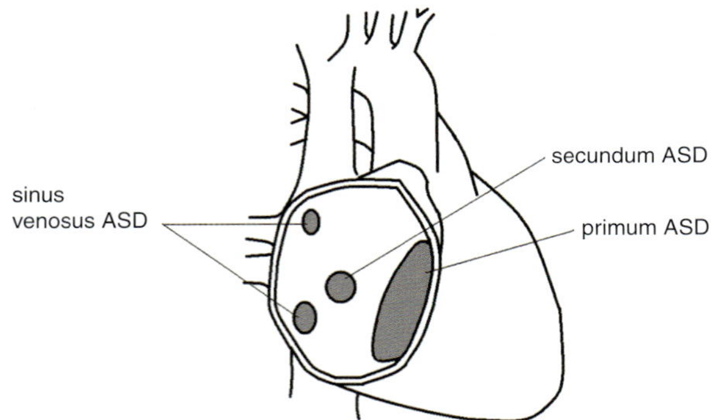

Fig. 14.7 This is a schematic diagram showing the three common types of atrial septal defects (*ASD*)

defect, the most common type of atrial septal defect [6]. The best imaging window is one that allows the ultrasound beam to have an orthogonal relationship with the atrial septum. This is usually the subcostal window, particularly in younger patients (Fig. 14.12). In older patients and those in whom subcostal views are suboptimal, a low parasternal window can be useful. The objective is to image the defect in the atrial septum with clear visualization of the rim. The problem of dropout should be borne in mind particularly if the atrial septum is imaged tangentially.

Demonstration of shunting at the defect by color flow imaging is helpful for diagnosis. This must be differentiated from flow entering from the vena cava which is usually directed to the foramen ovale. Demonstration of flow convergence in the left atrium prior to its entrance into the right atrium in the setting of left to right shunt is an important feature of atrial shunting and differentiates this from the caval flow on to the foramen ovale (Fig. 14.12). Color flow imaging can also help differentiate a small atrial septal defect from stretched patent foramen ovale with small left to right shunting. In the former, the shunt flow is perpendicular to the atrial septum, while in the later, the shunt flow runs parallel to the atrial septum (Fig. 14.13).

The best view to image primum atrial septum is the apical four-chamber view in which the internal crux is clearly seen (Fig. 14.10). The sensitivity of transthoracic echocardiography exceeds 90% in the detection of this condition. Other associated findings such as mitral valve cleft are frequently present, as will be discussed in the section under atrioventricular septal defect.

Sinus venosus type of defect can be difficult to detect by transthoracic echocardiography, since both the

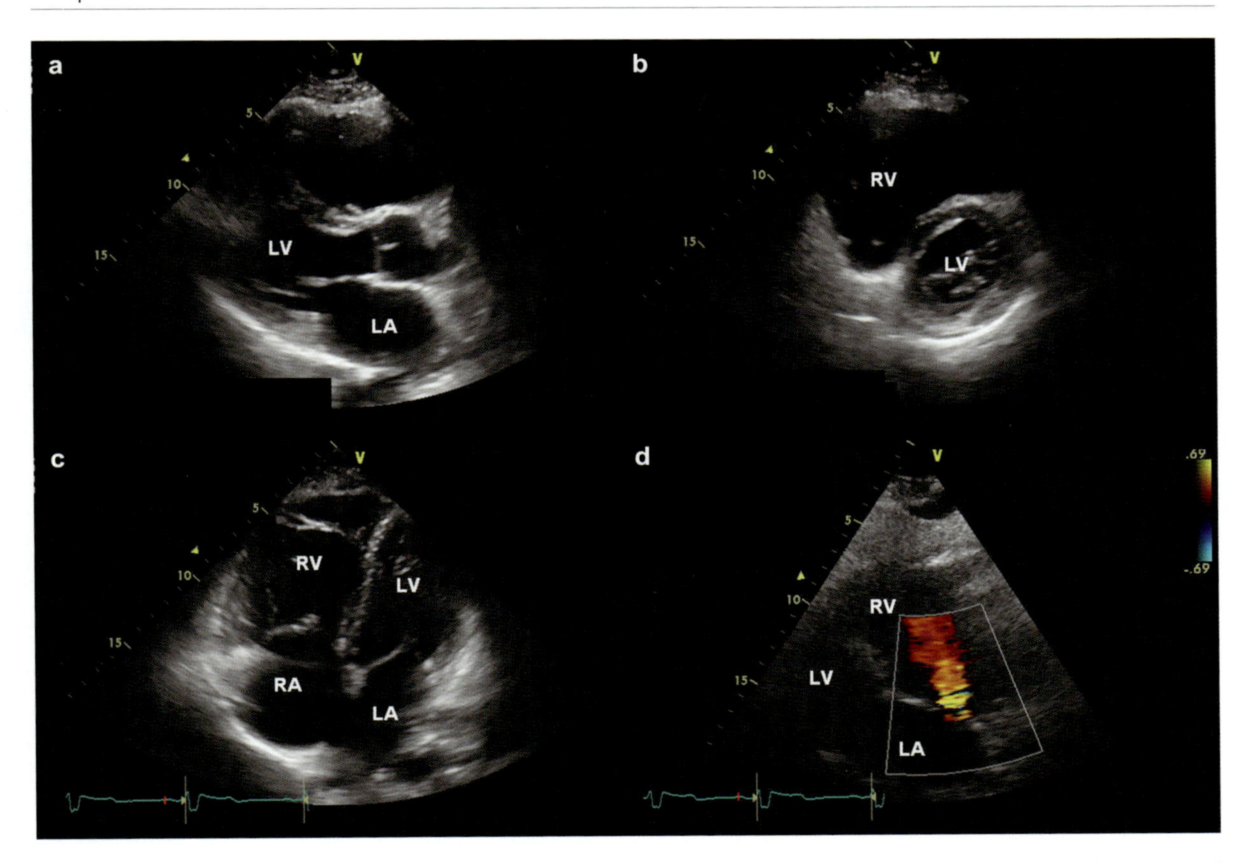

Fig. 14.8 The typical echocardiographic findings of a patient with a large secundum atrial septal defect are shown. In the parasternal long-axis (**a**), short-axis (**b**), and apical four-chamber (**c**) views, right ventricular volume overload is evident by a dilated right ventricle. In real time imaging, the ventricular septum usually shows paradoxical motion. The atrial septal defect is best seen in the subcostal view (**d**). Color flow imaging shows left to right shunting across the atrial septal defect

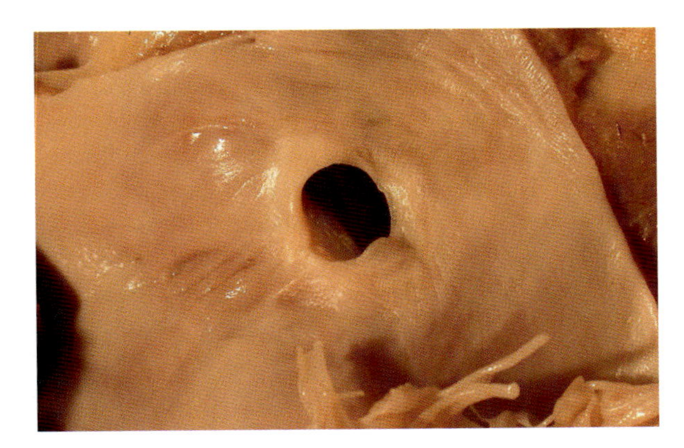

Fig. 14.9 Secundum type atrial septal defect in the midinteratrial septum (*left* atrial view)

superior and inferior vena cavae are not well imaged by this approach [6]. The overall sensitivity is about 50% for defects located just beneath the entrance of the superior vena cava. The sensitivity for defects located just above the entrance of the inferior vena cava is not well determined and likely quite low. [7] The subcostal window is the optimal one to image these defects (Fig. 14.11). The imaging plane needs to be tilted anteriorly to visualize the superior vena cava so as to image the superior portion of the atrial septum. A common associated abnormal finding is the presence of an anomalous pulmonary vein. This is usually difficult to diagnose with certainty by the transthoracic approach.

Transesophageal echocardiography provides an excellent assessment of the atrial septum and has a very high sensitivity (over 95%) in detecting all three types of atrial septal defect (Figs. 14.14–14.16). It also allows the identification of anomalous pulmonary veins. In patients with an inferior sinus venosus atrial septal defect, care needs to be taken to image the atrial septum all the way down to the entrance of the inferior

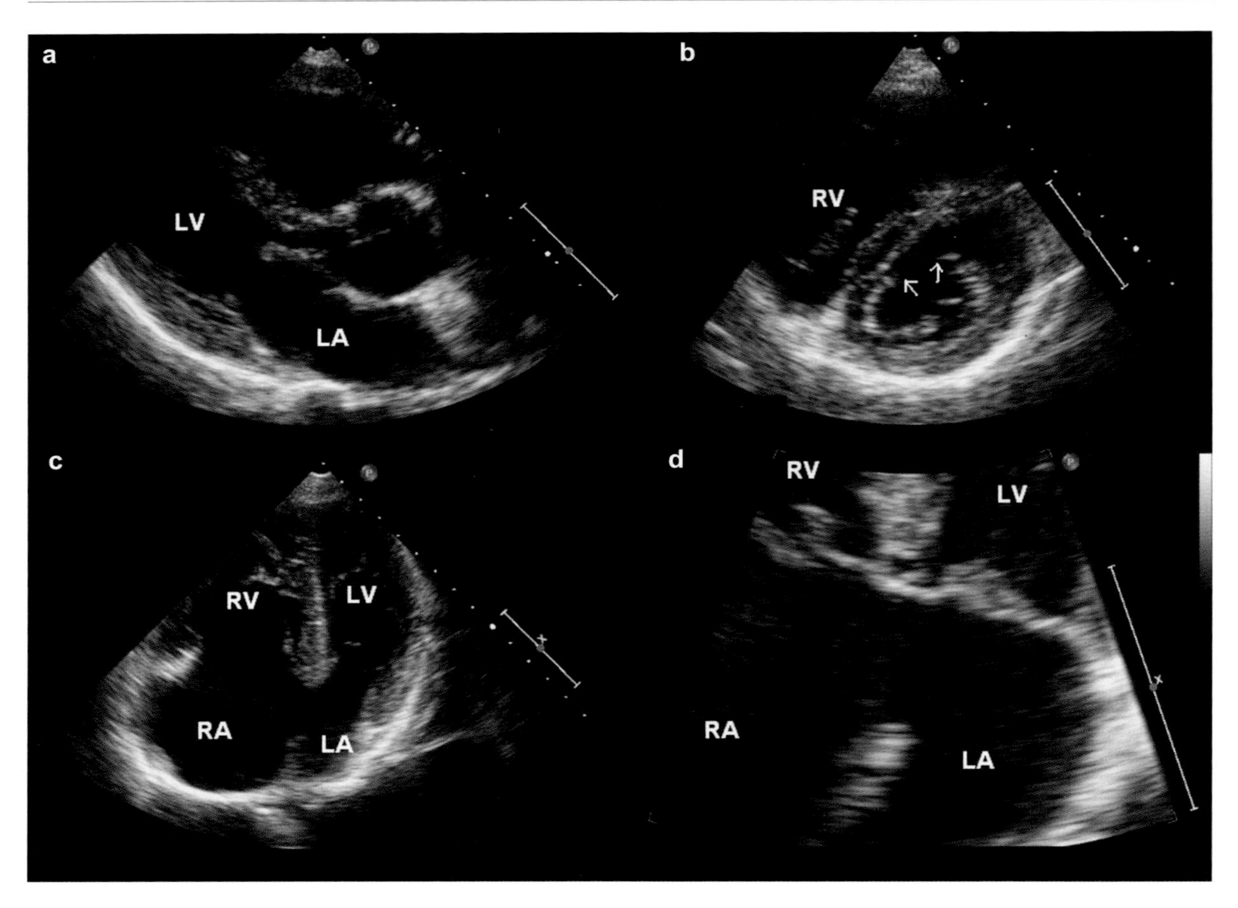

Fig. 14.10 This is a 23-year-old man with partial atrioventricular septal defect. The parasternal long-axis view (**a**) shows a narrow left ventricular outflow tract, common in this condition. The parasternal short-axis view (**b**) shows that there is a cleft in the anterior mitral leaflet. The apical four-chamber view (**c**) shows the large primum atrial septal defect. This zoomed view (**d**) shows the large primum atrial septal defect, as well as the abnormal orientation of the atrioventricular valves. *LA* left atrium, *LV* left ventricle, *RA* right atrium, *RV* right ventricle

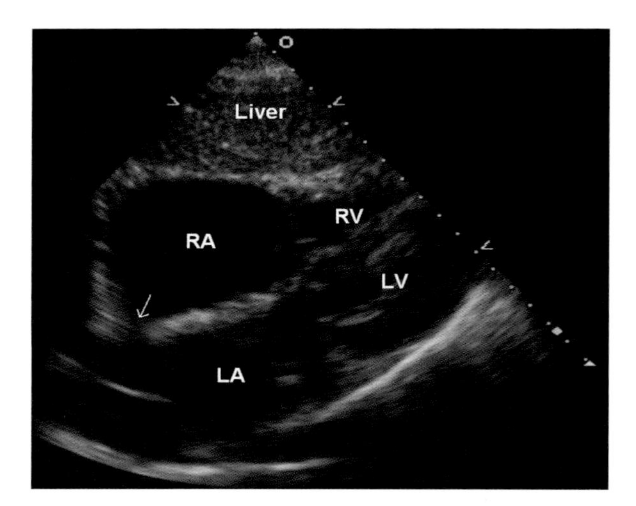

Fig. 14.11 The subcostal view shows the presence of a sinus venosus atrial septal defect (*arrow*). *LA* left atrium, *LV* left ventricle, *RA* right atrium, *RV* right ventricle

vena cava. Associated findings of right ventricular volume overload are present with all three types of atrial septal defect if they are associated with significant shunting. The presence of a clearly dilated right ventricle indicates the presence of shunting > 2:1.

Ventricular Septal Defects

There are several classifications for ventricular septal defects (VSD) [8]. Our institution prefers classifying ventricular septal defects into membranous, inlet, outlet, and trabecular types (Fig 14.17) [9]. The smooth-walled inlet is divided from the outlet septum by the inferior limb of the septal band, and it transitions into the apical trabecular septum at the insertions of the papillary muscles. The outlet septum is also smooth-walled

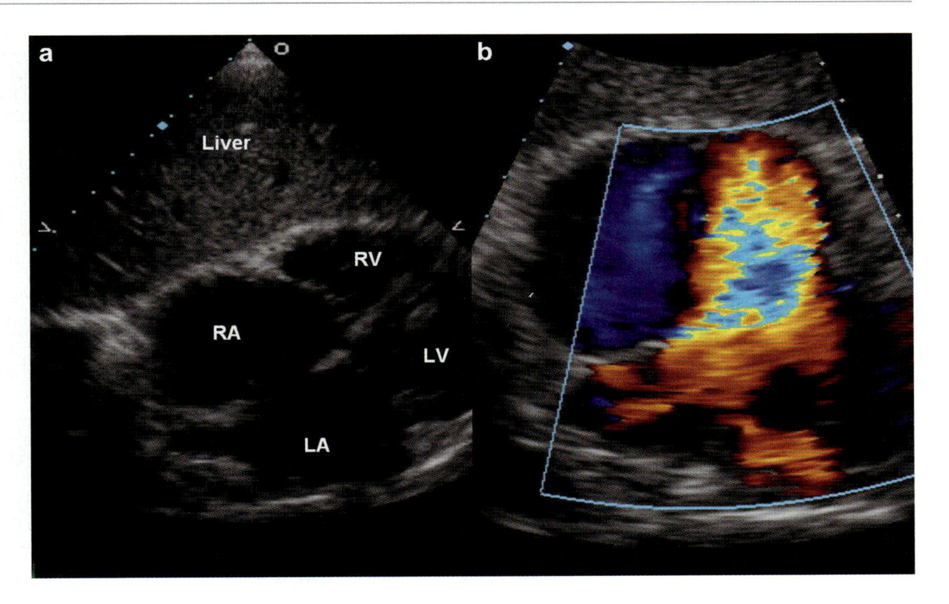

Fig. 14.12 The large secundum atrial septal defect is shown in the subcostal view (**a**). The color flow image (**b**) confirms a large left to right shunt across the defect. *LA* left atrium, *LV* left ventricle, *RA* right atrium, *RV* right ventricle

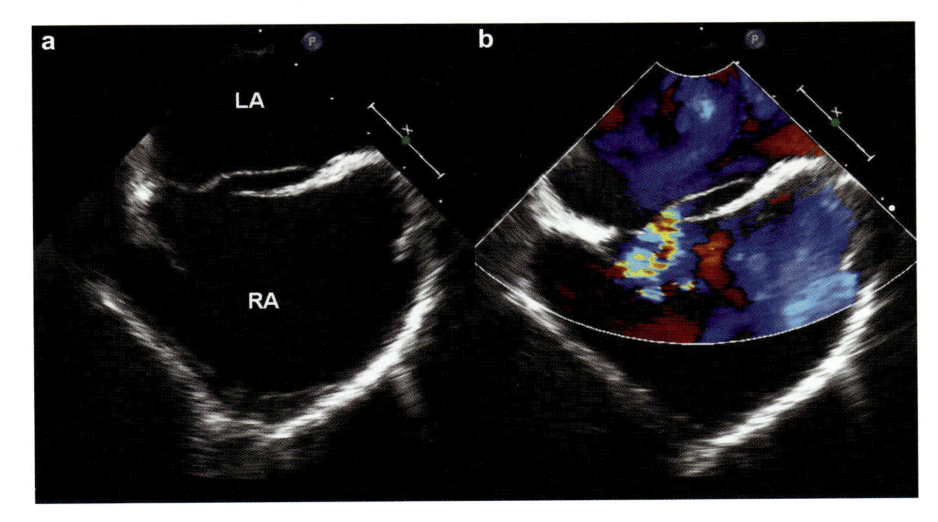

Fig. 14.13 The transesophageal bicaval view (**a**) shows the presence of patent foramen ovale with significant overlap of the primum atrial septum with the secundum atrial septum such that the left to right shunt flow runs parallel to the atrial septum as shown in the color image (**b**). *LA* left atrium, *RA* right atrium

and is divided by the superior limb of the septal band from the anteroapical trabecular septum. The membranous ventricular septal defect is best assessed by the parasternal long and short-axis views, bearing in mind its close relationship to the aortic root and septal tricuspid leaflet. Frequently, a small aneurysm can be seen at this region (Figs. 14.18–14.20). The inlet ventricular septal defects are muscular abnormalities and can be single or multiple. A septal defect involving the basal inlet region is part of the atrioventricular septal defect complex. The trabecular ventricular septal defects also involve the muscular septum. The outlet ventricular septal defect can be associated with aortic valve cusp prolapse into the defect resulting in aortic valve regurgitation (Fig. 14.21). This type of VSD can be well visualized using the parasternal short-axis view, as this defect is in close proximity to the pulmonic valve. With the trabecular ventricular septal defect, the actual defect can be difficult to image due to the trabeculated nature of this portion of the ventricular septum, and thus color flow imaging is essential in the detection of these types of defects (Fig. 14.22).

Doppler interrogation of the flow across a ventricular septal defect can provide important information, as it can give an assessment of the pressure in the right ventricle. Careful examination of the spectral Doppler signal indicates that the shunting is indeed continuous with low velocity flow in diastole reflecting the higher

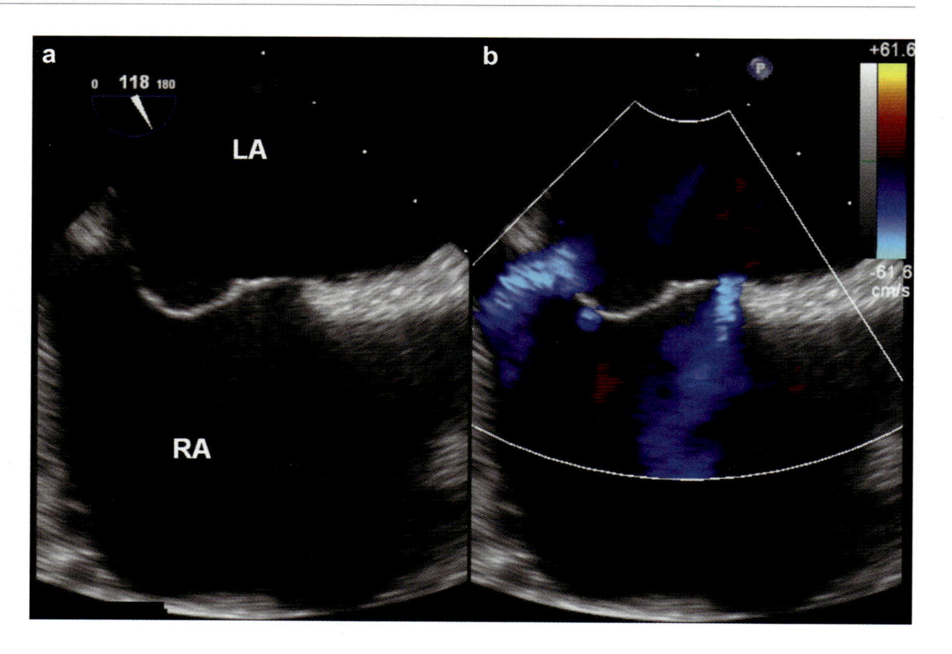

Fig. 14.14 The transesophageal bicaval view shows multiple small secundum atrial septal defects (**a**), and a small degree of left to right shunting through these defects by color-flow imaging (**b**). *LA* left atrium, *RA* right atrium

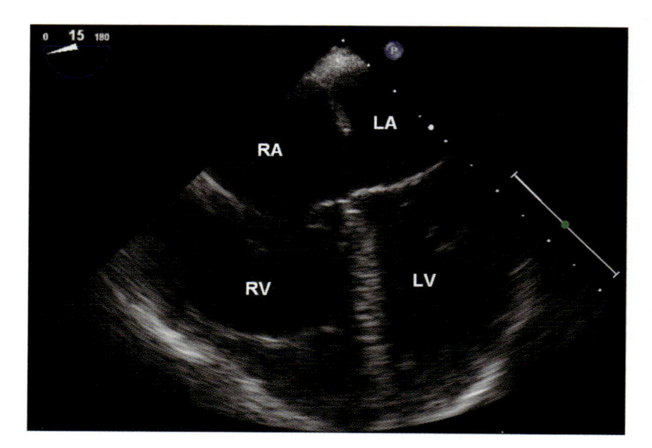

Fig. 14.15 This transesophageal four-chamber view shows the presence of a large primum atrial septal defect, associated with dilatation of the right atrium and right ventricle. *LA* left atrium, *LV* left ventricle, *RA* right atrium, *RV* right ventricle

diastolic pressure in the left ventricle as compared to the right ventricle (Fig. 14.23).

Atrioventricular Septal Defect

This congenital defect has multiple components, and is termed "complete" when all the components are present, and "partial" when all the components are not present. [5] The components include an atrial septal defect of the primum variety, ventricular septal defect of the inlet variety, and abnormal atrioventricular valves, including the cleft anterior mitral leaflet (Fig. 14.24). When any one of these components is detected, it is important to look for the presence of the other components. In addition, the left ventricular outflow tract is unusually elongated producing the "goose-neck" appearance, as described by contrast ventriculography. The papillary muscles may be closer than normal. A parachute mitral valve and double orifice mitral valve are seen with higher frequency in this condition. Pulmonary hypertension changes may be detected.

The defect involving the atrial septum and the upper ventricular septum are best seen with the four-chamber view. In this view, the tricuspid and mitral valves are seen to arise at the same level, which is a very useful diagnostic feature particularly in patients with partial atrioventricular septal defect and in whom the echocardiographic findings may be more subtle (it should be remembered that normally, the mitral valve inserts higher on the crux as seen on the four-chamber view) (Fig. 14.10). A cleft of the mitral valve is best seen using the short-axis view at the level of the mitral leaflet. The cleft typically points to the midpoint of the ventricular septum. In the patient with an isolated mitral cleft, which is a different entity, the mitral cleft points anteriorly. The depth of the cleft is difficult to appreciate by two-dimensional echo, but can be better seen by three-dimensional echocardiography (Fig. 14.25). Overriding of the valves and straddling of

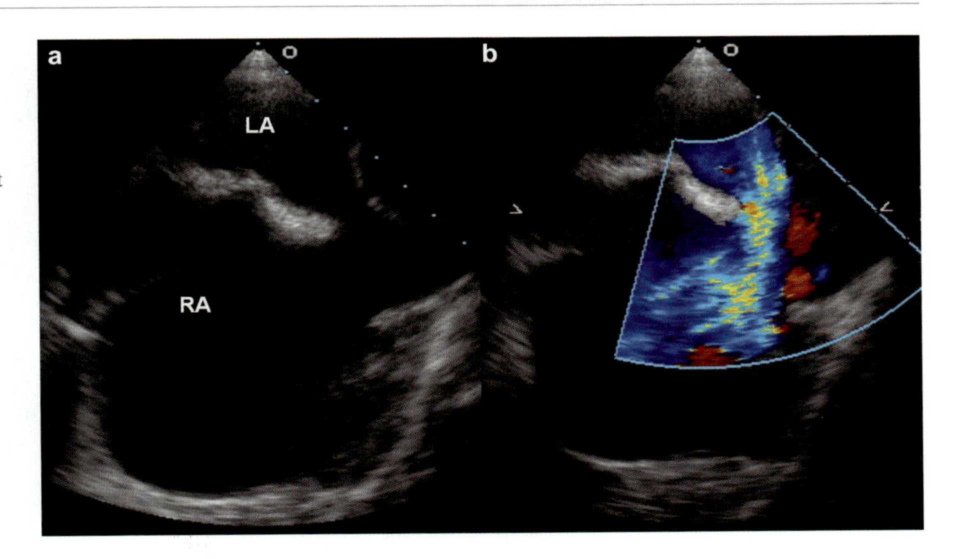

Fig. 14.16 A sinus venosus atrial septal defect located just under the entrance of the superior vena cava is shown in the transesophageal bicaval view (**a**). Left to right shunting is demonstrated by color flow imaging (**b**). *LA* left atrium, *RA* right atrium

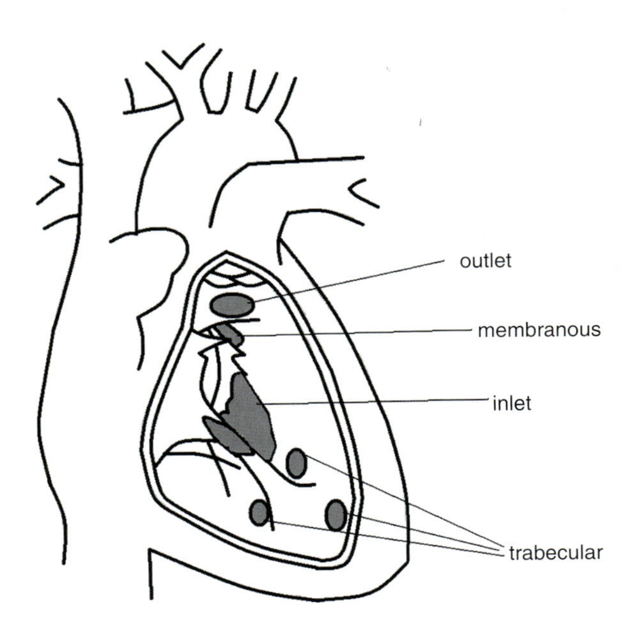

Fig 14.17 This is a schematic diagram showing the different types of ventricular septal defects

the chordae over the defect are important to detect as these features are important for the planning of surgical repair (Figs. 14.26, 14.27).

Patent Ductus Arteriosus

The ductus arteriosus, between the left pulmonary artery and the aorta, is a vital fetal circulation structure that normally closes shortly after birth and becomes the ligamentum arteriosum (Fig. 14.28). Occasionally, the ductus may remain open to provide circulation to the lungs (in conditions such as pulmonary atresia with VSD) and medication may be used to keep it open. Patent ductus arteriosus (PDA) refers to a state in which the ductus remains open pathologically [10]. PDA can be best imaged using the parasternal short-axis view showing the pulmonary bifurcation and the suprasternal view with slight leftward and posterior tilt to show the proximal left pulmonary artery (Figs. 14.29, 14.30). It is difficult to show both ends of the ductus with the same view. To image patent ductus arteriosus by transesophageal echo, we start with the distal aortic arch in short axis using a vertical imaging plane. The transesophageal probe is then gently advanced to show the proximal left pulmonary artery just under the aortic arch and further slight rotation right to left will usually bring out the ductus. Color flow imaging generally facilitates this process.

Coarctation

Coarctation refers to the narrowing of the aorta usually at the region of the ligamentum arteriosum, near the origin of the left subclavian artery (Figs. 14.31, 14.32). The aortic arch needs to be imaged from the suprasternal and high right and left parasternal windows to image the distal ascending aorta, transverse aorta, and proximal isthmus just distal to the left subclavian artery. A bright discrete shelf may be visualized, and

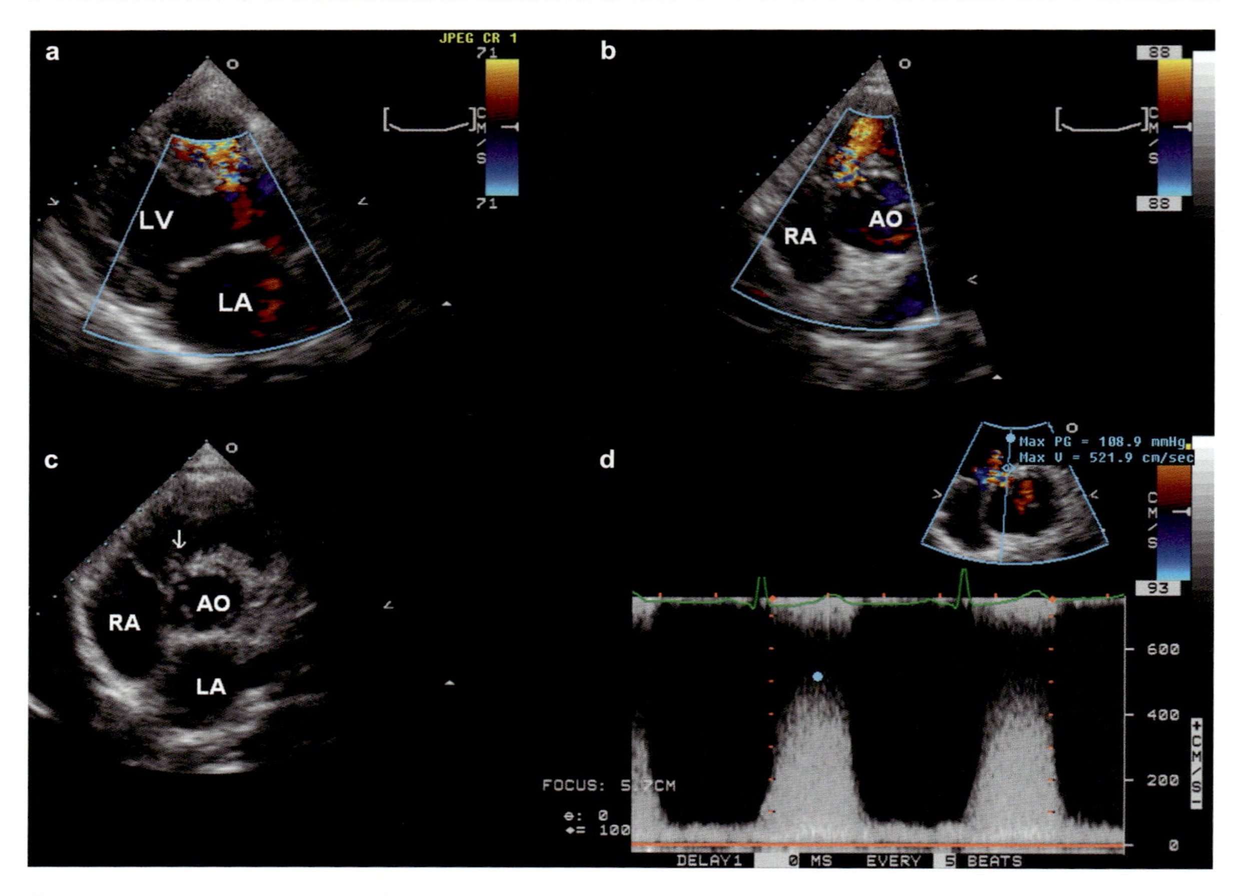

Fig. 14.18 A small membranous ventricular septal defect in a 28-year-old woman is shown with the use of color imaging in the parasternal long-axis (**a**) and short-axis (**b**) views. The short-axis view in (**c**) shows a small ventricular septal aneurysm at the membranous septum (*arrow*). Continuous wave Doppler confirms a high velocity jet across the ventricular septal defect (**d**). *Ao* aorta, *LA* left atrium, *LV* left ventricle, *RA* right atrium

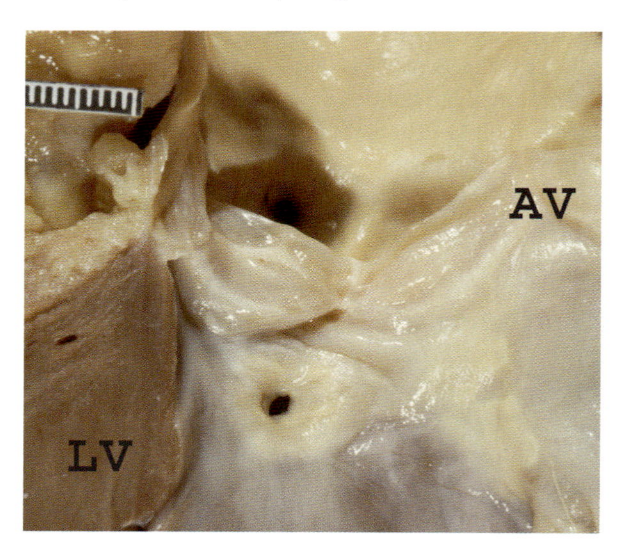

Fig. 14.19 Membranous ventricular septal defect is seen below the aortic valve (*AV*). *LV* left ventricle

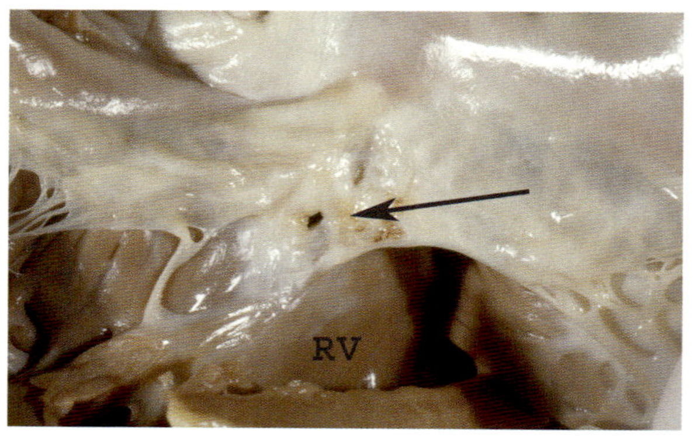

Fig. 14.20 Right ventricle (*RV*) and tricuspid valve from same patient as Fig. 14.19. The tricuspid valve is often attached or slightly aneurysmal in the area on the right side of the ventricular septal defect (*arrow*). The leaflet may actually seal the defect

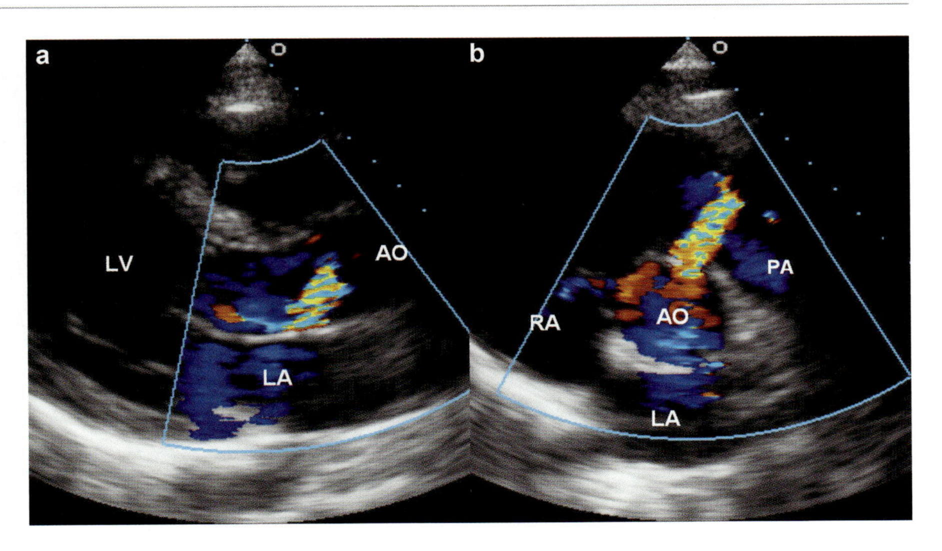

Fig. 14.21 An outlet ventricular septal defect in a 23-year-old man is demonstrated with the aid of color flow imaging in the parasternal short-axis view (**b**). The defect is located just under the pulmonic valve. The parasternal long-axis view (**a**) shows mild aortic regurgitation, which is frequently seen with this type of ventricular septal defect. *Ao* aorta, *LA* left atrium, *LV* left ventricle, *PA* pulmonary artery, *RA* right atrium

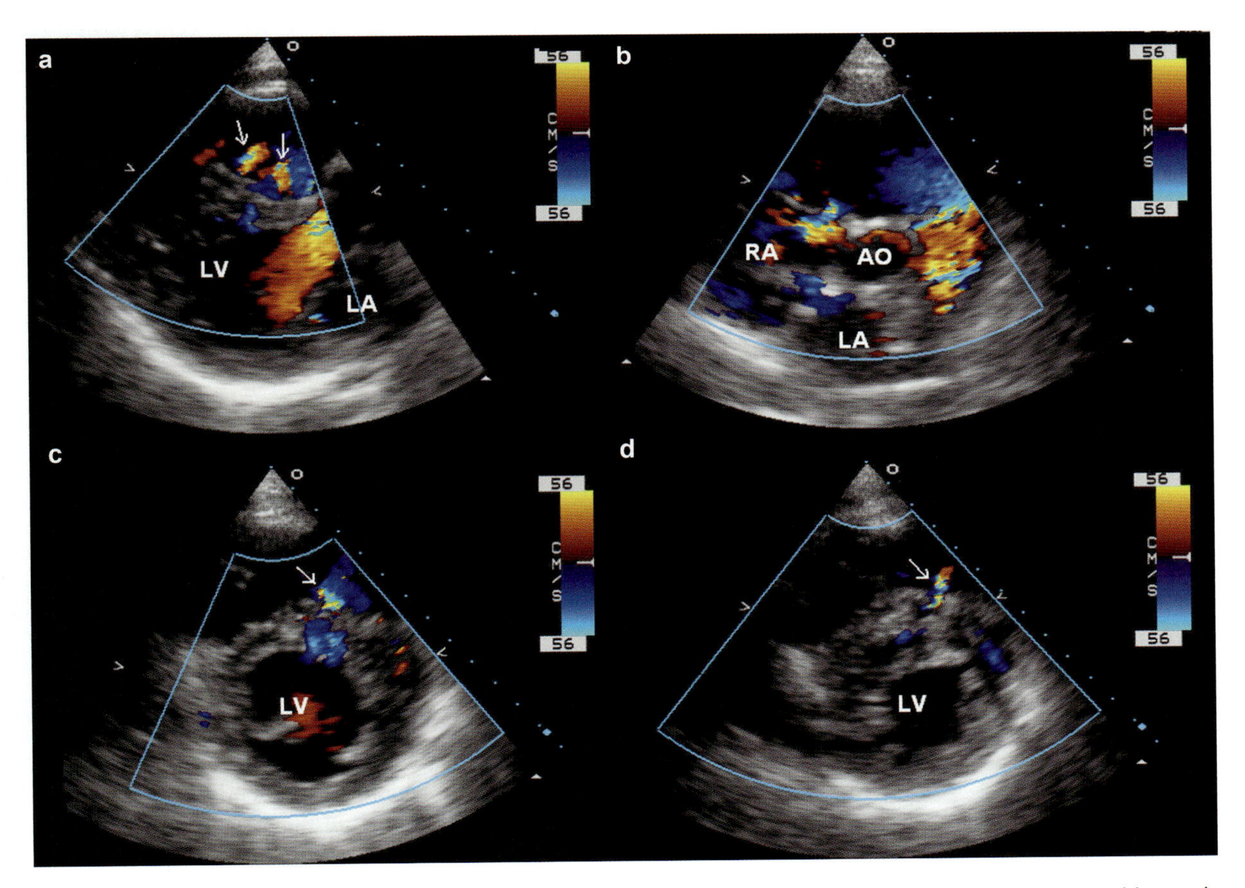

Fig. 14.22 Multiple trabecular ventricular septal defects (*arrows*) in a 27-year-old woman are shown in the parasternal long-axis (**a**) and multiple parasternal short-axis (**b–d**) views. In (**b**), the membranous ventricular septum is shown with no defect. A small jet of tricuspid regurgitation is present. *Ao* aorta, *LA* left atrium, *LV* left ventricle, *RA* right atrium

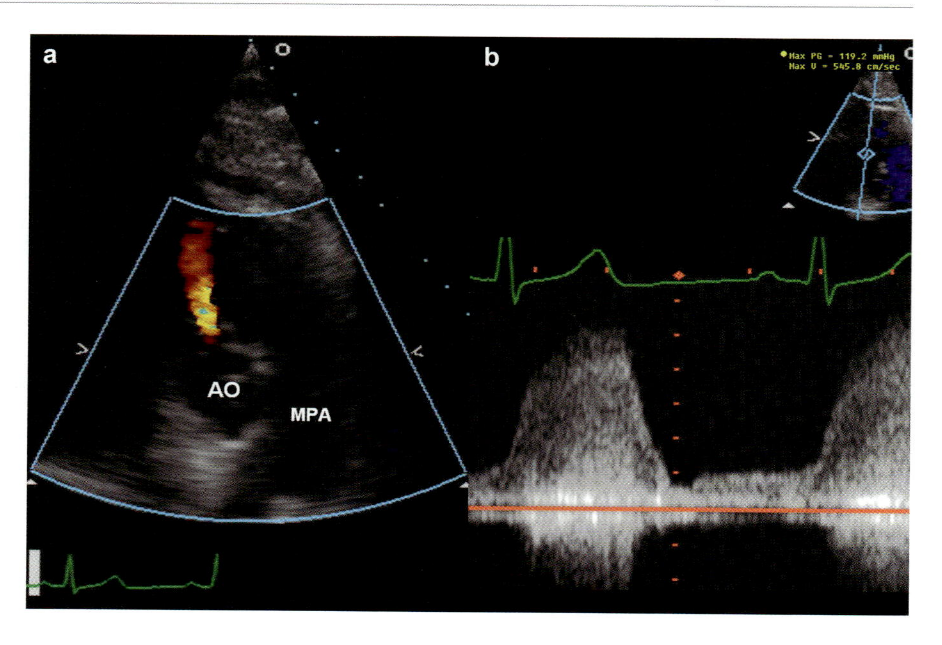

Fig. 14.23 A small membranous ventricular septal defect is shown in the color flow image of the parasternal short-axis view (**a**). Continuous wave Doppler shows a high systolic flow in systole, as well as low velocity diastolic flow reflecting the higher diastolic pressure in the left ventricle compared to the right ventricle (**b**). *Ao* aorta, *MPA* main pulmonary artery

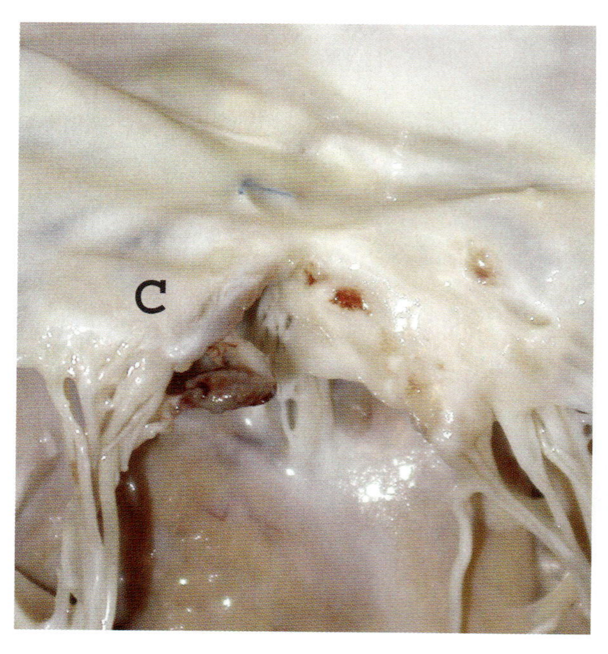

Fig. 14.24 Young woman who had prior repair of complete atrioventricular septal defect. Sutures still visible from the patch. She still has a mitral valve cleft (*C*). Unfortunately, she developed thrombus (red material) in the cleft which embolized to her coronary arteries and caused her to have sudden death

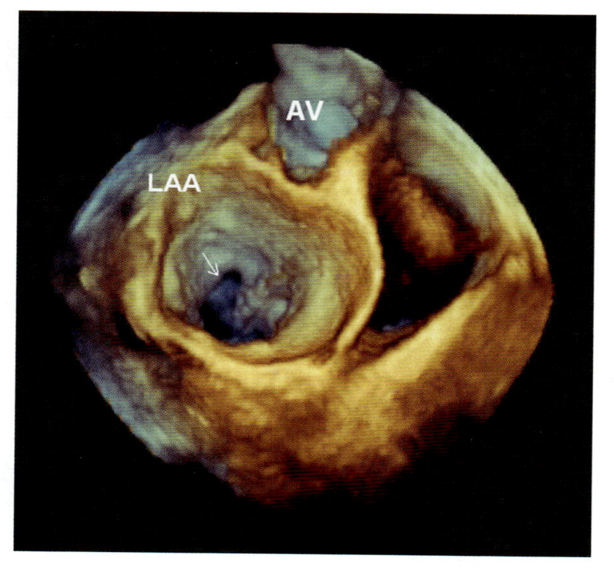

Fig. 14.25 The 3D image from the perspective of the left atrium shows a deep cleft (*arrow*) involving the anterior mitral leaflet in a 41-year-old woman with partial atrioventricular defect. *AV* aortic valve, *LAA* left atrial appendage

frequently associated with a hypoplastic small transverse aorta and aortic isthmus. (Fig. 14.33) [11]. In adult patients, the coarctation is usually of the "simple" variety. This means that it is not associated with other intracardiac anomalies except congenitally bicuspid aortic valve, which is a frequently associated finding present in about half of the patients.

If the coarctation is severe and has escaped detection until adulthood, extensive collaterals around the coarctation are likely present. Systemic arterial hypertension is common and can be difficult to manage. The optimal

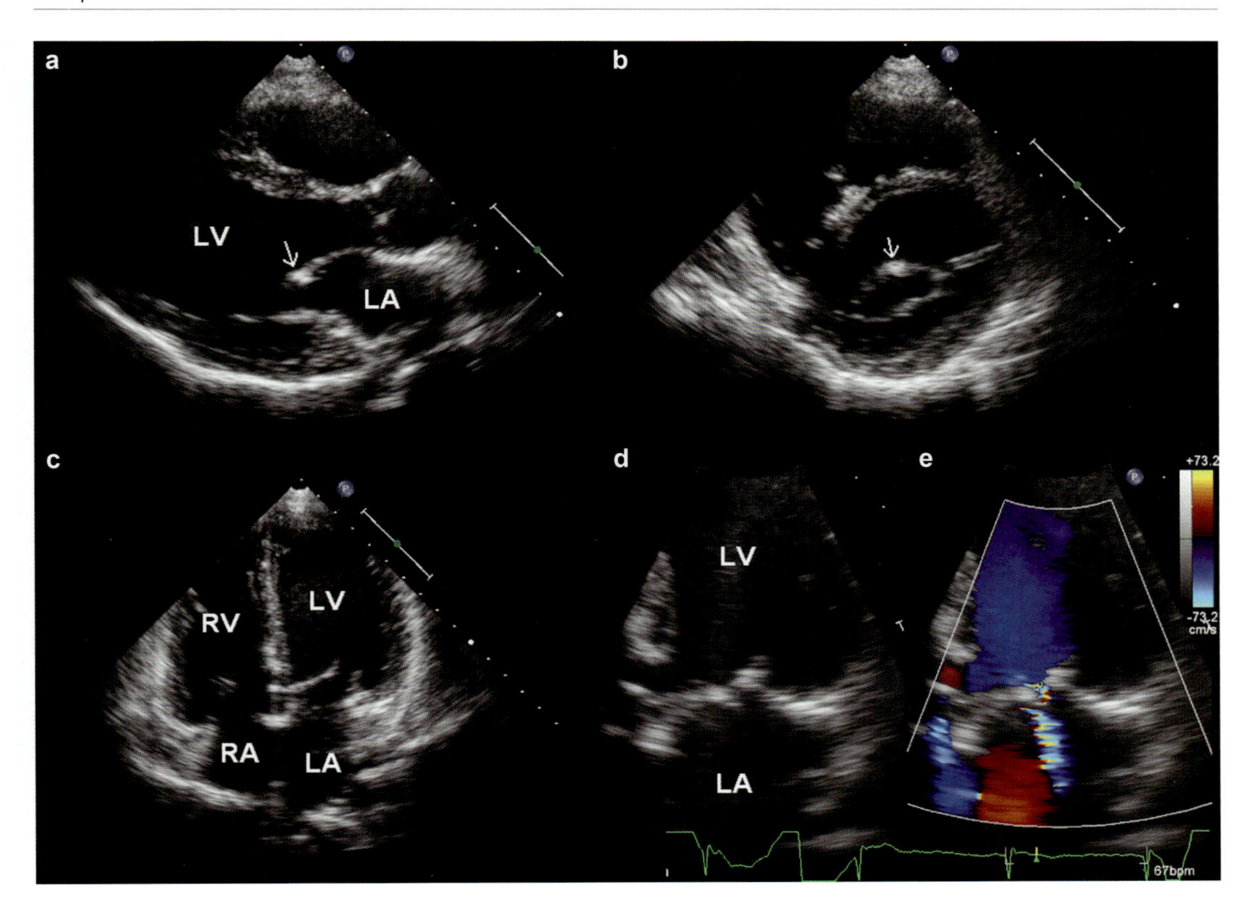

Fig. 14.26 This 19-year-old woman has had surgery for complete atrioventricular septal defect. The parasternal long-axis view (**a**) shows that the tip of the anterior mitral leaflet is thickened (*arrow*) consistent with suture repair of a mitral valve cleft. This is confirmed (*arrow*) in the parasternal short-axis view (**b**). The apical four-chamber view (**c**) shows echo brightness at the internal crux of the heart consistent with surgical patch repair of the primum atrial septal defect and ventricular septal defect. The close-up views of the mitral valve (**d, e**) show that there is mitral regurgitation arising away from the coaptation of the mitral leaflet indicating that the mitral regurgitation originates from the mitral leaflet cleft which has not been completely repaired

treatment remains unclear in an otherwise asymptomatic patient with severe aortic coarctation. In patients who have had surgery or stenting for coarctation, the repaired aortic segment needs to be assessed and followed, since long-term complications such as restenosis and pseudoaneurysm may occur (Fig. 14.34).

Left Superior Vena Cava

Normally, the right cardinal vein contributes to the formation of the superior vena cava. The left cardinal vein contributes to the formation of the coronary sinus. Persistent left superior vena cava represents persistence of the left anterior cardinal vein with drainage into a dilated coronary sinus [12]. Indeed, persistent left superior vena cava is the most common cause of a dilated coronary sinus (>10 mm in diameter in the parasternal long-axis view) (Fig. 14.35). Other causes of a dilated coronary sinus include anomalous pulmonary venous drainage into the coronary sinus, coronary artery fistula draining into the coronary sinus, and severe tricuspid regurgitation with dilated right atrium.

Persistent left superior vena cava has a prevalence of 0.5% in the general population and the prevalence is higher in patients with congenital cardiac anomalies. It can be readily detected by saline contrast injection in the left antecubital vein, showing early contrast in the coronary sinus before opacification in the right atrium.

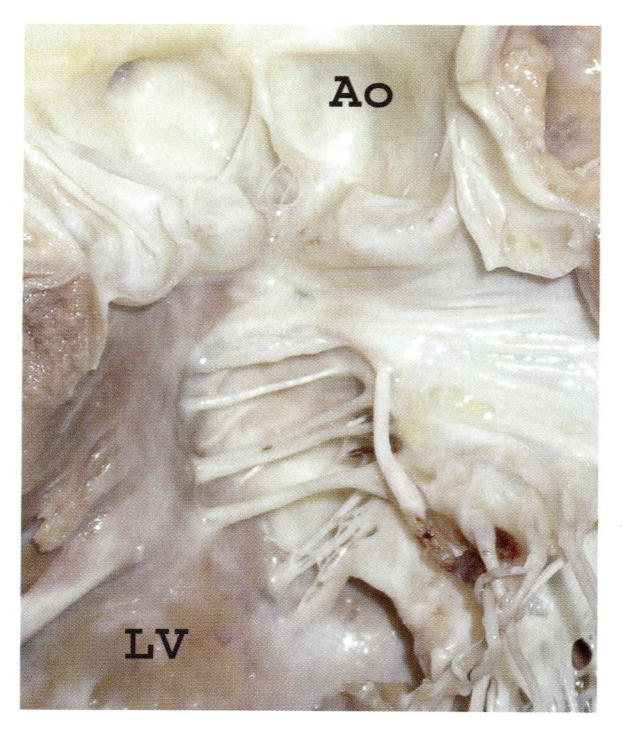

Fig. 14.27 Left ventricular outflow tract in a patient with prior repair of complete atrioventricular septal defect. This is the same patient as in Fig. 14.24. The "mitral" left-sided valve is in continuity with the aortic valve. Note the septal chordal attachments which are remnants of straddling chordae. *Ao* aorta, *LV* left ventricle

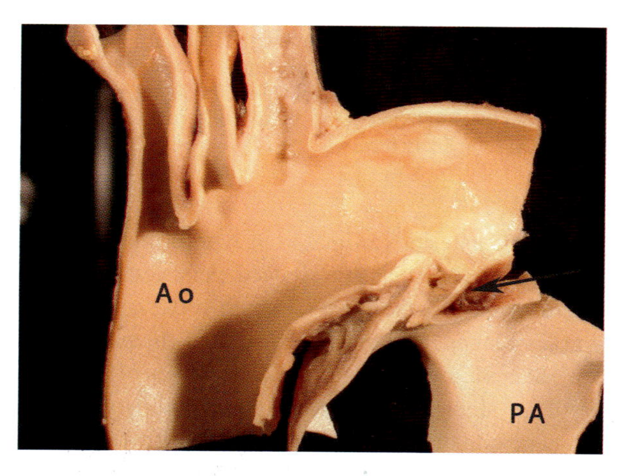

Fig. 14.28 Patent ductus arteriosus (*arrow*) connecting the aorta (*Ao*) and the pulmonary artery (*PA*)

Color flow imaging from the suprasternal window can identify a vertical vein to the left of the aortic arch, but imaging its connection to the coronary sinus is difficult. As it approaches the coronary sinus, the left superior vena cava can be visualized as a circular vascular structure between the left atrial appendage and the left upper pulmonary vein (Fig. 14.36). When the coronary sinus is severely dilated (>2.5 cm in diameter), concomitant atresia of the right superior vena should be suspected, and saline injection into the right antecubital vein will show early opacification of the coronary sinus before the right atrium, similar to the effect of saline contrast injection into the left antecubital vein in the same patient [13]. Persistent superior vena cava is a benign condition as it carries minimal hemodynamic consequences. Its presence is an important factor when interventions, such as pacemaker implantation, are contemplated.

Congenital Sinus of Valsalva Aneurysm

This is an uncommon finding, although the true prevalence is difficult to determine as unruptured sinus of Valsalva aneurysms are not associated with symptoms and generally unrecognized. If detected, for example, a right sinus aneurysm may be detected as a mass in the right ventricular outflow tract, mimicking a neoplasm or a thrombus. On the other hand, a ruptured sinus of Valsalva aneurysm has a dramatic presentation of chest pain, acute onset of heart failure, and a loud continuous murmur. The parasternal long and short-axis views are most useful in identifying the location and hemodynamic consequences [14]. It can be differentiated from ventricular septal aneurysm by its location in the aortic sinus beyond the aortic annulus. Ruptured aneurysm of the noncoronary sinus usually drains into the right atrium; ruptured aneurysm of the left coronary sinus into the left atrium; but ruptured aneurysm of the right coronary sinus may lead to fistula communication between the aorta and the right atrium, or between the aorta and the right ventricle. Surgical repair of this condition is highly successful with good long-term results (Figs. 14.37–14.39).

Postsurgical Conditions

Patients who have had complete correction for tetralogy of Fallot, intraatrial baffle for transposition of the great arteries, and Fontan procedure for lesions such as

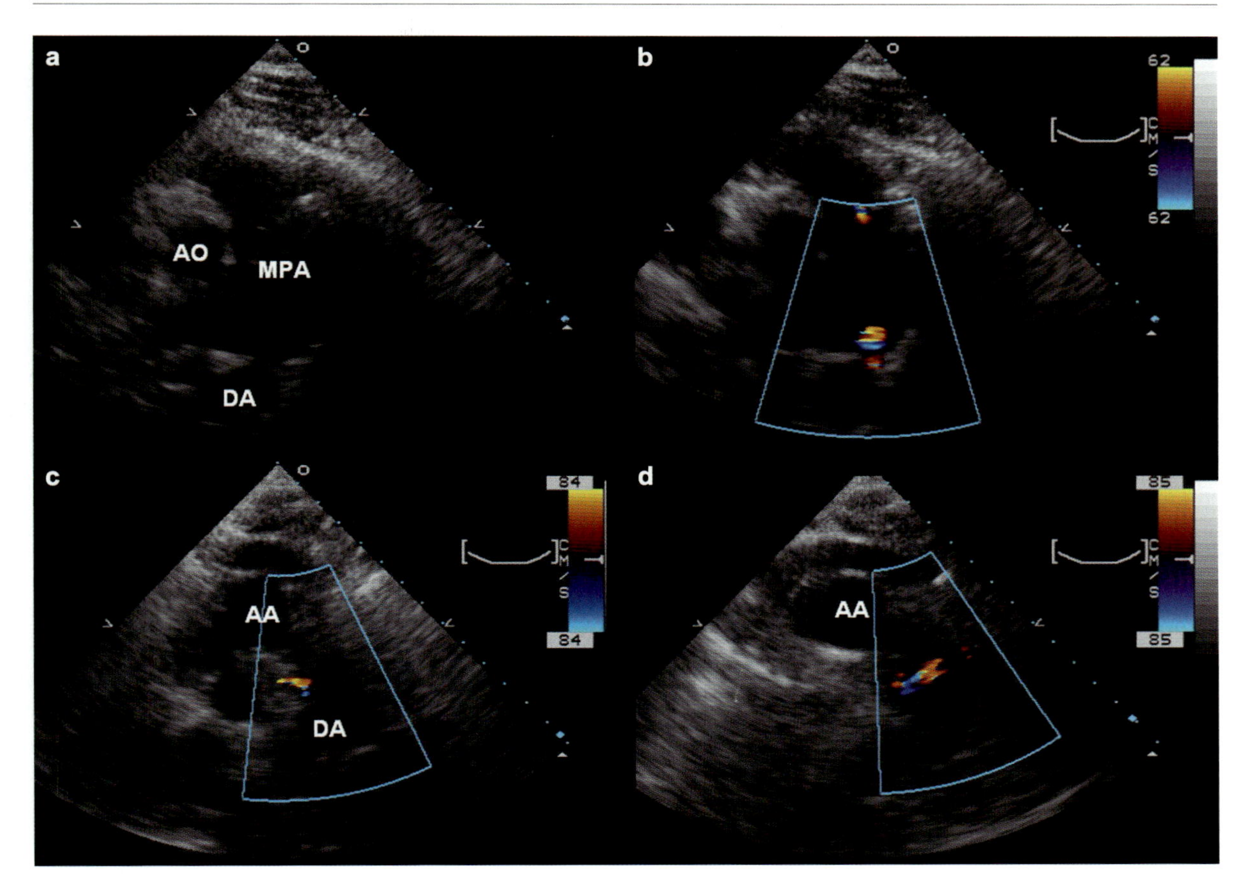

Fig. 14.29 A small patent ductus arteriosus in a 44-year-old man is shown in the parasternal short-axis view (**a**) with the aid of color flow imaging (**b**), the suprasternal long-axis (**c**) and the suprasternal short axis (**d**) views. The color flow images confirm a small degree of shunting which arises from the undersurface of the proximal descending aorta just distal to the take off of the left subclavian artery and drains into the pulmonary artery near the origin of the left pulmonary artery

tricuspid atresia generally survive into adulthood and are the common surgically repaired complex congenital heart diseases that are encountered in the adult echocardiographic laboratory. These patients derive obvious benefits from the surgery, but in the vast majority of these patients, the surgery does not restore normal intracardiac hemodynamics and they are subject to long-term sequelae.

Tetralogy of Fallot Postrepair

The underlying abnormalities of tetralogy of Fallot include a large ventricular septal defect, pulmonic stenosis (usually infundibular), overriding aorta, and right ventricular hypertrophy [15]. The underlying causative defect is an anterior deviation of the infundibular septum. Pulmonary valvotomy or creation of systemic pulmonary shunt (such as a Blalock-Taussig shunt) may be palliative. Complete repair consists of patch closure of the ventricular septal defect and relief of the pulmonic stenosis by resection of muscle from the infundibulum, possible pulmonary valve surgery, and patch enlargement of the infundibulum and/or pulmonary artery (Figs. 14.40, 14.41). The long-term sequelae following complete repair are shown in Table 14.3.

The most common long-term sequela is severe pulmonic regurgitation, either related to pulmonary valvotomy or the use of a transannular patch to enlarge the pulmonary artery and the infundibulum. Ventricular arrhythmias from right ventricular outflow tract surgical scar are also important [16]. Color flow assessment of the severity of pulmonary regurgitation can be difficult.

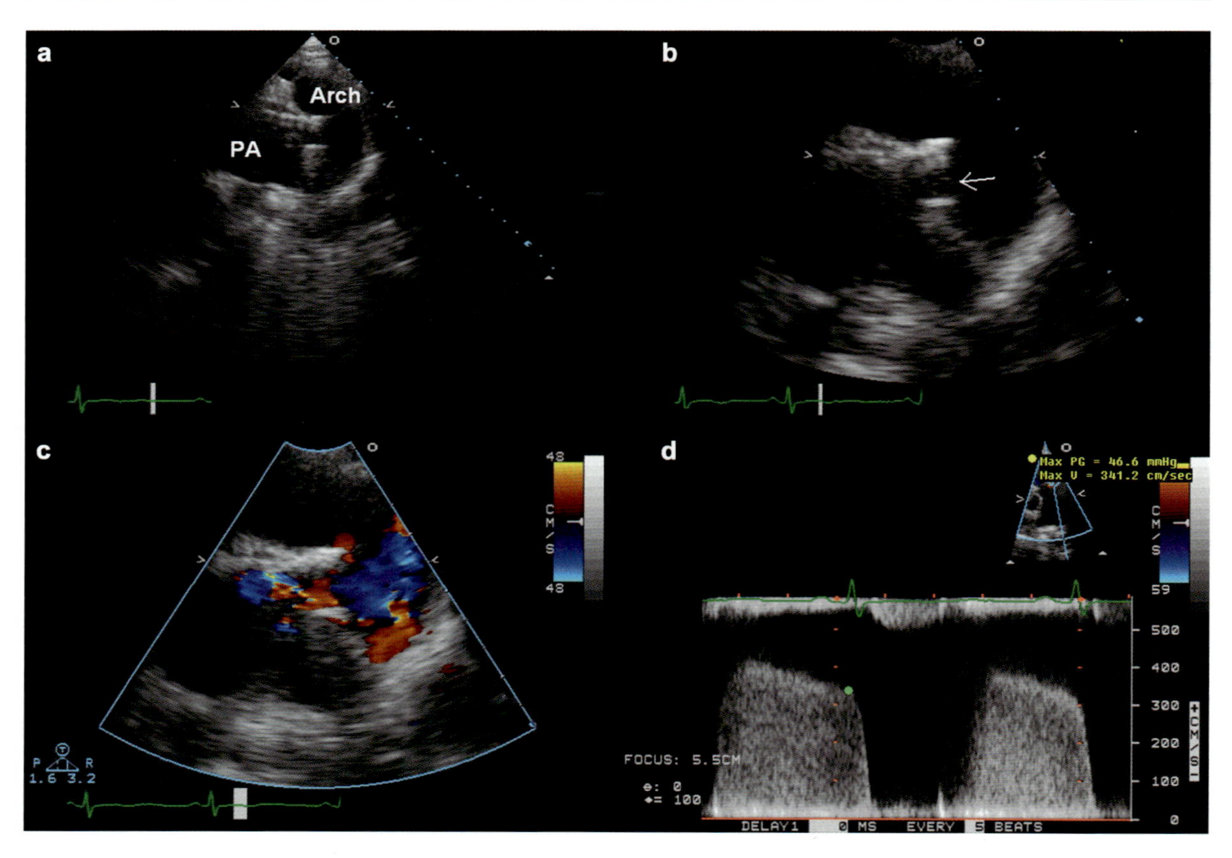

Fig. 14.30 A large patent ductus arteriosus with Eisenmenger physiology in a 45-year-old woman is shown in the suprasternal long-axis view (**a–c**). This is a large ductus (*arrow*) and color flow imaging shows low velocity flow across the ductus indicating the presence of severe pulmonary hypertension, which is confirmed by the high pulmonary regurgitation velocity shown in (**d**)

Continuous wave or pulsed wave Doppler shows a dense signal with low velocity and rapid drop-off [17] (Fig. 14.42). The regurgitation results in a dilated and dysfunctional right ventricle. It is a clinical dilemma to decide the optimum time to perform repeat surgery to eliminate pulmonic regurgitation so as to avoid irreversible right ventricular dysfunction. [18] (Figs. 14.43, 14.44). Left ventricular dysfunction is sometimes present, but the cause is uncertain.

Complete Transposition of the Great Arteries Post Repair

Complete transposition of the great arteries is a condition in which the aorta arises from the morphologic right ventricle and the pulmonary artery from the morphologic left ventricle (termed ventricular-arterial discordance). These patients can survive to adulthood following surgical procedures to correct the direction of intracardiac blood flow. Most adult patients who have had surgery for this condition would have had an atrial baffle or switch procedure such as the Mustard procedure or the Senning procedure. A small but growing group of younger patients would have had an arterial switch (Jantene) procedure [19].

In patients who have had atrial switch, the intraatrial baffle needs to be carefully examined to detect obstruction or leak (Fig. 14.45). The baffle obstruction usually involves the systemic venous limbs of the baffle. In some of these patients, percutaneous intervention with stent placement may alleviate the obstruction (Fig. 14.46). In these patients, the anatomic right ventricle is the systemic ventricle and worsening ventricular dysfunction with heart failure is a long-term concern. The tricuspid

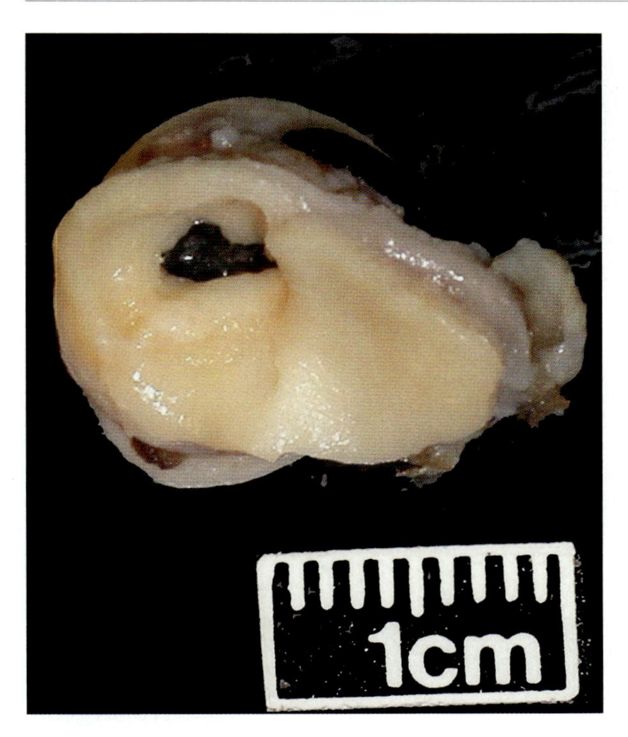

Fig. 14.31 Coarctation of the aorta. Cross section of the aorta demonstrates that the lumen narrows to a small hole

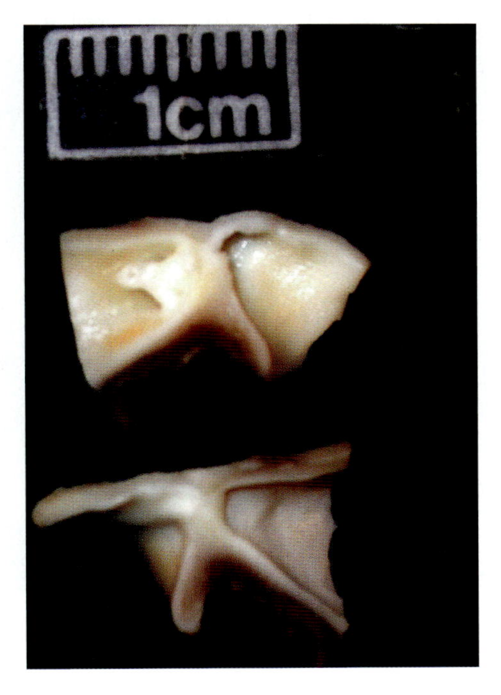

Fig. 14.32 Aortic coarctation - longitudinal cut demonstrating the hour glass-shaped aorta with the narrowed segment in the middle. This was surgically resected with graft placement

valve, the systemic atrioventricular valve, may be dysplastic with features suggestive of Ebstein's anomaly. The presence of significant tricuspid regurgitation may further accelerate the deterioration of the systemic right ventricle. Early tricuspid valve repair or replacement may be considered to preserve the ventricular function. Arrhythmia is a common long-term complication. Atrial flutter, atrial tachycardia, and sinus node dysfunction occur in about half of these patients.

In patients who have had an arterial switch procedure, the arterial anastomotic sites should be assessed, particularly the pulmonary artery, as supravalvular pulmonic stenosis can develop at this region. The development and progression of new aortic valve regurgitation can occur. Coronary artery anastomoses should also be evaluated.

Fontan Operation

This procedure diverts all the systemic venous return directly into the pulmonary arteries, generally without a subpulmonary ventricle. This operation was initially developed for patients with tricuspid atresia, but has since been used for other forms of single ventricle circulation. There are many modifications to the operation. The classic approach uses a direct atrio-pulmonary anastomosis of the right atrial appendage with the main pulmonary artery. The atrio-pulmonary connection is generally difficult to image by transthoracic echocardiography (Fig. 14.47). Transesophageal echocardiography is frequently employed to assess the patency of this anastomosis and to detect thrombus within the dilated right atrium [20] (Fig. 14.48). An extracardiac conduit diverting the vena caval flow directly into the pulmonary arteries has gained popularity, and such connections are even more difficult to assess with echocardiography. Other imaging modalities such as computed tomography and magnetic resonance imaging should be used in these patients.

Summary

Congenital heart diseases encompass a wide range of conditions ranging from the simple to the complex. The simple congenital cardiac lesions may escape

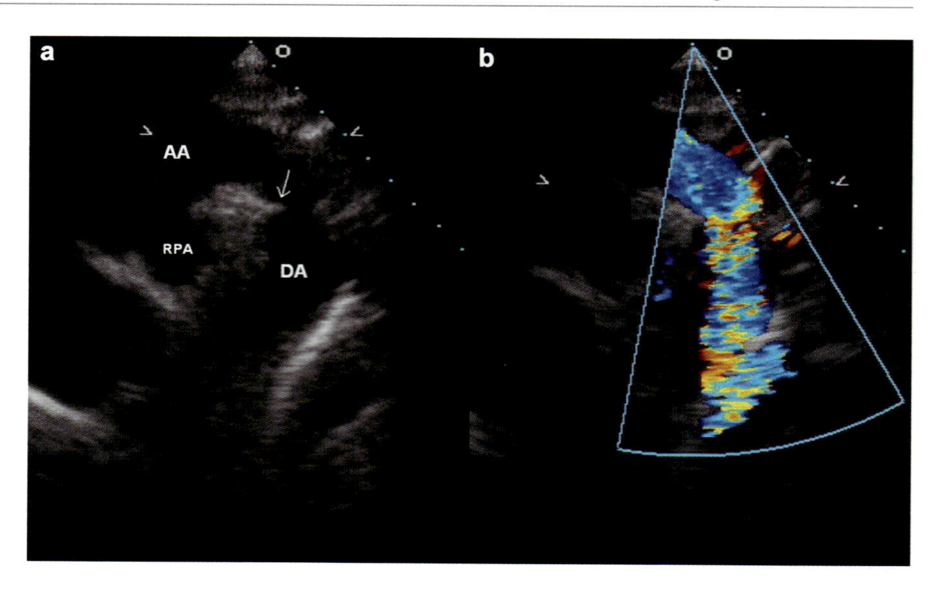

Fig. 14.33 This suprasternal long-axis (**a**) view in a 57-year-old woman who has had previous surgery for coarctation shows that there is a small residual shelf at the undersurface of the proximal descending thoracic aorta consistent with mild coarctation. Flow acceleration at this region is demonstrated by color flow imaging (**b**). *AA* aortic arch, *DA* descending aorta, *RPA* right pulmonary artery

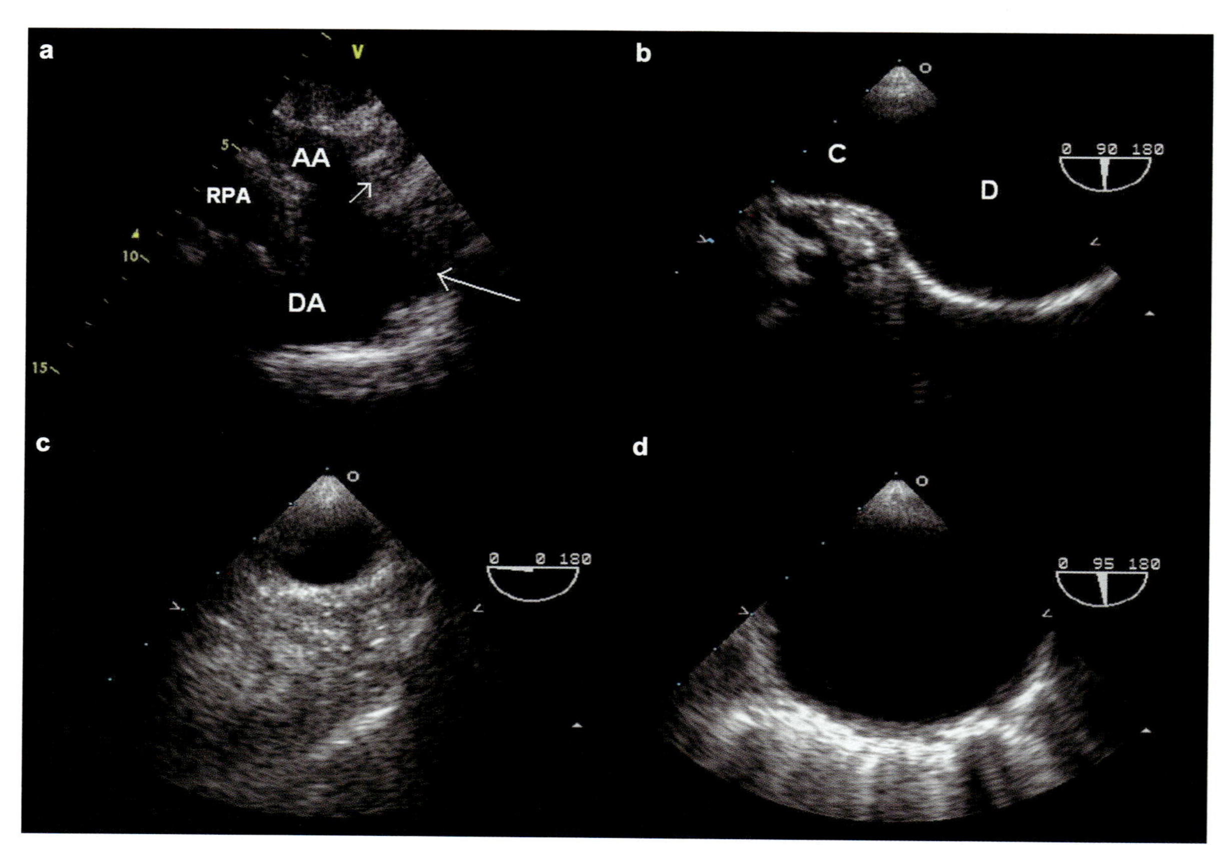

Fig. 14.34 This 20-year-old man has had previous surgical repair for coarctation using a Dacron patch. The suprasternal long-axis view (**a**) shows localized aneurysmal dilatation involving the proximal descending thoracic aorta (*arrow*) at the site of previous patch repair. Transesophageal echocardiogram confirms localized aneurysmal dilatation of the descending thoracic aorta (**b–d**). The relatively normal-sized descending thoracic aorta is illustrated by the aortic segment shown in (**c**). The aneurysmal segment is shown in its short-axis in (**d**). At repeat surgery, pseudoaneurysm formation due to dehiscence of the Dacron patch was identified. *AA* aortic arch, *DA* descending aorta, *RPA* right pulmonary artery

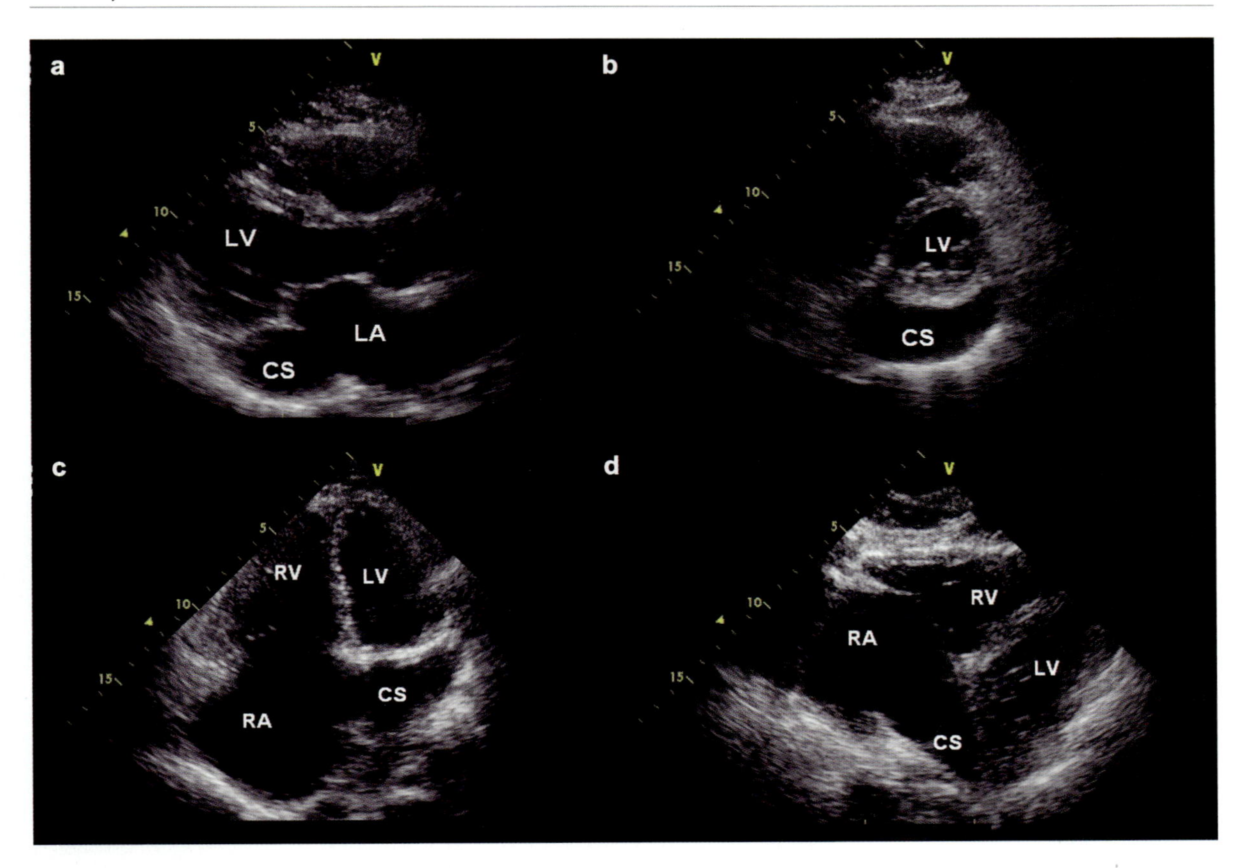

Fig. 14.35 This is a 36-year-old man with a dilated coronary sinus due to the presence of a persistent left superior vena cava draining into the coronary sinus. The dilated coronary sinus is shown in the parasternal long-axis (**a**), short-axis (**b**), apical (**c**) and subcostal (**d**) views. To visualize the coronary sinus from the apical window, the imaging plane needs to be tilted posteriorly. *CS* coronary sinus, *LA* left atrium, *LV* left ventricle, *RA* right atrium, *RV* right ventricle

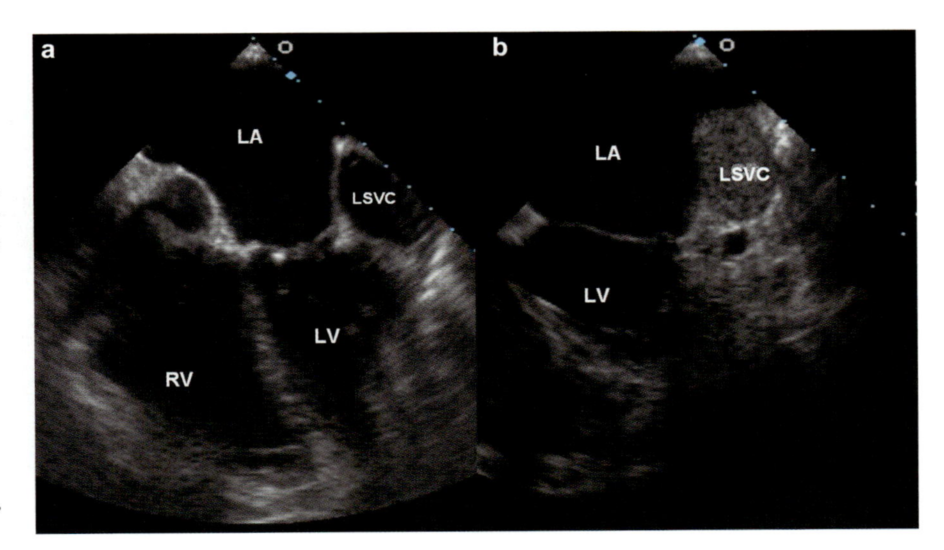

Fig. 14.36 The left superior vena cava can be readily demonstrated using transesophageal echocardiography. In (**a**), the left superior vena cava can be identified as a vascular structure located anterior to the left-sided pulmonary veins and posterior to the left atrial appendage, and it can be enhanced by injection of agitated saline into the left antecubital vein (**b**). *LA* left atrium, *LV* left ventricle, *LSVC* left superior vena cava, *RV* right ventricle

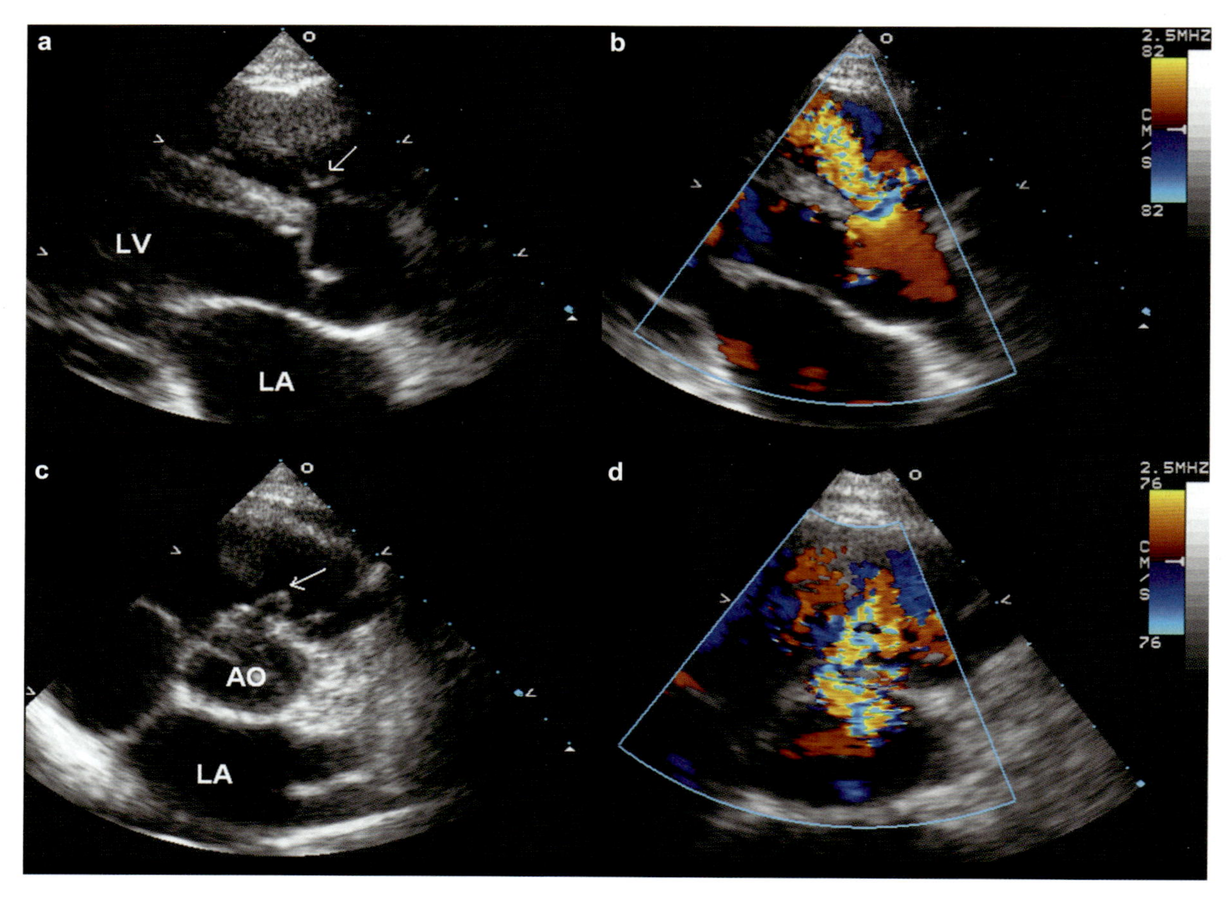

Fig. 14.37 A ruptured aneurysm of the right aortic sinus in an 18-year-old woman is demonstrated in the parasternal long-axis (**a, b**) and parasternal short-axis (**c, d**) views. The sinus of Valsalva aneurysm has a typical windsock appearance (*arrow*). Color flow imaging shows that there is continuous flow between the aorta and the right ventricle via the ruptured aneurysm. *Ao* aorta, *LA* left atrium, *LV* left ventricle

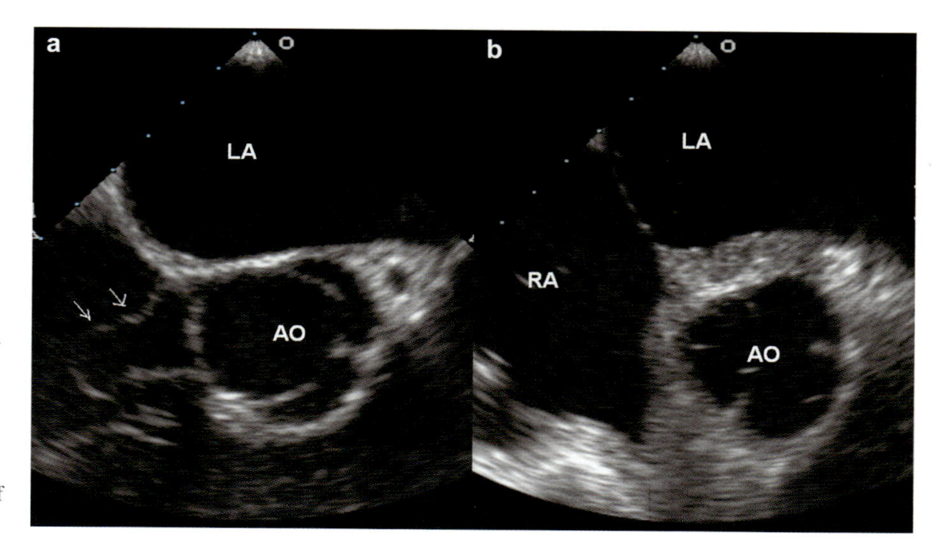

Fig. 14.38 This patient had a ruptured sinus of Valsalva aneurysm arising from the noncoronary sinus (*arrows*) draining into the right atrium (**a**). He underwent successful surgical repair with ligation of the aneurysm (**b**).

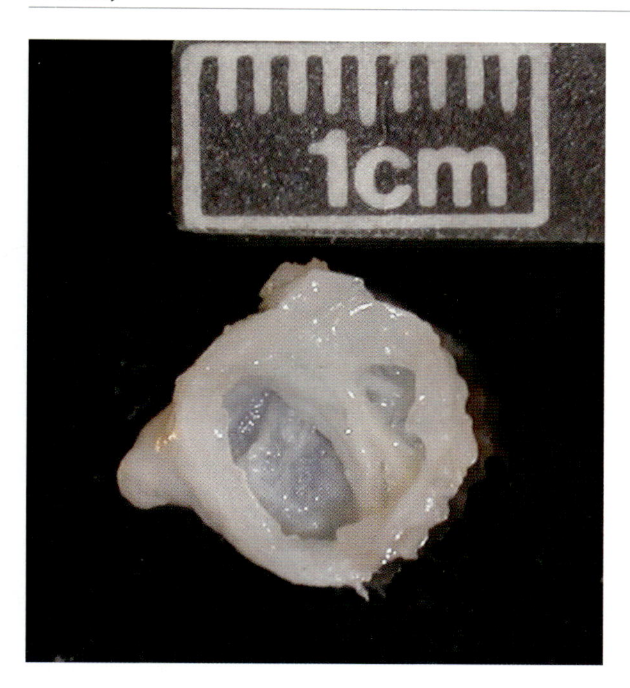

Fig. 14.39 This surgically excised Sinus of Valsalva aneurysm is a thin-walled fibrous structure. This one had not ruptured

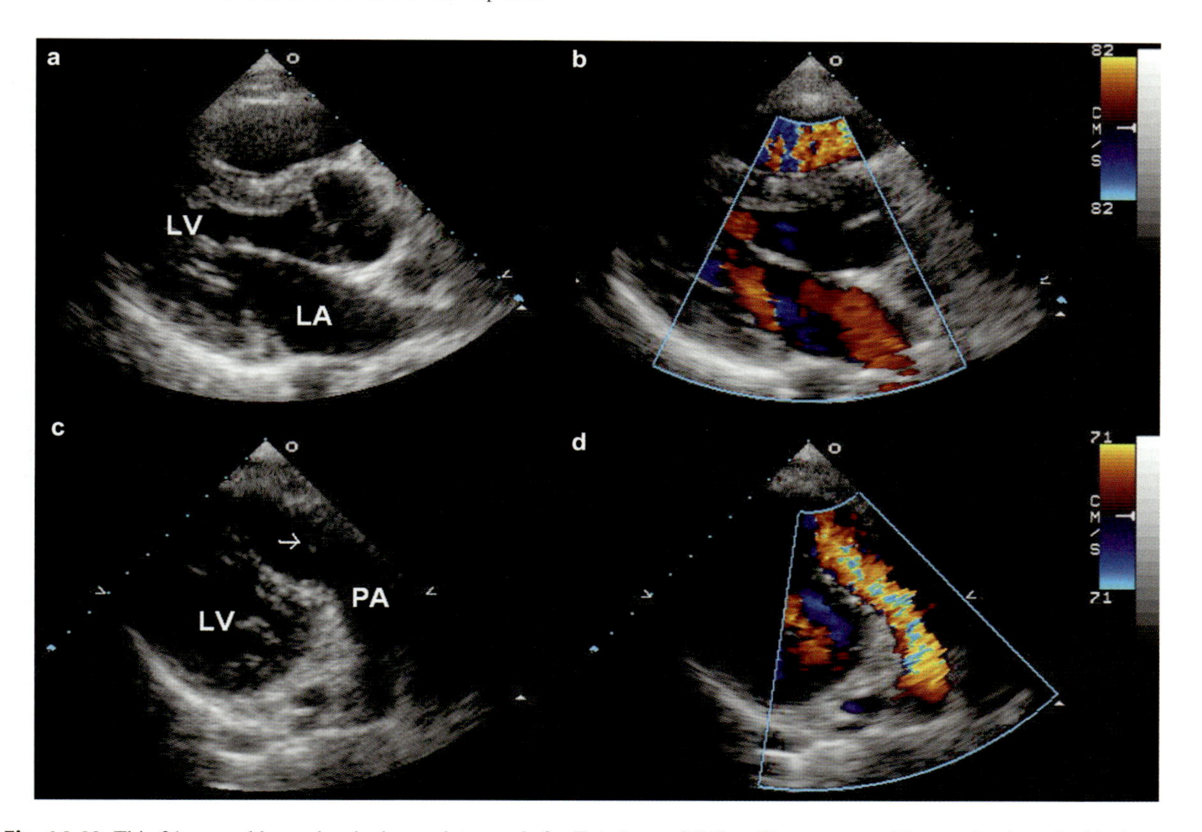

Fig. 14.40 This 21-year-old man has had complete repair for Tetralogy of Fallot. The parasternal long-axis views (**a, b**) show no residual ventricular septal defect. Parasternal short-axis (**c**) shows that the right ventricular outflow tract was widely patent and residual pulmonic valvular tissue is detected (*arrow*). Color flow image (**d**) shows severe pulmonic regurgitation which is a common sequela in these patients. *LA* left atrium, *LV* left ventricle, *PA* pulmonary artery

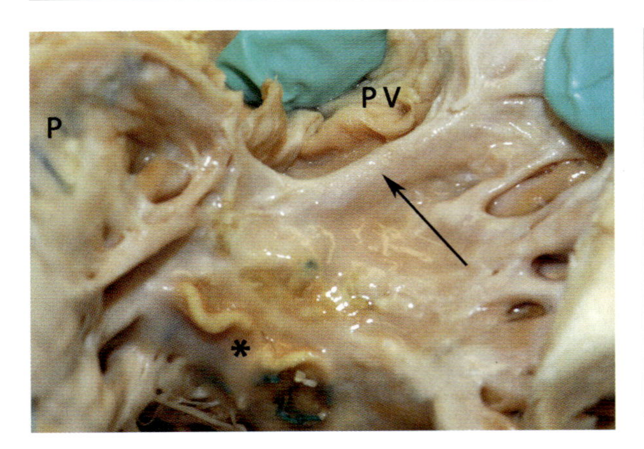

Fig. 14.41 This young patient had sudden death. He had complete repair of tetralogy of Fallot with right ventricle outflow patch (*P*) enlargement and infundibular resection. At autopsy, the outflow tract had a subvalvular ridge (*arrow*) and was restenotic. *PV* pulmonary valve, * = VSD patch

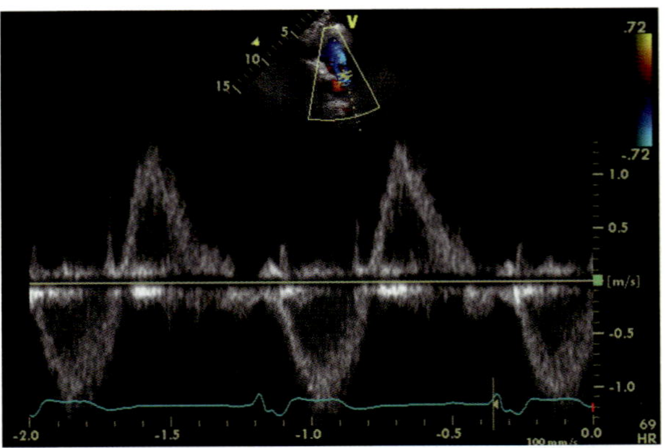

Fig 14.42 The pulsed Doppler demonstrates the typical spectral signal of severe pulmonic regurgitation in a patient who has had complete repair of tetralogy of Fallot. The pulmonic regurgitation has a lower velocity and a rapid drop off

Table 14.3 Common postoperative sequelae and complications in tetralogy of Fallot following surgical correction

Sequelae and complications	Risk factors
Arrhythmia	Residual hemodynamic abnormalities and ventricular scar
PA distortion	Prior systemic pulmonary shunt
RVOT obstruction	Inadequate infundibular resection or contraction of RVOT pericardial patch
RVOT aneurysm	Severe pulmonary regurgitation
Pulmonary regurgitation	Transannular patch
Tricuspid regurgitation	RV dilatation
Aortic root dilatation	Underlying aortopathy
LV dysfunction	Suboptimal cardiac protection during surgery

LV left ventricle, *PA* pulmonary artery, *RV* right ventricle, *RVOT* right ventricular outflow tract

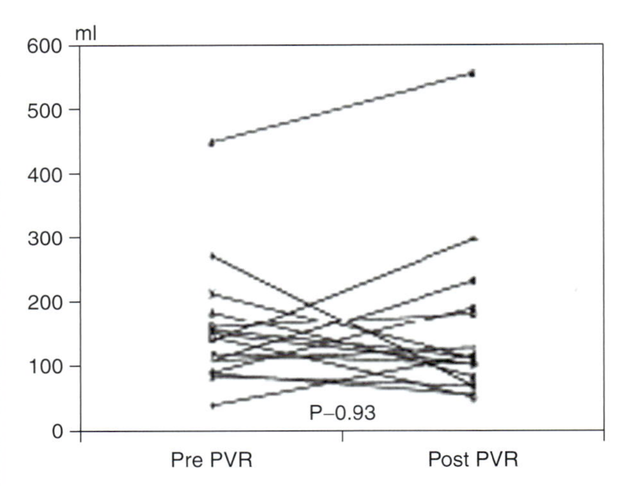

Fig. 14.43 Right ventricular end-systolic volume at rest, before and after pulmonary valve replacement (*PVR*), in patients with tetralogy of Fallot who had severe pulmonary regurgitation following surgical correction. In many of these patients, right ventricle volume remains elevated despite PVR (Reproduced from Therrien et al. [18]. With permission)

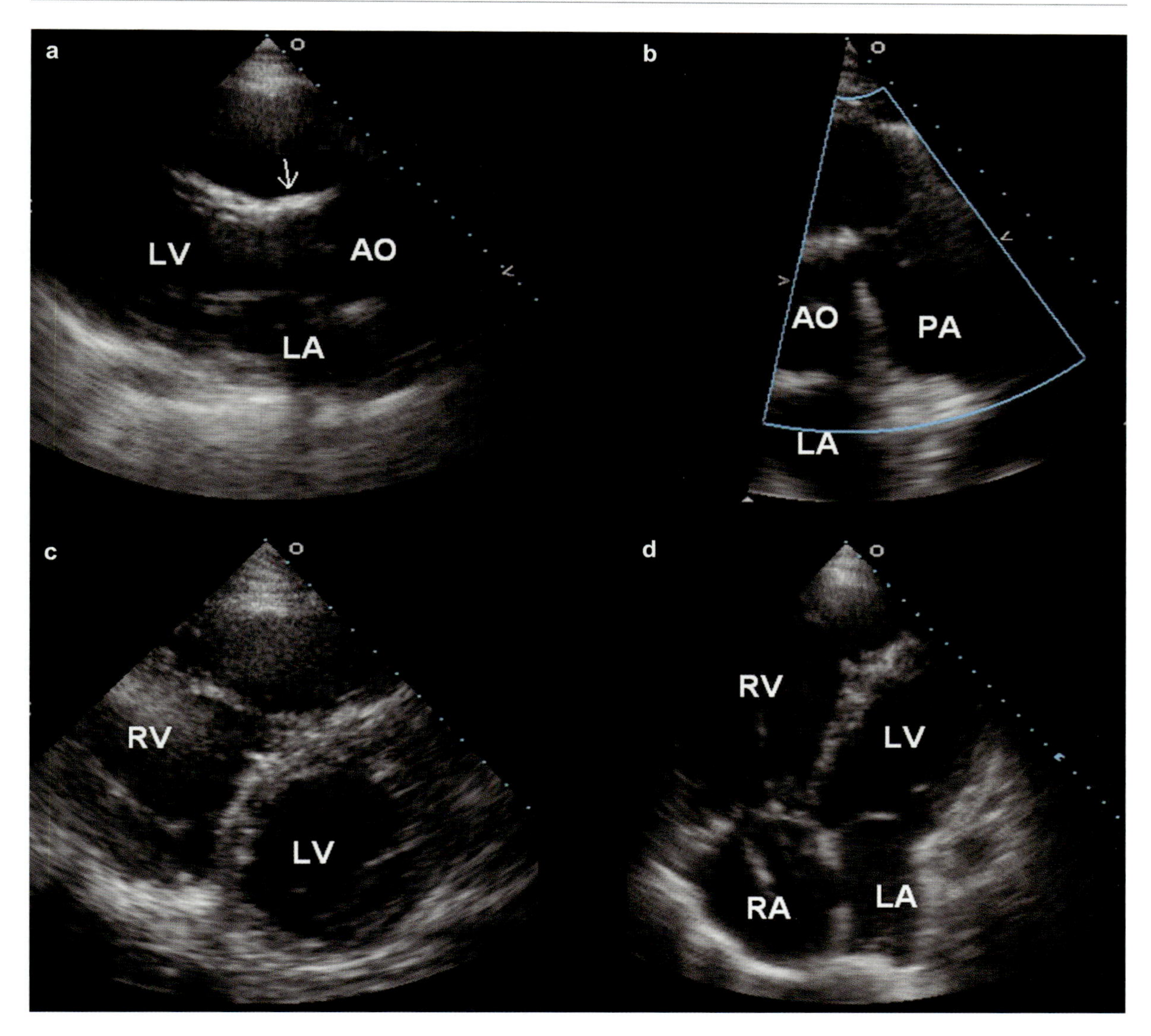

Fig. 14.44 This 40-year-old man had complete repair for tetralogy of Fallot and a repeat operation with implantation of a bioprosthetic valve to correct severe pulmonic regurgitation. The parasternal long-axis view (**a**) shows that the ventricular septal patch is intact (*arrow*). The parasternal short-axis view (**b**) shows the presence of a bioprosthetic valve in the pulmonic position. Despite elimination of pulmonic regurgitation, the right ventricle continues to be dilated and hypokinetic, as shown in the parasternal short-axis (**c**) and apical four-chamber (**d**) views. A pacemaker lead is seen in the right atrium and right ventricle (**d**). *Ao* aorta, *LA* left atrium, *LV* left ventricle, *RA* right atrium, *RV* right ventricle

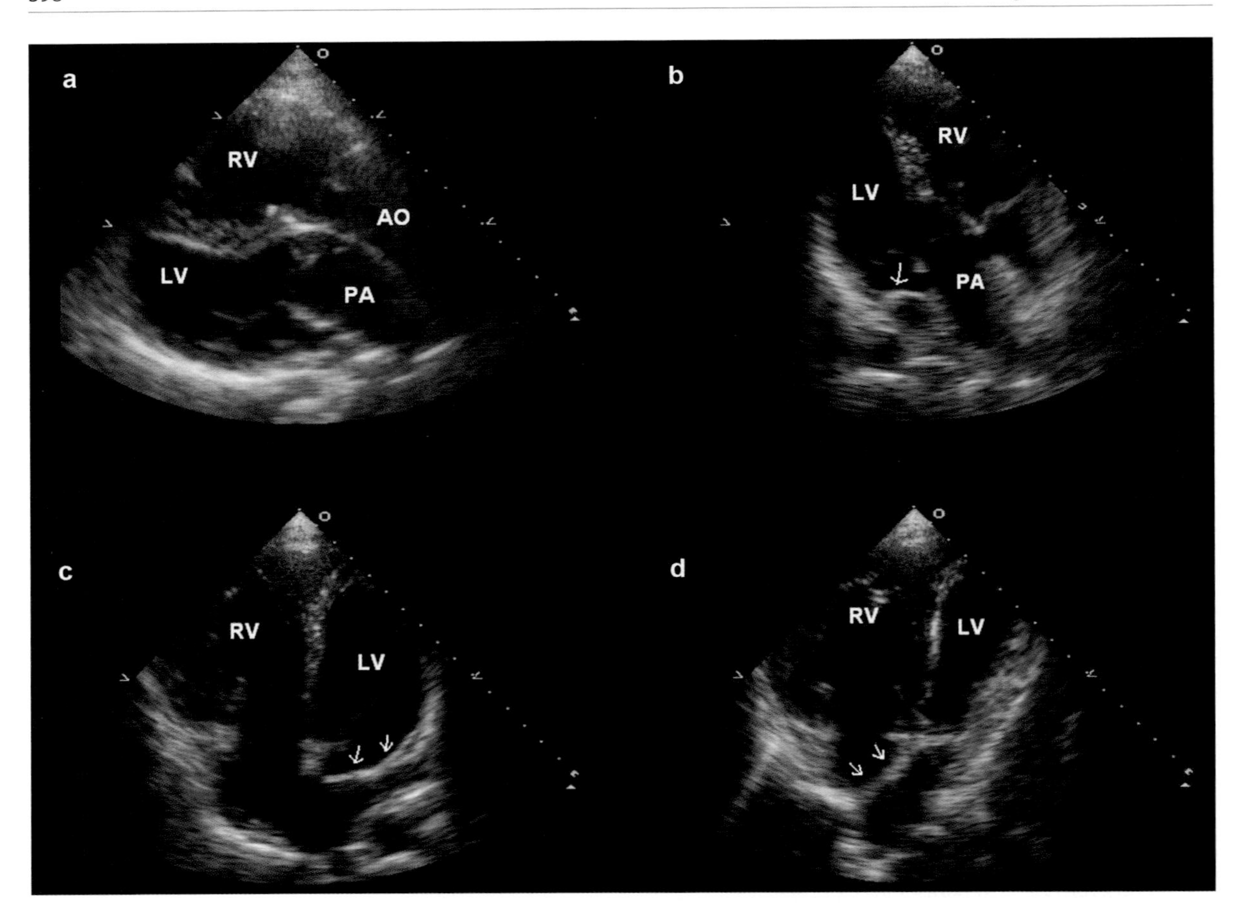

Fig. 14.45 This 30-year-old man had a Mustard procedure for complete transposition of the great arteries. The parasternal long-axis view (**a**) shows that the aorta is anterior to the pulmonary artery confirming transposition. The atrial baffle (*arrows*) is seen in the apical views (**b–d**). In (**c**), the pulmonary venous end of the baffle is shown and is widely patent. In (**d**), the baffle (*arrows*) diverting the blood flow from the inferior vena cava into the morphologic left ventricle is shown. *Ao* aorta, *LV* left ventricle, *PA* pulmonary artery, *RV* right ventricle

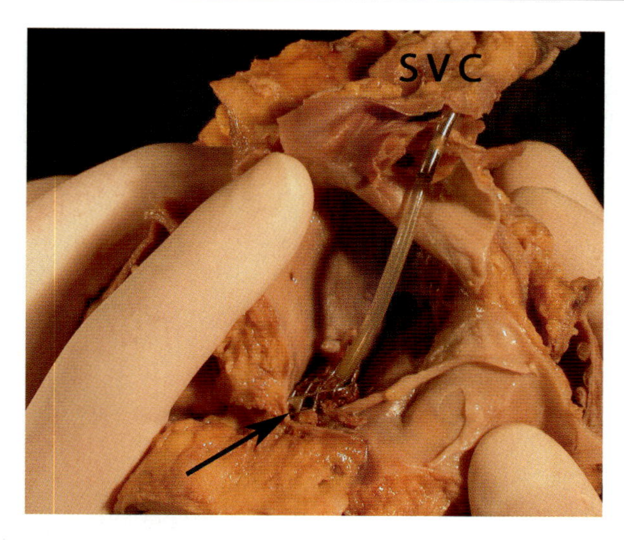

Fig. 14.46 Patient with complete transposition of the great arteries treated with a Mustard atrial baffle procedure. His systemic baffle had become obstructed and a stent (*arrow*) was successfully inserted. A defibrillator lead passed from the superior vena cava (*SVC*), through the stent and ended in the left ventricle

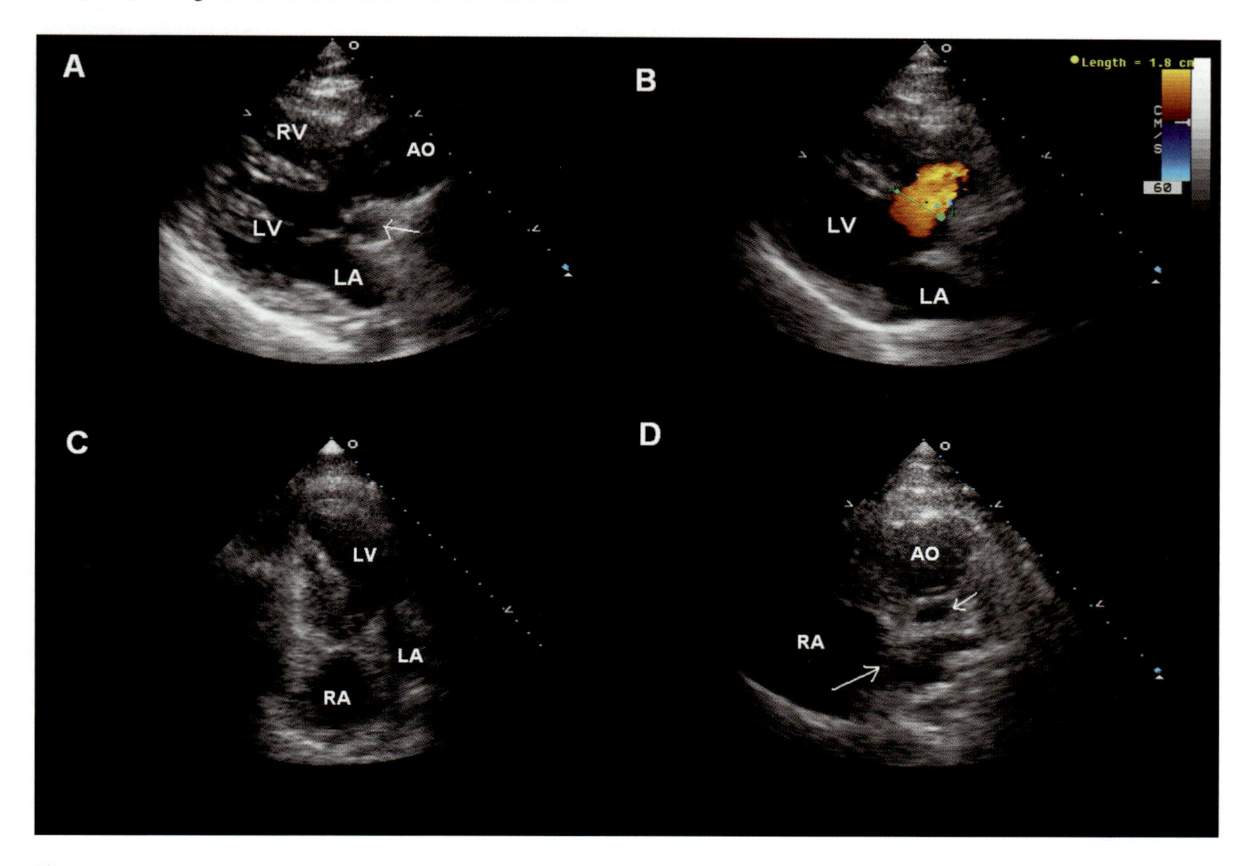

Fig. 14.47 This 25-year-old woman with complete transposition of the great arteries, nonrestrictive ventricular septal defect, and subpulmonic stenosis had undergone a Fontan operation. The parasternal long-axis views (**a, b**) show transposition, disconnected hypoplastic main pulmonary artery (*arrow*), and a large nonrestrictive ventricular septal defect. The tricuspid valve is atretic as shown in (**c**). In a high parasternal short-axis view (**d**), the conduit anastomosis (*long arrow*) from the right atrium to the pulmonary artery is shown, posterior to the disconnected hypoplastic main pulmonary artery (*short arrow*)

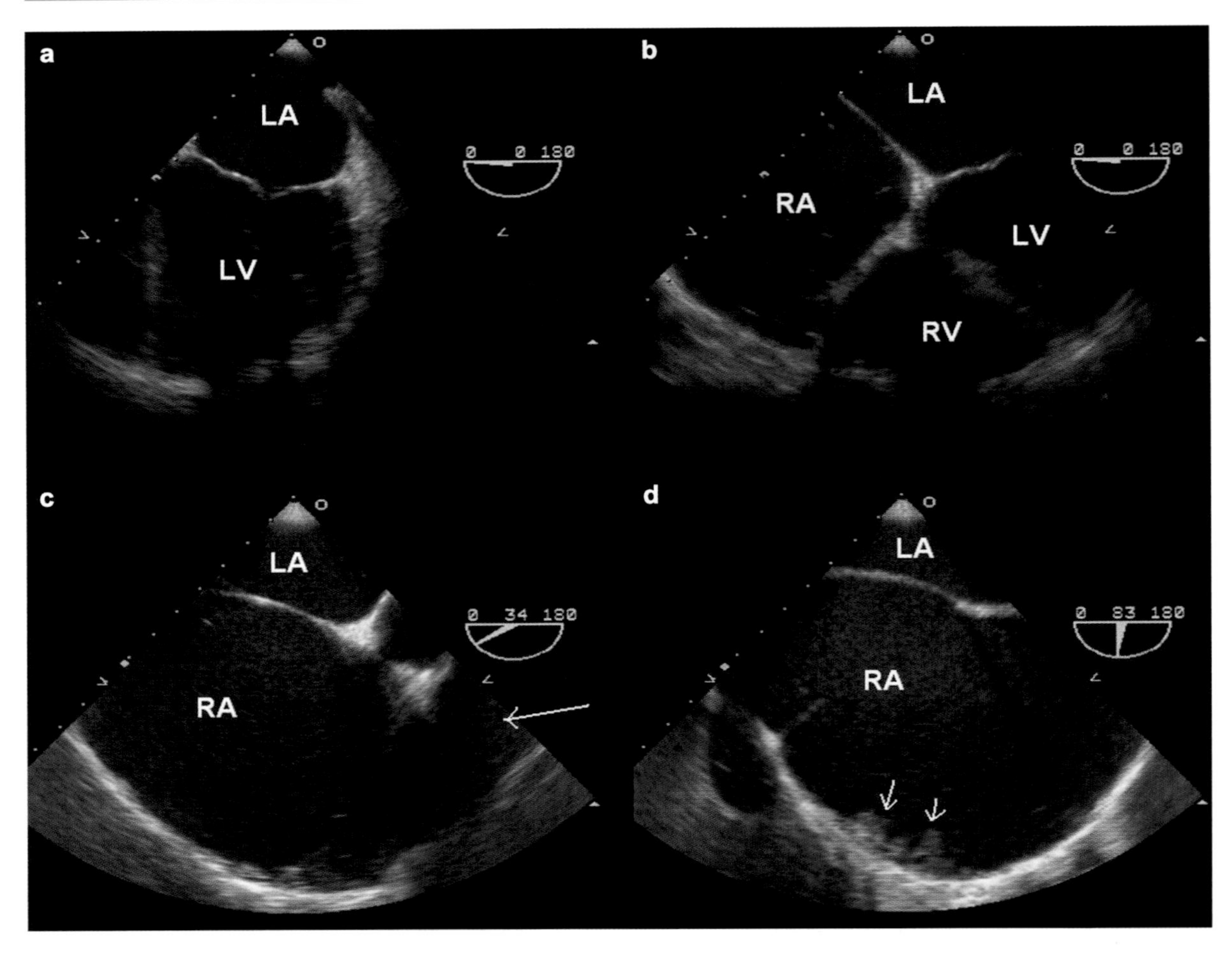

Fig. 14.48 Transesophageal echocardiograms in this 21-year-old woman who had a Fontan operation. A dilated left ventricle is shown in (**a**). The tricuspid valve is atretic (**b**). The Fontan conduit is shown in (**c**) (*arrow*). The right atrium is severely dilated (**c, d**). Masses suggestive of thrombi (*arrows*) are detected in the dilated right atrium (**d**)

early detection and present for the first time in the adult age. Serious complications, such as severe pulmonary hypertension, may occur in some patients with the simple lesions. Patients with complex congenital cardiac lesions generally require surgical intervention during childhood, and frequently have long-term sequelae and complications which require an in-depth understanding of the intracardiac anatomic and hemodynamic abnormalities for proper management. Such an understanding can be obtained using a systematic echocardiographic approach in examining these patients. Since the cardiac anatomy can be highly variable, the transducer position and imaging plane should not be limited to the standard windows, but should be modified as needed to provide the maximum information.

References

1. Sanders SP. Echocardiography and related techniques in the diagnosis of congenital heart defects. Part I. *Echocardiography*. 1984;1:185-217.
2. Sanders SP. Echocardiography and related techniques in the diagnosis of congenital heart defects. Part II. Echocardiography 1984;1:333-391.
3. Sanders SP. Echocardiography and related techniques in the diagnosis of congenital heart defects. Part III. Echocardiography 1984;1:443-493.
4. Horn KD, Devine WA. An approach to dissecting the congenitally malformed heart in the forensic autopsy: the value of sequential segmental analysis. *Am J Forensic Med Pathol*. 2001 Dec;22(4):405-11.
5. Webb G, Gatzoulis MA. Atrial septal defects in the adult - Recent progress and overview. *Circulation*. 2006;114(15): 1645-1653.

6. Shub C, Dimopoulos IN, Seward JB, et al. Sensitivity of two-dimensional echocardiography in the direct visualization of atrial septal defect utilizing the subcostal approach: experience with 154 patients. *J Am Coll Cardiol.* 1983 Jul;2(1):127-35.
7. Fagan S, Veinot JP, Chan KL. Residual sinus venosus atrial septal defect after surgical closure of atrial septal defect. *J Am Soc Echocardiogr.* 2001 Jul;14(7):738-741.
8. Minette MS, Sahn DJ. Ventricular septal defects. *Circulation.* 2006;114(20):2190-2197.
9. Hagler DJ, Edwards WD, Seward JB, Tajik AJ. Standardized nomenclature of the ventricular septum and ventricular septal defects, with applications for two-dimensional echocardiography. *Mayo Clin Proc.* 1985 Nov;60(11):741-752.
10. Schneider DJ, Moore JW. Patent ductus arteriosus. *Circulation.* 2006;114(17):1873-1882.
11. Smallhorn JF, Huhta JC, Adams PA, Anderson RH, Wilkinson JL, Macartney FJ. Cross-sectional echocardiographic assessment of coarctation in the sick neonate and infant. *Br Heart J.* 1983 Oct;50(4):349-361.
12. Hibi N, Fukui Y, Nishimura K, Miwa A, Kambe T, Sakamoto N. Cross-sectional echocardiographic study on persistent left superior vena cava. *Am Heart J.* 1980 Jul;100(1):69-76.
13. Chan KL, Abdulla A. Images in cardiology. Giant coronary sinus and absent right superior vena cava. *Heart.* 2000 Jun;83(6):704.
14. Engel PJ, Held JS, Van dB-K, Spitz H. Echocardiographic diagnosis of congenital sinus of Valsalva aneurysm with dissection of the interventricular septum. *Circulation.* 1981 Mar;63(3):705-711.
15. Bashore TM. Adult congenital heart disease - Right ventricular outflow tract lesions. *Circulation.* 2007;115(14):1933-1947.
16. Deanfield JE, Ho SY, Anderson RH, McKenna WJ, Allwork SP, Hallidie-Smith KA. Late sudden death after repair of tetralogy of Fallot: a clinicopathologic study. *Circulation.* 1983 Mar;67(3):626-631.
17. Silversides CK, Veldtman GR, Crossin J, et al. Pressure half-time predicts hemodynamically significant pulmonary regurgitation in adult patients with repaired tetralogy of fallot. *J Am Soc Echocardiogr.* 2003 Oct;16(10):1057-62.
18. Therrien J, Siu SC, McLaughlin PR, Liu PP, Williams WG, Webb GD. Pulmonary valve replacement in adults late after repair of tetralogy of Fallot: are we operating too late? *J Am Coll Cardiol.* 2000 Nov 1;36(5):1670-1675.
19. Warnes CA. Transposition of the great arteries. *Circulation.* 2006;114(24):2699-2709.
20. Fyfe DA, Kline CH, Sade RM, Gillette PC. Transesophageal echocardiography detects thrombus formation not identified by transthoracic echocardiography after the Fontan operation. *J Am Coll Cardiol.* 1991 Dec;18(7):1733-1737.

15 Cardiac Source of Embolism

Stroke is the third leading cause of death after heart disease and cancer. Its prevalence increases with age, affecting about 5% of people over 65 years of age. Stroke is frequently associated with severe long-term disability. There are multiple causes of stroke, and determination of the etiology of stroke is important for the acute management and the prevention of recurrent events. About 20% of strokes are believed to be embolic in nature related to cardiac abnormalities [1]. Another 30% are considered cryptogenic with no clear etiology. Many cryptogenic strokes may also be embolic in nature [2]. Thus, assessment for cardiac sources of embolism should be an integral part of the investigation of patients who have had a stroke.

Diagnostic Difficulties

The clinical history and physical findings have long been used to determine the etiology of stroke. A history of cardiac disease such as myocardial infarction and valvular heart diseases increases the likelihood of the stroke being cardioembolic in nature. Findings of irregular heartbeats, valvular abnormalities, or ventricular dysfunction suggest the presence of intracardiac thrombus which can embolize. In embolic stroke, the onset of symptoms is usually sudden and may be associated with Valsalva maneuver such as cough and sneeze. An embolic stroke tends to involve a large intracranial arterial territory or multiple territories simultaneously with significant neurological deficit which may improve spontaneously with break up and distal embolization of the embolus [3]. These clinical findings are helpful but are not sufficiently reliable to establish the etiology of stroke [4].

In many patients with stroke believed to be cardioembolic in nature, the diagnosis of stroke mechanism is circumstantial and largely made by excluding other mechanisms such as atherosclerotic disease or lacunar infarcts. In order to have a firm diagnosis, early arteriography is required to show evidence of embolic arterial occlusion of the arterial bed responsible for the stroke, but this is seldom performed. Many of the patients with presumed cardioembolic strokes have atherosclerotic risk factors and many have clinical evidence of atherosclerosis. Furthermore, risk factors for cardiac embolism are present in about 15% of patients with lacunar stroke [5]. It is important to underscore that the presence of a potential cardioembolic source does not necessarily mean that it is the cause of the stroke or that the stroke is cardioembolic in nature. We believe that it is more helpful to consider cardioembolic stroke as a syndrome with diverse potential causes rather than a single entity [4]. The importance of any potential cardiac source of embolism should be carefully adjudicated in the context of the clinical setting.

Diagnostic Approach

Since clinical features lack specificity in establishing the etiology of stroke, a systematic approach is required to investigate patients with stroke [6]. Neuroimaging and cardiac investigations should be considered in many of these patients (Fig. 15.1). Structural heart disease is likely present if there is a history of prior myocardial infarction, heart failure, or valve surgery. Clinical findings of fever, heart failure, cardiomegaly, or heart murmur also suggest structural heart disease and require further investigation. Transthoracic echocardiography (TTE) should be performed in these patients even when

K.-L. Chan and J.P. Veinot, *Anatomic Basis of Echocardiographic Diagnosis*,
DOI: 10.1007/978-1-84996-387-9_15, © Springer-Verlag London Limited 2011

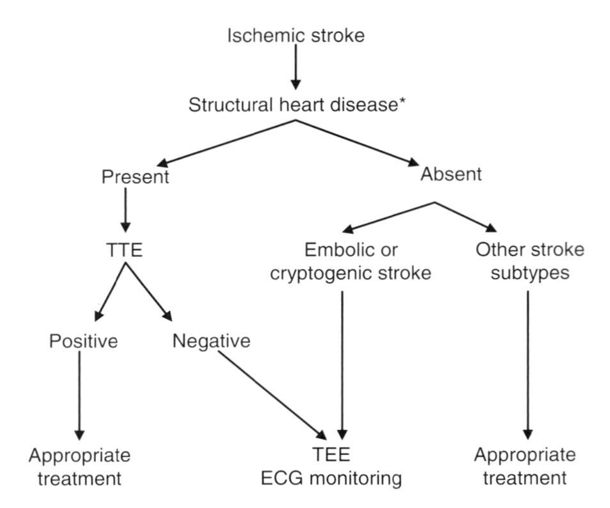

Fig. 15.1 Cardiac investigations in patients with ischemic stroke.*This is determined by clinical history and physical examination. Structural heart disease is present if there is a history of prior heart disease, such as myocardial infarction or valve surgery, or if there are physical findings suggestive of myocardial or valvular dysfunction. *ECG* electrocardiogram, *TEE* transesophageal echocardiography, *TTE* transthoracic echocardiography

the stroke is not believed to be cardioembolic in nature, as the clinical determination of stroke etiology is imprecise and TTE findings may alter management. In patients with embolic stroke or cryptogenic stroke, transesophageal echocardiography (TEE) may be preferred due to its higher diagnostic yield as compared to TTE. For instance, the sensitivity of TEE in detecting left atrial thrombi is 95–100% as compared to 39–73% with TTE [7, 8]. TEE is semiinvasive and associated with a very small but definite risk of complications [9].

In our echocardiographic laboratory, assessment for potential cardiac source of embolism is one of the most common reasons for referral for TEE, accounting for about 20% of the referrals [10]. Younger patients are more likely to be referred for TEE, but many older patients are also referred for this reason. Many TEE findings have been associated with embolic events, but a definitive cause effect relationship is difficult to establish. Although echocardiography, particularly TEE, is frequently used to evaluate patients with presumed embolic stroke, the clinical utility of TEE remains to be determined. It is essential to interpret the echo findings in the clinical context of each individual patient, as a given echo finding may impact on management in one patient and not in another. For instance, calcific aortic valve disease does not merit serious consideration in the evaluation of mechanism of a stroke in a 78-year-old man with hypertension and peripheral vascular disease, but should be looked at with high suspicion in a 50-year-old man who has suffered sudden blindness due to retinal arterial occlusion by a calcific embolus.

Occult atrial fibrillation should be sought, as atrial fibrillation is a known risk factor for stroke and anticoagulation treatment reduces the risk of stroke [11]. The implicit assumption is that the increased stroke risk in atrial fibrillation is due to embolization of left atrial thrombus, although other mechanisms are possible (Fig. 15.2) [12]. Extended electrocardiographic monitoring may be needed to detect atrial fibrillation which can be transient and intermittent. Holter monitoring for 24–48 h detects atrial fibrillation in < 5% of unselected

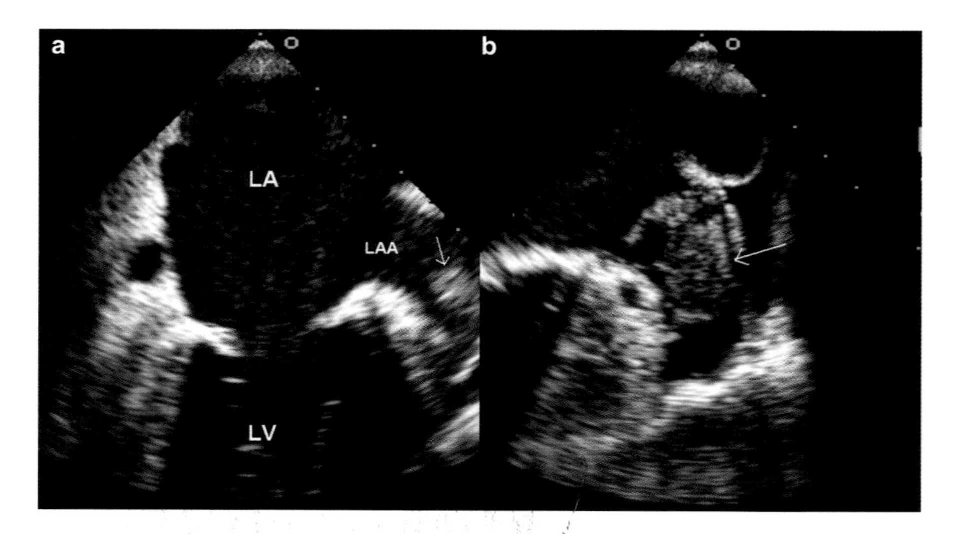

Fig. 15.2 (**a**) Transesophageal echocardiogram in a patient with aortic stenosis and atrial fibrillation shows a dilated left atrium and left atrial appendage with mild spontaneous contrast and suggestion of a mass (*arrow*) within the left atrial appendage. (**b**) The thrombus (*arrow*) is clearly demonstrated when the left atrial appendage is optimally imaged. *LA* left atrium, *LAA* left atrial appendage, *LV* left ventricle

stroke patients [13]. On the other hand, a recent study showed that extended monitoring revealed paroxysmal atrial fibrillation in 23% of patients with cryptogenic stroke or transient ischemic attack [14]. Thus extended electrocardiographic monitoring should be considered in patient groups with a higher yield of occult atrial fibrillation and no other indications for anticoagulation. These include patients with structural heart disease and negative TTE, patients with a high likelihood of embolic stroke, and possibly patients with cryptogenic stroke.

Diagnostic Yield versus Therapeutic Yield

The diagnostic yield of TEE is superior to TTE and dependent on the patient population. The yield is higher in older patients and patients in atrial fibrillation. TEE can detect potential cardiac sources of embolism in more than 50% of patients with ischemic stroke and without clinically overt heart disease [15], but it is important to examine the significance of the cardiac abnormalities detected by TEE and to determine whether these impact on patient management. In many of the studies examining the role of TEE in stroke patients, the patient population was not well defined and the studies were retrospective in nature with inherent limitations [16–20]. Clearly, certain findings such as vegetation, tumor, or thrombus are significant and affect the management, but they account for a small minority of the TEE findings in these studies. Many findings have dubious significance, as they can be detected by the clinical history such as prosthetic heart valves, or they have no impact on management such as mitral valve prolapse, or they have uncertain relevance such as patent foramen ovale. The therapeutic impact of echocardiography (TTE or TEE) is therefore much less than the diagnostic yield may suggest [21, 22]. Strandberg et al. reviewed TEE findings in 441 patients with ischemic stroke or transient ischemic attack within 31 days of the events and no history of heart disease [23]. In 286 patients in sinus rhythm and no history of heart disease, a major cardiac source was detected in 5% of patients and a minor cardiac source in 39%. The minor cardiac sources were largely accounted for by patent foramen ovale and aortic plaque, while the major cardiac sources were left atrial thrombus or aortic thrombus. The clinical impact attributed to the TEE findings was the initiation of anticoagulation therapy in 8% of patients. It can be argued that TEE is not necessary in the patients already on anticoagulation or those who have an indication for anticoagulation.

A high diagnostic yield of TEE is misleading, since many of the findings are unlikely to influence management. The therapeutic yield of TEE is modest and needs to be better defined, despite the widespread use of TEE in this clinical setting. Lacking is an evidence-based and cost-effective approach in the evaluation of patients with ischemic stroke [24]. Our approach shown in Fig. 15.1 is pragmatic and should be modified depending on the clinical scenario. For instance, in a patient already having an indication for anticoagulation therapy, echocardiography (TTE or TEE) may not be necessary.

Echocardiographic Findings

There are many echocardiographic findings that have been implicated as potential cardiac sources of embolism (Fig. 15.3). Some of these findings clearly have important clinical significance as they are likely the cause of the embolic event, while other findings are weakly associated with embolic events and likely have little impact on management. Controversy surrounds certain findings such as a patent foramen ovale [25]. Ongoing research is needed to provide a proper perspective of the significance of many of these findings.

Many echocardiographic findings have been associated with an increased rate of embolic events. The associated risks of embolic events are different among these different echocardiographic findings, which can be categorized into three groups according to the estimated annual rate of thromboembolic events (Table 15.1) [15, 25].

High-Risk Findings

The high-risk category refers to findings that are associated with greater than 10 % annual risk of embolism. They include intracardiac thrombus (left atrial, left ventricular, and valvular thrombi), left atrial myxoma, mitral stenosis (with or without atrial fibrillation), and

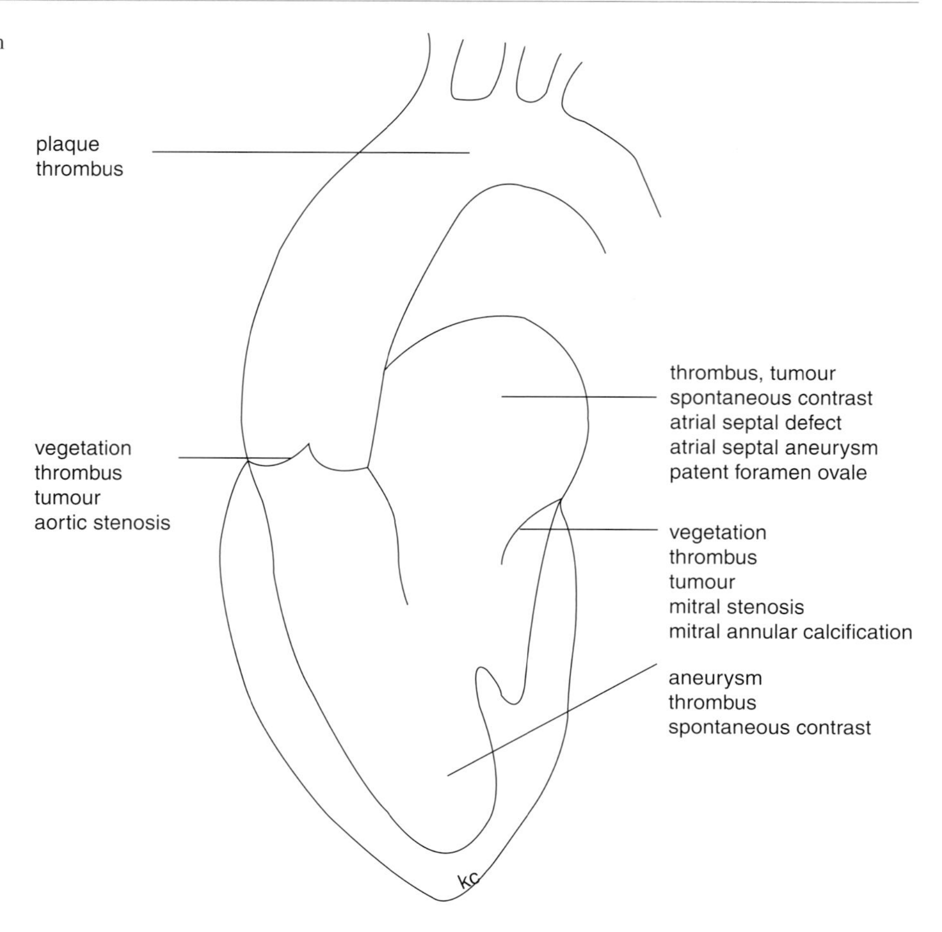

Fig. 15.3 Schematic diagram showing the cardiac and extracardiac conditions that have been associated with thromboembolic events

valvular vegetations (Figs. 15.4, 15.5). When any of these findings is detected by echocardiography, it is reasonable to assume that it is the likely source of embolism. The echocardiographic features of these entities have been discussed in detail in the previous chapters. An embolus in transit is a rare situation in which a large thrombus from the deep veins in the lower extremities migrates into the right atrium and crosses a coexisting patent foramen ovale (Fig. 15.6) [26]. Patients with this unusual finding not only have evidence of pulmonary embolism, but are also at a very high risk of systemic embolism. Surgical removal is the preferred treatment option in many of these patients.

Atrial Fibrillation

Systemic embolization is a major complication of nonvalvular atrial fibrillation, and the risk can be estimated on the basis of associated clinical risk factors including age, congestive heart failure, hypertension, diabetes mellitus, and a history of stroke [11]. The prevalence of atrial fibrillation increases with age, and the incidence of stroke associated with atrial fibrillation also increases with age [27, 28].

Anticoagulation therapy has been shown to reduce the risk of stroke, particularly in high-risk individuals [11]. In low-risk people, the risk of stroke should be balanced with the risk of bleeding associated with anticoagulation therapy.

Mitral Stenosis

Mitral stenosis is associated with a high risk of thromboembolic events with or without atrial fibrillation [25]. Patients with mitral stenosis should be on anticoagulation therapy, with the possible exception of

Table 15.1 Potential cardiac sources of embolism

High-risk findings
• Atrial fibrillation with multiple risk factors
• LA thrombus
• LV thrombus
• Endocarditis (infective or marantic [nonbacterial thrombotic])
• Mitral stenosis
• Myxoma
• Complex aortic arch plaques
Moderate-risk findings
• Recent myocardial infarction with LV dysfunction or aneurysm
• Severe LV dysfunction (EF < 35%)
• Prosthetic heart valves on anticoagulation
• Atrial fibrillation with absent or few clinical risk factors
• LA spontaneous contrast
• Mitral annular calcification with a mobile mass
Uncertain, likely low-risk findings
• Mild to moderate LV dysfunction (EF > 35%)
• Chronic LV aneurysm without thrombus
• Aortic stenosis
• Mitral valve prolapse
• Mitral annular calcification
• Patent foramen ovale
• Intrapulmonary shunt
• Atrial septal aneurysm
• Lambl's excrescence, valvular strands, fibroelastoma

EF ejection fraction, *LA* left atrium, *LV* left ventricle

patients with mild mitral stenosis, sinus rhythm, and normal left atrial size.

Aortic Plaque

The thromboembolic risks in patients with aortic plaque appear to be related to the severity and complexity of the plaque (Figs. 15.7, 15.8). In patients with severe aortic arch plaque exceeding 4 mm in thickness, the cerebral thromboembolic risk increases by several fold as compared to controls [29]. However, optimal management remains unclear. The SPAF-III study suggests that anticoagulation may reduce the embolic risks in this setting although only high-risk patients with atrial fibrillation were included in this study and hence this observation may not be generalizable to other populations [12]. Treatment with statins may be useful [30]. Surgical removal of complex plaques does not appear to be a good option since this procedure is associated with a high risk of perioperative cerebrovascular event [31].

Descending aortic plaques should not be a risk factor for cerebral embolization, but their presence suggests that similar changes may affect the ascending aorta and arch which should be carefully assessed for aortic

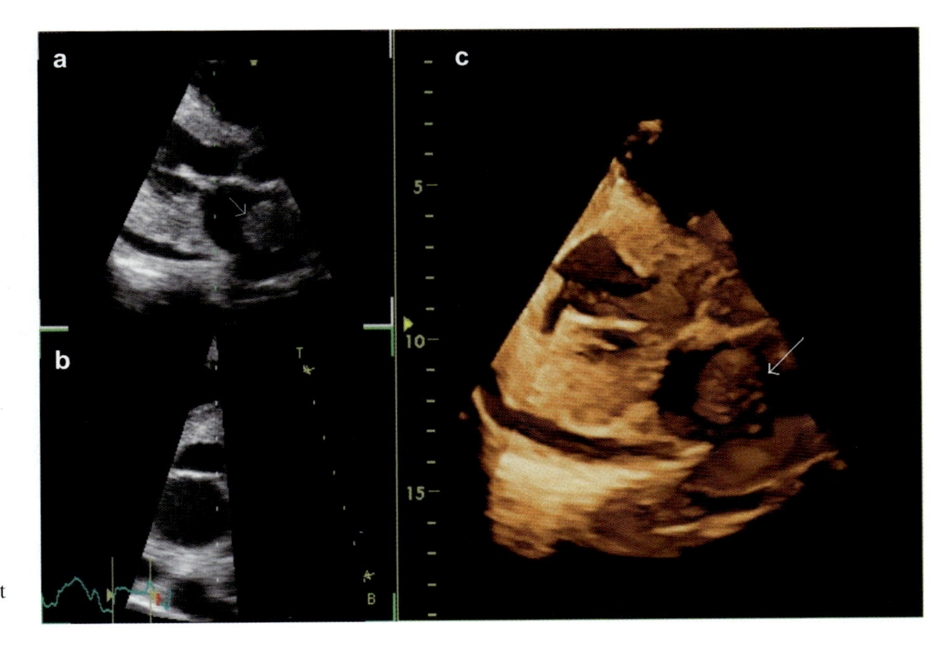

Fig. 15.4 The parasternal long-axis (**a**), short-axis (**b**) and the 3D (**c**) views show the presence of a large free-flowing ball valve thrombus (*arrow*) in a patient with amyloid heart disease

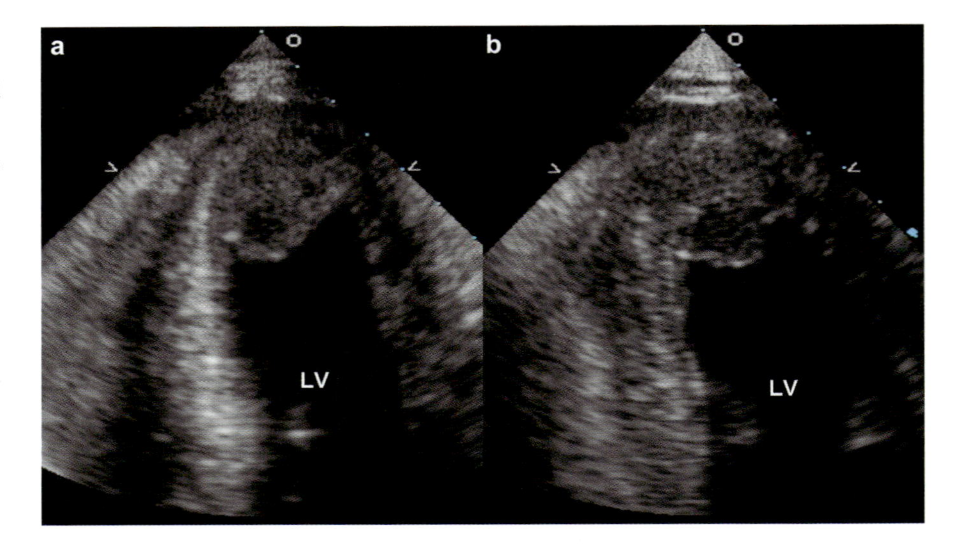

Fig. 15.5 A large thrombus is present within the left ventricular apex in the apical four-chamber (**a**) and two-chamber (**b**) views in a patient with a recent anterior wall myocardial infarction. *LV* left ventricle

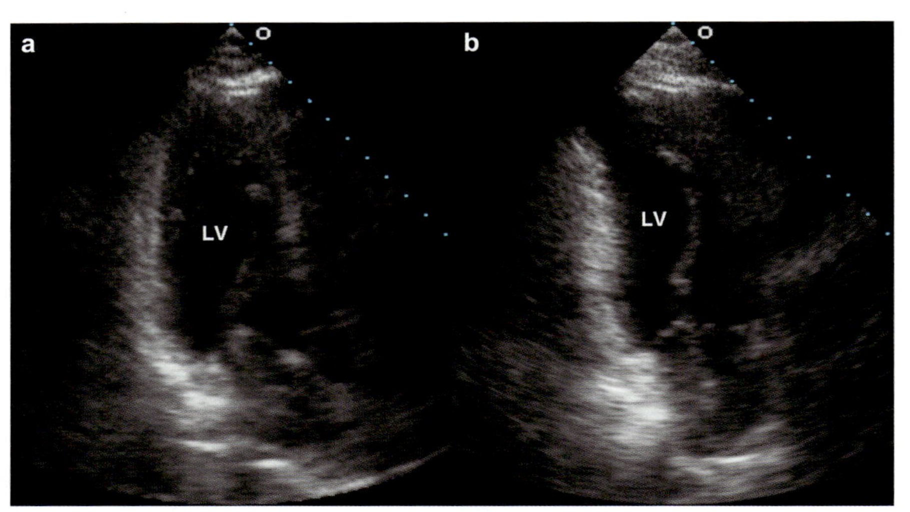

Fig. 15.6 The apical long-axis (**a**) and two-chamber (**b**) views in a 39-year-old truck driver with chest pain show a long sausage-like mass within the left atrium protruding into the left ventricle. Other views (not shown) showed that the mass was trapped at the foramen ovale with part of it in the right atrium. This was a large thrombus arising from the leg veins which had embolized into the right heart and traversed into the left heart via a patent foramen ovale. These findings were confirmed at surgery. *LV* left ventricle

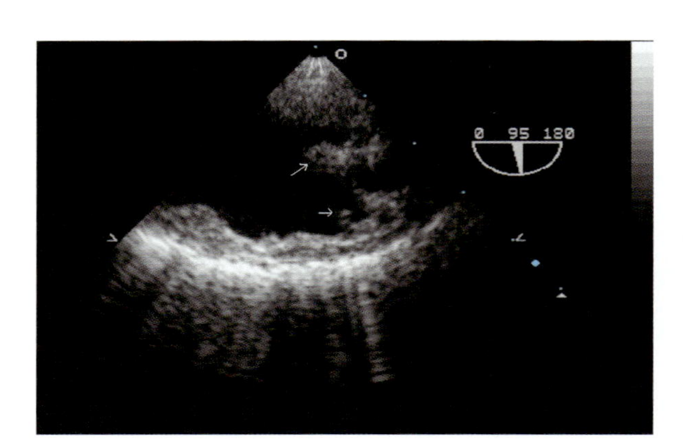

Fig. 15.7 Transesophageal echocardiogram of the aortic arch shows diffuse involvement with complex aortic plaques. Some of the plaques (*arrows*) are mobile

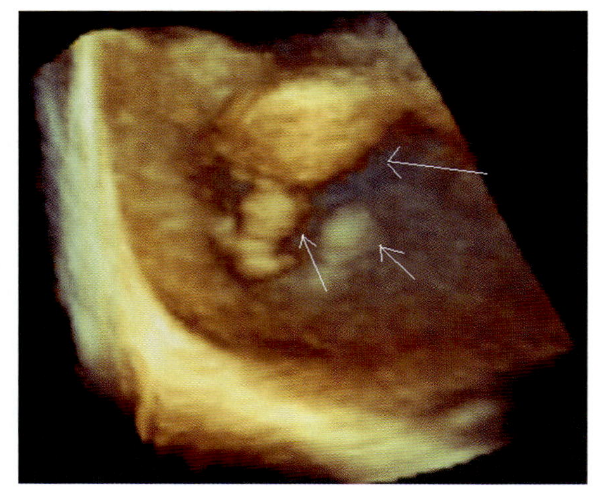

Fig. 15.8 Transesophageal 3D view of the proximal descending aorta shows multiple aortic plaques of varying sizes (*arrows*)

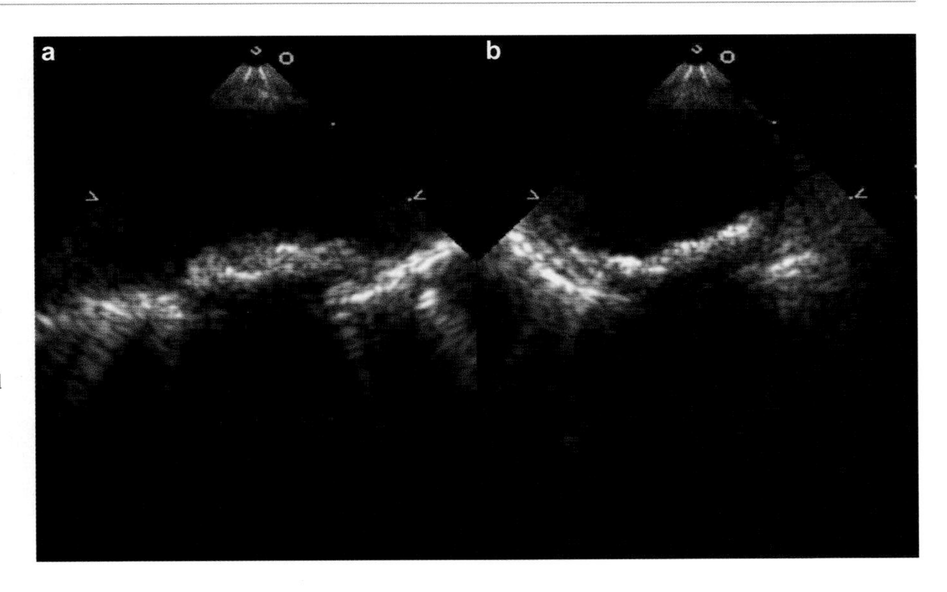

Fig. 15.9 Transesophageal longitudinal (**a**) and transverse (**b**) views of the proximal descending aorta show a large plaque with some degree of calcification, as demonstrated by the shadowing in the far field. The presence of complex plaques in the descending aorta increases the likelihood that similar findings are present in the aortic arch and ascending aorta which should be carefully examined

plaques (Fig. 15.9) [12]. In a small subset of patients, a large mobile thrombus can occur in the ascending aorta or arch and be associated with cerebral embolic events [32]. The underlying aortic wall may be normal or may have a small plaque. The exact mechanism for the formation of a large thrombus in these patients remains unclear. Both anticoagulation therapy and surgery have been used in this setting with favorable outcome.

Moderate-Risk Findings

The second category includes conditions with a moderate risk of embolism (annual risk of embolic events between 1–10%). Acute left ventricular aneurysm post myocardial infarction with no thrombus, atrial fibrillation with no or few risk factors, and dense left atrial spontaneous contrast belong to this category.

Myocardial Infarction and Left Ventricular Dysfunction

Left ventricular thrombus can occur in patients with myocardial infarction or dilated cardiomyopathy. This can be readily detected by TTE, and anticoagulation therapy for 3–6 months is indicated to reduce the risk of embolic events. Acute myocardial infarction is associated with an increased risk of stroke (about 1–2.5%) within the first 4 weeks, and the risk is higher in anterior wall myocardial infarction (Fig. 15.10) [33]. The use of anticoagulation therapy for 3–6 months can be considered in patients with anterior wall myocardial infarct with significant left ventricular dysfunction in the absence of left ventricular thrombus. In patients with dilated cardiomyopathy, the risk of stroke is increased but low and anticoagulation therapy is usually not recommended. Future trials will provide more data in this patient group [34].

Prosthetic Valves

Both bioprosthetic and mechanical heart valves are associated with an increased risk of stroke, even with a therapeutic level of anticoagulation (Fig. 15.11) [35]. The risk is higher with early generation valves, prosthetic valves in the mitral position, mechanical valves, and concomitant atrial fibrillation. When a presumed embolic event occurs despite therapeutic anticoagulation, investigations should be performed to exclude bleeding as a cause for the event. This can be followed by the consideration of adding an antiplatelet agent or intensifying the anticoagulation level.

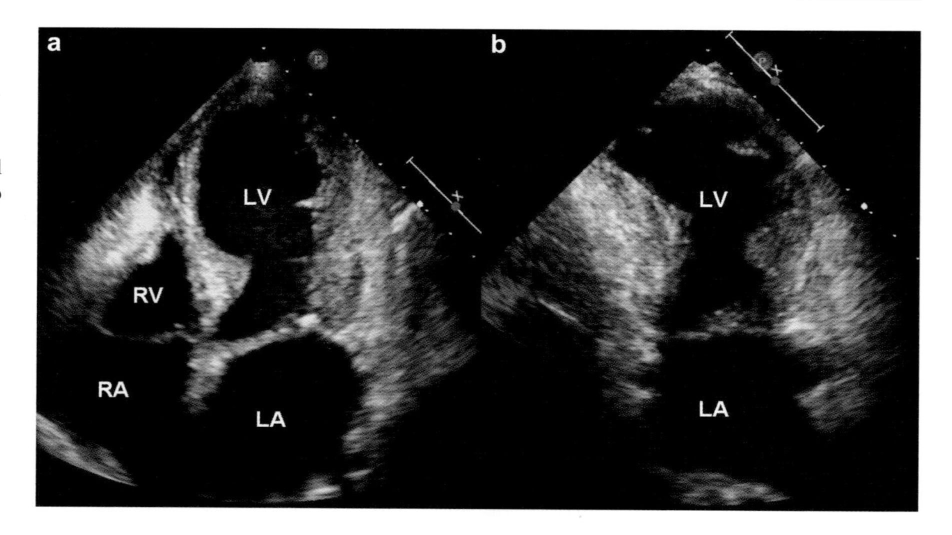

Fig. 15.10 Apical four-chamber (**a**) and two-chamber (**b**) views in an 84-year-old woman with anterior wall myocardial infarction show a large apical left ventricular aneurysm. No definite thrombus is seen within the aneurysm. *LA* left atrium, *LV* left ventricle, *RA* right atrium, *RV* right ventricle

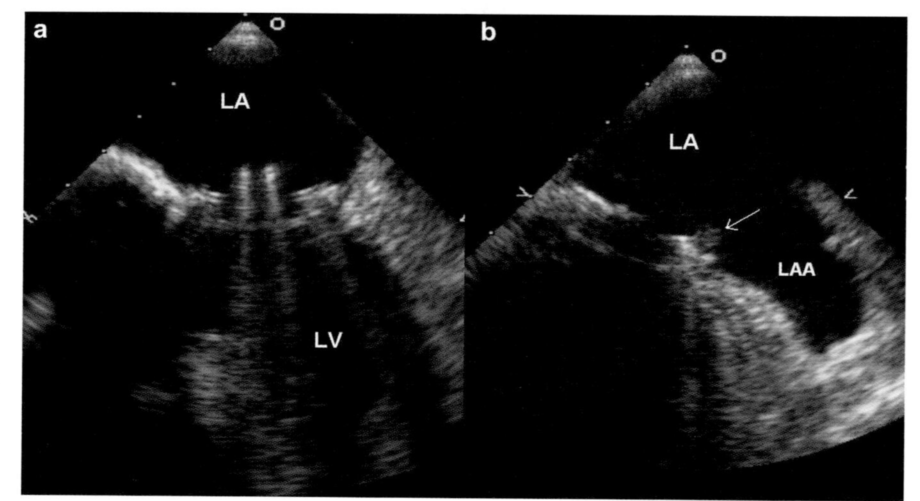

Fig. 15.11 Transesophageal transverse (**a**) and longitudinal (**b**) views of a bileaflet mitral mechanical prosthetic valve show that there is a small mass (*arrow*) consistent with thrombus on the atrial surface of the anterior aspect of the sewing ring. *LA* left atrium

Spontaneous Echo Contrast

Spontaneous echo contrast describes the phenomenon of slow-moving smoke-like echo density in area of stasis. Its swirling pattern resembles smoke from a chimney. It reflects stagnant blood flow and is best seen in the left atrial appendage (Figs. 15.12, 15.13) [36]. It is associated with mitral stenosis and atrial fibrillation, although it is sometimes detected in the absence of valve disease and in sinus rhythm. Dense spontaneous contrast is strongly associated with left atrial thrombus and increases the risk of thromboembolic events by more than threefold in patients with atrial fibrillation (Fig. 15.14) [12]. Anticoagulation therapy is effective in reducing the thromboembolic risks associated with the spontaneous contrast in the left atrium. In patients

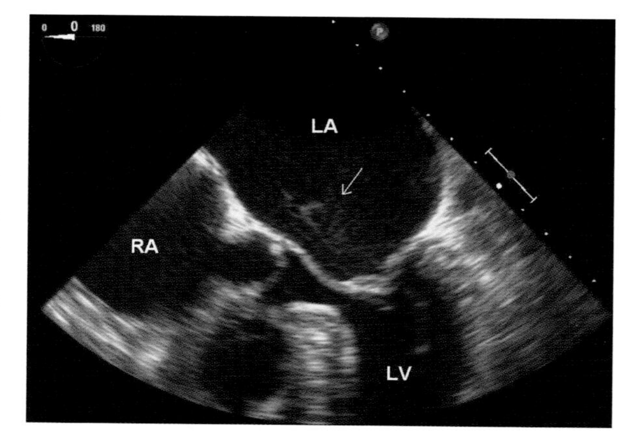

Fig. 15.12 Transesophageal echocardiogram shows mild left atrial spontaneous contrast (*arrow*) in a patient with mitral stenosis and a dilated left atrium. *LA* left atrium, *LV* left ventricle, *RA* right atrium

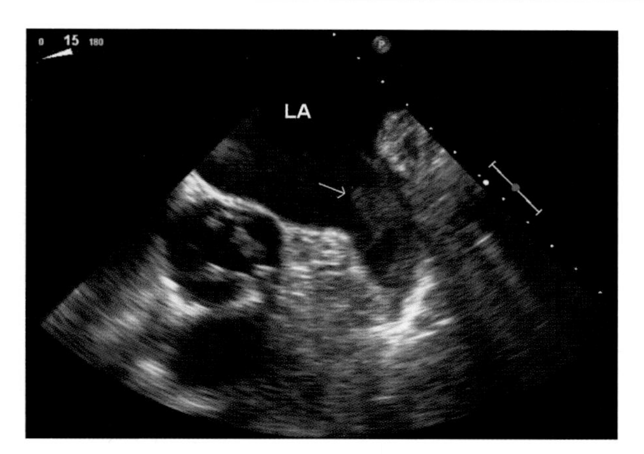

Fig. 15.13 Transesophageal echocardiogram of the left atrial appendage showing dense spontaneous contrast (*arrow*) within the left atrial appendage. This is the same patient as in Fig. 15.12

with mild degree of spontaneous contrast and no history of thromboembolic events, the usefulness of anticoagulation therapy is unknown.

Uncertain, Likely Low-Risk Findings

Although the following echocardiographic findings have been associated with ischemic stroke, their clinical significance is uncertain and the annual embolic event rate is relatively low at about 1% per year or less. Chronic left ventricular aneurysm, simple aortic plaques, and patent foramen ovale belong to this category.

Chronic Left Ventricular Aneurysm

Chronic left ventricular aneurysm is a source of stasis leading to the formation of left ventricular endocardial thrombus. The optimal management of patients with this condition remains unclear, although chronic anticoagulation therapy may be reasonable if the anticipated risk of bleeding is low. In one retrospective study of 69 patients with this condition, not on anticoagulation therapy, one thromboembolic event was reported in a follow-up of 288 patient-years [37].

Patent Foramen Ovale

Patent foramen ovale (PFO) can be a normal finding and is present in up to 30% of young adults [38, 39]. Due to its high prevalence in patients free of cardiac symptoms, convincing supportive evidence should be present before this condition is accepted to have a role in the development of embolic events. Contrast echocardiography using agitated saline is the preferred way to detect PFO by demonstrating right to left atrial shunting within three cardiac cycles following the intravenous injection of saline contrast (Figs. 15.15, 15.16). The shunting can be present at rest, but more frequently detected during cough or the release phase of the Valsalva maneuver. A large PFO is one with shunting at rest, persistent separation > 2 mm, and large shunt > 50 bubbles (Figs. 15.17–15.19) [15]. The hypothesis is

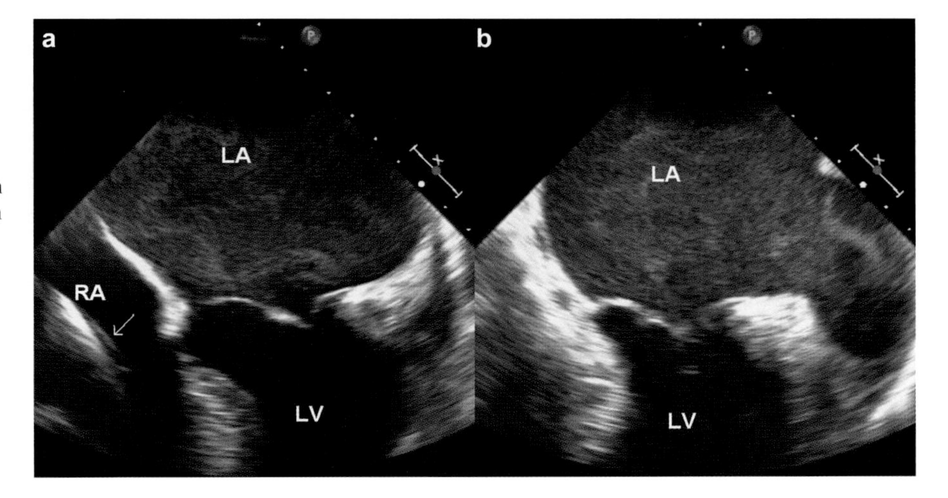

Fig. 15.14 Transesophageal transverse (**a**) and longitudinal (**b**) views in a patient with longstanding atrial fibrillation show a severely dilated left atrium with dense spontaneous contrast. Dense spontaneous contrast is frequently associated with thrombus, which is not present in this patient. A pacemaker lead (*arrow*) is present in the right atrium and right ventricle

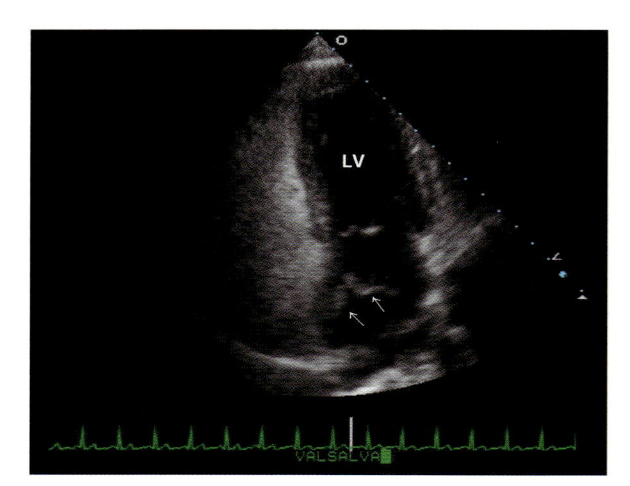

Fig. 15.15 Intravenous injection of agitated saline is performed to demonstrate the presence of atrial shunting. The apical four-chamber view is preferred for this purpose. Good opacification of the right atrium and right ventricle is achieved, and during the release phase of the Valsalva maneuver, contrast is seen coming from the right atrium into the left atrium (*arrows*) indicating the presence of patent foramen ovale. *LV* left ventricle

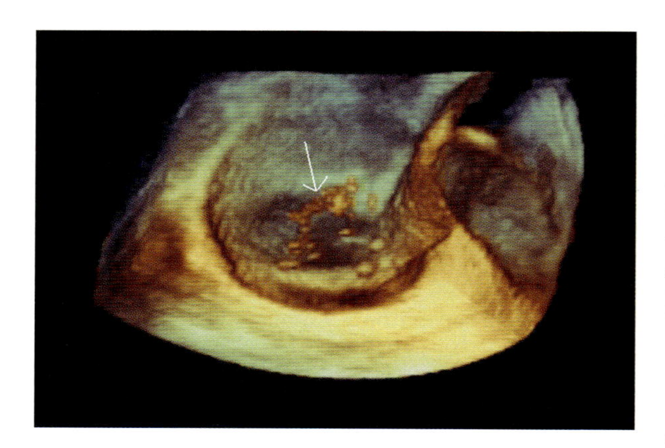

Fig. 15.16 Transesophageal 3D view of a patent foramen ovale following intravenous contrast injection with agitated saline shows bubbles (*arrow*) crossing from the right atrium into the left atrium

that PFO allows paradoxic embolization which is the passage of thrombus originating from the deep veins to get into the systematic circulation resulting in a stroke. However, deep vein thrombosis is infrequently found in patients suspected to have paradoxic embolization [38]. Population studies suggest that PFO is a benign finding in most individuals. There is variability in the diagnosis of this condition and in grading the size of the shunting. We have demonstrated that spontaneous contrast can develop in the left atrium during cough or the release phase of the Valsalva maneuver. This spontaneous contrast appears to emanate from the pulmonary veins and can be detected without contrast injection [40]. Awareness of this phenomenon is important so as not to confuse it with right to left shunting via a PFO during contrast injection.

The prevalence of PFO is higher in patients with cryptogenic stroke than in patients with other stroke subtypes [41, 42]. Two randomized trials have shown that PFO did not confer an increased risk of recurrent stroke [42, 43]. In one study, the presence of PFO and atrial septal aneurysm was associated with an increased risk of recurrent strokes, although this involved a small number of patients with a wide confidence interval [42]. There is insufficient evidence to support any medical treatment or invasive intervention. Anticoagulation therapy is reasonable in a young patient with a large PFO and a history of stroke that has been associated with the Valsalva maneuver. Percutaneous device closure of PFO may be considered in patients who are unable to tolerate anticoagulation treatment or are at an increased risk of bleeding associated with the long-term use of anticoagulation therapy.

Although controversies surround the importance of PFO as a key component for systemic embolic events, there has been a persistent and at times enthusiastic willingness to close a PFO to prevent presumed embolic events [44]. This is particularly the case in young patients with no other apparent source for the development of a presumed embolic event. Properly conducted trials are crucial to clarify the appropriate therapy in these patients.

Atrial Septal Aneurysm

Atrial septal aneurysm is defined as bulging of the atrial septum in part or in whole. The bulging is usually into the right atrium and at least 10 mm from the normal atrial septal plane (Fig. 15.20) [45]. Frequently, it is associated with excessive mobility with the atrial septum flopping back and forth between the left and right atria. It is associated with a higher prevalence of PFO and atrial septal defect (Figs. 15.21, 15.22). In one study, the combination of atrial septal aneurysm and PFO was associated with a much higher risk of embolic events [42]. Physiologically, it is difficult to explain why atrial septal aneurysm should be a risk factor for embolic events, since it is usually highly mobile and unlikely to

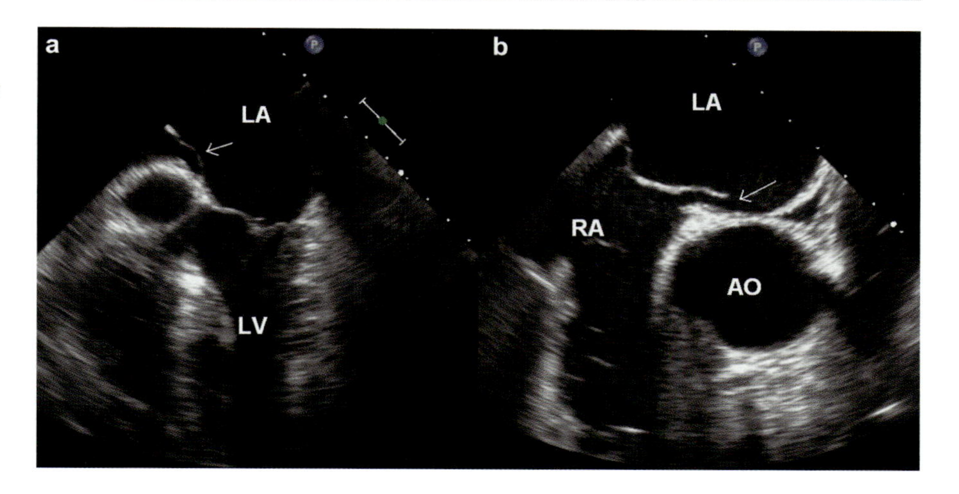

Fig. 15.17 Transesophageal views (**a, b**) of the atrial septum show the relationship of the atrial septum with the aortic root. In (**b**), persistent separation (*arrow*) is present indicating the presence of a large foramen ovale. *Ao* aorta, *LA* left atrium, *LV* left ventricle, *RA* right atrium

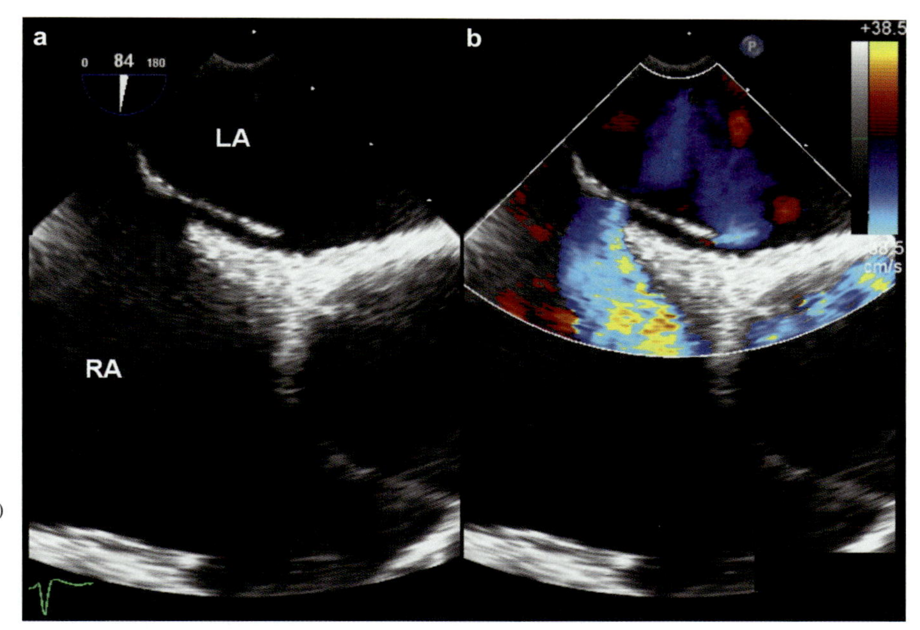

Fig. 15.18 Transesophageal view of the atrial septum (**a**) shows persistent separation consistent with large foramen ovale, and color flow image (**b**) shows resting shunt, which is also a sign of a large patent foramen ovale. *LA* left atrium, *RA* right atrium

be an area of stasis. We have not observed a single case of atrial thrombus located in an atrial septal aneurysm.

Intrapulmonary Shunt

Pulmonary arteriovenous malformation can lead to intrapulmonary shunting and therefore is a potential conduit for paradoxic embolization [46]. They can be detected echocardiographically by the late appearance of contrast in the left heart in three to five cardiac cycles after the opacification of the right heart with saline contrast. This condition may be associated with an increased risk of stroke, but the risk is not well defined. Endovascular occlusion has been successfully used to close these malformations.

Valvular Strands, Lambl's Excrescences, Fibroelastoma

Mobile filaments attached to the valve leaflets or cusps can be detected in about 5% of TEE studies

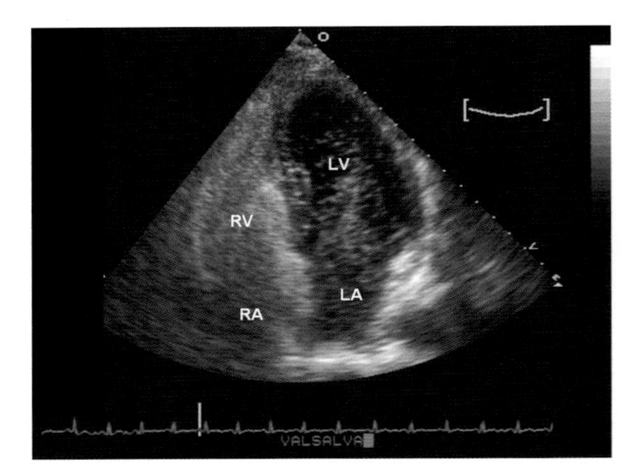

Fig. 15.19 Apical four-chamber view shows the presence of a large degree of contrast in the left atrium and left ventricle during the release phase of the Valsalva maneuver indicating a large shunt consistent with a large patent foramen ovale

(Figs. 15.23–15.27) [47, 48]. Available histologic studies show a hyalinized amorphous stromal core with loose connective tissue and a single layer of endothelium. Indeed, valvular strands, Lambl's excrescences, and fibroelastoma overlap macroscopically and microscopically, so that these findings may be clinically similar [48]. These valvular filaments are usually benign and asymptomatic [49]. With current harmonic imaging, spontaneous contrast emanating from leaflet closure in the setting of native valve can be observed. Extreme care must be taken to differentiate this type of spontaneous contrast from valvular strands. Association with thromboembolic events has been reported, but the therapeutic strategy of patients with these valvular abnormalities remains unclear [47]. Based on case reports, antiplatelet therapy as well as anticoagulation may be effective [48]. In patients with very large lesions and recurrent thromboembolic events, surgical excision may be necessary.

Valve Diseases

Early studies suggested an association of mitral valve prolapse with stroke, but recent studies have not confirmed this association [50]. Mitral annular calcification is common in the elderly who frequently have other risk factors for stroke, and is unlikely to have a significant role in the causation of the stroke (Fig. 15.28). However, mobile masses sometimes seen arising from the mitral annular calcification are associated with an increased risk of stroke. They are likely thrombi arising from denuded area of the mitral annulus, and anticoagulation therapy is an effective treatment and should be used in these patients [51].

Embolic stroke is an uncommon occurrence in patients with aortic stenosis, although subclinical events may be common after invasive attempts in crossing the aortic valve to measure the transvalvular gradient. The embolic material is usually calcific in nature and thus anticoagulation is unlikely to reduce the risk of recurrence.

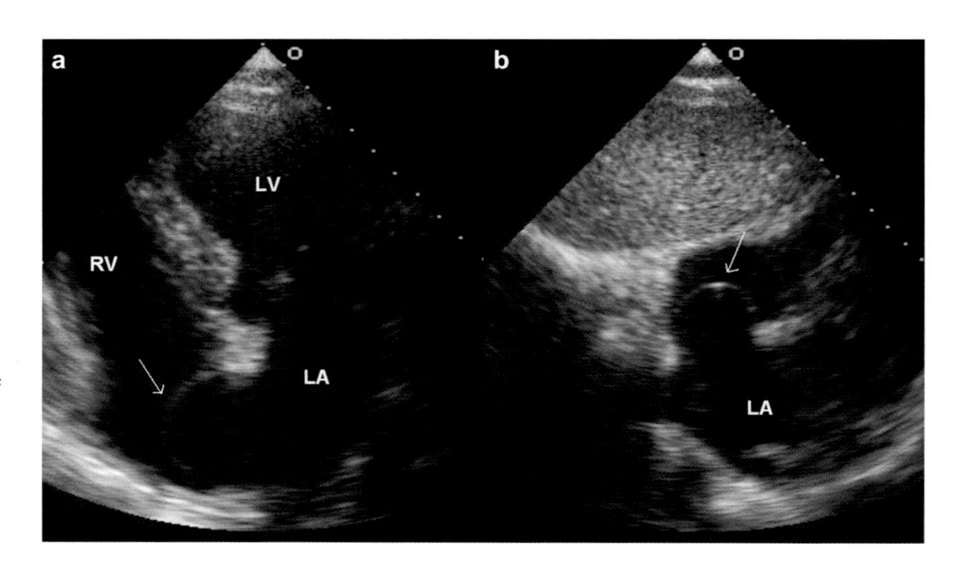

Fig. 15.20 Apical four-chamber (**a**) and subcostal (**b**) views show the presence of an atrial septal aneurysm with a marked degree of bulging (*arrow*) into the right atrium. *LA* left atrium, *LV* left ventricle, *RV* right ventricle

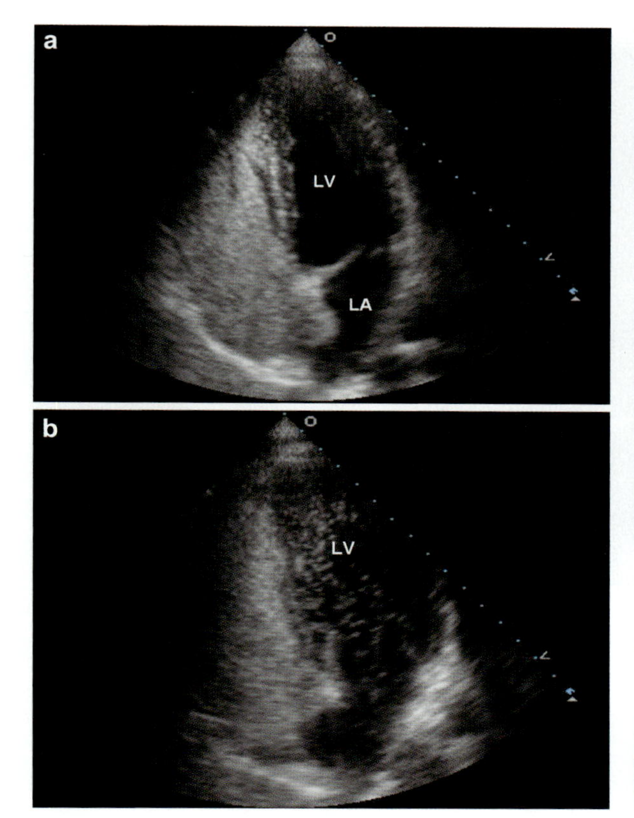

Fig. 15.21 (**a**) Intravenous contrast injection with agitated saline in the four-chamber view shows that the atrial septal aneurysm bulges into the left atrium at the very beginning of the release phase of the Valsalva maneuver. *LA* left atrium, *LV* left ventricle. (**b**) During the later part of the release phase of the Valsalva maneuver, the atrial septal aneurysm bulges into the right atrium and there is a large degree of contrast opacification of the left atrium and left ventricle consistent with the presence of patent foramen ovale. Atrial septal aneurysm and patent foramen ovale frequently coexist in the same patient. *LV* left ventricle

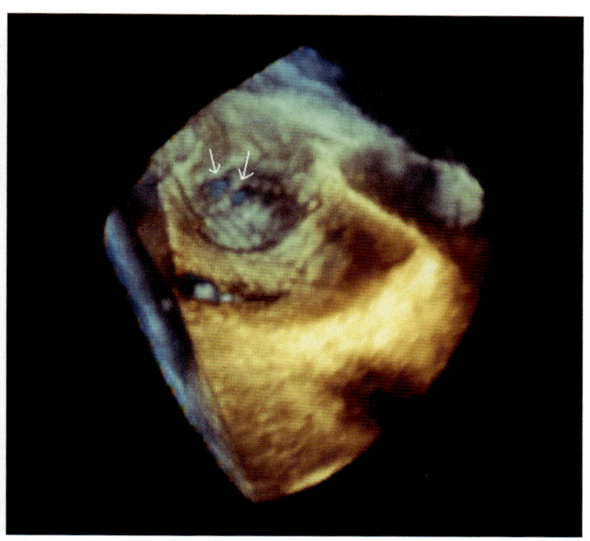

Fig. 15.22 Transesophageal 3D view from the left atrial perspective shows the presence of atrial septal aneurysm and the presence of two small atrial septal defects (*arrows*)

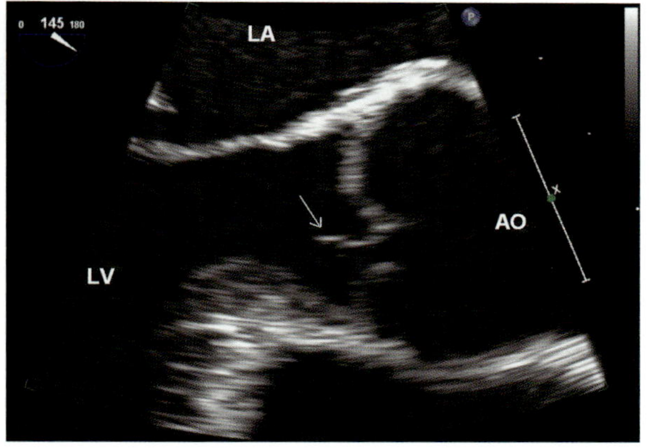

Fig. 15.23 Transesophageal echocardiogram of the left ventricular outflow tract in a 52-year-old man shows the presence of a linear density (*arrow*) attached to the aortic valve consistent with valvular strand. *Ao* aorta, *LA* left atrium, *LV* left ventricle

Summary

Embolic stroke pathoetiology cannot be confidently determined by clinical findings alone. A systematic approach is important to evaluate the etiology of ischemic stroke. Transthoracic echocardiography is a low-yield procedure in the identification of potential cardiac source of embolism. The yield is higher in high-risk patients such as those with a positive cardiac history or in those with abnormal cardiac findings. In the presence of atrial fibrillation, echocardiographic studies are unlikely to alter management. Compared to TTE, TEE produces a higher yield of echo findings that are associated with an increased risk of embolic events, although the therapeutic yield may be limited as the significance of many of these findings remains uncertain. We need to curb our enthusiasm to intervene or correct many of these findings until more convincing data become available from future trials.

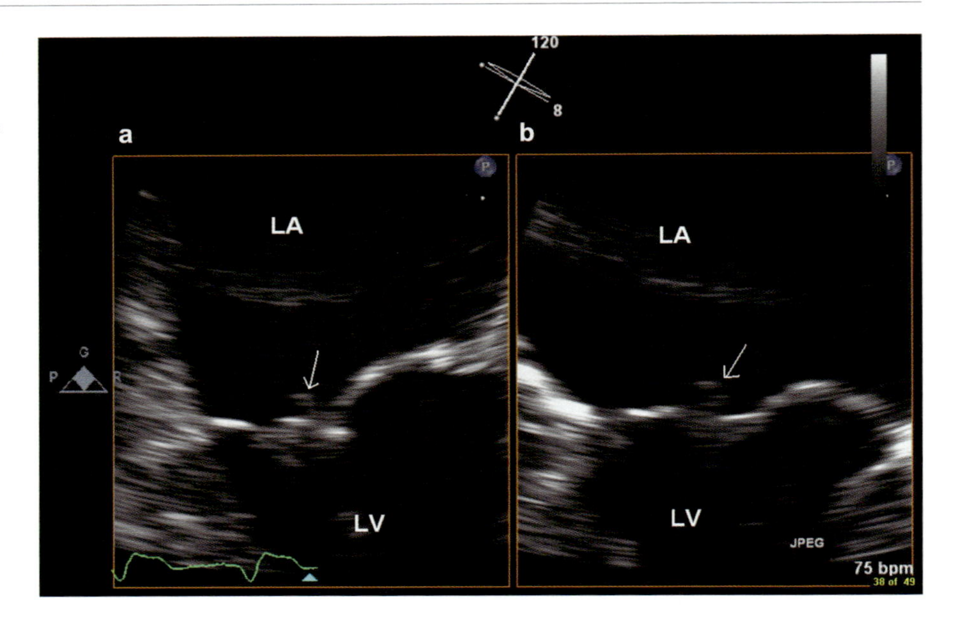

Fig. 15.24 Transesophageal views (**a**, **b**) of the mitral valve in systole in a 72-year-old woman show the presence of linear strand (*arrow*) attached to the closing margins of the mitral leaflets. *LA* left atrium, *LV* left ventricle

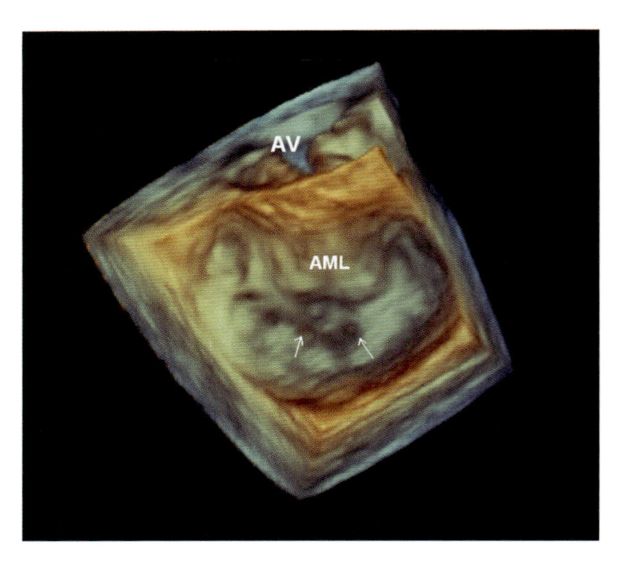

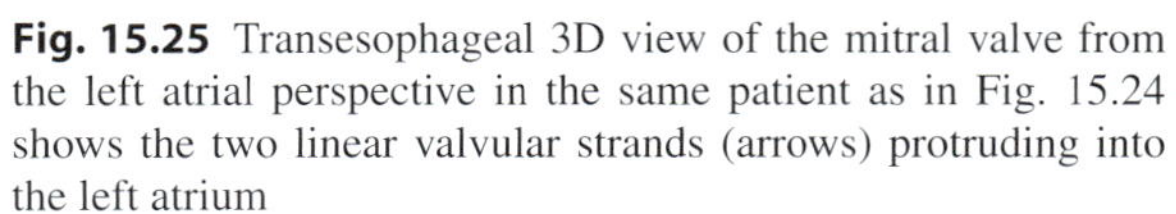

Fig. 15.25 Transesophageal 3D view of the mitral valve from the left atrial perspective in the same patient as in Fig. 15.24 shows the two linear valvular strands (arrows) protruding into the left atrium

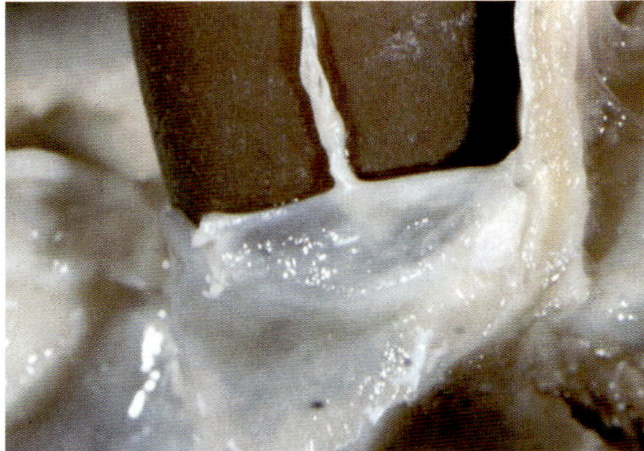

Fig. 15.26 Aortic valve with long fibrous strand that extends from the mid cusp location

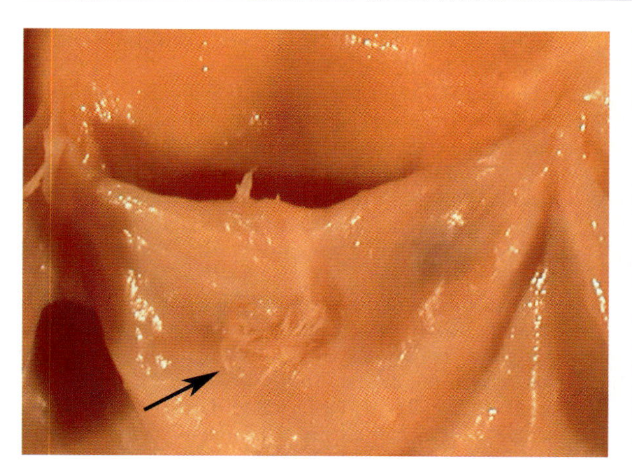

Fig. 15.27 Aortic valve cusp with Lambl's excrescences (*arrow*). These are whisker-like multiple fronds that are located along the line of valve closure and often, as in this case, are in the center of the cusp

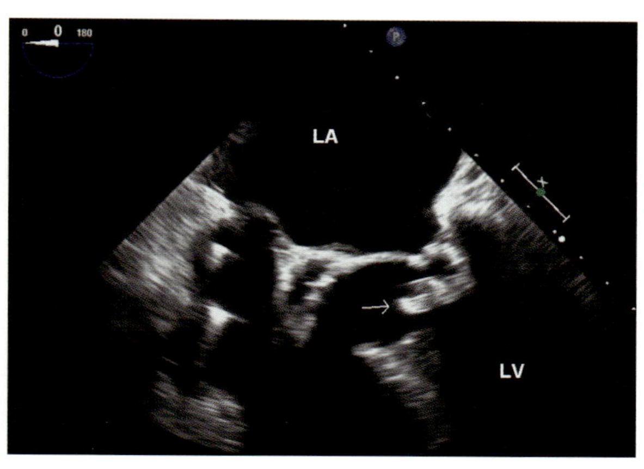

Fig. 15.28 Transesophageal echocardiogram in an 80-year-old man shows the presence of mitral annular calcification and an echo-mobile density (*arrow*) with attachment to the mitral annular calcification protruding into the left ventricular outflow tract. This mass is likely an organized thrombus and is associated with an increased thromboembolic risk

References

1. Albers GW, Amarenco P, Easton JD, Sacco RL, Teal P. Antithrombotic and thrombolytic therapy for ischemic stroke: the Seventh ACCP Conference on Antithrombotic and Thrombolytic Therapy. *Chest*. 2004 Sep;126(3 Suppl): 483S-512S.
2. Sacco RL, Ellenberg JH, Mohr JP, et al. Infarcts of undetermined cause: the NINCDS Stroke Data Bank. *Ann Neurol*. 1989 Apr;25(4):382-390.
3. Minematsu K, Yamaguchi T, Omae T. 'Spectacular shrinking deficit': rapid recovery from a major hemispheric syndrome by migration of an embolus. *Neurology*. 1992 Jan; 42(1):157-162.
4. Freeman WD, Aguilar MI. Stroke prevention in atrial fibrillation and other major cardiac sources of embolism. *Neurol Clin*. 2008 Nov;26(4):1129-1160.
5. Horowitz DR, Tuhrim S, Weinberger JM, Rudolph SH. Mechanisms in lacunar infarction. *Stroke*. 1992 Mar;23(3): 325-327.
6. Ramirez-Lassepas M, Cipolle RJ, Bjork RJ, et al. Can embolic stroke be diagnosed on the basis of neurologic clinical criteria? *Arch Neurol*. 1987 Jan;44(1):87-89.
7. Egeblad H, Andersen K, Hartiala J, et al. Role of echocardiography in systemic arterial embolism. A review with recommendations. *Scand Cardiovasc J*. 1998;32(6):323-342.
8. Peterson GE, Brickner ME, Reimold SC. Transesophageal echocardiography: clinical indications and applications. *Circulation*. 2003 May 20;107(19):2398-2402.
9. Chan KL, Cohen GI, Sochowski RA, Baird MG. Complications of transesophageal echocardiography in ambulatory adult patients: analysis of 1500 consecutive examinations. *J Am Soc Echocardiogr*. 1991 Nov;4(6):577-582.
10. Yvorchuk KY, Sochowski RA, Chan KL. A prospective comparison of the multiplane probe with the biplane probe in structure visualization and Doppler examination during transesophageal echocardiography. *J Am Soc Echocardiogr*. 1995 Mar;8(2):111-120.
11. Laupacis A, Albers G, Dalen J, Dunn MI, Jacobson AK, Singer DE. Antithrombotic therapy in atrial fibrillation. *Chest*. 1998 Nov;114(5 Suppl):579S-589S.
12. Anonymous. Transesophageal echocardiographic correlates of thromboembolism in high-risk patients with nonvalvular atrial fibrillation. *Ann Intern Med*. 1998 Apr 15;128(8):639-647.
13. Liao J, Khalid Z, Scallan C, Morillo C, O'Donnell M. Noninvasive cardiac monitoring for detecting paroxysmal atrial fibrillation or flutter after acute ischemic stroke: a systematic review. *Stroke*. 2007 Nov;38(11):2935-40.
14. Tayal AH, Tian M, Kelly KM, et al. Atrial fibrillation detected by mobile cardiac outpatient telemetry in cryptogenic TIA or stroke. *Neurology*. 2008 Nov 18;71(21):1696-1701.
15. Doufekias E, Segal AZ, Kizer JR. Cardiogenic and aortogenic brain embolism. *J Am Coll Cardiol*. 2008 Mar 18; 51(11):1049-59.
16. Pearson AC, Labovitz AJ, Tatineni S, Gomez CR. Superiority of transesophageal echocardiography in detecting cardiac source of embolism in patients with cerebral ischemia of uncertain etiology. *J Am Coll Cardiol*. 1991 Jan;17(1):66-72.
17. Lee RJ, Bartzokis T, Yeoh TK, Grogin HR, Choi D, Schnittger I. Enhanced detection of intracardiac sources of cerebral emboli by transesophageal echocardiography. *Stroke*. 1991 Jun;22(6):734-739.
18. Aschenberg W, Schluter M, Kremer P, Schroder E, Siglow V, Bleifeld W. Transesophageal two-dimensional echocardiography for the detection of left atrial appendage thrombus. *J Am Coll Cardiol*. 1986 Jan;7(1):163-166.
19. Cujec B, Polasek P, Voll C, Shuaib A. Transesophageal echocardiography in the detection of potential cardiac source of embolism in stroke patients. *Stroke*. 1991 Jun;22(6): 727-733.
20. Pop G, Sutherland GR, Koudstaal PJ, Sit TW, de Jong G, Roelandt JR. Transesophageal echocardiography in the detection of intracardiac embolic sources in patients with transient ischemic attacks. *Stroke*. 1990 Apr;21(4):560-565.
21. Harloff A, Handke M, Reinhard M, Geibel A, Hetzel A. Therapeutic strategies after examination by transesophageal echocardiography in 503 patients with ischemic stroke. *Stroke*. 2006 Mar;37(3):859-864.
22. de Bruijn SF, Agema WR, Lammers GJ, et al. Transesophageal echocardiography is superior to transthoracic echocardiography in management of patients of any age with transient ischemic attack or stroke. *Stroke*. 2006 Oct;37(10):2531-2534.
23. Strandberg M, Marttila RJ, Helenius H, Hartiala J. Transoesophageal echocardiography in selecting patients for anticoagulation after ischaemic stroke or transient ischaemic attack. *J Neurol Neurosurg Psychiatry*. 2002 Jul;73(1):29-33.
24. Morris JG, Duffis EJ, Fisher M. Cardiac workup of ischemic stroke: can we improve our diagnostic yield? *Stroke*. 2009 Aug;40(8):2893-2898.
25. Kapral MK, Silver FL. Preventive health care, 1999 update: 2. Echocardiography for the detection of a cardiac source of embolus in patients with stroke Canadian Task Force on Preventive Health Care CMAJ. 1999 Oct 19;161(8):989-996.
26. Meacham RR III, Headley AS, Bronze MS, Lewis JB, Rester MM. Impending paradoxical embolism. *Arch Intern Med*. 1998 Mar 9;158(5):438-448.
27. Feinberg WM, Blackshear JL, Laupacis A, Kronmal R, Hart RG. Prevalence, age distribution, and gender of patients with atrial fibrillation. Analysis and implications. *Arch Intern Med*. 1995 Mar 13;155(5):469-473.
28. Wolf PA, Abbott RD, Kannel WB. Atrial fibrillation as an independent risk factor for stroke: the Framingham Study. *Stroke*. 1991 Aug;22(8):983-988.
29. The French Study of Aortic Plaques in Stroke Group. Atherosclerotic disease of the aortic arch as a risk factor for recurrent ischemic stroke. *N Engl J Med*. 1996 May 9; 334(19):1216-1221.
30. Tunick PA, Nayar AC, Goodkin GM, et al. Effect of treatment on the incidence of stroke and other emboli in 519 patients with severe thoracic aortic plaque. *Am J Cardiol*. 2002 Dec 15;90(12):1320-1325.
31. Messe SR, Silverman IE, Kizer JR, et al. Practice parameter: recurrent stroke with patent foramen ovale and atrial septal aneurysm: report of the Quality Standards Subcommittee of the American Academy of Neurology. *Neurology*. 2004 Apr 13;62(7):1042-1050.
32. Choukroun EM, Labrousse LM, Madonna FP, Deville C. Mobile thrombus of the thoracic aorta: diagnosis and treatment in 9 cases. *Ann Vasc Surg*. 2002 Nov;16(6):714-22.
33. Witt BJ, Brown RD Jr, Jacobsen SJ, Weston SA, Yawn BP, Roger VL. A community-based study of stroke incidence

after myocardial infarction. *Ann Intern Med.* 2005 Dec 6;143(11):785-792.

34. Pullicino P, Thompson JL, Barton B, Levin B, Graham S, Freudenberger RS. Warfarin versus aspirin in patients with reduced cardiac ejection fraction (WARCEF): rationale, objectives, and design. *J Card Fail.* 2006 Feb;12(1):39-46.
35. Stein PD, Alpert JS, Dalen JE, Horstkotte D, Turpie AG. Antithrombotic therapy in patients with mechanical and biological prosthetic heart valves. *Chest.* 1998 Nov;114(5 Suppl):602S-610S.
36. Mugge A, Kuhn H, Nikutta P, Grote J, Lopez JA, Daniel WG. Assessment of left atrial appendage function by biplane transesophageal echocardiography in patients with nonrheumatic atrial fibrillation: identification of a subgroup of patients at increased embolic risk. *J Am Coll Cardiol.* 1994 Mar 1;23(3):599-607.
37. Lapeyre AC III, Steele PM, Kazmier FJ, Chesebro JH, Vlietstra RE, Fuster V. Systemic embolism in chronic left ventricular aneurysm: incidence and the role of anticoagulation. *J Am Coll Cardiol.* 1985 Sep;6(3):534-538.
38. Kizer JR, Devereux RB. Clinical practice. Patent foramen ovale in young adults with unexplained stroke. *N Engl J Med.* 2005 Dec 1;353(22):2361-2372.
39. Hagen PT, Scholz DG, Edwards WD. Incidence and size of patent foramen ovale during the first 10 decades of life: an autopsy study of 965 normal hearts. *Mayo Clin Proc.* 1984 Jan;59(1):17-20.
40. Kim HH, Tam JW, Chan KL. A prospective transesophageal echocardiographic study to assess a new type of left atrial spontaneous contrast at rest and during respiratory manoeuvres. *Can J Cardiol.* 1999 Nov;15(11):1217-1222.
41. Handke M, Harloff A, Olschewski M, Hetzel A, Geibel A. Patent foramen ovale and cryptogenic stroke in older patients. *N Engl J Med.* 2007 Nov 29;357(22):2262-2268.
42. Mas JL, Arquizan C, Lamy C, et al. Recurrent cerebrovascular events associated with patent foramen ovale, atrial septal aneurysm, or both. *N Engl J Med.* 2001 Dec 13;345(24):1740-1746.
43. Homma S, Sacco RL, Di Tullio MR, Sciacca RR, Mohr JP. Effect of medical treatment in stroke patients with patent foramen ovale: patent foramen ovale in Cryptogenic Stroke Study. *Circulation.* 2002 Jun 4;105(22):2625-31.
44. Maisel WH, Laskey WK. Patent foramen ovale closure devices: moving beyond equipoise. *JAMA.* 2005 Jul 20;294(3):366-369.
45. Agmon Y, Khandheria BK, Meissner I, et al. Frequency of atrial septal aneurysms in patients with cerebral ischemic events. *Circulation.* 1999 Apr 20;99(15):1942-1944.
46. Moussouttas M, Fayad P, Rosenblatt M, et al. Pulmonary arteriovenous malformations: cerebral ischemia and neurologic manifestations. *Neurology.* 2000 Oct 10;55(7):959-964.
47. Freedberg RS, Goodkin GM, Perez JL, Tunick PA, Kronzon I. Valve strands are strongly associated with systemic embolization: a transesophageal echocardiographic study. *J Am Coll Cardiol.* 1995 Dec;26(7):1709-1712.
48. Wolf RC, Spiess J, Vasic N, Huber R. Valvular strands and ischemic stroke. *Eur Neurol.* 2007;57(4):227-231.
49. Veinot JP, Walley VM. Focal and patchy cardiac valve lesions: a clinicopathological review. *Can J Cardiol.* 2000 Dec;16(12):1489-1507.
50. Gilon D, Buonanno FS, Joffe MM, et al. Lack of evidence of an association between mitral-valve prolapse and stroke in young patients. *N Engl J Med.* 1999 Jul 1;341(1):8-13.
51. Sia YT, Dulay D, Burwash IG, Beauchesne LM, Ascah K, Chan KL. Mobile ventricular thrombus arising from the mitral annulus in patients with dense mitral annular calcification. *Eur J Echocardiogr.* 2010 Mar;11(2):198-201.

Assessment of Diastolic Function

16

Heart failure has become an increasingly important medical problem. It is one of the major reasons for hospitalization and is associated with increased mortality. The prevalence of heart failure is expected to rise with the aging of the population. About half of the patients with heart failure have preserved left ventricular systolic function, and heart failure in these patients is frequently ascribed to diastolic dysfunction. The common causes of diastolic dysfunction in the setting of preserved systolic function are listed in Table 16.1. A good understanding of the pathophysiology underlying heart failure in these patients should lead to a more reasoned approach to its management [1–5].

Diastole is closely coupled with systole such that inadequate diastolic filling inevitably results in reduced stroke volume or elevated filling pressures despite a normal left ventricular systolic function. During diastole, large volume changes occur with relatively small changes in pressure, and the peak flow velocity through the mitral valve during diastole exceeds that through the aortic valve during systole. Yet, a small increase in pressure, for instance, from a mean left atrial pressure of 10 mmHg to a mean left atrial pressure of 20 mmHg, can result in heart failure symptoms. The intracardiac pressure and its rate of change are governed by intrinsic properties of the myocardium and the loading conditions. Myocardial relaxation is an active process best measured by Tau which is an expression of the exponential fall in left ventricular pressure following left ventricular ejection. Compliance refers to the increase in pressure with a given increase in volume.

Diastole can be divided into four phases – isovolumic relaxation, rapid filling, slow filling, and atrial contraction (Fig. 16.1). Left ventricular relaxation is an active process resulting in a rapid decline in left ventricular pressure during isovolumic relaxation. This generates a diastolic pressure gradient between the left atrium and the left ventricle. Rapid filling ensues following opening of the mitral valve, with blood flowing from the left atrium into the left ventricle with rapid propagation to the left ventricular apex. The most widely accepted measure of the rate of left ventricular relaxation is Tau, which is a measure of the mono-exponential pressure decay, but Tau can be reliably measured invasively only by using high fidelity pressure measuring catheters. When relaxation is impaired, as is invariably present in patients with left ventricular systolic dysfunction, the pressure decay is slow leading to a delay in mitral valve opening. This may be detected by a prolonged isovolumic relaxation time, which is the time interval between aortic valve closure and mitral valve opening. This can be readily detected by continuous wave Doppler.

The rate of left ventricular filling is driven by the pressure gradient between the left atrium and left ventricle, such that the lower the left ventricular diastolic pressure, the higher is the pressure gradient and the diastolic filling rate. Thus a normally low early diastolic left ventricular pressure allows the transfer of a large volume into the left ventricle without the necessity of an elevated left atrial pressure. In patients with a variety of heart diseases including ischemic heart disease, left ventricular relaxation is impaired such that the early diastolic gradient between the left atrium and left ventricle is reduced. This can be compensated for by an increase in left atrial pressure. Indeed, the inability to achieve normal left ventricular filling without an elevation in filling pressure is a sensitive indication of myocardial dysfunction. Near the end of the rapid filling phase, the left ventricular pressure may be higher than the left atrial pressure for a brief period of time. During the slow filling phase, there is very little

K.-L. Chan and J.P. Veinot, *Anatomic Basis of Echocardiographic Diagnosis*,
DOI: 10.1007/978-1-84996-387-9_16, © Springer-Verlag London Limited 2011

Table 16.1 Causes of left ventricular diastolic dysfunction with preserved systolic function

- Aging
- Hypertension
- Aortic stenosis
- Hypertrophic cardiomyopathy
- Ischemic heart disease
- Infiltrative cardiomyopathy, e.g., amyloid, myocarditis

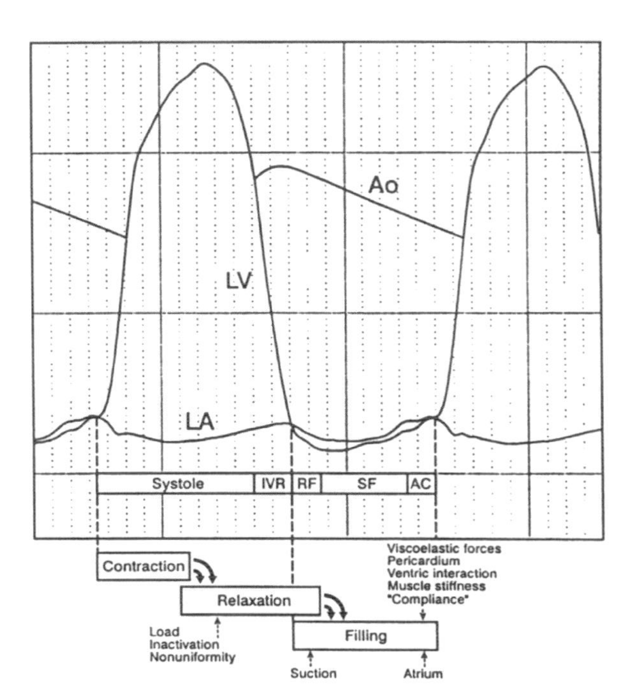

Fig. 16.1 These pressure curves from a patient with hypertrophic cardiomyopathy show the four phases of diastole which comprise isovolumic relaxation (*IVR*), rapid filling (*RF*), slow filling (*SF*), and atrial contraction (*AC*). An alternate approach is to view the cardiac cycle in three related phases which are contraction, relaxation, and filling (Reproduced from (5). With permission)

diastolic filling as the pressure in the left atrium and left ventricle have equalized. This is followed by atrial contraction which drives blood into the left ventricle from the left atrium by generating a second pressure gradient between the two chambers. Upon atrial relaxation, the pressure gradient falls and the mitral valve starts to drift closed. Mitral valve closure occurs when the ventricular pressure rises to exceed left atrial pressure at the onset of ventricular systole.

Echo-Doppler Measures of Diastolic Function

The usefulness of many echo-Doppler variables has been investigated over the past decade [6–9]. Many of these variables describe different aspects of left ventricular filling and some reflect intrinsic myocardial properties. A careful analysis of the interplay of these variables can tell us about diastolic filling, which is linked to diastolic filling pressure, but not the pressure per se. There are technical limitations to a number of these variables [10–13] (Table 16.2). Adequate pulmonary venous signals that allow reliable measurement of the retrograde A wave duration can be obtained only in about half of the patients in our experience. The flow propagation velocity has a great degree of variability from beat to beat and from study to study, although it can be readily obtained. Some of the new measures such as time duration between the onset of mitral E wave and onset of annular E velocity require meticulous care that the cycle length is identical, and more validation studies are required.

Among the variables, mitral inflow velocities remain the cornerstone in the assessment of diastolic function. This can be obtained in almost all patients, but care is required to optimize the signal to allow for accurate analysis. Color-flow imaging is useful to show the orientation of the mitral inflow jet. In a dilated left ventricle, the mitral inflow jet is frequently oriented posterolaterally as a result of the tethering of the mitral leaflets. Moving the location of the transducer to obtain a parallel alignment of the sample volume with the

Table 16.2 Doppler measures in the assessment of left ventricular diastolic function

Measures	Limitations
Mitral inflow velocities E, A, DT	• Affected by multiple variables including preload and heart rate
IVRT	• Affected by heart rate
Pulmonary vein velocities	• Not obtainable in about one third of patients
Propagation velocity	• Variability in measurements
Mitral annular velocities	• Only relatively independent of preload
A_{PV}-A_{MV} duration	• Difficult to obtain optimal measurements
Onset of E′ to E duration	• Variable cycle length; requires more validation

mitral inflow should be attempted in every case. A sample volume of 1–3 mm is placed at the mitral leaflet tips during diastole to obtain the maximum E and A waves. Moving the sample volume to the annulus level gives a cleaner display of the A wave and should allow for a more accurate measurement of the A duration. In our laboratory, pulmonary venous flow signal is always attempted by placing a sample volume of 2–3 mm well into the pulmonary vein in the apical four-chamber view. It is only with routine practice that adequate pulmonary venous signal can be obtained in the majority of cases (Fig. 16.2).

Annular tissue velocities have gained popularity because they can be reliably obtained from almost all patients using present day technology [8]. Pulsed-wave tissue Doppler imaging detects the high intensity, lower velocities of the myocardium by minimizing the wall filter and maximizing the low velocity scale. Multiple velocities can be obtained, and the waves that should be consistently measured are the systolic, early diastolic, and late diastolic velocities (Fig. 16.3). The annular E′ wave is a measure of myocardial diastolic lengthening and less influenced by preload. The ratio of mitral E wave to annular E′ wave has been shown to predict left ventricular filling pressures. Indeed, regression formula incorporating this ratio to calculate left ventricular filling pressure has become a part of the clinical and research practices in some laboratories (Fig. 16.4). Algorithms have also been proposed to be used in classifying patients into different diastolic dysfunction categories, or those with normal or elevated filling pressure (Fig. 16.5). The clinical context and the effect of age should be considered in applying any of these algorithms.

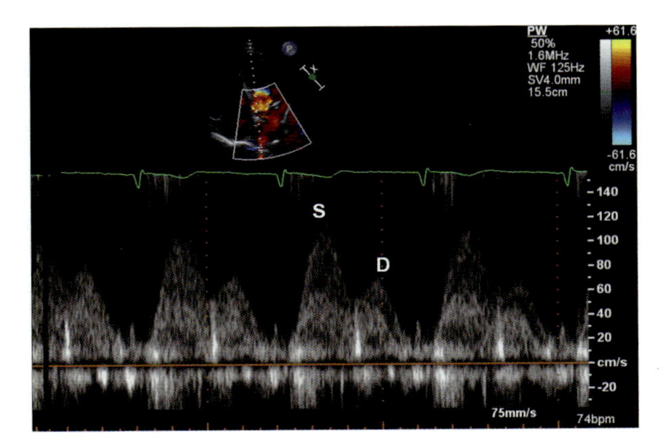

Fig. 16.2 This is a pulmonary venous flow recording showing a prominent systolic component (*S*) compared to the diastolic component (*D*). The atrial reversal flow is not well displayed and likely has a low velocity

The E/E′ ratio is easy to use but a number of issues need to be borne in mind. Although studies have shown good correlation between this ratio and filling pressures such as the pulmonary capillary wedge pressure, the correlation is not a very tight one such that by itself the E/E′ ratio does not reliably differentiate patients with normal filling pressure from those with abnormal filling pressures [6, 9] (Fig. 16.4). The situation is further compounded by technical differences. Some laboratories preferentially use the septal annular velocity, while others use the lateral annular velocity. An average of the septal and lateral annular velocities may be a reasonable compromise when there is a large discrepancy between the two velocities. Different ratios such as 10, 12, or 15 have been used in various studies. Using a lower ratio gives a higher sensitivity but less specificity, whereas using a higher ratio gives lower sensitivity but higher specificity. Definition of elevated filling pressure has not been uniform, with some studies using a cut-off value of 12 mmHg and some using a cut-off value as high as 20 mmHg.

We believe that the assessment of diastolic function should include evaluation of clinical factors, echo features as well as the Doppler findings during the Valsalva maneuver [1, 5] (Fig. 16.6). The age and symptomatic state of the patient should be taken into consideration. Age impacts on all the parameters, and the normal values for the different age-groups have wide confidence limits making proper interpretation difficult (Table 16.3). In asymptomatic patients, caution needs to be exercised to minimize the risks of labeling. There are many echo findings that need to be integrated in the assessment of diastolic function. The essential ones are left ventricular systolic function, left ventricular hypertrophy, and left atrial size. Other useful but less common echo findings include the B bump, early cut off sign on the mitral regurgitation spectral signal, atrial septal motion, aortic regurgitation spectral signal, and pulmonic regurgitation spectral signal (Fig. 16.7). A qualitative rather than a quantitative approach should be taken. When the findings are discordant, the effect of the Valsalva maneuver can be helpful [9, 10]. The change in the mitral inflow signal with Valsalva should be observed. In general, a drop of the mitral E wave by 20 cm/s during the strain phase indicates an adequate Valsalva maneuver. A decrease

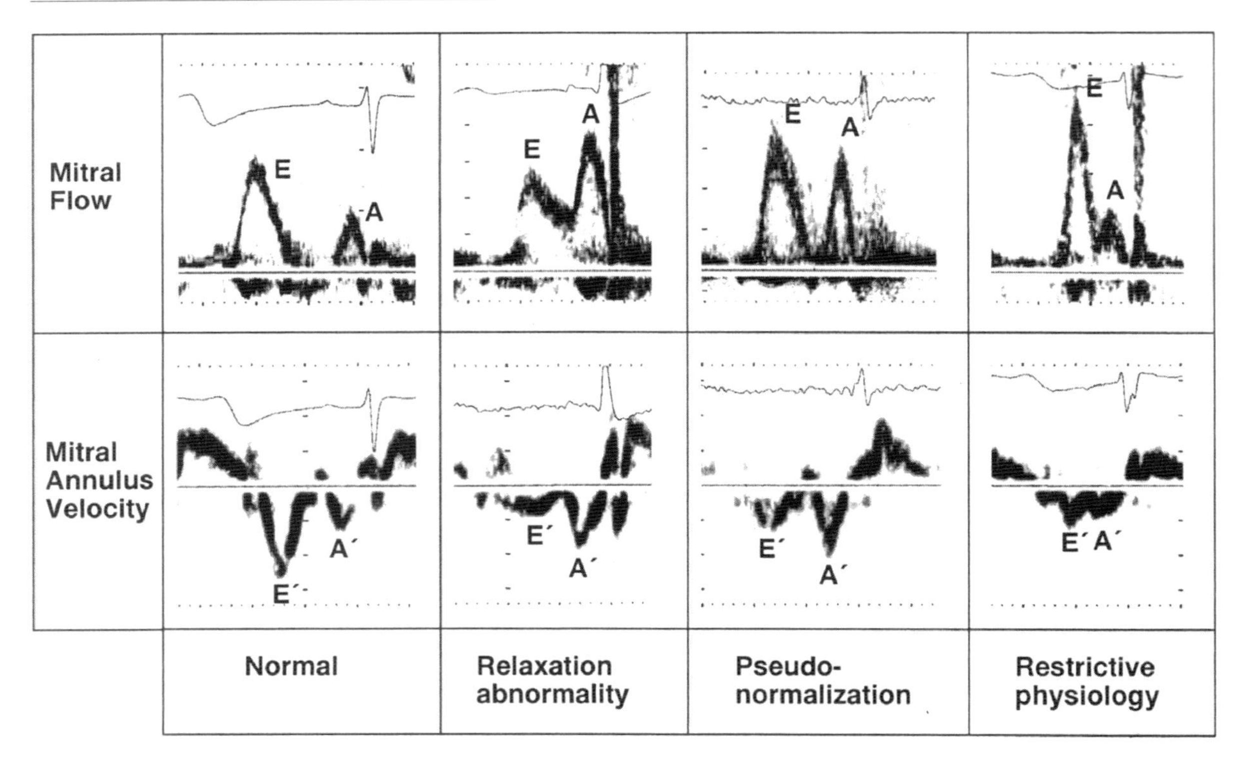

Fig. 16.3 The mitral annulus velocities are useful in the assessment of the severity of diastolic dysfunction. The pseudonormalization pattern of mitral flow can be easily differentiated from normal (Reproduced from (8). With permission)

of greater than 40% of the E/A ratio during the strain phase is predictive of elevated left ventricular filling pressure. The magnitude (>35 cm/s) and duration (> mitral A duration) of the pulmonary venous A wave can also be useful [10].

Assessment of atrial size should be an integral part of the assessment of diastolic function. Atrial enlargement is associated with diastolic dysfunction and is usually present in patients with moderate or severe diastolic dysfunction, such that the diagnosis of diastolic dysfunction should be reexamined if the atrial size is normal [14]. Atrial enlargement can be considered a marker of the severity and duration of diastolic dysfunction, in the absence of significant valvular regurgitation. Left atrial volume has recently gained acceptance as a more reliable means to assess atrial size than the one-dimensional atrial dimension [15]. Indeed, a recent study showed that atrial volume predicted all-cause mortality in a general population, although it was not an independent predictor after adjusting for diastolic dysfunction [14].

Normal Diastolic Function

Interpretation of diastolic function starts with the mitral flow velocities which can be readily obtained. Although mitral velocities reflect the diastolic filling characteristics of the left ventricle, they are affected by many other factors including age, heart rate, and loading conditions. Assessment of diastolic function should take these factors into consideration. Published values for different age-groups should be used when interpreting these velocities. In healthy individuals less than 60 years of age, E velocity is dominant and E/A ratio is greater than 1 (Figs. 16.8, 16.9). The pulmonary vein flow shows that the early diastolic flow is dominant and the velocity of atrial reversal is low (less than 35 cm/s). Optimal spectral signal of the atrial reversal velocity may be difficult to obtain. The early diastolic mitral annular velocities (E′) should exceed 10 cm/s, and the velocities at the lateral annulus are usually higher than those at the septal annulus.

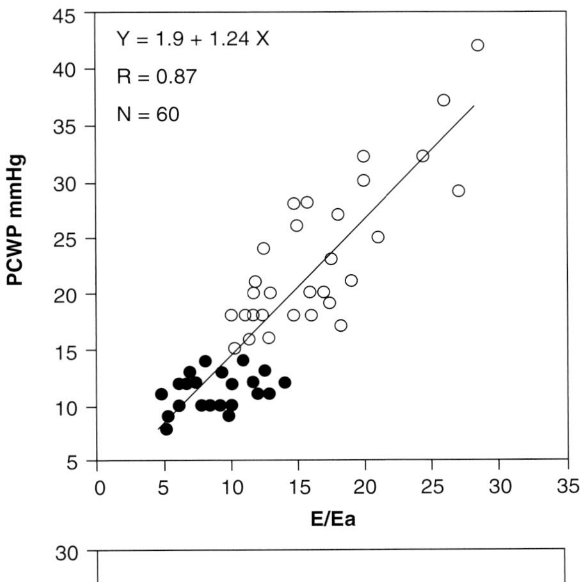

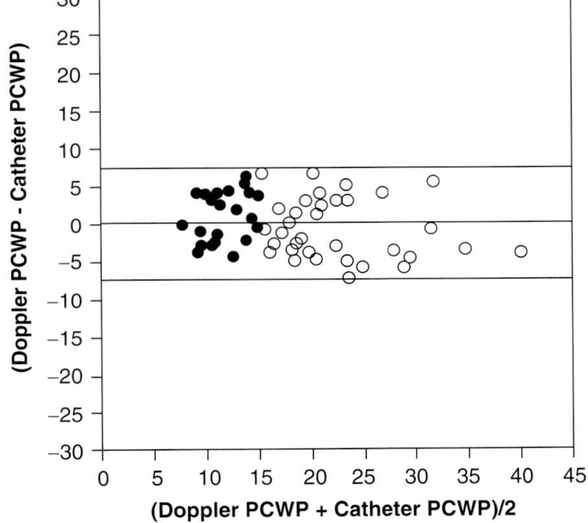

Fig. 16.4 The plot shows the relation of E/Ea to pulmonary capillary wedge pressure (*PCWP*) in the top panel. The difference between Doppler-estimated and catheter-measured PCWP versus the average of both observations is shown in the bottom panel. Solid circles are patients with impaired relaxation and open circles are patients with pseudonormalization mitral inflow pattern (Reproduced from (6). With permission)

Mild Diastolic Dysfunction

In patients with mild diastolic dysfunction, there is mild impairment in left ventricular relaxation resulting in a lower left atrium to left ventricle pressure gradient. The early diastolic flow rate is reduced which is reflected by a lower mitral E wave (Figs. 16.10, 16.11). Similarly, the early diastolic annular wave E′ is also reduced. The mitral deceleration time is prolonged, also due to the delay in relaxation. There is compensatory increase in flow rate during atrial contraction which delivers a greater proportion of diastolic filling resulting in a tall A wave. The E/A ratio is generally less than 1. With the more complete emptying of the left atrium after atrial contraction, there is increased filling of the left atrium during ventricular systole which is manifested by a tall S wave in the pulmonary venous signal. The E/E′ ratio is less than 15. In this setting, the mean left atrial pressure is normal, although the left ventricular end diastolic pressure may be elevated.

Moderate Diastolic Dysfunction

When left ventricular relaxation is more severely impaired, the left atrial pressure is elevated in order to maintain diastolic filling by maintaining the left atrium to left ventricle pressure gradient (Figs. 16.12, 16.13). In this setting, the mitral E wave is increased and the deceleration time will be decreased as the left ventricular operative compliance is reduced leading to an early equalization of pressure between the left atrium and the left ventricle. The mitral annular E wave is reduced reflecting the decrease in rate of diastolic lengthening. As a result the E/E′ ratio is increased. The E′ may also be delayed, occurring after the mitral E wave. The decreased operative compliance also explains the early termination of the mitral A wave compared to the pulmonary venous A wave. The velocity of the pulmonary venous A wave is increased. Mitral leaflet closure may also be significantly delayed compared to termination of the mitral A wave, again reflecting the decrease of the operative compliance of the left ventricle and likely a delay in isovolumic contraction. Patients with these features have impaired left ventricular relaxation and increased left atrial pressures.

Severe Diastolic Dysfunction

In this setting, relaxation is even slower associated with further increase in left atrial pressure. The mitral E wave becomes much more elevated and deceleration time

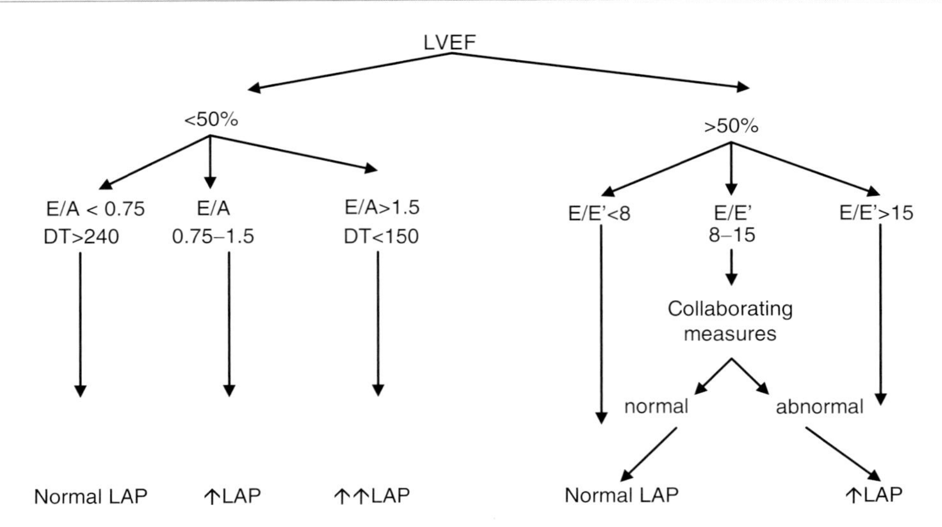

Fig. 16.5 This is a schema to assess left ventricular diastolic function depending on whether or not the systolic function is preserved. If the systolic function is impaired (EF<50%), the mitral inflow velocities are generally sufficient in assessing the left ventricular filling pressure or the left atrial pressure. In patients with preserved systolic function (EF>50%), the mitral annular velocities, particularly E′, are the preferred measures to categorize the left atrial pressure into normal or elevated, dependent on the E/E′ ratio. If E/E′ is clearly elevated (>15), the LA pressure is likely elevated; and if E/E′ is < 8, the LA pressure is likely normal. In patients with E/E′ between 8 and 15, other collaborating measures should be taken into consideration. These include the duration of pulmonary vein A wave exceeding the duration of mitral valve A wave by 30 ms, the response of mitral velocities to the Valsalva maneuver, and the left atrial volume. In patients with hypertrophic cardiomyopathy, the collaborating measures should always be considered because E/E′ ratio is less predictive

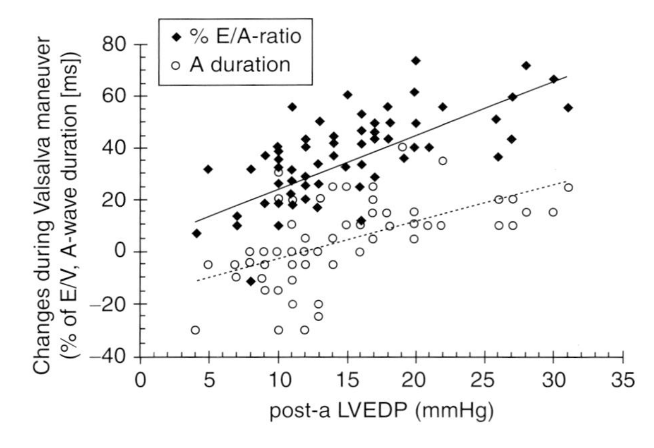

Fig. 16.6 Relation between changes during the Valsalva maneuver and the left ventricular filling pressure. E/A ratio, ratio of mitral early diastolic velocity to atrial flow velocity; *LVEDP* left ventricular end diastolic pressure (Reproduced from (10). With permission)

much abbreviated. E/A ratio is frequently > 2 and the deceleration time < 150 ms. (Figs. 16.14, 16.15). The mitral annular E wave is also further reduced and delayed. Thus the E/E′ ratio becomes even higher (much greater than 15:1). In addition to the slow relaxation, isovolumic contraction is also slowed in this setting leading to a short diastolic filling time which can be further compromised if there is first-degree AV block. This is one reason for improvement with artificial pacing in these patients, by programming a short AV delay to increase the diastolic filling time. The delay in the relaxation may sometimes result in a mid diastolic gradient which can manifest as an L-wave, and is more commonly seen with a slow heart rate (Fig. 16.16) [16].

In some of these patients, atrial contribution becomes minimal due to low left ventricular operative compliance and atrial dysfunction such that A wave may not be discernable. Despite little or no flow during slow filling and atrial contraction phases, the mitral valve remains open until the isovolumic contraction phase (Fig. 16.16). Diastolic mitral regurgitation may occur as a result. Table 16.4 summarizes the values of the Doppler measures useful in the classification of severity of diastolic dysfunction [17].

In addition to diagnosis, a comprehensive assessment using these echo-Doppler measures can provide useful insight into prognosis and management of patients with heart failure (Fig. 16.17). These measures

Table 16.3 Normal values for Doppler-derived diastolic measurements

Measurement	Age-group (years) 16–20	21–40	41–60	>60
IVRT(ms)	50 ± 9(32–68)	67 ± 8 (51–83)	74 ± 7 (60–88)	87 ± 7 (73–101)
E/A ratio	1.88 ± 0.45 (0.98–2.78)	1.53 ± 0.40 (0.73–2.33)	1.28 ± .25 (0.78–1.78)	0.96 ± 0.18(0.6–1.32)
DT(ms)	142 ± 19 (104–180)	166 ± 14 (138–194)	181 ± 19 (143–219)	200 ± 29 (142–258))
A duration(ms)	113 ± 17 (79–147)	127± 13(101–153)	133 ± 13(107–159)	138 ± 19 (100–176)
PV S/D ratio	0.82 ± 0.18 (0.46–1.18)	0.98 ± 0.32 (0.34–1.62)	1.21 ± 0.2 (0.81–1.61)	1.39 ± 0.47 (0.45–2.33)
PV Ar (cm/s)	16 ± 10 (1–36)	21 ± 8 (5–37)	23 ± 3 (17–29)	25 ± 9 (11–39)
PV Ar duration (ms)	66 ± 39(1–144)	96 ± 33 (30–162)	112 ± 15 (82–142)	113 ± 30 (53–173)
Septal e′ (cm/s)	14.9 ± 2.4 (10.1–19.7)	15.5 ± 2.7 (10.1–20.9)	12.2 ± 2.3 (7.6–16.8)	10.4 ± 2.1 (6.2–14.6)
Septal e′/a′ ratio	2.4*	1.6 ± 0.5 (0.6–2.6)	1.1 ± 0.3 (0.5–1.7)	0.85 ± 0.2 (0.45–1.25)
Lateral e′ (cm/s)	20.6 ± 3.8 (13–28.2)	19.8 ± 2.9 (14–25.6)	16.1 ± 2.3(11.5–20.7)	12.9 ± 3.5 (5.9–19.9)
Lateral e′/a′ ratio	3.1*	1.9 ± 0.6 (0.7–3.1)	1.5 ± 0.5(0.5–2.5)	0.9 ± 0.4 (0.1–1.7)

Data are expressed as mean ± SD (95% confidence interval)
Source: Reproduced from [1]. With permission

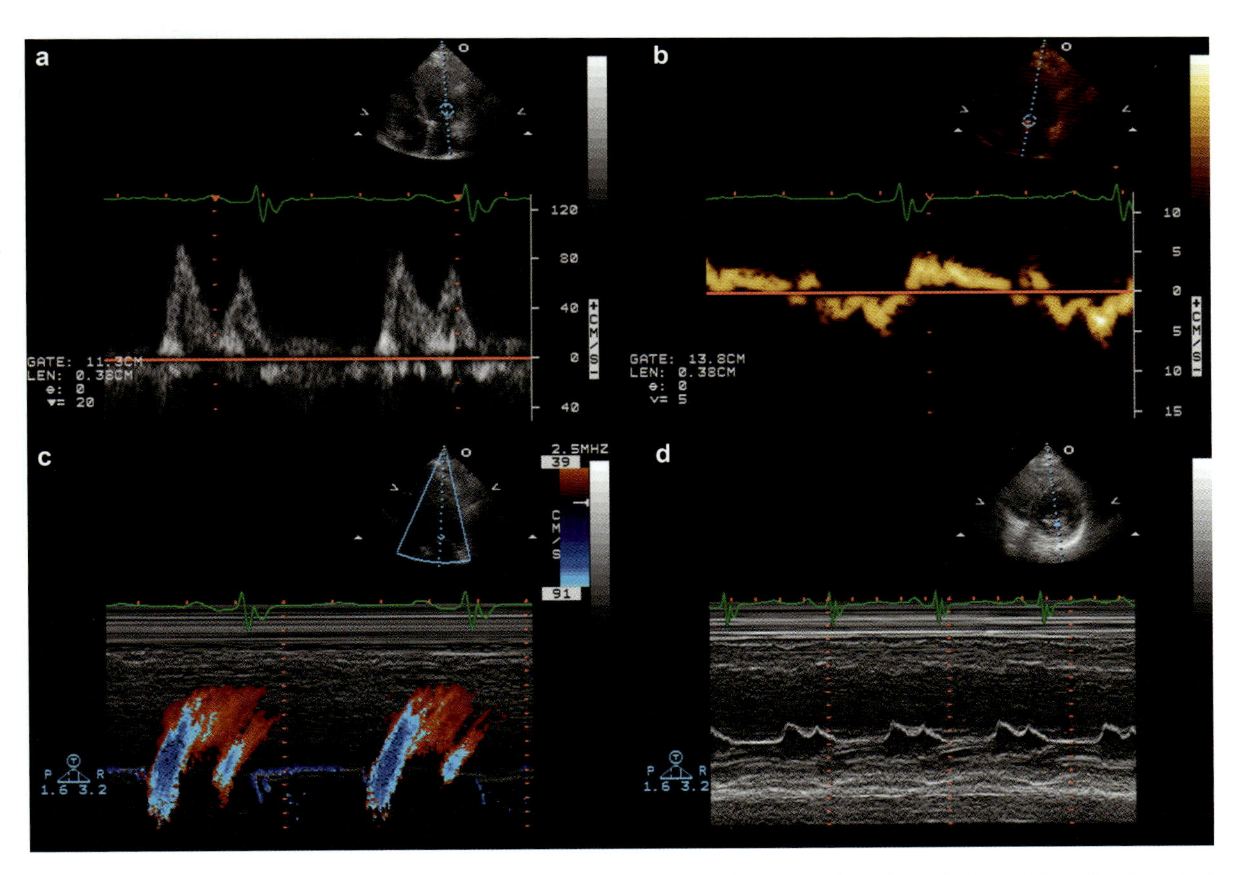

Fig. 16.7 The mitral inflow velocities are shown in **(a)**, septal annual velocities in **(b)**, propagation velocity in **(c)**, and M-mode of the mitral valve in **(d)**. Although the mitral inflow pattern appears normal, the low annular early diastolic velocity shows that it is pseudonormalization. This is further confirmed by the low propagation velocity and the presence of B bump on the mitral M-mode tracing

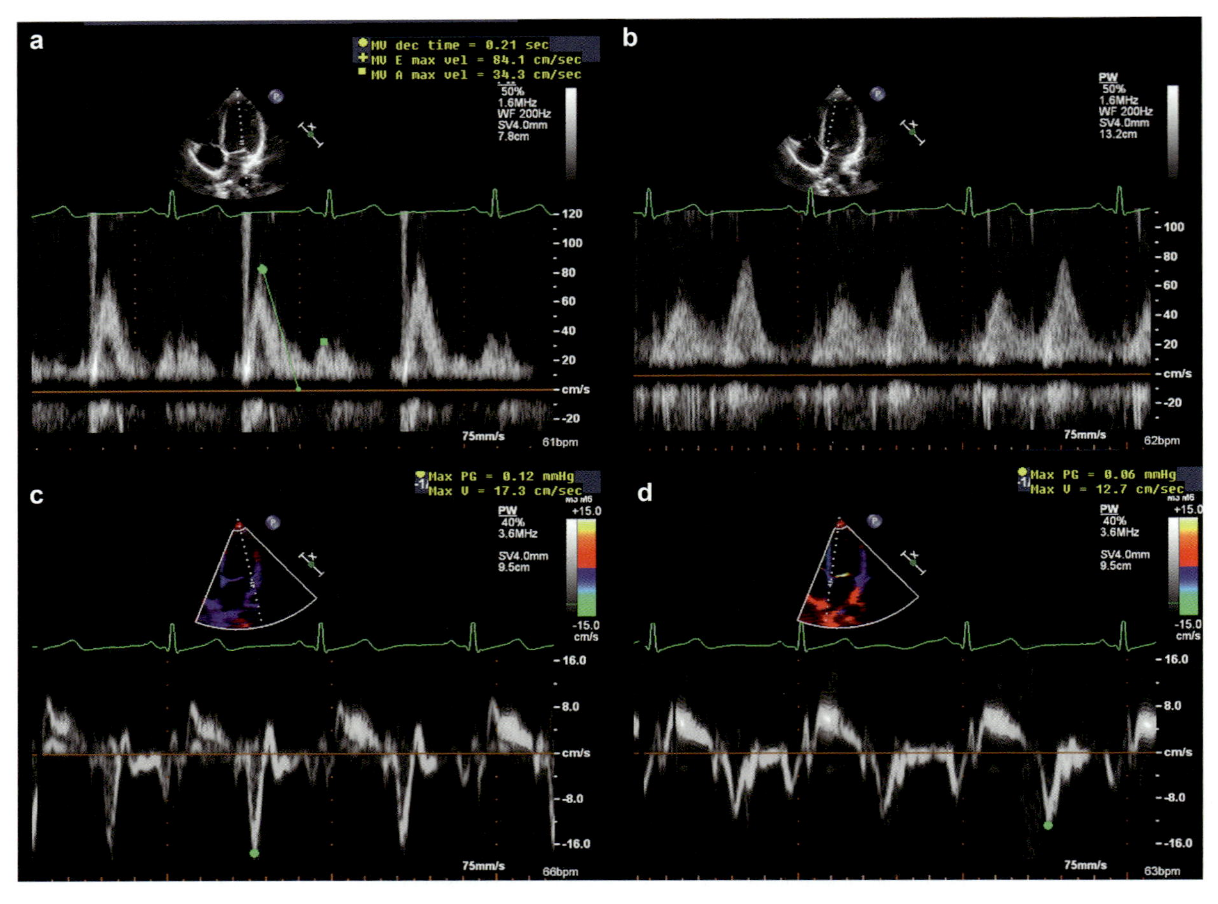

Fig. 16.8 The recordings are from a 21-year-old woman showing the mitral inflow in (**a**), pulmonary venous flow in (**b**), lateral annular velocities in (**c**), and septal annular velocities in (**d**). These measures are in keeping with normal diastolic function

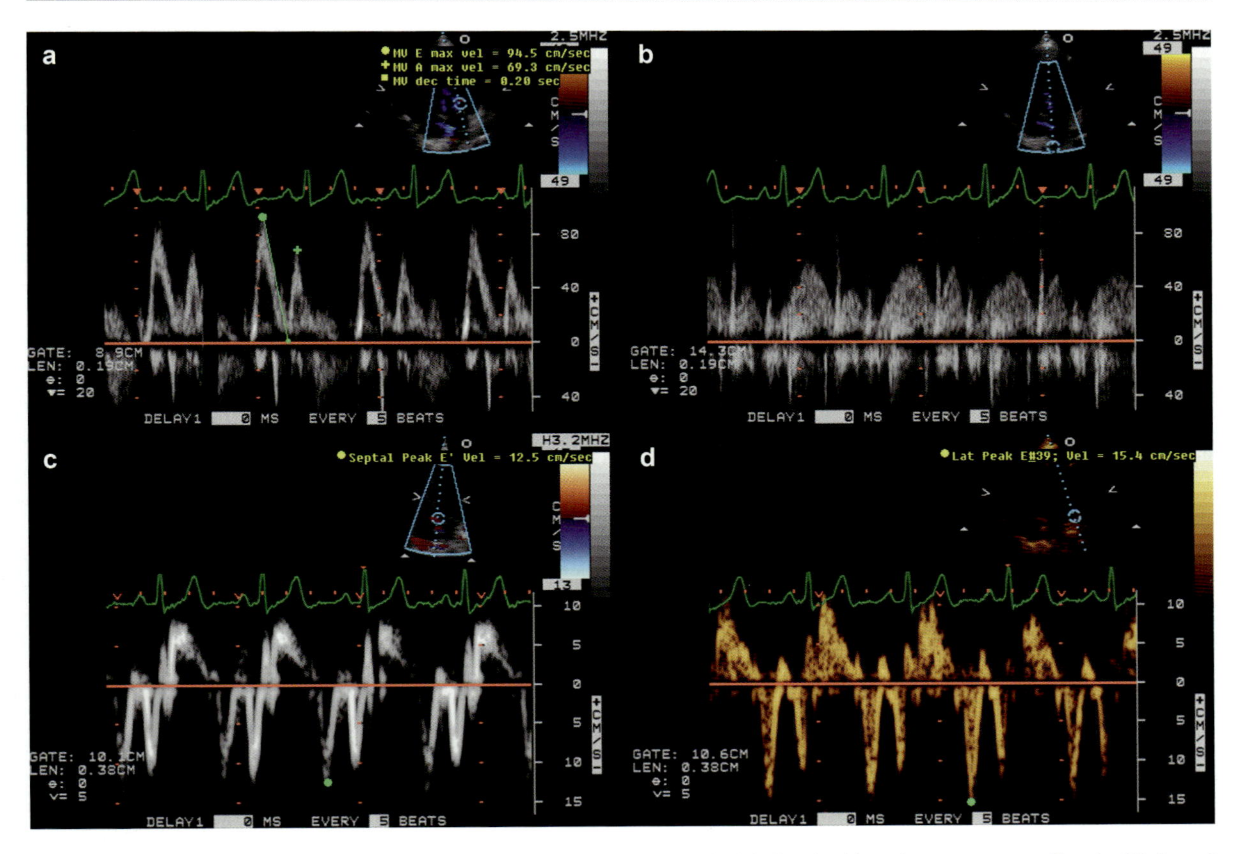

Fig. 16.9 These recordings are from a 48-year-old woman, showing the mitral inflow in **(a)**, pulmonary venous flow in **(b)**, lateral annular velocities in **(c)**, and septal annular velocities in **(d)**. These measures are in keeping with normal diastolic function. The effect of age is illustrated by the mitral E/A ratio of 1.4, compared to 2.5 in the much younger patient shown in Fig. 16.8

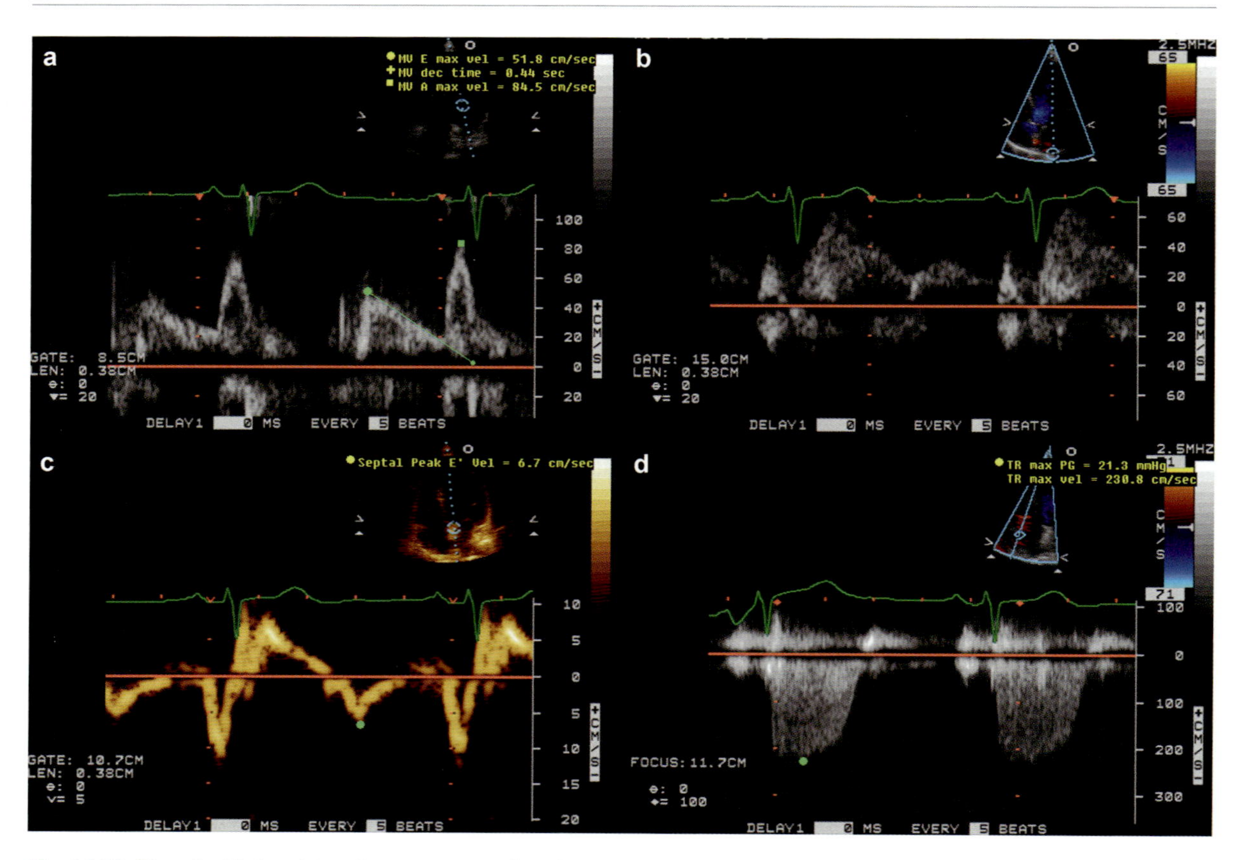

Fig. 16.10 The mitral inflow (**a**), pulmonary venous flow (**b**), the septal annular velocities (**c**), and the tricuspid regurgitation velocity (**d**) show that there is impaired relaxation as evidenced by the long mitral deceleration time and the low septal early diastolic velocity. The E/E′ is 7.7 and the right ventricular systolic pressure is normal, suggesting that the left atrial pressure is normal

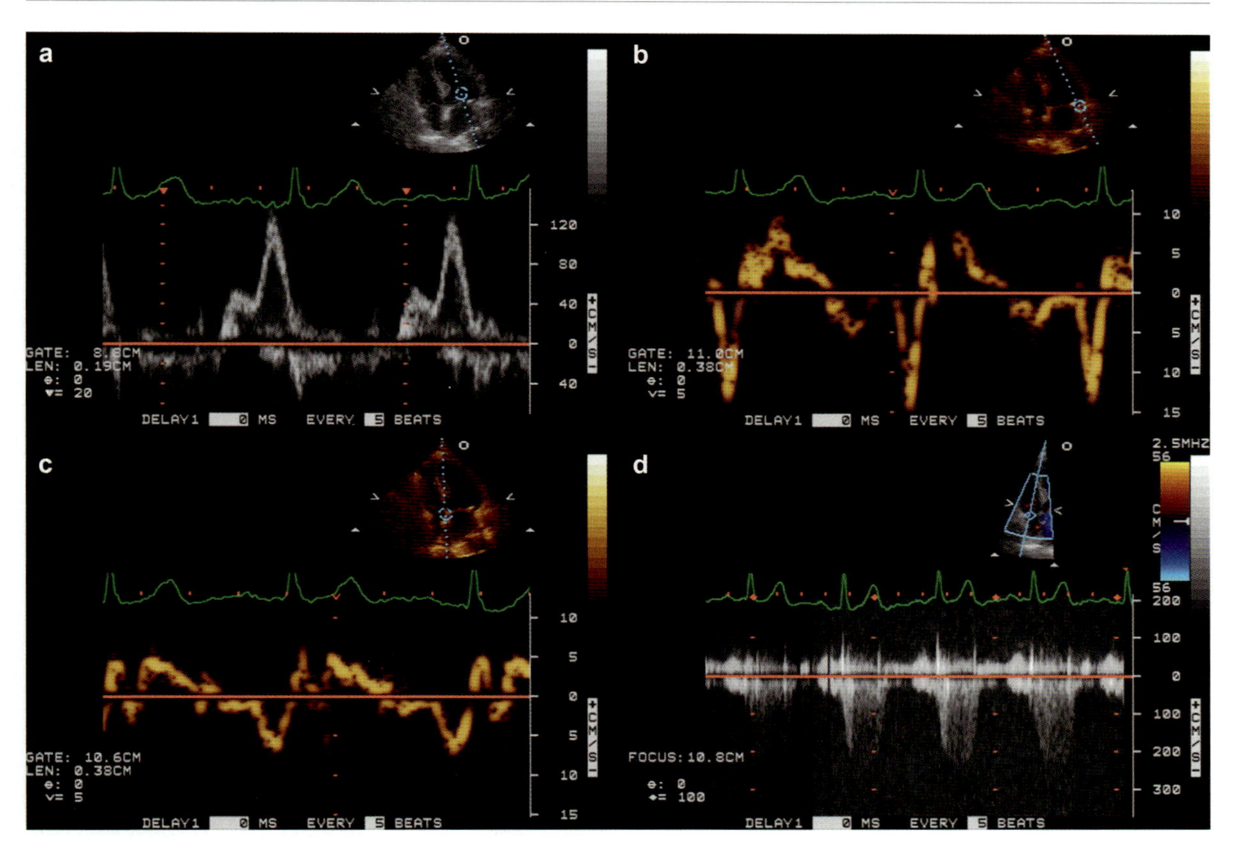

Fig. 16.11 The mitral inflow (**a**), the lateral annular velocities (**b**), the septal annular velocities (**c**), and the tricuspid regurgitation velocity (**d**). There is impaired relaxation with prominent mitral A and long deceleration time. The annular early diastolic velocities are also low. The mitral E velocity is 45 cm/s and the septal E′ is 2 cm/s giving a ratio of 22.5. Despite the high E/E′ ratio, the low mitral E (<50 cm/s) generally indicates that left atrial pressure is not elevated, and this is supported by the normal tricuspid regurgitation velocity

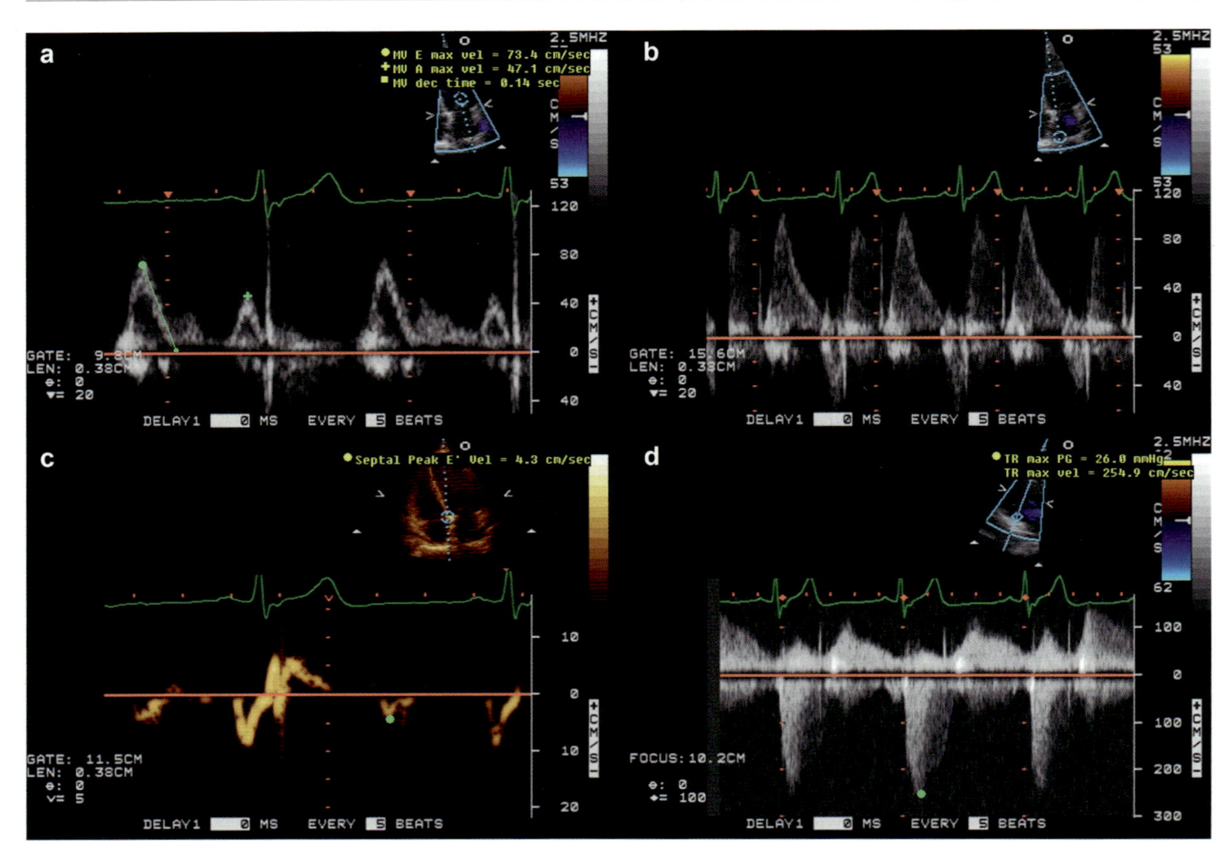

Fig. 16.12 The mitral inflow (**a**), pulmonary venous flow (**b**), the septal annular velocity (**c**), and the tricuspid regurgitation velocity (**c**) are shown. The E/A is 1.5, E/E′ 17, and a pulmonary atrial velocity 45 cm/s, all pointing to elevated LA pressure. The right ventricular systolic pressure is also elevated

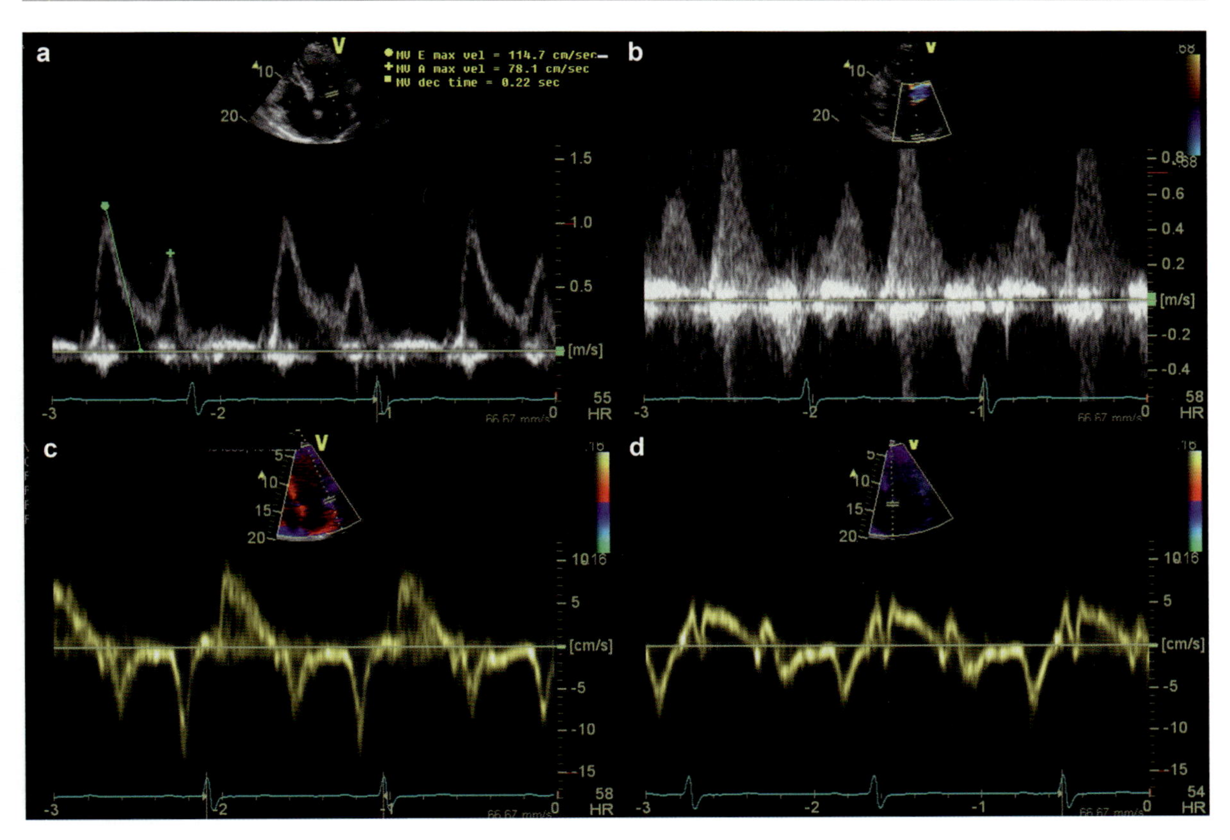

Fig. 16.13 The mitral inflow (**a**), pulmonary venous flow (**b**), the lateral annular velocities (**c**), and the septal annular velocities (**d**) show that E/A is 1.5 and E/E′ (septal) 23. The pulmonary atrial velocity is 40 cm/s and its duration exceed mitral A by 35 ms

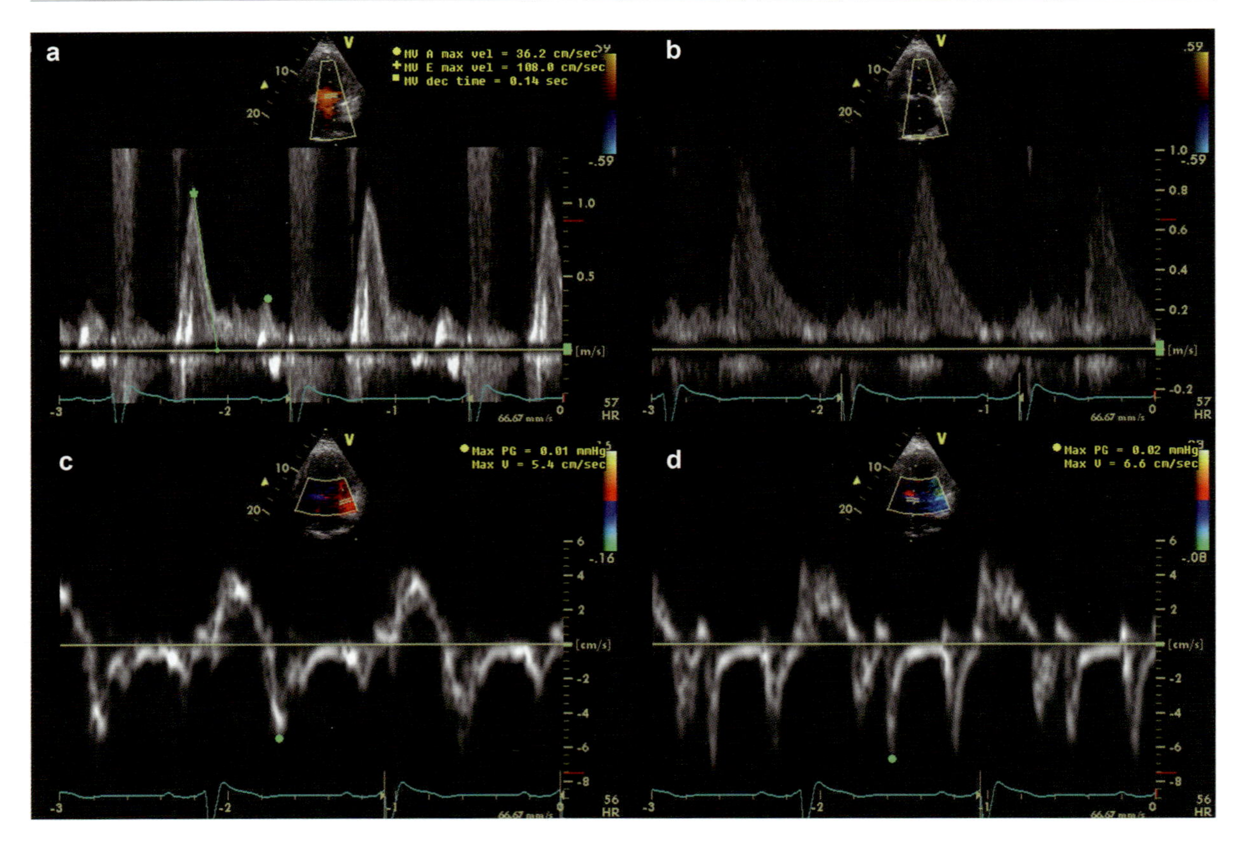

Fig. 16.14 The mitral inflow (**a**), pulmonary venous flow (**b**), the lateral annular velocities (**c**), and the septal annular velocities (**d**) are shown. The E/A is 3 and the deceleration time is 140 ms. The pulmonary venous flow shows prominent early diastolic velocity and low systolic antegrade velocity. The pulmonary atrial reversal is not clearly shown

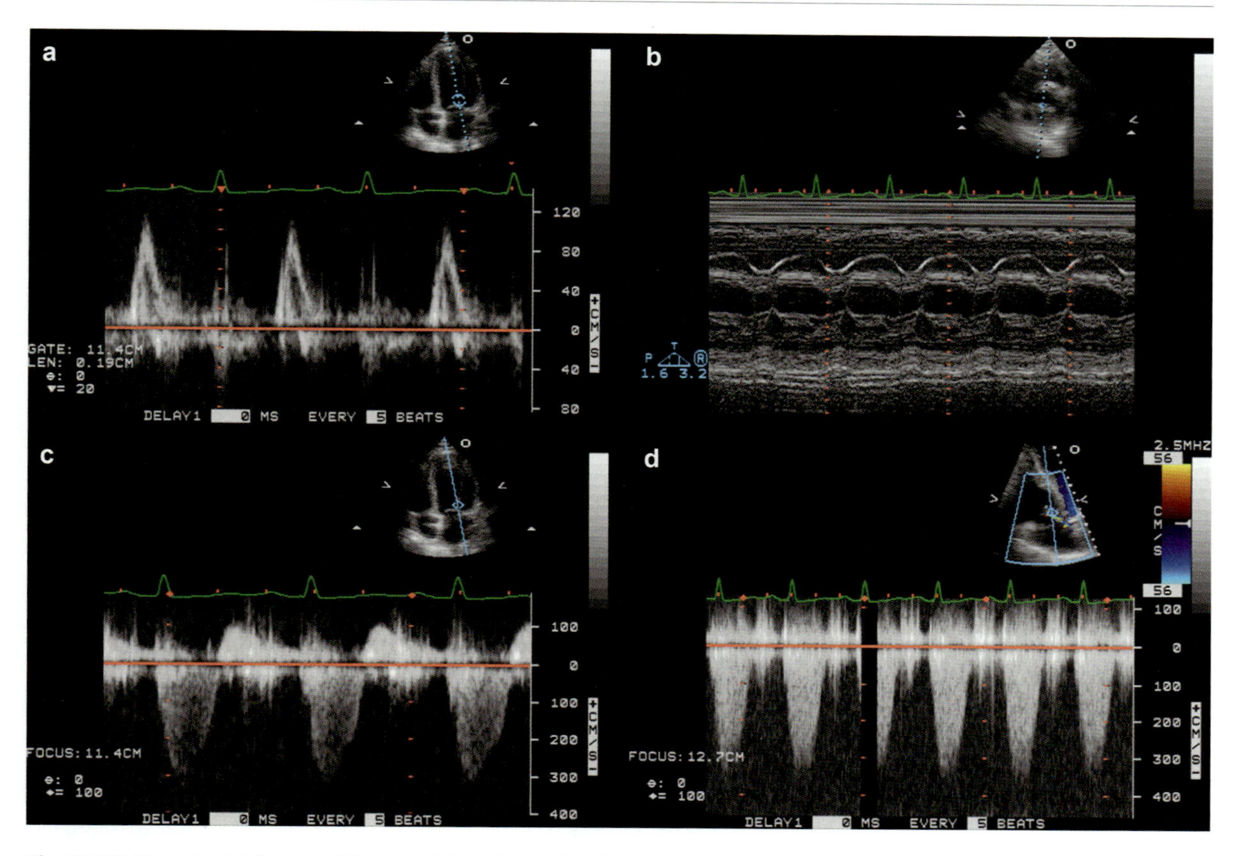

Fig. 16.15 The mitral inflow (**a**), M-mode of the mitral valve (**b**), the mitral regurgitation velocity (**c**), and the tricuspid regurgitation velocity (**d**) are shown. There is a prominent E and no distinct A, but mitral M-mode shows that the mitral valve remains open despite the fact that there is no significant antegrade flow from the left atrium into the left ventricle. The mitral regurgitation velocity is low consistent with systemic hypotension and elevated left atrial pressure. The tricuspid regurgitation velocity shows the pressure of pulmonary hypertension which is particularly significant in view of systemic hypotension indicated by the low mitral regurgitation velocity

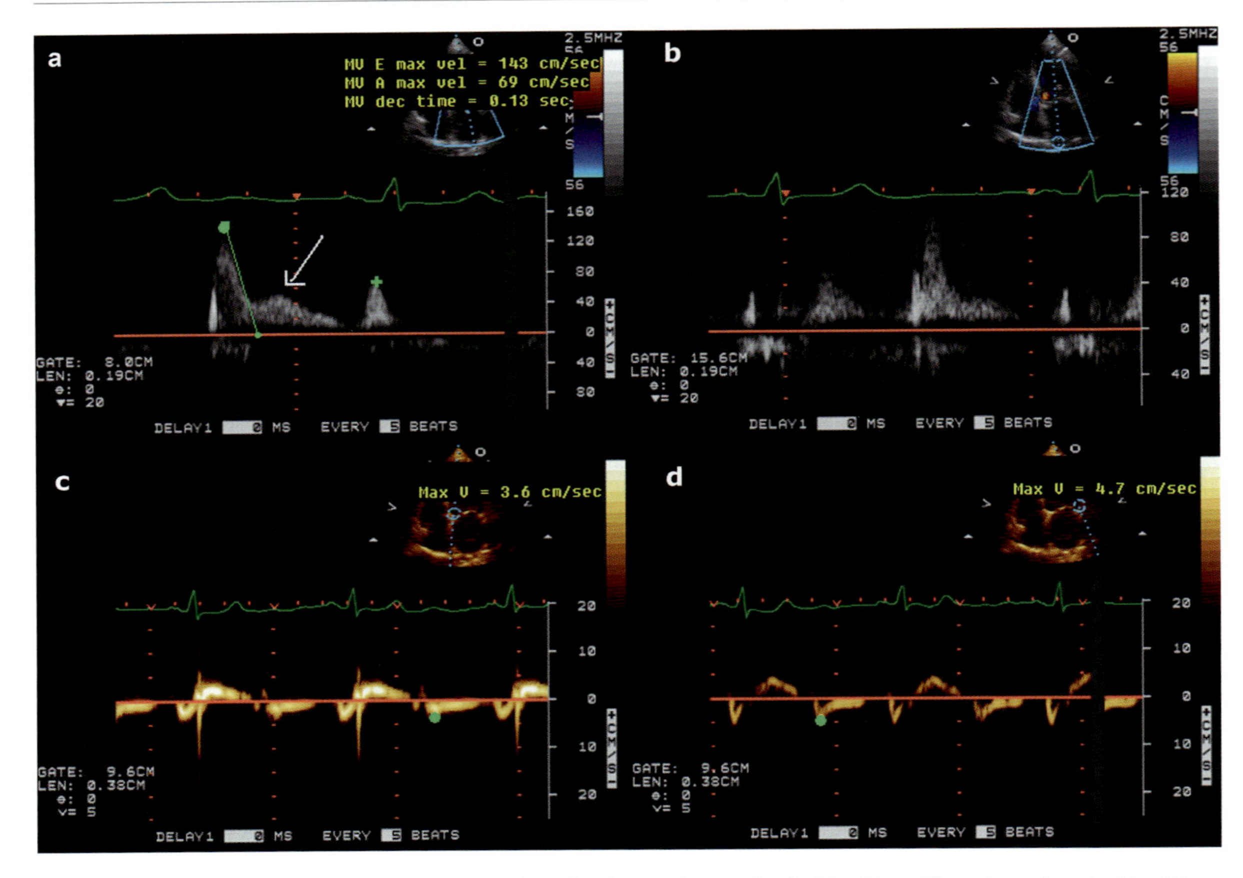

Fig. 16.16 The mitral inflow (**a**), pulmonary venous flow (**b**), the annular septal velocities (**c**), and lateral annular velocities (**d**) are shown. The mitral inflow shows a prominent mid diastolic velocity (50 cm/s) which reflects marked delay in left ventricular relaxation and elevated left atrial pressure. The presence of elevated left atrial pressure is supported by the high E/E′ ratio

Table 16.4 Doppler measures in different severities of diastolic dysfunction

	Normal	Abnormal relaxation	Pseudonormalization	Restriction
E/A ratio	1–1.5	<1	1–1.5	>2
DT (ms)	160–240	≥240	160–240	≤150
IVRT (ms)	60–100	≥110	60–100	<60
PV S/D ratio	~1[a]	>1	<1	<<1
A_r	<A	>A	>A	>A
A_r vel (cm/s)	<20	<35	>35	>25[b]
Ea (cm/s)	>8	<8	<8	<8
Vp (cm/s)	>45	<45	<45	<45

E/A mitral E/A ratio, *DT* deceleration time, *IVRT* isovolumic relaxation time, *PV S/D* pulmonary vein systolic and diastolic flow, *A*atrial reversal flow of pulmonary vein, *A* mitral A duration, *vel* velocity, *Ea* early mitral annular longitudinal tissue velocity, *Vp* velocity of transmitral flow propagation

[a]Young patients and athletes may have values of <1[b] <1. If atrial contractile failure is present, the value will be <25 cm/s

Source: Reproduced with permission from [17]

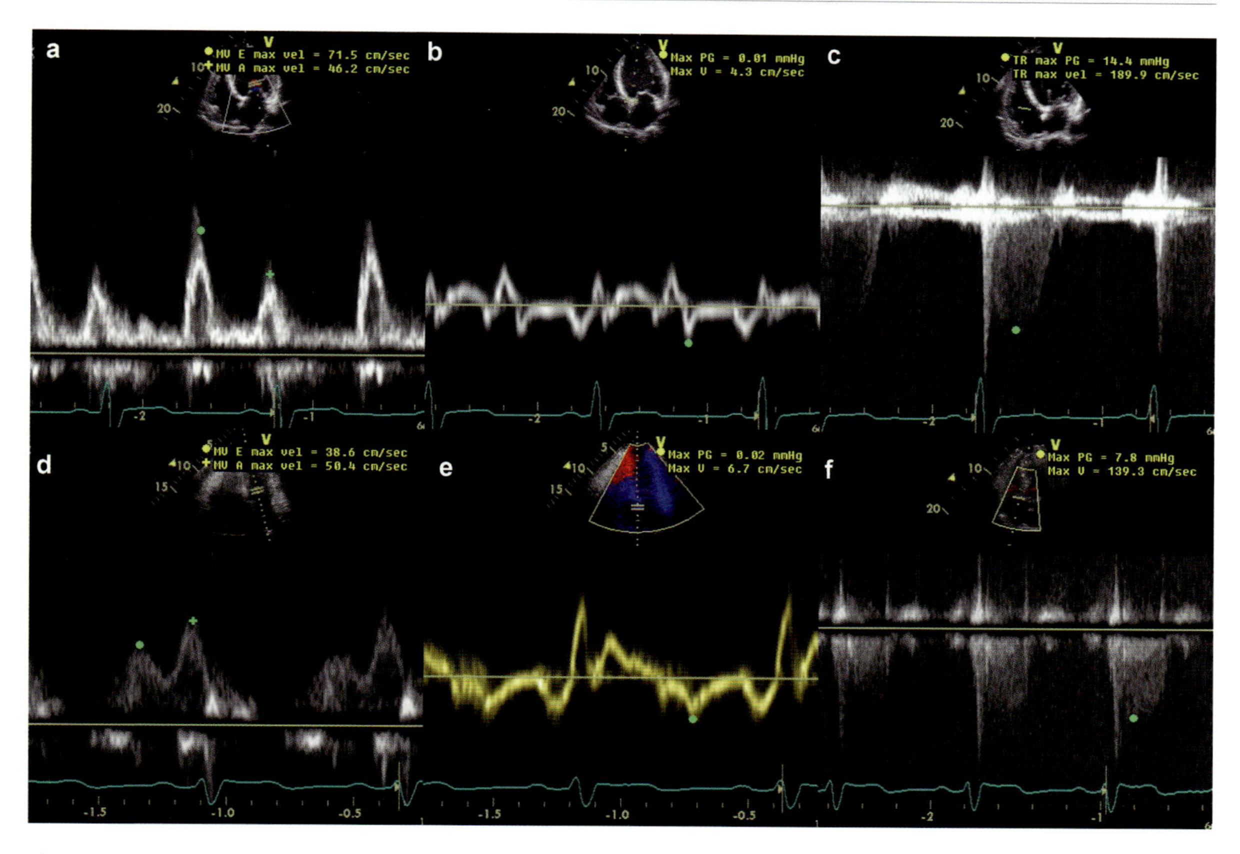

Fig. 16.17 This patient presents with heart failure and responds favorably to the medical treatment. The mitral inflow, the septal annular velocity, and the tricuspid regurgitation velocity before treatment are shown in **(a)**, **(b)**, and **(c)** respectively; and the similar recordings after treatment are shown in **(d)**, **(e)**, and **(f)**. The mitral inflow reverts to E/A < 1 and the tricuspid velocity also decreases. The tricuspid regurgitation velocity is low in this patient because of systemic hypotension and an elevated right atrial pressure

can be dynamic and correlate with the response to treatment. An improvement in the severity of diastolic dysfunction to treatment confers a more favorable prognosis [1].

Summary

Left ventricular diastolic filling is a complex process with multiple determinants. Many echo-Doppler findings are useful in assessing the diastolic function, but we should avoid reliance on any single measure. Currently, it is imprudent to provide a quantitative measure of left ventricular filling pressure on the basis of calculations utilizing some or all of these echo-Doppler variables. On the other hand, qualitative assessment is generally feasible based on a careful analysis of all the available clinical, echocardiographic, and Doppler findings.

References

1. Nagueh SF, Appleton CP, Dillebert TC, et al. Recommendations for the evaluation of left ventricular diastolic function by echocardiography. *J Am Soc Echocardiogr*. 2009;22:107-133.
2. Oh KJ, Hatle L, Tajik AJ, Little WC. Diastolic heart failure can be diagnosed by comprehensive two-dimensional and Doppler echocardiography. *J Am Coll Cardiol*. 2006;47:500-506.
3. Lam CSP, Roger VL, Rodeheffer RJ, Bursi F, Borlaug BA, Ommen SR. Cardiac structure and ventricular-vascular function in persons with heart failure and preserved ejection fraction: from Olmstead County, Minnesota. *Circulation*. 2007;115:1982-1990.
4. Yamamoto K, Nishimura RA, Chaliki HP, Appleton CP, Holmes DR Jr, Redfield MM. Determination of left ventricular

Table 17.1 Systemic diseases with frequent cardiac manifestations

Connective tissue disease
Metabolic diseases
Nutritional deficiencies
Hematologic disorders
Endocrine disorders
Infectious diseases
Neoplastic diseases
Sarcoid
Drug and physical toxicities

Table 17.2 Pathognomonic echocardiographic findings of systemic diseases

Disease entity	Pathognomonic findings
Carcinoid	"Frozen" tricuspid and pulmonic valves
Marfan syndrome	Pear shape aortic root
Ankylosing spondylitis	Subaortic ridge
Kawasaki	Proximal coronary aneurysm
Takotsubo	Apical ballooning
Takayasu	"rat tail" aorta
Sarcoid	Basal septal involvement and small mouth LV aneurysm
RV cardiomyopathy	Focal RV aneurysm
LV non-compaction	Heavily trabeculated LV

LV left ventricle, *RV* right ventricle

Small mouth left ventricular aneurysms, particularly involving the basal left ventricular free wall, should raise the possible diagnosis of cardiac sarcoidosis, but such aneurysms are a rare finding. More common findings include thinning and brightness of the basal septum, involvement of the posteromedial papillary muscle leading to mitral regurgitation, and myocardial involvement with restrictive physiology [11, 12]. In many systemic diseases, pathognomonic findings may be relatively uncommon. Thus the presence of pathognomonic findings can be used to help make the diagnosis of the underlying systemic diseases, but their absence should not be used to exclude these diseases.

Nonspecific Findings Are More Common

Although pathognomonic findings can be useful in making the diagnosis of the underlying disease, they may be relatively uncommon in many systemic diseases. Nonspecific findings are usually much more common. For instance, pericardial effusion may be a manifestation of many connective tissue diseases (Table 17.3) [13]. In patients with systemic lupus erythematosus, cardiac involvement can be detected in over half of these patients and is the third leading cause of death after infection and renal failure. Valvular involvement is common, occurring in about three quarters of these patients, but the type of valvular involvement is nonspecific with the most frequent finding being valve thickening, particularly of the mitral valve [14, 15] (Figs. 17.7, 17.8). Valvular regurgitation is more common than valvular stenosis. Pericardial effusion is also a common finding present in about 50% of the patients. Recognition of these nonspecific findings may not necessarily lead to the diagnosis of the underlying disease, but can provide useful information for the management of the patient.

Any Part of the Cardiovascular System May Be Affected

The discussion of systemic lupus makes it clear that any components of the cardiovascular system can be affected, including the pericardium, myocardium, valves, conduction system, the coronary arteries, and the great arteries (Fig. 17.9). In cardiac sarcoidosis, granulomatous involvement of the basal anterior septum affects the conduction system leading to heart block.

The coronary arteries may be selectively affected in Kawasaki disease, an acute systemic vasculitis of unknown cause (Fig. 17.10). Kawasaki presents as mucocutaneous lymph node syndrome, mainly in children under the age of 5. Although it has a high prevalence in Japan, this condition has been reported worldwide. It is believed that vasculitis of the coronary vasa vasora (small adventitial blood vessels that supply the coronary arteries themselves) results in coronary artery aneurysms, which are present in 15–20% of the affected individuals and are responsible for most of the mortality

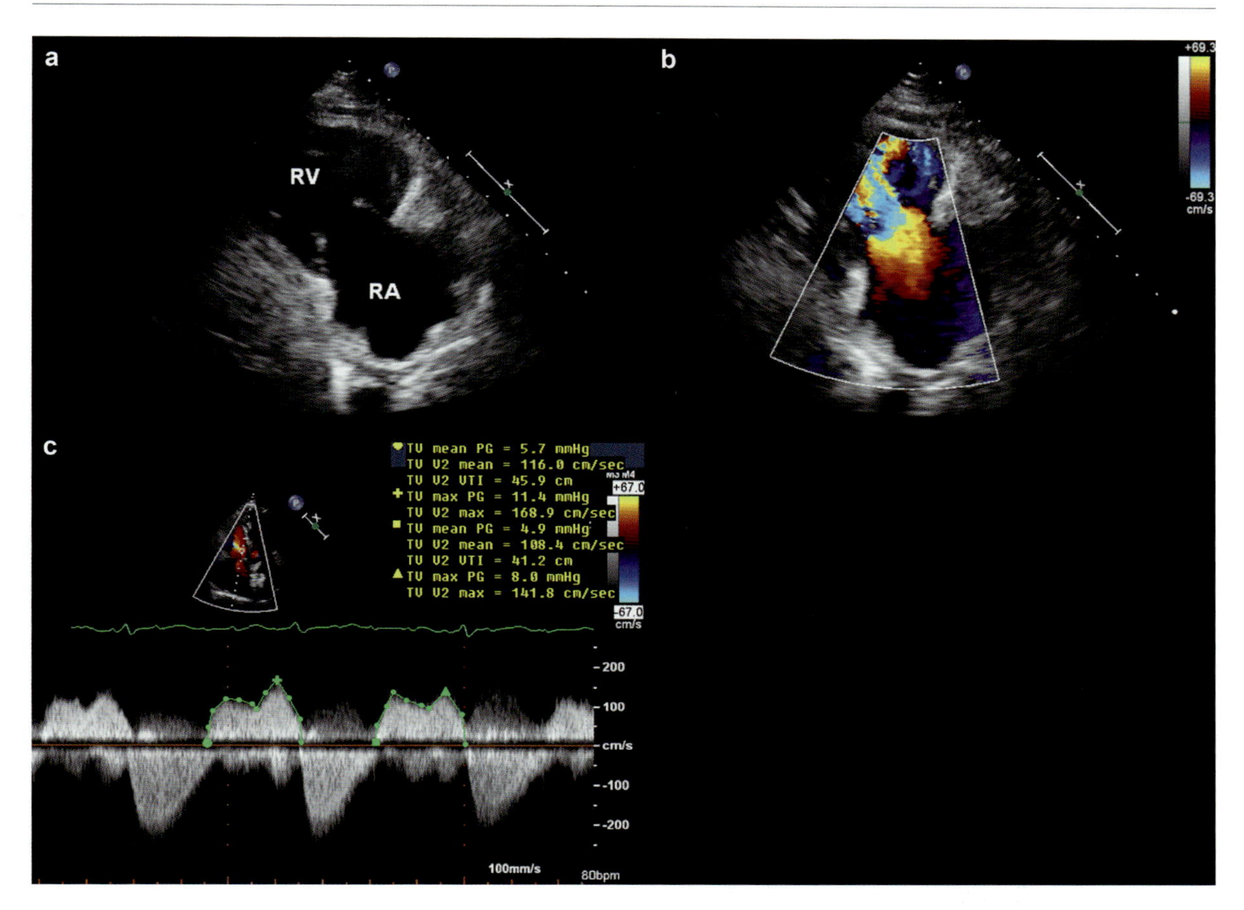

Fig. 17.1 This is a 67-year-old woman with a carcinoid tumor. The right ventricular inflow view in diastole (**a**) shows that both the right atrium and right ventricle are dilated. The tricuspid valve is thickened and restricted in excursion. Color-flow image (**b**) in the same view shows that there is flow acceleration across the tricuspid valve consistent with some degree of tricuspid stenosis. The continuous wave Doppler across the tricuspid valve (**c**) confirms that there is tricuspid stenosis with a mean tricuspid diastolic gradient of 4.9 mmHg. The Doppler signal also shows that there is severe tricuspid regurgitation as evidenced by the dense systolic signal, which is low in velocity and has a rapid deceleration consistent with rapid equalization of pressures between the right atrium and right ventricle. *RA* right ventricle, *RV* right ventricle

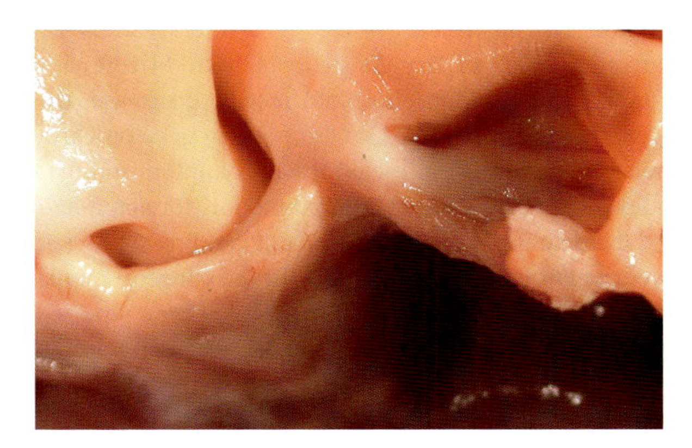

Fig. 17.2 This is an opened pulmonary valve with carcinoid disease-related valve changes. There is cusp thickening and commissural fusion from the white endocardial plaques. These fibromuscular plaques fix the valves so that it is stenotic and regurgitant

[16, 17]. Usually, only the proximal coronary artery segments are affected. The coronary artery aneurysms may resolve or progress to thrombosis with time. Proximal focal coronary aneurysms are a pathognomonic finding for Kawasaki disease. Other findings of cardiac involvement in Kawasaki disease include pericardial effusion, mitral regurgitation, and left ventricular dysfunction.

In patients with systemic diseases, predilection to any specific cardiac structure should be kept in mind and a comprehensive assessment of all the different components of the cardiovascular system should be performed, since any one component or multiple components of the cardiovascular systems can be affected.

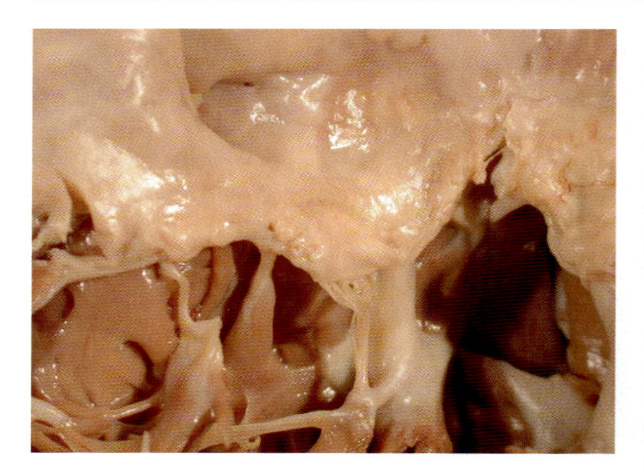

Fig. 17.3 This is a severely diseased tricuspid valve with thickened leaflets and chords from fibromuscular endocardial plaques typical of carcinoid disease. These plaques make the leaflets immobile and the valve is regurgitant. Note the chordal thickening and obliteration of the normal space between the chords, the leaflets and the papillary muscle

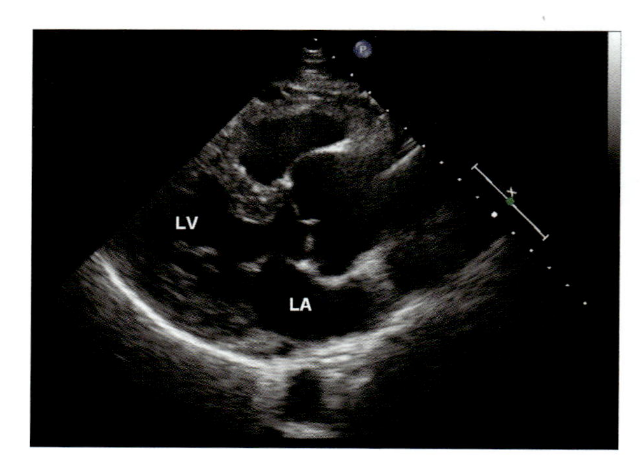

Fig. 17.4 This is a 51-year-old man with Marfan syndrome. This parasternal long-axis shows the typical enlargement of the aortic root giving the aorta a pear shape. *LA* left atrium, *LV* left ventricle

The Cardiac Involvement Can Be Focal or Diffuse

In Kawasaki disease, the vasculitis is usually focal and involves the proximal coronary segments. This is not the case with other forms of vasculitis such as Behcet syndrome, giant cell arteritis or Takayasu arteritis [18, 19]. Giant cell arteritis is characterized by granulomatous inflammation of large and medium sized arteries (Figs. 17.11, 17.12). It tends to affect the elderly with similar demographics to patients with polymyalgia rheumatica. Clinically evident aortitis occurs in about 15% of cases. Correct diagnosis and prompt treatment with corticosteroids can improve the outcome.

Takayasu arthritis is an idiopathic large vessel vasculitis in young people who are generally less than 40 years of age (Fig. 17.13). The involvement may be widespread involving the aorta and many of its major branches leading to vascular stenosis, occlusion, or aneurysm formation [20, 21]. In patients with suspected vasculitis, the entire arterial tree should be imaged. In addition to echocardiography, computed tomography or magnetic resonance scan should be considered.

Myocardial Involvement is Common in Neuromuscular Diseases

With advances in supportive care, patients with neuromuscular diseases are surviving into adulthood. It has also become clear that cardiac involvement is common not only in patients with clinically evident neuromuscular disease, but also in carriers of the genetic mutations without overt evidence of the disease (Table 17.4) [22–26]. The most common cardiac manifestation is myocardial dysfunction, which can be regional or global (Figs. 17.14, 17.15). When the involvement is regional, typically the posterior and inferior walls are affected (Fig. 17.16). In patients with Friedreich's ataxia, which is an autosomal recessive disease, the genetic mutation resides on the frataxin gene on chromosome 9 [27]. The mean age of symptom onset is about 12 years. Cardiac failure accounts for about half of the deaths. Cardiac involvement can present as left ventricular hypertrophy, usually of the concentric type (Fig. 17.17). Subaortic stenosis has also been reported [28–31]. Dilated cardiomyopathy is less common but reported. Friedreich's ataxia patients are also prone to the development of arrhythmias, particularly atrial fibrillation.

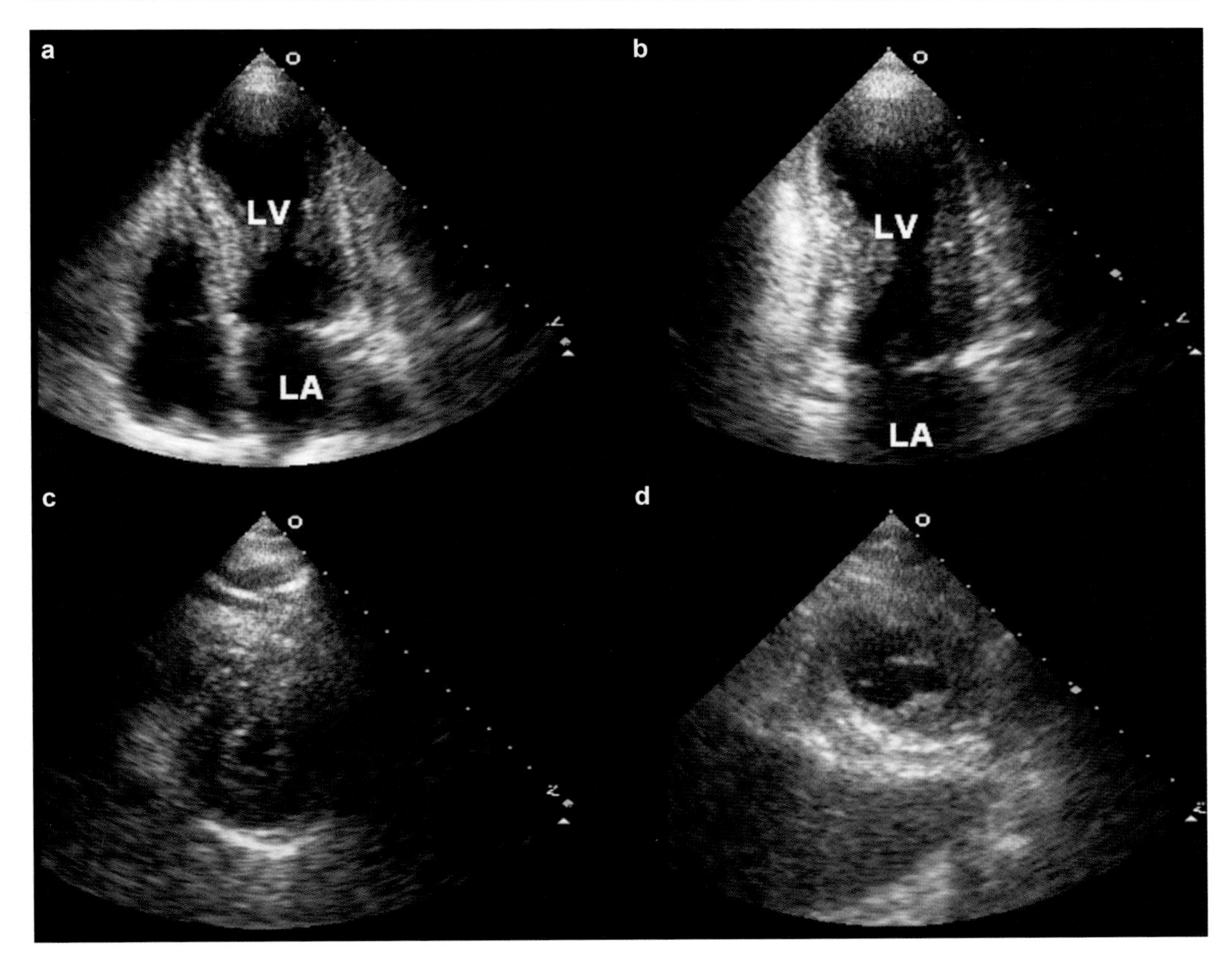

Fig. 17.5 This 65-year-old woman had a seizure while traveling on an airplane. She then became extremely dyspneic. The admission electrocardiogram showed diffuse ST segment elevation and emergent coronary angiogram showed no significant coronary artery disease. The echocardiogram was performed when she was in the Coronary Care Unit. Both the apical four-chamber (**a**) and two-chamber (**b**) views show that the left ventricular apex is enlarged and dyskinetic. The mid-ventricular segments and basal left ventricular segments were normal. The parasternal short-axis view at the level of the papillary muscle (**c**) shows that the left ventricle at this level had normal internal dimension and normal wall thickness, but the short-axis view of the left ventricular apex (**d**) shows that the apex was enlarged with a thin wall. These morphologic features are typical of Takotsubo cardiomyopathy

Systemic Disease Can Be a Cause of Cardiomyopathy

All of the different forms of cardiomyopathy (dilated, hypertrophic, and restrictive) may be caused by an underlying systemic disease. As previously mentioned, patients with Friedreich's ataxia can have findings of hypertrophic cardiomyopathy or dilated cardiomyopathy. Conversely patients with cardiomyopathy, be it hypertrophic, dilated, or restrictive, should be screened for underlying systemic disease. This is particularly the case in young patients with unexplained cardiomyopathy.

In patients with restrictive cardiomyopathy, a search for an underlying condition is likely to be fruitful since primary restrictive cardiomyopathy is rare. Diseases that may cause restrictive cardiomyopathy are listed in the Table 17.5. Among the underlying conditions, amyloidosis is a common underlying condition, and recent understanding of this condition has led to

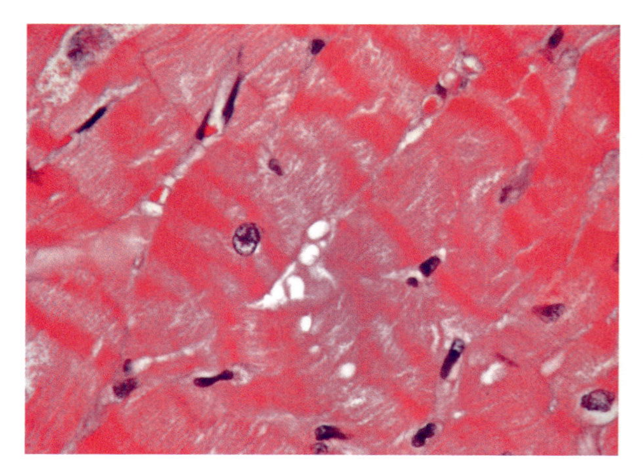

Fig. 17.6 This patient was an elderly postmenopausal female with anxiety who fell. She did not injure herself severely but became anxious and presented to emergency in cardiogenic shock. Despite resuscitation she died shortly thereafter. She had echocardiography suggestive of Takotsubo cardiomyopathy. The image is of her myocardium at autopsy. She had no underlying heart disease and normal coronary arteries. Widespread contraction band necrosis was noted in all her heart chambers consistent with stress cardiomyopathy

advances in treatment that may improve the prognosis (Fig. 17.18). Amyloidosis is a heterogeneous group of diseases with the common feature being the deposition of amyloid in multiple organs (Fig. 17.19). The different forms are characterized by different amyloid fibril proteins. In primary AL amyloid the protein is composed of portions of the immunoglobulin light chains. Cardiac involvement with heart failure is common and present in about 50% of the patients [32–34]. Cardiac complications are the most common cause of death in these patients. They include atrial fibrillation, conduction disturbance, valvular insufficiency, pericardial effusion, and myocardial dysfunction. The echocardiographic findings of amyloid heart disease are listed in the Table 17.6 [35, 36]. Transthyretin type amyloid may be age related or hereditary in younger patients. The age-related amyloid has a better prognosis than the AL type and the pathologist can aid in immunotyping the biopsy specimen. Secondary AA amyloid protein, deposited in inflammatory diseases, does not often involve the heart.

Suspect Congenital Syndromes or Chromosomal Diseases in the Setting of Cardiac Malformations

When congenital cardiac malformations, particularly multiple malformations, are present, congenital syndromes or chromosomal abnormalities should be suspected as cardiac manifestations are common in the setting of chromosomal abnormalities and have been well described in congenital syndromes (Table 17.7) [37–44]. In the patients with Fragile X syndrome, the dysplastic and myxomatous mitral valve, with marked degree of prolapse, is usually present (Fig. 17.20) [45]. The tricuspid valve can also be myxomatous with severe prolapse. In 20% of these patients, dilated aortic root can also be observed. Fragile X syndrome is an X-linked condition, which commonly causes mental retardation. Up to 20% of the affected males may be asymptomatic and a third of the women who are carriers have some degree of mental retardation. In patients with known congenital syndromes or chromosomal diseases, a comprehensive echocardiographic examination is crucial to look for cardiac malformations. Conversely when malformations, particularly multiple cardiac malformations, are present, congenital syndromes or chromosomal abnormalities should be sought in these patients.

Table 17.3 Relative frequencies of cardiac manifestations in connective tissue diseases

Disease entity	Pericardial involvement	Cardiomyopathy	Conduction disease	Valvular disease	Pulmonary hypertension	Aortitis
Lupus erythematosus	+++	++	+	+++	++	+
Rheumatoid arthritis	+++	+	+	+	+	++
Ankylosing spondylitis	+	+	+++	++	+	+++
Scleroderma	+++	+	+++	+	+++	-
Polymyositis	+	++	++	-	-	-

Source: Modified after Mandell and Hoffman in Heart Disease 6th ed. 2001 (46)
+++, frequently present; ++, sometimes present; +, rare; -, absent

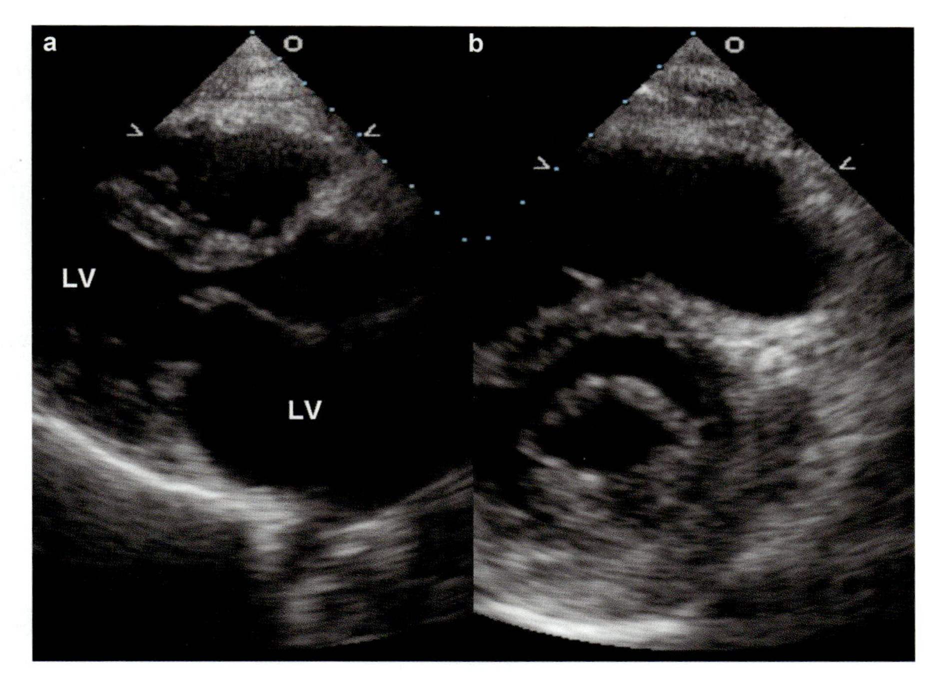

Fig. 17.7 This 36-year-old woman had a long history of systemic lupus erythematosus and had been noted to have a heart murmur for several years. The parasternal long-axis (**a**) and short-axis (**b**) views in diastole show that the mitral leaflets are diffusely thickened with mild restriction in excursion, but there is no commissural fusion

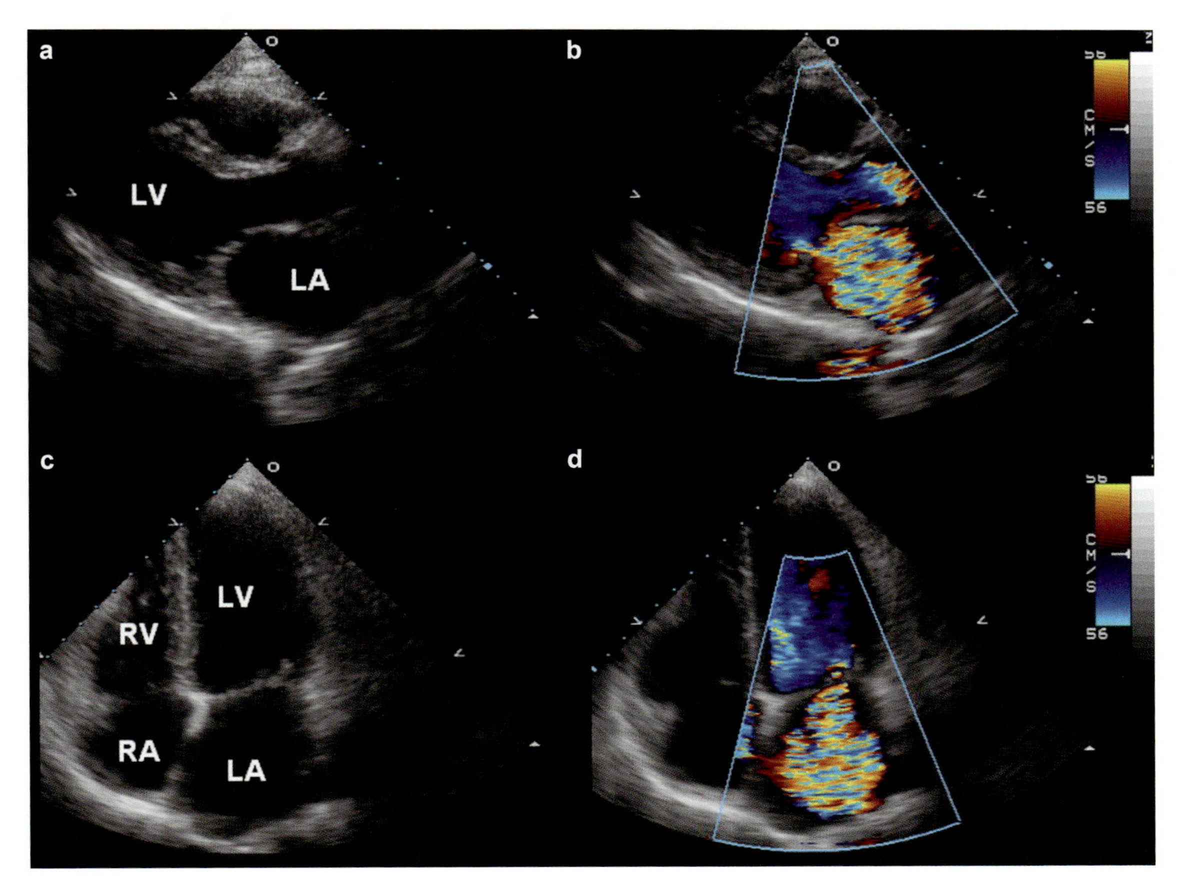

Fig. 17.8 This is the same patient as in Fig. 17.7. The parasternal long-axis (**a, b**) and the apical four-chamber (**c, d**) views are shown in systole. The mitral leaflets are diffusely thickened. Color-flow images (**b, d**) show the presence of severe mitral regurgitation

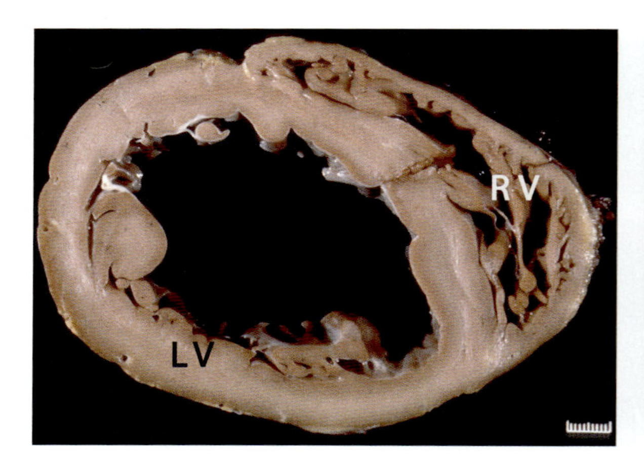

Fig. 17.9 This is a cross section of a heart from a young woman with severe systolic congestive heart failure. She had long standing lupus. Biventricular dilatation is prominent. There was no significant coronary artery disease or valve disease. *LV* left ventricle, *RV* right ventricle

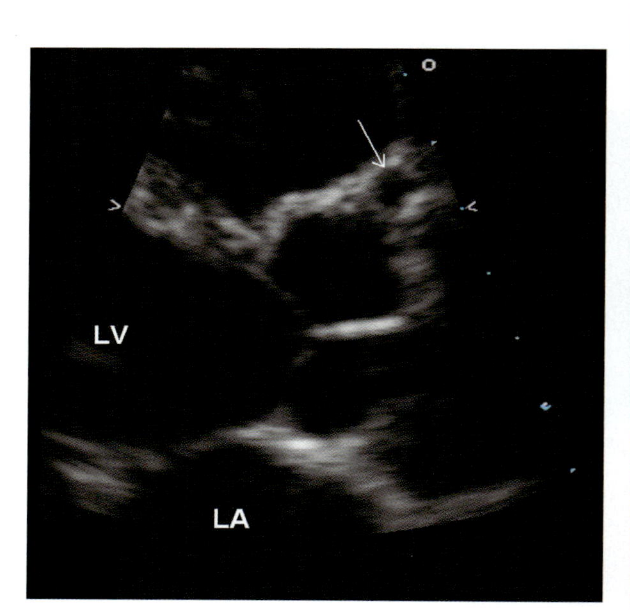

Fig. 17.10 This is a 20-year-old man with a history of Kawasaki disease during childhood. This zoomed parasternal long-axis view shows that the proximal right coronary artery (*arrow*) is dilated and measured about 7 mm in diameter. The left coronary artery (not shown) is normal in size

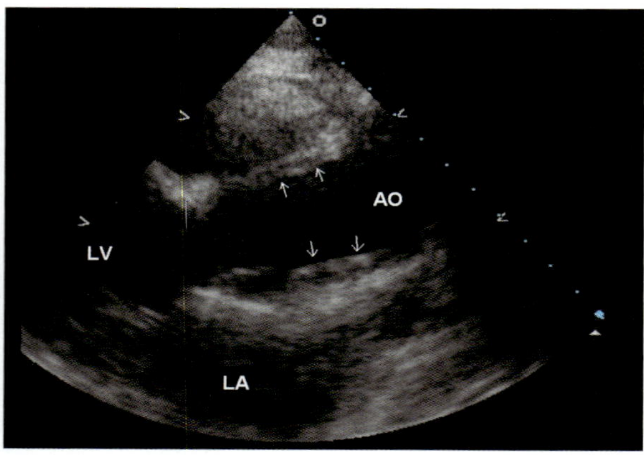

Fig. 17.11 This is a 57-year-old woman with giant cell arteritis. The parasternal long-axis view focuses on the ascending aorta showing that there is diffuse increase in thickness of the aortic wall (*arrows*) consistent with aortitis

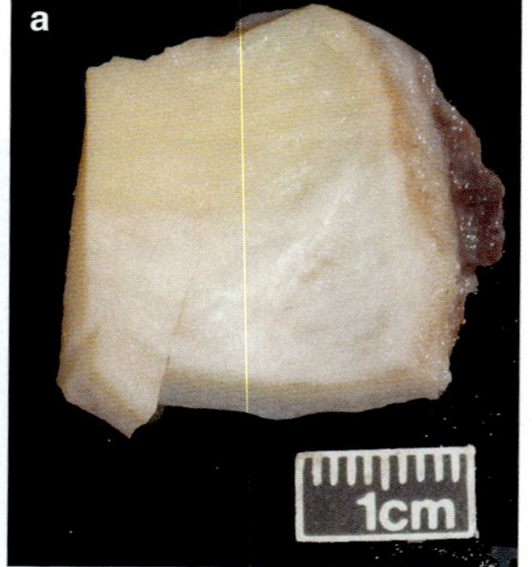

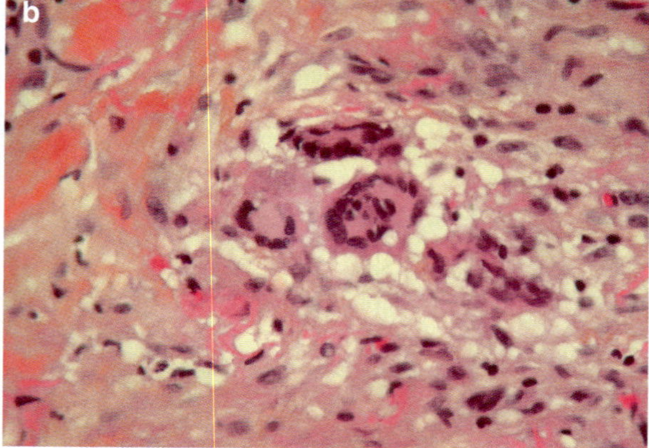

Fig. 17.12 (**a**) This is a segment of excised ascending aorta from an elderly patient with an ascending aortic aneurysm. The wall is thickened and the intima is white and discolored. (**b**) Microscopic examination revealed giant cell aortitis with medial destruction and the presence of numerous giant cells. Serology for syphilis was negative, as was serology for autoimmune diseases

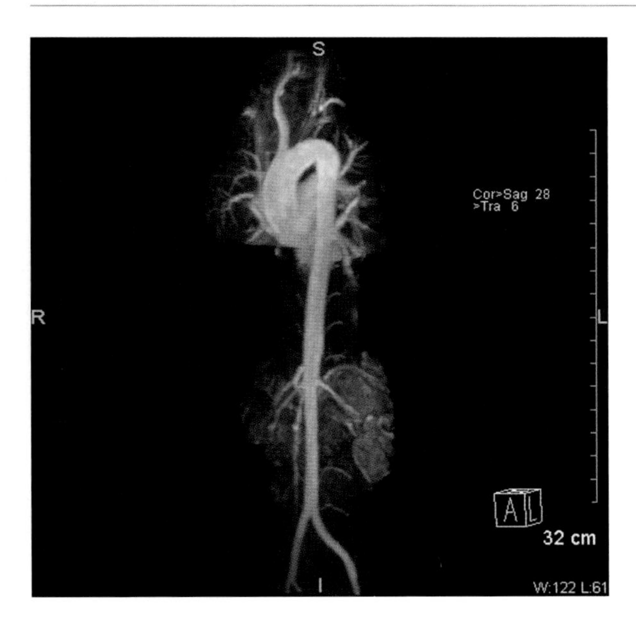

Fig. 17.13 This is a 36-year-old woman with Takayasu arteritis. The MRI view of the entire aorta shows mildly dilated ascending aorta, mild diffuse narrowing of the abdominal aorta beyond the renal arteries, severely stenotic left common carotid artery and absent right and left subclavian arteries

Table 17.4 Relative frequencies of cardiac manifestations in the common neuromuscular diseases

Disease entity	Genetic inheritance	Myocardial involvement	Valve involvement	Conduction disease	Arrhythmia
Duchenne	X-linked	+++	+	+	++
Becker[a]	X-linked	++	+	+	+
Myotonic	Autosomal dominant (chromosome 19)	+	+	+++	+
Friedreich's ataxia	Autosomal recessive (chromosome 9)	+++	-	-	+

[a]Association with left ventricular noncompaction has been reported
+++, frequently present; ++, sometimes present; +, rare; -, absent

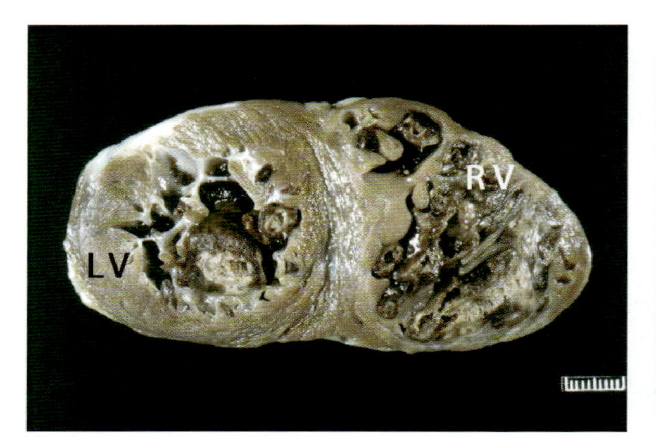

Fig. 17.14 This is a cross section of the heart of a young man with Becker's muscular dystrophy. He had bilateral large ventricular thrombi and died of pulmonary thromboemboli. Severe biventricular systolic dysfunction had been present. *LV* left ventricle, *RV* right ventricle

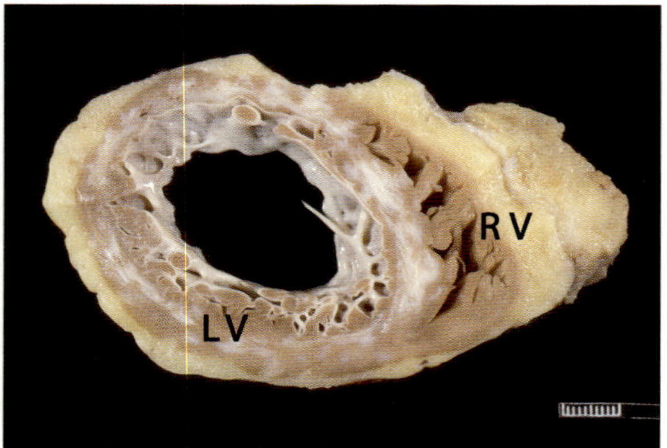

Fig. 17.15 This is a cross section of the heart of a patient with myotonic dystrophy. The myocardium has numerous patchy white fibrous scars. He had congestive heart failure. *LV* left ventricle, *RV* right ventricle

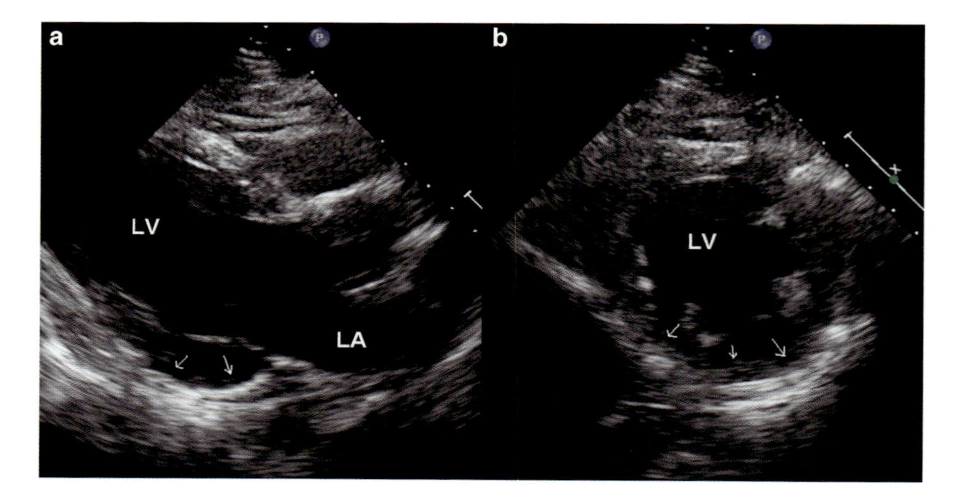

Fig. 17.16 This is a 19-year-old man with Duchenne muscular dystrophy. He was wheelchair bound but had no cardiac symptoms. The parasternal long-axis (**a**) and short-axis (**b**) views show that the left ventricle is dilated and there is localized thinning consistent with scar involving the basal and mid-posterior walls and inferior walls (*arrows*). *LA* left atrium, *LV* left ventricle

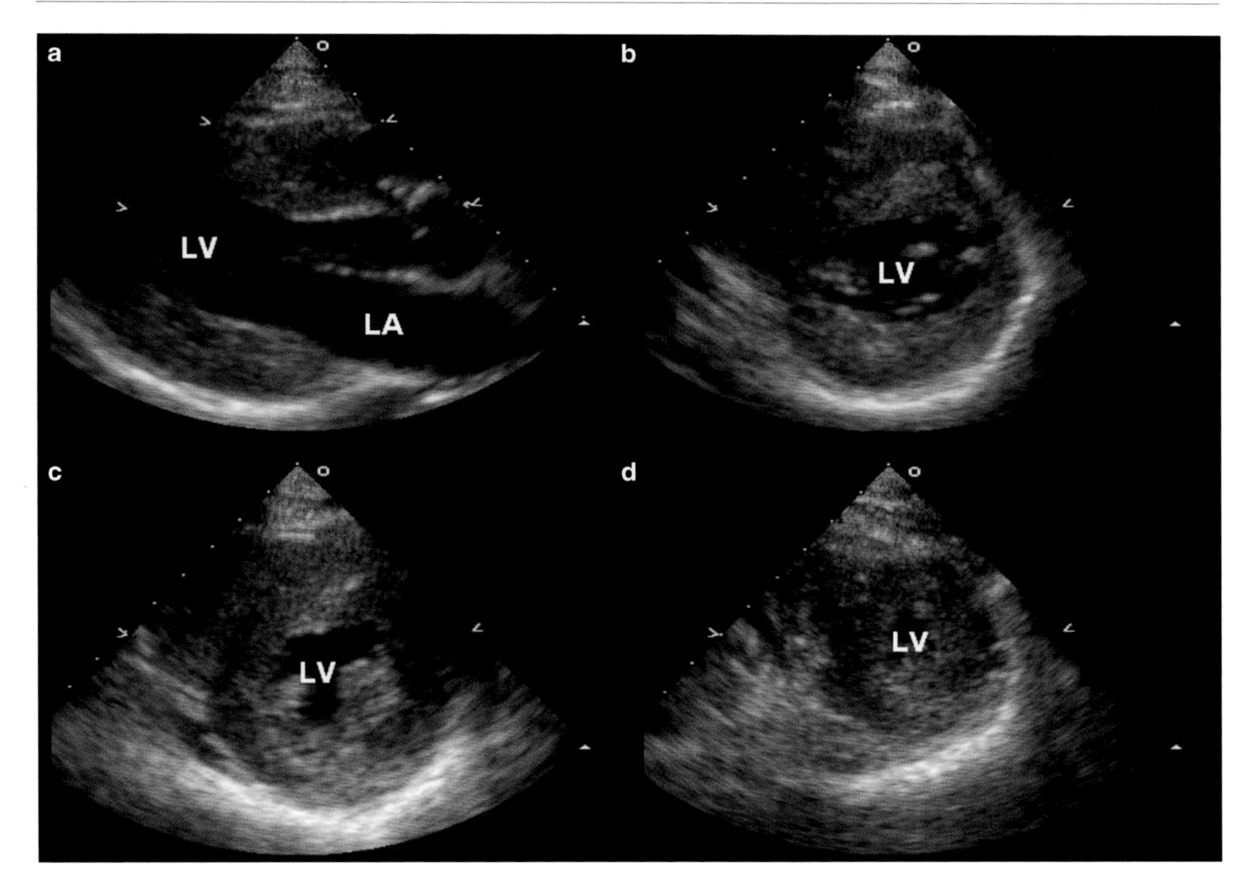

Fig. 17.17 This is a 27-year-old woman with Friedreich's ataxia. She has been using a wheelchair for ambulation for 3 years. The parasternal long-axis view (**a**) and short-axis views at multiple levels (**b–d**) show the diffuse hypertrophy involving the left ventricle

Table 17.5 Causes of restrictive cardiomyopathy

Infiltrative diseases
Amyloidosis
Sarcoidosis
Gaucher's disease
Hurler disease
Hemochromatosis
Fabry disease
Glycogen storage disease
Endomyocardial diseases
Endomyocardial fibrosis
Hypereosinophilic syndrome
Carcinoid
Radiation
Drug toxicity (e.g., anthracycline)

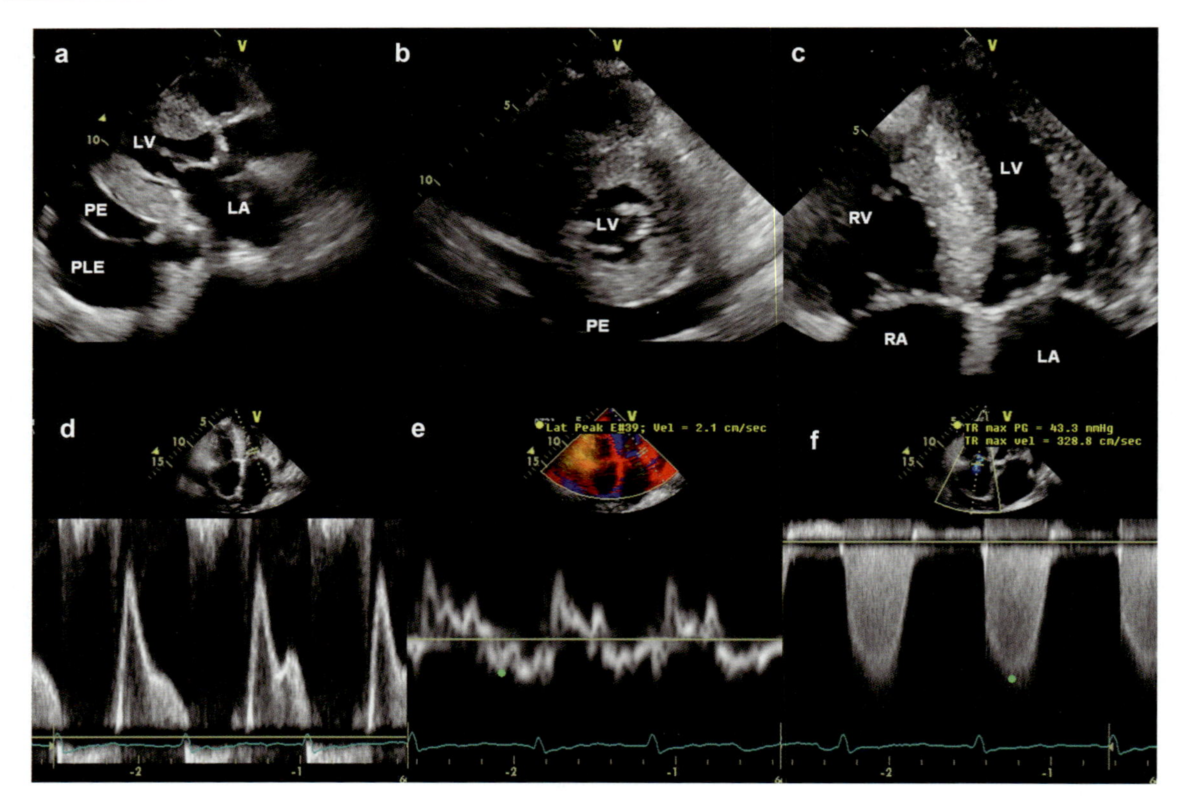

Fig. 17.18 This is a 92-year-old woman with advanced amyloid heart disease. The parasternal long-axis (**a**), short-axis (**b**), and apical four-chamber (**c**) views are shown. The left ventricle is normal in size with severe concentric hypertrophy. The cardiac valves are mildly thickened. A small circumferential pericardial effusion is present. There is also a moderate size left pleural effusion seen in the parasternal long-axis view (**a**). The mitral inflow pattern (**d**) shows a prominent E wave with a short deceleration time consistent with restrictive physiology. Annular tissue Doppler (**e**) shows reduced early diastolic velocity consistent with severe impaired relaxation. The tricuspid velocity (**f**) is high, consistent with pulmonary hypertension. These Doppler findings are in keeping with severe diastolic dysfunction

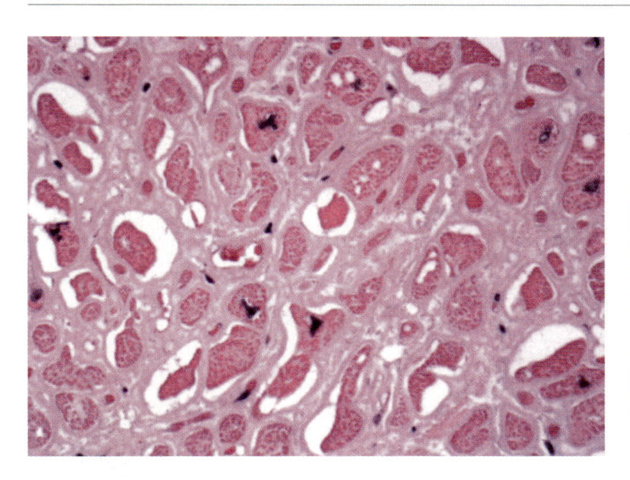

Fig. 17.19 Photomicrograph of myocardium from a patient with severe cardiac amyloid. This patient had diastolic heart failure. The amyloid is seen as pink material between the cardiac myocytes, which are red color and have nuclei. The amyloid was typed as AL type and subsequent investigation found plasma cell malignancy. In amyloid, the heart may be small, normal sized, or enlarged. The myocardium may appear normal, but is abnormally stiff

Table 17.6 Echocardiographic findings of amyloid heart disease

Increased LV and RV wall thickness
Increased myocardial echogenicity
Decreased LV systolic function
Regional wall motion abnormalities
Abnormal diastolic filling measurements
Valvular thickening and regurgitation
Atrial and/or ventricular thrombi
Pericardial effusion

LV left ventricle, *RV* right ventricle

Table 17.7 Cardiac anomalies in patients with chromosomal abnormalities

Chromosomal abnormality	Incidence of cardiac anomaly (%)	Typical cardiac anomaly
Trisomy 21	50	VSD, PDA, AVSD
Trisomy 22	65	ASD, VSD
Trisomy 13	90	VSD, PDA, dextrocardia
Trisomy 18	100	VSD, PDA, PS
Turners XO	35	Coarctation, AS, ASD

AS aortic stenosis, *ASD* atrial septal defect, *AVSD* atrioventricular septal defect, *PDA* patent ductus arteriosus, *PS* pulmonary stenosis, *VSD* ventricular septal defect

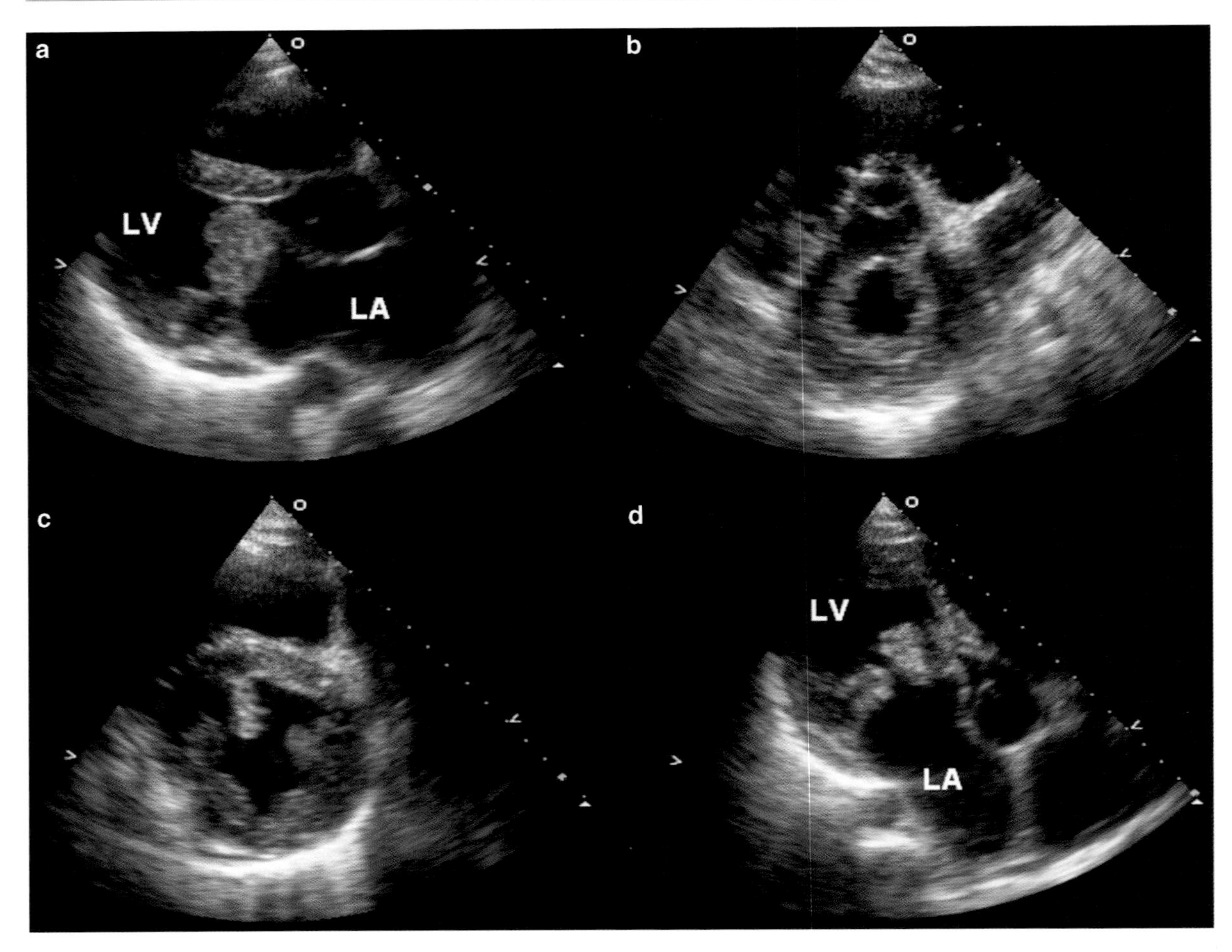

Fig. 17.20 This is a 26-year-old man with Fragile X syndrome. The parasternal long-axis (**a**) short-axis (**b, c**) and apical long-axis (**d**) views are shown. The mitral leaflets are extremely redundant and appear to have nodular masses in the freeze frames (**a, c, d**). The short-axis of the mitral leaflet tip level in diastole clearly shows that there is diffuse thickening involving the tips of both leaflets. The severe myxomatous appearance of the mitral valve is typical for this syndrome

Conclusion

There is a wide range of cardiac manifestations in patients with systemic diseases, making it difficult to provide a comprehensive listing of all the findings. We believe that a systematic approach based upon the principles discussed in this chapter is more useful to the echocardiographer who needs to integrate the myriad findings to help in making the diagnosis. The illustrated cases are used to explain these principles, and many of these cases highlight several of the principles at the same time.

References

1. Simula DV, Edwards WD, Tazelaar HD, Connolly HM, Schaff HV. Surgical pathology of carcinoid heart disease: a study of 139 valves from 75 patients spanning 20 years. *Mayo Clin Proc*. 2002;77:139-147.
2. Fox DJ, Khattar RS. Carcinoid heart disease: presentation, diagnosis, and management. *Heart*. 2004 Oct;90(10):1224-1228.
3. Pellikka PA, Tajik AJ, Khandheria BK, et al. Carcinoid heart disease. Clinical and echocardiographic spectrum in 74 patients. *Circulation*. 1993;87:1188-1196.
4. Callahan JA, Wroblewski EM, Reeder GS, Edwards WD, Seward JB, Tajik AJ. Echocardiographic features of carcinoid heart disease. *Am J Cardiol*. 1982 Oct;50(4):762-768.
5. Chan KL, Callahan JA, Seward JB, Tajik AJ, Gordon H. Marfan syndrome diagnosed in patients 32 years of age or older. *Mayo Clin Proc*. 1987 Jul;62(7):589-594.
6. Dean JCS. Management of Marfan syndrome. *Heart*. 2002 Jul;88(1):97-103.
7. Gott VL, Cameron DE, Alejo DE, et al. Aortic root replacement in 271 Marfan patients: a 24-year experience. *Annals Thoracic Surg*. 2002 Feb;73(2):438-443.
8. von Kodolitsch Y, Robinson PN. Marfan syndrome: an update of genetics, medical and surgical management. *Heart*. 2007;93(6):755-760.
9. Akashi YJ, Goldstein DS, Barbaro G, Ueyama T. Takotsubo cardiomyopathy: a new form of acute, reversible heart failure. *Circulation*. 2008;118(25):2754-2762.
10. Nef HM, Mollmann H, Elsasser A. Tako-tsubo cardiomyopathy (apical ballooning). *Heart*. 2007;93(10):1309-1315.
11. Butany J, Bahl NE, Morales K, et al. The intricacies of cardiac sarcoidosis: a case report involving the coronary arteries and a review of the literature. *Cardiovasc Pathol*. 2006;15(4):222-227.
12. Roberts WC, McAllister HA Jr, Ferrans V. Sarcoidosis of the heart: a clinicopathologic study of 35 necropsy patients (Group I) and review of 78 previously described necropsy patients (Group II). *Am J Med*. 1977;63:86-108.
13. Little WC, Freeman GL. Pericardial disease. *Circulation*. 2006 Mar 28;113(12):1622-1632.
14. Cervera R, Font J, Parë C, et al. Cardiac disease in systemic lupus erythematosus: prospective study of 70 patients. *Ann Rheum Dis*. 1992;51:156-159.
15. Cujec B, Sibley J, Haga M. Cardiac abnormalities in patients with systemic lupus erythematosus. *Can J Cardiol*. 1991;7:343-349.
16. Albat B, Missov E, Leclercq F, Grolleau R, Thevenet A. Adult coronary aneurysms related to Kawasaki disease. *J Cardiovasc Surg*. 1994;35:57-60.
17. Landing BH, Larson EJ. Pathological features of Kawasaki disease (mucocutaneous lymph node syndrome). *Am J Cardiovasc Pathol*. 1987;1:218-229.
18. Virmani R, Burke A. Pathological features of aortitis. *Cardiovasc Pathol*. 1994;3:205-216.
19. Lantuejoul S, Barbour A, Brambilla E, Nicholson AG, Sheppard MN. Idiopathic and non-idiopathic giant cell aortitis: a clinicopathological study of 43 cases. *Mod Pathol*. 2007;20:59A.
20. Graor RA. Takayasu's Disease. *Curr Probl Cardiol*. 1990;5:679-682.
21. Sharma BK, Jain S, Radotra BD. An autopsy study of Takayasu arteritis in India. *Int J Cardiol*. 1998 Oct 1; 66(Suppl):85-90.
22. Benditt DG, Dunnigan A, Milstein S, Limas C. Coexistence of skeletal muscle abnormalities in cardiomyopathy. *J Am Coll Cardiol*. 1989 Nov 15;14(6):1474-1475.
23. Posada RI, Gutierrez-Rivas E, Cabello A. [Cardiac involvement in neuromuscular diseases]. *Rev Esp Cardiol*. 1997 Dec;50(12):882-901.
24. Kinoshita H, Goto Y, Ishikawa M, et al. A carrier of Duchenne muscular dystrophy with dilated cardiomyopathy but no skeletal muscle symptom. *Brain Dev*. 1995 May; 17(3):202-205.
25. Brodsky GL, Muntoni F, Miocic S, Sinagra G, Sewry C, Mestroni L. Lamin A/C gene mutation associated with dilated cardiomyopathy with variable skeletal muscle involvement. *Circulation*. 2000 Feb 8;101(5):473-476.
26. Anastasakis A, Karandreas N, Stathis P, et al. Subclinical skeletal muscle abnormalities in patients with hypertrophic cardiomyopathy and their relation to clinical characteristics. *Int J Cardiol*. 2003 Jun;89(2–3):249-256.
27. Isnard R, Kalotka H, Durr A, et al. Correlation between left ventricular hypertrophy and GAA trinucleotide repeat length in Friedreich's ataxia. *Circulation*. 1997;95(9):2247-2249.
28. Boyer SH, Chisholm AW, McKusick VA. Cardiac aspects of Friedreich's ataxia. *Circulation*. 1962 Mar;25:493-505.
29. Osterziel KJ, Bit-Avragim N, Bunse M. Cardiac hypertrophy in Friedreich's ataxia. *Cardiovasc Res*. 2002 Jun; 54(3):694-696.
30. Alboliras ET, Shub C, Gomez MR, et al. Spectrum of cardiac involvement in Friedreich's ataxia: clinical, electrocardiographic and echocardiographic observations. *Am J Cardiol*. 1986 Sep 1;58(6):518-524.
31. Child JS, Perloff JK, Bach PM, Wolfe AD, Perlman S, Kark RA. Cardiac involvement in Friedreich's ataxia: a clinical study of 75 patients. *J Am Coll Cardiol*. 1986 Jun;7(6):1370-1378.
32. Cueto-Garcia L, Reeder GS, Kyle RA, et al. Echocardiographic findings in systemic amyloidosis: spectrum of cardiac involvement and relation to survival. *JACC*. 1985;6: 737-743.

33. Walley VM, Kisilevsky R, Young ID. Amyloid and the cardiovascular system: a review of pathogenesis and pathology with clinical correlations. *Cardiovas Pathol*. 1995;4:79-102.
34. Falk RH. Diagnosis and management of the cardiac amyloidoses. *Circulation*. 2005;112(13):2047-2060.
35. Klein AL, Hatle LK, Taliercio CP, et al. Serial Doppler echocardiographic follow-up of left ventricular diastolic function in cardiac amyloidosis. *J Am Coll Cardiol*. 1990;16:1135-1141.
36. Klein AL, Tajik AJ. Doppler assessment of diastolic function in cardiac amyloidosis. *Echocardiography*. 1991;8:233-251.
37. Hyett J, Moscoso G, Nicolaides K. Abnormalities of the heart and great arteries in first trimester chromosomally abnormal fetuses. Am J Med Genet 1997;69(2):207–16.
38. Marino B, Digilio MC. Congenital heart disease and genetic syndromes: specific correlation between cardiac phenotype and genotype. *Cardiovasc Pathol*. 2000 Nov;9(6):303-315.
39. Tennstedt C, Chaoui R, Korner H, Dietel M. Spectrum of congenital heart defects and extracardiac malformations associated with chromosomal abnormalities: results of a seven year necropsy study. *Heart*. 1999 Jul;82(1):34-39.
40. Richards AA, Santos LJ, Nichols HA, et al. Cryptic chromosomal abnormalities identified in children with congenital heart disease. *Pediatr Res*. 2008 Oct;64(4):358-363.
41. Song MS, Hu A, Dyhamenahali U, et al. Extracardiac lesions and chromosomal abnormalities associated with major fetal heart defects: comparison of intrauterine, postnatal and postmortem diagnoses. *Ultrasound Obstet Gynecol*. 2009 May; 33(5):552-559.
42. Schwanitz G, Zerres K, Gembruch U, Bald R, Gamerdinger F, Hansmann M. Prenatal detection of heart defects as an indication for chromosome analysis. *Ann Genet*. 1990;33(2): 79-83.
43. Digilio MC, Marino B, Giannotti A, Novelli G, Dallapiccola B. Conotruncal heart defects and chromosome 22q11 microdeletion. *J Pediatr*. 1997 Apr;130(4):675-677.
44. Johnson MC, Hing A, Wood MK, Watson MS. Chromosome abnormalities in congenital heart disease. *Am J Med Genet*. 1997 Jun 13;70(3):292-298.
45. Sreeram N, Wren C, Bhate M, Robertson P, Hunter S. Cardiac abnormalities in the fragile X syndrome. *Br Heart J*. 1989 Mar;61(3):289-291.
46. Mandell BF, Hoffman GS. Rheumatic diseases and the cardiovascular system. In Baknwald E, Zipes DP, Libby P ed. Heart disease-a text book of cardiovascular medicine. 6th ed. Saunders 2001:2199-2210.

Interventional Procedures

18

Technological advancements in cardiology have been proceeding at a rapid pace over the past two decades. Many surgical procedures can now be performed using a percutaneous approach. Echocardiography plays an important role in these procedures for selecting the appropriate patients, monitoring the procedure to avoid complications, assessing the result, and detecting long-term complications. These procedures can vary from a relatively straightforward insertion of pacemaker leads to the implantation of a left ventricular assist device. A good understanding of the impact of these intracardiac devices on cardiac structure and function is a prerequisite in the assessment of patients who have undergone these procedures.

Permanent Pacemaker and Internal Defibrillator Leads

It is important to recognize that currently multiple leads are usually inserted for cardiac pacing. The number and locations of the pacemaker leads need to be clearly determined during the echocardiographic examination. The right ventricular lead can be readily assessed using the right ventricular inflow view and the apical four-chamber view. The atrial lead is more difficult to image by the transthoracic approach but can readily be seen by the transesophageal approach. The right atrial lead usually resides in the right atrial appendage which can be imaged using the transesophageal bicaval view or the short-axis aortic valve view with rightward rotation to optimize the right atrial appendage (Figs. 18.1, 18.2). Venous thrombosis after the implantation of pacemaker leads may occur in up to 40% of patients, but this is generally clinically silent due to the development of venous collaterals [1, 2]. Adherent masses on the intracardiac pacemaker leads can be of varying sizes and they are located at specific locations, most commonly on the atrial portion of the leads (Fig. 18.3). We reported a 25% prevalence of lead-related thrombi in 185 patients who received defibrillator leads [3]. Many of the masses were strand-like and not associated with

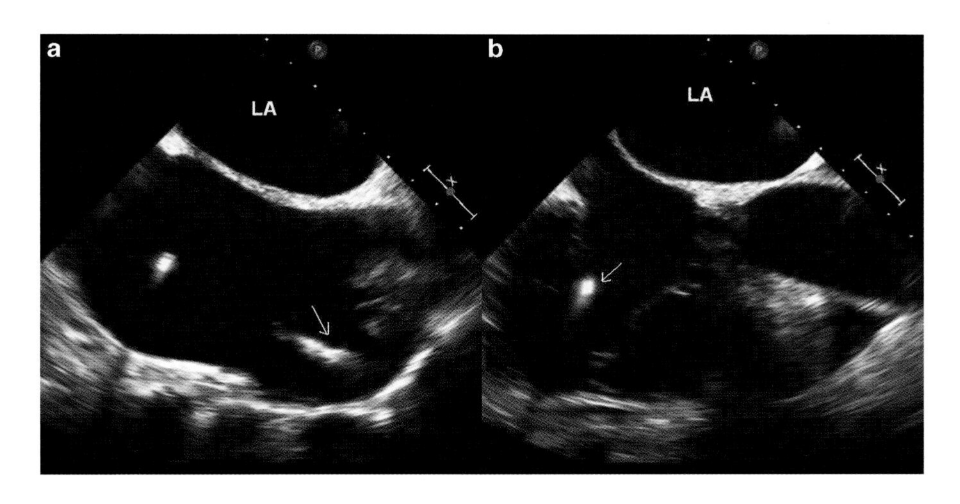

Fig. 18.1 Transesophageal views of a patient with a dual-chamber pacemaker showing the atrial lead (*arrow*) terminating in the right atrial appendage (**a**) and the ventricular lead (*arrow*) passing through the tricuspid valve (**b**). *LA* left atrium

K.-L. Chan and J.P. Veinot, *Anatomic Basis of Echocardiographic Diagnosis*,
DOI: 10.1007/978-1-84996-387-9_18, © Springer-Verlag London Limited 2011

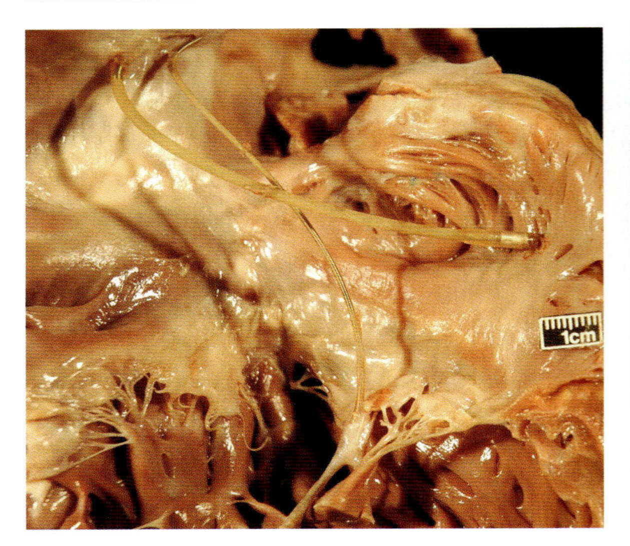

Fig. 18.2 Opened right atrium and right ventricle with a lead attached to the right atrial appendage area and another in the right ventricular apex

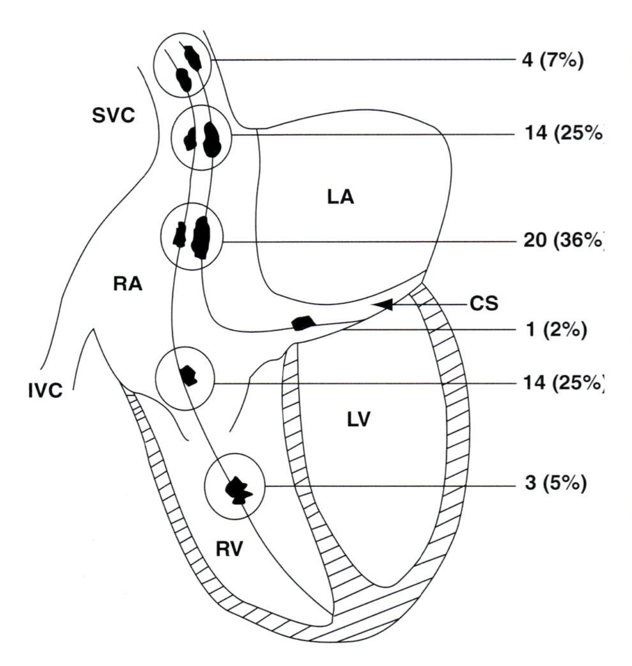

Fig. 18.3 Schematic diagram showing the typical locations of lead-related fibrin or thrombi. *RVC* right ventricular cavity, *LA* left atrium, *LV* left ventricle, *RA* right atrium, *RV* right ventricle, *SVC* superior vena cava (Reproduced from [3]. With permission)

symptoms (Fig. 18.4). Large lead-related atrial thrombi are uncommon, but can cause hemodynamic compromise by causing pulmonary embolism or obstruction

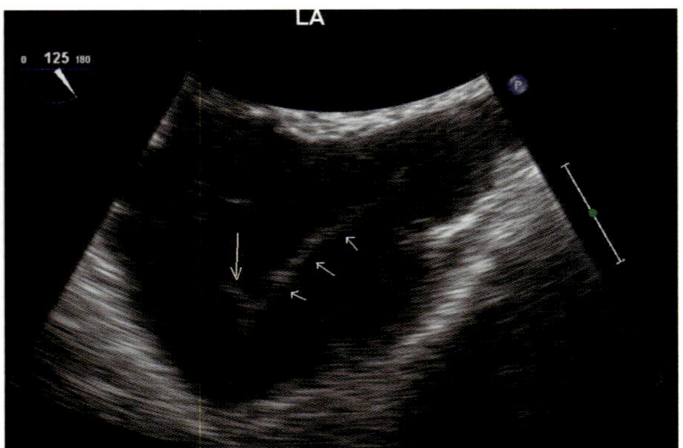

Fig. 18.4 Transesophageal views of the intra-atrial portion of the pacemaker lead (*short arrows*) showing a mobile strand (*long arrow*) on the lead. *LA* left atrium

of the vena cava (Fig. 18.5, 18.6) [4, 5]. When these large masses are present, anticoagulation therapy should be considered. If there is severe hemodynamic compromise, surgery or thrombolytic therapy may need to be considered [6]. Leads eventually encapsulate and there is severe surrounding fibrosis [7, 8]. Pacemaker-related infected vegetations should always be suspected if the masses are large and there are clinical findings of infective endocarditis (Fig. 18.7, 18.8).

The course of the pacemaker lead across the tricuspid valve and right ventricular cavity to terminate in the right ventricular apex should be clearly defined. Ventricular perforation should be considered if the tip of the pacemaker lead can be clearly visualized to protrude through the apex of the right ventricle (Fig. 18.9). Although the pacemaker lead generally does not affect tricuspid valvular function, it may be responsible for improper leaflet coaptation leading to severe tricuspid regurgitation in a small proportion of patients [9]. This may be due to excessive tension or unusual orientation of the pacemaker lead at the tricuspid annulus interfering with the leaflet excursion (Fig. 18.10). It is also possible for the pacemaker lead to transverse into the left atrium and the left ventricle via a patent foramen ovale (Fig. 18.11). The electrocardiogram shows a right bundle branch block pattern instead of the usual left bundle branch block pattern. This situation needs to be recognized early following implantation, so that the pacemaker lead can be removed from the systemic circulation to prevent systemic thromboembolic events.

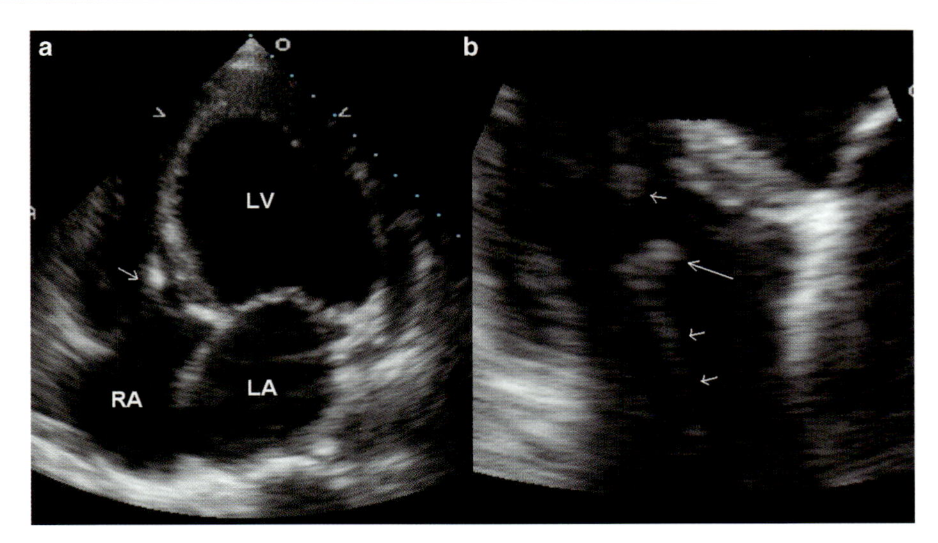

Fig. 18.5 Apical four-chamber view (**a**) in a patient with dilated cardiomyopathy and a right ventricular pacemaker lead (*arrow*). The zoomed view (**b**) shows a nodular mass (*long arrow*) on the pacemaker lead (*short arrows*). *LA* left atrium, *LV* left ventricle, *RA* right atrium

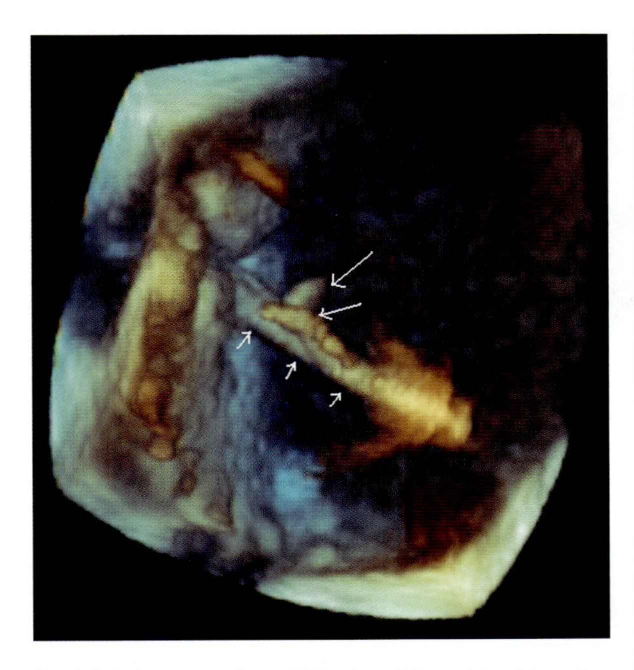

Fig. 18.6 A transesophageal 3D view of the right atrial portion of a pacemaker lead (*short arrows*) showing two thrombi (*long arrows*) on the lead

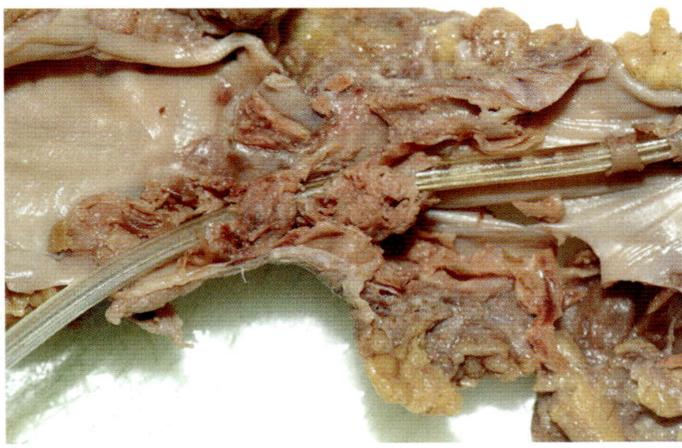

Fig. 18.7 Pacemaker lead infective endocarditis. The lead in the superior vena cava is surrounded by large amounts of shaggy infected thrombus

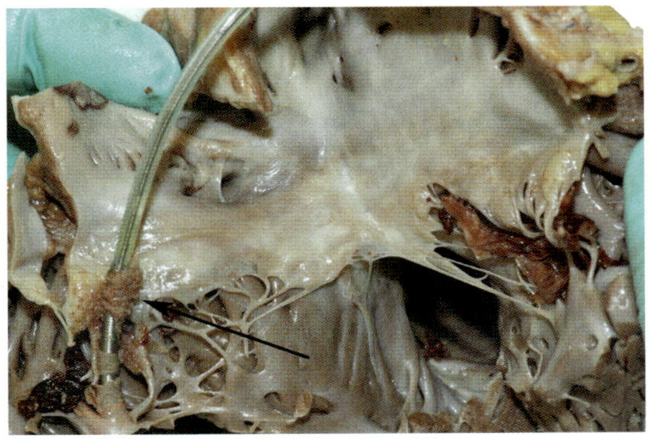

Fig. 18.8 Pacemaker lead infection. This is the same patient as in Fig. 18.7. The lead attached to the right ventricle has attached infected thrombus material (*arrow*)

Cardiac Resynchronization

Cardiac resynchronization (CRT) requires electronic pacing at multiple sites in the heart particularly the left ventricle, and has proven to be an effective treatment in patients with severe heart failure. About a third of

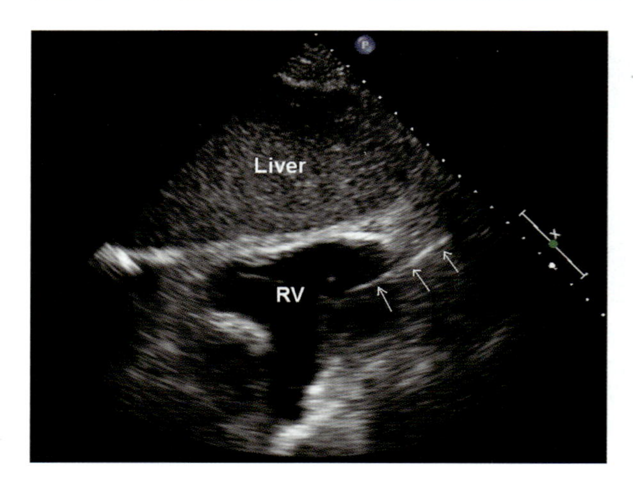

Fig. 18.9 Subcostal view of the right ventricle in a patient who developed chest pain following permanent pacemaker implantation shows that the tip of the ventricular lead (*arrows*) protrudes beyond the right ventricular apex consistent with perforation

the patients do not respond to this therapy [10, 11]. Detection and quantitation of mechanical dyssynchrony should identify patients who will respond to CRT, which improves contraction dyssynchrony by biventricular pacing. Multiple echocardiographic and Doppler measures of atrioventricular, interventricular, and intraventricular dyssynchrony have been studied (Table 18.1). Most of the studies have focused upon the assessment of intraventricular dyssynchrony [12–16]. Tissue Doppler velocity-based measures have been relied upon in many of the early studies to predict response to CRT. In a study using tissue Doppler imaging (TDI) to measure the lateral-septal contraction delay, which is the difference in duration from onset of QRS to the peak of the S-wave of the septal versus the lateral annulus, Bax et al. showed that a cut-off value of 65 ms predicted good response to CRT with reverse remodeling at 6 months (Fig. 18.12) [12]. The usefulness of the

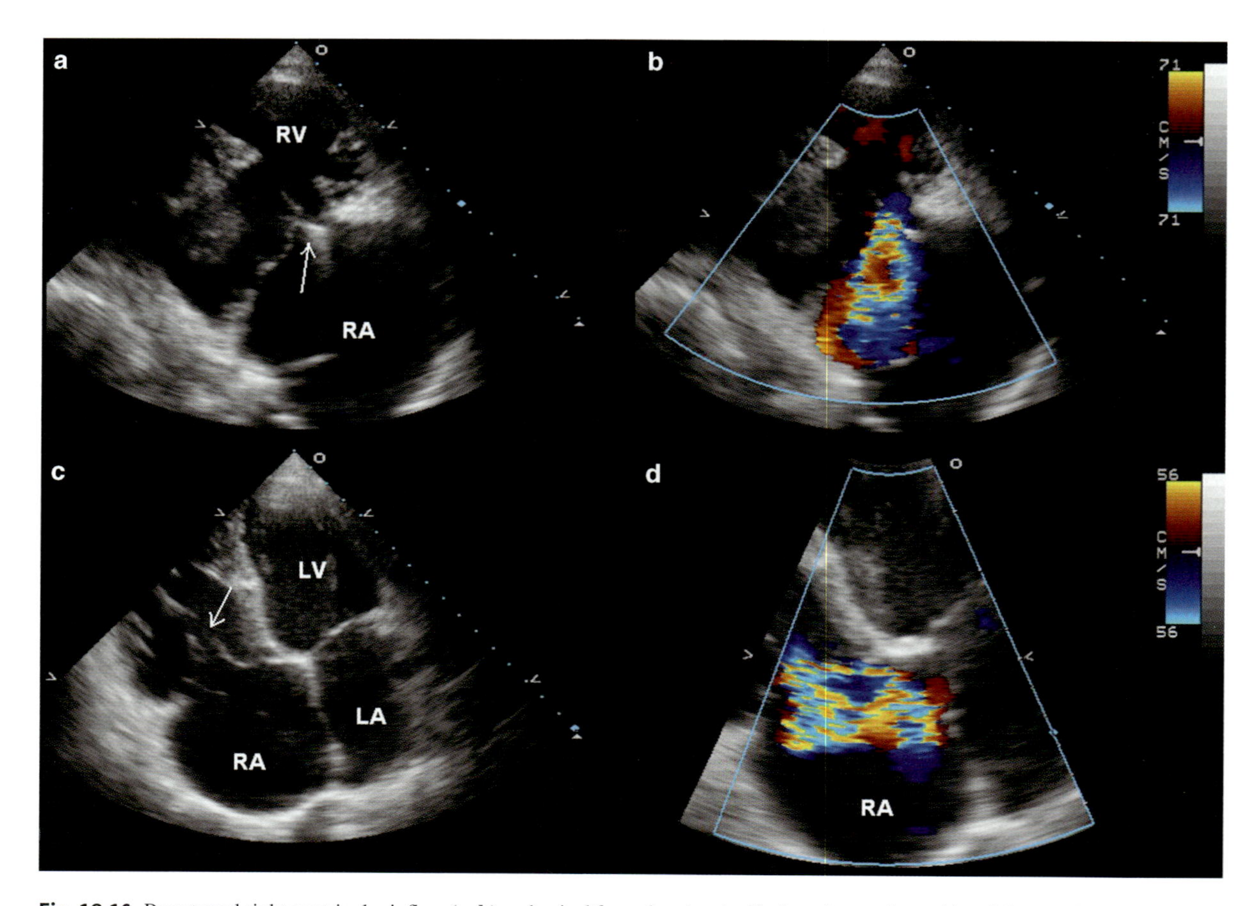

Fig. 18.10 Parasternal right ventricular inflow (**a, b**) and apical four-chamber (**c, d**) views in a patient with a right ventricular pacemaker lead shows that there was lack of coaptation of the tricuspid leaflets (*arrow*) best seen in the four-chamber view (**c**). The color-flow images (**b, d**) confirmed severe tricuspid regurgitation. *LA* left atrium, *LV* left ventricle, *RA* right atrium, *RV* right ventricle

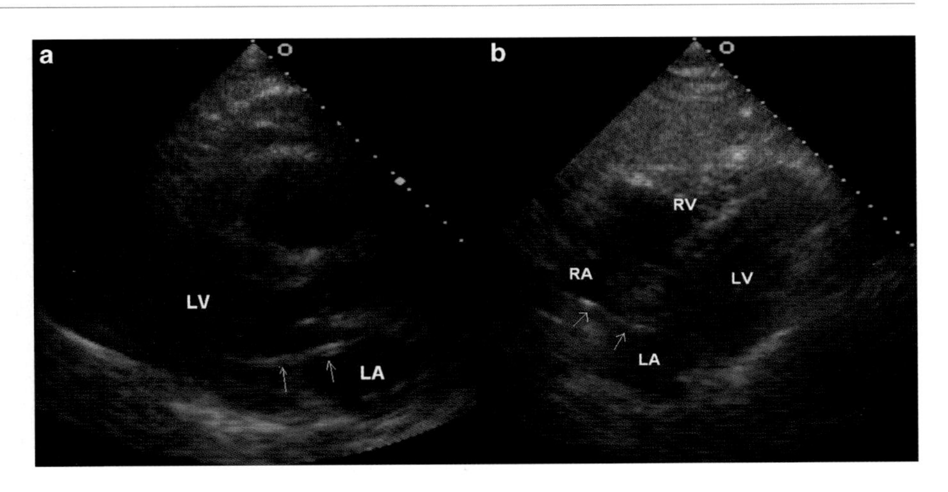

Fig. 18.11 Parasternal long-axis (**a**) and subcostal four-chamber (**b**) views in a patient shortly following permanent pacemaker implantation. The pacemaker lead (*arrows*) traverses the atrial septum via a patent foramen ovale (**b**). The lead (*arrows*) protrudes into the left atrium and left ventricle (**a**). *LA* left atrium, *LV* left ventricle, *RA* right ventricle, *RV* right ventricle

Table 18.1 Echo-Doppler measures in predicting the response to cardiac resynchronization therapy

Atrioventricular synchrony
• LV filling time fraction – Filling time to R-R interval ≤ 40%
Interventricular Dyssynchrony • Interventricular mechanical delay – Difference in pre-ejection times at LVOT and RVOT ≥ 40 ms
Intraventricular Dyssynchrony • Septal to posterior wall motion delay – Difference in onset of QRS to peak excursion of septum and posterior wall ≥ 130 ms • Pre-ejection time – Onset of QRS to onset of aortic ejection ≥ 140 ms • Regional contraction delay – Onset of QRS to peak of S wave by TDI at lateral wall versus septum ≥ 60 ms – Standard deviation of onset of QRS to peak S wave in 16 LV segments ≥ 32 ms – ≥ 65 ms between opposing walls by tissue synchronization imaging – Onset of QRS to minimal systolic volume between 12 segments by 3D echo > 8.35%

LV left ventricle, *LVOT* left ventricular outflow tract, *RVOT* right ventricular outflow tract, *TDI* tissue Doppler imaging

systolic asynchrony index is supported by the studies of Yu et al. The index is calculated as the standard deviation of the time to the peak of the S-wave by TDI in 12 myocardial segments. A cut-off value ≥ 32 ms identified responders to CRT [15, 16]. There are recent studies reporting the use of tissue synchronization imaging, which is easy to use, and 3D regional volume-time curves, which are more time consuming [17–20].

The echo Doppler measures of dyssynchrony have been evaluated in the PROSPECT study, a multicenter nonrandomized observation study to prospectively assess the value of the echo Doppler indices in predicting clinical outcome in heart failure patients receiving CRT [21]. Positive response to CRT was defined as improved clinical composite score and ≥ 15% reduction in left ventricular end-diastolic volume at 6 months (Fig. 18.13). None of the 12 echo Doppler measures had sufficiently high sensitivity and specificity in predicting the outcome to be clinically useful. There was also large variability in the analysis of these measures. At present the selection of patients for CRT should be based upon clinical criteria such as QRS duration and ejection fraction reported in the clinical trials. Dyssynchrony measurements by echocardiography are only one of many measures that can be useful in predicting the response to CRT (Table 18.2) [22].

Echocardiography may be more useful in guiding the settings of resynchronization therapy following the procedure. Optimal atrioventricular delay is indicated by maximal diastolic filling time with separation of the mitral E and A waves and that the A wave is not truncated [23]. The most reliable but time-consuming method is to assess the stroke volume response to different settings of atrioventricular and interventricular delays. New modalities such as strain and strain rate may be useful in the selection of patients for the procedure and fine tuning of the device settings following the procedure [24, 25]. More studies are clearly needed in this area.

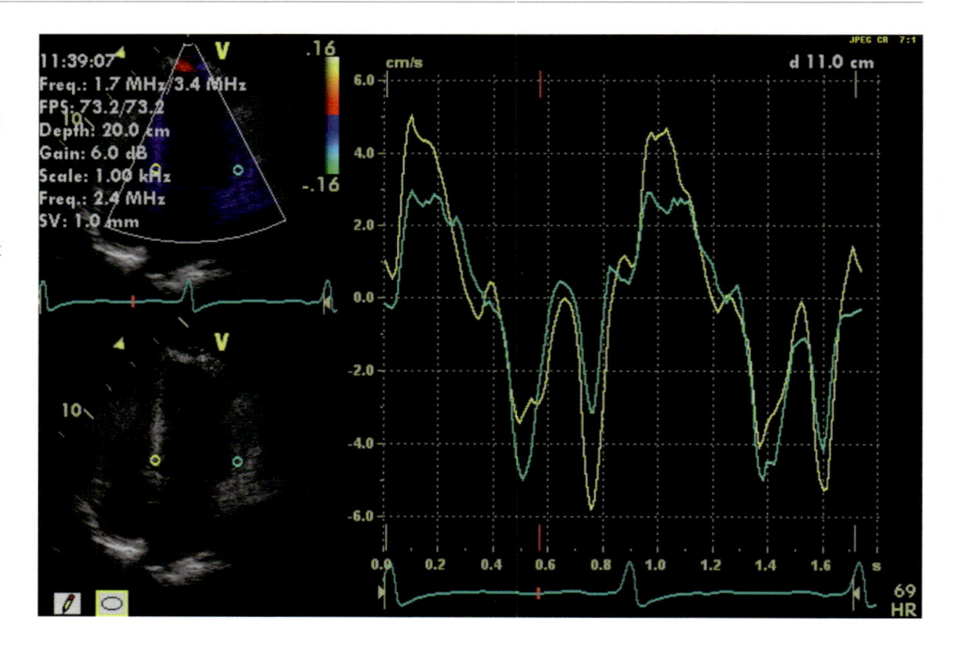

Fig. 18.12 Apical four-chamber view shows sample volume placements at the base of the septum and lateral wall with spectral velocity wave forms at each site. There is no significant time delay between the peaks of systolic velocities at the two myocardial segments, indicating no significant dyssynchrony

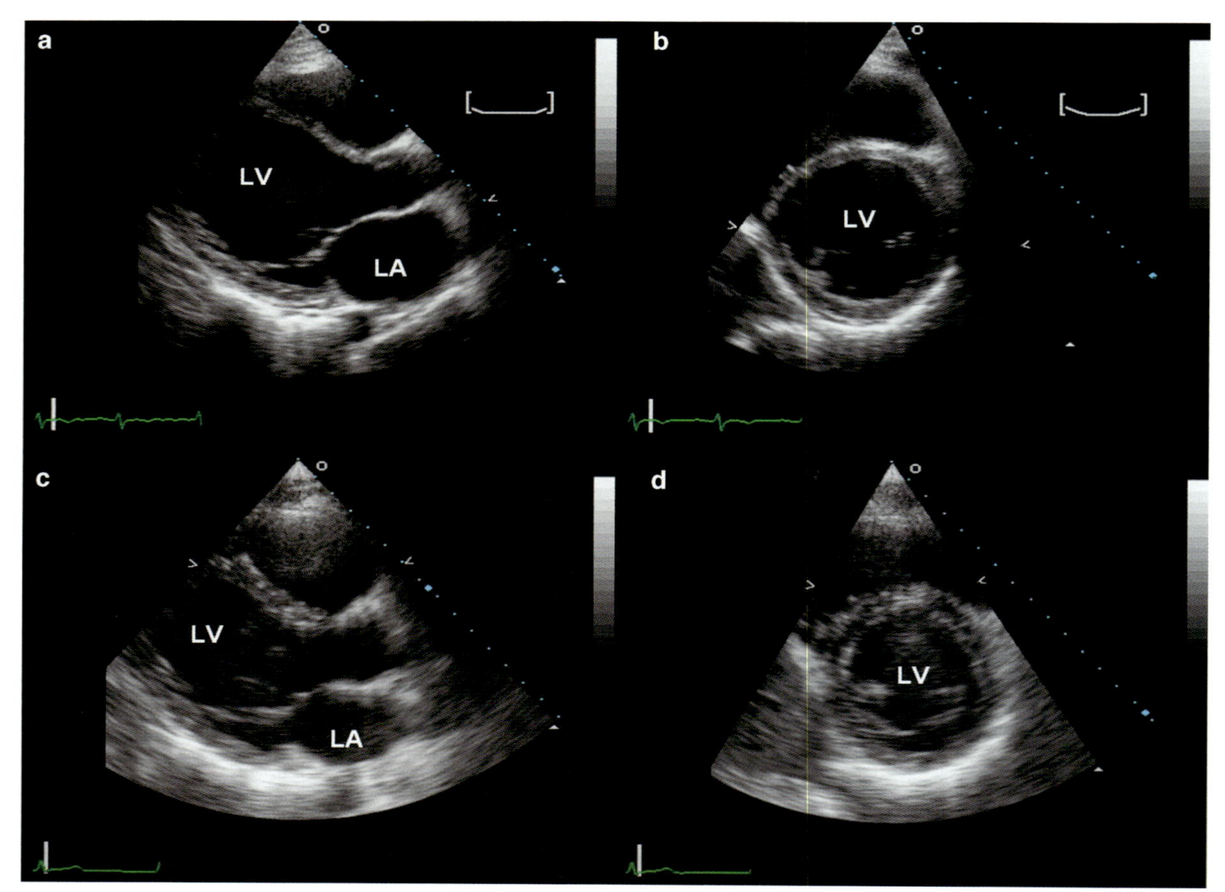

Fig. 18.13 Parasternal long and short-axis views in a patient before (**a, b**) and after (**c, d**) cardiac resynchronization therapy show a positive response to treatment with a marked decrease in left ventricular size and improvement in function. *LA* left atrium, *LV* left ventricle

Table 18.2 Factors predicting the likelihood of response to cardiac resynchronization therapy.

Low likelihood
• Ischemic etiology
• Very low EF (<20%)
• QRS < 120 ms
• No viability
• Large scar burden on MRI
• No dyssynchrony by echo Doppler measures
• Anterior lead location
High likelihood
• Non-ischemic etiology
• Moderate ↓ EF
• QRS > 120 ms
• Viability is present
• Small or no scar on MRI
• Dyssynchrony by multiple echo Doppler measures
• Postero-lateral lead location

The response to cardiac resynchronization therapy is a continuum and not an all or none phenomenon. The likelihood of response is higher if more of the positive predictors are present
EF ejection fraction, *MRI* cardiac magnetic resonance imaging
Source: Modified after Santaurlaria-Tomas, Abraham [22]

Table 18.3 Contraindications for device closure of atrial septal defects (*ASD*)

• Small, hemodynamically insignificant ASD
• Large ASD (>35 mm)
• Deficient rim
• Sinus venosus ASD
• Primum ASD
• Associated anomalies such as anomalous pulmonary veins
• Severe pulmonary hypertension
• Severe LV dysfunction

ASD atrial septal defect, *LV* left ventricle

Device Closure of Intracardiac Defects

Atrial Septal Defect

Atrial septal defect (ASD) is a well-tolerated condition, and many patients with ASD are asymptomatic when the condition is diagnosed. Closure of ASD is largely to prevent future complications such as heart failure, pulmonary hypertension, and atrial arrhythmia, although it can also improve exercise capacity and may even improve survival [26, 27]. This should be considered in patients with a hemodynamically significant defect which is ≥10 mm in diameter by TEE and has associated right ventricular enlargement. A Qp:Qs shunt ratio of >1.5 should be present at cardiac catheterization, although the shunt run is no longer routinely performed. Although device closure has rapidly become the procedure of choice over surgery in the treatment of patients with ASD, there are situations where device closure is not appropriate (Table 18.3). For the secure placement of the ASD device, there needs to be an adequate rim to minimize the risk of device embolization and residual shunt. In the setting of primum ASD, device closure of the ASD will certainly compromise the mitral and tricuspid leaflets. When there are associated cardiac anomalies, such as the presence of anomalous pulmonary veins, surgery will be more appropriate to correct both abnormalities. In patients with severe pulmonary hypertension and little shunting across the ASD, closing the ASD may eliminate a potential route to unload the failing right ventricle. Similarly, unloading the failing left ventricle via the ASD may not be possible after ASD closure.

Transesophageal echocardiography (TEE) is used to assess the size of the defect and to exclude other cardiac findings, such as anomalous pulmonary veins. TEE or intracardiac echocardiography can be used to monitor the procedure (Fig. 18.14). The most commonly used closure device is the Amplatzer device [28]. The size of the device is usually 1–2 mm larger than the stretched balloon diameter determined during the procedure. The slight oversizing ensures that adequate defect occlusion is achieved. Two devices have been used to close two defects in the same patient. At an early stage following device deployment, slight degree of shunt can be detected by TEE color-flow imaging. As the device remodels and flattens out, this slight degree of shunt usually disappears (Figs. 18.15–18.17).

Studies have shown that there is a very high success rate with no significant shunting in over 90% of patients following this procedure [29]. The new development of pericardial effusion following the procedure should be viewed with caution, as cardiac perforation due to the device can occur months or even years after the procedure [30]. This may be related to oversizing of the device and a deficient antero-superior rim just behind the aortic root. The overall incidence of this serious complication is very low (<0.1%). Another complication is thrombus formation on the device in about 1% of

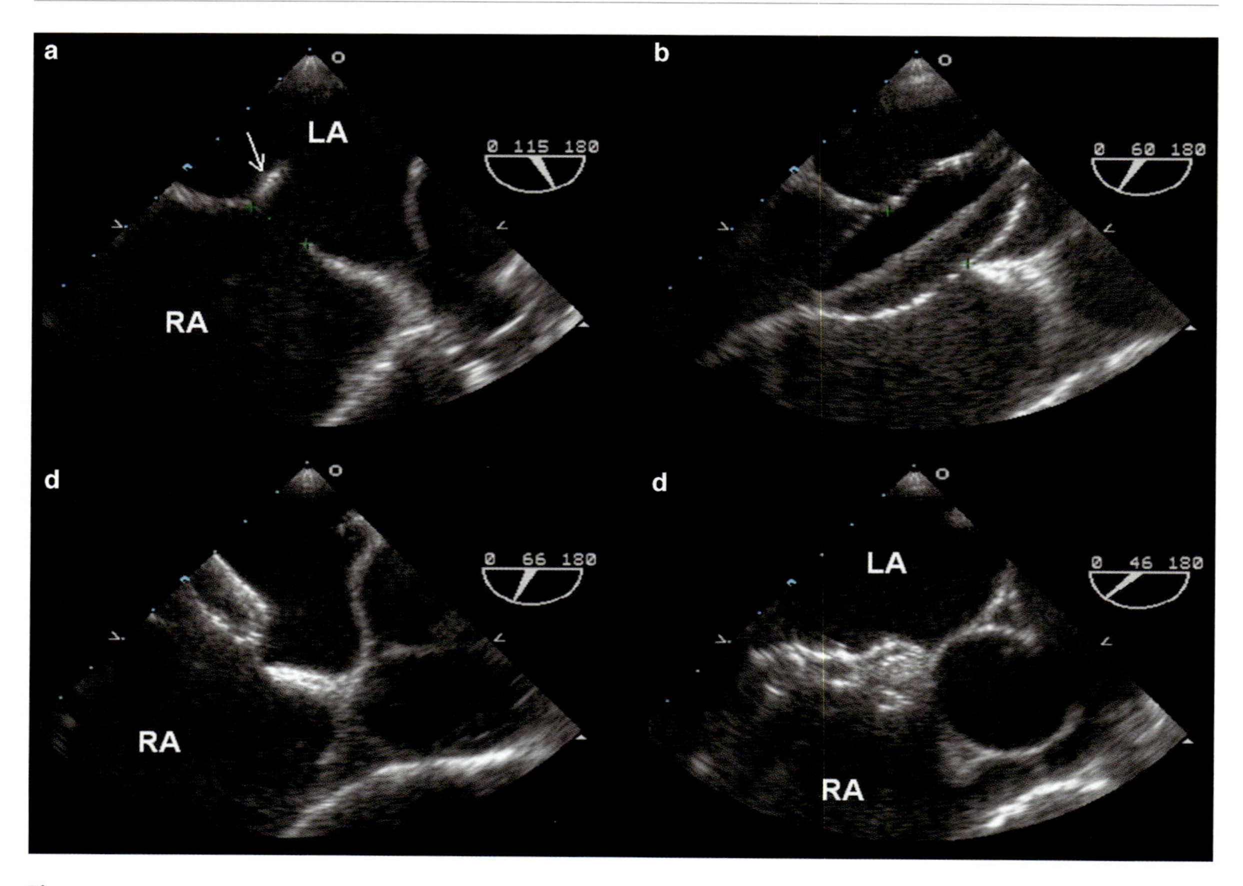

Fig. 18.14 Device closure of a secundum atrial septal defect is monitored by transesophageal echocardiography. In (**a**), the guide wire (*arrow*) is passed through the atrial septal defect into the left atrium. In (**b**), the stretched diameter of the defect is assessed by balloon inflation. In (**c**), the left atrial portion of the Amplatzer device is deployed. In (**d**), the Amplatzer device is completely deployed. *LA* left atrium, *RA* right atrium

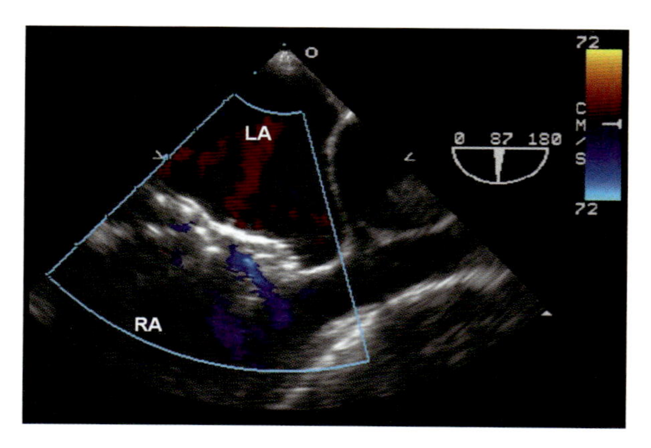

Fig. 18.15 Transesophageal color-flow imaging immediately following implantation of the Amplatzer device shows the presence of small degree of residual shunt. *LA* left atrium, *RA* right atrium

patients [31]. Antiplatelet therapy is usually prescribed for the first 3 months following implantation of the ASD device to prevent this complication. Other complications include device embolization, arrhythmia, and residual shunt (Fig. 18.18). Intense headache has also been reported following ASD device closure [32].

Patent Foramen Ovale

The role of device closure for patent foramen ovale (PFO) remains controversial as there is no accepted guideline for its use. It is frequently used in young patients with presumed embolic stroke and yet there is

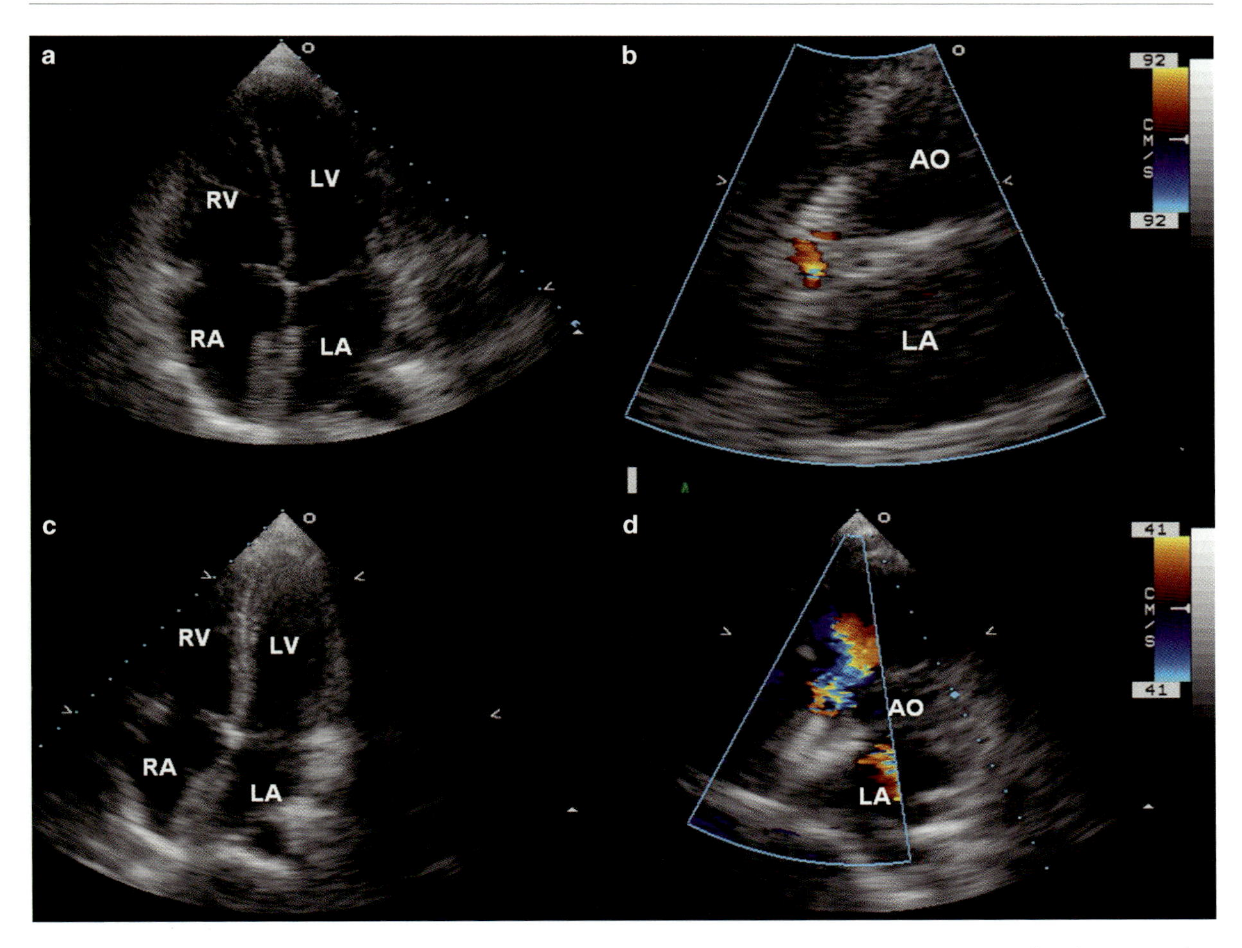

Fig. 18.16 Apical four-chamber views of a patient one day post (**a, b**) and 1 month post (**c, d**) a device closure for a large secundum atrial septal defect show that there is remodeling of the closure device such that by 1month it has a more streamline appearance. Color-flow images (**b, d**) show persistent mild residual shunting

no clear data that the rate of recurrent systemic embolism is reduced following the procedure. This is discussed in greater detail in Chap. 15. Transcatheter closure of PFO is also used in the treatment of platypnea orthodeoxia, which is a condition of arterial desaturation related to posture, and can be diagnosed with intravenous injecting of saline contrast showing right to left atrial shunting related to posture [33]. The role of PFO closure in the treatment of migraine is controversial and results from future trials are eagerly awaited [34, 35]. Transesophageal echocardiography can be used to assess the size of the PFO by looking at the size of the shunt flow by the degree of right to left shunting during saline contrast injection. Associated findings such as atrial septal aneurysm can complicate the procedure.

There are several different closure devices used for PFO closure. Transcatheter device deployment is generally performed using the femoral approach, and TEE or intracardiac echocardiography is not usually necessary. In our experience, residual shunting following the procedure is common (about 30–40%) early on following device implantation, as well as during long-term follow-up. Thrombus formation on the devise is a known complication and appears more frequent with the CardioSEAL device (6–22%) than with the Amplatzer device (<1%). Other rare complications include device embolization, air embolism, and cardiac perforation [31].

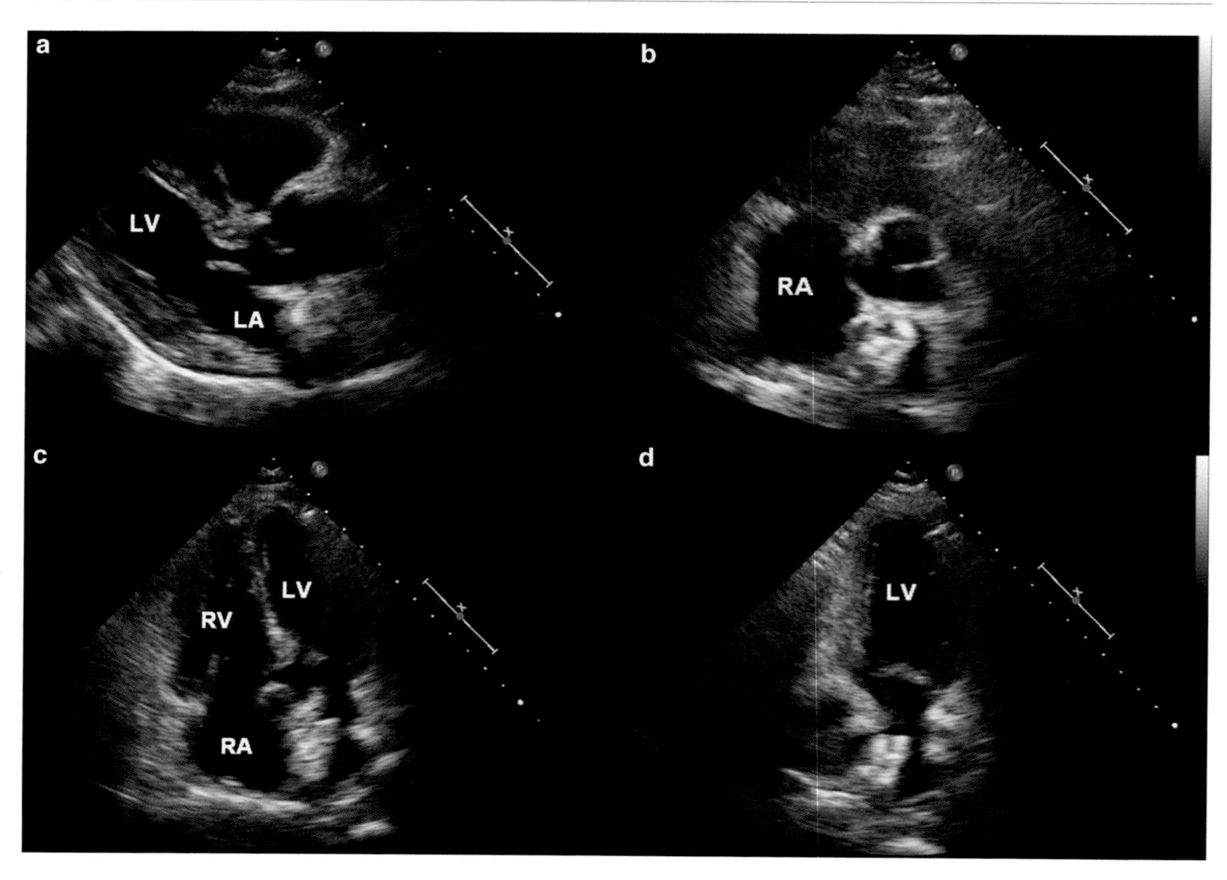

Fig. 18.17 In this patient following device closure for atrial septal defect, the Amplatzer device can be seen in multiple views including the parasternal long-axis (**a**), short-axis (**b**), apical four-chamber (**c**), and apical two-chamber (**d**) views. *LA* left atrium, *LV* left ventricle, *RA* right atrium, *RV* right ventricle

Ventricular Septal Defect

In the adult population, closure of postinfarction ventricular septal defect (VSD) has been reported using an investigational Amplatzer VSD closure device, which has a long waist and a large waist diameter. This is a technically challenging procedure as postinfarction VSD frequently has a serpiginous tract and it is difficult to cross the VSD using a retrograde approach from the left side [36]. Residual shunting following VSD closure is common. Procedural complications include device embolization, arrhythmia, valvular regurgitation, perforation, heart block, and hemolysis (Fig. 18.19).

Perivalvular Regurgitation

Perivalvular regurgitation is common following prosthetic valve implantation [37, 38]. It may be related to local dehiscence due to suture breaks, poor annular tissue (calcification or necrosis), or from endocarditis (at the time of active infection or as a consequence of a past infection) (Fig. 18.20). When the degree of regurgitation is small, it is well tolerated; but it can result in hemolysis and congestive heart failure. Since many of these patients are at high risk for repeat valve replacement surgery due to comorbidities, device closure of perivalvular regurgitation is a reasonable

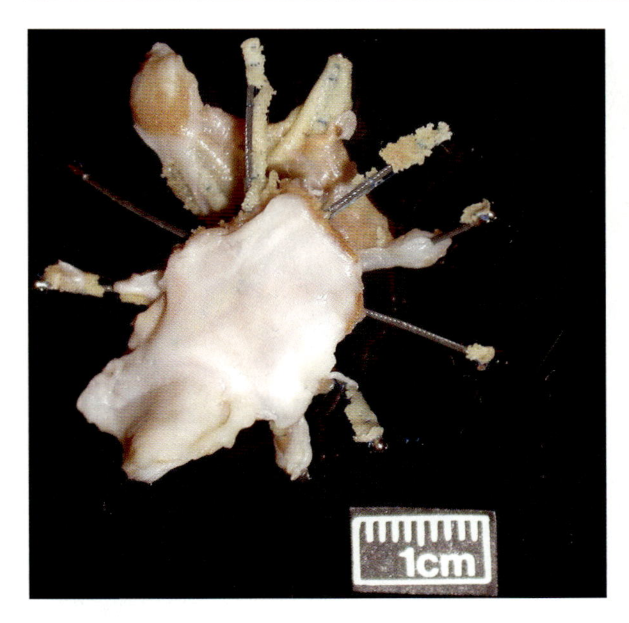

Fig. 18.18 Excised atrial septal defect (*ASD*) closure device. The device had not sealed well and a patch was subsequently placed. Note the thick white endocardial thickening that has covered the device

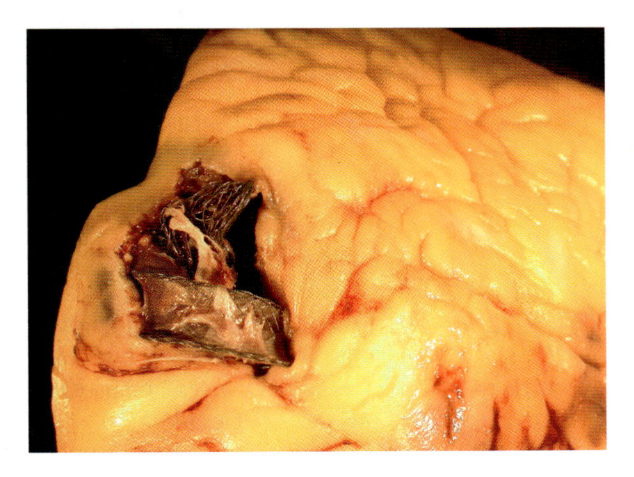

Fig. 18.19 Attempted closure of post-myocardial infarct ventricular septal defect (*VSD*). The procedure was complicated by ventricular rupture. The protruding device can be seen

alternative. TEE has an important role in determining the number and locations of the perivalvular defects, for monitoring the procedure to aid localizing the defect with the guide wire, and to ensure that the closure device does not interfere with the proper function

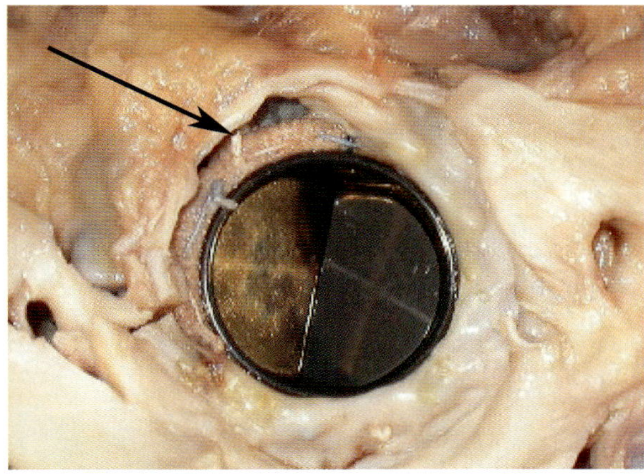

Fig 18.20 Paravalvular leak of a mitral prosthesis. At the valve ring a small defect can be seen (*arrow*). A probe could be passed easily between the left atrium and the left ventricle beside the valve

of the prosthetic valve (Fig. 18.21). The recent development of 3D TEE imaging may further facilitate the process (Fig. 18.22) [39]. The Amplatzer device is generally used for this purpose. The retrograde approach is used when dealing with perivalvular aortic regurgitation. Either the retrograde or the antegrade approach with transeptal puncture can be used with perivalvular mitral regurgitation. Early experience so far suggests that this procedure can be performed with reasonable success rate (about 80%). Clinical improvement can be expected in at least half of the patients despite some degree of residual perivalvular regurgitation [40, 41].

Percutaneous Aortic Valve Implantation

Symptomatic patients with severe aortic stenosis have a poor prognosis and should be considered for aortic valve replacement. Some of these patients may not be surgical candidates due to coexisting medical conditions such as renal failure and porcelain aorta. The development of percutaneous aortic valve implantation provides a viable treatment for these patients. There are two catheter-based valve models for this purpose. They are the Edwards Sapien valve and the Core Valve ReValving System [42–44]. The former is a balloon-expandable bioprosthesis and the latter is a

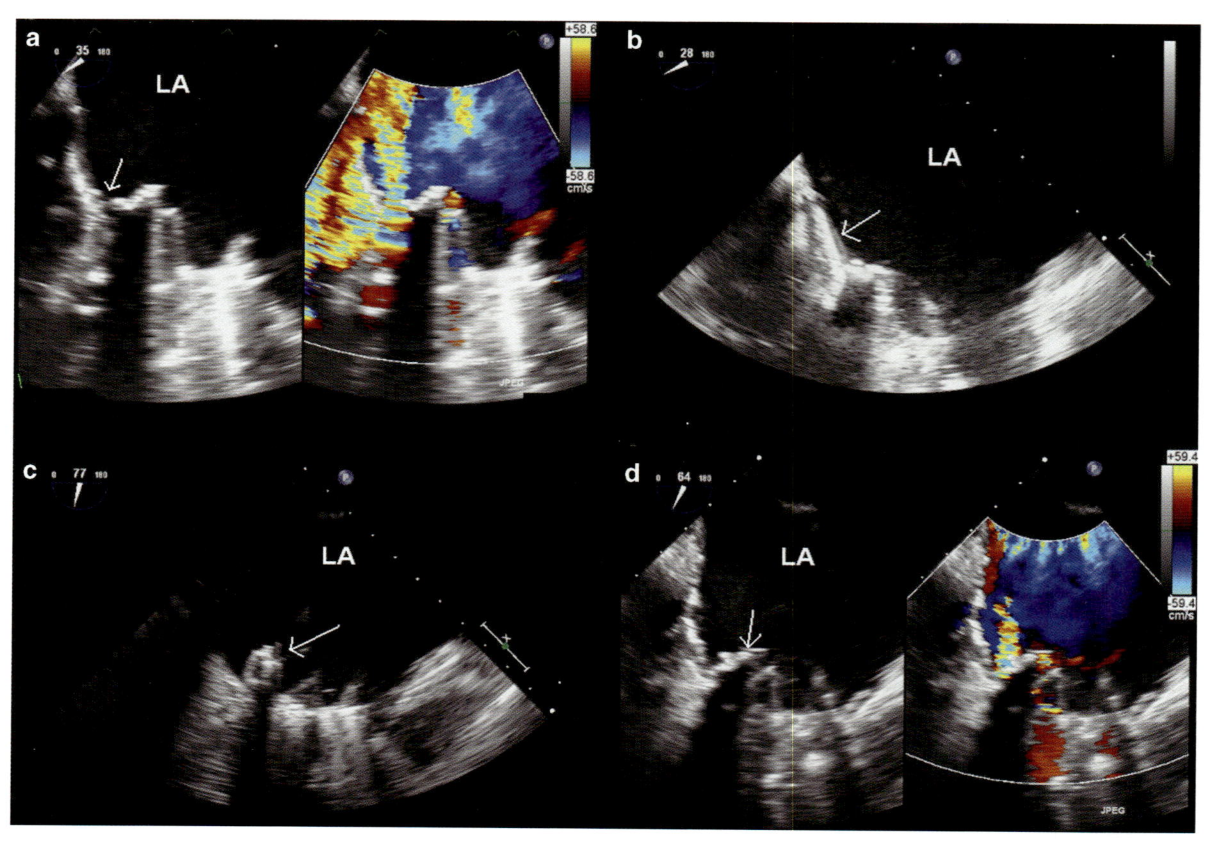

Fig. 18.21 (**a**) In this patient with a bileaflet mitral mechanical prosthetic valve, there is a large paravalvular regurgitant jet located at the posterior sewing ring (*arrow*). (**b**) A guidewire (*arrow*) is successfully passed through the defect using the retrograde approach. (**c**) The atrial component (*arrow*) of the closure device is deployed. (**d**) After deployment of the device (*arrow*) there is significant reduction in paravalvular regurgitation, although mild residual regurgitation is still present. *LA* left atrium

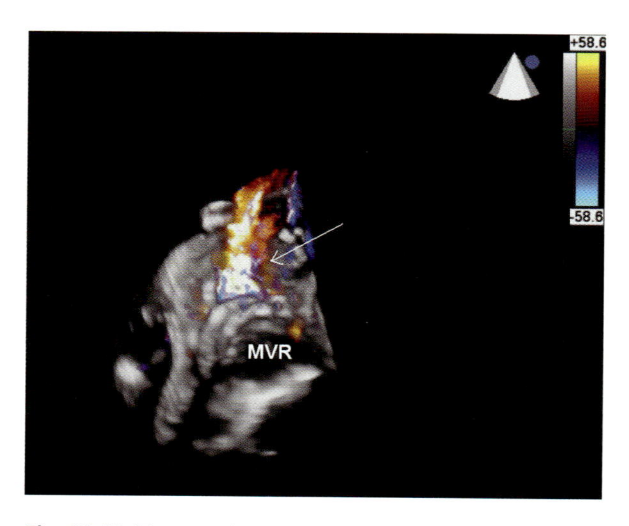

Fig. 18.22 Transesophageal 3D view from the left atrial perspective of a mitral mechanical valve showing the presence of paravalvular regurgitation (*arrow*) emanating outside of the sewing ring. *MVR* mitral prosthetic valve

bioprosthesis in a self-expanding Nitinol frame. In our center, our experience is with the Core Valve ReValving System (Fig. 18.23, 18.24). The percutaneous valves have lower transvalvular gradients, but a high incidence of perivalvular regurgitation, as compared to surgically implanted prosthetic valves [45].

Echocardiography has an essential role in percutaneous aortic valve implantation [44]. Accurate measurement of the aortic annulus is crucial due to the limited sizes of the percutaneous valves. Significant regurgitation may occur if there is a significant mismatch of the implant valve and the aortic annulus. The risk of valve embolization is increased when the aortic annulus is too large for the implant valve. The presence of severe localized calcific nodule may prevent proper apposition of the percutaneous valve leading to significant perivalvular regurgitation. During the procedure, TEE is used to monitor the placement of the guide wire and the valve [44].

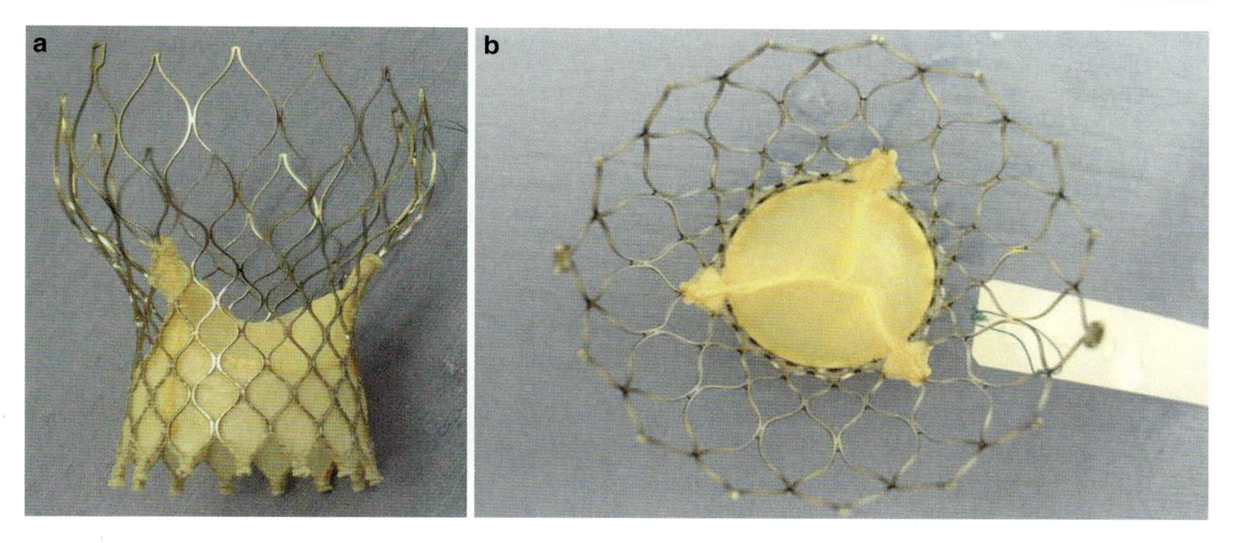

Fig. 18.23 (**a**) The CoreValve system is shown. A porcine valve is embedded inside a Nitinol frame. (**b**) This is the en-face view of the CoreValve system from the aortic perspective

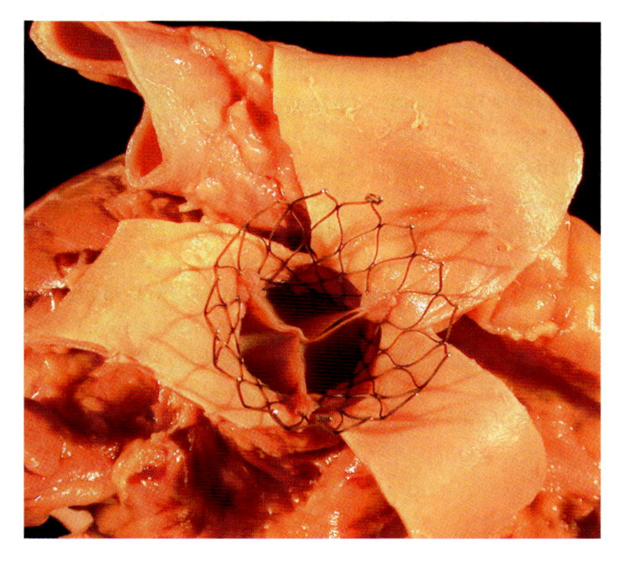

Fig. 18.24 CoreValve in place in the aortic valve area. The aorta has been opened showing the valve and the expanded wire framework that rests on the aorta

Immediately following valve implantation, it is common to have small degree of perivalvular regurgitation with small perivalvular regurgitant jets (Figs. 18.25–18.27). With time the Nitinol frame of the Core Valve will expand to better abut the annulus such that perivalvular regurgitation may diminish (Fig. 18.28). Significant aortic regurgitation is more common in patients with nodular valvular calcification or a dilated aortic annulus such that the percutaneous aortic valve may be undersized. Cardiac perforation is rare but can occur early on following the implantation. Development of pericardial effusion shortly after the procedure should be carefully followed. Other complications include device embolization and various forms of vascular or cardiac injuries (Fig. 18.29) [46].

Percutaneous Mitral Valve Repair

In patients with degenerative mitral regurgitation, surgical mitral valve repair has excellent result with low perioperative mortality in experienced centers. A percutaneous approach to correct degenerative mitral regurgitation has recently been developed, and involves the edge to edge repair with a clip akin to the Alfieri procedure (Fig. 18.30). The short-term results showed that the procedural success rate was high and the severity of mitral regurgitation was reduced [47]. The durability of the procedure and long-term outcome of this approach need to be better defined.

Left Ventricular Assist Device

Left ventricular assist devices (LVAD) are used in patients with acute decompensated heart failure not responding to medical treatment. There are two main

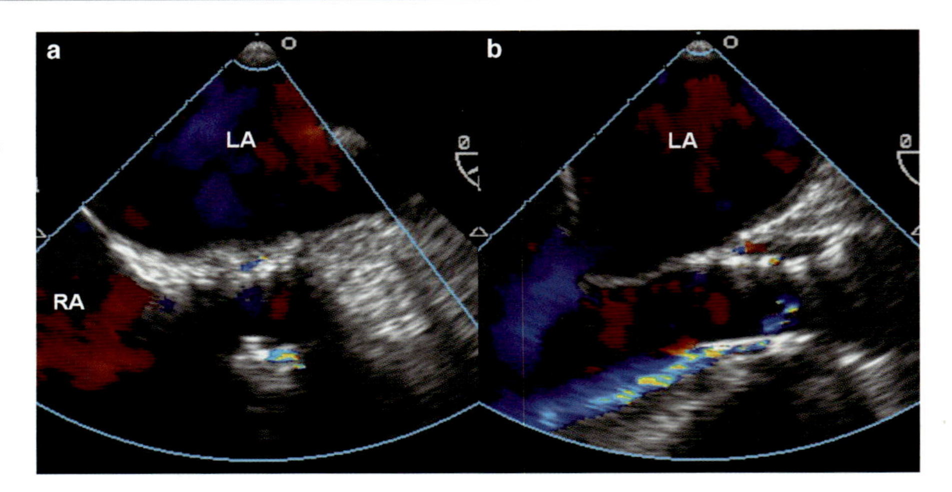

Fig. 18.25 Transesophageal view of the CoreValve in short-axis (**a**) and long-axis (**b**) views show that there are at least two jets of paravalvular regurgitation with a dominant jet located anteriorly

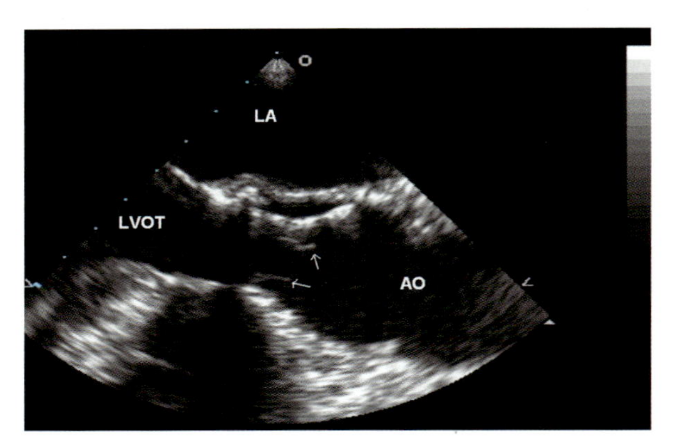

Fig. 18.26 Transesophageal longitudinal view showing the mobile aortic leaflets (arrows) within the Nitinol frame of the CoreValve. *Ao* aorta, *LA* left atrium, *LVOT* left ventricular outflow tract

types of assist device – the pulsatile flow pump and the continuous axial flow pump [48, 49]. With the pulsatile device, the inflow cannula is usually placed at the left ventricular apex and the outflow cannula into the right lateral aspect of the ascending aorta in an end to side fashion (Figs. 18.31–18.34). Echocardiography has a useful role before and after LVAD insertion (Table 18.4). With proper functioning of the device, the aortic valve remains closed with the cardiac output being delivered by the assist device. Aortic valve cusp fusion can occur [50]. In some patients, improvement of left ventricular function can occur, resulting in some degree of forward flow through the aortic valve. Thus, aortic valve opening while the patient is being supported by the assist device is an indication that there is recovery in left ventricular function. The flow patterns at the inflow and outflow cannulae are dependent on the type of LVAD and the device settings, and can be assessed by pulsed-wave, continuous wave and color-flow Doppler imaging. The axial propulsion flow device such as Heart Mate II shows a pulsatile pattern synchronous with the electrocardiogram superimposed on a continuous flow throughout the device cycle. The peak velocity is generally between 1 and 2 m/s (Fig. 18.35). On the other hand, the pulsatile device such as Thoratec gives a pulsatile pattern, which is asynchronous with the electrocardiogram and the flow can appear turbulent. Spectral Doppler of the inflow and outflow cannulae shows high velocity flow reaching velocity of $\geq$3 m/s depending on the setting of the device (Fig. 18.36). Serial follow-up of these velocities can provide an early indication of cannular obstruction if there is a sudden increase in the flow velocity [51, 52].

The continuous axial flow devices can be placed during surgery or percutaneously. The device traverses across the aortic valve to provide active support by transvalvular assistance (Fig. 18.37) [53]. There may be a guidewire in the distal tip to ensure proper position of the device (Fig. 18.38). The spinning motor within the device produces a characteristic artifact on color-flow imaging and should not be confused with the velocity of flow generated by the device. This type of device is contraindicated in patients with aortic stenosis, severe aortic regurgitation, or aortic mechanical prosthetic valves.

Dysfunction of the left ventricular assist device should be suspected when the pump flow rate is lower than expected. Obstruction of the inflow cannula can be caused by thrombi, papillary muscles or trabeculations.

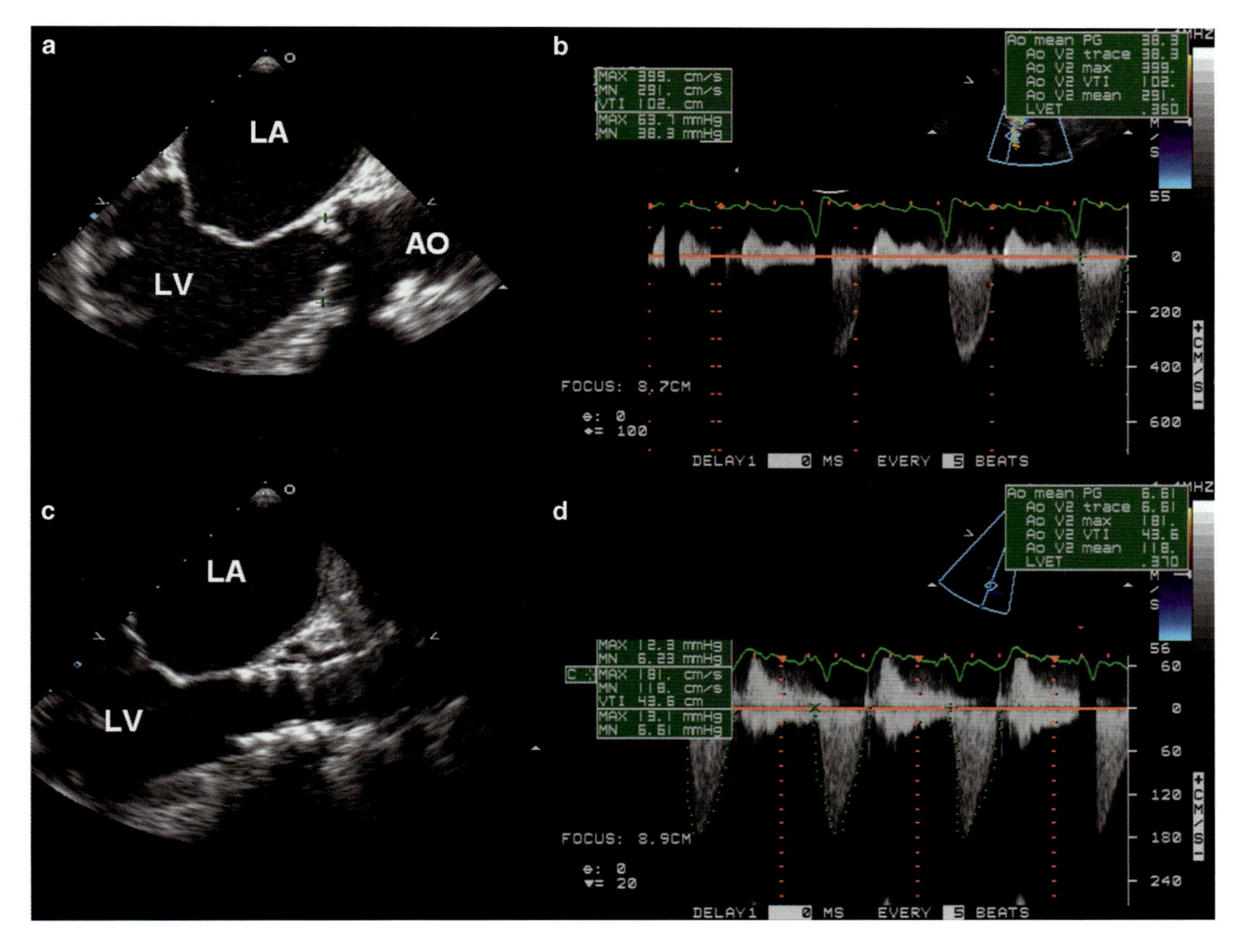

Fig. 18.27 Transesophageal views before (**a, b**) and after (**c, d**) the implantation of the CoreValve showing the improvement in aortic stenosis gradients after the procedure. *Ao* aorta, *LA* left atrium, *LV* left ventricle

When this happens, there is an increased velocity at the cannula associated with inadequate emptying of the left ventricle which can be recognized by an increased left ventricular volume with bulging of the ventricular septum into the right ventricle. Underfilling of the left ventricle can be a result of hypovolemia, sepsis, an excessive high rotor setting, or severe right ventricular dysfunction. The inflow cannula can be secondarily obstructed by the adjacent trabeculations or papillary muscles. In this setting, volume replacement or turning down the rotor setting may relieve the obstruction.

Adequate right ventricular function is essential to the delivery of the necessary preload to the left cardiac chambers. In assessing patients for LVAD, right ventricular function needs to be carefully evaluated. The presence of right ventricular dysfunction increases the perioperative mortality of the procedure, although right ventricular dysfunction may improve with LVAD if the right ventricular dysfunction is largely secondary to left ventricular dysfunction. However, if there is severe intrinsic right ventricular disease such as extensive right ventricular infarction, right ventricular dysfunction may worsen with LVAD and devices that provide biventricular assist are more appropriate in this setting.

LVAD is associated with an increased risk of bleeding, which can collect posteriorly and compress the adjacent cardiac chambers (Fig. 18.39). Other complications include thrombus formation on the inflow or outflow cannulas, endocarditis, and aortic injury such as dissection [54]. These complications are not unique to LVAD and are covered in greater detail in other chapters.

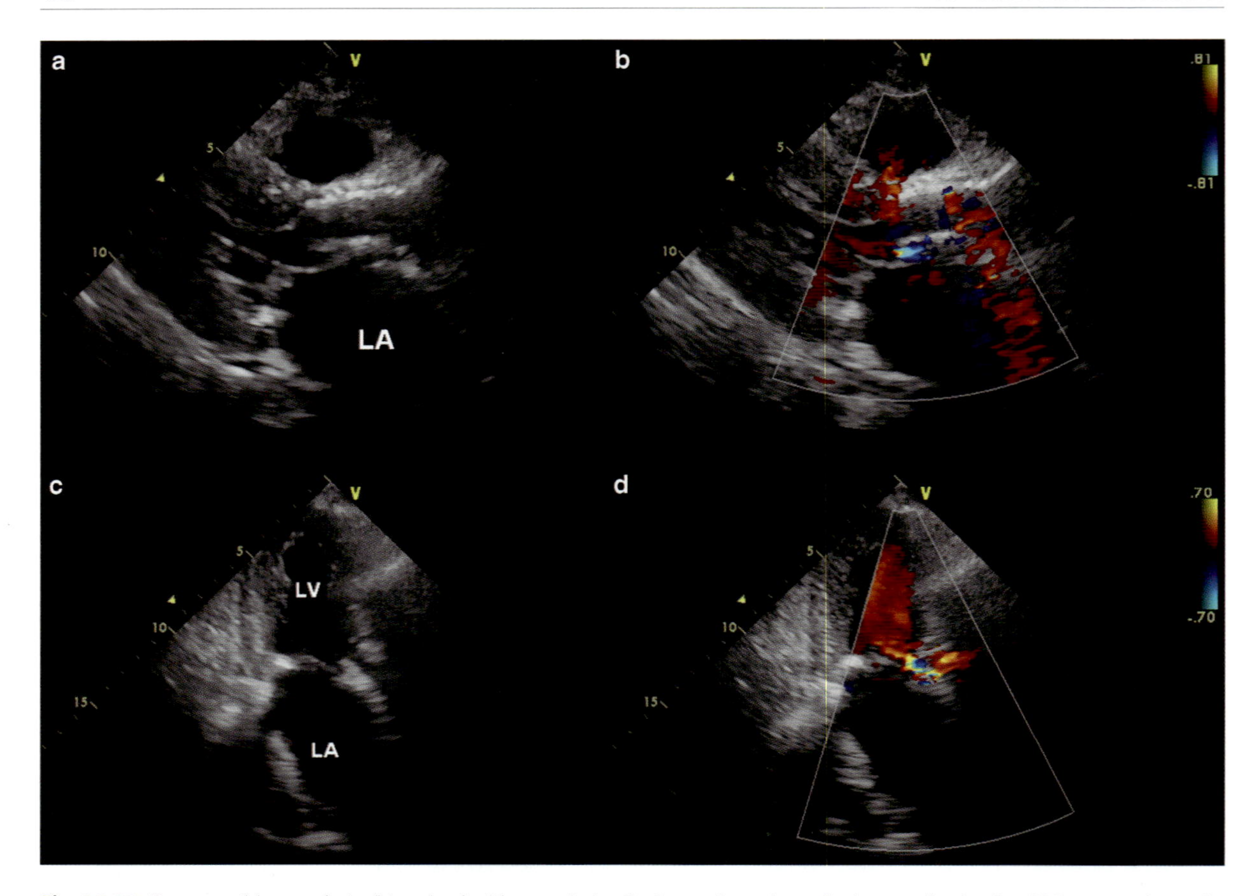

Fig. 18.28 Parasternal long-axis (**a, b**) and apical long-axis (**c, d**) views of a patient who has received a CoreValve several months previously show mild paravalvular regurgitation which is a common finding following this procedure. *LA* left atrium, *LV* left ventricle

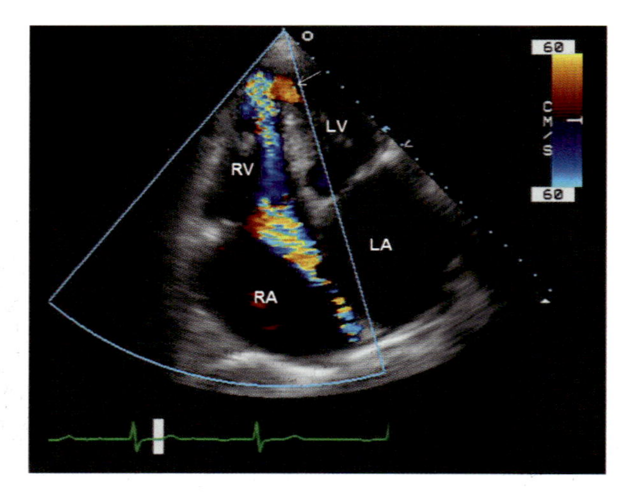

Fig. 18.29 Apical four-chamber view in a patient who has had implantation of the CoreValve shows the presence of iatrogenic ventricular septal defect (*arrow*) at the left ventricular apex. Tricuspid regurgitation is also present

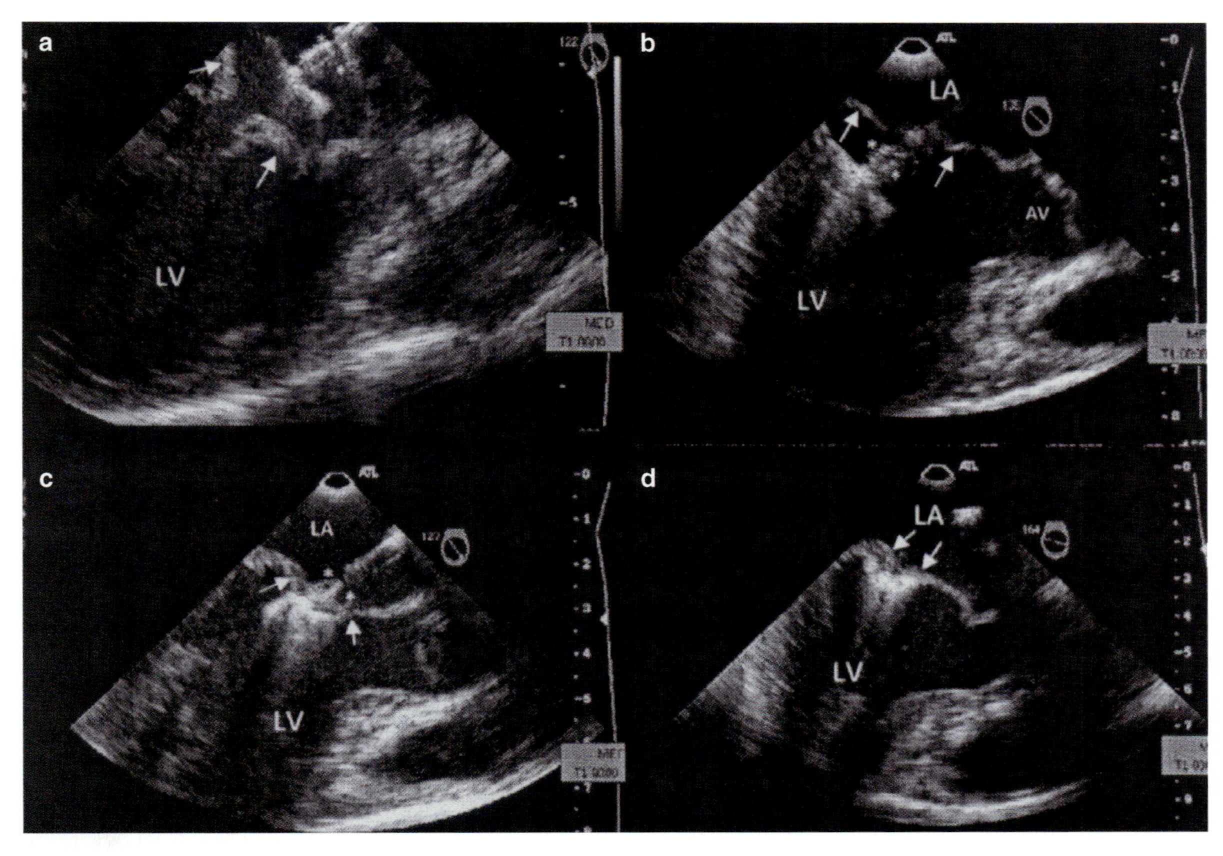

Fig. 18.30 Transesophageal views show the different stages of Evalve edge to edge repair. In (**a**), the open arms of the device are seen. In (**b**), the device with its open arms is advanced into the ventricle. In (**c**), the arms of the device are closed bringing together the anterior and posterior mitral leaflets. In (**d**), the anterior and posterior mitral leaflets are tethered together by the released clip. *LA* left atrium, *LV* left ventricle (Reproduced from Naqvi [44]. With permission.)

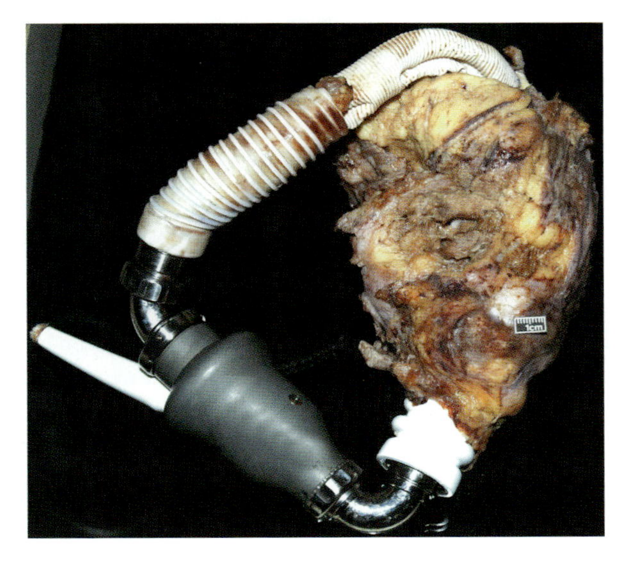

Fig. 18.31 HeartMate II left ventricular assist device placed with apical and aortic conduits

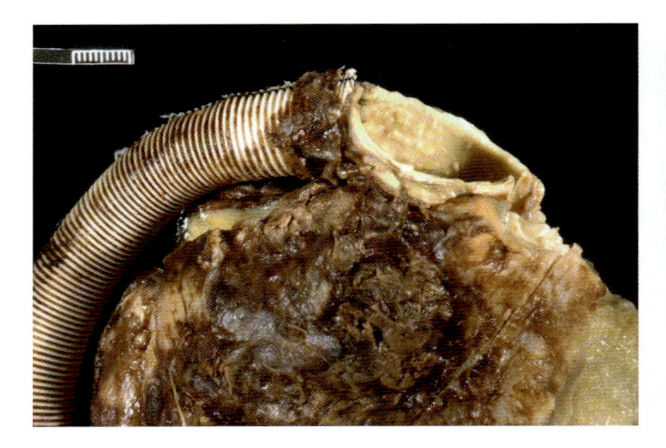

Fig. 18.32 Left ventricular assist device outflow aortic conduit with anastomosis of the graft to the side of the aorta

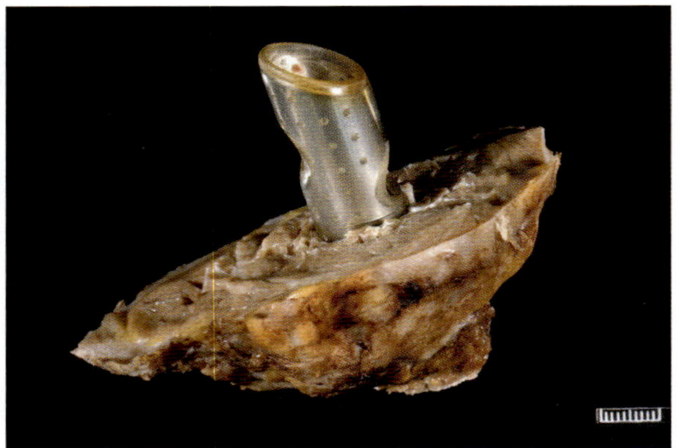

Fig. 18.33 Left ventricular assist device inflow ventricular conduit in the apex of the heart

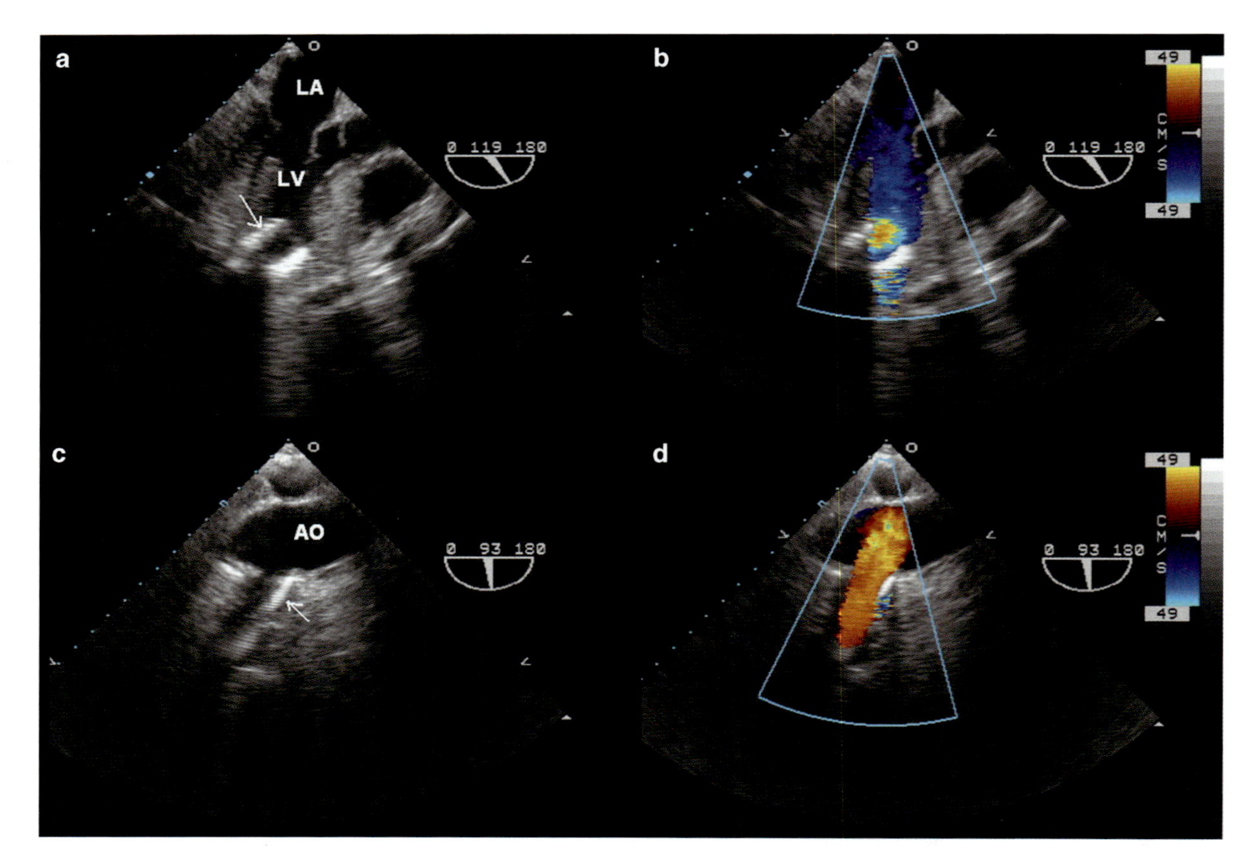

Fig. 18.34 Transesophageal views in a patient with an axial propulsion device (HeartMate II) show the inflow cannula (*arrow*) at the left ventricular apex (**a**, **b**) and the outflow cannula (*arrow*) connected to the anterior surface of the aortic root (**c, d**). *Ao* aorta; *LA* left atrium, *LV* left ventricle

Table 18.4 Echocardiographic assessment of left ventricular assist device

Before implantation
• RV function
• Valvular dysfunction such as aortic stenosis, aortic regurgitation, mitral stenosis, and tricuspid regurgitation
• Ascending aortic pathology
• LV thrombus
• Intracardiac shunt
Post implantation
• Intracardiac shunt
• Cannula location and alignment
• Cannula flow pattern by pulsed-wave, continuous wave, and color-flow Doppler imaging
• Effect of LV unloading
• RV function
• Extrinsic pericardial hematoma or effusion

Source: Modified after Chunnanvej et al. [54]

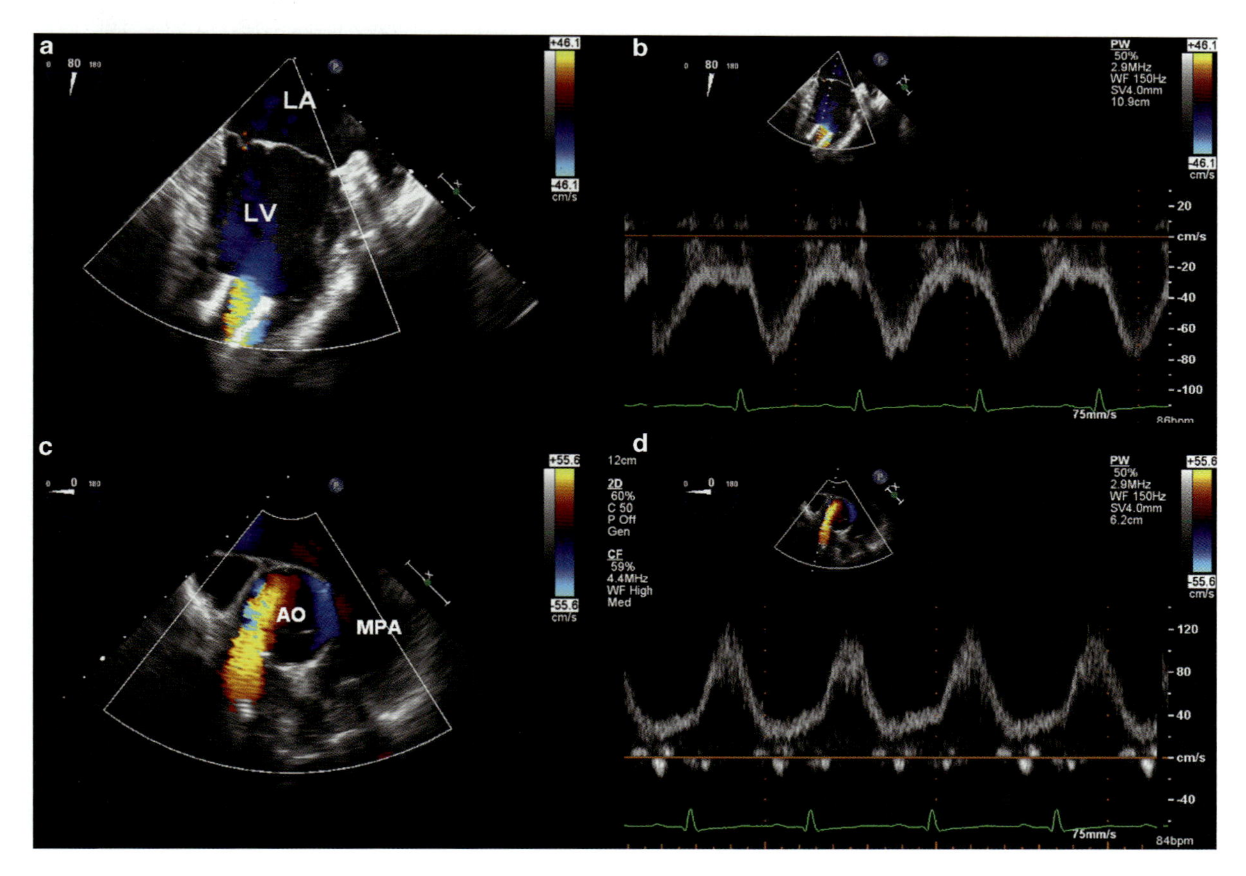

Fig. 18.35 Transesophageal views show the typical flow at the inflow cannula (**a, b**) and the outflow cannula (**c, d**) in a patient with the HeartMate II device. This axial propulsion device provides low velocity (1–2 m/s) pulsatile flow superimposed on continous flow throughout the device cycle. *Ao* aorta, *LA* left atrium, *LV* left ventricle, *MPA* main pulmonary artery

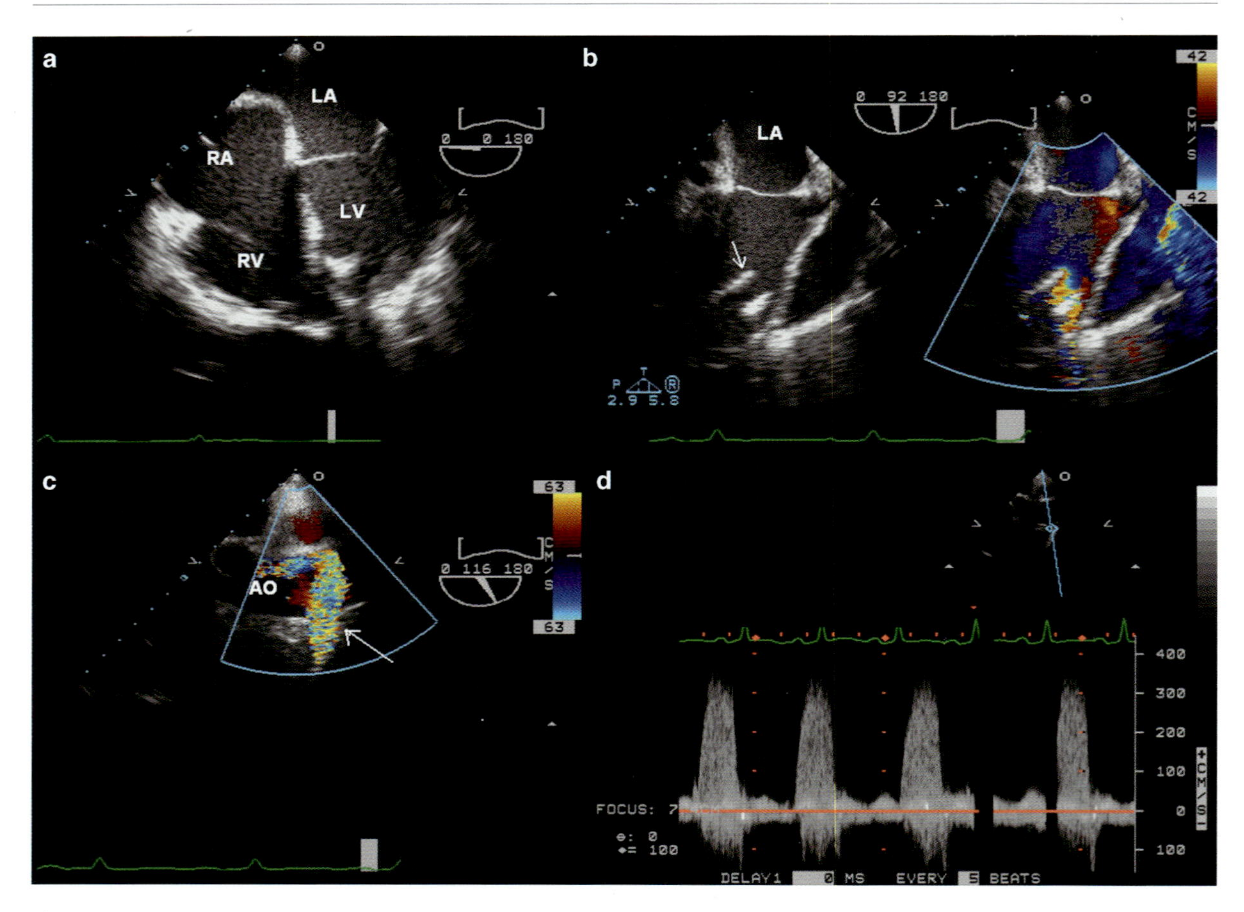

Fig. 18.36 Transesophageal views (**a, b**) in this patient with a pulsatile left ventricular assist device (Thoratec) show the inflow cannula in the left ventricular apex (*arrow*). At the outflow cannula (*arrow*) in (**c**), a turbulent flow is present. This is confirmed by continuous wave Doppler (**d**) showing high velocity flow exceeding 3 m/s which is asynchronous with the electrocardiogram

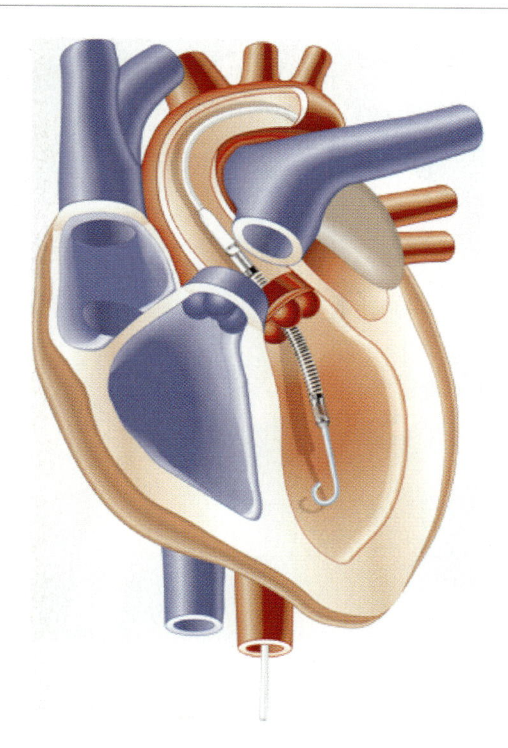

Fig. 18.37 Schematic diagram showing the position of an axial flow device across the aortic valve into the left ventricle (Reproduced from Thiele H et al. [53]. With permission)

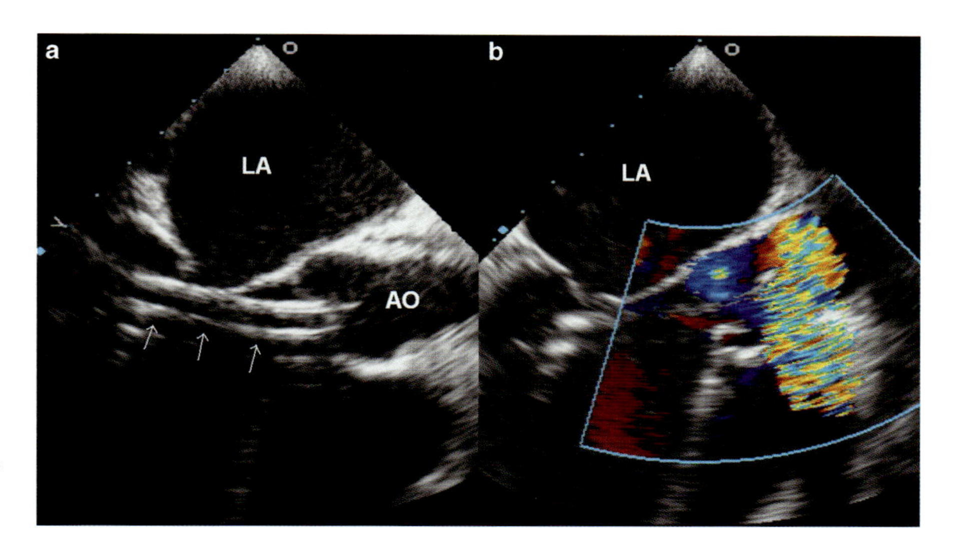

Fig. 18.38 (**a**) Transesophageal view of a continuous axial flow device (Impella) shows that the device (*arrows*) traverses the aortic valve with a portion of the device in the ascending aorta and a portion in the left ventricle. (**b**) Color-flow image shows color artifact produced by the spinning motor which should not be confused with blood flow. *Ao* aorta, *LA* left atrium, *LV* left ventricle

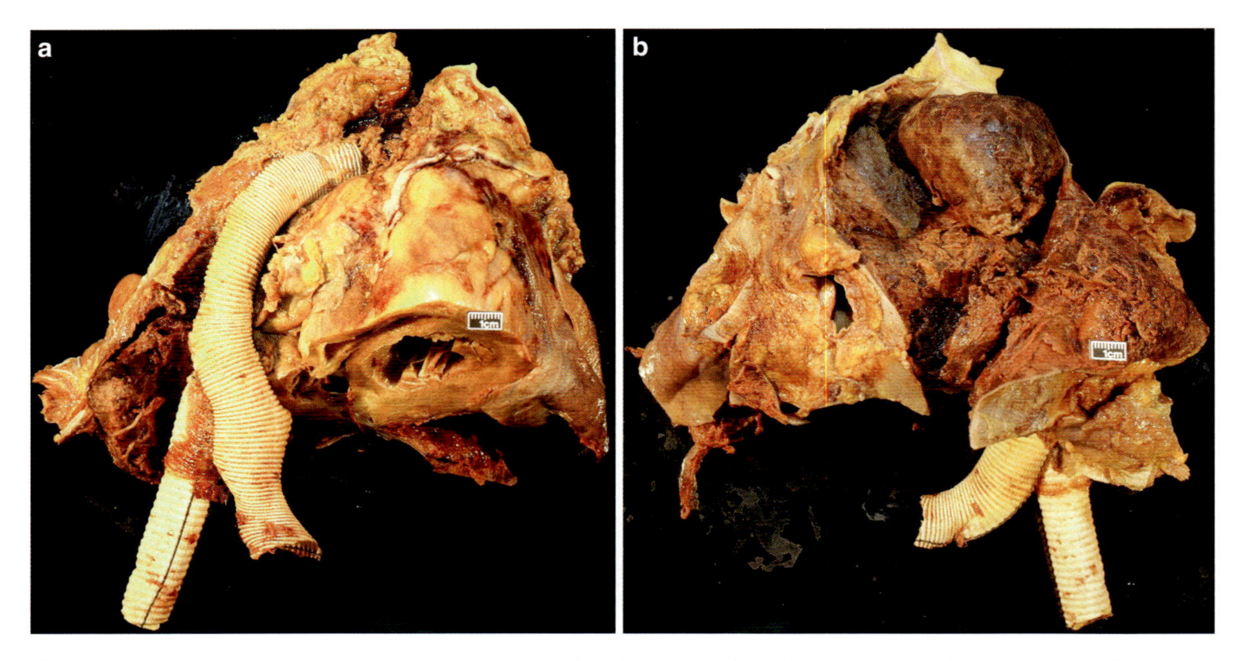

Fig. 18.39 Anterior (**a**) and posterior (**b**) views of a heart with a left ventricular assist device attached. There was poor function. A large amount of clot and hematoma was found behind the heart as seen in (**b**). This material compressed the right heart

Summary

Interventional cardiac procedures have proliferated over the past decade. We now have the ability to percutaneously close an ASD or implant a prosthetic valve. In order to select patients for these procedures and to follow them after the procedure, it is essential to have an in-depth understanding of the cardiac conditions and the characteristics of the intracardiac devices. Future trials will provide a proper perspective of the role of many of these devices.

References

1. Oginosawa Y, Abe H, Nakashima Y. The incidence and risk factors for venous obstruction after implantation of transvenous pacing leads. *Pacing Clin Electrophysiol*. 2002 Nov;25(11):1605-1611.
2. van Rooden CJ, Molhoek SG, Rosendaal FR, Schalij MJ, Meinders AE, Huisman MV. Incidence and risk factors of early venous thrombosis associated with permanent pacemaker leads. *J Cardiovasc Electrophysiol*. 2004 Nov;15(11): 1258-1262.
3. Chow BJ, Hassan AH, Chan KL, Tang AS. Prevalence and significance of lead-related thrombi in patients with implantable cardioverter defibrillators. *Am J Cardiol*. 2003 Jan 1; 91(1):88-90.
4. Torbicki A, Galie N, Covezzoli A, Rossi E, De RM, Goldhaber SZ. Right heart thrombi in pulmonary embolism: results from the International Cooperative Pulmonary Embolism Registry. *J Am Coll Cardiol*. 2003 Jun 18;41(12): 2245-2251.
5. Carda R, Almeria C, Lennie V, Serra V, Zamorano JL. What to do with an atrial thrombus? *Eur J Echocardiogr*. 2008 Jan;9(1):204-205.
6. Chartier L, Bera J, Delomez M, et al. Free-floating thrombi in the right heart: diagnosis, management, and prognostic indexes in 38 consecutive patients. *Circulation*. 1999 Jun 1;99(21):2779-2783.
7. Epstein AE, Kay GN, Plumb VJ, Dailey SM, Anderson PG. Gross and microscopic pathological changes associated with non-thoracotomy implantable defibrillator leads. *Circulation*. 1998 Oct 13;98(15):1517-1524.
8. Candinas R, Duru F, Schneider J, Luscher TF, Stokes K. Postmortem analysis of encapsulation around long-term ventricular endocardial pacing leads. *Mayo Clin Proc*. 1999 Feb;74(2):120-125.
9. Kim JB, Spevack DM, Tunick PA, et al. The effect of transvenous pacemaker and implantable cardioverter defibrillator lead placement on tricuspid valve function: an observational study. *J Am Soc Echocardiogr*. 2008 Mar;21(3):284-287.
10. Leclercq C, Faris O, Tunin R, et al. Systolic improvement and mechanical resynchronization does not require electrical synchrony in the dilated failing heart with left bundle-branch block. *Circulation*. 2002 Oct 1;106(14):1760-1763.
11. Abraham WT, Fisher WG, Smith AL, et al. Cardiac resynchronization in chronic heart failure. *N Engl J Med*. 2002 Jun 13;346(24):1845-1853.
12. Bax JJ, Ansalone G, Breithardt OA, et al. Echocardiographic evaluation of cardiac resynchronization therapy: ready for

routine clinical use? A critical appraisal. *J Am Coll Cardiol*. 2004 Jul 7;44(1):1-9.
13. Bax JJ, Bleeker GB, Marwick TH, et al. Left ventricular dyssynchrony predicts response and prognosis after cardiac resynchronization therapy. *J Am Coll Cardiol*. 2004 Nov 2;44(9):1834-1840.
14. Bax JJ, Marwick TH, Molhoek SG, Bleeker GB. van EL, Boersma E, et al. Left ventricular dyssynchrony predicts benefit of cardiac resynchronization therapy in patients with end-stage heart failure before pacemaker implantation Am J Cardiol. 2003 Nov 15;92(10):1238-1240.
15. Yu CM, Fung WH, Lin H, Zhang Q, Sanderson JE, Lau CP. Predictors of left ventricular reverse remodeling after cardiac resynchronization therapy for heart failure secondary to idiopathic dilated or ischemic cardiomyopathy. *Am J Cardiol*. 2003 Mar 15;91(6):684-688.
16. Yu CM, Gorcsan J III, Bleeker GB, et al. Usefulness of tissue Doppler velocity and strain dyssynchrony for predicting left ventricular reverse remodeling response after cardiac resynchronization therapy. *Am J Cardiol*. 2007 Oct 15; 100(8):1263-1270.
17. Yu CM, Zhang Q, Fung JW, et al. A novel tool to assess systolic asynchrony and identify responders of cardiac resynchronization therapy by tissue synchronization imaging. *J Am Coll Cardiol*. 2005 Mar 1;45(5):677-684.
18. Gorcsan J III, Kanzaki H, Bazaz R, Dohi K, Schwartzman D. Usefulness of echocardiographic tissue synchronization imaging to predict acute response to cardiac resynchronization therapy. *Am J Cardiol*. 2004 May 1;93(9):1178-1181.
19. Kapetanakis S, Kearney MT, Siva A, Gall N, Cooklin M, Monaghan MJ. Real-time three-dimensional echocardiography: a novel technique to quantify global left ventricular mechanical dyssynchrony. *Circulation*. 2005 Aug 16;112(7): 992-1000.
20. Burgess MI, Jenkins C, Chan J, Marwick TH. Measurement of left ventricular dyssynchrony in patients with ischaemic cardiomyopathy: a comparison of real-time three-dimensional and tissue Doppler echocardiography. *Heart*. 2007 Oct;93(10):1191-1196.
21. Chung ES, Leon AR, Tavazzi L, et al. Results of the Predictors of Response to CRT (PROSPECT) trial. *Circulation*. 2008 May 20;117(20):2608-2616.
22. Santaularia-Tomas M, Abraham TP. Criteria predicting response to CRT: is more better? *Eur Heart J*. 2009 Dec; 30(23):2835-2837.
23. Waggoner AD, Agler DA, Adams DB. Cardiac resynchronization therapy and the emerging role of echocardiography (part 1): indications and results from current studies. *J Am Soc Echocardiogr*. 2007 Jan;20(1):70-75.
24. Yu CM, Zhang Q, Chan YS, et al. Tissue Doppler velocity is superior to displacement and strain mapping in predicting left ventricular reverse remodelling response after cardiac resynchronisation therapy. *Heart*. 2006 Oct;92(10): 1452-1456.
25. Mele D, Pasanisi G, Capasso F, et al. Left intraventricular myocardial deformation dyssynchrony identifies responders to cardiac resynchronization therapy in patients with heart failure. *Eur Heart J*. 2006 May;27(9):1070-1078.
26. Brochu MC, Baril JF, Dore A, Juneau M, De GP, Mercier LA. Improvement in exercise capacity in asymptomatic and mildly symptomatic adults after atrial septal defect percutaneous closure. *Circulation*. 2002 Oct 1;106(14):1821-1826.
27. Murphy JG, Gersh BJ, McGoon MD, et al. Long-term outcome after surgical repair of isolated atrial septal defect. *N Engl J Med*. 1990;323:1646-1650.
28. Thomson JD, Aburawi EH, Watterson KG, Van DC, Gibbs JL. Surgical and transcatheter (Amplatzer) closure of atrial septal defects: a prospective comparison of results and cost. *Heart*. 2002 May;87(5):466-469.
29. Webb G, Gatzoulis MA. Atrial septal defects in the adult - Recent progress and overview. *Circulation*. 2006;114(15): 1645-1653.
30. Divekar A, Gaamangwe T, Shaikh N, Raabe M, Ducas J. Cardiac perforation after device closure of atrial septal defects with the Amplatzer septal occluder. *J Am Coll Cardiol*. 2005 Apr 19;45(8):1213-1218.
31. Krumsdorf U, Ostermayer S, Billinger K, et al. Incidence and clinical course of thrombus formation on atrial septal defect and patient foramen ovale closure devices in 1, 000 consecutive patients. *J Am Coll Cardiol*. 2004 Jan 21;43(2):302-309.
32. Sharifi M, Dehghani M, Mehdipour M, Al-Bustami O, Emrani F, Burks J. Intense migraines secondary to percutaneous closure of atrial septal defects. *J Interv Cardiol*. 2005 Jun;18(3):181-183.
33. Guerin P, Lambert V, Godart F, et al. Transcatheter closure of patent foramen ovale in patients with platypnea-orthodeoxia: results of a multicentric French registry. *Cardiovasc Intervent Radiol*. 2005 Mar;28(2):164-168.
34. Schwerzmann M, Nedeltchev K, Meier B. Patent foramen ovale closure: a new therapy for migraine. *Catheter Cardiovasc Interv*. 2007 Feb 1;69(2):277-284.
35. Tepper SJ, Cleves C, Taylor FR. Patent foramen ovale and migraine: association, causation, and implications of clinical trials. *Curr Pain Headache Rep*. 2009 Jun;13(3):221-226.
36. Martinez MW, Mookadam F, Sun Y, Hagler DJ. Transcatheter closure of ischemic and post-traumatic ventricular septal ruptures. *Catheter Cardiovasc Interv*. 2007 Feb 15; 69(3):403-407.
37. ÓRourke DJ, Palac RT, Malenka DJ, Marrin CA, Arbuckle BE, Plehn JF. Outcome of mild periprosthetic regurgitation detected by intraoperative transesophageal echocardiography. *J Am Coll Cardiol*. 2001 Jul;38(1):163-166.
38. Ionescu A, Fraser AG, Butchart EG. Prevalence and clinical significance of incidental paraprosthetic valvar regurgitation: a prospective study using transoesophageal echocardiography. *Heart*. 2003 Nov;89(11):1316-1321.
39. Becerra JM, Almeria C, de Isla LP, Zamorano J. Usefulness of 3D transoesophageal echocardiography for guiding wires and closure devices in mitral perivalvular leaks. *Eur J Echocardiogr*. 2009 Dec;10(8):979-981.
40. Sorajja P, Cabalka AK, Hagler DJ, et al. Successful percutaneous repair of perivalvular prosthetic regurgitation. *Catheter Cardiovasc Interv*. 2007 Nov 15;70(6):815-823.
41. Alonso-Briales JH, Munoz-Garcia AJ, Jimenez-Navarro MF, et al. Closure of perivalvular leaks using an Amplatzer occluder. *Rev Esp Cardiol*. 2009 Apr;62(4):442-446.
42. Cribier A, Eltchaninoff H, Tron C, et al. Treatment of calcific aortic stenosis with the percutaneous heart valve: mid-term follow-up from the initial feasibility studies: the French experience. *J Am Coll Cardiol*. 2006 Mar 21;47(6):1214-1223.
43. Grube E, Laborde JC, Gerckens U, et al. Percutaneous implantation of the CoreValve self-expanding valve prosthesis in high-risk patients with aortic valve disease: the Siegburg first-in-man study. *Circulation*. 2006 Oct 10;114(15):1616-1624.